THE WASHINGTON MANUAL OF OUTPATIENT INTERNAL MEDICINE

Second Edition

Executive Editor

Thomas M. De Fer, MD
Professor of Medicine
Director, Internal Medicine Clerkship and the ACES Program
Division of Medical Education, Department of Medicine
Washington University School of Medicine
Saint Louis, Missouri

Editor

Heather F. Sateia, MD
Instructor of Medicine
Division of Medical Education, Department of Medicine
Washington University School of Medicine
Saint Louis, Missouri

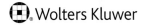

Philadelphia • Baltimore • New York • London
Buenos Aires • Hong Kong • Sydney • Tokyo

Executive Editor: Rebecca S. Gaertner
Product Development Editor: Kristina Oberle
Editorial Coordinator: Katie Sharp
Marketing Manager: Stephanie Kindlick
Production Project Manager: Bridgett Dougherty
Design Coordinator: Teresa Mallon
Manufacturing Coordinator: Beth Welsh
Prepress Vendor: SPi Global

Second edition

9 8 7 6 5 4 3 2 1

Printed in China

Library of Congress Cataloging-in-Publication Data
The Washington manual of outpatient internal medicine / [executive editor] Thomas M. De Fer ; editor, Heather Sateia. — Second edition.
     p. ; cm.
  Manual of outpatient internal medicine
  Complemented by: Washington manual of medical therapeutics.
  Includes bibliographical references and index.
  ISBN 978-1-4511-4327-0 (alk. paper)
  I. De Fer, Thomas M., editor. II. Sateia, Heather F., editor. III. Washington University (Saint Louis, Mo.). Department of Medicine, issuing body. IV. Washington manual of medical therapeutics. Complemented by (work): V. Title: Manual of outpatient internal medicine.
  [DNLM: 1. Ambulatory Care—Handbooks. 2. Internal Medicine—methods—Handbooks. WB 39]
  RC55
  362.12—dc23

                               2014048408

Contributors

Sophia Airhart, MD
Resident
Division of Medical Education

Enrique Alvarez, MD
Fellow
Department of Neurology

Adam Anderson, MD
Fellow
Division of Pulmonary and Critical Care Medicine

Milan J. Anadkat, MD
Associate Professor of Medicine
Division of Dermatology

Ananth Arjunan, MD
Instructor in Medicine
Division of Hospitalist Medicine

Jeffrey J. Atkinson, MD
Assistant Professor of Medicine
Division of Pulmonary and Critical Care Medicine

Sylvia Awadalla, MD
Professor of Neurology
Department of Neurology

Nusayba Bagegni, MD
Instructor in Medicine
Division of Hospitalist Medicine

Maria Q. Baggstrom, MD
Associate Professor of Medicine
Division of Medical Oncology

Ernie-Paul Barrette, MD, FACP
Associate Professor of Medicine
Division of Medical Education

Scott Biest, MD
Associate Professor of Obstetrics and Gynecology
Department of Obstetrics and Gynecology

Melvin Blanchard, MD
Associate Professor of Medicine
Division of Medical Education

Morey A. Blinder, MD
Professor of Medicine
Division of Hematology

Benjamin Bogucki, MD
Fellow
Division of Dermatology

Anthony Boyer, MD
Fellow
Division of Pulmonary and Critical Care Medicine

Richard D. Brasington, MD
Professor of Medicine
Division of Rheumatology

Jared G. Breyley, MD
Resident
Division of Medical Education

Jonathan Byrd, MD
Instructor in Clinical Medicine
Washington University Clinical Associates

Luigi R. Cardella, MD
Instructor in Psychiatry
Department of Psychiatry

David B. Carr, MD
Professor of Medicine
Division of Geriatrics and Nutritional Science

Mario Castro, MD, MPH
Professor of Medicine
Division of Pulmonary and Critical Care Medicine

Murali M. Chakinala, MD
Associate Professor of Medicine
Division of Pulmonary and Critical Care Medicine

Alexander Chen, MD
Assistant Professor of Medicine
Division of Pulmonary and Critical Care Medicine

Steven Cheng, MD
Associate Professor of Medicine
Division of Renal Diseases

Youngjee Choi, MD
Instructor in Medicine
Division of Medical Education

Courtney Chrisler, MD
Instructor in Medicine
Division of Infectious Diseases

Matthew A. Ciorba, MD
Assistant Professor of Medicine
Division of Gastroenterology

Enrique Cornejo Cisneros, MD
Resident
Division of Medical Education

William E. Clutter, MD
Associate Professor of Medicine
Division of Medical Education

Maria C. Dans, MD
Assistant Professor of Medicine
Division of Hospitalist Medicine

Thomas M. De Fer, MD
Professor of Medicine
Division of Medical Education

Shaun C. Desai, MD
Instructor in Otolaryngology
Department of Otolaryngology

Dayna S. Early, MD
Professor of Medicine
Division of Gastroenterology

Charles S. Eby, MD
Professor of Pathology and Immunology
Department of Pathology and Immunology

Brian F. Gage, MD
Professor of Medicine
Division of General Medical Sciences

Arvind K. Garg, MD
Fellow
Division of Nephrology

Nsangou Ghogomu, MD
Assistant Professor of Otolaryngology
Department of Otolaryngology

Luis A. Giuffra, MD, PhD
Professor of Clinical Psychiatry
Department of Psychiatry

Anuradha Godishala, MD
Resident
Division of Medical Education

Anne C. Goldberg, MD
Associate Professor of Medicine
Division of Endocrinology, Metabolism, and Lipid Research

Seth Goldberg, MD
Associate Professor of Medicine
Division of Renal Diseases

Parul J. Gor, MD
Resident
Division of Medical Education

Diptesh Gupta, MD
Fellow
Division of Renal Diseases

C. Prakash Gyawali, MD
Professor of Medicine
Division of Gastroenterology

Cynthia J. Herrick, MD
Instructor in Medicine
Division of Endocrinology, Metabolism, and Lipid Research

Ronald Jackups Jr., MD, PhD
Assistant Professor of Pathology and Immunology
Department of Pathology and Immunology

Mohammad A. Kizilbash, MD
Assistant Professor of Medicine
Division of Cardiology

Derek S. Larson, MD
Fellow
Division of Renal Diseases

Susana M. Lazarte, MD
Instructor in Medicine
Division of Medical Education

Brian R. Lindman, MD
Assistant Professor of Medicine
Division of Cardiology

Mauricio Lisker-Melman, MD
Professor of Medicine
Division of Gastroenterology

Janet B. McGill, MD
Professor of Medicine
Division of Endocrinology, Metabolism, and Lipid Research

Claire Meyer, MD
Fellow
Division of Gastroenterology

Jason D. Meyers, MD
Fellow
Division of Cardiology

Jonathan J. Miner, MD
Fellow
Division of Rheumatology

Arya B. Mohabbat, MD
Fellow
Division of Gastroenterology

Clare E. Moynihan, MD
Fellow
Division of Endocrinology, Metabolism,
  and Lipid Research

Nima Naimi, DO
Fellow
Division of Renal Diseases

Scott A. Norris, MD
Assistant Professor of Neurology
Department of Neurology

M. Allison Ogden, MD
Associate Professor of Otolaryngology
Department of Otolaryngology

Amit Patel, MD
Fellow
Division of Gastroenterology

Jayendrakumar S. Patel, MD
Instructor in Medicine
Division of Medical Education

Ian Pitha, MD
Resident
Department of Ophthalmology and Visual
  Sciences

Thomas Regenbogen, MD
Fellow
Division of Hematology and Oncology

Hilary E. L. Reno, MD, PhD
Assistant Professor of Medicine
Division of Infectious Diseases

Michael W. Rich, MD
Professor of Medicine
Division of Cardiology

Jessica R. Rosenstock, MD
Resident
Department of Obstetrics and Gynecology

Tonya Russell, MD
Associate Professor of Medicine
Division of Pulmonary and Critical Care
  Medicine

Kiran Sarikonda, MD
Fellow
Division of Pulmonary and Critical Care
  Medicine

Gregory Sayuk, MD
Assistant Professor of Medicine
Division of Gastroenterology

Joel D. Schilling, MD, PhD
Assistant Professor of Medicine
Department of Cardiology

Jeffrey Sharon, MD
Fellow
Department of Otolaryngology

Amy Sheldahl, MD
Assistant Professor of Medicine
Division of Hospitalist Medicine

Ajay Sheshadri, MD
Postdoctoral Research Scholar
Division of Pulmonary and Critical Care
  Medicine

Arsham Sheybani, MD
Assistant Professor
Department of Ophthalmology and Visual
  Sciences

Adrian Shifren, MD
Assistant Professor of Medicine
Division of Pulmonary and Critical Care
  Medicine

Sagar R. Shroff, MD
Fellow
Division of Gastroenterology

Timothy W. Smith, MD, PhD
Associate Professor of Medicine
Division of Cardiology

Sandeep S. Sodhi, MD
Fellow
Division of Cardiology

Shelby Sullivan, MD
Assistant Professor of Medicine
Division of Gastroenterology

Melissa Sum, MD
Instructor in Medicine
Division of Medical Education

Michael J. Tang, MD
Instructor in Medicine
Division of Hospitalist Medicine

James A. Tarbox, MD
Fellow
Division of Allergy and Immunology

Linda Tsai, MD
Associate Professor
Department of Ophthalmology and Visual
  Sciences

Peter G. Tuteur, MD
Associate Professor of Medicine
Division of Pulmonary and Critical Care
  Medicine

Babac Vahabzadeh, MD
Resident
Division of Medical Education

Benjamin A. Voss, MD
Instructor in Clinical Medicine
BJC Associated Internists

Tzu-Fei Wang, MD
Fellow
Division of Hematology and Oncology

Megan E. Wren, MD
Associate Professor of Medicine
Division of Medical Education

Arielle Yang, MD
Resident
Division of Medical Education

Lauren M. Young, MD
Fellow
Division of Geriatrics and Nutritional Science

Roger D. Yusen, MD, MPH
Associate Professor of Medicine
Division of Pulmonary and Critical Care
  Medicine

Preface

Welcome to the second edition of *The Washington Manual of Outpatient Internal Medicine*. This book is intended to serve as a companion to the 34th edition of *The Washington Manual of Medical Therapeutics* and allows for a more in-depth focus on the practice of medicine in the ambulatory setting. We are, as ever, indebted to the editors and authors of previous editions who created such a strong foundation upon which to build this new edition.

The focus of *The Washington Manual of Outpatient Internal Medicine* is to provide a reference that covers common ambulatory problems encountered in each medical subspecialty. Recognizing that many of the presentations seen in the outpatient setting fall outside of the traditional internal medicine subspecialties, we have included chapters on topics such as dermatology, neurology, ophthalmology, otolaryngology, and psychiatry written by specialists in these fields. In keeping with the tradition of other *Washington Manual* publications, all chapters are authored by the outstanding house staff and faculty at Barnes-Jewish Hospital and Washington University School of Medicine—we are humbled by their passion, skill, and dedication to this, and all, *Washington Manual* publications.

The second edition has been updated to reflect the most current literature and medical practices. We have continued to use a standard chapter template with a bulleted style that incorporates tables and figures for easy reference. Online and mobile access to this edition is available through Inkling electronic books. This provides readers with an interactive and fully searchable version of the text.

As always, the editors are deeply indebted to the staff at Wolters Kluwer/Lippincott Williams & Wilkins for their unwavering support and guidance. In particular, we would like to thank Rebecca Gaertner and Kristina Oberle for their limitless patience. Within our division, Katie Sharp works tirelessly with editors and authors to ensure an outstanding product, and we are profoundly grateful for her contribution. We have also received tremendous support from within the Department of Medicine—specifically, the Chairman of Medicine, Vicky Fraser, and Melvin Blanchard, the Chief of the Division of Medical Education.

Heather F. Sateia, MD
Thomas M. De Fer, MD

Contents

Contributors iii
Preface vii

General

1 Approach to the Ambulatory Patient 1
Benjamin A. Voss

2 Care of the Surgical Patient 11
Anuradha Godishala and Thomas M. De Fer

3 Women's Health 46
Jessica R. Rosenstock and Scott Biest

4 Men's Health 69
Melvin Blanchard

5 Screening and Adult Immunizations 89
Megan E. Wren

Cardiovascular

6 Hypertension 130
Arielle Yang and Thomas M. De Fer

7 Ischemic Heart Disease 158
Jayendrakumar S. Patel, Sandeep S. Sodhi, Anuradha Godishala, and Mohammad A. Kizilbash

8 Heart Failure and Cardiomyopathy 182
Sophia Airhart, Joel D. Schilling, and Michael W. Rich

9 Valvular Heart Disease 206
Jared G. Breyley and Brian R. Lindman

10 Arrhythmia and Syncope 218
Jason D. Meyers and Timothy W. Smith

11 Dyslipidemia 250
Clare E. Moynihan and Anne C. Goldberg

Hematologic

12 Disorders of Hemostasis 265
Tzu-Fei Wang, Charles S. Eby, and Ronald Jackups Jr.

13 Hematologic Diseases 284
Thomas Regenbogen and Morey A. Blinder

14 Venous Thromboembolism and Anticoagulant Therapy 309
Roger D. Yusen and Brian F. Gage

Pulmonary

15 Common Pulmonary Complaints 327
Adam Anderson, Peter G. Tuteur, and Adrian Shifren

16 Chronic Obstructive Pulmonary Disease and Asthma 341
Kiran Sarikonda, Ajay Sheshadri, Mario Castro, and Jeffrey J. Atkinson

17 Interstitial Lung Diseases and Pulmonary Hypertension 371
Anthony Boyer and Murali M. Chakinala

18 Sleep Disorders 389
Tonya Russell

19 Pleural Effusion and Solitary Pulmonary Nodule 400
Alexander Chen

Endocrine

20 Diabetes Mellitus 412
Cynthia J. Herrick and Janet B. McGill

21 Endocrine Diseases 431
William E. Clutter

22 Nutrition and Obesity 455
Melissa Sum and Shelby Sullivan

Nephrology

23 **Laboratory Assessment of Kidney and Urinary Tract Disorders** 480
Nima Naimi and Seth Goldberg

24 **Acute Kidney Injury, Glomerulopathy, and Chronic Kidney Disease** 488
Diptesh Gupta, Derek S. Larson, and Seth Goldberg

25 **Hematuria and Nephrolithiasis** 508
Arvind K. Garg and Steven Cheng

Infectious Disease

26 **General Infectious Diseases** 517
Enrique Cornejo Cisneros and Susana M. Lazarte

27 **HIV Infection and Sexually Transmitted Diseases** 566
Youngjee Choi, Courtney Chrisler, and Hilary E. L. Reno

Gastroenterology

28 **Common Gastrointestinal Complaints** 584
Babac Vahabzadeh and Dayna S. Early

29 **Gastroesophageal Reflux Disease** 607
C. Prakash Gyawali and Amit Patel

30 **Hepatobiliary Diseases** 617
Claire Meyer, Amit Patel, and Mauricio Lisker-Melman

31 **Inflammatory Bowel Disease** 642
Arya B. Mohabbat and Matthew A. Ciorba

32 **Irritable Bowel Syndrome** 650
Sagar R. Shroff and Gregory Sayuk

Rheumatology

33 **Rheumatologic Diseases** 658
Jonathan J. Miner and Richard D. Brasington

34 Musculoskeletal Complaints 687
Ananth Arjunan and Ernie-Paul Barrette

Cancer

35 Care of the Cancer Patient 725
Maria Q. Baggstrom

Palliative Care and Pain Management

36 Palliative Care and Hospice Medicine 748
Jonathan Byrd and Maria C. Dans

37 Pain Management 758
Nusayba Bagegni, Amy Sheldahl, and Maria C. Dans

Subspecialty Topics

38 Geriatrics 772
Lauren M. Young and David B. Carr

39 Allergy and Immunology 793
Michael J. Tang, Parul J. Gor, and James A. Tarbox

40 Otolaryngology 819
Shaun C. Desai, Nsangou Ghogomu, Jeffrey Sharon, and M. Allison Ogden

41 Dermatology 842
Benjamin Bogucki and Milan J. Anadkat

42 Psychiatry 869
Luigi R. Cardella and Luis A. Giuffra

43 Neurologic Disorders 906
Scott A. Norris, Enrique Alvarez, and Sylvia Awadalla

44 Ophthalmology 940
Ian Pitha, Arsham Sheybani, and Linda Tsai

45 Smoking Cessation 956
Megan E. Wren

46 Alcohol Abuse and Dependence 970
Luigi R. Cardella and Luis A. Giuffra

Index 979

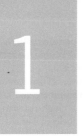

1 Approach to the Ambulatory Patient

Benjamin A. Voss

Ambulatory care is medical care provided to an outpatient. Disease prevention, health promotion, medical decision-making, and acute illness management are all performed in the ambulatory setting. The goals of an office visit will vary from visit to visit, and not every issue can or should be addressed at each visit.

PREVENTION OF FUTURE HEALTH PROBLEMS

- **Primary prevention** limits disease from occurring by removing the cause (e.g., immunizations). Primary prevention often takes place at the community level with efforts such as fluorination of water.
- **Secondary prevention** entails screening for asymptomatic disease while in an early, treatable phase. This includes screening for common cancers using modalities such as Papanicolaou (Pap) smears, colonoscopies, or mammograms.
- **Tertiary prevention** refers to those activities and interventions that prevent worsening of a disease or further complications, for example, using statins in patients with known coronary disease.
- **The periodic health exam**, also known as the "annual physical exam," is often used to address these preventive issues, and more time is typically allotted for these visits.

THE PERIODIC HEALTH EXAMINATION

- Covering all the issues that need to be covered as part of a periodic health exam in one visit is challenging. Many insurance companies may not cover a "routine visit." Therefore, addressing health maintenance and chronic disease management in an ongoing manner is necessary.
- Preventive medicine requires an individualized assessment tailored to each patient's age, gender, risk factors, and chronic illnesses.
- Counseling about a healthy lifestyle is a critical component of health care at any age.

Adolescents and Young Adults

- Adolescents and young adults are at risk for serious morbidity and even mortality related to the **risky behaviors** that are common in this age group.
- The clinician should maintain an open and nonjudgmental attitude to encourage the adolescent to speak frankly.
- **Confidentiality** is critical and should be assured.
- Topics to discuss include the avoidance of smoking, alcohol abuse, and illicit drug use; the use of bike helmets and car seatbelts; firearm safety; depression and suicide; the potential consequences of sexual activity and how to avoid them; and healthy dietary habits, eating disorders, and appropriate exercise. **Unintentional injury** is the leading cause of death among adolescents.
- Family history is an important part of the history in this age group.

- The physical examination should include height, weight, blood pressure (BP), cardiac, musculoskeletal, and testicular examinations. Routine internal pelvic examinations are not recommended in this age group but may be performed when indicated.
- Laboratory tests should include Pap smear (if the patient is over 21), screening for *Chlamydia trachomatis* and *Neisseria gonorrhoeae* in sexually active women, and targeted screening for HIV and other sexually transmitted diseases (STDs) in high-risk patients.
- Preventive measures include updating immunizations, especially rubella in women, hepatitis A virus (HAV), hepatitis B virus (HBV), human papillomavirus (HPV), tetanus, pertussis, and annual influenza vaccination.
- Women of childbearing age should take a daily vitamin with 0.4-mg folic acid to reduce the risk of neural tube defects in their offspring.

Midlife Adults

- Important topics to discuss include continued reinforcement of the importance of healthy habits, especially diet, exercise, avoidance of tobacco, alcohol abuse, and drugs.
- Physical and laboratory examinations should include height, weight, BP, cardiac exam, and **screening** for dyslipidemia and common treatable cancers.
- In most women, annual mammography should begin at age 40 (see Chapter 5).
- Men can be offered screening for prostate cancer beginning at age 50 (see Chapter 4).
- All patients should be screened for colorectal cancer beginning at age 50. Patients with high-risk factors, including a family history of disease, need more aggressive screening (see Chapter 5).
- Perimenopausal women should be counseled and should be offered screening for osteoporosis (see Chapter 3).

Older Adults

- Important topics to discuss include continued reinforcement of the importance of healthy habits, especially diet, exercise, and avoidance of tobacco, alcohol abuse, and drugs.
- Reviewing medication lists is critical for avoidance of **polypharmacy** and surveillance for side effects, drug interactions, and the need for dose adjustments (see Chapter 38).
- Physical and laboratory examinations generally continue as for younger adults with additional screening for deficits in vision, hearing, and mobility. **Fall risk** assessment and dementia screening are important (see Chapter 38).
- Patients should be monitored to ensure their ability to perform activities of daily living, including driving and taking medications accurately.
- Preventive measures include offering pneumococcal, zoster, and annual influenza vaccinations (see Chapter 5).
- Many elderly patients benefit from a daily multivitamin to prevent nutritional deficiencies.
- Few guidelines exist regarding the decision as to what age to cease routine cancer screening. Therefore, the decision must be individualized and based on patient preferences, age, comorbidities, functional status, and estimated life expectancy.
- Family and community resources can provide support to enable the aging patient to remain as independent and active as possible.
- End-of-life care and establishing a living will should be discussed on an ongoing basis with patients and their families.

SCREENING FOR DISEASE

- The benefit of screening depends on the prevalence of the disease, the sensitivity and specificity of the screening test, the ability to change the natural course of disease with treatment, and the acceptability of the test to the patient. See also Chapter 5.
- Various professional organizations have made recommendations regarding screening for disease; these guidelines apply only to **asymptomatic patients at average risk**, and they must be individualized.

○ The U.S. Preventive Services Task Force (USPSTF) usually takes a conservative standpoint and does not recommend screening without relatively clear evidence for a meaningful change in outcome (http://www.uspreventiveservicestaskforce.org/, last accessed July 18, 2013). Table 1-1 lists screening activities currently recommended by the USPSTF specifically for asymptomatic patients at average risk.

TABLE 1-1	Screening and Preventive Measures Recommended by the USPSTF for *Asymptomatic Average Risk* Individuals

Abdominal aortic aneurysm screening
    Ultrasound once for men only between ages 65 and 75 who have ever
    smoked
Breast cancer screening
    Mammography in women ages 50–74
BRCA mutation screening
    Women whose family history is associated with an increased risk for deleterious mutations in *BRCA* genes should be referred for genetic counseling and evaluation for *BRCA* testing.
Cervical cancer screening
    Pap smear every 3 years for women ages 21–65
Chlamydia screening
    Sexually active women age <24 years old and older women at increased risk
Cholesterol screening
    Men >35 and women >45 years old
    Start at age 20 if at increased risk for coronary heart disease.
Colorectal cancer screening
    Fecal occult blood testing, sigmoidoscopy, or colonoscopy ages 50–75
Depression screening
    When supports are in place to assure accurate diagnosis, effective treatment and follow-up
Diabetes mellitus (type 2) screening
    Adults with blood pressure (treated or untreated) >135/80
Gonorrhea screening
    All sexually active women if they are at increased risk
Hepatitis B screening
    All pregnant women at their first prenatal visit
HIV screening
    All adolescents and adults at increased risk
Hypertension screening
    All adults ages 18 and older
Iron deficiency anemia screening
    All pregnant women
Obesity screening
    All adults
Osteoporosis
    Women >65 and younger women whose fracture risk is equal to 65-year-old white woman without other risk factors
Syphilis screening
    All pregnant women and persons at increased risk
Tobacco use screening
    All adults

USPSTF, United States Preventive Services Task Force.

- ○ Disease-specific and subspecialty groups often advocate for more aggressive screening, such as prostate and lung cancer screening.
- ○ Other groups, such as the American College of Physicians (ACP), generally take the middle ground.
- **Many areas of controversy exist**, including ages to start and stop screening, frequency of screening, which tests to use, and potential harms in screening.
- There is a lack of definitive research regarding the effect of screening on morbidity and mortality for many diseases.

Cancer Screening

- Cancer screening recommendations have been issued by many organizations, including the American Cancer Society (ACS; http://www.cancer.org, last accessed July 18, 2013), the National Cancer Institute (http://www.nci.nih.gov, last accessed July 18, 2013), the American College of Physicians (ACP; http://www.acponline.org, last accessed July 18, 2013), the United States Preventive Services Task Force (USPSTF; http://www.uspreventiveservicestaskforce.org/, last accessed July 18, 2013), and many specialty societies.
- As with screening for other conditions, the approach much be individualized.

CURRENT DISEASE MANAGEMENT

- The clinician should evaluate the status of chronic diseases and any potential new problems.
- **Not every problem can be analyzed exhaustively at each visit**.
- The average office visit is scheduled for approximately 15 minutes, so **prioritization must occur** and is usually based on the patient's chief complaint and what the clinician feels is the most serious problem.
- Explanation of disease and relief of symptoms are keys to the patient's satisfaction. Symptom relief does not always require prescription drug therapy but may include lifestyle changes, physical therapy, or over-the-counter medications.
- Reassurance that a symptom is not indicative of a more serious illness is important.
- Screening for risk factors and treating chronic conditions known to produce cardiovascular disease are critical components of ambulatory care.

Hypertension

High BP is the most common primary diagnosis in the United States and is often referred to as "the silent killer" because it is generally asymptomatic. See also Chapter 6.

- The relationship between BP and cardiovascular events is continuous, consistent, and independent of other risk factors.
- All adults should have their BP measured at least every 2 years, and more frequently if elevated, but the optimum screening interval is unknown.
- Persons should be seated quietly for at least 5 minutes in a chair, with feet on the floor and arm supported at heart level. At least two measurements should be made with an appropriate-sized cuff.
- Ambulatory BP monitoring provides more detailed information and can evaluate for "white coat" hypertension.
- Normal BP is <120/80.
- Prehypertension is defined by a systolic BP of 120 to 139 or a diastolic BP of 80 to 89 mm Hg. Prehypertensives are at high risk of developing hypertension, and early intervention can decrease the rate of progression to hypertension.
- A systolic BP >140 or diastolic BP of >90 mm Hg (measured on more than one reading) is considered hypertension. in patients younger than 65-years-old. For patients over age 65, the definition of hypertension is BP >150/90 mm Hg.

- Antihypertensive therapy has been associated with a 40% reduction in stroke, 25% reduction in myocardial infarction, and 50% reduction in heart failure.
- Initial therapy includes counseling on weight loss, aerobic exercise, limiting alcohol intake, and reduction of sodium intake. The decision as to whether to start drug therapy should depend on the severity of hypertension, the presence of other disease, and evidence of end organ damage.[1]

Dyslipidemia

Research from many different sources indicates that elevated LDL cholesterol is a major cause of coronary artery disease (CAD). See also Chapter 11.

- **Cholesterol screening is recommended at least every 5 years for all adults older than 20 years of age.**
- Screening is best performed with a lipid profile (total cholesterol, LDL cholesterol, HDL cholesterol, and triglycerides) obtained after a 12-hour fast.
- Individual patient risk assessment and classification is critical for determining treatment goals and therapeutic options.
- Initial therapy for patients with elevated cholesterol includes counseling to decrease consumption of fats and to promote weight loss in overweight patients.
- Clinical trials demonstrate that LDL-lowering therapy reduces risk for CAD.[2,3]

Diabetes Mellitus

- Diabetes mellitus (DM) requires continuing medical care and ongoing patient self-management education and support to prevent acute complications and to reduce the risk of long-term complications. See also Chapter 20.
- The American Diabetes Association standards of care are as follows:
  - For decades, the diagnosis of DM was based on either fasting plasma glucose (FPG) or the 2-hour oral glucose tolerance test (OGTT).
  - In 2009, an international expert committee recommended the use of the A1C test to diagnose DM, with a threshold of $\geq 6.5\%$.
  - The established glucose criteria for the diagnosis of DM remain valid. FPG ≥ 126 mg/dL, 2-hour plasma glucose ≥ 200 mg/dL during an OGTT, and a random plasma glucose ≥ 200 mg/dL with classic symptoms of hyperglycemia or hyperglycemic crisis are all diagnostic.
- Asymptomatic adults with sustained BP (treated or untreated) >135/80 mm Hg should be screened for diabetes.
- Screen overweight (body mass index [BMI] ≥ 25 kg/m^2) adults who have additional risk factors (presented in Table 1-2).
- Patients with prediabetes should be referred to an effective ongoing support program targeting weight loss and increasing physical activity.[4]

Obesity

- Periodic height and weight measurements are recommended for all patients. See also Chapter 22.
- The BMI is calculated as weight in kilograms divided by the height in meters squared.
  - BMI ≥ 25 kg/m^2 is considered overweight.
  - BMI ≥ 30 kg/m^2 is considered obese.
  - BMI ≥ 40 kg/m^2 is considered severely obese.
- More than one-third of US adults are obese.
- Obesity increases the risk of many health conditions including heart disease, stroke, diabetes, and certain cancers.
- Diet and exercise are the cornerstones of weight loss, though medications and bariatric surgery can be considered when lifestyle changes fail.[5]

TABLE 1-2	Criteria for Testing for DM in Asymptomatic Adults

1. Test all adults who are overweight (BMI ≥25 kg/m^2) and have at least one additional risk factor:
   - Physical inactivity
   - First-degree relative with DM
   - High-risk ethnicity (e.g., African American, Latino, Native American, Asian American, Pacific Islander)
   - Women who delivered a baby weighing >9 pounds or who were diagnosed with gestational DM
   - Hypertension
   - HDL <35 mg/dL and/or a triglyceride level >250 mg/dL
   - Women with polycystic ovary syndrome
   - A1C ≥5.7%, impaired glucose tolerance, or impaired fasting glucose on previous testing
   - Other clinical conditions associated with insulin resistance (e.g., severe obesity, acanthosis nigricans)
   - History of cardiovascular disease
2. In the absence of the above criteria, testing should begin at age 45 years.
3. If results are normal, testing should be repeated at least at 3-year intervals. Prediabetics should be tested yearly.

Modified from American Diabetes Association. Standards of medical care in diabetes—2012. *Diabetes Care* 2012;35:S11–S63.

Tobacco Abuse

- An estimated 45.3 million (19.3%) US adults smoke cigarettes. See also Chapter 45.[6]
- Cigarette smoking is the leading cause of preventable death in the United States, accounting for one of every five deaths each year.
- Although only approximately 7% of patients are able to quit long term on their own, it is estimated that counseling and appropriate pharmacotherapy can increase the quit rate to 15% to 30%.
- A widely accepted approach to brief office-based counseling and pharmacotherapy was published by the U.S. Public Health Service in 2008.[7]
- Brief counseling should be provided to all smokers at every visit. Even short interventions can increase quit rates significantly.

LIFESTYLE COUNSELING

- The most important interventions for promoting good health center on changing personal health behaviors and habits rather than specific clinical interventions or medications.
- **Regular physical activity** is important at all ages. Patients should be encouraged to be physically active with a goal of accumulating 30 minutes of moderate to vigorous activity on most days of the week. There is strong evidence that exercise protects against CAD. Cardiac risks of physical activity can be diminished by appropriate screening, counseling, and adopting a staged approach to exercise. Frequent follow-up and physician support are vital components of a successful exercise program. Physicians should attempt to present themselves as positive role models to patients by maintaining their own physical fitness.[8]
- All patients should be counseled regarding a prudent low-fat **diet** with abundant fruits, vegetables, and whole grains. Some patients may benefit from decreased sodium intake. Women at risk for osteoporosis should be counseled to consume daily calcium and

vitamin D. Women of childbearing age should consume at least 0.4-mg folic acid daily by diet or supplements.
- Patients should be advised to use **seat belts** for themselves and their passengers, to use **safety helmets** when riding motorcycles or bicycles, and to avoid alcohol or sedating medications when driving.
- Other areas for counseling and screening include alcohol use, dental health, domestic violence, unintended pregnancy, and STDs.
- Alternative health care practices, including herbal medicines, chiropractic care, acupuncture, or hypnosis, should be inquired about in a nonjudgmental manner.

PATIENT SAFETY

- Patient safety and medical errors are pertinent topics in the ambulatory setting. Adverse drug events can account for hospital admissions and significantly contribute to increased morbidity and mortality. Steps must be routinely taken to reduce the number of errors.
- **Make patients active participants in their care**.
  - This helps avoid misinterpretation of diagnostic or therapeutic plans and problems with compliance or follow-up. Involving other members of the health care team, including family, nurses, dietitians, and therapists, is vital.
  - Ensure that the patient leaves with a clear comprehensible written plan and contact information if he or she has any questions.
- **Medication reconciliation is mandatory.**
  - Request patients bring all of the medicines and supplements they are currently taking to each visit to ensure an accurate ongoing list of all medications.
  - Make sure they know what the medication is prescribed for, the dosing schedule, how long they should take it, interactions with other medications and alcohol, any monitoring or screening that may be necessary, and the importance of compliance with the medication.
  - Inquire about any new allergies or adverse reactions.
- **Electronic medical records (EMRs) are helpful**.
  - EMRs serve to limit errors due to illegible handwriting.
  - Automatic allergy alerts to prescription medications are beneficial.
  - Reminder and alert systems help minimize systemic errors in practice.
  - Lack of product functionality can be frustrating for physicians.

ADHERENCE

- Assessment of adherence requires a nonjudgmental attitude and acknowledgment of the many challenges to compliance.
  - Open-ended questions actively involve the patient.
  - Pill counts are rarely useful and may be insulting to the patient. However, encouraging patients to bring medications to their visits can help both patients and physicians maintain accurate medication lists.
  - The patient's pharmacy can provide information on refill patterns.
  - Low serum drug levels may represent failure to take the medication, poor absorption, rapid metabolism, and/or large volume of distribution.
  - Cost of medications is a common barrier to compliance. Generic alternatives should be considered when possible.
- Noncompliance must be distinguished from ineffectiveness of treatment. Presumed non-adherence should be approached as any other clinical symptom by forming a differential diagnosis of possible etiologies.

Strategies to Enhance Adherence

- **Educate** the patient about the medical condition, the risks and benefits of therapy, and alternatives using understandable language.
- **Consider the patient's perspective and keep a nonjudgmental attitude**. The patient's health belief model includes acceptance of diagnosis, perceived seriousness of condition, supposed benefits of treatment, apparent barriers, readiness for change, and the level of confidence in the physician and treatment plan.
- **Maintain contact** through follow-up visits and telephone calls.
- **Keep care as simple and inexpensive** as possible by using generic medications, once-daily or combination formulations, and drugs that are not affected by meals.
- **Give written instructions**. Have the patient repeat the instructions to assess understanding.
- **Encourage self-monitoring** so that the patient feels a sense of control over his/her own health (e.g., home BP, blood sugar, food diary, exercise log).
- **Identify and address barriers**, which can include limitations of time, money, transportation, functional illiteracy, social isolation or conflict, depression, mental illness, substance abuse, or cognitive dysfunction.
- **Focus on the positive benefits** of treatment and reinforce the patient's efforts. Set small specific goals that are achievable. Take a problem-solving approach to analyze causes and work out alternative strategies if failure occurs.
- **Discuss adherence strategies** such as the use of medication log sheets, alarms, calendars, or daily pillboxes.

DIFFICULT DOCTOR-PATIENT INTERACTIONS

- The "difficult patient" refers to those patients with whom a physician has trouble forming a normal therapeutic relationship.[9]
- A more comprehensive definition is "a person who does not assume the patient role expected by the healthcare professional, who may have beliefs and values or other personal characteristics that differ from those of the caregiver, and who causes the caregiver to experience self-doubt."[10]
- Nearly one in six outpatient visits is considered difficult. These visits lead to physician burnout and lower work satisfaction.[11]
- One great advantage of an ongoing physician-patient relationship is that it allows an opportunity to become familiar with all of a patient's problems and understand them in the context of the patient's personality and life circumstances. Hopefully, for most patients, mutual understanding and trust will grow as a therapeutic relationship develops.
- Improved communication between the physician and patient can result in better patient outcomes, improved satisfaction of both parties, decreased litigation, and less physician burnout.
- **Do not lose sight of the contributions the clinician makes to the doctor-patient relationship, even when it is difficult.**
- Consider the interaction itself "difficult" rather than the actual patient.
- Patients who interrupt a caregiver's established routines and make extra work are often considered difficult patients.
- **Patient-related characteristics** that appear to be associated with difficult doctor-patient interactions include[12]
  - Mental disorder
  - Multisomatoform disorder
  - Panic disorder
  - Dysthymia
  - Generalized anxiety
  - Major depression

- ○ Alcohol abuse or dependence
- ○ High health care utilization
- ○ More acute and chronic problems
- ○ Tendency to bring up new symptoms at the last moment
- ○ Demanding/controlling
- Potentially contributory **physician factors** include[13]
  - ○ Less experienced
  - ○ Younger
  - ○ Poorer psychosocial attitudes
  - ○ Work more hours
  - ○ Higher stress
- Given the fiduciary nature of the doctor-patient relationship, it is generally accepted that the physician has a greater responsibility to resolve relationship issues and to ensure that the interactions are as productive as possible.
- Potentially helpful recommendations include[14]:
  - ○ Recognize when an interaction is not going well and acknowledge this to yourself and to the patient.
  - ○ Remember that you are not required to solve every problem in a single visit.
  - ○ **Carefully consider how your own responses to certain patient characteristics are contributing to the interaction**.
  - ○ Try to understand the patient's perspective, consider any cross-cultural issues, and be willing to work with different personality types.
  - ○ Be empathetic regarding displays of sadness and fear.
  - ○ Always **keep in mind your fundamental responsibilities to the patient**. Be sure to take a history, perform an exam, make an assessment, and offer your best medical advice in clear, nonjudgmental terms.
  - ○ Set clear expectations/limits and maintain boundaries. "Agreeing to disagree" can be a respectful way to summarize a challenging interaction.
  - ○ Do not prescribe a medication or order a study that you do not think the patient needs just to satisfy the patient's wishes.
  - ○ Self-reflection is critical after a difficult interaction. Analyze what barriers led to the difficult visit and try to learn from them.

REFERENCES

1. Chobanian AV, Bakris GL, Black HR, et al. National High Blood Pressure Education Program Coordinating Committee on Prevention, Detection, Evaluation, and Treatment of High Blood Pressure: the JNC 7 report. *JAMA* 2003;289:2560–2572.
2. Expert Panel on Detection, Evaluation, and Treatment of High Blood Cholesterol in Adults. Executive Summary of the Third Report of the National Cholesterol Education Program (NCEP) Expert Panel on Detection, Evaluation, and Treatment of High Blood Cholesterol in Adults (Adult Treatment Panel III). *JAMA* 2001;285:2486–2497.
3. Grundy SM, Cleeman C, Merz NB, et al. Implications of recent clinical trials for the National Cholesterol Education Program Adult Treatment Panel III Guidelines. *Circulation* 2004;110:227–239.
4. American Diabetes Association. Standards of medical care in diabetes—2012. *Diabetes Care* 2012;35:S11–S63.
5. Ogden CL, Carroll MD, Kit BK, et al. Prevalence of obesity in the United States, 2009–2010. *NCHS Data Brief* 2012;(82):1–8.
6. Centers for Disease Control and Prevention. Vital signs: current cigarette smoking among adults aged ≥18 years—United States, 2005–2010. *Morb Mortal Wkly Rep* 2011;60(33):1207–1212.

7. Fiore MC, Jaen CR, Baker TB, et al. *Treating Tobacco Use and Dependence: 2008 Update. Clinical Practice Guideline.* Washington, DC: Public Health Service, U.S. Department of Health and Human Services; 2008.
8. Metkus T, Baughman K, Thompson P. Exercise prescription and primary prevention of cardiovascular disease. *Circulation* 2010;121:2601–2604.
9. Simon JR, Dwyer J, Goldfrank LR. The difficult patient. *Emerg Med Clin North Am* 1999;17:353–370.
10. Macdonald M. Seeing the cage: stigma and its potential to inform the concept of the difficult patient. *Clin Nurse Spec* 2003;17:305.
11. An PG, Rabatin JS, Manwell LB, et al. Burden of difficult encounters in primary care: data from the minimizing error, maximizing outcomes study. *Arch Intern Med* 2009;169:410.
12. Hahn SR. Physical symptoms and physician-experienced difficulty in the physician-patient relationship. *Ann Intern Med* 2001;134:897.
13. Krebs EE, Garrett JM, Konrad TR. The difficult doctor? Characteristics of physicians who report frustration with patients: an analysis of survey data *BMC Health Serv Res* 2006;6:128.
14. Coulehan JL, Block MR. *The Medical Interview: Mastering Skills for Clinical Practice,* 5th ed. Philadelphia, PA: F. A. Davis Company; 2006.

2 Care of the Surgical Patient

Anuradha Godishala and Thomas M. De Fer

General Considerations

- The role of the primary physician in preoperative assessment is to risk stratify patients, determine the need for further evaluation, and recommend interventions to mitigate risk.
- Although preoperative evaluation often focuses on cardiac risk, it is essential to remember that poor outcomes can result from significant disease in other organ systems. Evaluation of the entire patient is necessary to provide optimal perioperative care.
- Approximations of risk are derived from the temporal necessity of a procedure, clinical factors, type of anesthesia, and inherent surgical risk. Patients are considered to be at low or elevated risk for perioperative complications based on a combination of these factors.
- It is important to remember that no patient is ever truly "cleared for surgery," as there will always be some risk of perioperative morbidity and mortality.

Elective versus Emergent

- Elective surgery carries less risk of perioperative complications compared to urgent or emergent surgery. An elective procedure by definition can be postponed for up to a year, allowing time for optimization of a patient's general medical condition and treatment of cardiovascular and pulmonary disease.
- **Emergent surgeries are often associated with serious medical comorbidities,** but the disadvantages of delaying surgery may outweigh the benefits in stabilizing the patient. Life or limb is threatened if the patient is not in the operating room in approximately 6 or less hours.[1]
- **Urgent** procedures threaten life or limb if the patient is not in the operating room within 6 to 24 hours.
- **Time-sensitive** procedures may allow time for evaluation and management up to 1 to 5 weeks.

Routine Preoperative Laboratory Testing

- Preoperative laboratory testing is not routinely indicated, but selective testing may be warranted in specific circumstances, including for patients with known underlying diseases or risk factors that affect operative management and certain high-risk procedures.[2]
- The evidence suggests that 60% to 70% of preoperative testing is unnecessary if a proper history and physical exam are performed. While the cost of individual tests may be low, the aggregate costs can be substantial. Furthermore, the likelihood of a false-positive test increases with the number of tests ordered. **The frequency of unanticipated abnormalities that ultimately change management is too low to justify routine labs for all patients.**[3–6]
- Three randomized trials of preoperative medical testing before cataract surgery failed to show a significant difference in the rate of adverse perioperative events between the testing group and the no-testing group.[6] Selective ordering of tests is safer and more efficient.

• **Complete blood cell count**
  ○ The subject of preoperative anemia and particularly transfusion is controversial. The prevalence of preoperative anemia is estimated at 0% to 30% depending on age, sex, and comorbid medical conditions. Nevertheless, a complete blood cell count (CBC) is not typically warranted unless the patient is undergoing major surgery with significant blood loss expected (more than 500 mL) or the history and physical exam indicate it.
  ○ A retrospective study published in 2007 using the VA National Surgical Quality Improvement Program (NSQIP) database (over 300,000 patients) showed that mild preoperative anemia or polycythemia was associated with increased 30-day postoperative mortality and cardiac events in older male veterans undergoing noncardiac surgery.[7]
  ○ A more recent and very large study (nearly 575,000 cases) also using the NSQIP database demonstrated, after adjustment for multiple other variables, a weak association between preoperative anemia and 30-day mortality (odds ratio 1.24 [1.10 to 1.40]) in noncardiac surgical patients.[8] In patients undergoing vascular and cardiac procedures, increased morbidity and mortality appears to be related to increasing degrees of anemia.[9,10]
  ○ There is accumulating evidence that restricting blood transfusions improves outcomes. A liberal approach to transfusions in anemic patients (goal ≥10 g/dL) has not been associated with significant differences in adverse events or mortality compared with a more restrictive strategy. Therefore, in the absence of other prevailing risk factors, a restrictive approach to transfusions in the perioperative period is recommended (i.e., a transfusion trigger or threshold of 7 to 8 g/dL).[11–14]

• **Serum electrolytes**
  ○ The goal of preoperative testing is to detect abnormalities that will alter management and lead to better outcomes. The frequency of unexpected electrolyte abnormalities is low, and the relationship between most electrolyte disturbances and operative morbidity is unclear.
  ○ A 1988 study suggested that hypokalemia is not associated with adverse events or perioperative arrhythmias.[15] However, a larger 1999 study in patients undergoing coronary artery bypass graft (CABG) surgery did reveal a relationship between potassium <3.5 mEq/L, arrhythmias, and the need for cardiopulmonary resuscitation (CPR).[16] Therefore, a selective approach to preoperative testing based on clinical indications is again emphasized.

• **Renal function tests**
  ○ Renal impairment is a major predictor of postoperative complications in cardiac and noncardiac surgery and is a component of both the Revised Cardiac Risk Index (RCRI) and the NSQIP Surgical Risk Calculator.[17,18] Renal insufficiency also necessitates dosage adjustment of many medications that are used perioperatively.
  ○ Unlike other clinical conditions, mild to moderate renal insufficiency is typically asymptomatic. Thus, some experts advocate preoperative renal function testing in patients with the following risk factors: age >50 years, diabetes mellitus (DM), hypertension, cardiac disease, nephrotoxic medications (e.g., angiotensin-converting enzyme [ACE] inhibitors), or major surgical procedures likely to cause hypotension.[4]

• **Coagulation studies**
  ○ Tests of hemostasis should be performed only in those patients currently anticoagulated or whose history and physical examination suggest the presence of a bleeding disorder.
  ○ The prothrombin time (PT) and activated partial thromboplastin time (aPTT) are not predictive of perioperative hemorrhage.[4,19–21]

• **Urinalysis**
  ○ Physicians often order a preoperative urinalysis to detect asymptomatic bacteriuria, due to a purported relationship between urinary tract infections (UTIs) and wound infections, particularly with prosthetic surgery. However, the utility of routine preoperative urinalysis remains unproven, and is not currently recommended.[4,22]

○ A study failed to find any difference in the frequency of wound infection between patients with normal and abnormal urinalysis undergoing orthopedic, nonprosthetic knee procedures.[23] Another found a higher risk of postoperative wound infection in those with asymptomatic UTI, whether it was treated or not.[24]

Anesthesia Modality

• The four main classifications of anesthesia are local anesthesia, regional anesthesia (including peripheral nerve and neuraxial blockade), monitored anesthesia care (MAC), and general anesthesia. The modality of anesthesia is an often-debated aspect of preoperative assessment for which **there is no absolute consensus.**
• Multiple individual studies and meta-analyses have produced conflicting results. Patient comorbidities, preferences, and the type of surgery are crucial in determining risk.[25–31]
• Whether or not regional anesthesia reduces postoperative morbidity and mortality compared to general anesthesia is still unclear. However, a reduced risk of deep venous thrombosis is a fairly consistent finding.

Preoperative Cardiovascular Risk Assessment

GENERAL PRINCIPLES

• Of the millions of patients undergoing noncardiac surgery annually, 1% to 6% (depending on the population studied and diagnostic criteria used) will suffer **a major adverse cardiac event (MACE).** Patients with underlying cardiovascular disease (CVD), including coronary heart disease (CHD), transient ischemic attack (TIA)/cerebrovascular accident (CVA), and peripheral arterial disease (PAD), have an increased risk of perioperative cardiac complications.
• Cardiac complications constitute the most common cause of perioperative morbidity and mortality. More than 50,000 perioperative myocardial infarctions (MIs) and 1 million other cardiovascular complications occur each year.[32] Of those who have a perioperative MI (PMI), the risk of in-hospital mortality is estimated at 10% to 15%.[33]
• Patients who have noncardiac complications are more likely to develop cardiac complications and vice versa.[34]
• Traditionally, MI was defined by the World Health Organization criteria, ECG criteria, and cardiac enzymes. Cardiac troponin assays have changed this definition. The recent universal definition of MI is based on a rise of cardiac biomarkers (preferably troponin) in the setting of myocardial ischemia: cardiac symptoms, ECG changes, or imaging findings.[35]
• Defining PMI is more difficult since most occur without symptoms in anesthetized or sedated patients, and ECG changes are often subtle or transient. Studies using serial troponin measurements demonstrate that most PMIs start within 24 to 48 hours of surgery.[36,37]
• Two distinct mechanisms may lead to PMI: acute coronary syndrome (ACS) and prolonged myocardial oxygen supply-demand imbalance, designated type 1 and type 2 MI, respectively.[35] This distinction is important to therapeutic considerations.
• ACS occurs when an unstable plaque undergoes rupture leading to acute coronary thrombosis, ischemia, and infarction. Based on autopsy studies and angiographic evidence, it is likely that plaque instability plays an integral role in a significant number of these events, just as in nonperioperative infarcts.[38] Evidence suggests, however, the incidence of type 1 PMI is much lower than that of type 2 PMI. Tachycardia is the most common cause of postoperative oxygen supply-demand imbalance, but hypotension, hypertension, anemia, hypoxemia, and systolic and diastolic dysfunction can all aggravate ischemia, leading to type 2 infarction.[38]

DIAGNOSIS

Clinical Presentation

History

- The objective of the history is to identify comorbid conditions or other factors that affect perioperative risk.
- Different classification schemas have incorporated slightly different sets of risk factors.
- **The most current guidelines** are those of the American College of Cardiology (ACC) and the American Heart Association (AHA), which focus on the identification of active cardiovascular conditions, risk factors for coronary artery disease (CAD), as well as assessment of the urgency of surgery and procedure-specific risk.[1]
- The perioperative risk of a MACE is estimated as low or elevated on the basis of combined clinical/surgical risk.
  - Vascular surgeries are generally among those with the highest perioperative risk of MACE. Procedures not involving significant fluid shifts or stress, such as plastic surgery and cataract surgery, are associated with low risk of cardiac complications.
  - **A low-risk procedure is one in which the combined surgical and patient characteristics predict a risk of a MACE of death or MI of <1%.** A patient with a low risk of MACE does not require additional testing and may proceed to surgery.[1]
  - **Procedures with a risk of a MACE of ≥1% are considered elevated risk.** If a patient is at elevated risk of MACE, further evaluation is typically necessary.[1]
- The history should also seek to elucidate validated independent predictors of major cardiac complications (MI, pulmonary edema, complete heart block, ventricular fibrillation, or cardiac arrest) using validated tools.
  - **RCRI** (Table 2-1).[17] Patients with 0 or 1 predictors of risk have a low risk of MACE, whereas those with ≥2 predictors have elevated risk.
  - Two newer tools have been created by the American College of Surgeons, the NSQIP MICA (MI or cardiac arrest) risk prediction rule and the NSQIP Surgical Risk Calculator, to assess the risk of perioperative MACE.[18,39] The former incorporates five factors (age, creatinine, American Society of Anesthesia [ASA] class [Table 2-2], preoperative functional capacity, and type of procedure [there are 20 categories]) and is readily accessible via the internet, http://www.surgicalriskcalculator.com/miorcardiacarrest, accessed 1/19/15. The latter is more complex, including 21 specific patient factors, urgency of the surgery (i.e., emergency or not), and the specific procedure being performed. It is available at http://www.riskcalculator.facs.org/ (accessed 1/19/15).
  - Each of these multivariate risk models has advantages and limitations, and none is particularly favored in the most recent ACC/AHA guidelines.
- Prior iterations of the ACC/AHA guidelines have included minor predictors (e.g., age >70 years, certain abnormal ECG findings, uncontrolled hypertension). Although potentially suggestive of a higher risk of CAD, the minor predictors are no longer part of the current guidelines. However, some of them are included in the risk prediction tools above.
- Obesity is not a risk factor for most adverse perioperative outcomes including MACE, with the exception of venous thromboembolism (VTE), wound dehiscence, and wound infection. In cardiac surgery, however, some studies have demonstrated higher complication rates for obese patients. Extreme obesity and being underweight may be associated with increased risk.[40–44]
- A crucial part of the history is assessment of exercise and functional capacity. Functional status is a reliable predictor of perioperative and long-term cardiac events. If a patient has not had a recent exercise test before noncardiac surgery, functional status can usually be estimated from activities of daily living.

TABLE 2-1	Revised Cardiac Risk Index

High-risk surgery
  Intraperitoneal
  Intrathoracic
  Suprainguinal vascular procedures
History of ischemic heart disease
  History of MI (not acute or recent)
  ECG with pathologic Q waves
  History of a positive exercise stress test
  Stable angina
  Nitrate therapy
History of compensated or prior HF
  History of HF
  History of pulmonary edema
  History of paroxysmal nocturnal dyspnea
  Bilateral rales
  S3 gallop
  Chest radiograph showing pulmonary vascular redistribution
  History of cerebrovascular disease
Stroke
  TIA
  Insulin therapy for diabetes
  Preoperative serum creatinine >2.0 mg/dL

Associated major cardiac complication rate

No risk factor/Class I, 0.4%–0.5%
One risk factor/Class II, 0.9%–1.3%
Two risk factors/Class III, 3.6%–6.6%
Three or more risk factors/Class IV, 9.1%–11%

HF, heart failure; ECG, electrocardiogram; MI, myocardial infarction; TIA, transient ischemic attack.
Data from Lee TH, Marcantonio ER, Mangione CM, et al. Derivation and prospective valida-tion of a simple index for prediction of cardiac risk of major noncardiac surgery. *Circulation* 1999;100:1043–1049.

TABLE 2-2	American Society of Anesthesiologists Physical Status Classification

Physical status 1	A normal healthy patient
Physical status 2	A patient with mild systemic disease
Physical status 3	A patient with severe systemic disease
Physical status 4	A patient with severe systemic disease that is a constant threat to life
Physical status 5	A moribund patient who is not expected to survive without the operation
Physical status 6	A declared brain-dead patient whose organs are being removed for donor purposes

- ○ Functional capacity is often expressed in terms of metabolic equivalents (METs). 1 MET is the resting or basal oxygen consumption of a 40-year-old, 70-kg man. Functional capacity is classified as excellent (>10 METs), good (7 to 10 METs), moderate (4 to 6 METs), poor (<4 METs), or unknown based on patient report (Table 2-3).[45,46]
  - ○ Functional status can also be assessed more formally by activity scales, such as the **Duke Activity Status Index** (DASI) and the Specific Activity Scale.[47]
  - ○ The likelihood of a MACE is inversely related to baseline functional status. Patients with reduced functional status preoperatively are at increased risk of major perioperative complications, and vice versa. In general, asymptomatic patients with moderate functional status (>4 METs) are at relatively low risk.
- Patients should be asked about all prescribed medications, over-the-counter agents, nutritional supplements, and complementary/alternative treatments.
- A history of substance use/abuse should be sought from all patients.
- Elderly patients, particularly those with underlying dementia, are at increased risk for postoperative agitation and delirium. Careful attention should therefore be paid to the medical factors that may contribute to altered mental status (e.g., sedative or alcohol abuse, other medications, and infection).

Physical Examination
- A complete physical examination is essential.
- Specific attention should be paid to the following:
  - ○ Vital signs, particularly blood pressure (BP). Systolic blood pressure (SBP) of <180 mm Hg and diastolic blood pressure (DBP) of <110 mm Hg are generally considered acceptable. The management of SBP >180 mm Hg or DBP >110 mm Hg is controversial. Postponing elective surgery to allow adequate BP control in this setting is reasonable but poorly studied. The appropriate length of time to wait after treatment is instituted is also unclear.

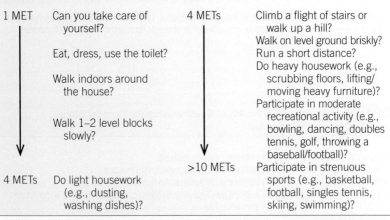

TABLE 2-3	Estimated Metabolic Equivalents (METs) of Various Activities		
1 MET	Can you take care of yourself?	4 METs	Climb a flight of stairs or walk up a hill?
			Walk on level ground briskly?
	Eat, dress, use the toilet?		Run a short distance?
			Do heavy housework (e.g., scrubbing floors, lifting/moving heavy furniture)?
	Walk indoors around the house?		
			Participate in moderate recreational activity (e.g., bowling, dancing, doubles tennis, golf, throwing a baseball/football)?
	Walk 1–2 level blocks slowly?		
		>10 METs	Participate in strenuous sports (e.g., basketball, football, singles tennis, skiing, swimming)?
4 METs	Do light housework (e.g., dusting, washing dishes)?		

Data from Hlatky MA, Boineau RE, Higginbotham MB, et al. A brief self-administered questionnaire to determine functional capacity (the Duke Activity Status Index). *Am J Cardiol* 1989;64:651–654; Fletcher GF, Balady G, Froelicher VF, et al. Exercise standards: statement for healthcare professionals from the American Heart Association. *Circulation* 1992;86:340–344; Fleisher LA, Beckman JA, Brown KA, et al. ACC/AHA 2007 guidelines on perioperative cardiovascular evaluation and care for noncardiac surgery. *Circulation* 2007;116:e418–e499.

○ Murmurs suggestive of significant valvular stenosis or regurgitation.
○ Evidence of heart failure (HF) (jugular venous distension, crackles, S3 gallop, peripheral edema).
- A thorough preoperative neurologic examination may identify patients with baseline cognitive impairment or dementia who are at increased risk for delirium, and serves as a useful comparison if there is a question of altered mental status perioperatively.

Diagnostic Criteria

Figure 2-1 presents an overview of the 2014 ACC/AHA guidelines on perioperative cardiovascular assessment and management of patients undergoing noncardiac surgery.[1]

Step 1
- **Determine the urgency of surgery—emergent or not.**
- If truly emergent, proceed to surgery.
- Perioperative monitoring and management should be based on the presence of or clinical risk factors for CAD.

Step 2
- **For urgent or elective surgery, determine if an ACS is present.**
- If the patient has an **ACS,** postpone surgery, evaluate, and treat based on guideline-directed medical therapy (GDMT).

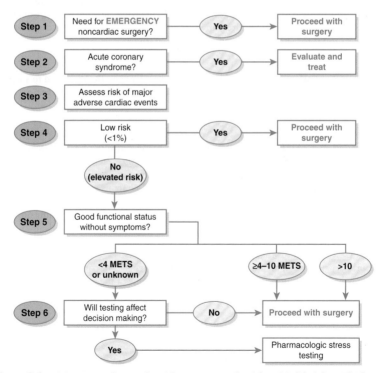

Figure 2-1 ACC/AHA cardiovascular risk assessment algorithm. Modified from Fleisher LA, Fleischmann KE, Auerbach AD, et al. 2014 ACC/AHA guideline on perioperative cardiovascular evaluation and management of patients undergoing noncardiac surgery. *J Am Coll Cardiol* 2014;64:e77–e137.

Step 3

Estimate perioperative risk of a MACE based on combined clinical/surgical risk. This estimate can be generated by incorporating the RCRI with an estimation of surgical risk or by using the NSQIP risk calculator (http://www.surgicalriskcalculator.com (accessed 1/19/15).[17,18]

Step 4

If the patient has a low risk of a MACE (<1%), no additional testing is required and the patient may proceed to surgery.

Step 5

• **If the patient is at elevated risk of a MACE (≥1%), determine functional capacity by either patient report or objective measure such as the DASI.**[45-47]
• If the patient has a functional capacity of ≥4 METs without symptoms, then proceed to surgery without further evaluation.

Step 6

• **A patient with poor (<4 METs) or unknown functional capacity may need additional testing, but only if it will impact patient decision making (i.e., willingness to undergo percutaneous coronary intervention [PCI] or CABG depending on the results of the test) or perioperative care.**
• Stress testing is appropriate in this context. If the stress test is abnormal, coronary angiography and revascularization should be pursued. Following this, the patient can either proceed to surgery or consider alternative strategies, such as noninvasive treatment or palliative care. If the stress test is normal, proceed to surgery.

Step 7

If testing will not affect decision making or perioperative care, then proceed to surgery with optimal medical management or consider alternate strategies as above.

Diagnostic Testing

12-Lead Electrocardiogram
• The current ACC/AHA guidelines recommend a preoperative resting 12-lead ECG for patients with known CHD, significant arrhythmia, PAD, cerebrovascular disease, or structural heart disease, except for those undergoing low-risk surgery.[1]
  ○ In patients with established CHD, the baseline ECG contains prognostic information relating to short- and long-term morbidity and mortality.
  ○ Although no data exist regarding the optimal time interval between obtaining an ECG and elective surgery, general consensus suggests 1 to 3 months is adequate.
• Preoperative resting ECG may also be considered for asymptomatic patients without known CHD, except for those undergoing low-risk surgery.
• The primary utility of a preoperative ECG in most patients is for comparison with ECGs that may be obtained postoperatively. Therefore, the value of the baseline ECG increases with the risk of the surgical procedure.

Resting Echocardiogram
• Several studies have demonstrated an association between reduced left ventricular (LV) systolic function and perioperative complications, particularly postoperative HF, with the greatest risk in patients with an left ventricular ejection fraction (LVEF) of <35%. Assessment of EF by echocardiogram has relatively high specificity for predicting perioperative cardiac events, but only modest incremental predictive power over clinical risk factors.[48]
• Indications for preoperative echocardiography are no different than in the nonoperative setting, and is not routinely recommended.[1]

- Auscultated murmurs suggestive of significant underlying valvular disease should be evaluated by echocardiography, as should occur in a nonoperative setting. Of significant note, the surgical risk of asymptomatic severe aortic stenosis is no longer considered prohibitively high as to be an absolute contraindication to elective noncardiac surgery.[1]
- The most recent ACC/AHA guidelines recommend preoperative evaluation of LV function with resting echocardiogram for the following[1]:
  ○ Patients with dyspnea of unknown origin.
  ○ Patients with known HF and worsening dyspnea or other change in clinical status.
  ○ In patients with a prior history of LV dysfunction, reassessment of LV function may be considered if more than a year has elapsed since the last evaluation.

Noninvasive Stress Testing
- **Routine stress testing of all patients undergoing surgery is not warranted.** The decision to pursue a stress evaluation should be guided by assessment of perioperative risk and functional capacity, as detailed above.
- Importantly, **stress testing should not be performed unless the patient is willing to undertake subsequent clearly indicated treatments.**
- Noninvasive stress testing is not routinely indicated for patients at low risk for noncardiac surgery.
- The 2014 ACC/AHA guidelines additionally recommend the following[1]:
  ○ Noninvasive stress testing (exercise or pharmacologic) for patients who are at an elevated risk of MACE and have either poor (<4 METs) or unknown functional capacity, if it will change management.
  ○ For patients with elevated risk and excellent (>10 METs) functional capacity, it is reasonable to forgo further exercise testing and proceed to surgery.
  ○ Consider noninvasive stress testing for patients with elevated risk and moderate (4 to 6 METs) or good (7 to 10 METs) functional capacity, only if it will alter perioperative care.

Coronary Angiography
- **Routine preoperative coronary angiography in all patients is not recommended.**[1]
- The indications for preoperative coronary angiography do not differ from those identified in the nonoperative setting. Patients with a clear indication for angiography on clinical grounds, apart from perioperative risk stratification, should be managed according to standard guidelines.
- The use of coronary computerized tomography angiography and calcium scoring to determine the presence and extent of CAD is a less invasive and lower risk alternative to cardiac catheterization. However, its utility in preoperative risk assessment has not been fully established.[49]

TREATMENT

Medications
β-Blockers
- Multiple, earlier, small trials suggested that perioperative β-blocker therapy improves cardiovascular outcome and reduces mortality.[50–53]
- More recent data, however, have questioned the purported benefits of perioperative β-blockade.[54–57]
  ○ In particular, the large POISE trial, which confirmed a decrease in cardiac events (e.g., ischemia, atrial fibrillation, need for coronary interventions) with aggressive perioperative β-blockade, but also demonstrated a higher overall mortality, related to an increased rate of stroke and death from noncardiac complications.[56]

- ○ An important difference between the studies showing effectiveness of perioperative β-blocker therapy and the POISE trial was the β-blocker regimen used. The POISE trial employed a relatively high dose of extended-release metoprolol beginning on the day of surgery. Prior studies, however, started a long-acting β-blocker days to weeks before surgery and titrated the dose preoperatively.
- The most recent ACC/AHA guidelines have incorporated the newer results into the recommendations regarding perioperative β-blocker use.[1,58]
  - ○ **β-blockers should be continued in patients receiving them chronically** for clear indications. Abrupt withdrawal of long-term β-blockade is harmful.[59]
  - ○ In patients with three or more RCRI risk factors (e.g., DM, HF, CAD, renal insufficiency, CVA) or intermediate- to high-risk myocardial ischemia noted on preoperative testing, it may be reasonable to begin perioperative β-blockade.
  - ○ It is preferred that β-blocker therapy is **initiated more than 1 day before surgery** in order to assess clinical effectiveness, safety, and tolerability. The need for dose titration is controversial.[60] **β-blockers should not be started on the day of surgery.**

α_2-Agonists

- Previous data suggested that prophylactic use of α_2-adrenergic agonists such as clonidine and mivazerol could reduce the risk of perioperative myocardial ischemia and death.[61–63]
- POISE-2, a recent large randomized clinical trial (RCT), failed to show any benefit of clonidine in decreasing perioperative morbidity or mortality. Clonidine did, however, increase the rate of nonfatal cardiac arrest and clinically significant hypotension.[64]
- The current ACC/AHA guidelines recommend against α_2-agonists for the prevention of cardiac events.[1]

Angiotensin-Converting Enzyme Inhibitors

- At present, there are insufficient data regarding specific surgery types or patient subgroups that are most likely to benefit from holding ACE inhibitors perioperatively.
- A meta-analysis of available trials demonstrated more frequent transient intraoperative hypotension in patients taking ACE inhibitors or angiotensin-receptor blockers (ARBs), but no difference in perioperative cardiovascular events.[65] A large retrospective study failed to find an association between ACE inhibitor use and hemodynamic findings.[66] A very recent study supports the concern for hypotension and also suggests the possibility for an association with acute kidney injury.[67] On the other hand, there is some evidence for poor outcomes in patients whose ACE inhibitors are discontinued abruptly and not resumed.[68,69]
- Continuation of ACE inhibitors or ARBs in the perioperative period is reasonable at present but new data are likely to refine this recommendation.[1] The optimal timing of the last dose before surgery and the first postoperative is uncertain at this time.

Statins

- Observational data support a reduced rate of MACE in patient undergoing noncardiac surgery.[70–73]
- The effect may be more notable in those undergoing vascular surgery.[74–76] It is reasonable to initiate statin therapy for anyone prior to vascular surgery.[1]
- Perioperative initiation of statins may also be considered in patients with clinical indications who are scheduled for elevated risk procedures.[1]
- Statin therapy should be continued in those currently taking statins.[1]

Revascularization

- The utility of preoperative revascularization in reducing perioperative cardiac complications continues to be uncertain. The combined morbidity and mortality of coronary revascularization and the planned noncardiac surgery must be considered in the context of a patient's overall health, functional status, and long-term prognosis before proceeding with either.[1]

- Revascularization before vascular surgery has not demonstrated improved outcomes in RCTs.[77-79] This includes the controversial DECREASE-V study.[78,79] Left main disease may be an exception.[80]
- According to the most recent ACC/AHA guidelines, revascularization before noncardiac surgery should be **limited to patients for whom revascularization is clinically indicated based on existing practice guidelines.**[1]
- **If preoperative PCI is necessary,** the urgency of the noncardiac surgery, as well as the risk of bleeding and ischemic events, including stent thrombosis, associated with the surgery in a patient taking dual antiplatelet therapy (DAPT) is important to consider in determining optimal timing, stent, and antiplatelet strategy.
- The ACC/AHA recommends DAPT with aspirin (ASA) 81 mg daily and a $P2Y_{12}$ receptor blocker (clopidogrel 75 mg daily, prasugrel 5 to 10 mg daily, or ticagrelor 90 mg bid) for a minimum duration of:[1,81]
  - At least 1 month in patients receiving bare metal stents (BMS).
  - 12 months in patients receiving drug-eluting stents (DES).
- BMS and DES have similar rates of early stent thrombosis, and the risk is greatest in the first 4 to 6 weeks following implantation.[82,83] This is largely attributed to the cessation of DAPT in the perioperative period. The risk of in-stent restenosis, however, is higher with BMS than DES.[84,85]
- Elective procedures with significant risk of bleeding should be postponed until patients have completed the minimum duration of DAPT. Some data suggest that in newer-generation DES, the risk of stent thrombosis is stabilized by 6 months after implantation.[1] However, 12 months is still preferred due to the risk, albeit low, of very late stent thrombosis.
- If noncardiac surgery is time sensitive or the risk of bleeding is high, consideration should be given to balloon angioplasty or BMS placement. If coronary revascularization is imperative prior to urgent or emergent surgery, CABG may also be considered.[1] For angioplasty alone, 2 to 4 weeks delay is recommended, though the event rates appear to be considerably lower.[86,87]
- For patients who have received coronary stents and must undergo procedures that mandate the discontinuation of $P2Y_{12}$ receptor blocker therapy, it is recommended to continue ASA if possible and to restart DAPT as soon as feasible after surgery.[1]
- DAPT should not be discontinued without first consulting the patient's cardiologist. See Figure 2-2 for an algorithm for antiplatelet management in patients with PCI and noncardiac surgery.[1]

SPECIAL CONSIDERATIONS

Hypertension

- DBP <110 mm Hg is does not appear to be an independent predictor of perioperative MACE, though evidence is limited.[88] A specific statement cannot be made about SBP due to a lack of data.
- Higher preoperative BPs are thought to be associated with exaggerated BP responses to anesthesia, reactions to noxious stimuli, and overall BP lability. Weak data also suggest an association with MI, arrhythmias, and other complications. Whether or not lowering BP preoperatively mitigates this risk is unclear at this time.
- Patients receiving antihypertensive agents for longitudinal indications are generally advised to remain on their current medication regimen in the perioperative period.[1]
  - Patients chronically on β-blockers should continue therapy to avoid tachycardia and rebound hypertension.
  - Maintaining continuity of ACE inhibitors or ARBs in the setting of treatment for hypertension or HF is also recommended. If held on the day of surgery, these medications should be resumed as soon as clinically feasible postoperatively.[65-69]

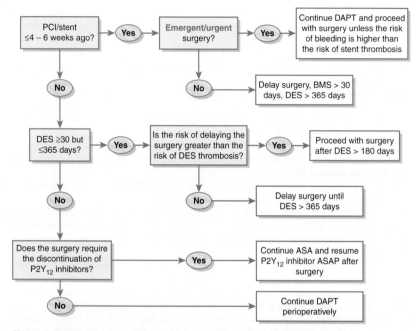

Figure 2-2 **Perioperative antiplatelet therapy for patients with PCI.** Modified from Fleisher LA, Fleischmann KE, Auerbach AD, et al. 2014 ACC/AHA guideline on perioperative cardiovascular evaluation and management of patients undergoing noncardiac surgery. *J Am Coll Cardiol* 2014;64:e77–e137.

Valvular Heart Disease

- Patients with preoperative suspicion for moderate to severe valvular abnormalities should be evaluated by echocardiography (if one has not been done in the past 1 year).[1]
- Symptomatic stenotic lesions are potentially more problematic than regurgitant lesions. Time permitting (i.e., the planned surgery is elective) therapy should follow established guidelines, including valvular repair or replacement as appropriate.[1,89] Transcatheter aortic valve replacement may be an option for some patients felt to be poor candidates for standard surgical aortic valve replacement.[1]
- The perioperative risks associated with severe aortic and mitral stenosis are currently felt to be less than indicated by prior studies, which demonstrated a very high incidence of MACE.[90–93] Therefore, these valvular abnormalities are no longer considered an absolute contraindication to urgent/emergent surgery.
- In patients with asymptomatic severe aortic or mitral stenosis, it may be acceptable to proceed with surgery and with appropriate intraoperative and postoperative hemodynamic monitoring.[1]
- Endocarditis prophylaxis is warranted only in specific clinical contexts (see Endocarditis Prophylaxis section).

Pacemakers and Implantable Cardioverter Defibrillators

- A major concern in the perioperative management of patients with cardiac implantable electronic devices (CIEDs) is the potential for interaction between the pacemaker or implantable cardioverter defibrillator (ICD) and monopolar electrocautery.
- Various errors may occur, ranging from resetting of the device to inadvertent reprogramming to unintentional discharge. Optimally, the device should be interrogated preoperatively and again postoperatively to ensure proper function.

- The most important precaution to take is direct communication between the physician managing the implanted device and the surgical team. In particular, they should discuss any electromagnetic interference that may occur during the planned procedure.[1,94]
- Continuous cardiac monitoring during the procedure should be done when an ICD has had its tachytherapy functions deactivated. A transcutaneous defibrillator must be available and the ICD must be reprogrammed after the surgery.[1,94]

Congestive Heart Failure

- Acute decompensated HF is a contraindication to surgery. Medical treatment for HF should be carefully optimized prior to elective noncardiac surgery (see Chapter 8).
- In a cohort study of 38,047 consecutive patients, perioperative morbidity and mortality was shown to be significantly higher in those with active HF compared to those with atrial fibrillation or CAD.[95] Lower ejection fraction appears to be associated with increased risk.

Preoperative Pulmonary Evaluation

GENERAL PRINCIPLES

- Postoperative pulmonary complications contribute significantly to overall perioperative morbidity and mortality and are as common as cardiac complications.[40,96]
- A cost analysis performed by the NSQIP found pulmonary complications to be the most expensive of major perioperative medical complications, including cardiac, infectious, and thromboembolic, and also resulted in the longest length of stay.[97]
- The most significant complications include **atelectasis, pulmonary infection, exacerbation of underlying lung disease, prolonged mechanical ventilation, and respiratory failure.**
- The American College of Physicians practice guideline recognizes the following patient-related factors that increase the risk of postoperative pulmonary complications.[40,96]
  - Age > 60
  - History of chronic obstructive pulmonary disease (COPD)
  - Congestive HF
  - ASA class >II (Table 2-2)[98]
  - Functional dependence
- Other data support the following as additional patient-related risk factors: smoking, HF, malnutrition, obstructive sleep apnea (OSA), and pulmonary hypertension.[99–102]
- Factors that have not been consistently shown to be associated with postoperative pulmonary complications include controlled asthma and obesity.[40]
- Procedure-related risk factors include the following[40,96,99–101]:
  - Surgical site: aortic, vascular, neurosurgery, head and neck, thoracic, and abdominal. Patients undergoing aortic aneurysm repair are at the highest risk for perioperative pulmonary complications. Low-risk procedures include hip surgery and gynecologic or urologic procedures.
  - Emergency surgery.
  - Prolonged surgery (>2.5 to 4 hours).
  - General anesthesia.
  - Use of long-acting neuromuscular blockers.

DIAGNOSIS

Clinical Presentation

- The focus should be on identifying the presence of patient-related risk factors.
- A thorough respiratory and smoking history should be obtained.

- Any current upper respiratory tract infection symptoms should be ascertained but they are not an absolute contraindication to surgery.
- Patients should be questioned about their general functional status and exercise tolerance.
- Attention should be paid to evidence of chronic lung disease such as increased antero-posterior dimensions of the chest, hyperresonance, diminished breath sounds, and the presence of adventitious lung sounds such as crackles, rhonchi, or wheezing.
- Signs of HF should also be sought, including rales, extra heart sounds, jugular venous distention, and peripheral edema.
- Body habitus may suggest the possibility of OSA and obesity hypoventilation syndrome. How aggressively to screen for OSA is an open question at present.

Diagnostic Criteria

- In contrast to the relatively well-defined risk assessment strategy for cardiovascular complications described above, there is no single, evidence-based algorithmic approach for perioperative pulmonary risk stratification for noncardiac surgery.
- The **postoperative pneumonia risk index** is presented in Table 2-4.[99]

TABLE 2-4	Postoperative Pneumonia Risk Index		
Risk factor	**Point value**	**Risk factor**	**Point value**
Type of surgery		Weight loss >10% in past 6 months	7
AAA repair	15	History of COPD	5
Thoracic	14	General anesthesia	4
Upper abdominal	10	Impaired sensorium	4
Neck	8	History of CVA	4
Neurosurgical	8	BUN (mg/dL)	
Vascular	3	<8	4
Age (years)		22–30	2
≥80	17	≥30	3
70–79	13	Transfusion >4 units	3
60–69	9	Emergency surgery	3
50–59	4	Chronic steroid use	3
Functional status		Current smoker with 1 year	3
Totally dependent	10	>2 drinks/day in past 2 weeks	2
Partially dependent	6		

Risk class	Risk of pneumonia
1 (0–15 points)	0.2%
2 (16–25 points)	1.2%
3 (26–40 points)	4.0%
4 (41–55 points)	9.4%
5 (>55 points)	15.3%

AAA, abdominal aortic aneurysm; BUN, blood urea nitrogen; COPD, chronic obstructive pulmonary disease; CVA, cerebrovascular accident.
Modified from Arozullah AM, Khuri SF, Henderson WG, et al.; Participants in the National Veterans Affairs Surgical Quality Improvement Program. Development and validation of a multifactorial risk index for predicting postoperative pneumonia after major noncardiac surgery. *Ann Intern Med* 2001;135:847–857.

TABLE 2-5	Respiratory Failure Risk Index

Predictor	Points
Type of surgery	
Abdominal aortic aneurysm	27
Thoracic	21
Neurosurgical, upper abdomen, peripheral vascular	14
Neck	11
Emergency surgery	11
Albumin <3.0 mg/dL	9
BUN >30 mg/dL	8
Partially of fully functionally dependent status	7
History of COPD	6
Age	
60–69	4
≥70	6

Class	Points	Risk of postoperative respiratory failure
1	≤10	0.5%
2	11–19	1.8%–2.1%
3	20–27	4.2%–5.3%
4	28–40	10.1%–11.9%
5	>40	26.6%–30.9%

Modified from Arozullah AM, Daley J, Henderson WG, et al. Multifactorial risk index for predicting postoperative respiratory failure in men after major noncardiac surgery. The National Veterans Administration Surgical Quality Improvement Program. *Ann Surg* 2000; 232:242–253.

- The **respiratory failure risk index** of Arozullah et al.[103] is a validated model that can assist in predicting the rate of postoperative respiratory failure (Table 2-5). An analysis of a larger more representative sample of surgical patients resulted in the respiratory risk index that is predictive of ≥48 hours of ventilator dependence or unplanned reintubation. It consists of 28 independently associated variables and, therefore, is not likely to be used frequently in routine clinical practice.[100]
- The Canet Risk Index was more recently developed to help determine the incidence of perioperative pulmonary complications of any severity. This index, based on seven, independent risk factors, was derived from a relatively small cohort study, however, and has the disadvantage of including outcomes of minor clinical significance (e.g., new wheezing treated with bronchodilators).[104]
- Regardless of how risk is determined, those at increased risk are reasonable targets for strategies intended to mitigate the risk of postoperative pulmonary complications.

Diagnostic Testing
Laboratory Studies
- A decreased **serum albumin level** is a potent predictor of pulmonary risk.[40,96]
  - A level <3.5 mg/dL appears to be indicative of increased risk. It is recommended to measure albumin in patients clinically suspected to have hypoalbuminemia as well as those with one or more risk factors for perioperative pulmonary complications.

- ○ At present, however, there is no conclusive evidence that enteral or parenteral nutritional supplementation decreases this risk.
- Elevated **blood urea nitrogen** (BUN) and creatinine have been associated with pulmonary complications. Preoperative renal function testing is therefore reasonable.
- It is unclear whether **arterial blood gas** (ABG) results contribute to the estimate of perioperative pulmonary risk beyond the aforementioned clinically derived variables.
  - ○ There are no proven abnormal levels beyond which surgery is contraindicated.
  - ○ A preoperative ABG is only justified if otherwise clinically necessary.
  - ○ The primary purpose in most patients will be to serve as a baseline comparison for ABGs that may be obtained in the postoperative period.

Imaging
- Many chest radiography (CXR) findings deemed abnormal are chronic and do not generally affect management.[4,40,96,101,105,106] Furthermore, abnormal preoperative CXRs are often predicted based on the history and physical examination, and CXR only rarely provides unexpected information that influences perioperative management.
- **Routine preoperative CXR in all patients is not recommended.**
- Limited evidence suggests that preoperative CXR may be beneficial for patients with known cardiopulmonary disease, and those >50 years of age who are undergoing upper abdominal, thoracic, or abdominal aortic aneurysm surgery.[96]

Diagnostic Procedures
- The value of **pulmonary function testing** before lung resection and in determining candidacy for CABG is generally well accepted but no consensus exists on the utility of routine spirometry before extrathoracic surgery.[40,96,101]
- Preoperative spirometry may identify patients at higher risk of pulmonary complications. However, the data are mixed and spirometry has not been shown to be superior to history and physical examination in predicting perioperative risk.
- No prohibitive spirometric threshold has been established below which the risk of surgery is unacceptable.
- Pulmonary function testing is warranted for patients with a suspected but yet undiagnosed pulmonary condition for which evaluation would have also been indicated outside the context of surgery.

TREATMENT

Smoking Cessation
- Smoking is associated with an increased occurrence of postoperative pulmonary complications.[40,101,102]
- A clear benefit has been shown if patients abstain from smoking at least 4 weeks prior to scheduled surgery.[101,107–109]
- Previous concerns about a paradoxical increase in complications appear unwarranted, so all patients should be counseled to stop smoking even if <8 weeks from surgery.[108]
- Smoking cessation is discussed in detail in Chapter 45.

Obstructive Lung Disease Therapy
- Medical therapy should be optimized and elective surgery postponed, if possible, in the setting of acute exacerbations of COPD or asthma.
- The treatment of COPD and asthma is discussed in Chapter 16.
- See Perioperative Corticosteroid Management regarding COPD or asthma patients taking systemic steroids.

Postoperative Interventions

- **Lung expansion maneuvers** (i.e., incentive spirometry, deep breathing exercises, and continuous positive airway pressure [CPAP]) may reduce the risk of postoperative pulmonary complications.[101,107] However, two recent meta-analyses have questioned the effectiveness of incentive spirometry and CPAP.[110,111]
- Patients with diagnosed OSA on CPAP therapy should continue it up to the day of surgery and during the hospitalization.
- A strategy of selective nasogastric tube placement after abdominal surgery rather than routine use has also been shown to decrease the risk of pulmonary complications.[107,112]

Perioperative Consideration in Liver Disease

GENERAL PRINCIPLES

- Patients with end-stage liver disease undergoing surgery are at high risk for perioperative morbidity and mortality.
- Likely related to decreased hepatic perfusion during anesthesia, patients with advanced liver disease have substantial risk of acute hepatic decompensation postoperatively.[113]
- The systemic effects of liver dysfunction can subsequently result in an increased frequency of other major complications as well, including severe coagulopathy, encephalopathy, acute respiratory distress syndrome, acute renal failure, and sepsis.

DIAGNOSIS

- Since significant liver disease is usually suspected clinically and the prevalence of unexpected liver enzyme abnormalities is low, **routine laboratory screening for hepatic dysfunction is not recommended.**[114]
- Patients with known or suspected liver disease should undergo a thorough evaluation of liver function including hepatic enzyme levels, albumin and bilirubin measurements, and tests of hemostasis.
- In patients with cirrhosis, higher **Child-Pugh scores** correlate with greater degrees of hepatic dysfunction and increasing perioperative morbidity and mortality.[115]
- Studies indicate that the **Model of End-Stage Liver Disease (MELD) score** may also be a reliable predictor of postoperative complications and mortality. The MELD score is discussed in detail in Chapter 30. Data suggest that a MELD score >14 more accurately predicts poor outcomes than does a Child class C.[116]

TREATMENT

- Elective surgery is contraindicated in patients with acute viral or alcoholic hepatitis, and should be delayed until recovery is documented. Patients with chronic hepatitis but without evidence of hepatic decompensation generally tolerate surgery well.
- The AGA Institute recommends the following management in cirrhotic patients[116]:
  - For those with a MELD score <11, the postoperative mortality is adequately low to justify the risks of surgery.
  - Patients with a MELD score of 12 to 19 should complete liver transplant evaluation prior to elective surgery so that they may proceed to urgent liver transplantation if necessary.
  - Elective procedures should be postponed until after liver transplantation in patients with a MELD score ≥20.
  - Others have suggested similar ranges, MELD <10, 10 to 15, and >15.[117]

- Based on the high perioperative mortality rates in patients with advanced cirrhosis, nonsurgical alternatives should be strongly considered.
- For patients requiring surgery, steps should be taken to optimize the preoperative status including coagulopathy, thrombocytopenia, renal and electrolyte abnormalities, volume status, ascites, and encephalopathy. These subjects are discussed in detail in Chapter 30.

Perioperative Consideration in Kidney Disease

- Chronic kidney disease (CKD) is an independent risk factor for perioperative MACE, so patients with renal disease need appropriate cardiac risk stratification.[1,11,18,39]
- End-stage renal disease (ESRD) patients undergoing surgery possess a substantial risk of morbidity and mortality.[118]
- Most general anesthetic agents have no appreciable nephrotoxicity or effect on renal function other than that mediated through hemodynamic changes.[119]
- Every effort should be made to achieve euvolemia preoperatively in order to reduce the incidence of volume-related complications in the perioperative period.[120]
  ○ Although this usually entails removing fluid, some patients may be hypovolemic and require hydration.
  ○ Patients with CKD may need diuretic therapy before surgery.
  ○ ESRD patients on dialysis should receive dialysis preoperatively. This is typically performed on the day prior to surgery but can be done on the day of surgery as well. The potential for transient electrolyte abnormalities, fluid shifts, and hemodynamic changes postdialysis must be considered, however.
- Hyperkalemia in the preoperative setting should be treated according to standard practice, particularly since the tissue breakdown occurring with surgery is likely to elevate the potassium level further (see Chapter 24).
- Platelet dysfunction is associated with uremia.
  ○ The ability of preoperative bleeding time to predict postoperative hemorrhagic complications is questionable.[121] Assessment of bleeding time prior to surgery is not routinely recommended in patients with CKD or ESRD.
  ○ Patients with evidence of perioperative bleeding, however, should receive further evaluation and treatment (see Chapter 12).

Perioperative Consideration in Diabetes Mellitus

GENERAL PRINCIPLES

- **Hospitalized patients with diabetes and hyperglycemia are at increased risk for poor outcomes.**[122]
- Data from critically ill/intensive care unit (ICU) patients initially suggested improved outcome with tight glycemic control. More recent trials using very stringent targets (e.g., 80 to 110 mg/dL) have failed to demonstrate a mortality benefit, possibly due to difficulty achieving these goals without raising the risk of severe hypoglycemia.[123–126]
- Although it is uncertain if improving glucose control in the non-ICU setting decreases morbidity or mortality, the robust association between hyperglycemia and surgical complications such as poor wound healing still makes glycemic control a priority in the perioperative setting.[122]
- **Severe hypoglycemia (<40 mg/dL) is independently associated with in-hospital mortality and should be scrupulously avoided.**[127,128]

TREATMENT

- **Elective surgery in patients with uncontrolled DM should preferably be delayed until acceptable glycemic control has been achieved.**
- Whenever possible, procedures should be scheduled for early morning to minimize prolonged fasting.
- **Frequent monitoring of blood glucose levels is essential in all situations.**
- **Hypoglycemia must be avoided with the same vigor as hyperglycemia.**

Target Glucose Levels

- The current American Diabetes Association inpatient guidelines take into account the most recent trial data regarding tight glycemic control and the risk of hypoglycemia.[122]
- For **critically ill patients,** therapy should be initiated for persistent hyperglycemia (threshold no >180 mg/dL) with a target glucose range of **140 to 180 mg/dL.** Targets <110 mg/dL are not recommended. **Insulin infusion protocols are preferred in such situations.**
- In noncritically ill hospitalized patients, a preprandial goal of <140 mg/dL and random blood glucose levels <180 mg/dL is recommended.
- The optimal glucose range in postsurgical patients is uncertain but likely to be in a very similar range (e.g., 150 to 200 mg/dL). More stringent targets are ineffective (i.e., do not lower the rate of infection, cardiovascular events, renal failure, or death) and associated with increased episodes of hypoglycemia.[129]
- The publically reported Surgical Care Improvement Project (SCIP) quality metric for patients undergoing cardiac surgery is glucose <200 mg/dL at 6 AM, the morning following surgery.

Type 1 Diabetes

- **Some form of basal insulin is required at all times.**
- On the evening prior to surgery, the regularly scheduled basal insulin dose should be continued. If taken in the morning, it is still recommended to give the basal insulin without dose adjustment.
- IV glucose (i.e., 5% dextrose-containing fluids) may need to be administered in the perioperative period to avoid hypoglycemia while the patient is NPO and until tolerance of oral intake is observed.
- For complicated surgeries or procedures requiring prolonged NPO status, a continuous insulin infusion will likely be necessary.
- **Caution should be exercised with the use of subcutaneous insulin in the intraoperative and critical care settings, as alterations in tissue perfusion may result in variable absorption.**

Type 2 Diabetes

- **Diet controlled**
  - These patients can generally be managed without insulin therapy.
  - Glucose values should be checked regularly. Elevated levels (>180 mg/dL) can be treated with intermittent doses of short-acting insulin.
- **Managed with oral therapy**
  - Short-acting sulfonylureas, as well as most other oral diabetic agents, should be **held on the day of surgery.**
  - Metformin and long-acting sulfonylureas (e.g., glimepiride) should be **withheld 1 day before scheduled surgical procedures.**
  - Metformin is generally held for at least 48 hours postoperatively. **Renal function should be normal or at baseline prior to resuming metformin.**

○ **Other oral diabetic agents can be resumed once patients are tolerating their preprocedure diet.** This recommendation assumes such patients will be discharged from the hospital shortly; otherwise, **oral hypoglycemic medications are generally inappropriate for most inpatients.**

○ As in the diet-controlled type 2 diabetics, blood sugar should be checked regularly and short-acting insulin therapy initiated if persistent hyperglycemia (>180 mg/dL) is noted.

○ Most of these patients can be managed without an insulin infusion.

• **Managed with insulin**

○ **So-called sliding scale insulin is often ineffective as monotherapy.**

○ If it is anticipated that the patient will be able to eat postoperatively, basal insulin should be given on the morning of surgery.

  ▪ If given as long-acting insulin (e.g., glargine insulin) and the patient usually takes the dose in the morning, 80% to 90% of the routine dose can be given.

  ▪ If the patient uses intermediate-acting insulin (e.g., NPH), half to two-thirds of the usual morning dose is given to avoid periprocedural hyperglycemia.

○ Patients undergoing major procedures may require an insulin infusion perioperatively. In these cases, glucose-containing IV fluids with supplemental potassium should be administered concomitantly to avoid hypoglycemia and hypokalemia, respectively.

○ The baseline insulin regimen can typically be resumed once oral intake is reestablished.

Perioperative Antiplatelet and Anticoagulation Management

ANTIPLATELET AGENTS

• Patients taking ASA for secondary prevention may continue it if having a minor dental, dermatologic, or cataract procedures.[130]

• Early use of ASA improves outcomes after PCI and CABG.[131] For patients undergoing PCI or CABG, ASA should be continued without interruption.[130]

• For patients undergoing CABG who are taking DAPT, the $P2Y_{12}$ receptor blocker should be held 5 to 7 days before surgery.[130]

• If possible, ASA and a $P2Y_{12}$ receptor blocker (clopidogrel, prasugrel, or ticagrelor) should be continued perioperatively in **patients with recent coronary stents** and who are undergoing noncardiac surgery. If surgery can be safely postponed until the minimal period of DAPT is complete (4 to 6 weeks BMS, 12 months DES), it should be.[1,81,130] Refer to the Revascularization section above for a detailed discussion. If the minimum time as has elapsed and the patient continues DAPT, then the $P2Y_{12}$ receptor blocker can be stopped starting 5 to 7 days preoperatively.

• The most recent American College of Chest Physicians (ACCP) guidelines recommend continuing ASA in patients who are at moderate to high risk for cardiovascular events.[130] But this recommendation came before the results of the POISE-2 trial. ASA is not indicated for patients at low risk.

• The recent **POISE-2 trial** enrolled over 10,000 patients at risk for cardiovascular complications who were going to undergo noncardiac surgery.

○ Inclusion criteria selected for those with CVD (i.e., history of CAD, PAD, CVA, or the need for major vascular surgery) or with several factors known to increase risk. Those within 1 year or 6 weeks of receiving a DES or BMS, respectively, were excluded. Very few patients who had a prior stent and few with a history of CAD were included.

○ Nearly half of the patients were already on a daily ASA regimen, which they stopped taking at least 3 days before surgery per the study protocol. In those patients who were randomized to the placebo group, there **was no associated increase in thrombotic events related to sudden withdrawal of ASA.**

- Patients were randomized to receive either ASA or placebo just before surgery and for 30 days after.
- There was **no difference in the primary outcome of death or nonfatal MI** between the ASA and placebo groups. There was, however, **a higher rate of major bleeding** in the ASA group.[132]
- These results suggest that patients at risk for CVD who are taking ASA for prevention of cardiovascular events should discontinue it at least 3 days prior to surgery.[132] Because the number of patients who had previously undergone PCI is small, it is difficult to draw firm conclusions about this group.[133]

- The ACC/AHA guideline, which does include the results of the POISE-2 trial, states that it still may be reasonable to continue ASA in patients at high risk for CAD or CVA when the risk of cardiovascular events outweighs the potential risk of increased bleeding, particularly those with a prior stent (Fig. 2-2).[1]

ANTICOAGULANTS

- In determining an appropriate anticoagulation strategy, the benefit of continued treatment must be weighed against the risk of bleeding for each individual patient and procedure.
- Proceeding directly to surgery is generally acceptable if the INR ≤ 1.5.
- Some procedures may be safely performed with an INR of 2.0 to 3.0 (e.g., endoscopy without biopsy, dental procedures, and skin biopsies). For dental procedures, the antifibrinolytic oral mouthwash tranexamic acid may be used.[130]
- If interruption of warfarin therapy is necessary, it should be discontinued 4 to 5 days before the procedure, allowing the INR to drift below 1.5.[130,134] Warfarin should then be resumed 12 to 24 hours after surgery and when there is adequate hemostasis.[130]
- With regard to the novel oral anticoagulants (NOACs), including the direct thrombin inhibitor dabigatran and the factor Xa inhibitors rivaroxaban and apixaban, there are no data available to guide perioperative management.[130] Given the lack of a specific reversal agent, however, discontinuation of NOACs ≥48 hours prior to surgery is recommended.[1]
- If a temporary interruption of anticoagulation is unacceptable (e.g., mechanical heart valve, atrial fibrillation, or high/moderate risk VTE), parenteral **bridging anticoagulation** (i.e., low molecular weight heparin [LMWH] or unfractionated heparin [UFH]) is warranted but should be discontinued 4 to 24 hours before the procedure, depending on the half-life of the drug.[130]
  - LMWH is favored over UFH in patients with normal renal function since it is easier to administer and does not require routine testing of PT, aPTT, or anti-Xa levels.
  - Following **high-bleeding-risk surgery** bridging anticoagulation can be resumed in approximately 48 to 72 hours. This would include urologic, cardiac, intracranial, and spinal procedures; surgery on highly vascular organs (e.g., kidney, spleen, liver); bowel resection; major surgery with extensive tissue injury (e.g., joint arthroplasty, cancer procedures, reconstructive plastic surgery); pacemaker and ICD placement; and resection of colonic polyps (usually sessile polyps >1 to 2 cm long).
  - Following **non–high-bleeding-risk surgery,** anticoagulation can be resumed at 24 hours.

Perioperative Corticosteroid Management

GENERAL PRINCIPLES

- Surgery is a potent activator of the hypothalamic-pituitary axis (HPA). Patients with adrenal insufficiency may lack the ability to respond appropriately to surgical stress.
- Additionally, patients on chronic corticosteroid therapy for indications other than adrenal dysfunction are at risk of developing perioperative adrenal insufficiency.

- The subtype of adrenal insufficiency has implications on management.
  - **Tertiary adrenal insufficiency** due to exogenous corticosteroid administration is the most common adrenal problem encountered. These patients should have intact mineralocorticoid function and therefore require only glucocorticoid supplementation.
  - Likewise, **secondary adrenal insufficiency** should not result in mineralocorticoid deficiency. The possibility of deficits in other hormones due to pituitary disease should be considered.
  - **Primary adrenal insufficiency** requires replacement of both mineralocorticoids and glucocorticoids.
- The dose and duration of exogenous corticosteroids required to produce clinically significant tertiary adrenal insufficiency is highly variable, but general principles can be outlined[135]:
  - Daily therapy with ≤5 mg of prednisone (or equivalent), alternate day corticosteroid therapy (<10 mg of prednisone), and any dose given for <3 weeks **should not result in clinically significant adrenal suppression.** Testing is not necessary in these patients and supplemental perioperative steroids are not warranted.
  - Patients currently receiving >20 mg/day of prednisone (or equivalent) for >3 weeks, as well as those cushingoid in appearance, can be **expected to have suppression of adrenal responsiveness,** and, therefore, testing is not necessary.
  - The function of the HPA **cannot be readily predicted** in patients currently taking prednisone doses of 5 to 20 mg for >3 weeks or who have received >5 mg/day for >3 weeks anytime within the prior year. These patients **should be tested for adrenal responsiveness.**
  - While uncommon, HPA suppression can occur with high-dose inhaled corticosteroids. One can consider testing adrenal responsiveness in patients taking >800 μg of fluticasone/day or >1,500 μg/day of another inhaled corticosteroid.[136,137]

DIAGNOSIS

- For patients in whom clinical prediction of adrenal function is difficult, a morning (AM) cortisol or a cosyntropin stimulation test can be performed.
- An AM cortisol level of >10 μg/dL is indicative of a very low likelihood of HPA suppression, while an AM cortisol level of <5 μg/dL (>24 hours after the last dose of exogenous steroid) is suggestive of significant suppression. Values between 5 and 10 μg/dL are nondiagnostic and require further investigation with a cosyntropin stimulation test.[138]
- The short cosyntropin stimulation test is as follows: 250 μg IV or IM cosyntropin is given and plasma cortisol is measured 30 minutes later. The normal response is a stimulated plasma cortisol >20 μg/dL.

TREATMENT

- It is generally agreed that patients with known or expected adrenal insufficiency undergoing more than minor surgery should be treated with perioperative glucocorticoids.
- If HPA axis status is uncertain and there is inadequate time to perform a cosyntropin stimulation test, preoperative corticosteroids should be administered empirically.
- The following guidelines are based on extrapolation from small studies in the literature, expert opinion, and clinical experience[135]:
  - **Minor surgical stress** (e.g., colonoscopy, cataract surgery, or inguinal hernia repair): Give 25 mg hydrocortisone or 5 mg methylprednisolone IV on the day of the procedure only. Some suggest that no so-called stress doses steroids are needed in these circumstances and the patient should simply take their usual morning dose of steroids.

- **Moderate surgical stress** (e.g., cholecystectomy, hemicolectomy, or joint replacement): Give 50 to 75 mg hydrocortisone or 10 to 15 mg methylprednisolone IV on the day of surgery and taper quickly over 1 to 2 days to the usual dose.
- **Major surgical stress** (e.g., cardiothoracic surgery, aortic aneurysm repair, or Whipple procedure): Give 100 to 150 mg hydrocortisone or 20 to 30 mg methylprednisolone IV on the day of the procedure and taper to the usual dose over the next 1 to 2 days.
- **Critically ill patients requiring emergent surgery** (e.g., septic or cardiogenic shock): Give 50 to 100 mg hydrocortisone IV every 6 to 8 hours or 0.18 mg/kg/hour as a continuous infusion plus 0.05 mg/day of fludrocortisone until shock resolves. Then gradually taper the dose, monitoring vital signs and serum electrolytes closely.

- Additional mineralocorticoid supplementation for patients with primary adrenal insufficiency may or may not be necessary, depending on the dose and mineralocorticoid potency of the corticosteroid given.
- A recent systematic review, including nine small studies, suggested that stress dose steroids may not be routinely required in the perioperative period for patients on therapeutic doses, so long as they continue to receive their usually daily dose.[139]

Other Medication Adjustments in Perioperative Period

THYROID HORMONE REPLACEMENT

- Patients with hypothyroidism who appear clinically euthyroid and are receiving thyroxine treatment can safely skip this medication for several days owing to its long half-life.
- Patients should restart therapy once they can take PO.
- In patients who are unable to resume oral intake within 5 to 7 days, IV thyroxine should be given at approximately 80% of the oral dose.[140]

ANTICONVULSANTS

- Elective surgery is generally avoided in patients with poorly controlled seizures.
- If surgery is necessary, anticonvulsants should be given parenterally until the patient is able to resume taking medications by mouth.
- When IV or IM preparations are unavailable, substitutes such as phenytoin, levetiracetam, or phenobarbital may be used, depending on seizure type.
- Phenytoin has a relatively long half-life and therefore a single dose may be held safely.

PSYCHIATRIC MEDICATIONS

- **Benzodiazepines** should be continued postoperatively in patients chronically receiving them, given the risk for acute, life-threatening withdrawal with abrupt cessation.
- **Selective serotonin reuptake inhibitors** (SSRIs) can safely be given in the perioperative period. Observational studies suggest an association of SSRIs with a very small increased risk of bleeding, but whether this should impact perioperative medication management is unknown.[141]
- **Tricyclic antidepressants** (TCAs) have significant anticholinergic and α-adrenergic blocking properties, in addition to a high potential for drug-drug interactions. It is preferable to hold TCAs several days prior to elective surgery.
- **Monoamine oxidase inhibitors** (MAOIs) have the potential for severe drug interactions, and, therefore, must be stopped at least 2 weeks prior to elective surgery.
- **Antipsychotics** can typically be continued without adverse effects. However, the clinician should be mindful of the QT prolongation that can occur with these medications and should consider discontinuation if a preoperative ECG demonstrates a prolonged QT interval.

- **Lithium** has a narrow therapeutic window. Serious toxicity can occur when overdosed. Lithium can cause fluid and electrolyte abnormalities and prolong the effects of anesthetic and neuromuscular blocking agents. Lithium should be held 1 to 2 days preoperatively and restarted once the patient is reliably taking PO.

HERBAL MEDICATIONS

- It is important to ask patients specifically about the use of alternative or herbal preparations, as many will not report these when asked for a medication list.
- All of the following herbal remedies should be stopped before surgery[142-144]:
  - **Feverfew, ginger, and gingko** can cause platelet dysfunction and increase the risk of perioperative bleeding.
  - **Valerian root** potentiates the effects of sedatives and anxiolytics.
  - **St. John's wort** may have MAOI-like activity.
  - Toxic effects of **ma huang** include hypertension, arrhythmias, and myocardial ischemia.

Prophylactic Measures

VENOUS THROMBOEMBOLISM PROPHYLAXIS

- VTE prophylaxis is generally relevant only in the inpatient setting. However, because of its importance, the topic will be briefly covered here.
- VTE encompasses both deep vein thrombosis (DVT) and pulmonary embolism (PE). Prophylaxis is of paramount concern as DVT/PE remains the leading cause of preventable in-hospital mortality.
- The 2012 ACCP guidelines divide patients undergoing surgery into very low, low, moderate, or high risk groups.[145,146] Although there have been many attempts to accurately quantitate these risks, no single method has been found to be universally acceptable. The Caprini VTE risk scoring model is presented in Table 2-6.[145,147] The Patient Safety in Surgery Study score can also be used but pertains only to surgical patients and includes factors generally outside the purview of the internist (e.g., wound class and surgical relative value units).[148] Regardless of the model used, **the risk of VTE increases with the number of risk factors** and point total.
- As seen in Table 2-6, patients at very low risk do not require specific prophylaxis. Those at low risk should receive mechanical prophylaxis. Those at high risk should receive pharmacologic and mechanical prophylaxis.[145] A validation study of the Caprini model in a surgical population indicates that those with >8 points are at especially high risk of VTE, with mean risk >6%.[149]
- A number of pharmacologic agents are available for VTE prevention in surgical patients, including UFH, LMWH, fondaparinux, warfarin, dabigatran, rivaroxaban, and apixaban. The selection of an appropriate prophylactic agent depends on its efficacy and safety, the risk of bleeding, as well as patient comorbidities and preferences.
- VTE prophylaxis should commence either before or shortly after surgery, and at minimum be continued until the patient is ambulatory.
- Of note, extended VTE prophylaxis (usually between 10 and 35 days) is offered postoperatively to patients at highest risk for DVT/PE, particularly those who have undergone major orthopedic, oncologic, or abdominal surgery.[147,149]

ENDOCARDITIS PROPHYLAXIS

- In 2007, the AHA released its most recent guideline regarding infective endocarditis (IE) prophylaxis, which contains major changes compared to prior iterations.[150]

TABLE 2-6 Caprini VTE Risk Scoring Model and the Risk of VTE

1 Point	2 Points	3 Points	5 Points
Age 41–60	Age 61–74	Age ≥75	Stroke <1 month ago
Minor surgery	Arthroscopic surgery	Personal history of VTE	Hip, pelvis, or leg fracture
BMI >25 kg/m^2	Open or laparoscopic surgery >45 minutes	Family history of thrombosis	Elective lower extremity arthroplasty
Leg edema, current	Malignancy (present or previous)	Heparin-induced thrombocytopenia	Spinal cord injury <1 month ago
Varicose veins	Confined to bed >72 hours	Prothrombin 20210A	Multiple trauma
Acute myocardial infarction	Immobilizing plaster cast <1 month	Elevated anticardiolipin antibodies	
Medical patient on bed rest	Central venous access	Factor V Leiden	
Heart failure, <1 month		Positive lupus anticoagulant	
Sepsis <1 month		Elevated serum homocysteine	
History of IBD		Other congenital or acquired thrombophilia	
Prior surgery <1 month ago			
Serious lung disease, including pneumonia <1 month			
Abnormal pulmonary function			
Pregnant or postpartum			
OCP or HRT			
History of unexplained or recurrent spontaneous abortion			

(Continued)

TABLE 2-6 Caprini VTE Risk Scoring Model and the Risk of VTE (*Continued*)

1 Point	2 Points	3 Points	5 Points

Risk stratification and interpretation

VTE risk category	Score	Estimated baseline risk in the absence of mechanical or pharmacologic prophylaxis (%)	Recommendation for thromboprophylaxis
Very low	0	<0.5	No specific prophylaxis other than early ambulation
Low	1–2	1.5	Mechanical prophylaxis[a]
Moderate	3–4	3.0	Pharmacologic[b] OR mechanical prophylaxis
High	≥5	6.0	Pharmacologic[b] AND mechanical prophylaxis

[a]Intermittent pneumatic compression favored over graduated compression stockings.

[b]Presuming the patient is not at high risk for major bleeding complications. Low molecular weight heparin generally preferred over unfractionated heparin. Warfarin and other oral anticoagulants alternatives for total knee and hip replacement.

BMI, body mass index; IBD, inflammatory bowel disease; OCP, oral contraceptive pills; HRT, hormone replacement therapy; VTE, venous thromboembolism.

Data from Gould MK, Garcia DA, Wren SM, et al. Prevention of VTE in nonorthopedic surgical patients: antithrombotic therapy and prevention of thrombosis, 9th ed.: American College of Chest Physicians evidence-based clinical practice guidelines. *Chest* 2012;141:e227S–e277S; Caprini JA. Risk assessment as a guide for the prevention of the many faces of venous thromboembolism. *Am J Surg* 2010;199:S3–S10.

- There is a notable lack of data supporting the use of antibiotic prophylaxis to prevent IE in the setting of dental, gastrointestinal (GI), and genitourinary (GU) procedures.
- To date, there has been no prospective, placebo-controlled, multicenter, randomized, double-blind study of the efficacy of IE antibiotic prophylaxis.
- Based on a synthesis of available data, the cumulative risk for IE is much greater from repeated bacteremias induced by daily activities (e.g., chewing, brushing, flossing) than dental procedures. Although the absolute risk for IE from a dental procedure is difficult to measure precisely, best available estimates suggest it is exceedingly low.
- Accordingly, only an extremely small number of cases of IE might be prevented even if antibiotic prophylaxis were 100% effective. Put differently, a large number of prophylactic doses would be needed to prevent a single case of IE.
- While the risks of single-dose antibiotic prophylaxis are minimal, they do exist (e.g., increased antibiotic resistance and rare cases of anaphylaxis).
- The AHA, therefore, suggests placing **greater emphasis on oral health and dental care in patients with underlying cardiac conditions that predispose to the acquisition of IE** and are associated with the highest risk of adverse outcomes from IE.
- The guidelines conclude that antibiotic prophylaxis is recommended **only in very few clinical situations.**
- Prophylaxis is recommended only for patients undergoing certain dental procedures and who have one of the cardiac conditions listed in Table 2-7.[150] **Patients with mitral valve prolapse are no longer included.**
  - Antibiotic prophylaxis is reasonable for **dental procedures that involve manipulation of the gingival tissue or periapical region** (i.e., near the roots) of the teeth, or perforation of the oral mucosa.
  - Tooth extractions and cleanings are included. In these instances, prophylactic antibiotics should be directed against viridans streptococci.
- Despite known resistance patterns, the recommended regimens for IE prophylaxis prior to dental procedures are as follows[150]:
  - **Amoxicillin 2 g PO taken 30 to 60 minutes before the procedure.**
  - **If unable to take PO,** ampicillin 2 g IM/IV **OR** cefazolin 1 g IM/IV **OR** ceftriaxone 1 g IM/IV 30 to 60 minutes before the procedure.
  - **If allergic to penicillin,** cephalexin 2 g PO (avoid if there is a history of anaphylaxis) **OR** azithromycin/clarithromycin 500 mg PO **OR** clindamycin 600 mg PO **30 to 60** minutes before the procedure. A different first- or second-generation cephalosporin can be substituted for cephalexin, if dose equivalent.

TABLE 2-7	Cardiac Conditions with the Highest Risk of Adverse Outcome from Infective Endocarditis

Prosthetic valve or prosthetic material used for valve repair
Previous infective endocarditis
Congenital heart disease (CHD)
Unrepaired cyanotic CHD, including palliative shunts and conduits
Completely repaired CHD with prosthetic material or device, whether placed by surgery or by catheter intervention, during the first 6 months after the procedure
Repaired CHD with residual defects at the site or adjacent to the site of a prosthetic patch or prosthetic device which inhibit endothelialization)
Cardiac transplantation recipients who develop cardiac valvulopathy

Data from Wilson W, Taubert KA, Gewitz M, et al. Prevention of infective endocarditis: guidelines from the American Heart Association. *Circulation* 2007;116:1736–1754.

○ For patients who are **penicillin-allergic AND cannot take PO,** cefazolin/ceftriaxone 1 g IM/IV (do not use if there is a history of anaphylactoid reactions) **OR** clindamycin 600 mg IM/IV 30 to 60 minutes before the procedure.

• While there are no conclusive data, the ACC/AHA guideline states that IE prophylaxis is also reasonable for high-risk patients (i.e., those with the conditions in Table 2-7) having **procedures on the respiratory tract involving incision or biopsy of the respiratory mucosa.** The same regimens recommended above for dental procedures can be used.[150]

• Prior to **procedures on infected skin, skin structures, or musculoskeletal tissue,** antibiotic prophylaxis may be reasonable in patients with the cardiac conditions shown in Table 2-7. It is likely that the treatment for the infection itself will be active against staphylococci and β-hemolytic streptococci; that is, an antistaphylococcal penicillin or cephalosporin. For patients allergic to penicillin, or who are suspected or known to have a methicillin-resistant *Staphylococcus aureus* infection, vancomycin or clindamycin should be used.[150]

• Antibiotic prophylaxis solely to prevent IE is **no longer recommended** for any patient undergoing **GI (including endoscopy) or GU procedures.**

REFERENCES

1. Fleisher LA, Fleischmann KE, Auerbach AD, et al. 2014 ACC/AHA guideline on perioperative cardiovascular evaluation and management of patients undergoing non-cardiac surgery. *J Am Coll Cardiol* 2014;64:e77–e137.
2. Garcia-Miguel FJ, Serrano-Aguilar PG, Lopez-Bastida J. Preoperative assessment. *Lancet* 2003;362:1749–1757.
3. Johnson RK, Mortimer AJ. Routine pre-operative blood testing: is it necessary? *Anaesthesia* 2002;57:914–917.
4. Smetana GW, Macpherson DS. The case against routine preoperative laboratory testing. *Med Clin North Am* 2003;87:7–40.
5. Dzankic S, Pastor D, Gonzalez C, et al. The prevalence and predictive value of abnormal preoperative laboratory tests in elderly surgical patients. *Anesth Analg* 2001;93:301–308.
6. Keay L, Lindsley K, Tielsch J, et al. Routine preoperative medical testing for cataract surgery. *Cochrane Database Syst Rev* 2012;(3):CD007293.
7. Wu WC, Schifftner TL, Henderson WG, et al. Preoperative hematocrit levels and postoperative outcomes in older patients undergoing noncardiac surgery. *JAMA* 2007;297:2481–2488.
8. Saager L, Turan A, Reynolds LF, et al. The association between preoperative anemia and 30-day mortality and morbidity in noncardiac surgical patients. *Anesth Analg* 2013;117:909–915.
9. Dunkelgrun M, Hoeks SE, Welten GM, et al. Anemia as an independent predictor of perioperative and long-term cardiovascular outcome in patients scheduled for elective vascular surgery. *Am J Cardiol* 2008;101:1196–1200.
10. Gupta PK, Sundaram A, Mactaggart JN, et al. Preoperative anemia is an independent predictor of postoperative mortality and adverse cardiac events in elderly patients undergoing elective vascular operations. *Ann Surg* 2013;258:1096–1102.
11. Carson JL, Terrin ML, Noveck H, et al. Liberal or restrictive transfusion in high-risk patients after hip surgery. *N Engl J Med* 2011;365:2453–2462.
12. Carson JL, Brooks MM, Abbott JD, et al. Liberal versus restrictive transfusion thresholds for patients with symptomatic coronary artery disease. *Am Heart J* 2013;165:964–971.

13. Salpeter SR, Buckley JS, Chatterjee S. Impact of more restrictive blood transfusion strategies on clinical outcomes: a meta-analysis and systematic review. *Am J Med* 2014;127:124–131.

14. Carson JL, Carless PA, Hebert PC. Transfusion thresholds and other strategies for guiding allogeneic red blood cell transfusion. *Cochrane Database Syst Rev* 2012;(4):CD002042.

15. Hirsch IA, Tomlinson DL, Slogoff S, et al. The overstated risk of preoperative hypokalemia. *Anesth Analg* 1988;67:131–136.

16. Wahr JA, Parks R, Boisvert D, et al. Preoperative serum potassium levels and perioperative outcomes in cardiac surgery patients. Multicenter Study of Perioperative Ischemia Research Group. *JAMA* 1999;281:2203–2210.

17. Lee TH, Marcantonio ER, Mangione CM, et al. Derivation and prospective validation of a simple index for prediction of cardiac risk of major noncardiac surgery. *Circulation* 1999;100:1043–1049.

18. Gupta PK, Gupta H, Sundaram A, et al. Development and validation of a risk calculator for prediction of cardiac risk after surgery. *Circulation* 2011;124:381–387.

19. Houry S, Georgeac C, Hat JM, et al. A prospective multicenter evaluation of preoperative hemostatic screening tests. The French Associations for Surgical Research. *Am J Surg* 1995;170:19–23.

20. Chee YL, Crawford JC, Watson HG, et al. Guidelines on the assessment of bleeding risk prior to surgery or invasive procedures. British Committee for Standards in Haematology. *Br J Haematol* 2008;140:496–504.

21. Seicean A, Schiltz NK, Seicean S, et al. Use and utility of preoperative hemostatic screening and patient history in adult neurosurgical patients. *J Neurosurg* 2012;116:1097–1105.

22. Lawrence VA, Kroenke K. The unproven utility of preoperative urinalysis: clinical use. *Arch Intern Med* 1988;148:1370–1373.

23. Koulouvaris P, Sculco P, Finerty E, et al. Relationship between perioperative urinary tract infection and deep infection after joint arthroplasty. *Clin Orthop Relat Res* 2009;467:1859–1867.

24. Ollivere BJ, Ellahee N, Logan K, et al. Asymptomatic urinary tract colonization predisposes to superficial wound infection in elective orthopedic surgery. *Int Orthop* 2009;33:847–850.

25. Urwin SC, Parker MJ, Griffiths R. General versus regional anaesthesia for hip fracture surgery: a meta-analysis of randomized trials. *Br J Anaesth* 2000;84:450–455.

26. Rodgers A. Walker N, Schug S, et al. Reduction of postoperative mortality and morbidity with epidural or spinal anesthesia: results from overview of randomized trials. *BMJ* 2000;321:1493–1497.

27. Parker MJ, Handoll HH, Griffiths R. Anaesthesia for hip fracture surgery in adults. *Cochrane Database Syst Rev* 2004;(4):CD000521.

28. Mauermann WJ, Shilling AM, Zuo Z. A comparison of neuraxial block versus general anesthesia for elective total hip replacement: a meta-analysis. *Anesth Analg* 2006;103:1018–1025.

29. Hu S, Zhang ZY, Hua YQ, et al. A comparison of regional and general anaesthesia for total replacement of the hip or knee: a meta-analysis. *J Bone Joint Surg Br* 2009;91:935–942.

30. Macfarlane AJ, Prasad GA, Chan VW, et al. Does regional anaesthesia improve outcome after total hip arthroplasty? A systematic review. *Br J Anaesth* 2009;103:335–345.

31. Macfarlane AJ, Prasad GA, Chan VW, et al. Does regional anesthesia improve outcome after total knee arthroplasty? *Clin Orthop Relat Res* 2009;467:2379–2402.

32. Fleisher LA, Eagle KA. Clinical practice. Lowering cardiac risk in noncardiac surgery. *N Engl J Med* 2001;345:1677–1682.

33. Adesanya AO, de Lemos JA, Greilich NB, et al. Management of perioperative myocardial infarction in noncardiac surgical patients. *Chest* 2006;130:584–596.
34. Fleischmann KE, Goldman L, Young B, et al. Association between cardiac and noncardiac complications in patients undergoing noncardiac surgery: outcomes and effects on length of stay. *Am J Med* 2003;115:515–520.
35. Thygesen K, Alpert JS, White HD; for the Joint ESC/ACCF/AHA/WHF Task Force for the Redefinition of Myocardial Infarction. Universal definition of myocardial infarction. *J Am Coll Cardiol* 2007;50:2173–2195.
36. Kikura M, Oikawa F, Yamamoto K, et al. Myocardial infarction and cerebrovascular accident following non-cardiac surgery: differences in postoperative temporal distribution and risk factors. *J Thromb Haemost* 2008;6:742–748.
37. Badner NH, Knill RL, Brown JE, et al. Myocardial infarction after noncardiac surgery. *Anesthesiology* 1998;88:572–578.
38. Landesberg G, Beattie WS, Mosseri M, et al. Perioperative myocardial infarction. *Circulation* 2009;119:2936–2944.
39. Cohen ME, Ko CY, Bilimoria KY, et al. Optimizing ACS NSQIP modeling for evaluation of surgical quality and risk: patient risk adjustment, procedure mix adjustment, shrinkage adjustment, and surgical focus. *J Am Coll Surg* 2013;217:336–346.
40. Smetana GW, Lawrence VA, Cornell JE; American College of Physicians. Preoperative pulmonary risk stratification for noncardiothoracic surgery: systematic review for the American College of Physicians. *Ann Intern Med* 2006;144:581–595.
41. Yap CH, Zimmet A, Mohajeri M, et al. Effect of obesity on early morbidity and mortality following cardiac surgery. *Heart Lung Circ* 2007;161:31–36.
42. Herrera FA, Yanagawa J, Johnson A, et al. The prevalence of obesity and postoperative complications in a Veterans Affairs Medical Center general surgery population. *Am Surg* 2007;73:1009–1012.
43. Tyson GH, Rodriguez E, Elci OC, et al. Cardiac procedures in patients with a body mass index exceeding 45: outcomes and long-term results. *Ann Thorac Surg* 2007;84:3–9.
44. Engel AM, McDonough S, Smith JM. Does an obese body mass index affect hospital outcomes after coronary artery bypass graft surgery? *Ann Thorac Surg* 2009;88:1793–1800.
45. Reilly DF, McNeely MJ, Doerner D, et al. Self reported exercise tolerance and the risk of serious perioperative complications. *Arch Intern Med* 1999;159:2185–92.
46. Fleisher LA, Beckman JA, Brown KA, et al. ACC/AHA 2007 guidelines on perioperative cardiovascular evaluation and care for noncardiac surgery. *Circulation* 2007;116:e418–e499.
47. Hlatky MA, Boineau RE, Higginbotham MB, et al. A brief self-administered questionnaire to determine functional capacity (the Duke Activity Status Index). *Am J Cardiol* 1989;64:651–654.
48. Rohde LE, Polanczyk CA, Goldman L, et al. Usefulness of transthoracic echocardiography as a tool for risk stratification of patients undergoing major noncardiac surgery. *Am J Cardiol* 2001;87:505–509.
49. Ahn JH, Park JR, Min JH, et al. Risk stratification using computed tomography coronary angiography in patients undergoing intermediate-risk noncardiac surgery. *J Am Coll Cardiol* 2014;61:661–668.
50. Mangano DT, Layug EL, Wallace A, et al. Effect of atenolol on mortality and cardiovascular morbidity after noncardiac surgery. *N Engl J Med* 1996;335:1713–1720.
51. Wallace A, Layug B, Tateo I, et al. Prophylactic atenolol reduces postoperative myocardial ischemia. McSPI Research Group. *Anesthesiology* 1998;88:7–17.
52. Stevens RD, Burri H, Tramèr MR. Pharmacologic myocardial protection in patients undergoing noncardiac surgery: a quantitative systematic review. *Anesth Analg* 2003;97:623–633.

53. McGory ML, Maggard MA, Ko CY. A meta-analysis of perioperative beta blockade: what is the actual risk reduction? *Surgery* 2005;138:171–179.

54. Juul AB, Wetterslev J, Bluud C, et al. Effect of perioperative beta blockade in patients with diabetes undergoing major non-cardiac surgery: randomized placebo controlled, blinded multicenter trial. *BMJ* 2006;332:1482–1488.

55. Yang H, Raymer K, Butler R, et al. The effects of perioperative beta-blockade: results of the Metoprolol after Vascular Surgery (MaVS) study, a randomized controlled trial. *Am Heart J* 2006;152:983–990.

56. POISE Study Group; Devereaux PJ, Yang H, et al. Effects of extended-release metoprolol succinate in patients undergoing non-cardiac surgery (POISE trial): a randomised controlled trial. *Lancet* 2008;371:1839–1847.

57. Bangalore S, Wetterslev J, Pranesh S, et al. Perioperative beta blockers in patients having non-cardiac surgery: a meta-analysis. *Lancet* 2008;372:1962–1976.

58. Wijeysundera DN, Duncan D, Nkonde-Price C, et al. Perioperative beta blockade in noncardiac surgery: a systematic review for the 2014 ACC/AHA guideline on perioperative cardiovascular evaluation and management of patients undergoing noncardiac surgery. *J Am Coll Cardiol* 2014;64:2406–2425.

59. Rangno RE, Langlois S. Comparison of withdrawal phenomena after propranolol, metoprolol, and pindolol. *Am Heart J* 1982;104:473–478.

60. Biccard BM, Sear JW, Foex P. Meta-analysis of the effect of heart rate achieved by perioperative beta-adrenergic blockade on cardiovascular outcomes. *Br J Anaesth* 2008;100:23–28.

61. Nishina K, Mikawa K, Uesugi T, et al. Efficacy of clonidine for prevention of perioperative myocardial ischemia: a critical appraisal and meta-analysis of the literature. *Anesthesiology* 2002;96:323–329.

62. Wijeysundera DN, Naik JS, Beattie WS. Alpha-2 adrenergic agonists to prevent perioperative cardiovascular complications: a meta-analysis. *Am J Med* 2003;114:742–752.

63. Wallace AW, Galindex D, Salahieh A, et al. Effect of clonidine on cardiovascular morbidity and mortality after noncardiac surgery. *Anesthesiology* 2004;101:284–293.

64. Devereaux PJ, Sessler DI, Leslie K, et al. Clonidine in patients undergoing noncardiac surgery. *N Engl J Med* 2014;370:1504–1513.

65. Rosenman DJ, McDonald FS, Ebbert JO, et al. Clinical consequences of withholding versus administering renin-angiotensin-aldosterone system antagonists in the preoperative period. *J Hosp Med* 2008;3:319–325.

66. Turan A, You J, Shiba A, et al. Angiotensin converting enzyme inhibitors are not associated with respiratory complications or mortality after noncardiac surgery. *Anesth Analg* 2012;114:552–560.

67. Nielson E, Hennrikus E, Lehman E, et al. Angiotensin axis blockade, hypotension, and acute kidney injury in elective major orthopedic surgery. *J Hosp Med* 2014;9:283–288.

68. Drenger B, Fontes ML, Miao Y, et al. Patterns of use of perioperative angiotensin-converting enzyme inhibitors in coronary artery bypass graft surgery with cardiopulmonary bypass: effects on in-hospital morbidity and mortality. *Circulation* 2012;126:261–269.

69. Mudumbai SC, Takemotos S, Cason BA, et al. Thirty-day mortality risk associated with the postoperative nonresumption of angiotensin-converting enzyme inhibitors: a retrospective study of the Veterans Affairs Healthcare System. *J Hosp Med* 2014;9:289–296.

70. Lindenauer PK, Pekow P, Wang K, et al. Lipid-lowering therapy and in-hospital mortality following major noncardiac surgery. *JAMA* 2004;291:2092–2099.

71. Kennedy J, Quan H, Buchan AM, et al. Statins are associated with better outcomes after carotid endarterectomy in symptomatic patients. *Stroke* 2005;36:2072–2076.

72. Desai H, Aronow WS, Ahn C, et al. Incidence of perioperative myocardial infarction and of 2-year mortality in 577 elderly patients undergoing noncardiac vascular surgery treated with and without statins. *Arch Gerontol Geriatr* 2010;51:149–151.
73. Raju MG, Pachika A, Punnam SR, et al. Statin therapy in the reduction of cardiovascular events in patients undergoing intermediate-risk noncardiac, nonvascular surgery. *Clin Cardiol* 2013;36:456–461.
74. Durazzo AE, Machado FS, Ikeoka DT, et al. Reduction in cardiovascular events after vascular surgery with atorvastatin: a randomized trial. *J Vasc Surg* 2004;39:967–976.
75. Schanzer A, Hevelone N, Owens CD, et al. Statins are independently associated with reduced mortality in patients undergoing infrainguinal bypass graft surgery for critical limb ischemia. *J Vasc Surg* 2008;47:774–781.
76. de Bruin JL, Baas AF, Heymans MW, et al. Statin therapy is associated with improved survival after endovascular and open aneurysm repair. *J Vasc Surg* 2014;59:39–44.
77. McFalls EO, Ward HB, Moritz TE, et al. Coronary-artery revascularization before elective major vascular surgery. *N Engl J Med* 2004;351:2795–2804.
78. Poldermans D, Schouten O, Vidakovic R, et al.; DECREASE Study Group. A clinical randomized trial to evaluate the safety of a noninvasive approach in high-risk patients undergoing major vascular surgery: the DECREASE-V Pilot Study. *J Am Coll Cardiol* 2007;49:1763–1769.
79. Schouten O, van Kuijk JP, Flu WJ, et al.; DECREASE Study Group. Long-term outcome of prophylactic coronary revascularization in cardiac high-risk patients undergoing major vascular surgery (from the randomized DECREASE-V Pilot Study). *Am J Cardiol* 2009;103:897–901.
80. Garcia S, Moritz TED, Ward HB, et al. Usefulness of revascularization of patients with multivessel coronary artery disease before elective vascular surgery for abdominal aortic and peripheral occlusive disease. *Am J Cardiol* 2008;102:809–813.
81. Levine GN, Bates ER, Blankenship JC, et al. 2011 ACCF/AHA/SCAI guideline for percutaneous coronary intervention. *Circulation* 2011;124:e574–e651.
82. Kaluza GL, Joseph J, Lee JR, et al. Catastrophic outcomes of noncardiac surgery soon after coronary stenting. *J Am Coll Cardiol* 2000;35:1288–1294.
83. Wilson SH, Fasseas P, Orford JL, et al. Clinical outcome of patients undergoing noncardiac surgery in the two months following coronary stenting. *J Am Coll Cardiol* 2003;42:234–240.
84. Wijeysundera DN, Wijeysundera HC, Yun L, et al. Risk of elective major noncardiac surgery after coronary stent insertion: a population-based study. *Circulation* 2012;126;1355–1362.
85. Hawn MT, Graham LA, Richman JS, et al. Risk of major adverse cardiac events following noncardiac surgery in patients with coronary stents. *JAMA* 2013;310:1462–1472.
86. Brilakis ES, Orford JL, Fasseas P, et al. Outcome of patients undergoing balloon angioplasty in the two months prior to noncardiac surgery. *Am J Cardiol* 2005;96:512–514.
87. Leibowitz D, Cohen M, Planer D, et al. Comparison of cardiovascular risk of noncardiac surgery following coronary angioplasty with versus without stenting. *Am J Cardiol* 2006;97:1188–1191.
88. Goldman L, Caldear DL. Risks of general anesthesia and elective operation in the hypertensive patient. *Anesthesiology* 1979;50:285–292.
89. Nishimura RA, Otto CM, Bonow RO, et al. 2014 AHA/ACC Guideline for the management of patients with valvular heart disease: a report of the American College of Cardiology/American Heart Association Task Force on Practice Guidelines. *Circulation* 2014;129:e521–e643.
90. Zahid M, Sonel AF, Saba S, et al. Perioperative risk of noncardiac surgery associated with aortic stenosis. *Am J Cardiol* 2005;96:436–438.

91. Calleja AM, Dommaraju S, Gaddam R, et al. Cardiac risk in patients aged >75 years with asymptomatic, severe aortic stenosis undergoing noncardiac surgery. *Am J Cardiol* 2010;105:1159–1163.

92. Agarwal S, Rajamanickam A, Bajaj NS, et al. Impact of aortic stenosis on postoperative outcomes after noncardiac surgeries. *Circ Cardiovasc Qual Outcomes* 2013;6:193–200.

93. Andersson C, Jørgensen ME, Martinsson A, et al. Noncardiac surgery in patients with aortic stenosis: a contemporary study on outcomes in a matched sample from the Danish health care system. *Clin Cardiol* 2014;37:680–686.

94. Crossley GH, Poole JE, Rozner MA, et al. The Heart Rhythm Society (HRS)/ American Society of Anesthesiologists (ASA) Expert Consensus Statement on the perioperative management of patients with implantable defibrillators, pacemakers and arrhythmia monitors. *Heart Rhythm* 2011;8:1114–1154.

95. Van Diepen S, Bakal JA, McAlister FA, et al. Mortality and readmission of patients with heart failure, atrial fibrillation, or coronary artery disease undergoing noncardiac surgery: an analysis of 38,047 patients. *Circulation* 2011;124:289–296.

96. Qaseem A, Snow V, Fitterman N, et al. Risk assessment for and strategies to reduce perioperative pulmonary complications for patients undergoing noncardiothoracic surgery: a guideline from the American College of Physicians. *Ann Intern Med* 2006;144:575–580.

97. Dimick JB, Chen SL, Taheri PA, et al. Hospital costs associated with surgical complications: a report from the private-sector National Surgical Quality Improvement Program (NSQIP). *J Am Coll Surg* 2004;199:531–537.

98. Khuri SF, Daely J, Henderson W, et al. Risk adjustment of the postoperative mortality rate for the comparative assessment of the quality of surgical care: results of the National Veterans Affairs Surgical Risk Study. *J Am Coll Surg* 1997;185:315–327.

99. Arozullah AM, Khuri SF, Henderson WG, et al.; Participants in the National Veterans Affairs Surgical Quality Improvement Program. Development and validation of a multifactorial risk index for predicting postoperative pneumonia after major noncardiac surgery. *Ann Intern Med* 2001;135:847–857.

100. Johnson RG, Arozullah AM, Neumayer L, et al. Multivariable predictors of postoperative respiratory failure after general and vascular surgery: results from the patient safety in surgery study. *J Am Coll Surg* 2007;204:1188–1198.

101. Bapoje SR, Whitaker JF, Schulz T, et al. Preoperative evaluation of the patient with pulmonary disease. *Chest* 2007;132:1637–1645.

102. Grønkjær M, Eliasen M, Skov-Ettrup LS, et al. Preoperative smoking status and postoperative complications: a systematic review and meta-analysis. *Ann Surg* 2014;259:52–71.

103. Arozullah AM, Daley J, Henderson WG, et al. Multifactorial risk index for predicting postoperative respiratory failure in men after major noncardiac surgery. The National Veterans Administration Surgical Quality Improvement Program. *Ann Surg* 2000;232:242–253.

104. Canet J, Gallart L, Gomar C, et al. Prediction of postoperative pulmonary complications in a population-based surgical cohort. *Anesthesiology* 2010;113:1338–1350.

105. Archer C, Levy AR, McGregor M. Value of routine preoperative chest X-rays: a meta-analysis. *Can J Anaesth* 1993;40:1022–1027.

106. Joo HS, Wong J, Naik VN, et al. The value of screening preoperative chest X-rays: a systematic review. *Can J Anaesth* 2005;52:568–574.

107. Lawrence VA, Cornell JE, Smetana GW. Strategies to reduce postoperative pulmonary complications after noncardiothoracic surgery: systematic review for the American College of Physicians. *Ann Intern Med* 2006;144:596–608.

108. Barrera R, Shi W, Amar D, et al. Smoking and timing of cessation: impact on pulmonary complications after thoracotomy. *Chest* 2005;127:1977–1983.

109. Mills E, Eyawo O, Lockhart I, et al. Smoking cessation reduces postoperative complications: a systematic review and meta-analysis. *Am J Med* 2011;124:144–154.
110. do Nascimento JP, Módolo NS, Andrade S, et al. Incentive spirometry for prevention of postoperative pulmonary complications in upper abdominal surgery. *Cochrane Database Syst Rev* 2014;(2):CD006058.
111. Ireland CJ, Chapman TM, Mathew SF, et al. Continuous positive airway pressure (CPAP) during the postoperative period for prevention of postoperative morbidity and mortality following major abdominal surgery. *Cochrane Database Syst Rev* 2014;(8):CD008930.
112. Nelson R, Edwards S, Tse B. Prophylactic nasogastric decompression after abdominal surgery. *Cochrane Database Syst Rev* 2007;(3):CD004929.
113. Wiklund RA. Preoperative preparation of patients with advanced liver disease. *Crit Care Med* 2004;32:S106–S115.
114. Rizvon MK, Chou CL. Surgery in the patient with liver disease. *Med Clin North Am* 2003;87:211–227.
115. Mansour A, Watson W, Shayani V, et al. Abdominal operations in patients with cirrhosis: still a major surgical challenge. *Surgery* 1997;122:730–735.
116. Teh SH, Nagorney DM, Stevens SR, et al. Risk factors for mortality after surgery in patients with cirrhosis. *Gastroenterology* 2007;132:1261–1269.
117. Hanje AJ, Patel T. Preoperative evaluation of patients with liver disease. *Nat Clin Pract Gastroenterol Hepatol* 2007;4:266–276.
118. Kellerman PS. Perioperative care of the renal patient. *Arch Intern Med* 1994;154:1674–1688.
119. Wagener G, Brentjens TE. Renal disease: the anesthesiologist's perspective. *Anesthesiol Clin* 2006;24:523–547.
120. Joseph AJ, Cohn SL. Perioperative care of the patient with renal failure. *Med Clin North Am* 2003;87:193–210.
121. Lind SE. The bleeding time does not predict surgical bleeding. *Blood* 1991;77:2547–2552.
122. Moghissi ES, Korytkowski MT, DiNardo M, et al. American Association of Clinical Endocrinologists and American Diabetes Association consensus statement on inpatient glycemic control. *Diabetes Care* 2009;32:1119–1131.
123. Arabi YM, Dabbagh OC, Tamim HM, et al. Intensive versus conventional insulin therapy: a randomized controlled trial in medical and surgical critically ill patients. *Crit Care Med* 2008;36:3190–3197.
124. Finfer S, Chittock DR, Su SY, et al.; NICE-SUGAR Study Investigators. Intensive versus conventional glucose control in critically ill patients. *N Engl J Med* 2009;360:1283–1297.
125. Finfer S, Liu B, Chittock DR, et al.; NICE-SUGAR Study Investigators. Hypoglycemia and risk of death in critically ill patients. *N Engl J Med* 2012;367:1108–1118.
126. Griesdale DE, de Souza RJ, van Dam RM, et al. Intensive insulin therapy and mortality among critically ill patients: a meta-analysis including NICE-SUGAR study data. *CMAJ* 2009;180:821–827.
127. Turchin A, Matheny ME, Shubina M, et al. Hypoglycemia and clinical outcomes in patients with diabetes hospitalized in the general ward. *Diabetes Care* 2009;32:1153–1157.
128. Garg R, Hurwitz S, Turchin A, et al. Hypoglycemia, with or without insulin therapy, is associated with increased mortality among hospitalized patients. *Diabetes Care* 2013;36:1107–1110.
129. Buchleitner AM, Martinez-Alonso M, Hernández M, et al. Perioperative glycaemic control for diabetic patients undergoing surgery. *Cochrane Database Syst Rev* 2012;(9):CD007315.

130. Douketis JD, Spyropoulos AC, Spencer FA, et al. Perioperative management of antithrombotic therapy: Antithrombotic Therapy and Prevention of Thrombosis, 9th ed.: American College of Chest Physicians Evidence-Based Clinical Practice Guidelines. *Chest* 2012;141:e326S–e350S.

131. Mangano DT. Aspirin and mortality from coronary bypass surgery. *N Engl J Med* 2002;347:1309–1317.

132. Devereaux PJ, Mrkobrada M, Sessler DI, et al.; POISE-2 Investigators. Aspirin in patients undergoing noncardiac surgery. *N Engl J Med* 2014;370:1494–1503.

133. Vaishnava P, Eagle KA. The yin and yang of perioperative medicine. *N Engl J Med* 2014;370;1554–1555.

134. White RH, McKittrick T, Hutchinson R, et al. Temporary discontinuation of warfarin therapy: changes in the international normalized ratio. *Ann Intern Med* 1995;122:40–42.

135. Coursin DB, Wood KE. Corticosteroid supplementation for adrenal insufficiency. *JAMA* 2002;287:236–240.

136. Lipworth BJ. Systemic adverse effects of inhaled corticosteroid therapy: a systematic review and meta-analysis. *Arch Intern Med* 1999;159:941–955.

137. Masoli M, Weatherall M, Holt S, et al. Inhaled fluticasone propionate and adrenal effects in adult asthma: systematic review and meta-analysis. *Eur Respir J* 2006;28:960–967.

138. Schmidt IL, Lahner H, Mann K, et al. Diagnosis of adrenal insufficiency: evaluation of the corticotropin-releasing hormone test and basal serum cortisol in comparison to the insulin tolerance test in patients with hypothalamic-pituitary-adrenal disease. *J Clin Endocrinol Metab* 2003;88:4193–4198.

139. Marik PE, Varon J. Requirement of perioperative stress doses of corticosteroids: a systematic review of the literature. *Arch Surg* 2008;143:1222–1226.

140. Fish LH, Schwartz HL, Cavanaugh J. Replacement dose, metabolism, and bioavailability of levothyroxine in the treatment of hypothyroidism. *N Engl J Med* 1987;316:764–770.

141. Serebruany VL. Selective serotonin reuptake inhibitors and increased bleeding risk: are we missing something? *Am J Med* 2006;119:113–116.

142. Ang-Lee MK, Moss J, Yuan C. Herbal medicines and perioperative care. *JAMA* 2001;286:208–216.

143. Miller LG. Herbal medicinals: selected clinical considerations focusing on known or potential drug-herb interactions. *Arch Intern Med* 1998;158:2200–2211.

144. Lee A, Chui PT, Aun CST, et al. Incidence and risk of adverse perioperative events among surgical patients taking traditional Chinese herbal medicines. *Anesthesiology* 2006;105:454–461.

145. Gould MK, Garcia DA, Wren SM, et al. Prevention of VTE in nonorthopedic surgical patients: antithrombotic therapy and prevention of thrombosis, 9th ed.: American College of Chest Physicians evidence-based clinical practice guidelines. *Chest* 2012;141:e227S–e277S.

146. Falck-Ytter Y, Francis CW, Johanson NA, et al. Prevention of VTE in orthopedic surgery patients: antithrombotic therapy and the prevention of thrombosis, 9th ed.: American College of Chest Physicians evidence-based clinical practice guidelines. *Chest* 2012;141(2):e278S–e325S.

147. Caprini JA. Risk assessment as a guide for the prevention of the many faces of venous thromboembolism. *Am J Surg* 2010;199:S3–S10.

148. Rogers SO Jr, Kilaru RK, Hosokawa P, et al. Multivariable predictors of postoperative venous thromboembolic events after general and vascular surgery: results from the patient safety in surgery study. *J Am Coll Surg* 2007;204:1211–1221.

149. Bahl V, Hu HM, Henke PK, et al. A validation study of a retrospective venous thromboembolism risk scoring method. *Ann Surg* 2010;251:344–350.

150. Wilson W, Taubert KA, Gewitz M, et al. Prevention of infective endocarditis: guidelines from the American Heart Association. *Circulation* 2007;116:1736–1754.

3 Women's Health

Jessica R. Rosenstock and Scott Biest

Osteoporosis

GENERAL PRINCIPLES

- Peak bone mineral density (BMD) is attained by 19 years of age and is determined primarily by genetic factors.[1]
- Osteoporosis can have serious consequences on quality of life:
  - Possible manifestations include pain, permanent disfigurement, loss of height, loss of self-esteem, and increased risk of hip fracture.
  - Only one-third of patients who experience a hip fracture are able to return to their prefracture level of function.
  - Half of all women who have a hip fracture spend time in a nursing home.
  - The 1-year mortality after a hip fracture has been reported to be as high as 27%, although recent data indicate this rate may be decreasing.[2,3]
- Osteoporosis is clinically silent until the first fracture occurs; therefore, it is imperative that those at risk for this disease are identified early and that steps are taken to prevent bone loss and fracture.

Definition

Osteoporosis is defined as a disease of low bone mass and microarchitectural deterioration of bone tissue that leads to enhanced bone fragility and a consequent increase in fracture risk.[4]

Risk Factors

- **Low bone mass is the single most accurate predictor of fracture.**
- Risk factors for low bone density (Table 3-1) have limited value in estimating a woman's actual bone density.[5]
- Risk factors for fracture that are independent of BMD are presented in Table 3-1.
- Significant ethnic variation exists: BMD is highest in African American women, lower in Mexican American women, and lowest in Caucasian women.[6]
- Ten-year fracture risk can be estimated using the **World Health Organization (WHO) Fracture Risk Assessment Tool (FRAX)** available at http://www.shef.ac.uk/FRAX (last accessed 2/20/14).[7]

DIAGNOSIS

Clinical Presentation

History

- Risk factor screening is a useful tool in the evaluation of patients with osteoporosis, as it allows the physician to recognize factors that can influence bone density and fracture risk (Table 3-1).
- Essential historical information includes the following:
  - Height at age 30 years and any loss of height
  - Medications, including heparin, thyroid medications, diuretics, hormone replacement/oral contraceptive pills (OCPs), phenytoin/phenobarbital, prednisone, calcium, calcitonin, vitamins, raloxifene, or bisphosphonates

TABLE 3-1	Risk Factors for an Osteoporotic Fracture or Low Bone Density

Associated with increased risk of fracture independent of BMD	Associated with low BMD
Advanced age	Female sex
History of fracture during adulthood	Caucasian or Asian ethnicity
Family history of an osteoporotic fracture	Prolonged calcium deficit
Prolonged use of corticosteroids	Vitamin D deficiency
Low body weight (<127 pound/58 kg)	Sedentary lifestyle
Smoking	Early menopause (before 45 years of age)
Excessive alcohol intake	Prolonged amenorrhea
	Bilateral oophorectomy
	History of gastric surgery
	Many medical conditions (including endocrine, gastrointestinal, rheumatologic, bone/marrow-related, and genetic disorders; organ transplantation)
	Drugs (e.g., corticosteroids, immunosuppressants, anticonvulsants, heparin, chemotherapy, thyroid hormone)

- ○ Dietary history, specifically calcium intake
- ○ Fractures or falls as an adult
- ○ Family history of fractures or osteoporosis
- ○ Physical activity
- ○ Menstrual history
- ○ Pain and functional limitations of activities of daily living

Physical Examination
- A complete physical examination should be performed on each patient, with emphasis on accurate measurement of height and weight.
- A spinal examination should be included, noting evidence of kyphosis, pain, and muscle spasm.
- Gait stability and fall risk should be assessed including balance, proprioception, and muscle strength.

Diagnostic Testing

Laboratories
- Laboratory studies should be limited and directed by the history and physical examination.
- Fractures in relatively young postmenopausal women or those with BMD lower than expected for her age may necessitate a workup for secondary causes of osteoporosis.[8]
- **Comprehensive biochemical profile** provides a simple screen for secondary causes, such as calcium-phosphorus ratio for hyperparathyroidism, total protein-albumin ratio for myeloma, and screening for liver and kidney disease.
- **Thyroid-stimulating hormone (TSH)** should be measured in patients with symptoms of thyroid dysfunction or those who are receiving thyroid replacement.
- **25-Hydroxyvitamin D** screens for body stores of vitamin D (desirable ≥30 ng/mL).
- Additional studies can be considered for those with very low bone mass or those who continue to lose bone despite antiresorptive therapy. These studies include parathyroid

TABLE 3-2	Indications for Bone Mineral Densitometry, Bone Mass Measurement Act of 1998

- An estrogen-deficient women at clinical risk of osteoporosis as determined by a physician or qualified nonphysician practitioner based on her medical history and other findings
- Postmenopausal women deciding whether to begin ERT or other osteoporosis therapy
- Radiologically suspected osteopenia
- Receiving or expecting to receive glucocorticoids ($\geq$7.5 mg/day for $\geq$3 months)
- Primary hyperparathyroidism
- Serial monitoring to follow therapy

hormone (PTH) battery, 24-hour urine for calcium excretion, serum protein electrophoresis (SPEP), cortisol levels, estradiol levels in women, testosterone levels in men, screening for celiac disease, and bone biopsy (rarely required).

Imaging
- Bone densitometry has improved the diagnosis and treatment of osteoporosis. It allows the clinician to diagnose low bone mass before a fracture occurs. Bone mass measurement is an accurate predictor of fractures.[9]
- The indications for bone mineral densitometry according to the **Bone Mass Measurement Act of 1998** are presented in Table 3-2 and those of the **National Osteoporosis Foundation** (NOF) in Table 3-3.[10]
- All bone mass measurement techniques are valuable for making the diagnosis of osteoporosis and predicting fracture risk.
  - The most widely available methods are single x-ray absorptiometry, dual x-ray absorptiometry (DXA), quantitative computed tomography, and ultrasound densitometry.
  - Techniques vary in terms of precision, cost, radiation exposure, and ability to follow changes over time.
  - The most common method of measuring bone mass and currently the gold standard is DXA.

TABLE 3-3	National Osteoporosis Foundation Indications for Bone Mineral Density Testing

- All women 65 years of age and older
- All men 70 years of age and older
- Postmenopausal women <65 years old in whom there is a concern for osteoporosis based on clinical risk profile
- Men 50–69 years old in whom there is a concern for osteoporosis based on clinical risk profile
- Perimenopausal women with a specific risk factor associated with increased fracture risk (Table 3-1)
- Adults who have a fracture after the age of 50
- Adults with a medical condition or taking a medication associated with low BMD
- Anyone being considered for pharmacologic therapy for osteoporosis
- Anyone being treated for osteoporosis, to monitor treatment effect
- Anyone not receiving therapy in whom evidence of bone loss would lead to treatment

TABLE 3-4	World Health Organization Criteria for the Diagnosis of Osteoporosis
Category	**T score**
Normal	<−1 SD from peak bone mass
Low bone mass/osteopenia	−1 SD to −2.5 SD from peak bone mass
Osteoporosis	≤−2.5 SD from peak bone mass
Severe osteoporosis	≤−2.5 SD with fragility fracture

Diagnostic guidelines developed for postmenopausal women.
SD, standard deviation.

- For the diagnosis of osteoporosis, the bone density of a patient is compared with the mean young adult normal reference range (the T score).
- The WHO has developed **diagnostic criteria** for osteoporosis using **T scores** (Table 3-4)[11]:
  - A T score of −2.5 (2.5 standard deviations below the young-adult mean BMD) is defined as osteoporosis because more than half of osteoporotic fractures occur below that level.
  - Z scores, which compare a patient's BMD with that of age-matched controls, are also reported on bone mass measurement.
  - If the Z score is more than two standard deviations below age-matched subjects, a cause other than age-related bone loss should be considered, and a secondary cause of osteoporosis should be sought.
- Serial BMD measurements can be used to **monitor the effect of treatment or the clinical course of a specific medical condition.**
- The usefulness of serial measurements is dependent on the precision error of the measuring device used.

TREATMENT

Medications
- Regardless of the specific therapy for the prevention or treatment of osteoporosis, all patients should receive adequate calcium and vitamin D, engage in regular weight-bearing exercise, and stop smoking.
- According to the NOF, treatment should be strongly considered in postmenopausal women and men aged 50 years or older with the following[9]:
  - Hip or vertebral fracture
  - T score of ≤ −2.5 at the femoral neck or spine (after appropriate evaluation to exclude secondary causes)
  - Low BMD (T score of −1.0 to −2.5 at the femoral neck or spine) and a 10-year risk of hip fracture of ≥3% or a 10-year risk of any major osteoporotic fracture of ≥20% (based on the WHO FRAX algorithm, http://www.shef.ac.uk/FRAX, last accessed 2/20/14)

First Line
- **Bisphosphonates**
  - For most patients, bisphosphonates are first-line therapy. All increase the BMD and reduce the risk of fractures.
  - Bisphosphonates inhibit the action of osteoclasts.
  - The bisphosphonates alendronate, risedronate, ibandronate, and zoledronic acid are approved for the prevention and treatment of osteoporosis.
  - Orally administered bisphosphonates are poorly absorbed and therefore, should be taken first thing in the morning, on an empty stomach, with no liquid, food, or other medications taken for at least 30 minutes. Calcium supplements should not be taken for at least 1 hour afterwards.

- ○ When taken orally, bisphosphonates may cause esophagitis. Therefore, patients should sit or stand for at least 30 minutes after taking the drug with at least 8 oz of water. If taken properly, tolerance is excellent.[12] Less frequent administration may also improve gastrointestinal tolerability.[13]
- ○ There may also be a link between the administration of bisphosphonates and osteonecrosis (avascular necrosis) of the jaw. The level of risk is not precisely known but is most likely very small. Risk factors appear to be high-dose IV administration, cancer, and dental procedures.[14-18]
- ○ IV administration can result in flu-like symptoms (fever, arthralgias, myalgias, and headache) and transient hypocalcemia. The latter underscores the importance of calcium and vitamin D supplementation.
- ○ The maximal duration of bisphosphonate therapy is uncertain. However, some recommend discontinuation of therapy or a drug holiday after 5 years.
- ○ An increasing or stable BMD (generally measured every 2 years) is indicative of a positive treatment effect.
- ○ **Alendronate**
  - Alendronate has been shown to improve BMD in the spine by 8.8% and in the hip by 5.9% after 3 years of therapy.[19] A meta-analysis of 11 randomized trials found after 3 years of ≥10 mg of alendronate, a 7.48% increase in BMD of the lumbar spine and 5.60% of the hip.[20]
  - Women with osteoporosis treated with alendronate therapy for 3 years (2 years of 5 mg and 1 year of 10 mg) had a reduction in vertebral fractures by 47% and hip fractures by 51%.[21] The above-mentioned meta-analysis found a pooled relative risk (RR) of fracture of 0.52 for vertebral fractures and 0.51 for nonvertebral fractures.[20]
  - The recommended dosage for the treatment of osteoporosis in men and women is alendronate, 10 mg PO daily or 70 mg PO once weekly.[22]
  - The dosage for the prevention of osteoporosis in postmenopausal women is 5 mg/day or 35 mg once weekly.
  - The dose for the treatment of corticosteroid-induced osteoporosis is 5 mg/day, except in postmenopausal women not receiving estrogen, for whom the recommended dosage is 10 mg/day.
- ○ **Risedronate**
  - Risedronate has been shown to improve BMD in the spine by 4% to 6% and in the hip by 1% to 3%.[23]
  - The Vertebral Efficacy with Risedronate Trial (VERT) showed a 41% to 49% reduction in spinal fractures and a 39% reduction in nonvertebral fractures.[23,24] Women aged 70 to 79 years with confirmed osteoporosis had a 40% reduction in hip fractures with 5 mg/day.[25]
  - A meta-analysis of eight randomized trials found, after at least 1 year of 5 mg risedronate, an increase in BMD of 4.54% for the lumbar spine and 2.75% for the femoral neck. The RR of fracture after at least 1 year of ≥2.5 mg of risedronate was 0.64 for vertebral fractures and 0.73 for nonvertebral fractures.[26]
  - Recommended dosage for treatment and prevention of postmenopausal osteoporosis is risedronate, 5 mg PO daily. The dose for the prevention and treatment of corticosteroid-induced osteoporosis is 5 mg/day, or 35 mg once weekly,[27] or 75 mg on 2 consecutive days a month,[28] or 150 mg once monthly.[29]
- ○ **Ibandronate**
  - Ibandronate daily or intermittently has also been shown to significantly increase BMD and decrease fractures.[30-33]
  - The recommended dosage of ibandronate is 150 mg monthly.[34,35]
  - Ibandronate can also be administered IV, 3 mg every 3 months.[36,37] This regimen may be effective for those who cannot tolerate oral administration or who cannot follow oral dosing precautions.

○ **Zoledronic Acid**
  ▪ IV zoledronic acid is approved for the treatment and prevention of osteoporosis.
  ▪ Both once-yearly and intermittent administration **increase BMD**[38] and **reduce the risk of vertebral** (70%) **and hip fractures** (41%).[39]
  ▪ If given within 90 days after repair of a hip fracture, zoledronic acid reduces the risk of new fractures (35%) and improves survival (28%).[40]
  ▪ The recommended dosage for treatment of osteoporosis is 5 mg IV over at least 15 minutes annually. For prevention of osteoporosis, the recommended dose is 5 mg IV every 2 years.
  ▪ Zoledronic acid also has indications for hypercalcemia of malignancy, multiple myeloma, and bone metastases from solid tumors.

• **Raloxifene**
  ○ Raloxifene is a selective estrogen receptor (ER) modulator. It inhibits the loss of BMD but does not cause endometrial hyperplasia.
  ○ In the Multiple Outcomes of Raloxifene Evaluation (MORE) trial, 7,705 women were assigned to receive placebo or raloxifene at 60 or 120 mg. Treatment with raloxifene **increased the BMD** of the femoral neck and spine by 2.1% to 2.3% and 2.5% to 2.6%, respectively, compared with placebo.[41,42] During the 4-year continuation of a subset of MORE subjects (Continuing Outcome Relevant to Evista, CORE), differences in BMD between raloxifene and placebo were maintained.[43]
  ○ **Vertebral fractures were reduced by 30% to 50%.**[41,42,44]
  ○ **No data support reduction in nonvertebral fractures** at this time.[41–44]
  ○ The MORE trial revealed a **70% reduction in the development of invasive breast cancer** in patients who were treated with raloxifene and had no effect on the endometrium.[45] The Raloxifene Use for The Heart (RUTH) trial demonstrated a 43% reduction in invasive breast cancer.[46] During the combined MORE/CORE 8 years, there was a 66% reduction in invasive breast cancer and a 76% reduction in ER-positive invasive breast cancer.[47] There was no change in the incidence of ER-negative invasive breast cancer.
  ○ Total serum cholesterol and low-density lipoprotein cholesterol levels decreased significantly without change in high-density lipoprotein or triglyceride levels. Raloxifene 60 mg daily reduced the total cholesterol level by 6.4% and the low-density lipoprotein level by 10.1%.[48]
  ○ Raloxifene **does not appear to have a significant effect on the risk of coronary events.**[46,49]
  ○ **The risk of venous thromboembolism with raloxifene may be elevated:** MORE trial RR 2.1 to 3.1, CORE study RR 2.17, and RUTH trial hazard ratio (HR) 1.44.[41,46,47,49,50] The risk is probably less than that seen with tamoxifen.[51]
  ○ In the RUTH trial, raloxifene was associated with an **increased risk of fatal stroke** (HR 1.49) but not with total stroke or all-cause mortality.[46]
  ○ Other side effects include hot flashes and leg cramps.
  ○ The recommended dosage of raloxifene for prevention and treatment is 60 mg daily.

• **Calcitonin**
  ○ Salmon or human calcitonin can be given as an SC injection or as a nasal spray.
  ○ BMD increases by 1% to 2% in patients who are treated with 200 IU calcitonin nasal spray daily.
  ○ The Prevent Recurrence of Osteoporotic Fracture (PROOF) trial showed a reduction in vertebral fractures by 36% with the nasal spray in women who were 5 years postmenopausal with vertebral fractures. However, 59% of participants withdrew prematurely; therefore, results of this study should be interpreted cautiously. No significant reduction in hip fractures occurred.[52]
  ○ A meta-analysis showed a reduction in vertebral fractures (RR 0.46) and nonvertebral fractures (RR 0.52).[53]
  ○ Most consider calcitonin less effective than bisphosphonates.

  ○ Calcitonin has an analgesic effect when given as treatment for compression fractures.[54]
  ○ Recommended dosage for the treatment of women >5 years postmenopausal with low bone mass is one spray (200 IU) in one nostril daily. The patient should alternate nostrils each day. The SC dose is 100 IU/day.

• **Parathyroid Hormone**
  ○ PTH is considered to be an "anabolic" treatment, in that it stimulates bone formation rather than acting as an antiresorptive.
  ○ Intermittent PTH administration, as opposed to chronic elevations (as seen with chronic kidney disease or primary hyperparathyroidism), stimulates the maturation of osteoblasts and, therefore, bone formation. The explanation for this incongruity is not fully understood.
  ○ PTH affects trabecular bone more than cortical bone and qualitatively improves trabecular architecture.
  ○ PTH is usually given as recombinant human PTH amino acids 1 to 34, known as **teriparatide.** Intact PTH is also effective.[55]
  ○ In the Fracture Prevention Trial (FPT) of 1,637 postmenopausal women with a prior vertebral fracture randomized to placebo or 20 or 40 μg teriparatide daily, BMD increased in the spine and hip but not in the radial shaft.[56]
  ○ After a median treatment period of 21 months in the FPT, there was significant reduction in vertebral fractures (RR 0.31 to 0.35) and nonvertebral fractures (RR 0.46 to 0.47).[56] BMD increases before fracture reduction occurs.
  ○ Side effects include hypercalcemia, nausea, headache, leg cramps, and dizziness.
  ○ Animal studies suggest an increased risk of osteosarcoma. Teriparatide should not be given to patients with existing risk factors for osteosarcoma such as Paget disease, skeletal radiation therapy, or a history of bone malignancy.
  ○ The recommended dosage of teriparatide is 20 μg subcutaneously daily for a maximum of 2 years.
  ○ A bisphosphonate is typically given after completion of teriparatide.[57] However, concurrent administration of alendronate does not produce an additive effect and may actually reduce the effects of PTH.[58]

• **Estrogen Replacement Therapy (ERT)**
  ○ Estrogen therapy (ET) has been shown to slow down bone loss following menopause or to increase it by as much as 6%.[59]
  ○ Since the publication of the Women's Health Initiative (WHI) findings (excess coronary events, strokes, pulmonary emboli, and invasive breast cancer) and the availability of other effective drugs, ET is no longer considered appropriate for first-line therapy for the prevention and treatment of osteoporosis.[60]
  ○ Dosing is discussed in the "Menopause" section below.

• **Denosumab**
  ○ Denosumab is a human monoclonal antibody to receptor activator of nuclear factor kappaB ligand (RANKL), an osteoclast differentiating factor. It inhibits osteoclast formation, thereby decreasing bone resorption and increasing BMD.
  ○ Denosumab is approved for treatment of osteoporosis in postmenopausal women at high risk of fracture.
  ○ In the FREEDOM Trial, 7,868 women aged 60 to 90 with osteoporosis were randomly assigned denosumab or placebo every 6 months for 36 months. Denosumab reduced the risk of vertebral fracture by 68%, the risk of hip fracture by 40%, and the risk of nonvertebral fracture by 20%.[61]
  ○ Recommended dosing is 60 mg subcutaneously every 6 months.

Lifestyle/Risk Modification

Smoking cessation and alcohol intake reduction are important for those with or at risk for osteoporosis.

Diet

- **Diet therapy** is essential in the prevention and treatment of osteoporosis.
- Calcium supplementation alone has a small positive effect on BMD.[62]
- **Calcium intake for postmenopausal women should be 1,200 mg/day.**
- Examples of the elemental calcium content of various foods include the following: 8-oz glass of milk contains 300 mg, 1 oz of Swiss cheese contains 270 mg, and 1 cup of cooked broccoli contains 100 mg.[63]
- Eating calcium-fortified foods should be encouraged.
- **Calcium supplements:** Calcium carbonate is acceptable for most patients. It is cheap and has relatively few side effects. Guidelines for calcium supplementation:
  - Calcium is best absorbed in small amounts; consider dividing the daily dose if >500 mg.
  - Synthetic calcium supplements are optimal. Oyster shell calcium, dolomite, and bone meal can contain heavy metal contaminants.[64]
- **Vitamin D (800 to 1,000 IU PO daily)** is beneficial for patients with osteoporosis. Ambulatory men and women older than the age of 65 years who were given calcium carbonate and vitamin D had a significant reduction in nonvertebral fractures.[65] Patients with significant hypovitaminosis D require more aggressive repletion.

Activity

Exercise, including weight-bearing and muscle-strengthening exercise, should be encouraged in patients with osteoporosis as allowed by their functional status. <make this reference 115>

SPECIAL CONSIDERATIONS

Management of Corticosteroid-Induced Osteoporosis

- Skeletal effects of corticosteroids include decreased BMD and increased fracture risk and are related to dose and duration of therapy.
- Daily prednisone doses of ≥7.5 mg/day can result in significant bone loss. Lower doses can also have an effect on bone metabolism. Alternate-day regimens have not been shown to be superior.
- Bone densitometry should be considered for any patient who is presently receiving corticosteroids or if long-term therapy is initiated.
- Patients who are on corticosteroids should maintain adequate calcium (1,500 mg/day) and vitamin D (800 IU) intake.
- Weight-bearing exercise should be encouraged.
- **Alendronate** has been shown to prevent bone loss in patients receiving corticosteroids and to reduce the risk of fractures in postmenopausal women on corticosteroids.[66,67]
- **Risedronate and zoledronic acid** are similarly effective.[68–71]
- **Calcitonin** may preserve bone loss, but it has not been shown to prevent fractures in the setting of corticosteroid treatment.[72,73]
- **Teriparatide** may be more effective than alendronate in patients who have osteoporosis and have received corticosteroids for at least 3 months.[74]

Management of Osteoporosis in Men

- If a male patient presents with a fracture that is associated with mild-to-moderate trauma, BMD testing should be performed, and a search for secondary causes of bone loss should be considered.
- Evaluation should look for risk factors for osteoporosis including drugs that could affect BMD, such as corticosteroids or anticonvulsants; history of alcohol ingestion (>100 g/day); or nicotine use.
- Appropriate laboratory studies should be done including SPEP, complete blood cell count, calcium, phosphate, albumin, creatinine, alkaline phosphatase, PTH battery, TSH, free testosterone, 25-hydroxyvitamin D, 24-hour urine collection for calcium and creatinine excretion, and cortisol levels.

- Causes of hypogonadism, such as Klinefelter syndrome, hyperprolactinemia, anorexia nervosa, and hemochromatosis, should also be considered. Bone biopsy may be needed if no etiology is found.
- As with female patients, sufficient calcium and vitamin D is important. Patients should be encouraged to stop smoking and drinking alcohol.
- If a secondary cause is found, it should be treated.
- Hypogonadism is a relatively common cause, and testosterone replacement increases BMD.[75–77] **Alendronate** has been shown to maintain BMD and prevent fractures in men with osteoporosis, vertebral fracture (odds ratio [OR] 0.44) and nonvertebral fracture (OR 0.60).[78]
- **Risedronate** has been shown to reduce vertebral fractures and increase the bone mass in men treated with corticosteroids.[79–82]
- **Teriparatide** has also been shown to be effective in men.[83–85]

PATIENT EDUCATION

- Patient education is essential for the prevention and treatment of osteoporosis particularly with regard to **fall prevention**. Patients at risk should be instructed to:
  - Look for and remove throw rugs, loose carpets, slippery floors, cords and wires, or anything that can cause a patient to slip.
  - Inspect home for unstable furniture or clutter that can obstruct mobility.
  - Ensure adequate lighting, especially at night.
  - Have grab bars installed for the toilet and place a nonslip surface in the shower.
  - Wear properly fitting shoes.
  - Have irregular sidewalks and uneven surfaces repaired and have accumulated ice or snow removed.
- Correct vision and hearing problems.
- Eliminate causes of postural hypotension if possible. Otherwise, advise patients to get up slowly.
- **Hip protectors** may reduce hip fractures in nursing home patients.[86,87] Acceptance of and adherence to hip protectors is relatively low.

Menopause

GENERAL PRINCIPLES

- The menopausal transition period is typified by variation in menstrual cycle length and eventual skipped periods.
- Menopause is the cessation of menstrual periods, defined retrospectively after 12 months of amenorrhea.
- The average age of menopause is 50 to 51 years.[88]
- With ovarian failure, follicle-stimulating hormone and luteinizing hormone levels rise and estradiol levels fall.
- Other causes of amenorrhea and menopausal symptoms should be considered including excessive weight loss, concurrent medical illnesses, pregnancy, thyroid disease, pituitary disease, and medications.

DIAGNOSIS

Clinical Presentation

- Symptoms associated with menopause include the following:
  - Irregular bleeding
  - Hot flashes/night sweats

- ○ Sleep disturbance
- ○ Vaginal dryness/itching/dyspareunia
- ○ Sexual dysfunction
- ○ Urinary incontinence
- ○ Mood changes (inconsistent degree of association)
- Menopausal symptoms typically last for a few months but can persist for several years.[88]
- **Hot flashes** affect approximately 75% of menopausal women. They occur most frequently at night and are due to estrogen deficiency. It is believed that estrogen withdrawal lowers the temperature set point in the hypothalamus to reduce the body thermostat. As a result, vasodilatation of the vessels in the hands and upper body occurs so that the heat in the central organs is lost at the periphery.[89]
  - ○ Hot flashes are not synonymous with estrogen deficiency.
  - ○ Other causes of hot flashes should be considered, such as pheochromocytoma, carcinoid, pregnancy, thyroid disease, and panic disorder.
- Long-term effects in the postmenopausal period include osteoporosis and increased cardiovascular disease risk.

Diagnostic Testing

- Diagnostic testing is generally unnecessary.
- As noted, follicle-stimulating hormone and luteinizing hormone levels are high and estradiol levels are low.
- Other tests may be indicated to rule out other possible causes of amenorrhea.

TREATMENT

- **Hot flashes**
  - ○ **Estrogen therapy (ET)**
    - **ET is the most effective treatment.**[88,90,91]
    - However, the results of the WHI and the Heart and Estrogen/progestin Replacement Study (HERS) have greatly called into question the advisability of long-term (i.e., greater than approximately 5 years) or chronic indefinite ET, specifically with regard to combined estrogen and progestin treatment.[60,92] It is important to recognize that the direct applicability of these studies to all menopausal women is somewhat tenuous.[93]
    - Quality of life is also a very important consideration.[94]
    - The balance of risks and benefits appears to be more favorable for women who have had a hysterectomy receiving estrogen-only treatment in comparison with women with a uterus receiving combined estrogen-progestin treatment.
    - On balance, short-term (i.e., less than approximately 2 to 3 years) administration of the lowest effective dose of estrogen is a viable option for women with moderate-to-severe vasomotor symptoms who have no history of cardiovascular disease, breast cancer, endometrial cancer, or venous thromboembolism.[91,93,94]
    - Low-dose estrogen therapies include 0.3 mg oral conjugated estrogen, 0.25 to 0.5 mg micronized 17β-estradiol, and 0.025 mg transdermal 17β-estradiol patch.[93] Higher doses may be necessary in some patients for symptom control.
    - **A progestin must be added in women with an intact uterus.**[95]
    - Low-dose (i.e., containing 20 μg of ethinyl estradiol) OCPs are also a reasonable option for women less than approximately 50 years old.
    - ET can generally be tapered off gradually after a year or two. Some women may have recurrent hot flashes.
    - **Other side effects of estrogen** include abdominal bloating, cramps, breast tenderness, hypertriglyceridemia (oral estrogen only), breakthrough bleeding, weight changes, enlargement of benign tumors of the uterus, dry eyes, and skin changes.

- **Side effects of progestins** include breakthrough bleeding, edema, weight changes, rash, insomnia, and somnolence.
  ○ **Other treatments**
  - Simple **environmental changes,** including keeping the room cool and dressing in layers, may make hot flashes more tolerable.
  - **Serotonin reuptake inhibitors** (SSRIs, e.g., paroxetine and fluoxetine) and **serotonin-norepinephrine reuptake inhibitors** (SNRIs, e.g., venlafaxine) are effective for vasomotor symptoms but not as much as ET.[88,91,96]
  - **Gabapentin** appears to be effective at reducing the frequency of hot flashes.[88,91,97] Doses up to 900 mg/day may be required. Common side effects of gabapentin include dizziness/unsteadiness and fatigue/somnolence.
  - Studies regarding clonidine are of fairly low quality and conflicting.[88,96]
  - The effectiveness of soy foods, soy extracts, red clover extracts, and black cohosh is questionable.[88,91,96,98,99]
- **Genitourinary symptoms**
  ○ Vaginal atrophy presents with dyspareunia, vaginal dryness, itching, and irritation. Oral and vaginal estrogen is useful for symptoms associated with vaginal atrophy. Systemic effects of vaginal estrogen are probably quite low. Concomitant progestin therapy is not necessary for women with a uterus receiving topical vaginal estrogen.
  ○ The terminal urethra is embryonically related to the vagina. As it becomes thinner, there is more risk of infection and incontinence. Dysuria without evidence of infection is due to the thinning of the epithelium, allowing urine in close contact with the sensory nerves. Also, the normal urethral pressures created by the urethra and surrounding tissues are decreased. Topical estrogen in some studies has been shown to reduce the incidence of urinary tract infections.[88,100]

Cervical Cancer Screening

- Widespread screening with cervical cytology has dramatically reduced the incidence of and mortality from cervical cancer over the last three decades. Half of the women in the United States with invasive cervical carcinoma have never had a Pap smear, and another 10% have not had a Pap smear in 5 years.[101]
- Risk factors for developing cervical cancer include cigarette smoking, multiple sexual partners, early onset of sexual activity, history of sexually transmitted infection, increasing parity, prolonged use of OCPs, immunocompromise, and HIV infection.[102,103]
- **Human papillomavirus** (HPV) is the causative agent in almost all cases of cervical cancer. There are 15 to 18 subtypes of HPV that are considered "high risk" for causing cervical cancer. HPV-16 and 18 account for approximately 70% of all cases.[102]
- Cervical cancer screening with the Pap smear is recommended for all women who have a cervix. The American Cancer Society (ACS), United States Preventative Services Task Force (USPSTF), American Society for Colposcopy and Cervical Pathology (ASCCP), and American College of Obstetrics and Gynecology (ACOG) recently updated their joint guidelines for cervical cancer screening.
- Screening should begin at 21 years regardless of sexual history.
- **ACOG, ASCCP, USPSTF,** and **ACS** recommend the following:
  ○ For women aged 21 to 29, cervical cytology screening alone is recommended every 3 years.
  ○ Women aged 30 to 65 and older with negative results on three consecutive cervical cytology tests may be screened with cervical cytology and HPV cotesting every 5 years. Cytology alone every 3 years is also acceptable.
  ○ Women aged >65 years do not require screening after adequate negative prior screening results.

- ○ Women with a history of CIN 2, CIN 3, or adenocarcinoma in situ should continue routine age-based screening for at least 20 years.
  - ○ Women who have undergone hysterectomy for benign indications with previous history of advanced cervical dysplasia do not require screening.[102,104,105]
- **Cervical intraepithelial neoplasias** are usually divided into categories based on cytologic grades. The **Bethesda system** is the currently recognized reporting system. Included in this system is the pathologist's interpretation of the smear, including the presence of benign cellular changes, evidence of cellular atypia, or both. Infectious processes such as *Trichomonas*, *Candida*, *Actinomyces*, or cellular changes associated with herpes simplex virus are reported. Reactive (but benign) changes associated with inflammation, atrophy, radiation, or intrauterine contraceptive device are also reported. The four categories of squamous cell abnormalities are as follows:
  - ○ Atypical squamous cells (ASC): of undetermined significance (ASC-US) or cannot exclude HSIL (ASC-H)
  - ○ Low-grade squamous intraepithelial lesions (LSIL)
  - ○ High-grade squamous intraepithelial lesions (HSIL)
  - ○ Squamous cell carcinoma
- **ASC of undetermined significance (ASC-US)** are subjected to reflex HPV testing and are managed based on the presence or absence of high risk strains of HPV.
  - ○ Those with positive testing for high-risk HPV types should be referred for colposcopy.
  - ○ In those with negative testing, cytology should be repeated in 3 years.
- **ASC but HSIL cannot be ruled out (ASC-H)** should be evaluated with colposcopy.[106]
- **LSIL** should be further evaluated with colposcopy. In adolescents, however, repeat cytology at 12 months is recommended.[106] HPV testing is an option for postmenopausal women.
- **HSIL** must be further evaluated with colposcopy.[106]
- Women with positive HPV testing and negative cytology can be followed with repeat cotesting in 12 months or immediate HPV genotype-specific testing for HPV 16 or HPV 16/18. If positive, colposcopy is indicated.[102]
- **Glandular cell abnormalities** are another category of abnormal Pap smear results. These patients also require evaluation with colposcopy and endometrial biopsy if they are over age 35 or have risk factors for endometrial pathology such as obesity.
- **HPV vaccination** is recommended for all women aged 9 to 26 for primary prevention of cervical cancer.

Nipple Discharge

GENERAL PRINCIPLES

- Nipple discharge is common and mostly benign.
- Nipple discharge can be classified as lactation, physiologic (galactorrhea), or pathologic.
- **Galactorrhea** is bilateral, milky, involves multiple ducts, and occurs at least 1 year following cessation of breast-feeding or pregnancy.
  - ○ It is most commonly caused by **hyperprolactinemia**, also suggested by the presence of amenorrhea. Hyperprolactinemia may result from medications, pituitary tumors, or endocrine abnormalities.
  - ○ Hypothyroidism, chronic nipple stimulation, and renal insufficiency are less common causes of galactorrhea.[107]
  - ○ Medications associated with galactorrhea include antipsychotics, methyldopa, reserpine, Reglan, cimetidine, opioids, and antidepressants.[107–109]
- **Pathologic nipple discharge** is usually unilateral and localized to a single duct. It is spontaneous, intermittent, and persistent.
  - ○ The fluid can be serosanguineous, bloody, green, or clear.
  - ○ The most common cause of unilateral discharge is intraductal papilloma, followed by mammary duct ectasia.[108]

○ About 10% to 15% of cases are due to breast carcinoma.[108]

○ Purulent discharge can be caused by mastitis.

DIAGNOSIS

Clinical Presentation

- The history should include evaluation of menstrual pattern, recent pregnancy, infertility, medications, symptoms of hypothyroidism, breast stimulation or trauma, and presence of headaches or visual complaints.
- Medications associated with galactorrhea should be stopped, and pregnancy should be ruled out.
- Physical examination should include a complete breast examination and evaluation for signs of hypothyroidism or pituitary tumor.
- Try to determine if the discharge is from one or multiple ducts.

Diagnostic Testing

- If fluid is expressed and not grossly bloody, it should be evaluated for occult blood.
- Measurement of TSH, prolactin, creatinine, and a pregnancy test are indicated with discharge from multiple ducts.
- Mammography should be obtained in patients over 30 years of age with pathologic discharge. All patients should undergo periareolar ultrasound.
- Ductography, cannulation of the secreting duct followed by injection of contrast material, can be considered, but it is painful for patients and the technique is difficult. It has been reported to miss as many as 20% of ductal lesions.
- Magnetic resonance imaging and ductoscopy are also available diagnostic tests.
- Duct excision is indicated if abnormalities are identified on the above tests.[109]

TREATMENT

- Galactorrhea:
  ○ Patients with normal periods and normal prolactin levels do not require treatment.
  ○ Breast stimulation is discouraged.
  ○ If the patient is receiving a medication that is associated with galactorrhea, the dose can be decreased or the drug stopped and the patient followed.
  ○ The management of prolactinoma is discussed in Chapter 21.
- Patients with pathologic discharge should be referred for evaluation by a surgeon who is experienced with diseases of the breast for possible surgical intervention.

Breast Masses

GENERAL PRINCIPLES

Risk factors for breast cancer include female gender, increasing age, first-degree relative (mother or sister) with breast cancer (highest risk is if the relative was premenopausal and the cancer was bilateral), previous breast cancer, late age of first pregnancy, and nulliparity.

DIAGNOSIS

Clinical Presentation

History

- The patient should be questioned regarding any associated symptoms, such as pain and nipple discharge.
- Menstrual history should be obtained, as well as assessment of the possibility of pregnancy.

- Medications should be reviewed, and any history of trauma should be obtained.
- An accurate family history should be elicited. If a history of breast, ovarian, colon, or prostate cancer is found in numerous family members, genetic counseling should be considered.

Physical Examination
- Physical examination should include inspection and palpation of the breast with the patient seated and then lying flat. The breasts should be observed for skin dimpling or changes in contour.
- The breast should be palpated gently and circumferentially to the axilla, including the nipple, areola, and breast tissue.
- The nipple should be closely evaluated for discharge, and the character of the discharge should be noted. A ductal carcinoma may present with an isolated spontaneous serosanguineous discharge.
- The axillary and supraclavicular area should be palpated for evidence of a mass or enlarged lymph nodes.

Differential Diagnosis
- Differential diagnosis for a discrete nodule includes fibroadenoma, cyst, fibrocystic changes, malignancy, and trauma.
- A dominant nodule remains unchanged throughout the menstrual cycle.
- In fibrocystic disease, the palpable nodules frequently feel cystic and are subject to change during the menstrual cycle.
- Benign nodules have characteristics such as easy mobility, regular borders, and a soft or cystic feel. However, **physical examination alone cannot exclude malignancy;** therefore, other diagnostic tests are indicated.

TREATMENT

- **Women younger than 30 years** with a breast mass and no other symptoms can be observed through one menstrual cycle, and if it resolves, no further treatment is indicated. If the mass persists, ultrasound is a reasonable next step.
- **Women over 30 years old** should have a mammogram. Ultrasound may also be indicated.
- **Routine screening mammography** recommendations are discussed in Chapter 5.

VAGINITIS

- The presence of vaginal discharge is not always abnormal.
- Symptoms are usually nonspecific.
- The vagina has 25 bacterial species, and pH is usually 4.0 due to lactobacilli; however, semen, menses, and ectropion may alter the pH.
- Fifty percent of vaginitis is from bacterial vaginosis (BV), 25% from *Trichomonas* vaginitis, and 25% from *Candida* vaginitis.
- Management of sexually transmitted infections is discussed in Chapter 27.

Bacterial Vaginosis

GENERAL PRINCIPLES

- BV is thought to result from a polymicrobial alteration in the normal vaginal flora in which lactobacilli are replaced with high concentrations of anaerobes such as *Gardnerella*, *Mycoplasma*, and *Prevotella*.

- *Gardnerella vaginalis* may be cultured from 30% to 70% of healthy asymptomatic women.
- BV infection increases the risk of acquisition of some STIs (HIV, HSV-2, *Neisseria gonorrhoeae*, and *Chlamydia trachomatis*), gynecologic surgical complications, and pregnancy complications.[110]

DIAGNOSIS

- BV is characterized by malodorous vaginal discharge, with or without vaginal pruritus.
- The discharge is a homogeneous, nonviscous, grey-white fluid that coats the vagina and cervix.
- The presence of **"clue cells"** (epithelial cells with borders obscured by small bacteria) is an accepted criterion for diagnosis.
- **The vaginal pH should be >4.5.**
- Another common test **(whiff test)** involves the amine (fishy) odor released when the vaginal discharge is alkalinized by mixing with 10% KOH.
- No cultures are needed in clinical diagnosis of BV.

TREATMENT

- Treatment is recommended for symptomatic women.
- **Metronidazole** is the most effective antimicrobial for BV, with cure rates >90%.
  - ○ Standard treatment is metronidazole, 500 mg PO bid for 7 days.[110]
  - ○ Alternative treatments are metronidazole gel 0.75%, one application intravaginally every night for 5 nights or clindamycin cream 2%, one application intravaginally at night for 7 nights. Oral tinidazole or clindamycin are also alternatives.[110]
  - ○ Patients should be advised to avoid alcohol consumption during treatment with metronidazole due to a possible disulfiram-type reaction.
  - ○ Nausea and metallic taste are common side effects.[111]
- The effectiveness of probiotics is uncertain.[112]
- Relapses are relatively common after treatment.

Trichomonas Vaginitis

GENERAL PRINCIPLES

- *Trichomonas vaginalis* is a contagious protozoon that is acquired through sexual contact.
- It is often found in the presence of other sexually transmitted infections.
- Symptoms include diffuse, malodorous, yellow-green vaginal discharge, although many women are asymptomatic.
- *T. vaginalis* may also cause urethritis in men but is usually asymptomatic.

DIAGNOSIS

- Diagnosis can be made by microscopic detection of motile trichomonads on examination of a saline wet prep of vaginal or urethral secretions. The slide should be examined soon after preparation to detect motility. Organisms are detected in 60% to 70% of infected women.
- **The vaginal pH should be >4.5, and whiff test may be positive.**
- The "strawberry cervix" caused by cervical petechiae is a characteristic manifestation.
- The reliability of the Pap smear is quite variable.
- Culture is available but generally not necessary.

TREATMENT

- **Standard treatment is single-dose metronidazole** (2 g PO) or 500 mg PO bid for 7 days.[110,113] Patients should be warned not to drink alcohol during the course of treatment.
- Tinidazole 2 g PO ×1 is an alternative therapy.
- The cure rate is approximately 90% to 95% with metronidazole and 86% to 100% with tinidazole.
- Most physicians advocate treating all patients who have detectable organisms to reduce the sexual transmission of the organism.
- Treatment of male sexual partners is recommended.[110]

Vulvovaginal Candidiasis

GENERAL PRINCIPLES

- This "yeast infection" is suggested by the presence of vulvovaginal soreness, dyspareunia, vulvar pruritus, external dysuria, and thick or "cheesy" vaginal secretions.
- It is typically caused by *Candida albicans* but can sometimes be caused by other *Candida* spp.
- Factors that predispose to colonization and infection include diabetes, steroid therapy, pregnancy, antibiotics, obesity, OCPs, immunosuppressant drugs, and HIV infection.
- Candidiasis is usually not transmitted sexually.
- Ten to twenty percent of women normally have yeast colonized in the vagina; 75% of women have at least one episode of *Candida vaginitis*, and 45% have two or more episodes during their lifetime.

DIAGNOSIS

- Speculum examination may reveal candidal plaques adherent to the vaginal mucosa with erythema or edema of the introitus.
- **The vaginal pH is usually <4.5.**
- Diagnosis can be made by inspection of the typical vaginal lesions or by observation of fungal elements (budding yeast and pseudohyphae) in a KOH preparation.
- Cultures may be obtained for symptomatic women with negative KOH testing.
- It is justifiable to treat an apparent or suspected candidal vulvovaginitis even with a negative KOH preparation (only 40% to 80% sensitive).

TREATMENT

- Treatment is with one of the **imidazole antifungal drugs,** such as butoconazole, clotrimazole, miconazole, terconazole, or tioconazole. All are more effective than is nystatin.[110]
  - Courses of treatment range from single dose to 3 to 7 days depending on the agent and dose.
  - Most agents come in cream or suppository for intravaginal use.
- If the woman is menstruating, she should not use tampons, which may absorb the drug.
- **Single-dose oral fluconazole,** 150 mg, is an effective alternative.
- Recurrent candidal infections are common and can be distressing. All predisposing factors should be addressed. Each recurrent episode generally responds to topical treatment, but longer treatment may be indicated. Oral fluconazole 100 to 200 mg every third day for 3 doses followed by maintenance suppression with fluconazole 100 to 200 mg weekly for 6 months may be effective.[110,114]

REFERENCES

1. Baxter-Jones AD, Faulkner RA, Forwood MR, et al. Bone mineral accrual from 8 to 30 years of age: an estimation of peak bone mass. *J Bone Miner Res* 2011;26:1729–1739.
2. Miller CW. Survival and ambulation following hip fracture. *J Bone Joint Surg* 1978;60:930–934.
3. Brauer CA, Coca-Perraillon M, Cutler DM, et al. Incidence and mortality of hip fractures in the United States. *JAMA* 2009;302(14):1573–1579.
4. Consensus development conference: diagnosis, prophylaxis, and treatment of osteoporosis. *Am J Med* 1993;94:646–650.
5. Slemenda CW, Hui SL, Longcope C, et al. Predictors of bone mass in perimenopausal women. A prospective study of clinical data using photon absorptiometry. *Ann Intern Med* 1990;112:96–101.
6. Looker AC, Melton LJ III, Harris TB, et al. Prevalence and trends in low femur bone density among older US adults: NHANES 2005-2006 compared with NHANES III. *J Bone Miner Res* 2010;25:64–71.
7. *WHO Scientific Group on the Assessment of Osteoporosis at Primary Health Care Level.* Geneva, Switzerland: World Health Organization, 2007.
8. American College of Obstetricians and Gynecologists Women's Health Care Physicians. Osteoporosis. *Obstet Gynecol* 2012;129:718–734.
9. Cummings SR, Nevitt MC, Browner WS, et al. Risk factors for hip fracture in white women. Study of Osteoporotic Fractures Research Group. *N Engl J Med* 1995;332:767–773.
10. *Clinician's Guide to Prevention and Treatment of Osteoporosis.* Washington, DC: National Osteoporosis Foundation, 2008.
11. Kanis JA, Melton LJ III, Christiansen C, et al. The diagnosis of osteoporosis. *J Bone Miner Res* 1994;9:1137–1141.
12. Cryer B, Bauer DC. Oral bisphosphonates and upper gastrointestinal tract problems: what is the evidence? *Mayo Clin Proc* 2002;77:1031–1043.
13. Strampel W, Emkey R, Civitelli R. Safety considerations with bisphosphonates for the treatment of osteoporosis. *Drug Saf* 2007;30:755–763.
14. King AE, Umland EM. Osteonecrosis of the jaw in patients receiving intravenous or oral bisphosphonates. *Pharmacotherapy* 2008;28:667–677.
15. Pazianas M, Miller P, Blumentals WA, et al. A review of the literature on osteonecrosis of the jaw in patients with osteoporosis treated with oral bisphosphonates: prevalence, risk factors, and clinical characteristics. *Clin Ther* 2007;29:1548–1558.
16. Khan AA, Sándor GK, Dore E, et al.; Canadian Taskforce on Osteonecrosis of the Jaw. Bisphosphonate associated osteonecrosis of the jaw. *J Rheumatol* 2009;36:478–490.
17. Rizzoli R, Burlet N, Cahall D, et al. Osteonecrosis of the jaw and bisphosphonate treatment for osteoporosis. *Bone* 2008;42:841–847.
18. Woo SB, Hellstein JW, Kalmar JR. Narrative [corrected] review: bisphosphonates and osteonecrosis of the jaws. *Ann Intern Med* 2006;144:753–761.
19. Liberman UA, Weiss SR, Bröll J, et al. Effect of oral alendronate on bone mineral density and the incidence of fractures in postmenopausal osteoporosis. The Alendronate Phase III Osteoporosis Treatment Study Group. *N Engl J Med* 1995;333:1437–1443.
20. Cranney A, Wells G, Willan A, et al.; Osteoporosis Methodology Group and The Osteoporosis Research Advisory Group. Meta-analyses of therapies for postmenopausal osteoporosis. II. Meta-analysis of alendronate for the treatment of postmenopausal women. *Endocr Rev* 2002;23:508–516.
21. Black DM, Cummings SR, Karpf DB, et al. Randomised trial of effect of alendronate on risk of fracture in women with existing vertebral fractures. Fracture Intervention Trial Research Group. *Lancet* 1996;348:1535–1541.

22. Rizzoli R, Greenspan SL, Bone G III, et al.; Alendronate Once-Weekly Study Group. Two-year results of once-weekly administration of alendronate 70 mg for the treatment of postmenopausal osteoporosis. *J Bone Miner Res* 2002;17:1988–1996.

23. Harris ST, Watts NB, Genant HK, et al. Effects of risedronate treatment on vertebral and nonvertebral fractures in women with postmenopausal osteoporosis: a randomized controlled trial. Vertebral Efficacy with Risedronate Therapy (VERT) Study Group. *JAMA* 1999;282:1344–1352.

24. Reginster J, Minne HW, Sorensen OH, et al. Randomized trial of the effects of risedronate on vertebral fractures in women with established postmenopausal osteoporosis. Vertebral Efficacy with Risedronate Therapy (VERT) Study Group. *Osteoporos Int* 2000;11:83–91.

25. McClung MR, Geusens P, Miller PD, et al.; Hip Intervention Program Study Group. Effect of risedronate on the risk of hip fracture in elderly women. Hip Intervention Program Study Group. *N Engl J Med* 2001;344:333–340.

26. Cranney A, Tugwell P, Adachi J, et al.; Osteoporosis Methodology Group and The Osteoporosis Research Advisory Group. Meta-analyses of therapies for postmenopausal osteoporosis. III. Meta-analysis of risedronate for the treatment of postmenopausal osteoporosis. *Endocr Rev* 2002;23:517–523.

27. Harris ST, Watts NB, Li Z, et al. Two-year efficacy and tolerability of risedronate once a week for the treatment of women with postmenopausal osteoporosis. *Curr Med Res Opin* 2004;20:757–764.

28. Delmas PD, Benhamou CL, Man Z, et al. Monthly dosing of 75 mg risedronate on 2 consecutive days a month: efficacy and safety results. *Osteoporos Int* 2008;19:1039–1045.

29. Delmas PD, McClung MR, Zanchetta JR, et al. Efficacy and safety of risedronate 150 mg once a month in the treatment of postmenopausal osteoporosis. *Bone* 2008;42:36–42.

30. Delmas PD, Recker RR, Chesnut CH III, et al. Daily and intermittent oral ibandronate normalize bone turnover and provide significant reduction in vertebral fracture risk: results from the BONE study. *Osteoporos Int* 2004;15:792–798.

31. Chesnut CH III, Skag A, Christiansen C, et al.; Oral Ibandronate Osteoporosis Vertebral Fracture Trial in North America and Europe (BONE). Effects of oral ibandronate administered daily or intermittently on fracture risk in postmenopausal osteoporosis. *J Bone Miner Res* 2004;19:1241–1249.

32. Harris ST, Blumentals WA, Miller PD. Ibandronate and the risk of non-vertebral and clinical fractures in women with postmenopausal osteoporosis: results of a meta-analysis of phase III studies. *Curr Med Res Opin* 2008;24:237–245.

33. Cranney A, Wells GA, Yetisir E, et al. Ibandronate for the prevention of nonvertebral fractures: a pooled analysis of individual patient data. *Osteoporos Int* 2009;20:291–297.

34. Miller PD, McClung MR, Macovei L, et al. Monthly oral ibandronate therapy in postmenopausal osteoporosis: 1-year results from the MOBILE study. *J Bone Miner Res* 2005;20:1315–1322.

35. Reginster JY, Adami S, Lakatos P, et al. Efficacy and tolerability of once-monthly oral ibandronate in postmenopausal osteoporosis: 2 year results from the MOBILE study. *Ann Rheum Dis* 2006;65:654–661.

36. Delmas PD, Adami S, Strugala C, et al. Intravenous ibandronate injections in postmenopausal women with osteoporosis: one-year results from the dosing intravenous administration study. *Arthritis Rheum* 2006;54:1838–1846.

37. Eisman JA, Civitelli R, Adami S, et al. Efficacy and tolerability of intravenous ibandronate injections in postmenopausal osteoporosis: 2-year results from the DIVA study. *J Rheumatol* 2008;35:488–497.

38. Reid IR, Brown JP, Burckhardt P, et al. Intravenous zoledronic acid in postmenopausal women with low bone mineral density. *N Engl J Med* 2002;346:653–661.

39. Black DM, Delmas PD, Eastell R, et al.; HORIZON Pivotal Fracture Trial. Once-yearly zoledronic acid for treatment of postmenopausal osteoporosis. *N Engl J Med* 20073;356(18):1809–1822.
40. Lyles KW, Colón-Emeric CS, Magaziner JS, et al.; HORIZON Recurrent Fracture Trial. Zoledronic acid and clinical fractures and mortality after hip fracture. *N Engl J Med* 2007;357:1799–1809.
41. Ettinger B, Black DM, Mitlak BH, et al. Reduction of vertebral fracture risk in post-menopausal women with osteoporosis treated with raloxifene: results from a 3-year randomized clinical trial. Multiple Outcomes of Raloxifene Evaluation (MORE) Investigators. *JAMA* 1999;282:637–645.
42. Delmas PD, Ensrud KE, Adachi JD, et al.; Multiple Outcomes of Raloxifene Evaluation Investigators. Efficacy of raloxifene on vertebral fracture risk reduction in postmenopausal women with osteoporosis: four-year results from a randomized clinical trial. *J Clin Endocrinol Metab* 2002;87:3609–3617.
43. Siris ES, Harris ST, Eastell R, et al.; Continuing Outcomes Relevant to Evista (CORE) Investigators. Skeletal effects of raloxifene after 8 years: results from the continuing outcomes relevant to Evista (CORE) study. *J Bone Miner Res* 2005;20:1514–1524.
44. Cranney A, Tugwell P, Zytaruk N, et al.; Osteoporosis Methodology Group and The Osteoporosis Research Advisory Group. Meta-analyses of therapies for postmeno-pausal osteoporosis. IV. Meta-analysis of raloxifene for the prevention and treatment of postmenopausal osteoporosis. *Endocr Rev* 2002;23:524–528.
45. Cummings SR, Eckert S, Krueger KA, et al. The effect of raloxifene on risk of breast cancer in postmenopausal women: results from the MORE randomized trial. Multiple Outcomes of Raloxifene Evaluation. *JAMA* 1999;281:2189–2197.
46. Barrett-Connor E, Mosca L, Collins P, et al.; Raloxifene Use for The Heart (RUTH) Trial Investigators. Effects of raloxifene on cardiovascular events and breast cancer in postmenopausal women. *N Engl J Med* 2006;355:125–137.
47. Martino S, Cauley JA, Barrett-Connor E, et al.; CORE Investigators. Continuing outcomes relevant to Evista: breast cancer incidence in postmenopausal osteoporotic women in a randomized trial of raloxifene. *J Natl Cancer Inst* 2004;96:1751–1761.
48. Delmas PD, Bjarnason NH, Mitlak BH, et al. Effects of raloxifene on bone mineral density, serum cholesterol concentrations, and uterine endometrium in postmeno-pausal women. *N Engl J Med* 1997;337:1641–1647.
49. Collins P, Mosca L, Geiger MJ, et al. Effects of the selective estrogen receptor modula-tor raloxifene on coronary outcomes in the Raloxifene Use for The Heart trial: results of subgroup analyses by age and other factors. *Circulation* 2009;119:922–930.
50. Grady D, Ettinger B, Moscarelli E, et al.; Multiple Outcomes of Raloxifene Evaluation Investigators. Safety and adverse effects associated with raloxifene: multiple outcomes of raloxifene evaluation. *Obstet Gynecol* 2004;104:837–844.
51. Vogel VG, Costantino JP, Wickerham DL, et al.; National Surgical Adjuvant Breast and Bowel Project (NSABP). Effects of tamoxifen vs raloxifene on the risk of develop-ing invasive breast cancer and other disease outcomes: the NSABP Study of Tamoxifen and Raloxifene (STAR) P-2 trial. *JAMA* 2006;295:2727–2741.
52. Chesnut CH III, Silverman S, Andriano K, et al. A randomized trial of nasal spray salmon calcitonin in postmenopausal women with established osteoporosis: the prevent recurrence of osteoporotic fractures study. PROOF Study Group. *Am J Med* 2000;109:267–276.
53. Cranney A, Tugwell P, Zytaruk N, et al.; Osteoporosis Methodology Group and The Osteoporosis Research Advisory Group. Meta-analyses of therapies for postmeno-pausal osteoporosis. VI. Meta-analysis of calcitonin for the treatment of postmeno-pausal osteoporosis. *Endocr Rev* 2002;23:540–551.
54. Knopp JA, Diner BM, Blitz M, et al. Calcitonin for treating acute pain of osteoporotic vertebral compression fractures: a systematic review of randomized, controlled trials. *Osteoporos Int* 2005;16:1281–1290.

55. Greenspan SL, Bone HG, Ettinger MP, et al.; Treatment of Osteoporosis with Parathyroid Hormone Study Group. Effect of recombinant human parathyroid hormone (1–84) on vertebral fracture and bone mineral density in postmenopausal women with osteoporosis: a randomized trial. *Ann Intern Med* 2007;146:326–339.
56. Neer RM, Arnaud CD, Zanchetta JR, et al. Effect of parathyroid hormone (1–34) on fractures and bone mineral density in postmenopausal women with osteoporosis. *N Engl J Med* 2001;344:1434–1441.
57. Black DM, Bilezikian JP, Ensrud KE, et al.; PaTH Study Investigators. One year of alendronate after one year of parathyroid hormone (1–84) for osteoporosis. *N Engl J Med* 2005;353:555–565.
58. Black DM, Greenspan SL, Ensrud KE, et al.; PaTH Study Investigators. The effects of parathyroid hormone and alendronate alone or in combination in postmenopausal osteoporosis. *N Engl J Med* 2003;349:1207–1215.
59. Effects of hormone therapy on bone mineral density: results from the postmenopausal estrogen/progestin interventions (PEPI) trial. The Writing Group for the PEPI. *JAMA* 1996;276:1389–1396.
60. Rossouw JE, Anderson GL, Prentice RL, et al.; Writing Group for the Women's Health Initiative Investigators. Risks and benefits of estrogen plus progestin in healthy postmenopausal women: principal results From the Women's Health Initiative randomized controlled trial. *JAMA* 2002;288:321–333.
61. Cummings SR, Sam Martin J, McCLung MR, et al. Denosumab for prevention of fractures in postmenopausal women with osteoporosis. *N Engl J Med* 2009;361:756–765.
62. Shea B, Wells G, Cranney A, et al.; Osteoporosis Methodology Group and The Osteoporosis Research Advisory Group. Meta-analyses of therapies for postmenopausal osteoporosis. VII. Meta-analysis of calcium supplementation for the prevention of postmenopausal osteoporosis. *Endocr Rev* 2002;23:552–559.
63. NIH Consensus Conference. Optimal calcium intake. NIH Consensus Development Panel on Optimal Calcium Intake. *JAMA* 1994;272:1942–1948.
64. Whiting SJ. Safety of some calcium supplements questioned. *Nutr Rev* 1994;52:95–97.
65. Dawson-Hughes B, Harris SS, Krall EA, et al. Effect of calcium and vitamin D supplementation on bone density in men and women 65 years of age or older. *N Engl J Med* 1997;337:670–676.
66. Saag KG, Emkey R, Schnitzer TJ, et al. Alendronate for the prevention and treatment of glucocorticoid-induced osteoporosis. Glucocorticoid-Induced Osteoporosis Intervention Study Group. *N Engl J Med* 1998;339:292–299.
67. Adachi JD, Saag KG, Delmas PD, et al. Two-year effects of alendronate on bone mineral density and vertebral fracture in patients receiving glucocorticoids: a randomized, double-blind, placebo-controlled extension trial. *Arthritis Rheum* 2001;44:202–211.
68. Cohen S, Levy RM, Keller M, et al. Risedronate therapy prevents corticosteroid-induced bone loss: a twelve-month, multicenter, randomized, double-blind, placebo-controlled, parallel-group study. *Arthritis Rheum* 1999;42:2309–2318.
69. Reid DM, Hughes RA, Laan RF, et al. Efficacy and safety of daily risedronate in the treatment of corticosteroid-induced osteoporosis in men and women: a randomized trial. European Corticosteroid-Induced Osteoporosis Treatment Study. *J Bone Miner Res* 2000;15:1006–1013.
70. Mok CC, Tong KH, To CH, et al. Risedronate for prevention of bone mineral density loss in patients receiving high-dose glucocorticoids: a randomized double-blind placebo-controlled trial. *Osteoporos Int* 2008;19:357–364.
71. Reid DM, Devogelaer JP, Saag K, et al.; HORIZON Investigators. Zoledronic acid and risedronate in the prevention and treatment of glucocorticoid-induced osteoporosis (HORIZON): a multicentre, double-blind, double-dummy, randomised controlled trial. *Lancet* 2009;373:1253–1263.

72. Montemurro L, Schiraldi G, Fraioli P, et al. Prevention of corticosteroid-induced osteoporosis with salmon calcitonin in sarcoid patients. *Calcif Tissue Int* 1991;49:71–76.
73. Luengo M, Pons F, Martinez de Osaba MJ, et al. Prevention of further bone mass loss by nasal calcitonin in patients on long term glucocorticoid therapy for asthma: a two year follow up study., *Thorax* 1994;49:1099–1102.
74. Saag KG, Shane E, Boonen S, et al. Teriparatide or alendronate in glucocorticoid-induced osteoporosis. *N Engl J Med* 2007;357:2028–2039.
75. Anderson FH, Francis RM, Faulkner K. Androgen supplementation in eugonadal men with osteoporosis-effects of 6 months of treatment on bone mineral density and cardiovascular risk factors. *Bone* 1996;18:171–177.
76. Katznelson L, Finkelstein JS, Schoenfeld DA, et al. Increase in bone density and lean body mass during testosterone administration in men with acquired hypogonadism. *J Clin Endocrinol Metab* 1996;81:4358–4365.
77. Behre HM, Kliesch S, Leifke E, et al. Long-term effect of testosterone therapy on bone mineral density in hypogonadal men. *J Clin Endocrinol Metab* 1997;82:2386–2390.
78. Sawka AM, Papaioannou A, Adachi JD, et al. Does alendronate reduce the risk of fracture in men? A meta-analysis incorporating prior knowledge of anti-fracture efficacy in women. *BMC Musculoskelet Disord* 2005;6:39.
79. Ringe JD, Faber H, Farahmand P, et al. Efficacy of risedronate in men with primary and secondary osteoporosis: results of a 1-year study. *Rheumatol Int* 2006;26:427–431.
80. Ringe JD, Farahmand P, Faber H, et al. Sustained efficacy of risedronate in men with primary and secondary osteoporosis: results of a 2-year study. *Rheumatol Int* 2009;29:311–315.
81. Boonen S, Orwoll ES, Wenderoth D, et al. Once-weekly risedronate in men with osteoporosis: results of a 2-year, placebo-controlled, double-blind, multicenter study. *J Bone Miner Res* 2009;24:719–725.
82. Majima T, Shimatsu A, Komatsu Y, et al. Effects of risedronate or alfacalcidol on bone mineral density, bone turnover, back pain, and fractures in Japanese men with primary osteoporosis: results of a two-year strict observational study. *J Bone Miner Metab* 2009;27:168–174.
83. Kurland ES, Cosman F, McMahon DJ, et al. Parathyroid hormone as a therapy for idiopathic osteoporosis in men: effects on bone mineral density and bone markers. *J Clin Endocrinol Metab* 2000;85:3069–3076.
84. Orwoll ES, Scheele WH, Paul S, et al. The effect of teriparatide [human parathyroid hormone (1–34)] therapy on bone density in men with osteoporosis. *J Bone Miner Res* 2003;18:9–17.
85. Finkelstein JS, Hayes A, Hunzelman JL, et al. The effects of parathyroid hormone, alendronate, or both in men with osteoporosis. *N Engl J Med* 2003;349:1216–1226.
86. Parker MJ, Gillespie WJ, Gillespie LD. Hip protectors for preventing hip fractures in older people. *Cochrane Database Syst Rev* 2005;(3):CD001255.
87. Sawka AM, Boulos P, Beattie K, et al. Do hip protectors decrease the risk of hip fracture in institutional and community-dwelling elderly? A systematic review and meta-analysis of randomized controlled trials. *Osteoporos Int* 2005;16:1461–1474.
88. Nelson HD. Menopause. *Lancet* 2008;371:760–770.
89. Bäckström T. Symptoms related to the menopause and sex steroid treatments. *Ciba Found Symp* 1995;191:171–186.
90. Maclennan AH, Broadbent JL, Lester S, et al. Oral oestrogen and combined oestrogen/progestogen therapy versus placebo for hot flushes. *Cochrane Database Syst Rev* 2004;(4):CD002978.
91. American College of Obstetricians and Gynecologists Women's Health Care Physicians. Vasomotor symptoms. *Obstet Gynecol* 2004;104(4 Suppl):106S–117S.

92. Hulley S, Grady D, Bush T, et al. Randomized trial of estrogen plus progestin for secondary prevention of coronary heart disease in postmenopausal women. Heart and Estrogen/progestin Replacement Study (HERS) Research Group. *JAMA* 1998;280:605–613.
93. North American Menopause Society. Estrogen and progestogen use in peri- and postmenopausal women: March 2007 position statement of The North American Menopause Society. *Menopause* 2007;14:168–182.
94. ACOG Task Force for Hormone Therapy American College of Obstetricians and Gynecologists Women's Health Care Physicians. Summary of balancing risks and benefits. *Obstet Gynecol* 2004;104(4 suppl):128S–129S.
95. American College of Obstetricians and Gynecologists Women's Health Care Physicians. Ovarian, endometrial, and colorectal cancers. *Obstet Gynecol* 2004;104 (4 suppl):77S–84S.
96. Nelson HD, Vesco KK, Haney E, et al. Nonhormonal therapies for menopausal hot flashes: systematic review and meta-analysis. *JAMA* 2006;295:2057–2071.
97. Toulis KA, Tzellos T, Kouvelas D, et al. Gabapentin for the treatment of hot flashes in women with natural or tamoxifen-induced menopause: a systematic review and meta-analysis. *Clin Ther* 2009;31:221–235.
98. Lethaby AE, Brown J, Marjoribanks J, et al. Phytoestrogens for vasomotor menopausal symptoms. *Cochrane Database Syst Rev* 2007;(4):CD001395.
99. Krebs EE, Ensrud KE, MacDonald R, et al. Phytoestrogens for treatment of menopausal symptoms: a systematic review. *Obstet Gynecol* 2004;104:824–836.
100. American College of Obstetricians and Gynecologists Women's Health Care Physicians. Genitourinary tract changes. *Obstet Gynecol* 2004;104(4 Suppl):56S–61S.
101. Spitzer M. Cervical screening adjuncts: recent advances. *Am J Obstet Gynecol* 1998;179:544–556.
102. Screening for cervical cancer. Practice Bulletin No. 131. American College of Obstetricians and Gynecologists. *Obstet Gynecol* 2012;131:1222–1238.
103. International Collaboration of Epidemiological Studies of Cervical Cancer. Comparison of risk factors for invasive squamous cell carcinoma and adenocarcinoma of the cervis: collaborative reanalysis of individual data on 8097 women with squamous cell carcinoma and 1374 women with adenocarcinoma from 12 epidemiological studies. *Int J Cancer* 2006;120:885–891.
104. Saslow D, Solomon D, Loawson HW et al. American Cancer Society, American Society for Colposcopy and Cervical Pathology, and American Society for Clinical Pathology screening guidelines for the prevention and early detection of cervical cancer. *CA Cander J Clin* 2012;62:147-172.
105. Moyer VA. Screening for cervical cancer: U.S. Preventive Services Task Force recommendation statement. U.S. Preventive Services Task Force. *Ann Intern Med* 2012;156:880–891.
106. Wright TC Jr, Massad LS, Dunton CJ, et al.; 2006 American Society for Colposcopy and Cervical Pathology-sponsored Consensus Conference. 2006 consensus guidelines for the management of women with abnormal cervical cancer screening tests. *Am J Obstet Gynecol* 2007;197:346–355.
107. Huang W, Molitch ME. Evaluation and management of galactorrhea. *Am Fam Phys* 2012;85(11):1074–1080.
108. Hussain AN, Policarpio C, Vincent MT. Evaluating nipple discharge. *Obstet Gynecol Surv* 2006;61:278–283.
109. Gray RJ, Pockaj BA, Karstaedt, PJ. Navigating murkey waters: a modern treatment algorithm for nipple discharge. *Am J of Surg* 2007;194:850–855.
110. Centers for Disease Control and Prevention, Workowski KA, Berman SM. Sexually transmitted diseases treatment guidelines, 2010. *MMWR Recomm Rep* 2010;59:56–63.

111. Oduyebo OO, Anorlu RI, Ogunsola FT. The effects of antimicrobial therapy on bacterial vaginosis in non-pregnant women. *Cochrane Database Syst Rev* 2009;(3):CD006055.

112. Senok AC, Verstraelen H, Temmerman M, et al. Probiotics for the treatment of bacterial vaginosis. *Cochrane Database Syst Rev* 2009;(4):CD006289.

113. Forna F, Gülmezoglu AM. Interventions for treating trichomoniasis in women. *Cochrane Database Syst Rev* 2003;(2):CD000218.

114. Sobel JD, Wiesenfeld HC, Martens M, et al. Maintenance fluconazole therapy for recurrent vulvovaginal candidiasis. *N Engl J Med* 2004;351:876–883.

115. Bonaiuti D, Shea B, Iovine R, et al. Exercise for preventing and treating osteoporosis in postmenopausal women. *Cochrane Database Syst Rev* 2002;(3):CD000333.

4 Men's Health
Melvin Blanchard

Prostate Cancer Screening

GENERAL PRINCIPLES

- Prostate cancer is the most common noncutaneous malignancy in older men and is the second most common cause of cancer mortality after lung cancer.
- Approximately 239,000 men will be diagnosed in 2013, and 29,000 will die from this malignancy.[1]
- The introduction of screening tests has led to intense debate and varying recommendations (also see Chapter 5).
  - The variable course of prostate cancer makes screening for the presence of disease a complicated decision. Some men have subclinical prostate cancer that progresses slowly and never contributes to mortality, whereas others have disease aggressive enough to cause premature death.
  - The American Cancer Society recommends screening and early detection programs for men at high risk for prostate cancer (first-degree relative diagnosed prior to age 65 or African American) starting as early as 40 to 45 years of age. The American Urological Society recommends an individualized approach for men 54 to 71 years old. However, the U.S. Preventive Services Task Force (USPSTF), Canadian Task Force on Preventive Health Care, and United Kingdom National Screening Committee all recommend against screening.
- Unfortunately, neither highly sensitive screening tests that detect cancers likely to be clinically significant nor highly specific tests that identify low-grade disease unlikely to cause death are available.
- Early detection and treatment are the only ways to decrease mortality from prostate cancer since it is incurable once spread beyond the capsule. Screening has effectively increased the identification of organ-confined and potentially curable cancer. However, the apparent gain in survival resulting from early detection may be due to **lead-time bias**, as men who would otherwise never be diagnosed or have any sequelae of prostate cancer are having it detected earlier.
- The benefit of treatment in clinically localized prostate cancer has not been definitively proven.
  - In observational studies of men with well- and moderately differentiated cancers, active surveillance or observation alone is associated with high prostate cancer–specific survival rates.[2–5]
  - The primary treatment modalities, radical prostatectomy and radiation therapy, are associated with significant rates of complications, including erectile dysfunction (ED), urinary incontinence, and urethral or rectal injury.
- Controversy persists as to whether screening for prostate cancer decreases its morbidity or mortality. Two large multicenter randomized prospective clinical trials, one conducted in Europe and another in the United States, reported conflicting results on this question.[6,7]
  - The European study reported a 20% decline in mortality, whereas the US study found no significant difference in death rate.
  - The initial results of the US study reported at 9 years persisted in follow-up analysis after 10 and 13 years.[8]

DIAGNOSIS

Digital Rectal Examination

- The digital rectal examination (DRE) is a nonstandardized examination of the prostate that reveals abnormalities in 3% to 12% of patients.[9] In fact, the interrater agreement among urologists for detecting prostate abnormalities is poor.[10]
- **An abnormal DRE** (asymmetric, nodular, or indurated) has a positive predictive value for cancer of 18% to 28%.[11] When abnormal, it necessitates a transrectal ultrasound-guided prostate biopsy. Therefore, **72% to 82% of patients with an abnormal DRE will have a prostate biopsy that is negative for malignancy**.

Prostate-Specific Antigen

- Prostate-specific antigen (PSA) is a 240-amino-acid serine protease secreted by prostatic epithelial cells that lyses the clotted ejaculate to enhance sperm motility. Some PSA naturally leaks into blood and does so to a greater extent in prostate cancer.
- Ejaculation and prostate manipulation raise PSA levels; **however, a routine DRE does not clinically change the results of PSA testing**.[12]
- Finasteride, a 5-α-reductase inhibitor, reduces total PSA (tPSA) by about 50% in 6 to 12 months.[13]
- The positive predictive value of a tPSA >4.0 ng/mL is about 30%, but it is a continuum, as the risk of prostate cancer increases significantly even within the normal range.[14] **The sensitivity of this cutoff is 70% to 80%, but the specificity is low,** as multiple conditions besides cancer can elevate tPSA (Table 4-1).

Prostate-Specific Antigen Velocity

- PSA velocity (PSAV), the rate of change in PSA over time, is **abnormal when it is >0.35 ng/mL/year (for tPSA <4 ng/mL) or >0.75 ng/mL/year (for tPSA >4)**.
- It correlates with prostate cancer diagnosis and is most reliable when three values are obtained at the same laboratory over at least 18 months. High PSAV, however, may be indicative of prostatitis.
- One study suggests that PSAV may be prognostic when obtained in the year before the diagnosis of prostate cancer.[15]

Free Prostate-Specific Antigen

- Percent-free PSA (fPSA), the ratio of free circulating to bound PSA in serum, is **lower in men with prostate cancer than in those with benign prostatic diseases.**
- It is most useful in deciding which patients with a mildly elevated PSA (4 to 10 ng/mL) should undergo biopsy.

TABLE 4-1	Processes That Affect Prostate-Specific Antigen (PSA) besides Prostate Cancer	
Increase PSA	**No effect on PSA**	**Decrease PSA**
Age	α-Blocker therapy	Finasteride therapy
Benign prostatic hyperplasia	Cystoscopy	Prostate resection
Prostate biopsy	Routine digital rectal examination	
Prostatitis	Testosterone replacement	
Recent ejaculation	Urethral catheterization	
Urinary tract infection		
Vigorous prostate massage		

- An **upper cutoff of 30%** significantly decreases the number of false-positive biopsies while maintaining a high level of sensitivity.[16]
- The complexed PSA (cPSA) is also measurable, but has no significant advantage over fPSA.

Prostate-Specific Antigen Density
- Defined as the PSA divided by prostate volume (measured by transrectal ultrasound or MRI) and compared with **age-/race-specific reference ranges**
- More costly and has less clear benefit on cancer detection rates. **Not currently a part of routine guidelines**

Screening

- **The decision as to whether to screen for prostate cancer must be individualized,** as the lack of evidence from clinical trials has led to very different recommendations on screening. Patients who request screening must be educated about the risks and benefits involved. (Fig. 4-1).
- The USPSTF 2012 update concludes that there is moderate certainty that the benefit of screening does not outweigh potential harm and recommends against PSA-based screening for prostate cancer. Men who request screening should be educated to enable an informed choice.
- The **American Cancer Society** recommends screening for men at age 50 if life expectancy is at least 10 years. The frequency should be annual if PSA is >2.5 ng/mL and every 2 years if PSA is <2.5 ng/mL. Men at high risk (African American men or men with one or more first-degree relatives with prostate cancer prior to age 65) should be offered screening starting at age 40 to 45.
- The **American Urological Association** recommends an individualized approach and shared decision making for men 55 to 69 years old.

Benign Prostatic Hyperplasia

GENERAL PRINCIPLES

- Benign prostatic hyperplasia (BPH) is defined histologically as hypertrophy of glandular and stromal tissue.
- It is present primarily in older men with functioning testicles. The **prevalence of BPH increases with age** from 8% among men in their fourth decade of life to 80% among those >80 years of age, with lower urinary tract symptoms (LUTS) in about 25% to 45% of men >70 years of age.[17]
- BPH may be complicated by recurrent urinary tract infections (UTIs), urinary bladder stones, and acute urinary retention.

DIAGNOSIS

Clinical Presentation

History
- Patients with LUTS complain of urgency, frequency, nocturia, weak stream, hesitancy, and incomplete emptying.
- The **American Urological Association Symptom Index** (AUA-SI) (Table 4-2), a standardized questionnaire that quantifies these symptoms, should be administered to all men with BPH.[18] The AUA-SI score is used to classify symptom severity, guide treatment recommendations, and follow response to therapy.
- The history should also assess for sexual dysfunction, neurogenic bladder; prior urethral trauma or urethritis; diabetes; hematuria; family history of BPH or prostate cancer; and drugs that decrease bladder function or increase tone at bladder neck (anticholinergics, sympathomimetic amines).

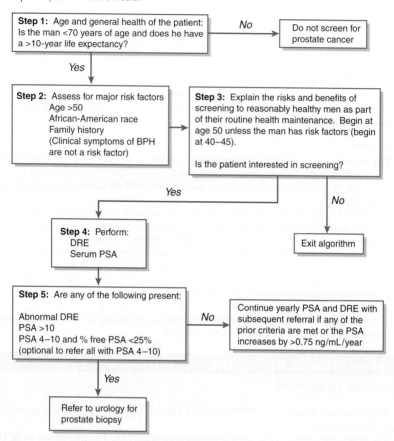

Figure 4-1 Prostate cancer screening algorithm. BPH, benign prostatic hyperplasia; DRE, digital rectal examination; PSA, prostate-specific antigen.

Physical Examination

The prostate should be palpated for nodules and an estimation of its size. Men with over-sized prostates are at increased risk of experiencing complications and undergoing prostate surgery.

Diagnostic Testing

Laboratories

- **Urinalysis** should be obtained to rule out infection and assess for complications (hematuria, UTI) and glycosuria.
- **Serum creatinine** should be obtained as it may indicate underlying kidney disease, which could contribute to LUTS.
- **Screening for prostate cancer is optional,** as its prevalence is not increased despite the fact that PSA is elevated in 25% to 30% of men with BPH.
- **PSA is predictive of prostate size,** as PSA values of >1.6, 2.0, and 2.3 correlate with 70% sensitivity and specificity to prostates >40 mL in size in men in their 50s, 60s, and 70s, respectively.[19]

TABLE 4-2 American Urological Association Symptom Index

During the past month, how often have you...	Not at all	Less than one time in five	Less than half the time	Half the time	More than half the time	Almost always
1. Had the sensation of not emptying your bladder completely after you finished urinating?	0	1	2	3	4	5
2. Had to urinate <2 hours after you finished urinating?	0	1	2	3	4	5
3. Found you stopped and started several times when you urinated?	0	1	2	3	4	5
4. Found it difficult to postpone urination?	0	1	2	3	4	5
5. Had a weak urinary stream?	0	1	2	3	4	5
6. Had to push or strain to begin urination?	0	1	2	3	4	5
7. Typically needed to get up to urinate from the time you went to bed at night until the time you got up in the morning?	None	1 (time)	2 (times)	3 (times)	4 (times)	5 (times)

0–7 points = mild symptoms
8–19 points = moderate symptoms
20–35 points = severe symptoms
Modified from Barry MJ, Fowler FJ Jr, O'Leary MP, et al. The American Urological Association Symptom Index for benign prostatic hyperplasia. The Measurement Committee of the American Urological Association. *J Urol* 1992;148:1549.

Imaging
Renal imaging (ultrasound or intravenous pyelography) should be performed in patients with complications such as hematuria, recurrent UTIs, or unexplained chronic kidney disease.

Diagnostic Procedures
Urodynamic testing (peak flow rate and pressure volume studies) should be reserved for patients with an unclear diagnosis, suspected neurogenic bladder dysfunction, or moderate to severe disease that fails to respond to initial therapy.

TREATMENT

- The major factors to consider in selecting a therapy are AUA-SI score and prostate size. The other factors to consider are age, concomitant hypertension, current medications, sexual history, and the degree to which the symptoms affect quality of life.
- **Watchful waiting** without treatment is **recommended for patients with mild symptoms (AUA-SI ≤7) and is an option for those with moderate symptoms who do not want to initiate lifelong medical therapy and do not have BPH complications** (urinary retention, renal insufficiency, or UTI).
- Patients should minimize fluids before bedtime and avoid medications with anticholinergic or sympathomimetic properties (including antihistamines, tricyclic antidepressants, and decongestants), caffeinated beverages, and alcohol.
- Many patients with mild symptoms have no change or improve without treatment; however, there is some concern that delay in treatment may result in bladder decompensation.[20]

Medications

Pharmacologic therapy is recommended for patients with moderate symptoms who request treatment and for those with severe symptoms.

First-Generation α-Blockers
- **Terazosin and doxazosin** are α_1-adrenergic blockers that relax smooth muscle cells in the prostate and lead to an improvement of symptoms (decrease of 4 to 6 points on AUA-SI) within weeks of initiating therapy.[21]
- Symptomatic improvement is maintained with long-term therapy, but α_1-blockers do not decrease prostate size, the rate of urinary retention, the need for surgery, or PSA.
- α_1-Blockers are effective in men with small and large prostates.
- These agents are possible choices for men with concomitant hypertension that requires treatment. Terazosin and doxazosin decrease blood pressure (BP) by approximately 10 to 15/10 to 15 mm Hg in men with elevated BP but have no clinically significant effect on BP in normotensive patients.[22] However, they should not be used at the expense of other drugs for overriding indications (see Chapter 6).
- Treatment is initiated at night with dose titration over 2 to 3 weeks to minimize side effects.
  - Terazosin is titrated weekly from 1 to 2 to 5 mg PO nightly and can subsequently be increased to 10 to 20 mg PO nightly.
  - Doxazosin is titrated from 1 to 2 to 4 mg PO nightly and can be subsequently increased to 8 to 16 mg PO nightly.
- Common side effects are dizziness, orthostatic hypotension, and fatigue. **Hypotension and orthostasis are exacerbated with concomitant use of phosphodiesterase inhibitors for ED** (e.g., sildenafil, vardenafil, tadalafil).
- The Food and Drug Administration (FDA) has posted a drug safety alert indicating that α_1-blockers increase the risk of floppy iris syndrome in patients with cataract surgery.

Second-Generation α-Blockers

- **Alfuzosin, silodosin, and tamsulosin are uroselective α_{1a}-blockers** with pharmacologic activity that is limited to the prostate with minimal systemic effects on BP. They are good choices for men who want rapid symptom relief and who are prone to orthostasis.
- The dose for alfuzosin is 10 mg PO daily, silodosin is 8 mg PO daily, and tamsulosin is 0.4 to 0.8 mg PO daily.
  - Dose titration and nocturnal dosing are unnecessary for these three agents.
  - The dose of silodosin should be halved for patients with a creatinine clearance of 30 to 49 mL/minute.
  - Both silodosin and alfuzosin should be avoided in patients with a creatinine clearance of <30 mL/minute.
- Common side effects of these agents are ejaculatory problems and dizziness.
- The FDA has posted a drug safety alert indicating that tamsulosin and other α_1-blockers increase the risk of floppy iris syndrome in patients with cataract surgery.

5α-Reductase Inhibitors

- **Finasteride and dutasteride** are 5α-reductase inhibitors that inhibit conversion of testosterone to dihydrotestosterone (DHT), reverse epithelial glandular hyperplasia, and shrink the prostate by approximately 15% to 30% within several months.
- Symptomatic improvement is sustained long term, and they are the only drug class that have been shown to decrease the rate of urinary retention and need for prostate surgery.[23–25]
- These agents are more **effective in men with prostates >40 mL in size.**[26]
- PSA can predict which patients are candidates for treatment with finasteride (see the Prostate-Specific Antigen section).
- The **symptomatic response to these agents is delayed** for 6 to 12 months.
- The dose **for finasteride** is 5 mg PO daily, and for dutasteride, it is 0.5 mg PO daily.
- The only common side effects are sexual, including ED, decreased libido, and ejaculatory dysfunction.
- After 6 months of therapy, finasteride decreases PSA by approximately 50%.
  - PSA may still be used as a screening test for prostate cancer provided that the PSA value is doubled.[27]
  - Free PSA is unchanged by treatment.
- Questions have been raised about the safety of these agents in the Prostate Cancer Prevention Trial. This 7-year study showed that, compared with placebo, finasteride reduced the risk of prostate cancer. However, participants who developed prostate cancer while on study drug were more likely to develop higher-grade cancers.[28,29] The FDA recommends that patients be assessed for prostate cancer before starting this class of drugs.

Combination Therapy

- Combination therapy with an α_1-blocker and finasteride makes theoretical sense for men with large prostates and is frequently attempted, but research study results are mixed.
- It is a general practice among many to use combination therapy in symptomatic men with large prostate and monotherapy (α_1-blockers) in patients with small gland size.[30,31]

Herbal Treatment

- Several different forms of herbal therapy, including saw palmetto (*Serenoa repens*), *Pygeum africanum*, Cernilton, and β-sitosterols, are available and self-prescribed by patients to treat BPH.
- These agents have been shown to be effective in the short term, but their mechanism of action and long-term efficacy are unknown.[32]
- **Saw palmetto** (160 mg PO bid) is the most commonly used herb in the United States, but is not FDA approved.

Surgical Management

- **Indications for referral to urology** include refractory LUTS, complications such as recurrent hematuria or recurrent UTIs, bladder stones, acute urinary retention and renal insufficiency with hydronephrosis, a rectal examination or PSA suspicious for prostate cancer, and an unclear diagnosis when urodynamic testing may be helpful.
- **Transurethral resection of the prostate (TURP),** the "gold standard" for BPH treatment, has a much greater benefit in reducing symptoms than medical therapy.
  - ○ TURP results in retrograde ejaculation and ED in a significant percentage of patients, and approximately 20% have unsatisfactory results and require further therapy.
  - ○ As TURP removes only central prostatic tissue, it does not eliminate the chance of developing prostate cancer.
  - ○ Several new **minimally invasive surgical procedures** have been introduced as alternatives to TURP.

Prostatitis

GENERAL PRINCIPLES

- Prostatitis is the most common urologic complaint among men <50 years of age.
- The prostatitis syndromes are classified by the acuity of presentation and findings on urinalysis and culture before and after prostatic massage.
- Prostatitis is classified as follows:
  - ○ Acute prostatitis
  - ○ Chronic bacterial prostatitis
  - ○ Chronic prostatitis/chronic pelvic pain syndrome:
    - ▪ Inflammatory
    - ▪ Noninflammatory
  - ○ Asymptomatic inflammation of the prostate
- **Only 5% to 10% of cases are due to bacterial causes.**[33]

DIAGNOSIS

Acute Bacterial Prostatitis

- Patients present with symptoms of a UTI (e.g., dysuria, frequency, urgency) and systemic symptoms such as fever, malaise, and lower abdominal or back pain. Risk factors include instrumentation and HIV.
- A gentle prostate examination might reveal an enlarged, warm, and very tender prostate. **Vigorous massage is contraindicated** as this could cause bacteremia and sepsis.
- Urinalysis and culture are positive, most often for *Escherichia coli* or other gram-negative organisms.
- An abdominal ultrasound or CT scan to rule out a prostatic abscess should be considered if initial treatment fails.

Chronic Prostatitis Syndromes

- Patients with the three chronic prostatitis syndromes present with similar symptoms, classically a triad of recurrent voiding symptoms, pain (pelvic, perineal, inguinal, back, penile, or scrotal), and ejaculatory symptoms (pain, hematospermia).
- Patients with **chronic bacterial prostatitis** are usually older, frequently have recurrent UTIs with the same organism, and may have a history of acute prostatitis.
- Patients with the two **chronic nonbacterial prostatitis syndromes** are often younger and do not have a history of recurrent UTIs.

TABLE 4-3	Diagnostic Prostate Massage Results		
Type of prostatitis	Prostate examination	Postmassage urinalysis	Postmassage culture
Acute bacterial (5%)	Warm, boggy, enlarged, tender	Vigorous massage contraindicated	Vigorous massage contraindicated
Chronic bacterial (5%–10%)	Can be mildly tender and boggy or can be normal	Positive[a]	Positive[b]
Inflammatory chronic nonbacterial (50%–60%)	Usually normal	Positive[a]	Negative
Noninflammatory chronic nonbacterial (prostatodynia) (30%–40%)	Usually normal	Negative	Negative

[a]A positive urinalysis is >10 to 15 WBCs/high-power field.
[b]A positive culture has a colony count that is at least 10-fold greater than the premassage culture.

- The predominant symptom of pain and predilection to occur in younger men distinguish it from BPH.
- Chronic nonbacterial prostatitis is the most common urologic diagnosis in men <50 years of age.
- The prostate examination is often normal in men with each of the chronic prostatitis syndromes. A **diagnostic prostate massage** comparing a midstream urine specimen (the second 10 mL of urine voided) with one after a vigorous prostate massage is the test of choice to correctly diagnose the three syndromes (Table 4-3). However, this is usually done after presumptive diagnosis fails to respond to treatment.

TREATMENT

Acute Bacterial Prostatitis

- Patients should be treated initially with broad-spectrum parenteral antibiotics followed by oral agents if they respond.
  - Potential oral regimens include **trimethoprim-sulfamethoxazole**, 1 DS tablet PO bid; **doxycycline**, 100 mg PO bid; **ciprofloxacin**, 500 mg PO bid; or **levofloxacin**, 500 mg PO daily for 4 to 6 weeks.
  - Severely ill patients with suspected bacteremia require admission for IV antibiotics.
- Supportive care with analgesics, stool softeners, and vigorous oral hydration may be beneficial.
- Because of the relatively high risk for urinary retention, bladder scanning should be done to assess the postvoid residual. For patients who require short-term drainage, a small urethral catheter may be sufficient; those who require long-term drainage will need a suprapubic catheter.

Chronic Bacterial Prostatitis

- **Prolonged courses of antibiotics** (4 to 6 weeks), preferably with a **fluoroquinolone** (excellent prostate penetration), are recommended.
- **α_1-Adrenergic blockers** (see the "Benign Prostatic Hyperplasia" section above) may provide additional symptomatic relief.
- Recurrences require retreatment.

Chronic Nonbacterial Prostatitis

- **Treatment of both types of chronic nonbacterial prostatitis is difficult** and often prolonged. Recommendations are based primarily on clinical experience, as controlled trial data are limited.[34]
- Patients with **inflammatory chronic nonbacterial prostatitis** should receive a trial of 4 to 6 weeks of antibiotics (fluoroquinolone or trimethoprim-sulfamethoxazole). This should be continued for 12 weeks if improvement occurs due to anecdotal evidence that links the syndrome to atypical pathogens. Doxycycline and azithromycin can be used to treat *Chlamydia trachomatis*.
- Treatment options for **noninflammatory chronic nonbacterial prostatitis** (prostatodynia) include α_1-adrenergic blockers, nonsteroidal anti-inflammatory drugs, "muscle relaxants" such as diazepam, and anticholinergic agents.[35]

Erectile Dysfunction

GENERAL PRINCIPLES

- ED is the **consistent** inability to attain or maintain an erection that is satisfactory for successful intercourse.[36]
- The prevalence increases with advancing age, and the impact on quality of life is substantial.[37]
- Many men are embarrassed to raise the subject, so it is important that primary care physicians initiate the conversation with their patients.
- The risk factors for ED are presented in Table 4-4.

DIAGNOSIS

Clinical Presentation

History

- A detailed **sexual history** should assess the severity, onset, duration, progression, and situational nature of the problem to confirm that the patient has erectile failure and not a problem with libido or ejaculation.
- A gradual progressive onset of ED with absence of nocturnal or morning erections suggests an **underlying medical cause.**
- ED that develops suddenly is likely either **psychogenic** or due to a **medication.**
- Risk factors for ED should be reviewed (Table 4-4).
- The **potential cardiovascular risk of intercourse** to the patient should be assessed, given the strong association between ED and coronary artery disease. Sexual activity is equivalent to walking 1 mile in 20 minutes, climbing two flights of stairs in 10 seconds, or 3 metabolic equivalents (METs) of activity.[38]
- Patients who can safely exercise to a level of five METs (see Chapter 2, Table 2-3) are at low risk for coronary ischemia during intercourse. Stress testing should be considered, before the initiation of therapy or resumption of intercourse, in sedentary men with multiple cardiac risk factors who cannot safely exercise to this level. Patients should complete 4 minutes on the Bruce treadmill protocol (5 to 6 METs) without symptoms, arrhythmias, or fall in blood pressure.[38]

TABLE 4-4	Common Risk Factors for Erectile Dysfunction

Category	Examples
Vascular disease	Coronary artery disease, diabetes, hyperlipidemia, hypertension, peripheral vascular disease
Neurologic disorders	Multiple sclerosis, Parkinson disease, spinal cord injury, stroke
Endocrine disorders	Hyperprolactinemia, hyperthyroidism, hypothyroidism, primary hypogonadism (testicular), secondary hypogonadism (CNS)
Chronic medical disorders	Chronic renal insufficiency, cirrhosis, COPD
Psychogenic	Anxiety disorder, depression, marital/relationship discord
Urologic disorders	Advanced prostate cancer, colorectal, bladder, or prostate surgery, pelvic trauma/fracture, Peyronie disease, radiation therapy
Medications	Antihypertensives (especially thiazide diuretics, beta-blockers, clonidine), psychiatric medications (anticholinergics, MAO inhibitors, phenothiazines, SSRIs, TCAs), antiandrogens (cimetidine, digoxin, estrogens, finasteride, ketoconazole, LHRH agonists, spironolactone)
Illicit substances	Alcohol, amphetamines, cocaine, marijuana, opiates, tobacco

CNS, central nervous system; COPD, chronic obstructive pulmonary disease; LHRH, luteinizing hormone–releasing hormone; MAO, monoamine oxidase; SSRIs, selective serotonin reuptake inhibitors; TCAs, tricyclic antidepressants.

Physical Examination

The physical examination should assess for evidence of vascular or neurologic disease, stigmata of hypogonadism (small testicles, gynecomastia), prostate abnormality (with DRE), and penile anatomic abnormalities (Peyronie disease).

Diagnostic Testing

- **Routine laboratory evaluation** should include serum glucose, renal function, complete blood count, and lipid analysis.
- A **PSA** should be considered if testosterone therapy needs to be initiated.
- Thyroid-stimulating hormone and liver function tests should be performed if the initial history or physical examination is suggestive of thyroid or liver disease.
- **Routine testosterone assessment in patients with ED is controversial.**
  - ○ Hypogonadism is the cause of ED in 5% to 10% of patients, but only approximately one-third of these patients improve with testosterone replacement.[39]
  - ○ Testing with morning total and free serum testosterone is initially recommended only for patients with low libido or evidence of hypogonadism.
  - ○ Testing should otherwise be deferred until patients have failed oral pharmacologic therapy.
  - ○ Abnormal initial testosterone levels should be repeated for confirmation along with serum luteinizing hormone (LH), follicle-stimulating hormone (FSH), and prolactin to determine the source of hypogonadism.
- **Urologic testing** with nocturnal penile tumescence or vascular studies is unnecessary in the primary care setting.

TREATMENT

- In 80% to 90% of men, erectile function should be restored with some form of therapy.
- Attempts should be made to **improve uncontrolled risk factors,** such as diabetes and hypertension, and to decrease the use of tobacco, alcohol, and other illicit substances.
- If possible, **potentially contributing medications** should be stopped or have their doses decreased.
- **Reassurance** may be curative in young men with psychogenic ED. Referral to a psychologist for **marital or couples counseling** may be helpful as an adjunctive form of therapy for psychogenic ED that has failed to respond to oral pharmacologic therapy.

Medications

Phosphodiesterase Inhibitors
- Phosphodiesterase inhibitors include **sildenafil, tadalafil, and vardenafil** (Table 4-5).
- These agents are the treatment of choice for ED and work by selectively inhibiting PDE5, which is found in high concentrations within the corpus cavernosum.

TABLE 4-5	**Phosphodiesterase Inhibitors for Erectile Dysfunction**			

Drug	Onset (duration) of action	Dose range	Food interaction	Comments
Vardenafil	1 hour (4 hours)	5 mg, 10 mg, 20 mg Dose adjustment not required for renal impairment. Not studied in dialysis patients	May take with or without food	Prolongs QT interval. Should not be prescribed to patients with congenital long QT syndrome or those taking antiarrhythmics (amiodarone, sotalol, procainamide, or quinidine)
Sildenafil	1 hour (4 hours)	25 mg, 50 mg, 100 mg Start with 25 mg if CrCl <30 mL/ minute or liver dysfunction	High fat Grapefruit juice may increase drug levels and toxicity.	
Tadalafil	1 hour (36 hours)	2.5 mg, 10 mg, 20 mg 2.5 mg used in once-daily dosing Dosing adjustment required when creatinine clearance is ≤50 mL/min or hepatic dysfunction	Grapefruit juice may increase drug levels and toxicity.	

- They require sexual stimulation to precipitate an erection and are **effective in all forms of organic and psychogenic ED,** but response rates are lower in patients with complete ED and diabetes and after radical prostatectomy.[40]
- They do not increase libido.
- **The three agents available are thought to have similar efficacy** (no head-to-head trials yet done).
- Side effects include headaches, flushing, dyspepsia, visual disturbance, rhinitis, priapism, and dizziness.
- Patients with symptoms of cardiac disease should be referred for cardiac evaluation before initiation of these agents.
- The PDE5 inhibitors **potentiate the effect of nitrates** causing severe and refractory hypotension, so the combination of these agents with nitrates in any form (oral, transdermal, IV) is **absolutely contraindicated.**[41]
- The combination **with α_1-adrenergic blockers can also cause orthostatic hypotension** and even severe hypotension. Alcohol potentiates the hypotensive effects of these agents.
- They are metabolized in the liver by cytochrome P450 CYP3A4, and thus, caution must be exercised when prescribing with inhibitors such as ketoconazole, itraconazole, protease inhibitors, and cimetidine.

Testosterone Replacement
- **Testosterone replacement is only indicated for men with documented hypogonadism**.
- Currently, there are no oral preparations of testosterone sold in the United States.
- Since prostate cancer is hormone sensitive, before initiating testosterone, it is necessary to ensure that the patient does not have prostate cancer. After starting testosterone replacement, PSA, prostate examination, testosterone levels, liver function tests, and cholesterol should be monitored.[42]
- **Intramuscular injections of testosterone enanthate** or **testosterone cypionate** are initiated at dosages of 150 to 200 mg IM every 2 to 3 weeks.
- **Testosterone patches** provide physiologic doses of hormone replacement. **Androderm, 2.5 to 7.5 mg,** is applied daily to clean, dry, non–hair-bearing areas.
- Several **testosterone gels are available (AndroGel, Testim, Foresta, Axiron).** They are applied to clean, dry skin via metered-dose device in a dosage range of 5 to 10 g/day.
- **One buccal form of testosterone is available (Striant).** It is dosed as 30 mg every 12 hours and applied to the gum area above the upper incisors.
- A subcutaneous testosterone pellet (Testopel), which is implanted under the skin, is administered every 3 to 6 months.
- Patients on testosterone replacement need to be monitored upon initiation, around dose changes (q2 to 3 months), and every 6 to 12 months while on a stable regimen.
- Adverse effects of testosterone include erythrocytosis, worsening of sleep apnea, and enlargement of the prostate.

Other Nonpharmacologic Therapies
- More invasive nonsurgical treatment options include **intracorporeal and intraurethral injections of alprostadil and external vacuum constriction devices.**
- Intracorporeal injections and vacuum devices are very effective but suffer from high dropout rates.
- These forms of therapy should be deferred to a urologist unless the primary care physician has undergone appropriate training in the administration of these modalities, which require significant office-based patient education and training.

REFERRAL

- Indications for referral to urology include a history of pelvic trauma, abnormal genital examination, contraindications to or intolerable side effects from oral pharmacologic therapy, and failure of oral therapy in patients who wish to try a more invasive modality.
- Priapism is an indication for an emergent urology consult.

Testicular Masses

GENERAL PRINCIPLES

- Patients with testicular masses may present with a painless lump or scrotal discomfort, ranging from a dull ache that worsens with exercise to severe testicular pain.
- **Benign causes** include fluid collections, infection (e.g., acute orchitis, focal or subacute orchitis, or postinflammatory scarring), infarction (idiopathic or secondary to torsion), and cysts.
  - A **hydrocele** is a collection of peritoneal fluid between the parietal and visceral layers of the tunica vaginalis, a potential space surrounding the testicle. A communicating hydrocele allows peritoneal fluid to pass between the peritoneal cavity and the layers of the tunica vaginalis. A noncommunicating hydrocele represents an imbalance in the secretory and absorptive capacities of the layers of the tunica vaginalis. This is most often due to injury or infection with resultant inflammatory reaction. A hydrocele may also accompany a testicular neoplasm or torsion. Hydroceles transilluminate, but hernias or other mass lesions do not. Ultrasound can be helpful, when the cause of the hydrocele is unclear. Simple aspiration of hydrocele usually leads to reaccumulation.
  - A **varicocele** is an abnormal tortuosity and dilation of the pampiniform venous plexus and internal spermatic vein. Varicoceles are found in 20% of men, more frequently on the left (because of the drainage of left gonadal vein). Patients are usually asymptomatic, but may report achy, dull pain exacerbated by standing. Varicoceles constitute the most common surgically correctable cause of male factor infertility (15% to 30% of infertile men), although the benefit of surgery is controversial.
  - A **spermatocele** is a painless cystic mass (2 to 5 cm) separate from the testis (<2 cm; this is called an epididymal cyst). These are located at the superior pole of the testes and can be diagnosed by physical examination, but ultrasound may be used to confirm the diagnosis if there is uncertainty.
- **Malignant causes** include primary testicular cancer and extratesticular malignancies such as leukemia or lymphoma.
  - **Testicular cancer** accounts for only 1% of all cancers in men but is the most common cancer in men 15 to 34 years of age.
  - A significantly increased number of testicular cancers are found in patients with cryptorchidism, with neoplasms developing in the undescended and the contralateral descended testis.[43-45] Other risk factors include family history (6- to 10-fold for first-degree relative), tobacco use (doubles risk), white race, and infertility.
  - **Lymphomas and leukemia are the most common extratesticular malignancies to involve the testicles.** Lymphoma accounts for 1% to 7% of all testicular tumors and is a frequent cause of testicular enlargement in men >50 years of age. Involvement is bilateral in 50% of cases either simultaneously or successively. Leukemic infiltration (50% have bilateral involvement) is usually seen in children, and the testis is the most common site of relapse of acute leukemia.

DIAGNOSIS

Clinical Presentation

History

- Men with **hydrocele** present with a painless scrotal swelling that can be transilluminated. The swelling may be small and soft on awakening but worsens during the day, becoming large and tense.
- Most **varicoceles** occur on the left side as the left testicular vein drains into the left renal vein, whereas the right testicular vein drains directly into the large inferior vena cava. Patients generally report a mass that lies posterior to and above the testis. The sudden onset of a left-sided varicocele in an elderly man may be indicative of a renal cell carcinoma and should be evaluated with a renal ultrasound. Sudden development of a right-sided varicocele may occur with inferior vena cava obstruction. The venous dilation is commonly decreased when the patient is supine and increases when he is upright.
- A painless testicular mass is suggestive of a **primary testicular tumor** but occurs only in a minority of patients. Most present with diffuse testicular pain, swelling, hardness, or some combination of these findings.[46]

Physical Examination

- The testes should be palpated for masses, volume, tenderness, and cryptorchidism.
- A testicle that is <4 cm long is considered small.
- All masses and swellings should be **transilluminated**. Solid tumors do not transmit light, whereas a **hydrocele** glows a soft red color.
- If a testicle cannot be palpated within the scrotum, the inguinal canals and lower abdomen should be examined.
- **The epididymis, spermatic cord, and vas deferens** are examined next.
  - The epididymis is located posterior to the testicle.
  - Have the patient perform the Valsalva maneuver while standing.
  - Palpate for a mass of dilated testicular veins in the spermatic cord, forming a varicocele above and behind the testis.
- The **inguinal canals** should be explored for hernias or cord tenderness. Inflammation of the cord structures can cause inguinal or scrotal pain, with a normal testis.
- Classically, a **varicocele** feels like a "bag of worms" above the testicle. Examine the patient in both upright and supine positions. Have him perform the Valsalva maneuver when standing, which accentuates the dilation.
- **Spermatoceles** are typically located superior and posterior to the testis, freely movable, and **transilluminate** easily. Aspiration of the contents usually reveals dead sperm.
- Evaluate men for the presence of **gynecomastia,** as 30% of Leydig cell tumors produce testosterone, which is converted to estrogen.
- Rarely, testicular tumors present with disseminated disease, such as supraclavicular lymphadenopathy or abdominal masses from retroperitoneal lymph node spread or as a result of a tumor that arises within an undescended intra-abdominal testis.

Diagnostic Testing

Laboratories

- **α-Fetoprotein** is produced by nonseminomatous germ cell tumors (embryonal carcinomas and yolk sac tumors). An elevated α-fetoprotein may be seen at any stage, although 40% to 60% of patients with metastases have increased serum concentrations.
- **β-Human chorionic gonadotropin** is increased in seminomatous and nonseminomatous tumors. Elevations occur in 40% to 60% of patients with metastatic nonseminomatous germ cell tumors and 15% to 20% of patients with metastatic seminomas.
- **Lactate dehydrogenase** elevation is nonspecific but has prognostic value in patients with advanced germ cell tumors. It is increased in 60% of patients with nonseminomatous germ cell tumors and 80% of those with seminomatous germ cell tumors.

Imaging

- Testicular **ultrasound** is a highly reliable way of differentiating intratesticular from extra-testicular lesions and should be the initial imaging study of choice.
- Gray-scale sonography of lymphomatous and leukemic testicular involvement reveals diffuse or multifocal decreased echogenicity, which can be more subtle and ill defined than the typical well-circumscribed hypoechoic mass of primary testicular cancer.
- Germ cell tumors are typically intratesticular and may produce one or more hypoechoic masses or show diffuse abnormalities with microcalcifications.
- **CT scans and MRI** of malignancy demonstrate a mass that is relatively isointense to the surrounding normal testicular parenchyma on T1-weighted images and exhibits brisk and early enhancement after IV gadolinium.

TREATMENT

Benign Masses

Hydrocele

- Management of hydrocele may require aspiration of the fluid (by a urologist) to be able to palpate the testis carefully.
- A scrotal ultrasound should always be considered if the diagnosis is in question, as a reactive hydrocele may occur with a testicular neoplasm.
- Generally, no therapy is needed except in the setting of discomfort from either a bulky mass or a tense hydrocele, which decreases circulation to the testis.
- Tense or uncomfortable hydroceles should always be aspirated.

Varicocele

- Not all varicoceles are associated with infertility and not all need to be corrected.
- If the patient has an abnormal semen analysis and is infertile or if the patient is symptomatic with a dull ache or feeling of heaviness in the testicle, the varicocele should be treated.
- Therapy consists of surgical ligation or sclerotherapy of the pampiniform plexus.

Malignant Masses

- Management of suspicious masses should be with urologic consultation.
- For lesions that are likely malignant, a radical orchiectomy with ligation of the spermatic cord at the internal ring is required.
- The primary lymphatic and vascular drainage of the testis is to the retroperitoneal lymph nodes and the renal or great vessels, respectively. Therefore, direct testicular biopsy through the scrotum is contraindicated.
- The staging workup includes CT scans of the abdomen and pelvis and a chest x-ray.

Priapism

- Priapism is a prolonged (>4 hours), usually painful, erection that is not initiated by sexual stimuli. It results from a disturbance in the normal regulatory mechanisms that initiate and maintain penile flaccidity.
- **Low-flow, or ischemic, priapism** is due to decreased penile venous outflow. The etiologies include hematologic dyscrasias (sickle cell disease, thalassemia, G6PD deficiency), tumor infiltrates, vasoactive erectile agents (papaverine, phentolamine), infectious (toxin mediated) such as scorpion sting and spider bites, hormones (testosterone), recreational drugs (alcohol, cocaine, marijuana), neurogenic (cauda equina compression, autonomic neuropathy, spinal cord injury), or idiopathic.
- **Low-dose, or arterial, priapism** produces painless, persistent semirigid to rigid erections that may still increase in tumescence in response to sexual stimuli. It results from

increased arterial inflow into the cavernous sinusoids, which overwhelms venous outflow. The etiology is usually groin or straddle trauma that causes injury to the internal pudendal artery or its branches. This establishes a direct arterial-to-cavernous shunt that bypasses the normally regulatory helicine arteries. A growing cause is vasoactive erectile agents/drugs.

- Patients with priapism should be **emergently managed in consultation with a urologist**. Evaluation may include blood gas assessment of cavernosal aspirate.
- Therapeutic options range from aspiration to embolization and surgical intervention.[47,48]

Androgenetic Alopecia

GENERAL PRINCIPLES

- Androgenetic alopecia is a hereditary thinning of the hair that is induced by androgens in genetically susceptible men. DHT, produced by action of the enzyme 5α-reductase on testosterone, is the most important androgen responsible for induction and promotion of alopecia. It is also known as **male pattern hair loss** or **common baldness.**
- Thinning of the hair usually begins between 12 and 40 years of age, and approximately 50% of men express this trait to some degree before the age of 50 years.
- The pattern of inheritance is polygenic.
- The onset is gradual, and the condition slowly develops over years.
- It is important to rule out other causes of alopecia, such as has hypo- or hyperthyroidism, iron deficiency, acute illness, and effects of drugs such as anticonvulsants.

TREATMENT

Medications

Topical Minoxidil
- Topical minoxidil, a potassium channel agonist and vasodilator, is able to increase survival time and delay senescence of cultured keratinocytes in vitro.
- After topical application, minoxidil increases the duration of the anagen phase, leading to production of hairs that are progressively thicker and longer. Cessation of the drug leads to loss of hair growth resulting from the treatment.
- Minoxidil lotion 2% or 5%, 1 mL should be applied twice per day to the affected scalp. Twice-daily application has no significant systemic side effects.
- The percentage of patients who show cosmetically acceptable hair regrowth after 1 year ranges from 40 to 60, depending on patient selection.
- Adverse effects include allergic contact dermatitis and reversible hypertrichosis.

Finasteride
- Low-dose oral finasteride, 1 mg/day, is FDA approved for androgenic alopecia.
- It is an oral 5α-reductase isoenzyme 2 inhibitor, which decreases DHT levels in scalp and blood by 60%.
- It may take 6 to 12 months to see the full effect of the drug, and it must be continued to maintain the new hair growth.
- Patients taking finasteride for androgenic alopecia have about 50% reduction in PSA. The FDA has issued warnings regarding the risk of high-grade prostate cancer among men who develop prostate cancer while taking finasteride.
- There is minimal effect on libido at the dose for alopecia when compared with effects seen at the higher BPH dose.[49–53]

Other Nonpharmacologic Therapies

Surgical options including hair transplantation, scalp flaps, and excision of bald scalp with or without tissue expansion are options to treat advanced androgenetic alopecia.

REFERENCES

1. Siegel R, Naishadham D, Jemal A. Cancer statistics, 2013. *CA Cancer J Clin* 2013;63:11–30.
2. Klotz L, Zhang L, Lam A, et al. Clinical results of long term follow-up of large, active surveillance cohort with localized prostate cancer. *J Clin Oncol* 2010;28:126–131.
3. Stattin P, Holmberg E, Bratt O, et al. Surveillance and deferred treatment for localized prostate cancer. Population based study in the National Prostate Cancer Register of Sweden. *J Urol* 2008;180:2423–2430.
4. Shappley WV III, Kenfield SA, Kasperzyk JL, et al. Prospective study of determinants and outcomes of deferred treatments or watchful waiting among men with prostate cancer in nationwide cohort. *J Clin Oncol* 2009;27:4980–4985.
5. Thompson I, Thrasher JB, Aus G, et al. Guideline for the management of clinically localized prostate cancer: 2007 update. *J Urol* 2007;177:2106–2131.
6. Schröder FH, Hugosson J, Roobol MJ, et al. Screening and prostate-cancer mortality in a randomized European study. *N Engl J Med* 2009;360:1320–1328.
7. Andriole GL, Crawford ED, Grubb RL III, et al. Mortality results from a randomized prostate-cancer screening trial. *N Engl J Med* 2009;360:1310–1319.
8. Andriole GL, Crawford ED, Grubb RL, et al. Prostate cancer screening in randomized Prostate, Lung, Colorectal, and Ovarian Cancer Screening Trial: mortality after 13 years follow-up. *J Natl Cancer Inst* 2012;104:125–132.
9. Thompson IM, Ankerst DP. Prostate-specific antigen in the early detection of prostate cancer. *CMAJ* 2007;176:1853–1858.
10. Smith DS, Catalona WJ, et al. Interexaminer variability of digital rectal examination in detecting prostate cancer. *Urology* 1995;45:70–74.
11. Wilbur J. Prostate cancer screening: the continuing controversy. *Am Fam Physician* 2008;78:1338.
12. Crawford ED, Schutz MJ, Clejan S, et al. The effect of digital rectal examination on prostate-specific antigen levels. *JAMA* 1992;267:2227–2228.
13. Roehrborn CG, Marks LS, Fenter T, et al. Efficacy and safety of dutasteride in the four-year treatment of men with benign prostatic hyperplasia. *Urology* 2004;63:709–715.
14. Gann PH, Hennekens CH, Stampfer MJ. A prospective evaluation of plasma prostate-specific antigen for detection of prostatic cancer. *JAMA* 1995;273:289–294.
15. D'Amico AV, Chen MH, Roehl KA, et al. Preoperative PSA velocity and the risk of death from prostate cancer after radical prostatectomy. *N Engl J Med* 2004;351:125–135.
16. Lee R, Localio AR, Armstrong K, et al. A meta-analysis of the performance characteristics of the free prostate-specific antigen test. *Urology* 2006;67:762–768.
17. Guess HA, Arrighi HM, Metter EJ, et al. Cumulative prevalence of prostatism matches the autopsy prevalence of benign prostatic hyperplasia. *Prostate* 1990;17:241–246.
18. Barry MJ, Fowler FJ Jr, O'Leary MP, et al. The American Urological Association Symptom Index for benign prostatic hyperplasia. The Measurement Committee of the American Urological Association. *J Urol* 1992;148:1549–1557.
19. Roehrborn CG, Boyle P, Gould AL, et al. Serum prostate-specific antigen as a predictor of prostate volume in men with benign prostatic hyperplasia. *Urology* 1999;53:581–589.
20. Flanigan RC, Reda DJ, Wasson JH, et al. 5-year outcome of surgical resection and watchful waiting for men with moderately symptomatic benign prostatic hyperplasia: a Department of Veterans Affairs cooperative study. *J Urol* 1998;160:12–16.
21. AUA Practice Guidelines Committee. AUA guideline on management of benign prostatic hyperplasia (2003). Chapter 1: diagnosis and treatment recommendations. *J Urol* 2003;170(2 Pt 1):530–547.
22. Lepor H, Kaplan SA, Klimberg I, et al. Doxazosin for benign prostatic hyperplasia: long-term efficacy and safety in hypertensive and normotensive patients. The Multicenter Study Group. *J Urol* 1997;157:525–530.

23. Thorpe A, Neal D. Benign prostatic hyperplasia. *Lancet* 2003;361:1359–1367.
24. McConnell JD, Bruskewitz R, Walsh P, et al. The effect of finasteride on the risk of acute urinary retention and the need for surgical treatment among men with benign prostatic hyperplasia. Finasteride Long-Term Efficacy and Safety Study Group. *N Engl J Med* 1998;338:557–563.
25. Roehrborn CG, Boyle P, Nickel JC, et al. Efficacy and safety of a dual inhibitor of 5-alpha-reductase types 1 and 2 (dutasteride) in men with benign prostatic hyperplasia. *Urology* 2002;60:434–441.
26. Lepor H, Williford WO, Barry MJ, et al. The impact of medical therapy on bother due to symptoms, quality of life and global outcome, and factors predicting response. Veterans Affairs Cooperative Studies Benign Prostatic Hyperplasia Study Group. *J Urol* 1998;160:1358–1367.
27. Andriole GL, Guess HA, Epstein JI, et al. Treatment with finasteride preserves usefulness of prostate-specific antigen in the detection of prostate cancer: results of a randomized, double-blind, placebo-controlled clinical trial. PLESS Study Group. Proscar Long-term Efficacy and Safety Study. *Urology* 1998;52:195–201.
28. Thomson IM, Goodman PJ, Tangen CM, et al. The influence of finasteride on development of prostate cancer. *N Engl J Med* 2003;349:215–224.
29. Andriole GL, Bostwick DG, Brawey OW, et al. Effect of dutasteride on the risk of prostate cancer. *N Engl J Med* 2010;362:1192–1202.
30. Lepor H, Williford WO, Barry MJ, et al. The efficacy of terazosin, finasteride, or both in benign prostatic hyperplasia. Veterans Affairs Cooperative Studies Benign Prostatic Hyperplasia Study Group. *N Engl J Med* 1996;335:533–539.
31. McConnell JD, Roehrborn CG, Bautista OM, et al. The long-term effect of doxazosin, finasteride, and combination therapy on the clinical progression of benign prostatic hyperplasia. *N Engl J Med* 2003;349:2387–2398.
32. Wilt TJ, Ishani A, Stark G, et al. Saw palmetto extracts for treatment of benign prostatic hyperplasia: a systematic review. *JAMA* 1998;280:1604–1609.
33. Benway BM, Moon TD. Bacterial prostatitis. *Urol Clin North Am* 2008;35:23–32.
34. McNaughton Collins M, MacDonald R, Wilt TJ. Diagnosis and treatment of chronic abacterial prostatitis: a systematic review. *Ann Intern Med* 2000;133:367–381.
35. Pontari MA. Chronic prostatitis/chronic pelvic pain syndrome. *Urol Clin North Am* 2008;35:81–89.
36. NIH Consensus Conference. Impotence. NIH Consensus Development Panel on Impotence. *JAMA* 1993;270:83–90.
37. Feldman HA, Goldstein I, Hatzichristou DG, et al. Impotence and its medical and psychosocial correlates: results of the Massachusetts Male Aging Study. *J Urol* 1994;151:54–61.
38. Nehra A, Jackson G, et al. The Princeton III Consensus recommendations for management of erectile dysfunction and cardiovascular disease. *Mayo Clin Proc* 2012;87:766–778.
39. Buvat J, Lemaire A. Endocrine screening in 1,022 men with erectile dysfunction: clinical significance and cost-effective strategy. *J Urol* 1997;158:1764–1767.
40. Cohan P, Korenman SG. Erectile dysfunction. *J Clin Endocrinol Metab* 2001;86:2391–2394.
41. Webb DJ, Freestone S, Allen MJ, et al. Sildenafil citrate and blood-pressure-lowering drugs: results of drug interaction studies with an organic nitrate and a calcium antagonist. *Am J Cardiol* 1999;83:21C–28C.
42. Petak SM, Nankin HR, Spark RF, et al. American association of clinical endocrinologists medical guidelines for clinical practice for the evaluation and treatment of hypogonadism in adult male patinets-2002 update. *Endocr Pract* 2002;8:440–456.
43. Bosl GJ, Motzer RJ. Testicular germ-cell cancer. *N Engl J Med* 1997;337:242–253.

44. Shaw J. Diagnosis and treatment of testicular cancer. *Am Fam Physician* 2008;77:469–474.
45. Tiemstra JD, Kapoor S. Evaluation of scrotal masses. *Am Fam Physician* 2008;78:1165–1170.
46. Wampler SM. Common Scrotal and Testicular Problems. *Prim Care* 2010; 37:613–626.
47. Burnett AL, Bivalacqua TJ. Priapism: current principles and practice. *Urol Clin North Am* 2007;34:631–642, viii.
48. Burnett AL, Bivalacqua TJ. Priapism: new concepts in medical and surgical management. *Urol Clin North Am* 2011;38:185–194.
49. Sinclair R. Male pattern androgenetic alopecia. *BMJ* 1998;317:865–869.
50. Price VH. Treatment of hair loss. *N Engl J Med* 1999;341:964–973.
51. Kaufman KD, Olsen EA, Whiting D, et al. Finasteride in the treatment of men with androgenetic alopecia. Finasteride Male Pattern Hair Loss Study Group. *J Am Acad Dermatol* 1998;39:578–589.
52. D'Amico AV, Roehrborn CG. Effect of 1 mg/day finasteride on concentrations of serum prostate-specific antigen in men with androgenic alopecia: a randomized controlled trial. *Lancet Oncol* 2007;8:21–25.
53. Otberg N, Finner AM, Shapiro J. Androgenetic alopecia. *Endocrinol Metab Clin North Am* 2007;36:379–398.

5 Screening and Adult Immunizations

Megan E. Wren

Screening for Disease

GENERAL PRINCIPLES

- The benefit of screening depends on the prevalence of the disease, the sensitivity and specificity of the screening test, the acceptability of the test to the patient, and, most importantly, the ability to change the natural course of disease with treatment.
- For many diseases, there is a lack of definitive evidence regarding the effect of screening on morbidity and mortality.
- Studies of the benefits of screening are susceptible to several forms of bias:
  - **Lead-time bias** refers to the overestimation of survival duration among screen-detected cases when survival is measured from the time of diagnosis.
  - **Length bias** refers to the fact that slow-growing cancers have a long period of time in which they are asymptomatic but potentially detectable by screening tests (preclinical period). Aggressive tumors have a shorter preclinical period, so they are less likely to be detected in a screening program. Therefore, screening programs tend to detect less aggressive disease.
  - **Overdiagnosis** is an extreme form of length bias in which the diagnosed cancer is so slowly progressive that it never would have become clinically evident (and therefore would not have required treatment).
  - **Volunteer bias** refers to the fact that people who sign up for screening studies are not necessarily representative of the general population. Some may have subtle symptoms or risk factors for the disease. Most study participants tend to be more concerned about their health, have healthier habits, and are more compliant with therapy, leading to improved outcomes.
- Statistics on screening efficacy are frequently misunderstood by both physicians and the public.[1,2] Because of the biases outlined above, "x-year survival" is a misleading measure of the benefit of screening. Mortality rates are a more appropriate measure of the effect of screening and treatment.
- Many areas of controversy exist, including ages to start and stop screening, which tests to use, or whether to screen at all.
- Various professional organizations have made recommendations regarding screening for disease; **these guidelines apply only to asymptomatic patients at average risk, and they must be individualized.** Some of the most widely cited organizations include the following:
  - The American Cancer Society (ACS, www.cancer.org, last accessed December 23, 2014).
  - The U.S. Preventive Services Task Force (USPSTF, www.ahrq.gov/clinic/uspstfix.htm, last accessed December 23, 2014).
  - The American College of Physicians (ACP, www.acponline.org/clinical/guidelines/?hp, last accessed December 23, 2014).
  - The National Cancer Institute (NCI, www.nci.nih.gov, last accessed December 23, 2014).
  - The American Congress of Obstetrics and Gynecology (ACOG, www.acog.org, last accessed December 23, 2014).
- Table 5-1 presents a simplified screening schedule.

TABLE 5-1	Simplified Screening Schedule for Asymptomatic Average-Risk Persons		
	Source		
Breast CA		**Ages 20–39:**	**Ages 40–49:**	**Ages ≥ 50:**
	ACS	CBE q3 yrs	CBE q1 yr + Mamms q1 yr	CBE q1 yr + Mamms q1 yr
	ACOG	CBE q3 yrs	CBE q1 yr + Mamms q1 yr	CBE q1 yr + Mamms q1 yr
	USPSTF	—	Indiv. decision	50–74: Mamms q2 yrs
		BSE is an option	BSE is an option	BSE is an option
Colorectal CA	Joint guideline	Age >50: Acceptable: gFOBT q1 yr, or FIT q1 yr, or stool DNA (interval unknown)		
		Preferred: FSIG q5 yrs or colonoscopy q10 yrs or ACBE q5 yrs or CT colonography q5 yrs		
	USPSTF	Age 50–75: FOBT, sigmoidoscopy, or colonoscopy (intervals unspecified)		
Prostate CA	ACS	Informed decision making age 50 (at 40–45 in higher-risk men)		
		If screening: PSA q1-2 yrs; stop if <10-year life expectancy		
	ACP	Informed decision making 50–69; only test if clear preference for screening		
	AUA	Shared decision making age 55–69 (high risk start age 40); if screen: PSA q2 yrs		
	USPSTF	Do not screen		
Lung CA	Various	Shared decision making: consider LDCT if age 55–74, at least 30-pack-years of smoking (current or quit <15 years)		
Cervical CA		**AFTER age 21:**		**Age ≥ 30:**	**Stop:**
	ACS	Pap q3 yrs		Pap + HPV-DNA q5 yrs	Age ≥ 65 IF adequate prior
	ACOG	(No HPV test)		(or Pap alone q3 yrs)	screening
	USPSTF	S/P total hysterectomy for benign disease: no cervical cancer screening			
		Continue screening if hx no/irregular screening, hx abnl Paps or CA, high-risk behavior, or immunocompromised (HIV, CA, meds), or hx prenatal DES exposure			

Testicular CA		Routine screening not recommended
Ovarian CA		Routine screening not recommended
Lipids	NCEP	Age ≥ 20: FLP q5 yrs (more frequent if risk factors)
	USPSTF	Screen men age ≥ 35, women age ≥ 45 (younger if risk factors)
HTN	JNC7	Q2 yrs (q1 yr if pre-HTN)
DM	ADA	Fasting plasma glucose or A1c q3 yrs in all adults age ≥ 45 Screen younger if BMI >25 + risk factors: preDM, HTN, low HDL, high TG, CVD, PCOS, gestational DM or baby >9lbs, FHx DM, physical inactivity, severe obesity, acanthosis nigricans, or use of glucocorticoids or antipsychotics
AAA	USPSTF	One-time screening for AAA by ultrasonography in men aged 65–75 who have ever smoked (not women)
Osteoporosis	NOF	Screen women age ≥ 65 and men age ≥ 70
	USPSTF	Screen postmenopausal women and men 50–70 yrs if risk factors Screen women aged ≥ 65 (age ≥ 60 if risk factors)
Hepatitis C	CDC and USPSTF	Screen everyone born in 1945–1965
HIV	CDC	Screen everyone age 13–64 (after notification) unless patient declines High-risk individuals should be screened at least annually Include in routine panel of prenatal screening tests for all pregnant women
	USPSTF	Screen all pregnant women, everyone age 15–65, anyone at increased risk
Other STDs	USPSTF	Screen pregnant women for hepatitis B, HIV, and syphilis Routinely screen women ≤24 for chlamydia and gonorrhea (pregnant or not)

CANCER SCREENING

Research evidence has often been inadequate to reach definitive conclusions regarding how, when, whom, and whether to screen for various cancers. The guidelines below are a synthesis of the recommendations of the major organizations.

Breast Cancer Screening

- Breast cancer is common in the United States.
  - ○ Breast cancer is the most commonly diagnosed invasive cancer in US women: Approximately one in eight (12.5%) will develop breast cancer by age 90.[3]
    - Conversely, 88% will not develop breast cancer.
    - Many women greatly overestimate their risk of breast cancer. In one study, 89% of women overestimated their risk with an average estimate of 46% lifetime risk (more than triple the actual risk).[4]
  - ○ Breast cancer mortality in US women is second only to lung cancer; approximately 1 in 36 (2.8%) will die of breast cancer.[3]
  - ○ African American women have a lower incidence of breast cancer than white women, but a higher mortality rate.[5]
- Breast cancer mortality has declined approximately 30% over the past two decades, but there is controversy about the relative roles of screening versus improved treatments.
- **Risk factors for breast cancer:**
  - ○ Sex—breast cancer is 100 times more common in women than men.
  - ○ Age—about 75% of breast cancers occur after age 50.
  - ○ Family history—the risk is approximately doubled with one affected first-degree relative. The risk rises if there are multiple affected family members, especially if they had early-onset breast and/or ovarian cancer (suggestive of BRCA mutations).
  - ○ Estrogen—exogenous estrogen, early menarche, late menopause, nulliparity, or late first childbirth.
  - ○ Dense breast tissue.
  - ○ History of atypical hyperplasia on biopsy.
  - ○ History of radiation therapy to the chest in childhood/adolescence.
  - ○ Obesity.
  - ○ Drinking >2 alcoholic drinks/day.
  - ○ Protective factors include parity, breast-feeding, and exercise.
  - ○ The Gail model to estimate risk is available at www.cancer.gov/bcrisktool (last accessed December 23, 2014); it is less accurate in women with a strong family history.
- The benefits of screening are best proven for mammography in women ages 50 to 69.
  - ○ Women aged 40 to 49 have a lower incidence of breast cancer and denser breasts (thus lower sensitivity and specificity of screening), leading to lower predictive values. The USPSTF review stated that "for biennial screening mammography in women aged 40 to 49 years, there is moderate certainty that the net benefit is small." They emphasized the lower incidence in this group and the adverse consequences of screening.[6,7]
  - ○ Data are limited for women ages 70 and over, and older women have competing causes of mortality, limiting the benefit of cancer screening.
- Potential harms from screening include the following:
  - ○ False positives leading to additional imaging.
  - ○ False positives leading to unnecessary biopsies (a decade of annual screening is estimated to result in almost 20% of women referred for a biopsy).[8]
  - ○ Overdiagnosis and subsequent treatment.
  - ○ Mammography is often uncomfortable and may be anxiety provoking.
- It has been shown in randomized trials that teaching breast self-examination (BSE) does not save lives.[9] Many groups now endorse teaching "breast self-awareness" rather than formal BSE teaching.[10]

- Clinical breast exam (CBE) may modestly improve cancer detection rates if experienced clinicians use very careful technique.[11]
- Recommendations of some major groups are as follows.
  - The USPSTF issued updated recommendations in 2009[12]:
    - Women aged 50 to 74 years should have mammography every 2 years.
    - Screening mammography should not be done "routinely" for women ages 40 to 49 years. Women and their doctors should base the decision to start mammography before age 50 years on the risk for breast cancer and preferences about the benefits and harms.
    - Current evidence is insufficient to assess the benefits and harms of CBE or screening mammography in women 75 years or older.
    - The USPSTF recommends against teaching patients BSE.
  - The ACS recommends the following[13]:
    - Ages 20 to 39: CBE every 3 years.
    - Ages 40 and over: annual CBE and annual mammography.
    - Optional BSEs.
    - No specific upper age limit is specified. "The decision to stop screening should be individualized based on the potential benefits and risks of screening within the context of overall health status and estimated longevity."
    - Women at very high risk (>20% lifetime risk) should undergo magnetic resonance imaging (MRI) screening and mammography every year. Women at moderately increased risk (15% to 20% lifetime risk) should talk to their physicians about the benefits and limitations of MRI screening in addition to yearly mammography.
  - The ACOG recommends the following[10]:
    - Ages 20 to 39: CBE every 1 to 3 years.
    - Ages 40 and over: annual CBE and annual mammography.
    - Over age 75, the decision to screen should be individualized.
    - "Breast self-awareness should be encouraged and can include breast self-examination."
    - Women at very high risk (>20% lifetime risk) should have "enhanced screening" with annual mammography, CBE every 6 to 12 months, instruction in BSE, and possibly MRI.

Cervical Cancer Screening

- The effectiveness of cervical cancer screening has never been studied in a randomized trial but is supported by strong epidemiologic evidence: the cervical cancer death rate falls in proportion to the intensity of screening. Most cases of cervical cancer occur in unscreened or inadequately screened women.
- Cervical cytologic screening may be done with the conventional Pap smear or with liquid-based tests (method does not change screening frequency).
- For some age groups, cotesting with cytology plus testing for human papillomavirus (HPV) is an option.
- **HPV vaccination does not change the screening guidelines**.
- The ACS, USPSTF, and ACOG have similar recommendations, as summarized below.
- **Do not begin screening until age 21 years** regardless of sexual history.
  - Under age 21, cervical cancer is quite rare (1 to 2 per million) while HPV infection is common and dysplasia may occur but both usually spontaneously remit.
  - Early screening may lead to anxiety, expense, and morbidity (excisional procedures on the cervix).
- **Women aged 21 to 29 years** should be screened every 3 years with cytology only. HPV testing would detect many transient infections without carcinogenic potential.
- **Women aged 30 and older** may be screened by cytology plus HPV cotesting every 5 years (preferred) or with cytology alone every 3 years.
- Women who have had a **total hysterectomy** (including removal of the cervix) for benign disease may stop cervical cancer screening.

- **Screening may be stopped at age 65** in women who have had adequate screening (three consecutive negative Pap tests or two consecutive negative HPV/Pap cotests within past 10 years and most recent test within 5 years).
- Risk factors and special cases:
  - In **women with HIV infection,** the Centers for Disease Control and Prevention (CDC) recommends cervical cytology screening twice in the 1st year after diagnosis and annually thereafter while the ACOG recommends annual cytology starting at age 21.[14]
  - ACOG recommends that women with a **history of high-grade dysplasia or cancer** should continue routine age-based testing for 20 years, even past age 65.
  - More frequent screening may be required in women with a history of prenatal exposure to diethylstilbestrol (DES) and women who are immunocompromised (such as organ transplantation).

Colorectal Cancer Screening

- Colorectal cancer (CRC) has a lifetime incidence of about 5%, and about one-third of those will die from it, making CRC the third leading cancer killer of men and of women (second for men and women combined).
- Screening for CRC is associated with decreases in incidence as well as mortality, due to removal of premalignant adenomatous polyps, but only about two-thirds of Americans have been screened adequately.[15]
- CRC is more common in men (35% higher than in women), in African Americans (25% higher than in Whites), and with advancing age (90% diagnosed after age 50).[5]
- Other risk factors include:
  - Personal history of CRC or adenomatous polyps (especially if polyps are multiple, large [>1 cm], or villous/tubulovillous).
  - Family history of polyps or CRC. The risk is doubled for those with one first-degree relative with CRC and further increased for those with multiple affected relatives or relatives with early-onset CRC (age <50).
  - Genetic syndromes including familial adenomatous polyposis (FAP) and the Lynch syndrome/hereditary nonpolyposis colorectal cancer (HNPCC) syndrome.
  - Inflammatory bowel disease, especially ulcerative colitis with pancolitis.
  - History of abdominal radiation therapy in childhood.
  - There may be an increased risk of CRC associated with obesity, alcohol consumption, smoking, physical inactivity, and dietary factors (red meat, low fiber, few fruits and vegetables, low dairy).
- Data suggest a protective effect for the use of aspirin and other nonsteroidal anti-inflammatory drugs.
- Screening strategies fall into 2 main categories:
  - Stool-based tests that primarily detect cancer: guaiac-based fecal occult blood testing (gFOBT), fecal immunochemical test (FIT), or stool DNA testing
  - Tests that detect both cancer and adenomatous polyps, thus permitting polyp removal for cancer prevention: flexible sigmoidoscopy (FSIG), colonoscopy, barium enema, or CT colonography
- For any test other than colonoscopy, **any abnormalities must be followed up with a full colonoscopy, not just repeat testing.**
- A brief summary of screening tests and recommended intervals includes:
  - Annual gFOBT with a high sensitivity test such as Hemoccult SENSA (not Hemoccult II):
    - Home collection of three specimens (**in-office rectal exam is not an acceptable stool test for CRC screening**).
    - Modest test sensitivity and specificity but has been shown in randomized controlled trials (RCTs) to lower CRC mortality.

- ○ Annual FIT, which detects human globin from lower GI bleeding (globin from upper GI sources is digested) and is therefore more specific.
- ○ Stool DNA test, interval uncertain.
- ○ FSIG every 5 years:
  - ▪ Requires a limited bowel prep; no sedation required.
  - ▪ Colonic perforation is rare (<1 in 20,000).
  - ▪ Only examines the distal colon but has been shown to lower CRC mortality.
- ○ Air contrast barium enema (ACBE) every 5 years:
  - ▪ Requires a full bowel prep; no sedation is used and the test may be uncomfortable.
  - ▪ Sensitivity is much lower than colonoscopy.
- ○ Computed tomography colonography (CTC) or "virtual colonoscopy" every 5 years:
  - ▪ Requires a full bowel prep and air insufflation.
  - ▪ Sensitivity is probably comparable to colonoscopy.
  - ▪ Patients with large polyps must be referred for colonoscopic resection, but uncertainty exists about management of small (<6 mm) polyps.
- ○ Colonoscopy every 10 years:
  - ▪ Requires a full bowel prep and sedation.
  - ▪ Regarded as the gold standard, but may miss 5% to 12% of lesions >1 cm.
  - ▪ Lesions can be resected during the procedure.
  - ▪ Risk of colonic perforation is about 1 in 1,000 and also can cause bleeding and cardiovascular complications.
- Current guidelines were published in 2012 by the ACP,[16] in 2008 by the USPSTF,[17] and in 2008 by a joint guideline[18] published by ACS, the US Multi-Society Task Force on Colorectal Cancer, and the American College of Radiology.
- The USPSTF recommendations include the following:
  - ○ Screen adults ages 50 to 75 using annual high-sensitivity gFOBT, or sigmoidoscopy every 5 years combined with high-sensitivity gFOBT every 3 years, or colonoscopy every 10 years.
  - ○ Do not routinely screen those aged 76 to 85 years, but there may be considerations that support screening in an individual patient.
  - ○ Screening is not recommended >85 years of age.
- The ACP recommends that
  - ○ Clinicians perform individualized assessment of risk for CRC in all adults.
  - ○ Average-risk adults should start CRC screening at age 50, using annual gFOBT, annual FIT, FSIG every 5 years, or colonoscopy every 10 years.
  - ○ High-risk adults should start screening with colonoscopy at age 40 or 10 years younger than the age at which the youngest affected relative was diagnosed with CRC.
  - ○ Screening should stop at age 75 or if life expectancy is <10 years.
- The joint guideline recommends that
  - ○ Screening for CRC in average risk, asymptomatic adults should begin at age 50.
  - ○ CRC screening is not appropriate if the patient is not likely to benefit from screening due to life-limiting comorbidity.
  - ○ Colon cancer prevention should be the primary goal of screening.
  - ○ Acceptable screening tests include annual gFOBT with a high sensitivity test, or annual FIT, or stool DNA test, interval uncertain.
  - ○ Preferred tests detect adenomatous polyps and can prevent cancer: FSIG every 5 years, ACBE every 5 years, CTC every 5 years, or colonoscopy every 10 years.
- **High-risk persons** need earlier and/or more frequent screening. These include those with a personal history of CRC or adenomatous polyps, inflammatory bowel disease, endometrial cancer before age 50, a hereditary CRC syndrome, or a strong family history of CRC or polyps.
  - ○ For those with CRC or adenomatous polyps in a first-degree relative <60 years or in two first-degree relatives of any age, they should be screened with colonoscopy every 5 years.

Screening should begin at age 40, or 10 years before the youngest case in the immediate family, whichever is earlier.

○ For those with CRC or adenomatous polyps in a first-degree relative at 60 or older, or two second-degree relatives with CRC, screening should begin at age 40 with any recommended form of testing at the usual intervals.

Lung Cancer Screening

- Lung cancer is the number one cause of cancer-related death in men and in women. Approximately 90% of cases occur in current or former smokers; **smoking cessation is the single most important factor in reducing lung cancer mortality**.
- Multiple randomized trials have demonstrated **no mortality benefit to screening with plain chest radiography (CXR), with or without sputum cytology**.
- Observational trials in the late 1990s showed that low-dose (2 mSv), single breath-hold, helical CT (LDCT) scans could detect early-stage lung cancers much more effectively than CXRs.
- The National Lung Screening Trial (NLST) published in 2011 was the first randomized trial to show a statistically significant benefit to CT screening for lung cancer.[19]
  ○ The trial compared annual LDCT to CXR for 3 years in more than 50,000 people ages 55 to 74; participants had at least 30 pack-years of smoking, including current smokers and former smokers who had quit within 15 years.
  ○ At a median follow-up of 6.5 years, there was a **relative mortality reduction of 20% for lung cancer deaths** and 6.7% reduction in all-cause mortality in the LDCT group.
  ○ To prevent one lung cancer death, the number needed to screen with LDCT was 320.
  ○ A substantial number of participants had an abnormal screening test (24% in the LDCT group and 6.9% in the CXR group), >90% of which were false positives. Most only required additional imaging, but some subjects required invasive procedures, including surgery. Complications from the diagnostic workup occurred at a low rate, about 1.5% of the participants who had abnormal screening tests.
- Lung cancer screening recommendations are in evolution. The USPSTF guidelines are undergoing review.
- A number of expert organizations have issued at least preliminary guidelines, including the ACS,[20] the National Comprehensive Cancer Network,[21] American College of Chest Physicians,[22] and others. In general, they **support LDCT screening in individuals similar to those in the NLST**:
  ○ Ages 55 to 74.
  ○ At least 30-pack-years of smoking.
  ○ Current smoker or quit within the past 15 years.
  ○ Screening is not appropriate for patients with severe comorbidities that limit life expectancy or would preclude potentially curative treatment.
  ○ The decision to start screening should be preceded by a process of informed and shared decision making, with discussion of the potential benefits, limitations, and harms associated with screening.

Prostate Cancer Screening

- Prostate cancer is the second leading cause of cancer-related death in US men and is the most commonly diagnosed cancer in US men, with a lifetime risk of about 1 in 6.
- The incidence increases with age. There is a higher incidence and earlier age of onset in African American men. The risk is higher in those with affected first-degree relatives or inherited cancer syndromes such as BRCA or Lynch syndrome (HNPCC).
- Although 17% of men will be diagnosed with prostate cancer, only 2.4% will die of it.
- Screening for prostate cancer is a controversial topic. Randomized controlled trials have shown small or no survival benefit in screened groups. Many men die "with" rather than

"of" prostate cancer. Treatment has potential harms, including erectile dysfunction, urinary incontinence, and bowel problems.

- **The USPSTF** recommends against **prostate-specific antigen (PSA) testing**, concluding that screening produces more harms than benefits.[23]
- **The ACS stresses the need for informed decision making** with adequate provision of information about the uncertainties, risks, and potential benefits associated with prostate cancer screening.[24]
  - This information should be provided starting at age 50 (at 40 to 45 in higher-risk men).
  - Men with <10-year life expectancy should not be offered prostate cancer screening. At age 75, only about half of men have a life expectancy of 10 years or more.
  - Key discussion points include the following:
    - Screening may be associated with a reduction in the risk of dying from prostate cancer; however, evidence is conflicting and experts disagree about the value of screening.
    - Not all men whose prostate cancer is detected through screening require immediate treatment. It is not currently possible to predict which men are likely to benefit from treatment.
    - Treatment for prostate cancer can lead to urinary, bowel, sexual, and other health problems. These problems may be significant or minimal, permanent, or temporary.
    - The PSA and digital rectal exam (DRE) may produce false-positive or false-negative results.
    - Abnormal results require prostate biopsies that can be painful, may lead to complications like infection or bleeding, and can miss clinically significant cancer.
  - If screening is elected, the ACS recommends PSA with or without DRE.
    - Initial PSA <2.5 ng/mL: screen every 2 years.
    - Initial PSA ≥2.5 ng/mL: screen annually.
    - PSA >4.0 ng/mL: refer for biopsy (2.5 to 4.0 ng/mL, individualized assessment).
- The **ACP recommends that PSA testing should only be done in patients with a clear preference for screening.**[25]
  - Clinicians should inform men ages 50 to 69 about the limited potential benefits and substantial harms of screening for prostate cancer.
  - Screening should not be done in average-risk men aged <50 or >69 nor those with a life expectancy of <10 to 15 years.
- The American Urological Association (AUA) published its guideline online in 2013.[26] Recommendations include:
  - Men <40 years of age should not be screened.
  - Average-risk men <55 years of age should not be routinely screened. For men 40 to 55 years of age who are at higher risk (family history or African American), decisions should be individualized.
  - For men ages 55 to 69, they strongly recommend shared decision making, based on a man's values and preferences after weighing the benefits against the known potential harms associated with screening and treatment. One prostate cancer death is averted for every 1,000 men screened for a decade.
  - Men should not be routinely screened if they are >70 years of age or have a life expectancy <10 to 15 years. Some men aged >70 years who are in excellent health may benefit from prostate cancer screening.
  - If men choose PSA screening, an interval of 2 years or more may be preferred over annual screening as it is expected that screening intervals of 2 years preserve the majority of the benefits and reduce overdiagnosis and false positives. Intervals for rescreening can be individualized by a baseline PSA level.
  - There is **no evidence that DRE is beneficial as a primary screening test.**

Ovarian Cancer Screening

- Ovarian cancer is uncommon (2% lifetime risk) but often lethal because only 15% are diagnosed while still localized to the ovary.[27] Detection is hampered by the deep anatomic location of the ovary and because ovarian cancer is often multifocal and extraovarian, even at early stages.
- Risk factors for ovarian cancer include:
  - Family history, especially the inherited cancer syndromes (BRCA, Lynch syndrome). The BRCA1 gene mutation conveys a lifetime risk of about 40%, and the BRCA2 gene mutation conveys a lifetime risk of about 20%.
  - Other risk factors include a history of infertility, polycystic ovarian syndrome, endometriosis, postmenopausal hormone replacement therapy, and cigarette smoking.
  - Protective factors include past use of oral contraceptives, history of breast-feeding >12 months, previous pregnancy, tubal ligation, and hysterectomy.
- **Pelvic examination is not effective for screening due to poor sensitivity and specificity.**
- Ovarian cancer is occasionally found incidentally on a Pap smear (sensitivity <30%).
- **The tumor marker CA 125 has limited sensitivity and specificity.**
  - Only about half of early ovarian cancers have elevated levels of CA 125.
  - False positives are too common (about 1%) for an effective screening test. Levels vary with the menstrual cycle, age, ethnicity, and smoking, and CA 125 can be increased with endometriosis, uterine leiomyomata, cirrhosis, ascites from any cause, and a variety of cancers.
  - Assessment of changes in CA 125 levels over time may have better test characteristics.
- **Transvaginal ultrasound (TVU) has limited sensitivity and specificity** for ovarian cancer screening.
- A large randomized trial in the US showed that screening with CA 125 and TVU did not improve ovarian cancer mortality (relative risk 1.18, screened vs. usual care).[28] Positive predictive value was only about 1%. For every screen-detected ovarian cancer, approximately 20 women underwent surgery; 20% of those surgeries resulted in major complications.
- **No organization recommends screening average-risk women for ovarian cancer.**
  - The USPSTF specifically recommends against screening due to lack of benefit and potential harms (unnecessary surgeries).[29]
  - ACOG concluded that currently, there is no effective strategy for ovarian cancer screening.[30] Clinicians should have a high index of suspicion when women present with symptoms commonly associated with ovarian cancer: pelvic or abdominal pain, increase in abdominal size or bloating, and difficulty eating or feeling full. High-risk women may be offered the combination of pelvic examination, TVU, and CA 125 testing.

Testicular Cancer

- USPSTF recommends against screening for testicular cancer in adolescent or adult males.
  - The incidence is low (approximately 1% of cancers in men).
  - Testicular germ cell tumors are one of the most curable solid neoplasms (overall cure rate >90%).
  - No evidence has shown that routine screening would improve health outcomes.
- The AUA recommends monthly testicular self-exams.

Screening for Other Cancers

- Routine population screening is not recommended for the following cancers: endometrial, testicular, bladder, thyroid, oral cavity, or skin. Clinicians should be vigilant for early symptoms of possible cancer in those sites.

• The ACS recommends that "the cancer-related checkup should include examination for cancers of the thyroid, testicles, ovaries, lymph nodes, oral cavity, and skin, as well as health counseling about tobacco, sun exposure, diet and nutrition, risk factors, sexual practices, and environmental and occupational exposures."

SCREENING FOR OTHER CONDITIONS

Hypertension

• The Seventh Report of the Joint National Committee on Prevention, Detection, Evaluation, and Treatment of High Blood Pressure (JNC 7) recommends that all patients should have their blood pressure (BP) measured every 2 years.[31] See Table 5-2 for the classification of BP levels. JNC 8 does not specifically address screening or classification.
• Lifestyle modification includes counseling on weight loss, aerobic exercise, limiting alcohol intake, and reduction in sodium intake.
• Treatment of hypertension is discussed in detail in Chapter 6.

Dyslipidemia

• The recent American College of Cardiology/American Heart Association (ACC/AHA) guidelines for cardiovascular risk assessment recommend screening those aged 20 to 79 years without atherosclerotic cardiovascular disease every 4 to 6 years and estimating the 10-year risk.[32] The risk calculator may be found at http://tools.cardiosource.org/ASCVD-Risk-Estimator/ (last accessed December 23, 2014).
• The USPSTF strongly recommends screening for lipid disorders starting at age 35 in men and age 45 in women. Younger adults should be screened if they have other risk factors for coronary heart disease (CHD).
• The treatment of dyslipidemia is discussed in detail in Chapter 11.

Diabetes Mellitus

• The American Diabetes Association annually updates recommendations for diabetes mellitus (DM) care. The 2013 guidelines that recommend screening are presented here.[33]
• The A1C, fasting plasma glucose, or 75-g 2-hour oral glucose tolerance test (OGTT) are all acceptable screening tests. Healthy adults should be tested starting at age 45.

TABLE 5-2	Classification, Follow-Up, and Treatment of Hypertension		
Blood pressure (mm Hg)	**Classification**	**Follow-up**	**Treatment**
<120/80	Normal	Recheck in 2 years	
120–139/80–89	Prehypertension	Recheck in 1 year	Recommend lifestyle modification
140–159/90–99	Stage 1 hypertension	Confirm within 2 months	Lifestyle modification and medications
≥160/100	Stage 2 hypertension	Start treatment	Lifestyle modification and medications

Data from Chobanian AV, Bakris GL, Black HR, et al. National High Blood Pressure Education Program Coordinating Committee on Prevention, Detection, Evaluation, and Treatment of High Blood Pressure: the JNC 7 report. *JAMA* 2003;289:2560-2572.

- Consider testing all adults who are overweight (BMI ≥25 kg/m²) and have additional risk factors: hypertension, HDL cholesterol <35 mg/dL or triglyceride level >250 mg/dL, cardiovascular disease, women with polycystic ovary syndrome, previous A1C ≥5.7%, impaired glucose tolerance or impaired fasting glucose, women who delivered a baby weighing >9 pounds or who were diagnosed with gestational DM, physical inactivity, first-degree relative with DM, high-risk ethnicity (e.g., African American, Latino, Native American, Asian American, Pacific Islander), and other risk conditions (e.g., severe obesity, acanthosis nigricans, or use of glucocorticoids or antipsychotics).
- If results are normal, testing should be repeated at least every 3 years, with consideration of more frequent testing depending on initial results and risk status.
- Those with prediabetes should be tested yearly:
  - A1C 5.7% to 6.4%
  - Fasting glucose 100 to 125 mg/dL
  - OGTT 2-hour value of 140 to 199 mg/dL

Abdominal Aortic Aneurysm

- The USPSTF recommends one-time screening for abdominal aortic aneurysm (AAA) by ultrasonography in men aged 65 to 75 years who are current or former smokers.[34]
- They make no recommendation for or against screening for AAA in patients with no smoking history.
- They recommend against routine screening for AAA in women.

Coronary Heart Disease

- The USPSTF recommends against routine screening with resting ECG or exercise treadmill test for the prediction of CHD in low-risk adults and found insufficient evidence to recommend for or against routine screening in adults at intermediate or high risk for CHD events.[35] The USPSTF found insufficient evidence to recommend for or against the use of nontraditional risk factors such as C-reactive protein (CRP), ankle-brachial index (ABI), coronary artery calcification (CAC) score on electron beam CT, homocysteine level, or lipoprotein(a) level.[36]
- As noted above, recent ACC/AHA guidelines for cardiovascular risk assessment recommend screening those ages 20 to 79 years without atherosclerotic cardiovascular disease every 4 to 6 years for risk factors and estimating the 10-year risk.[32] Additionally, if a risk-based treatment decision is unclear, high-sensitivity CRP (hs-CRP) (≥2 mg/L), CAC scoring (≥300 Agatston units or ≥75th percentile for age, sex, and ethnicity), or ABI (<0.9) may provide further guidance. Lipoprotein(a), albuminuria, renal function, cardiorespiratory fitness testing, and carotid intima-media thickness (CIMT) are of unclear or limited value.

Peripheral Arterial Disease

- The USPSTF recommends against routine screening for peripheral arterial disease (PAD) because there is little evidence that treatment of PAD at this asymptomatic stage of disease, beyond treatment based on standard cardiovascular risk assessment, improves health outcomes.[37]
- As noted, the ACC/AHA has said that measurement of the ABI is reasonable for cardiovascular risk assessment in asymptomatic adults for whom risk-based treatment decisions are unclear.[32]

Thyroid Disease

Screening for thyroid disease is not routinely recommended, but clinicians should keep a low threshold for measurement of thyroid-stimulating hormone for subtle or nonspecific symptoms, especially in older women (see Chapter 21).

Obesity

- Periodic height and weight measurements are recommended for all patients.
- The body mass index (BMI) is the body weight in kilograms divided by the square of the height in meters.
  - BMI 18.5 to 24.9 kg/m^2 is considered normal.
  - BMI >25 kg/m^2 is considered overweight.
  - BMI 30 to 34.9 kg/m^2 is class I obesity.
  - BMI 35 to 39.9 kg/m^2 is class II obesity.
  - BMI ≥40 kg/m^2 is class III or morbid obesity.
- BMI may overestimate the degree of obesity in extremely muscular individuals (such as professional athletes).
- For persons with a BMI of 25 to 35, it can be useful to measure the waist circumference. Increased morbidity is associated with waist >102 cm (40 inches) in men and 88 cm (35 inches) in women.

Osteoporosis

- The USPSTF recommends screening for osteoporosis in[38]:
  - Women age ≥65 years.
  - Women <65 years whose risk factors put them at a fracture risk equivalent to a 65-year-old white woman.
  - Evidence is insufficient to assess the balance of benefits and harms of screening for osteoporosis in men.
- National Osteoporosis Foundation (NOF) recommends[39]:
  - All postmenopausal women and men ≥50 should be evaluated for osteoporosis risk and risk for falling.
  - Bone mineral density (BMD) testing should be considered for
    - All women ≥65 and men ≥70
    - Persons with clinical risk factors for fracture if they are men ages 50 to 69 and post-menopausal or perimenopausal women
    - Adults with a fracture after age 50
    - Adults with a condition (e.g., rheumatoid arthritis) or taking a medication associated with bone loss (e.g., glucocorticoids equivalent to ≥5 mg/day prednisone for 3 or more months)

Sexually Transmitted Diseases

- The CDC website, www.cdc.gov (last accessed December 23, 2014), has up-to-date recommendations about screening for sexually transmitted disease (STD). Basic guidelines are as follows:
  - Sexually active men who have sex with men (MSM) should be screened annually for HIV (in uninfected patients) and for bacterial STDs, such as syphilis, gonorrhea, and chlamydia.
  - MSM who engage in higher-risk behaviors (such as multiple or anonymous partners, or sex in conjunction with illicit drug use) should be screened every 3 to 6 months.
  - Sexually active females aged ≤25 years should be screened for chlamydia testing annually and gonorrhea testing annually for those at risk.
- HIV screening:
  - HIV testing should be encouraged for adolescents who are sexually active and those who use injection drugs.
  - Individuals aged 13 to 64 should get tested at least once in their lifetimes and those with risk factors get tested at least annually.
  - The USPSTF also supports widespread HIV screening for persons aged 15 to 65 years (younger adolescents and older adults who are at increased risk should also be screened), and for all pregnant women.[40]

Hepatitis C

The CDC and USPSTF recommend that everyone born 1945–1965 be screened for hepatitis C.[41]

Alcohol Abuse and Dependence

- Screening for alcohol abuse and dependence is an important part of the routine checkup (see Chapter 46).
- Definitions (from the National Institute on Alcohol Abuse and Alcoholism at www.niaaa. nih.gov, last accessed December 23, 2014):
  - **Heavy or at-risk drinking** is diagnosed in the following group:
    - Men who consume >14 drinks per week or >4 drinks per occasion
    - Women who consume >7 drinks per week or >3 drinks per occasion
    - Elderly who consume >7 drinks per week or >3 drinks per occasion
  - **One drink** is 12 g ethanol, as in 12 oz of beer, 5 oz of wine, or 1.5 oz of distilled spirits.
  - **Alcohol abuse** is a maladaptive pattern of use; manifested by continued or recurrent use despite failure in major role obligations at work, school, or home; of use in physically hazardous situations, or of use despite alcohol-related legal, social, or interpersonal problems.
  - **Alcohol dependence** is marked by tolerance, the presence of withdrawal symptoms on cessation, impaired control (drinking more/longer than intended), persistent desire, and continued use despite physical or psychological problems related to alcohol.
- **The CAGE questions** are a useful screening tool for alcohol dependence. Two positive responses are considered a positive test and indicate further assessment is warranted.
  - Have you ever felt that you should **Cut down** on drinking?
  - Have people **Annoyed** you by criticizing your drinking?
  - Have you ever felt bad or **Guilty** about your drinking?
  - **Eye-opener:** Have you ever had a drink first thing in the morning to steady your nerves or to get rid of a hangover?

Adult Immunizations

GENERAL PRINCIPLES

- Guidelines are subject to change over time and according to local public health conditions.
- Each patient's clinical context should be considered and risks and benefits weighed.
- The following are general guidelines, and manufacturer's information should be consulted regarding individual products.
- Various professional organizations make recommendations regarding immunization practices. The official national policy is determined by the following:
  - The Department of Health and Human Services (HHS)
  - The Centers for Disease Control and Prevention (CDC)
  - The Advisory Committee on Immunization Practices (ACIP)
- The ACIP makes recommendations that are then reviewed by the director of the CDC and HHS. They become official policy when published in CDC's Morbidity and Mortality Weekly Reports.
- Table 5-3 lists abbreviations used in this chapter regarding immunizations.

RESOURCES FOR INFORMATION

Immunization guidelines are quite detailed and are periodically updated. Useful resources for accessible, up-to-date information include the following:

- The CDC vaccine information website (www.cdc.gov/vaccines, last accessed December 23, 2014) has extensive information including the General Recommendations on Immunization and recommendations for specific vaccines.

TABLE 5-3	Glossary of Vaccine-Related Abbreviations
ACIP	The Advisory Committee on Immunization Practices
DPT	Full dose of diphtheria and tetanus toxoids plus whole killed pertussis (pediatric use only, no longer available in the US)
DT	Full dose of diphtheria and tetanus toxoids (pediatric use only)
DTaP	Full dose of diphtheria and tetanus toxoids plus acellular pertussis (pediatric use only)
HAV	Hepatitis A vaccine
HB	Hepatitis B
HBIG	Hepatitis B immunoglobulin
HBsAg	Hepatitis B surface antigen
HBV	Hepatitis B virus
Hib	*Haemophilus influenzae* type B
HibCV	*Haemophilus influenzae* type B conjugated vaccine
HPV	Human papillomavirus
HRIG	Human rabies immunoglobulin
IG	Immunoglobulin
IM	Intramuscular
IPV	Inactivated (injected) polio vaccine
LAIV	Live attenuated intranasal influenza vaccine
MCV4	Tetravalent meningococcal conjugate vaccine
MMR	Measles, mumps, and rubella vaccine
MMRV	Measles, mumps, rubella, and varicella vaccine
OPV	Oral polio vaccine
PCV13	13-Valent pneumococcal conjugate vaccine, Prevnar
PPSV23	23-Valent pneumococcal polysaccharide vaccine, Pneumovax
Td	Full dose tetanus and reduced dose diphtheria toxoid (for persons over age of 7 years)
Tdap	Full dose tetanus and reduced dose diphtheria toxoid plus acellular pertussis (for adults and adolescents)
IIV	Inactivated influenza vaccine—the "flu shot"
VAERS	Vaccine Adverse Events Reporting System
VZV	Varicella zoster virus

- The CDC publishes an adult immunization schedule annually (www.cdc.gov/vaccines/schedules/hcp/adult.html, lasted accessed December 23, 2014).
- "The Pink Book: Epidemiology & Prevention of Vaccine-Preventable Diseases" contains a wealth of information and is available in PDF format at www.cdc.gov/vaccines/pubs/pinkbook/index.html (last accessed December 23, 2014).
- The Immunization Action Coalition (IAC) website has educational materials, camera-ready and copyright-free, at www.immunize.org. They also have many translated documents for non–English-speaking patients. They have comprehensive vaccine information for the public at www.vaccineinformation.org (last accessed December 23, 2014).

LEGAL RESPONSIBILITIES OF THE PROVIDER

- Serious or unusual adverse events must be reported to the Vaccine Adverse Events Reporting System (VAERS), whether or not the provider thinks they are causally associated. Forms are available from the Food and Drug Administration at www.fda.gov/cber/vaers/vaers.htm (last accessed December 23, 2014).

- Federally approved Vaccine Information Statement must be given to all patients prior to administering vaccines. Copies are available from the CDC or at www.immunize.org (last accessed December 23, 2014).
- Permanent vaccination records must be maintained by all vaccine providers.

TIMING OF ADMINISTRATION

- Specified times are minimum intervals.
  - Doses that are administered at shorter intervals may not result in adequate antibody response and should not be counted as part of a primary series.
  - Delay or interruption in the immunization schedule does **not** require starting over or extra doses.
- Simultaneous administration of multiple vaccines improves compliance.
  - In general, inactivated (killed) and most live vaccines can be administered at the same time at separate anatomic sites.
  - Live parenteral vaccines (see Table 5-4) and live intranasal influenza vaccine (LAIV) should be administered at the same visit or should be separated by at least 4 weeks.
  - Live oral vaccines (such as oral typhoid) may be given at any time before or after live parenteral vaccines or LAIV.
  - Tuberculin test response can be inhibited by live virus vaccines. Tuberculin skin testing can be done on the same day as the vaccination or 4 to 6 weeks later.
- Antibody-containing blood products can interfere with the response to live virus vaccines, particularly measles and varicella (but not the zoster vaccine). The interactions can be complex, so the clinician should consult the CDC website, specifically the Pink Book, Chapter 2.

DOCUMENTATION OF PRIOR VACCINATIONS

- If records cannot be located, an age-appropriate schedule of so-called catch-up immunizations should be started. Persons who have served in the military usually have been vaccinated against measles, rubella, tetanus, diphtheria, and polio.
- Self-reported doses of influenza vaccine and pneumococcal polysaccharide vaccine are acceptable.
- Vaccines received outside the US are usually of adequate potency. Foreign records are acceptable if they include written documentation of the date of vaccination, and the schedule (age and interval) was comparable with that recommended in the United States.

HYPERSENSITIVITY TO VACCINE COMPONENTS

- **Persons with a history of anaphylactic reactions to any vaccine component should not receive that vaccine**, except under the supervision of an experienced allergist. Vaccines may have traces of egg protein or antibiotics; the manufacturer's insert should be carefully checked.
- Contact dermatitis to neomycin is a delayed-type (cell-mediated) immune response, not anaphylaxis, and is therefore not a contraindication to vaccine use.
- Hypersensitivity to thimerosal is usually a local delayed-type or an irritant effect.
- Many vaccines may cause mild-to-moderate local or systemic adverse effects such as low-grade fever or injection site swelling, redness, or soreness. These are not a contraindication to future doses of the vaccine.

TABLE 5-4	Adult Immunizations				

Vaccine	Live?	Usual schedule[a]	Contraindications	Precautions
		Times are minimum intervals for adequate antibody response; longer intervals do NOT require extra doses.	**For ALL vaccines: Severe allergic reaction (e.g., anaphylaxis) after a previous dose or to a vaccine component is a contraindication.**	For ALL vaccines: Moderate or severe acute illness with or without fever is a precaution.
Haemophilus	No	1 dose		
Hepatitis A	No	0, 6 months		
Hepatitis B[b]	No	0, 1, 6 months		
HPV	No	0, 2, 6 months		
Influenza (IIV)	No	1 dose annually	• Anaphylaxis to eggs or vaccine components	• Administer in deltoid area only. • Pregnancy • Caution if GBS within 6 weeks of previous influenza vaccination • Persons who experience only hives with exposure to eggs should receive IIV with additional safety precautions (see text)
Influenza, intranasal (LAIV)	Yes	1 dose annually	• Anaphylaxis to eggs or vaccine components • Contraindicated in pregnancy or immune compromise	• Chronic medical conditions • Caution if GBS within 6 weeks of previous influenza vaccination • Receipt of antivirals (see text)
Measles, MMR	Yes	0, 1 month	• Contraindicated in pregnancy or immune compromise	• Receipt of antibody-containing blood product within 11 months (see text) • History of thrombocytopenia
Meningococcus	No	1 dose for most; If 2 doses: 0, 2 months		• Caution if GBS

(Continued)

TABLE 5-4 Adult Immunizations (Continued)

Vaccine	Live?	Usual schedule[a]	Contraindications	Precautions
Pneumococcus	No	See Table 5-5		• Caution if GBS within 6 weeks of previous tetanus vaccination
Tetanus, Td or Tdap	No	0, 1, 7–13 months; Booster every 10 years	• For pertussis-containing vaccines: encephalopathy not attributable to another cause <7 days after previous dose of Tdap, DTP, or DTaP	• Caution if history of Arthus reaction with tetanus vaccine • For pertussis-containing vaccines: progressive or unstable neurologic disorder
Varicella	Yes	0, 1–2 months	• Contraindicated in pregnancy or severe immune compromise	• Receipt of antivirals (see text) • Receipt of antibody-containing blood product within 11 months (see text)
Zoster	Yes	1 dose	• Contraindicated in pregnancy or severe immune compromise	• Receipt of antivirals (see text)

[a]First dose at time "0 month."

[b]See text for schedule for hemodialysis patients.

DTaP, full dose diphtheria/tetanus toxoid plus acellular pertussis (pediatric only); DTP, full dose diphtheria/tetanus toxoid plus whole killed pertussis (pediatric only, no longer available in US) HPV, human papillomavirus; GBS, history of Guillain-Barré syndrome; IM, intramuscularly; IIV, inactivated influenza vaccine (injected); LAIV, live attenuated intranasal influenza vaccine MMR, measles, mumps, and rubella; Tdap, tetanus and reduced dose diphtheria toxoid with acellular pertussis vaccine; Td, tetanus and reduced dose diphtheria toxoids.

SPECIFIC VACCINES AND IMMUNOBIOLOGIC AGENTS

See the Specific Patient Groups section for age-based checklists and recommendations for persons who have chronic illnesses, are immunocompromised, are pregnant or breast-feeding, or are health care workers or travelers. Table 5-4 provides an overview of the schedules and contraindications.

Measles, Mumps, and Rubella

Indications
- Ensure that all adults are immune to measles, mumps, and rubella (MMR). Documentation of physician-diagnosed disease is not adequate evidence of immunity.
- Adequate evidence of immunity to measles or mumps can include any of the following:
  ○ Documentation of at least 1 dose of live measles/mumps vaccine on or after the first birthday.
  ○ Serologic evidence of immunity.
  ○ Persons born before 1957 are considered immune, unless they are health care workers.
- Adequate evidence of immunity to rubella requires the following:
  ○ Documentation of at least 1 dose of rubella vaccine on or after the first birthday
  ○ Serologic evidence of immunity
- Nonimmune persons should receive 1 dose of MMR, especially women of childbearing years.
- A second dose of MMR (>1 month after first dose) is recommended for:
  ○ Prior recipients of a killed measles vaccine or an unknown type from 1963 to 1967
  ○ Health care workers (unless serologic evidence of immunity)
  ○ All students (unless serologic evidence of immunity)
  ○ Persons who travel outside the US
  ○ HIV-infected persons without immunity to measles, rubella, and mumps, if the CD4 lymphocytes are ≥15% and ≥200/μL for ≥6 months

Postexposure Prophylaxis
- Live measles vaccine may prevent disease if given within 72 hours of exposure.
- Immune globulin (IG) may prevent or modify disease and provide temporary protection if given within 6 days of exposure.
  ○ The dose is 0.25 mL/kg IM (maximum of 15 mL).
  ○ Immunocompromised persons, irrespective of evidence of measles immunity, should receive 0.5 mL/kg IM (maximum 15 mL).
  ○ After administration of IG, the passively acquired measles antibodies can interfere with the immune response to measles vaccination, so vaccination should be delayed for 6 months.

Contraindications, Side Effects, and Precautions
- MMR is a live attenuated virus and is therefore **contraindicated in pregnancy**. Pregnancy should be avoided for 3 months after MMR-containing vaccine. Close contact with a pregnant woman or immunocompromised person is **not** a contraindication to MMR vaccination (the vaccine is not shed).
- **MMR is generally contraindicated in immunocompromised hosts.** HIV-infected persons may be vaccinated with MMR if they lack evidence of measles immunity, are asymptomatic, and are not severely immunosuppressed (for adults CD4 lymphocytes ≥200/μL or >14%).
- Persons who have experienced a severe allergic reaction to a vaccine component or following a prior dose of measles vaccine should generally not be vaccinated with MMR.

○ In the past, persons with a history of anaphylaxis to eggs were considered to be at increased risk for serious reactions from measles or mumps vaccines. However, anaphylactic reactions to these vaccines are not associated with hypersensitivity to egg antigens but to other components of the vaccines (such as gelatin or neomycin).

○ **MMR may be administered to egg-allergic persons without prior routine skin testing or the use of special protocols.**[42]

• Moderate or severe acute illness with or without fever is a precaution. Mild acute illness and low-grade fever are not contraindications to immunization.

• Adverse reactions may include fever (5% to 15%), rash (5%), arthralgias (up to 25% of adult females), or rarely thrombocytopenia or lymphadenopathy.

• Because blood products can interfere with the antibody response, MMR administration should be delayed (consult the CDC for exact intervals). However, rubella-susceptible women should be vaccinated immediately postpartum even if anti-Rho(D) (RhoGAM, WinRho, etc.) or other blood products were administered during pregnancy or at delivery. Antibody levels should be measured 3 months later to assess response.

• Tuberculin test response can be inhibited by live virus vaccines; tuberculosis skin testing can be done on the same day as the vaccination or 4 to 6 weeks later.

Tetanus, Diphtheria, and Pertussis Vaccines

Indications

• All adults of any age should complete a primary series of 3 doses of Td if they have not done so during childhood or if the vaccination history is uncertain.

○ Tetanus vaccine was first widely used in the 1940s, so elderly persons may have never received a primary series.

○ Doses that are given as part of wound management do count toward the 3 doses needed.

• **A tetanus booster is recommended every 10 years, lifelong. Many adults are overdue for boosters.**

• Only about one-third of tetanus cases result from puncture wounds; other sources include minor wounds, burns, frostbite, bullet wounds, crush injuries, and even chronic wounds such as abscesses and chronic ulcers (14% of cases). Approximately 4% of patients with tetanus recall no antecedent wound.

• Because infection does not confer complete immunity, tetanus patients should be immunized after recovery.

• See Figure 5-1 for guidelines for postexposure prophylaxis.

Formulations

• Vaccine terminology can be confusing; all formulations contain a full dose of tetanus toxoid.

• DPT: **No longer available in the US**; pediatric use only and full dose of diphtheria toxoid plus whole killed pertussis.

• DTaP (Daptacel, Infanrix, and Tripedia brands): Pediatric use only, full dose of diphtheria toxoid plus acellular pertussis, and take care to avoid confusion with Tdap.

• DT: Pediatric use only; full dose of diphtheria toxoid.

• Td: For persons over age 7 years, reduced dose of diphtheria toxoid.

• Tdap (Adacel and Boostrix brands): for adults and children over age 10 (Boostrix) or 11 (Adacel) years; reduced dose of diphtheria toxoid plus acellular pertussis; and take care to avoid confusion with DTaP.

Tdap

• In 2005, a tetanus/diphtheria toxoid with acellular pertussis vaccine (Tdap) was approved for use in adolescents and adults.

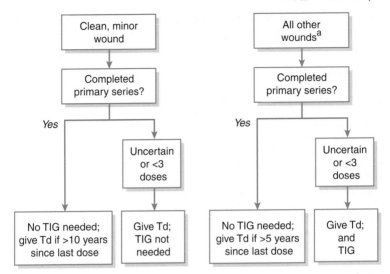

Figure 5-1 Guidelines for postexposure prophylaxis to prevent tetanus. [a]Tetanus-producing wounds are often not the classic puncture wounds but can include minor wounds, burns, frostbite, bullet wounds, crush injuries, and chronic wounds such as abscesses and chronic ulcers. TIG, tetanus immunoglobulin; Td, tetanus and diphtheria toxoids, adsorbed.

- **Many adults are susceptible to pertussis,** so the vaccine should help to reduce pertussis morbidity among adults and reduce the transmission of pertussis to infants and in health care settings.
- The ACIP recommends a single dose of Tdap in the following circumstances:
  - All adults who have not received Tdap previously or for whom vaccine status is unknown. Tdap can be administered regardless of interval since the most recent tetanus or diphtheria-containing vaccine.
  - Tdap is especially important for adults who are close contacts of infants <12 months of age (e.g., parents, grandparents, or child care providers).
  - Administer 1 dose to pregnant women during EACH pregnancy (ideally at 27 to 36 weeks' gestation).
  - Health care personnel with direct patient contact should receive a dose of Tdap.
  - Adults with unknown or incomplete history of completing a 3-dose primary series of tetanus vaccine should begin or complete a primary vaccination series. Tdap should be substituted for a single dose of Td in the series, preferably the first dose.
  - For wound management, Tdap is preferred to Td if the patient has not previously received Tdap.

Contraindications, Side Effects, and Precautions

- Severe allergic reaction (e.g., anaphylaxis) after a previous dose or to a vaccine component is a contraindication.
- Too frequent administration can produce increased rates of local or systemic reactions due to antigen-antibody complexes (Arthus-type reaction).
- Urticarial or anaphylactic reactions can occur but are rare. If such a history exists, then serologic testing to determine immunity to tetanus can be performed to evaluate the need for a booster dose. If additional doses are needed to ensure immunity, referral to an allergist is indicated.
- Local reactions are common and consist of erythema, induration, or tenderness.

- Moderate or severe acute illness with or without fever is a precaution. Mild acute illness and low-grade fever are not contraindications to immunization.

Influenza

- Influenza-associated deaths range from 3,000 to 49,000 per year. Persons most at risk for serious complications include the elderly, the very young, pregnant women, and persons with chronic illness.
- Antibodies from previous infections or vaccinations are not fully protective against new strains because the virus undergoes constant antigenic drift (point mutations) and occasional antigenic shift (change in subtype).
- Those who are at highest risk of the disease and its complications are also the least able to respond to vaccination. Overall, the vaccine is about 60% to 80% effective against vaccine-type viruses.
- Influenza vaccines available in the US include the following:
  ○ The inactivated influenza vaccine (IIV), trivalent or quadrivalent, the common flu shot.
  ○ High-dose IIV (Fluzone High-Dose, Sanofi Pasteur Inc.) contains four times the amount of antigen as regular IIV.
  ○ The intranasally administered live attenuated influenza vaccine (LAIV) (FluMist, MedImmune); formerly trivalent, the LAIV became quadrivalent in 2013.

Indications

- **Since 2010, the ACIP has recommended annual influenza vaccination for ALL persons age 6 months or older.**
- IIV may be used in anyone aged 6 months or more.
- LAIV is indicated for healthy, nonpregnant persons aged 2 to 49 years. Possible advantages of LAIV include its potential to induce a broad mucosal and systemic immune response and the acceptability of an intranasal rather than intramuscular route of administration.
- Adults aged 65 years or older can receive the standard dose IIV or the high-dose IIV (Fluzone High-Dose).

Contraindications, Side Effects, and Precautions

- A previous severe allergic reaction (anaphylaxis) to influenza vaccine, regardless of the component suspected to be responsible for the reaction, is a contraindication to future receipt of the vaccine.
- Persons who experience only hives with exposure to eggs should receive IIV (rather than LAIV) with additional safety precautions (health care provider should be familiar with the potential manifestations of egg allergy, and vaccine recipients should be observed for at least 30 minutes for signs of a reaction after administration of each vaccine dose).[43]
- Moderate or severe acute illness with or without fever is a precaution. Mild acute illness and low-grade fever are not contraindications to immunization.
- Side effects of the flu shot are usually limited to mild arm soreness. Placebo-controlled trials have demonstrated no increase in systemic symptoms.
- **The flu shot is not a live virus and cannot cause the flu,** but the live attenuated intranasal vaccine may cause rhinorrhea, nasal congestion, headache, or sore throat.
- **The intranasal LAIV should not be used in**
  ○ Those aged <2 or >50 years
  ○ Pregnant women
  ○ Persons with chronic health problems
  ○ Persons with a history of Guillain-Barré syndrome (GBS)
  ○ Persons with a history of hypersensitivity, including anaphylaxis, to any of the components of LAIV or to eggs
  ○ Children or adolescents receiving aspirin or other salicylates (because of the association of Reye syndrome with wild-type influenza virus infection)

○ Health care workers and others who have close contact with severely immunocom-promised persons who require protective environment (such as patients with stem cell transplants)
- GBS has not been associated with the influenza vaccine since the 1976 to 1977 swine flu vaccine (which was associated with approximately 5 to 10 excess cases of GBS/million vaccines).
- **Persons with a history of egg allergy who have experienced only hives after exposure to egg should receive influenza vaccine**, with the following additional safety measures:
  ○ The IIV should be used, not LAIV.
  ○ Vaccine should be administered by a health care provider who is familiar with the poten-tial manifestations of egg allergy.
  ○ Vaccine recipients should be observed for at least 30 minutes after administration of each vaccine dose.
- Persons who report having had severe reactions to egg (angioedema, respiratory distress, light-headedness, recurrent emesis, or who required medical intervention) should be referred to an experienced allergist for further risk assessment.

Pneumococcal Vaccine

- *Streptococcus pneumoniae* is a major cause of pneumonia, bacteremia, and meningitis and of over 4,000 deaths per year in the United States.
- Efficacy of the vaccine is controversial and is estimated at 50% to 80%. Because polysac-charide vaccines do not induce T-cell–dependent responses associated with immunologic memory, there is no true anamnestic response to additional doses of vaccine (although antibody levels will rise).

Formulations
- Pneumovax 23 (Merck) is a 23-valent polysaccharide vaccine (PPSV23), which contains polysaccharide antigen from 23 types of pneumococcal bacteria that cause 88% of bacte-remic pneumococcal disease.
- Prevnar 13 (Wyeth) is a 13-valent pneumococcal conjugate vaccine (PCV13). It is used for routine immunization of infants and for certain adults (see Indications for PSV13 below).

Indications for PPSV23
- When indicated, PPSV23 should be administered to patients who are uncertain of their vaccination status.
- When PCV13 is also indicated, the PCV13 should be given before the PPSV23.
- PPSV23 should be given to all healthy persons age 65 years or older if
  ○ Not previously vaccinated
  ○ Unknown vaccination status
  ○ Vaccinated 5 or more years ago and were <65 years old at first vaccination
- PPSV23 should be given to all adults aged 19 to 64 years with risk factors for invasive pneumococcal disease:
  ○ Chronic heart disease (excluding hypertension, but including congestive heart failure or cardiomyopathy)
  ○ Cigarette smoking
  ○ Chronic lung disease (including chronic obstructive pulmonary disease or asthma)
  ○ DM
  ○ Cerebrospinal fluid (CSF) leaks
  ○ Cochlear implant
  ○ Alcoholism
  ○ Chronic liver disease, including cirrhosis
  ○ Persons with functional or anatomic asplenia (including sickle cell disease, other hemo-globinopathies, splenectomy)

- Immunocompromised persons (a second dose of PPSV23 is recommended 5 years after the first dose for persons with functional or anatomic asplenia and for immunocompromised persons):
  - Congenital or acquired immunodeficiencies
  - HIV infection
  - Chronic renal failure or nephrotic syndrome
  - Hematologic malignancies (leukemia, lymphoma, Hodgkin disease, or multiple myeloma)
  - Generalized malignancy
  - Diseases requiring treatment with immunosuppressive drugs, including long-term systemic corticosteroids or radiation therapy
  - Solid organ transplantation

Revaccination

- Revaccination is not routinely recommended. ACIP does not recommend multiple revaccinations because of insufficient data regarding clinical benefit, particularly the degree and duration of protection, and safety.
- Revaccination is contraindicated if the patient had a severe reaction to the prior dose.
- A single revaccination should be considered after 5 years for those who are likely to have a rapid decline in antibody levels, including those with anatomic or functional asplenia, or those with immunocompromising conditions (see list above).

Indications for PCV13

- When indicated, PCV13 should be administered to patients who are uncertain of their vaccination status.
- In 2012, the ACIP recommended routine use PCV13 (Prevnar 13, Wyeth) for adults aged ≥19 years with the following[44]
  - Immunocompromising conditions (as per list above)
  - Functional or anatomic asplenia
  - CSF leaks
  - Cochlear implants
- For pneumococcal vaccine-naïve persons, ACIP recommends that adults with immunocompromising conditions, functional or anatomic asplenia, CSF leaks, or cochlear implants should receive a dose of PCV13 first, followed by a dose of PPSV23 at least 8 weeks later.
- Subsequent doses of PPSV23 should follow current PPSV23 recommendations for adults at high risk.
  - Specifically, a second PPSV23 dose is recommended 5 years after the first PPSV23 dose for persons aged 19 to 64 years with functional or anatomic asplenia and for persons with immunocompromising conditions.
  - Those who received PPSV23 before age 65 years for any indication should receive another dose of the vaccine at age 65 years, or later after at least 5 years have elapsed since their previous PPSV23 dose.
- Adults with immunocompromising conditions, functional or anatomic asplenia, CSF leaks, or cochlear implants, who did previously receive 1 or more doses of PPSV23 should be given a PCV13 dose ≥1 year after the last PPSV23 dose was received. For those who require additional doses of PPSV23, the first such dose should be given no sooner than 8 weeks after PCV13 and at least 5 years after the most recent dose of PPSV23.
- In late 2014 ACIP recommended PCV13 for all adults ≥65 years.
- See Table 5-5 for a summary.

Contraindications, Side Effects, and Precautions

- Pneumococcal vaccine is contraindicated in those with a severe reaction to a previous dose (anaphylaxis or local Arthus-type reaction).

TABLE 5-5 Pneumococcal Vaccine Guidelines

	NEVER had a pneumococcal vaccine	Previously had Pneumovax
Healthy	PPSV23 (Pneumovax) age 65	PPSV23 (Pneumovax) age 65
Chronic disease (including cardiac, pulmonary or liver disease, diabetes mellitus, smoking, alcohol abuse)	PPSV23 (Pneumovax) now PPSV23 (Pneumovax) age 65	(Nothing now) PPSV23 (Pneumovax) age 65
CSF leak or cochlear implant	PCV13 (Prevnar) now PPSV23 (Pneumovax) 8 weeks later PPSV23 (Pneumovax) age 65	PCV13 (Prevnar) now PPSV23 (Pneumovax) age 65
Asplenia (functional or anatomic) or immunocompromise (HIV, hematologic or generalized malignancy, immunosuppressant medications, organ transplant, chronic kidney disease, nephrotic syndrome)[a]	PCV13 (Prevnar) now PPSV23 (Pneumovax) 8 weeks later PPSV23 (Pneumovax) 5 years later PPSV23 (Pneumovax) age 65	PCV13 (Prevnar) now PPSV23 (Pneumovax) 5 years later PPSV23 (Pneumovax) age 65

[a]In late 2014 ACIP recommended PCV13 for all adults ≥65 years.
PCV13 is the 13-valent pneumococcal conjugate vaccine (Prevnar)
PPSV23 is the 23-valent pneumococcal polysaccharide vaccine (Pneumovax)

- Approximately half of patients experience injection site soreness, redness, or swelling; systemic symptoms are rare.
- Moderate or severe acute illness with or without fever is a precaution. Mild acute illness and low-grade fever are not contraindications to immunization.

Hepatitis A Vaccine and Immune Globulin

The levels of antibody following hepatitis A vaccine (HAV) or immunoglobulin (IG) administration are much lower than those following natural infection and are usually below the level of detection of most commercial assays but are protective against infection (>90% effective by 1 month).

Formulations

- Two inactivated HAVs are available: HAVRIX (GlaxoSmithKline) and VAQTA (Merck); both are available in pediatric and adult formulations. Adults 19 years of age and older should receive 1 dose of adult formulation with a booster dose at least 6 months later.
- There is also a combination of hepatitis A and hepatitis B vaccine (Twinrix, GlaxoSmithKline), which is administered in a 3-dose series at 0, 1, and 6 months for adults 18 or more years of age. Single-antigen HAV may be used to complete a series that begun with Twinrix and vice versa (for a total of 3 doses, on the Twinrix schedule).

Indications for Vaccination for Preexposure Prophylaxis

- In high-prevalence populations, it may be reasonable (but not necessary) to check serology before offering HAV vaccine.
- Target groups for vaccination include the following:
  - Persons traveling to/working in countries in which HAV is endemic.
  - Men who have sex with men.

- ○ Illicit drug users (injection or noninjection).
- ○ Persons with HIV infection.
- ○ Persons with an occupational risk (e.g., laboratory workers).
- ○ Persons with chronic liver disease or liver transplant recipients (no increased risk of acquiring infection, but complications would be more likely).
- ○ Persons who receive clotting factor concentrates.
- ○ Vaccination can also be considered for food handlers to reduce potential transmission.
- ○ Persons who anticipate close contact with an international adoptee during the first 60 days following arrival of the adoptee to the US from an endemic country. The first dose of the 2-dose HAV series should be administered as soon as adoption is planned, ideally 2 or more weeks before the arrival of the adoptee.

Travelers
- Travelers to Canada, Western Europe, Scandinavia, Australia, New Zealand, and Japan are at no greater risk for infection than in the US. Elsewhere, there is increased risk even if travelers observe precautions against enteric infection or stay in urban areas or luxury hotels.
- Ideally, travelers should receive HAV at least 4 weeks before travel. A second dose 6 to 12 months later is necessary for long-term protection.
- Unvaccinated adults >40 years of age, immunocompromised persons, and persons with chronic liver disease planning to travel in 2 weeks or sooner should receive the first dose of vaccine and also can receive immune globulin (IG, 0.02 mL/kg) at the same visit.
- Travelers who choose not to receive the vaccine should be administered a single dose of IG (0.02 mL/kg), which will provide protection for up to 3 months. For travel periods that exceed 2 months, the dose should be 0.06 mL/kg; administration must be repeated if the travel period exceeds 5 months.

Postexposure Prophylaxis
- In high-prevalence populations, it may be reasonable, but not necessary, to check serology before offering IG.
- The IG (0.02 mL/kg) should be given as soon as possible, but no later than 10 days to 2 weeks after exposure.
- Persons who received HAV vaccine at least 1 month before exposure do not need IG.
- Postexposure prophylaxis is indicated for household and sexual contacts of confirmed cases but not casual contacts.
- Day care center staff and attendees need prophylaxis if one or more cases are confirmed.
- If a food handler is diagnosed with hepatitis A, other food handlers at the same location need IG (and should consider vaccine). Transmission to patrons is unlikely, but prophylaxis can be considered if an infectious worker directly handled uncooked or previously cooked foods and had diarrhea or poor hygienic practices, and patrons can be contacted and treated within 2 weeks.

Contraindications, Side Effects, and Precautions
- Contraindications include history of a severe allergic reaction to a vaccine component, or hypersensitivity to alum or the preservative 2-phenoxyethanol.
- Moderate or severe acute illness with or without fever is a precaution. Mild acute illness and low-grade fever are not contraindications to immunization.
- The most frequent side effects are injection site erythema and soreness and mild systemic symptoms such as malaise or low-grade fever.
- Vaccine and IG should be administered with separate syringes at different anatomic sites.

Hepatitis B Vaccine and Immune Globulin
Efficacy and Postvaccination Testing
- The vaccine is 80% to 100% effective in preventing infection.
  - ○ Protection is essentially complete for those with an adequate antibody response (≥ 10 mIU/mL).

- Protective antibody titers are developed after 3 doses of the vaccine in >90% of young adults but in only 75% of those over age 60.
- Efficacy is lower in hemodialysis patients.
- Postvaccination testing for serologic response (1 to 6 months after completion of the vaccine series) is advised only for persons whose subsequent clinical management depends on knowledge of their immune status or those who are expected to have a suboptimal response (e.g., infants born to hepatitis B surface antigen [HBsAg]–positive mothers, sex partners of HBsAg-positive persons, dialysis patients and staff, persons over age 50, persons with HIV infection). Postvaccination testing should also be considered for persons at occupational risk.
- When nonresponders are revaccinated, 30% to 50% produce an adequate antibody response after three additional doses. Persons who fail to develop detectable anti-HBs after 6 doses should be tested for HBsAg as they may be chronically infected.
- Antibody levels decline over time, but protection against disease appears to persist despite undetectable antibody. Therefore, booster doses of vaccine are not recommended for immunocompetent adults.

Formulations and Schedules
- Two hepatitis B vaccines are available: Recombivax HB (Merck) and Engerix-B (GlaxoSmithKline Pharmaceuticals), both in pediatric and adult formulations. Engerix-B is also available in combination with hepatitis A as Twinrix (GlaxoSmithKline) for adults 18 or more years of age.
  - For adult dose schedules, the brands are interchangeable.
  - All are recombinant in origin and contain no potentially infectious virions.
  - Adults 20 or more years of age should receive 1 mL of any brand of HB vaccine.
  - Adolescents <20 years of age may receive any of the following:
    - Recombivax HB: pediatric or adult formulation at 0.5 mL (5 μg) per dose
    - Engerix-B: pediatric formulation 0.5 mL (10 μg) or adult formulation 1 mL (20 μg) per dose
- The usual schedule is 2 doses separated by no <4 weeks and a third dose 4 to 6 months after the second dose (i.e., at time 0, 1 month, and 5 to 6 months).
  - If an accelerated schedule is needed, the minimum interval between the first 2 doses is 4 weeks, and the minimum interval between the second and third doses is 8 weeks, with at least 16 weeks between the first and third doses.
  - Doses given at less than these minimum intervals should not be counted as part of the vaccination series.
  - Longer than minimum times are acceptable. **It is not necessary to restart the series or add doses because of an extended interval between doses.**
- Patients on hemodialysis require larger or increased number of doses, or both, to achieve adequate antibody levels. For dialysis patients aged ≥20 years, use either schedule:
  - Recombivax-B: use 3 doses of the special 40-μg/mL formulation (1 mL IM at 0, 1, and 6 months)
  - Engerix-B: use 4 double doses of the regular 20 μg/mL formulation (2 mL IM at 0, 1, 2, and 6 months)
  - Measure titers 1 to 6 months after immunization.
  - Antibody levels should be tested annually and a booster dose administered when <10 mIU/mL.

Indications
- Prevaccination serologic testing is usually cost-effective and should be considered for groups with a high risk of HBV infection:
  - All persons born in Africa, Asia, the Pacific Islands, or other regions with endemic HBV infection
  - Household, sex, and needle-sharing contacts of HBsAg-positive persons

- Men who have sex with men
- Injection drug users
- Incarcerated persons
- Certain persons receiving cytotoxic or immunosuppressive therapy
- There is no harm in vaccinating persons who are already immune.
- Hepatitis B vaccination is recommended for all unvaccinated adults at risk for HBV infection and for all adults requesting protection from HBV infection. Persons at risk for infection include the following:
  - Household contacts and sex partners of persons with chronic HBV infection.
  - Sexually active persons who are not in a long-term, mutually monogamous relationship.
  - Persons seeking evaluation or treatment for a STD.
  - Men who have sex with men.
  - Current or recent injection drug users.
  - Persons with HIV infection.
  - Household contacts of HBsAg-positive persons.
  - International travelers to regions of endemic HBV infection.
  - Residents and staff of facilities for developmentally disabled persons, or correctional facilities.
  - Health care and public safety workers with risk for exposure to blood or blood-contaminated body fluids.
  - Persons with end-stage renal disease, including predialysis or any form of dialysis.
  - Persons with chronic liver disease or liver transplant recipients (no increased risk of acquiring infection, but complications would be more likely).
  - Adults with DM type 1 or 2. In 2011, ACIP recommended that all previously unvaccinated adults aged 19 to 59 years with DM be vaccinated against hepatitis B as soon as feasible after a diagnosis of DM is made (and may be considered in those aged 60 or older). Persons with DM are at increased risk of HBV infection, probably because of breaches in infection control during assisted blood glucose monitoring (e.g., reuse of single patient finger stick devices).
- Vaccinate all adults requesting protection from HBV infection, without requiring them to acknowledge a specific risk factor.

Contraindications, Side Effects, and Precautions
- A severe allergic reaction (anaphylaxis) to a vaccine component or following a prior dose of hepatitis B vaccine is a contraindication to further doses of vaccine. Such allergic reactions are rare.
- Moderate or severe acute illness with or without fever is a precaution. Mild acute illness and low-grade fever are not contraindications to immunization.
- Pregnancy is not a contraindication.
- The most common adverse reactions are injection site pain or mild systemic complaints, such as fatigue or headache. Serious systemic adverse reactions are rare.

Postexposure Prophylaxis
- Hepatitis B immune globulin (HBIG) is used for postexposure prophylaxis in susceptible individuals (no vaccine or known nonresponder).
- Vaccine and HBIG can be administered at the same time, but at separate sites.
- After an occupational exposure to blood or body fluids, the source patient and the exposed person should be checked for HBsAg status; see Table 5-6 for the treatment algorithm.[45]
- In nonoccupational settings, HBV can be spread to household contacts, sexual partners, and needle-sharing contacts. Unvaccinated contacts should be tested for susceptibility to HBV infection and should receive the first dose of hepatitis B vaccine immediately after collection of blood for serologic testing.
  - Management of nonoccupational exposure to a source known to be HBsAg positive:
    - Persons with written documentation of a complete HB vaccine series but no postvaccination testing should receive a single HB vaccine booster dose.

TABLE 5-6 — Hepatitis B Prophylaxis Following Percutaneous Exposure to Blood

Exposed person is:	Treatment when source patient is:		
	HBsAg positive	HBsAg negative	Status unknown
Unvaccinated	HBIG ×1; initiate HB vaccine series	Initiate HB vaccine series	Initiate HB vaccine series
Previously vaccinated, known responder	No treatment	No treatment	No treatment
Previously vaccinated, known nonresponder after 3 doses	HBIG × 1 and initiate revaccination	No treatment	If known high-risk source, treat as if source were HBsAg positive
Previously vaccinated, known nonresponder after 6 doses	HBIG × 2 (1 month apart)	No treatment	If known high-risk source, treat as if source were HBsAg positive
Previously vaccinated, response unknown	Check anti-HBs level; if adequate[a], no treatment; if inadequate, HBIG × 1 plus HB vaccine booster dose	No treatment	Check anti-HBs level; if adequate[a] no treatment; if inadequate[a] initiate revaccination

[a]Adequate anti-HBsAg level is 10 SRU by radioimmunoassay or positive by enzyme immunoassay.
HB, hepatitis B; HBIG, hepatitis B immune globulin; HBsAg, hepatitis B surface antigen.

- Persons who are not fully vaccinated should receive HBIG and should complete the vaccine series.
- Unvaccinated persons should receive both HBIG and hepatitis B vaccine series as soon as possible after exposure (preferably within 24 hours).
  ○ Management of nonoccupational exposure to source with unknown HBsAg status:
    - Persons with written documentation of a complete HB vaccine series require no further treatment.
    - Persons who are not fully vaccinated should complete the vaccine series.
    - Unvaccinated persons should receive the HB vaccine series with the first dose administered as soon as possible after exposure, preferably within 24 hours.

Varicella (Chickenpox) Vaccine

- Approximately 10% of US adults are susceptible to the varicella-zoster virus (VZV) and its complications (bacterial infections of skin lesions, viral pneumonia, aseptic meningitis, encephalitis, thrombocytopenia, hepatitis and others). Prior to routine immunization, approximately 100 deaths occurred annually, mostly in healthy persons.
- Evidence of immunity to varicella in adults includes any of the following:
  ○ Documentation of 2 doses of varicella vaccine
  ○ Laboratory evidence of immunity or confirmation of disease (but commercial assays may yield false-negative results after vaccination)

   ○ Born in the US before 1980 (but not adequate evidence of immunity for health care providers or pregnant women)
   ○ A health care provider diagnosis of varicella disease or herpes zoster.

Efficacy
• In adolescents and adults, the seroconversion rate is 99% after 2 doses.
• Breakthrough infections in vaccinated persons are usually mild, with <50 lesions.
• The incidence of herpes zoster may be less after vaccination than after the natural disease.

Indications
Two doses of varicella vaccine are indicated for all susceptible adolescents and adults, with emphasis on the following groups:

• Susceptible adolescents
• Adults who live with young children
• All nonpregnant women of childbearing age
• Household contacts of immunocompromised persons
• Health care workers
• Workers in schools and day care centers
• Those who live in closed populations such as colleges or the military
• International travelers

Contraindications, Side Effects, and Precautions
• Severe allergic reaction (e.g., anaphylaxis) after a previous dose or to a vaccine component is a contraindication. All VZV vaccines contain tiny amounts of neomycin and hydrolyzed gelatin but do not contain egg protein or preservative.
• Moderate or severe acute illness with or without fever is a precaution. Mild acute illness and low-grade fever are not contraindications to immunization.
• Because it is a live attenuated virus vaccine, **varicella vaccine is contraindicated in pregnancy** (defer pregnancy 1 month after vaccination).
• Varicella vaccine is contraindicated in some immunocompromised individuals including those with leukemia, lymphoma, or generalized malignancy, immune deficiency disease, or on immunosuppressive therapy (including steroids at more than replacement dose).
• Varicella vaccine may be administered to persons with impaired humoral immunity (e.g., hypogammaglobulinemia), but the blood products used for treatment (IG) may interfere with the response to vaccination. Recommended spacing between administration of the blood product and receipt of varicella vaccine should be observed (consult CDC website).
• Approximately 25% to 33% of recipients had injection site soreness, swelling, erythema, or rash.
• In <1%, a diffuse rash developed with a median of five lesions, most caused by a coincidental wild-type virus.
• Vaccine-type virus from the varicella-like rash after immunization can infrequently be transmitted to susceptible contacts, but the secondary cases are subclinical or mild.

Herpes Zoster (Shingles) Vaccine
Latent VZV can cause herpes zoster, also known as shingles. About one in five cases of zoster leads to postherpetic neuralgia (increased incidence with aging), and rare complications include pneumonia, cranial nerve damage, or encephalitis.

Efficacy
• The zoster vaccine has an efficacy of about 50% in preventing herpes zoster and 66% in preventing postherpetic neuralgia. The efficacy declines with age.[46]
• The duration of protection is unknown, but is probably >4 years.

Indications
- The vaccine is FDA approved for use in adults >50 years of age, but ACIP recommends vaccination at age 60.
- Persons with a reported history of zoster can be vaccinated.
- Although both are made from live attenuated varicella zoster virus, **the varicella vaccine (Varivax) and the zoster vaccine (Zostavax) are not interchangeable**—the zoster vaccine is a much higher dosage (15×).

Contraindications, Side Effects, and Precautions
- The most common side effects are redness, pain and swelling at the injection site, and headache.
- Antiherpes medications (acyclovir, famciclovir, valacyclovir) might interfere with the response to the zoster vaccine; they should be discontinued 24 hours before administration of zoster vaccine, if possible. They may be restarted 14 days later.
- Because it is a live attenuated virus vaccine, **zoster vaccine is contraindicated in pregnancy and in most immunocompromised patients,** including those with hematologic malignancies, AIDS, HIV infection with CD4 cell count <200/μL, and more than 20 mg/day of prednisone (or equivalent).
- Other contraindications include a history of severe allergic reaction to gelatin, neomycin, or any component of the vaccine.
- The following are not contraindications:
  - Topical, inhaled, or intra-articular steroids or long-term alternate-day treatment with low to moderate doses of short-acting systemic corticosteroids.
  - Low doses of drugs used for the treatment of rheumatoid arthritis, inflammatory bowel disease, and other conditions, such as methotrexate, azathioprine, or 6-mercaptopurine, are also not considered sufficiently immunosuppressive to create safety concerns for zoster vaccine.
- The safety and efficacy of zoster vaccine administered concurrently with recombinant human immune mediators and immune modulators (such as the anti–tumor necrosis factor agents adalimumab, infliximab, and etanercept) is not known. It is preferable to administer zoster vaccine before, or 1 month after, treatment with these drugs. Otherwise, the immune status of the recipient should be assessed on a case-by-case basis.
- Blood products do not interfere with zoster vaccination because all persons with a history of varicella maintain high levels of antibody to VZV (comparable to those found in antibody-containing blood products).
- Moderate or severe acute illness with or without fever is a precaution. Mild acute illness and low-grade fever are not contraindications to immunization.

Meningococcal Vaccine

Formulations
- All US vaccines contain 4 purified bacterial capsular polysaccharides: A, C, Y, and W-135 but not serogroup B (serogroup B polysaccharide is poorly immunogenic in humans).
- Menomune (Sanofi Pasteur) is an older quadrivalent meningococcal polysaccharide vaccine (MPSV4) and is preferred for persons aged 56 and older.
- The newer quadrivalent meningococcal conjugate vaccines (MCV4) contain the same capsular polysaccharides, conjugated to proteins for enhanced immunogenicity. It is preferred for persons aged 55 and younger. Brands include Menactra (Sanofi Pasteur) and Menveo (Novartis).

Indications and Schedules
- For healthy adolescents, ACIP recommends routine vaccination with MCV4 at age 11 or 12 years, with a booster dose at age 16 years to maintain protective immunity through ages 16 to 21 years, when their risk for disease is greatest.

○ If the first dose was at ages 13 to 15, a booster dose should be administered at ages 16 to 18, before the peak in increased risk.
○ If the first dose was at age 16 or later, a booster is not needed.
○ First-year college students up through age 21 years who are living in residence halls should be vaccinated if they have not received a dose on or after their 16th birthday.
○ Routine vaccination of healthy persons is not recommended after age 21 years.
• Persons aged 2 to 54 years with reduced immune response should receive 2 doses of MCV4 administered 2 months apart and then a booster dose every 5 years. Indications include persistent complement component deficiencies and functional or anatomic asplenia.
• Other persons at increased risk for meningococcal disease (e.g., microbiologists, military recruits, or travelers to endemic areas) should receive a single dose of MCV4.
• If persons with HIV infection need meningococcal vaccination, they should receive 2 doses of MCV4.

Contraindications, Side Effects, and Precautions
• Severe allergic reaction (e.g., anaphylaxis) after a previous dose or to a vaccine component is a contraindication. MPSV4 contains thimerosal, but MCV4 does not.
• Moderate or severe acute illness with or without fever is a precaution. Mild acute illness and low-grade fever are not contraindications to immunization.
• Systemic reactions, such as headache and malaise, occur in up to 60% of recipients, and up to 5% of recipients develop a fever within 7 days of vaccination.
• Safety in pregnancy is unknown, but pregnancy is not considered a contraindication.
• GBS has been associated with receipt of MCV4; therefore, a history of GBS is a relative contraindication to receiving MCV4. The nonconjugated MPSV4 may be used for short-term protection (3 to 5 years).

Human Papillomavirus (HPV) Vaccine
• HPV infection is associated with anogenital warts (90% have HPV types 6 or 11), recurrent respiratory papillomatosis, cervical cancer (70% have HPV types 16 or 18), and other cancers (anal, vaginal, vulvar, penile, and some head and neck cancers).
• HPV infection is common among adolescents and young adults (prevalence up to 64% in adolescent girls).
• **Vaccination is not a substitute for routine cervical cancer screening** (Pap smears).

Formulations
• Two inactivated HPV vaccines are available in the US.
○ Quadrivalent HPV (HPV4) vaccine (Gardasil, Merck) contains types 16 and 18 (high risk) and types 6 and 11 (low risk). It is approved for females and males 9 to 26 years of age.
○ Bivalent HPV (HPV2) vaccine (Cervarix, GlaxoSmithKline) contains types 16 and 18 (high risk). It is approved for females 10 to 25 years of age (not males).
• For both vaccines, >99% of recipients developed an antibody response, and the vaccines showed >90% efficacy in preventing cervical neoplasia or genital warts related to the HPV types included in the vaccine. The vaccines had no therapeutic effect on existing infection or disease. Prior infection with one HPV type did not diminish efficacy of the vaccine against other vaccine HPV types.

Indications and Schedules
• The vaccine is administered as a 3-dose series at 0, 2, and 6 months.
• ACIP recommends routine vaccination of
○ Females 11 to 12 years of age (as young as 9 years at the clinician's discretion)
○ Catch-up vaccination for females 13 to 26 years of age
○ Males 11 to 12 years of age (as young as 9 years at the clinician's discretion)

- Catch-up vaccination for males 13 to 21 years of age (males age 22 to 26 may also be vaccinated)
- All immunocompromised males (including HIV infection) up to age 26
- Men who have sex with men up to age 26

Contraindications, Side Effects, and Precautions
- Severe allergic reaction (e.g., anaphylaxis) after a previous dose or to a vaccine component is a contraindication.
- Moderate or severe acute illness with or without fever is a precaution. Mild acute illness and low-grade fever are not contraindications to immunization.
- HPV vaccines are not recommended for use in pregnant women, but pregnancy testing is not needed before vaccination. If a woman is found to be pregnant after initiating the vaccination series, no intervention is needed; the remainder of the 3-dose series should be delayed until completion of pregnancy.
- Common adverse reactions include injection site pain, redness, or swelling. Systemic reactions are no more frequent than with placebo. Syncope has been reported among adolescents receiving vaccines, so recipients should be seated.

Haemophilus influenzae Type B (Hib) Conjugated Vaccine (HibCV)
- Most invasive *H. influenzae* disease occurs in very young children but can also occur in adults with chronic pulmonary disease and conditions that predispose to infections with encapsulated organisms.
- Most *H. influenzae* disease in adults is due to nontypeable strains, but HibCV can be considered for adults at increased risk for invasive Hib disease. Previously unvaccinated adults with one of these high-risk conditions should be given at least 1 dose of any Hib conjugated vaccine:
  - HIV infection
  - Functional or anatomic asplenia
  - Immunodeficiency (especially IgG2 subclass deficiency)
  - Immunosuppression from cancer chemotherapy
  - Leukemia or receipt of a hematopoietic stem cell transplant
- Side effects of injection site swelling, redness, and/or pain have been reported in 5% to 30% of children; systemic reactions are infrequent.
- Severe allergic reaction (e.g., anaphylaxis) after a previous dose or to a vaccine component is a contraindication.
- Moderate or severe acute illness with or without fever is a precaution. Mild acute illness and low-grade fever are not contraindications to immunization.

Polio
Indications
- Wild-type polio has been eradicated from the entire Western Hemisphere.
- The oral polio vaccine (OPV) is a live attenuated virus that can cause vaccine-associated paralytic poliomyelitis (approximate rate: one in 2 to 3 million) and is shed in the stool. It is now recommended that OPV should not be used in the US, even in healthy children. **Only inactivated (injected) polio vaccine (IPV) should be used**.
- US adults do not need polio vaccination unless they plan travel to endemic areas or have occupational exposure to poliovirus. **Unvaccinated adults who are at increased risk** should receive a primary vaccination series with IPV (3 doses at time 0, 1 to 2 months later, and 6 to 12 months after the second dose).
- Severe allergic reaction (e.g., anaphylaxis) after a previous dose or to a vaccine component is a contraindication (IPV contains trace amounts of streptomycin, polymyxin B, and neomycin).
- Moderate or severe acute illness with or without fever is a precaution. Mild acute illness and low-grade fever are not contraindications to immunization.

Rabies Vaccine and Immune Globulin

- Most reported cases of animal rabies in the US occur among carnivores, primarily raccoons, skunks, foxes, and bats. The majority of human rabies cases in the US have resulted from variants of rabies viruses associated with insectivorous bats.
- Worldwide, wild dogs account for most cases; some US cases of rabies originate from dog bites sustained abroad, even >1 year earlier. Rabies prophylaxis in foreign countries may be inadequate.
- Vaccines available in the US include human diploid cell vaccine (HDCV, Imovax Rabies, Sanofi Pasteur) and purified chick embryo cell vaccine (PCECV, RabAvert, Novartis Vaccines and Diagnostics).
  - A full 1-mL IM dose is used for both preexposure and postexposure prophylaxis regimens.
  - Rabies vaccines induce an active immune response that requires approximately 7 to 10 days to develop; rabies virus–neutralizing antibodies generally persist for several years.
- Severe allergic reaction (e.g., anaphylaxis) after a previous dose or to a vaccine component is a contraindication.
- Vaccine side effects include injection site soreness and erythema. Mild systemic symptoms (such as headache, nausea, myalgias) are common.
- Moderate or severe acute illness with or without fever is a precaution. Mild acute illness and low-grade fever are not contraindications to immunization.

Postexposure Prophylaxis

- After an exposure, all wounds require immediate and thorough washing with copious amounts of soap and water. Tetanus prophylaxis should also be considered.
- In all postexposure prophylaxis regimens, except for persons previously vaccinated, human rabies immune globulin (HRIG) should be administered concurrently with the first dose of vaccine.
- Use of HRIG provides a rapid, passive immunity that persists for a short time (half-life 21 days) for protection until the production of active immunity in response to vaccine administration. Two antirabies immune globulin formulations prepared from hyperimmunized human donors are available for use in the US: HyperRab S/D (Talecris Biotherapeutics) and Imogam Rabies-HT (Sanofi Pasteur).
- Previously immunized patients should receive 2 doses of vaccine: 1-mL IM in the deltoid on days 0 and 3.
- Persons not previously immunized should be treated with:
  - A single 20 IU/kg dose of HRIG, up to half infiltrated in the area of the wound and half IM. HRIG should be given immediately but can be administered up to the eighth day after vaccine was started.
  - Four doses of vaccine (1 mL IM in the deltoid on days 0, 3, 7, and 14).
- Immunocompromised persons should be tested for adequacy of antibody response.
- The local department of health should be notified.
- The decision to initiate postexposure prophylaxis should include the following considerations:
  - Bites to the head or neck can result in rabies in <1 week; therefore, immediate prophylaxis is indicated.
  - A healthy domestic dog, cat, or ferret should be held for observation for 10 days; if signs of illness develop in the animal, the human contact should be immediately treated with HRIG and vaccine while the animal is tested.
  - Bites from a suspected rabid dog or cat require immediate prophylaxis. Casual contact (petting) does not require prophylaxis.
  - Bats and wild carnivores should be regarded as rabid unless confirmed negative by laboratory tests.

- Bites by some animals, such as bats, can inflict very minor injury and thus be unde-tected. **A bat found in a room with a sleeping person is considered an exposure**.
- Small rodents (e.g., squirrels, hamsters, guinea pigs, gerbils, chipmunks, rats, and mice) and lagomorphs (rabbits and hares) are almost never found to be infected with rabies and have not been known to transmit rabies to humans.

Preexposure Prophylaxis
- Preexposure vaccination simplifies management of a rabies exposure by eliminating the need for HRIG and decreasing the number of doses of vaccine needed. It is indicated for persons whose jobs or hobbies bring them into contact with potentially rabid animals, such as the following:
  - Animal handlers, veterinarians, and their staff.
  - Rabies researchers and certain laboratory workers.
  - Animal control and wildlife officers in areas where animal rabies is enzootic.
  - International travelers if they are likely to come in contact with animals in areas where rabies is enzootic and immediate access to appropriate medical care might be limited.
- Preexposure vaccination consists of three 1-mL doses of HDCV or PCECV given IM on days 0, 7, and 21 or 28.
- Persons at ongoing risk of exposure to rabies virus should have periodic serum testing for rabies virus–neutralizing antibody. See CDC guidelines for details.

Specific Immunization Patient Groups

CHECKLISTS BY AGE

Young Adults (About 18 to 26 Years)
- Assure receipt of a primary series (3 doses) of tetanus (DPT, DTaP, or Tdap).
- Tetanus booster (Td) every 10 years; substitute Tdap for 1 dose of Td.
- Assure receipt of at least 1 dose of MMR.
  - Students and health care workers need to have received 2 doses of MMR.
  - Women of childbearing age should have laboratory evidence of immunity to rubella.
  - Health care workers should have laboratory evidence of immunity to MMR.
- Offer varicella vaccine (2 doses) to those who are susceptible (never had chickenpox or the vaccine).
- Ensure receipt of meningococcal vaccine for those up to age 21 (or with risk factors).
  - If the first dose was before age 13, give a booster at age 16.
  - If the first dose was at ages 13 to 15 years, give a booster at ages 16 to 18.
  - If the first dose was at age 16 or later, a booster is not needed.
- Offer HPV vaccine (Gardasil) for women and men up to age 26.
- Annual influenza vaccine is recommended for everyone over age 6 months.
- Assess risk factors that indicate the need for other vaccines: hepatitis A, hepatitis B, or pneumococcal vaccines.

Midlife Adults (About 27 to 49 Years)
- Assure receipt of a primary series (3 doses) of tetanus (DPT, DTaP, or Tdap).
- Tetanus booster (Td) every 10 years; substitute Tdap for 1 dose of Td.
- Assure receipt of at least 1 one dose of MMR.
  - Students and health care workers need to have received 2 doses of MMR.
  - Women of childbearing age should have laboratory evidence of immunity to rubella.
  - Health care workers should have laboratory evidence of immunity to MMR.
- Offer varicella vaccine to those who are susceptible (never had chickenpox or vaccine).

- Annual influenza vaccine.
- Assess risk factors that indicate the need for other vaccines: hepatitis A, hepatitis B, meningococcal, influenza, or pneumococcal vaccines.

Adults Ages 50 Years and Older

- Assure receipt of a primary series (3 doses) of tetanus (DPT, DTaP, or Tdap). Tetanus vaccine was first widely used in the 1940s; many older adults are not immune.
- Tetanus booster (Td) every 10 years; substitute Tdap for 1 dose of Td.
- Assure receipt of at least 1 dose of MMR.
  ○ Health care workers should have laboratory evidence of immunity to MMR.
  ○ Students and health care workers need to have received 2 doses of MMR.
  ○ Those born before 1957 generally are considered immune to measles and mumps.
- Annual influenza vaccination.
- A single dose of pneumococcal vaccine should be given at age 65.
- Offer varicella vaccine to those who are susceptible (never had chickenpox or vaccine).
- Offer zoster (shingles) vaccination to those aged 60 and older.
- Assess risk factors that indicate the need for other vaccines: hepatitis A, hepatitis B, meningococcal, or pneumococcal vaccines.

PREGNANCY AND BREAST-FEEDING

- **Pregnancy is a contraindication for live virus vaccines.** MMR and varicella may be administered to the children of a pregnant woman because these vaccines are not shed.
- All pregnant women should be tested for rubella antibodies; women who are susceptible to rubella should be vaccinated immediately after delivery.
- Influenza vaccine is recommended for all pregnant women.
- Administer 1 dose of Tdap in EACH pregnancy (ideally at 27 to 36 weeks' gestation).
- Pregnant women who are not fully immunized against tetanus should begin the primary series to prevent neonatal tetanus (Tdap for first dose, Td for others).
- Vaccines against hepatitis B, hepatitis A, pneumococcus, and meningococcus are indicated for pregnant women who are at high risk for these infections or their complications.
- Breast-feeding is not a contraindication for any vaccine for infant or mother (except for smallpox vaccine).

IMMUNOSUPPRESSED PATIENTS

- **Live vaccines are generally contraindicated in immunosuppressed patients**, such as those with congenital immunodeficiency, HIV infection, leukemia, lymphoma, generalized malignancy or therapy with alkylating agents, antimetabolites, radiation, or supraphysiologic doses of corticosteroids (such as prednisone at 20 mg/day or more for 14 days or longer).
- Killed (inactivated) vaccines can be safely administered, but the response may be suboptimal. Vaccination during (or within 2 weeks before) chemotherapy or radiation therapy results in a poor antibody response and therefore should be delayed or repeated 3 months after therapy is discontinued.
- Patients with immune compromise other than HIV should receive
  ○ Pneumococcal vaccines (PCV13 and PPSV23 as per Table 5-5)
  ○ Annual IIV (not LAIV)
  ○ One-time dose of Tdap for Td booster and then boost with Td every 10 yrs
  ○ HPV vaccine if <27 years of age
  ○ **Should NOT receive live vaccines including MMR, varicella, or zoster vaccines.**

- Persons with HIV infection who are not severely immunosuppressed (CD4 $\geq$200/μL) should receive
  - Pneumococcal vaccines (PCV13 and PPSV23 as per Table 5-5)
  - Annual IIV (not LAIV)
  - One-time dose of Tdap for Td booster and then boost with Td every 10 years
  - HPV vaccine if <27 years of age
  - Hepatitis B vaccine
  - May receive varicella vaccine or MMR if indicated
- Persons with HIV infection and severe immune compromise (CD4 <200/μL)
  - Should receive pneumococcal vaccines (PCV13 and PPSV23 as per Table 5-5)
  - Should receive annual IIV (not LAIV)
  - Should receive one-time dose of Tdap for Td booster and then Td every 10 years
  - Should receive HPV vaccine if <27 years of age
  - Should receive hepatitis B vaccine
  - **Must NOT receive live vaccines including MMR, varicella, or zoster vaccines**
  - If exposed to measles, they should receive immunoglobulin (0.25 mL/kg; maximum dose 15 mL), regardless of prior vaccination status.
- Hematopoietic cell transplant recipients require revaccination with inactivated vaccines, starting 6 months after transplant (see General Recommendations on Immunization for details).

PERSONS WITH CHRONIC ILLNESS

- **Persons with hemophilia, bleeding disorders, or taking anticoagulant medications** usually tolerate IM injections if a 23-gauge needle is used and firm pressure is applied to the site for at least 2 minutes without rubbing. If the patient receives factor replacement therapy, IM vaccination can be scheduled shortly after such therapy.
- In addition to routine use of influenza, Tdap/Td, MMR, HPV, varicella, and zoster vaccines, persons with chronic illnesses may need additional vaccines as follows:
  - **Persons with liver disease** are at increased risk of suffering complications and should be vaccinated against hepatitis A and hepatitis B. They also should receive pneumococcal vaccine PPSV23 (1 or 2 doses depending on age).
  - **Persons with chronic kidney disease and renal transplant recipients** should receive hepatitis B and pneumococcal vaccines (PCV13 and PPSV23 as per Table 5-4).
  - **Persons with DM** should receive hepatitis B and pneumococcal vaccines (PPSV23, 1 or 2 doses depending on age).
  - **Persons with splenic dysfunction**, including sickle cell disease, or anatomic asplenia should receive meningococcal and pneumococcal vaccines (PCV13 and PPSV23 as per Table 5-5). Those scheduled for elective splenectomy should receive these vaccines at least 2 weeks before the operation.

PERSONS WITH ACUTE ILLNESS

- Mild illnesses (such as otitis media, upper respiratory infections, and diarrhea) are **not** contraindications to vaccination.
- With few exceptions, use of an antimicrobial agent is not a contraindication to vaccination.
  - Oral typhoid vaccine should not be administered until 24 hours after the last dose of antibiotics.
  - Anti-influenza drugs can interfere with the response to live attenuated (intranasal) influenza vaccine. Antiviral drugs active against herpes viruses (such as acyclovir) might reduce the efficacy of live attenuated varicella and zoster vaccines. Live attenuated virus vaccines should not be administered until at least 2 days after related antiviral drugs. If feasible, antiviral medication should not be administered for 14 days after vaccination.

HEALTH CARE WORKERS

- Health care workers and first responders are at risk for exposure to and possible transmission of vaccine-preventable diseases.
- Hepatitis B is an occupational hazard for any worker with possible exposure to blood or bloody fluids.
- Annual influenza vaccine is recommended for all adults and is especially important for health care workers. Those who care for severely immunosuppressed persons who require a protective environment should not receive LAIV given the theoretical risk for transmission of the live attenuated vaccine virus.
- All health care workers should document immunity to MMR, and varicella.
- Health care workers of any age should receive a single dose of Tdap to reduce transmission of pertussis.
- Additional vaccines are indicated for veterinarians, laboratory technicians, animal handlers, and others who may have occupational exposure to rabies, poliovirus, smallpox virus, *Yersinia pestis* (plague), or *Bacillus anthracis* (anthrax).

MEN WHO HAVE SEX WITH MEN (MSM)

In addition to routine use of influenza, Tdap/Td, MMR, HPV, varicella, and zoster vaccines, MSM should be vaccinated against hepatitis A and B. Those <27 years of age should be offered HPV vaccine. Other vaccines are as indicated by risk factors (such as zoster or pneumococcal).

TRAVELERS

- The risk of acquiring illness during international travel depends on the areas to be visited and the extent to which the traveler is likely to be exposed to diseases.
- Influenza is present in the Southern Hemisphere from April through September and year-round in the tropics.
- Hepatitis A is a risk for travelers in most of the world except the US, Australia, Canada, Western Europe, Japan, or New Zealand.
- Travelers should be counseled about safe sex practices.
- Selected travelers may need immunization against yellow fever, cholera, typhoid, plague, meningococcus, rabies, hepatitis B, or hepatitis A.
- Resources for up-to-date information for travelers include the CDC website (http://wwwnc.cdc.gov/travel, last accessed December 23, 2014), which has detailed information about worldwide destinations, and the CDC's toll-free 24-hour Travelers' Health Automated Information Line, 877-394-8747 (877-FYI-TRIP).

REFERENCES

1. Wegwarth O, Schwartz LM, Woloshin S, et al. Do physicians understand cancer screening statistics? A national survey of primary care physicians in the United States. *Ann Intern Med* 2012;156:340–349.
2. Schwartz LM, Woloshin S, Black WC, et al. The role of numeracy in understanding the benefit of screening mammography. *Ann Intern Med* 1997;127:966–72.
3. http://www.cancer.org/research/cancerfactsstatistics/breast-cancer-facts-figures (last accessed December 23, 2014).
4. Fagerlin A, Zikmund-Fisher BJ, Ubel PA. How making a risk estimate can change the feel of that risk: shifting attitudes toward breast cancer risk in a general public survey. *Patient Educ Couns* 2005;57:294–299.

5. Siegel R, Deepa Naishadham D, Ahmedin Jemal A. Cancer statistics, 2013. *CA Cancer J Clin* 2013;63:11–30.

6. Humphrey LL, Helfand M, Chan BK, et al. Breast cancer screening: a summary of the evidence for the U.S. Preventive Services Task Force. *Ann Intern Med* 2002;137:347–360.

7. U.S. Preventive Services Task Force. Screening for breast cancer: U.S. Preventive Services Task Force recommendation statement. *Ann Intern Med* 2009;151:716–726.

8. Fletcher SW, Elmore JG. Clinical practice. Mammographic screening for breast cancer. *N Engl J Med* 2003;348:1672–1680.

9. Thomas DB, Gao DL, Ray RM, et al. Randomized trial of breast self-examination in Shanghai: final results. *J Natl Cancer Inst* 2002;94:1445–1457.

10. American College of Obstetricians-Gynecologists. Practice bulletin no. 122: breast cancer screening. *Obstet Gynecol* 2011;118(2 Pt 1):372–382.

11. Barton MB, Harris R, Fletcher SW. Does this patient have breast cancer? *JAMA* 1999;282:1270–1280.

12. U.S. Preventive Services Task Force. Screening for breast cancer: U.S. Preventive Services Task Force Recommendations. *Ann Intern Med* 2009;151:I44.

13. Smith RA, Durado Brooks D, Cokkinides V, et al. Cancer screening in the United States, 2013; a review of current American Cancer Society guidelines, current issues in cancer screening, and new guidance on cervical cancer screening and lung cancer screening. *CA Cancer J Clin* 2013;63:88–105.

14. Kaplan JE, Benson C, Holmes KH, et al. Guidelines for prevention and treatment of opportunistic infections in HIV-infected adults and adolescents: recommendations from CDC, the National Institutes of Health, and the HIV Medicine Association of the Infectious Diseases Society of America. Centers for Disease Control and Prevention (CDC); National Institutes of Health; HIV Medicine Association of the Infectious Diseases Society of America. *MMWR Recomm Rep* 2009;58(RR-4):1–207.

15. Winawer SJ, Zauber AG, Ho MN, et al. Prevention of colorectal cancer by colonoscopic polypectomy. The National Polyp Study Workgroup. *N Engl J Med* 1993;329:1977–1981.

16. Qaseem A, Denberg TD, Hopkins RH, et al.; for the Clinical Guidelines Committee of the American College of Physicians. Screening for colorectal cancer: a guidance statement from the American College of Physicians. *Ann Intern Med* 2012;156:378–386.

17. U.S. Preventive Services Task Force. Screening for colorectal cancer: U.S. Preventive Services Task Force recommendation statement. *Ann Intern Med* 2008;149:627–637.

18. Levin B, Lieberman DA, McFarland B, et al. Screening and surveillance for the early detection of colorectal cancer and adenomatous polyps, 2008: a joint guideline from the American Cancer Society, the US Multi-Society Task Force on Colorectal Cancer, and the American College of Radiology. *CA Cancer J Clin* 2008;58:130–160.

19. National Lung Screening Trial Research Team; Aberle DR, Adams AM, et al. Reduced lung-cancer mortality with low-dose computed tomographic screening. *N Engl J Med* 2011;365:395–409.

20. Wender R, Fontham ET, Barrera E Jr, et al. American Cancer Society lung cancer screening guidelines. *CA Cancer J Clin* 2013;63:107–117.

21. NCCN Clinical Practice Guidelines in Oncology. Lung cancer screening (version 1.2014). www.nccn.org/professionals/physician_gls/pdf/lung_screening.pdf (last accessed December 23, 2014).

22. Detterbeck FC, Mazzone PJ, Naidich DP, et al. Screening for lung cancer: diagnosis and management of lung cancer, 3rd ed: American College of Chest Physicians evidence-based clinical practice guidelines. *Chest* 2013;143:e78S–e92S.

23. Moyer VA, on behalf of the U.S. Preventive Services Task Force. Screening for prostate cancer: U.S. Preventive Services Task Force recommendation statement. *Ann Intern Med* 2012;157:120–134.

24. Wolf AMD, Wender RC, Etzioni RB, et al. American Cancer Society guideline for the early detection of prostate cancer: update 2010. *CA Cancer J Clin* 2010;60:70–98.

25. Qaseem A, Barry MJ, Denberg TD, et al.; for the Clinical Guidelines Committee of the American College of Physicians. Screening for prostate cancer: a guidance statement from the Clinical Guidelines Committee of the American College of Physicians. *Ann Intern Med* 2013;158:761–769.

26. Carter HB, Albertsen PC, Barry MJ, et al. Early detection of prostate cancer: AUA guideline. www.auanet.org. 2013;190:419–426. www.auanet.org/education/guidelines/prostate-cancer-detection.cfm (last accessed December 23, 2014).

27. Smith RA, Brooks D, Cokkinides V, et al. Cancer screening in the United States, 2013: a review of current American Cancer Society guidelines, current issues in cancer screening, and new guidance on cervical cancer screening and lung cancer screening. *CA Cancer J Clin* 2013;63:87–105.

28. Buys SS, Partridge E, Black A, et al.; PLCO Project Team. Effect of screening on ovarian cancer mortality: the prostate, lung, colorectal and ovarian (PLCO) cancer screening randomized controlled trial. *JAMA* 2011;305:2295–2303.

29. Moyer VA; on behalf of the U.S. Preventive Services Task Force. Screening for ovarian cancer: U.S. Preventive Services Task Force Reaffirmation recommendation statement. *Ann Intern Med* 2012;157:900–904.

30. American College of Obstetricians and Gynecologists Committee on Gynecologic Practice. Committee Opinion No. 477: the role of the obstetrician gynecologist in the early detection of epithelial ovarian cancer. *Obstet Gynecol* 2011;117:742–746.

31. Lenfant C, Chobanian AV, Jones DW, et al. Seventh report of the Joint National Committee on the prevention, detection, evaluation, and treatment of high blood pressure (JNC 7): resetting the hypertension sails. *Hypertension* 2003;41:1178–1179.

32. Goff DC Jr, Lloyd-Jones DM, Bennett G, et al. 2013 ACC/AHA guideline on the assessment of cardiovascular risk: a report of the American College of Cardiology/American Heart Association Task Force on Practice Guidelines. *Circulation* 2014;129:S49–S73.

33. Diabetes Care. Standards of Medical Care in Diabetes—2013. *Diabetes Care* 2013;36:S11–S66.

34. U.S. Preventive Services Task Force. Screening for abdominal aortic aneurysm: recommendation statement. *Ann Intern Med* 2005;143:198–202.

35. Moyer VA; on behalf of the U.S. Preventive Services Task Force. Screening for coronary heart disease with electrocardiography: U.S. Preventive Services Task Force recommendation statement. *Ann Intern Med* 2012;157:512–518.

36. U.S. Preventive Services Task Force. Using nontraditional risk factors in coronary heart disease risk assessment: U.S. Preventive Services Task Force recommendation statement. *Ann Intern Med* 2009;151:474–482.

37. U.S. Preventive Services Task Force. Screening for peripheral artery disease and cardiovascular disease risk assessment with the ankle-brachial index in adults: U.S. Preventive Services Task Force recommendation statement. *Ann Intern Med* 2013;159:342–348.

38. U.S. Preventive Services Task Force. Screening for osteoporosis: U.S. Preventive Services Task Force recommendation statement. *Ann Intern Med* 2011;154:356–364. www.uspreventiveservicestaskforce.org/uspstf/uspsoste.htm (last accessed February 25, 2014).

39. National Osteoporosis Foundation. Clinician's guide to prevention and treatment of osteoporosis. www.nof.org/hcp/clinicians-guide (last accessed December 23, 2014).

40. Moyer VA; on behalf of the U.S. Preventive Services Task Force. Screening for HIV: U.S. Preventive Services Task Force recommendation statement. *Ann Intern Med* 2013;159:51–60.

41. Moyer VA; on behalf of the U.S. Preventive Services Task Force. Screening for hepatitis C virus infection in adults: U.S. Preventive Services Task Force recommendation statement. *Ann Intern Med* 2013;159:349–357.

42. Watson JC, Hadler SC, Dykewicz CA, et al. Measles, mumps, and rubella—vaccine use and strategies for elimination of measles, rubella, and congenital rubella syndrome and control of mumps: recommendations of the Advisory Committee on Immunization Practices (ACIP). *MMWR Recomm Rep* 1998;47(RR-8):1–57.

43. Centers for Disease Control and Prevention. Prevention and control of influenza with vaccines: recommendations of the Advisory Committee on Immunization Practices (ACIP)—United States, 2012–13 Influenza Season. *MMWR Morb Mortal Wkly Rep* 2012;61:613–618.

44. Centers for Disease Control and Prevention Use of 13-Valent Pneumococcal Conjugate Vaccine and 23-Valent Pneumococcal Polysaccharide Vaccine for Adults with Immunocompromising Conditions: Recommendations of the Advisory Committee on Immunization Practices (ACIP). *MMWR Morb Mortal Wkly Rep* 2012;61:816–819.

45. U.S. Public Health Service. Updated U.S. Public Health Service guidelines for the management of occupational exposures to HBV, HCV, and HIV and recommendations for postexposure prophylaxis. *MMWR Recomm Rep* 2001;50(RR11):1–42.

46. Oxman MN, Levin MJ, Johnson GR, et al. A vaccine to prevent herpes zoster and postherpetic neuralgia in older adults. *N Engl J Med* 2005;352:2271–2284.

6 | Hypertension
Arielle Yang and Thomas M. De Fer

GENERAL PRINCIPLES

- Hypertension (HTN) is one of the most commonly encountered diseases in the outpatient setting, with an **estimated prevalence rate of 30%.**
- Starting from as low as 115/75 mm Hg, the mortality from cardiovascular disease (CVD) doubles for every increase of 20 mm Hg systolic or 10 mm Hg diastolic pressure, highlighting the tremendous burden that elevated blood pressure (BP) places on society as well as the importance of prompt recognition and treatment.[1]
- Although considerable progress has been made in raising awareness of HTN over the last few decades, current recognition of those affected is far from adequate. **Approximately 50% of patients with HTN have not achieved their treatment goal. Among these, an estimated 40% are not aware of their diagnosis and 90% have received health care in the past year.**[2]

Definition

- For epidemiologic and practical reasons, HTN is currently defined as a systolic blood pressure (SBP) of ≥140 mm Hg and/or a diastolic blood pressure (DBP) of ≥90 mm Hg. This is based upon the **average of two or more properly measured readings** at each of two or more visits following an initial screen.[3]
- However, BP is a continuously distributed trait with a correspondingly variable risk of CVD, so defining HTN in terms of numbers is somewhat arbitrary. HTN can perhaps be better described as a progressive cardiovascular (CV) syndrome characterized by the presence of BP elevation to a level that places patients at increased risk for target organ damage in multiple vascular beds.
- HTN is further stratified into stages of severity based on both systolic and diastolic pressure. Table 6-1 provides the classification scheme for adults aged 18 and older from the Seventh Report of the Joint National Committee on Prevention, Detection, Evaluation, and Treatment of High Blood Pressure (JNC 7).[3] Definitions and classification of HTN are not addressed specifically by the most recent JNC 8.[4]
- The term prehypertension was adopted to identify those at high risk of developing HTN in whom early intervention can decrease the rate of BP progression with age but does not denote a disease category.[3,5]

Epidemiology

- An estimated 66.9 million people, with an overall prevalence rate of 30.4%, have HTN based on 2003–2010 National Health and Nutrition Examination Survey (NHANES) data, a substantial increase from earlier estimates of 50 million from 1988 to 1994.[2]
- The growing prevalence is directly related to an **aging population and a higher rate of obesity.**
- HTN is more common in dark-skinned individuals of African descent and those with a family history of HTN. The prevalence is higher in men than in women until the age of 60, after which women are affected in greater numbers.
- HTN is a major risk factor for the development of CVD, chronic kidney disease (CKD), and dementia, with most affected patients dying from ischemic heart disease.

TABLE 6-1	Classification of Blood Pressure for Adults	
BP classification	SBP (mm Hg)	DBP (mm Hg)
Normal/optimal	<120	And <80
Prehypertension	120–139	Or 80–89
Stage 1 hypertension	140–159	Or 90–99
Stage 2 hypertension	≥160	Or ≥100
Isolated systolic hypertension	≥140	And <90
Isolated diastolic hypertension	<140	And ≥90

BP, blood pressure; DBP, diastolic blood pressure; SBP, systolic blood pressure.
Modified from Chobanian AV, Bakris GL, Black HR, et al. National High Blood Pressure Education Program Coordinating Committee on Prevention, Detection, Evaluation, and Treatment of High Blood Pressure: the JNC 7 report. *JAMA* 2003;289:2560–72.

- **Reversible risk factors** include prehypertension, being overweight or obese, excessive alcohol intake, a high-sodium low-potassium diet, and a sedentary lifestyle.
- Associated conditions include the metabolic syndrome, diabetes mellitus (DM), kidney disease, and obstructive sleep apnea (OSA).

Etiology

- **Essential/primary hypertension**
  - The most common cause of HTN affecting approximately 95% of patients
  - Thought to be due to a complex interplay of multiple factors including genetics, increased sympathetic and angiotensin II activity, insulin resistance, salt sensitivity, and environmental influences
- **Secondary hypertension**
  - Affects a much smaller minority (about 5%) of patients.
  - Secondary to a disease process with a specific identifiable structural, biochemical, or genetic defect resulting in elevated BP.
  - Some of the more common examples include renovascular disease, renal parenchymal disease, endocrinopathies, side effect of other drugs, and OSA. These entities are described further in the "Special Considerations" section.

Screening

- Elevated BP is usually discovered in asymptomatic patients during routine office visits and should, therefore, be checked as part of every health care encounter.
- **The U.S. Preventive Services Task Force strongly recommends HTN screening but the optimal screening interval for HTN is unknown.**[6] Current recommendations call for checking BP at least every 2 years in those with normal BP (<120/80 mm Hg) and annually for persons with prehypertension. Table 6-2 presents a suggested time frame for follow-up evaluations based on BP measurements.[3,7]
- If systolic and diastolic categories are different, follow recommendations for the shorter follow-up.
- The schedule may be modified based on reliable information about past BP measurements, other CV risk factors, and target organ damage.

DIAGNOSIS

- The diagnosis of HTN is established by documenting **SBP of ≥140 mm Hg and/or DBP of ≥90 mm Hg,** based on the average of two or more readings obtained on each of two or more office visits.

TABLE 6-2	Recommendations for Follow-Up Based on Initial Blood Pressure
Initial blood pressure	**Recommended follow up**
Normal	Recheck in 2 years
Prehypertension	Recheck in 1 year
Stage 1 hypertension	Confirm within 2 months
Stage 2 hypertension	Evaluate within 1 month
	For those with severely elevated blood pressure (i.e., >180/110 mm Hg), evaluate and treat immediately if the clinical situation warrants; otherwise reevaluate within 1 week

Modified from Chobanian AV, Bakris GL, Black HR, et al. National High Blood Pressure Education Program Coordinating Committee on Prevention, Detection, Evaluation, and Treatment of High Blood Pressure: the JNC 7 report. *JAMA* 2003;289:2560–72.

- A patient may be diagnosed on the basis of an elevated SBP alone, even if the DBP is normal (i.e., isolated systolic HTN).
- With extreme elevations of BP (>210/120 mm Hg), the diagnosis can usually be safely made without the need for serial evaluations. **In these circumstances, one should focus on the evaluation of end-organ damage and treatment of hypertensive urgency or emergency as indicated** (see "Hypertensive Urgencies and Emergencies").
- After the diagnosis of HTN has been made, there are three major objectives:
  ○ Assess lifestyle or other CV risk factors that may affect prognosis and guide treatment.
  ○ Reveal a cause of secondary HTN (most often not present).
  ○ Assess the presence or absence of target organ damage.
- The history, physical examination, and further diagnostic testing are the primary tools to achieve these objectives.

Clinical Presentation

History

- Determine additional **risk factors** that increase the risk for CV events: increased age (men >45, women >55), cigarette smoking, obesity (body mass index [BMI] >30 kg/m²), physical inactivity, dyslipidemia, DM, kidney disease, and family history of premature CVD (for men, age <55, for women, age < 65). Modifiable risk factors should be treated.
- Seek evidence of **end-organ damage** that may be either known or suggested by characteristic symptoms:
  ○ Coronary artery disease (CAD) or prior myocardial infarction (MI) (angina or exertional dyspnea)
  ○ Heart failure (HF) (symptoms of volume overload and/or dyspnea)
  ○ Prior transient ischemic attack (TIA) or stroke (dementia or focal deficits)
  ○ Peripheral artery disease (PAD, claudication)
  ○ Renal disease
- **Secondary HTN** should be considered when BP becomes severely elevated acutely in a previously normotensive individual, at extremes of age (<20 or >50), or if refractory to treatment with multiple medications. Other symptoms that may be helpful include muscle weakness, palpitations, diaphoresis, skin thinning, flank pain, snoring, or daytime somnolence. See the "Secondary Hypertension" section.
- Conduct a thorough evaluation of the patient's **medications,** as many agents have side effects of elevated BP. Common examples include oral contraceptives, nonsteroidal anti-inflammatory drugs (NSAIDs), and tricyclic antidepressants.

- Oral contraceptives induce sodium retention and potentiate the action of catecholamines.
- NSAIDs block the formation of vasodilating, natriuretic prostaglandins and interfere with the effectiveness of many antihypertensives.
- Tricyclic antidepressants inhibit the action of centrally acting agents (e.g., clonidine).
- Excess alcohol consumption and illicit substances such as cocaine can also raise BP.

Physical Examination
- **Blood pressure measurement**
  - Optimal detection of HTN depends on proper technique.[8]
  - BP should be measured while the patient is in the **seated position with the arm supported at the heart level.**
  - The patient should have avoided caffeine, exercise, and smoking for at least 30 minutes prior to measurement.
  - An **appropriately sized cuff** with the bladder encircling at least 80% of the arm circumference should be used to ensure accuracy.
  - The cuff should be inflated rapidly to 20 to 30 mm Hg past the level where the radial pulse is no longer felt and then deflated at a rate of 2 mm Hg/second.
  - The stethoscope should be placed lightly over the brachial artery.
  - SBP should be noted at the sound of the brachial pulse (Korotkov phase I) and DBP at the disappearance of the pulse (Korotkov phase V).
  - Two readings should be taken, ideally separated by at least 2 minutes.
  - Elevated values should be confirmed in both arms. If there is a disparity due to a unilateral arterial lesion, the reading from the arm with higher pressure should be used.
- **Ambulatory blood pressure monitoring**
  - In some situations, ambulatory blood pressure monitoring (ABPM) can be used to provide further information.[3] With ABPM, patients wear automated, lightweight devices that obtain multiple BP measurements at specific intervals throughout a 24- to 48-hour period. It more effectively reflects a patient's true diurnal variation in BP with lower values during sleep and higher values during wakefulness or activity.
  - By ABPM HTN can be defined as an average awake BP >135/85 and average sleep BP >120/75.[3]
  - Studies have suggested that values obtained with ABPM more closely correlate with end-organ complications than do values obtained in the physician's office.[9]
  - ABPM may be particularly useful in suspected cases of **white coat HTN** in which the anxiety of the physician encounter may falsely elevate BP while values outside of the office are often normal. The risk of CV events in patients with true white coat HTN is frequently debated but a meta-analysis of eight trials suggested there may be no excess risk over normotensive individuals.[10]
  - Ambulatory monitoring may also reveal **masked HTN** and nighttime **nondippers.** Masked HTN indicates patients with normal in-office BP but hypertensive readings during ABPM, and has a prevalence on the order of 10%.[11] It is associated with increased CV risk.[10,12] Currently, it is not clear whom should be screened for masked HTN. Patients receiving treatment for HTN may also display masked HTN with ABPM. Nocturnal HTN and nondipping (i.e., BP not falling by ≥10% during sleep) are also associated with increased CV events.[13,14]
  - ABPM may also be helpful in guiding treatment decisions in patients with borderline HTN, resistant HTN, or symptoms suggestive of hypotension on treatment.[3]
  - ABPM is often impractical due to cost and poor reimbursement. **Home blood pressure monitoring** (HBPM) with self-measurement of BP may serve as a more practical alternative in patients whose values are consistently <130/80 mm Hg despite an elevated office value.[3] It is also recommended as an adjuvant to HTN management.[15]
- After obtaining accurate BP measurements, the physical examination should be tailored to evaluate the presence and severity of target end-organ damage and any features that may suggest secondary HTN.

- **Cardiopulmonary exam:** S4 gallop suggesting left ventricular hypertrophy (LVH), murmurs, or rales suggesting HF.
- **Funduscopic exam:** papilledema, arteriolar narrowing, cotton wool spots, and microaneurysms.
- **Vascular exam:** bruits of major arterial vessels (carotids, femorals, and aorta), asymmetric or diminished distal pulses.
- **Neurologic exam:** altered mental status or focal findings suggestive of prior stroke.
- **Endocrine:** elevated BMI, thyroid enlargement, and Cushingoid features (e.g., buffalo hump, striae, and skin thinning).

Diagnostic Testing

- Routine laboratory tests recommended before initiating therapy include serum electrolytes, blood urea nitrogen (BUN), creatinine, blood glucose, hematocrit, lipoprotein profile, thyroid-stimulating hormone, and urinalysis.
- Measurement of microalbuminuria is recommended in those with DM or renal disease but is otherwise elective and may add to the overall assessment of CV risk.[16–18]
- An ECG should be obtained in all patients to assess for LVH and/or signs of previous infarct. Although echocardiography is more sensitive at diagnosing LVH, it is not recommended in all patients.
- A more detailed workup can be pursued for features suggestive of a secondary cause of HTN. Some of these are described in Table 6-3.

TREATMENT

- The goal of antihypertensive therapy is to reduce the morbidity and mortality of CVD attributable to HTN.
- **Patient education** is an essential component of the treatment plan and promotes better adherence. Physicians should stress the following:
  ○ Lifelong treatment is often required.
  ○ **Symptoms are an unreliable gauge of severity** (despite many patients' claims that they can "feel" when their BP is high).
  ○ Prognosis improves with effective management.
  ○ The importance of therapeutic lifestyle changes.
  ○ Adherence to medication therapy is critically important.
- **All patients with prehypertension or HTN should be counseled regarding therapeutic lifestyle changes.**[3,19,20] See "Other Nonpharmacologic Therapy".
- **For the general population of patients <60 years old the JNC 8 BP goal is <140/90.** This does not differ from the JNC 7 recommendations.[3,4]
- **For the general population of patients ≥60 years old the new JNC 8 goal is <150/90.** The prior JNC 7 goal had been <140/90. The JNC believes that the evidence most strongly support the SBP goal of <150 and points out that some data suggest that <140 adds no additional benefit.[3,4,21–24]

Medications

- Medication treatment is generally considered appropriate/indicated for.[4]
  ○ Patients <60 years with SBP >140 and/or DBP >90.
  ○ Patients ≥60 years with SBP >150 and/or DBP >90.
- Starting two drugs in patients with more marked elevation in BP (<60 years >160/100, ≥60 years >170/100) is reasonable.[3]
- Many factors should be taken into consideration when initiating drug therapy including the following: evidence of improved clinical outcomes, comorbid diseases and other CV risk factors, demographic differences in response, affordability, lifestyle issues, and the likelihood of adherence.

TABLE 6-3 Causes of Secondary Hypertension

Cause	Clinical presentation	Diagnosis	Treatment
Obstructive sleep apnea	Relatively common; daytime sleepiness, snoring, nonrestorative sleep, gasping or choking at night, witnessed apnea, morning headaches, obesity, large neck circumference, and crowded oropharyngeal airway	Polysomnography	Weight loss, CPAP
Renovascular disease (atherosclerotic and fibromuscular)	Relatively common; onset of hypertension at a young age, especially in women (fibromuscular); atherosclerotic disease associated with cigarette smoking, dyslipidemia, increasing age, CAD, other PAD, CKD, flash pulmonary edema and HF, and abdominal bruits	Elevated creatinine level (usually with bilateral renovascular disease), and sudden increase in creatinine level after treatment with an ACE inhibitor or ARB; disparate kidney size; digital subtraction angiography is the diagnostic gold standard but MRA, CTA, and duplex Doppler ultrasonography are potential alternatives	Renal revascularization is indicated for most patients with fibromuscular dysplasia; benefit is much less clear with atherosclerotic stenosis—those with atherosclerotic disease should be treated with aggressive secondary prevention measures
Renal parenchymal disease	Relatively common; in earlier stages there are minimal signs and symptoms; in later stages polyuria, nocturia, oliguria, edema, malaise, fatigue, anorexia, weight loss	Elevated BUN, creatinine, potassium, and phosphate levels; low calcium level; proteinuria; and anemia	ACE inhibitor/ARB if tolerated loop diuretic to control volume
Primary hyperaldosteronism (see Chapter 21)	Relatively common; hypokalemia (only present about 50% of the time), lack of edema, mild metabolic acidosis, mild hypernatremia, generalized muscle weakness	PRA (typically very low), PAC (elevated), PAC:PRA >30; aldosterone secretion does not suppress with sodium loading; adrenal CT to determine type (carcinoma, adenoma, hyperplasia); adrenal vein sampling often necessary if surgery is a potential course	If unilateral, adrenalectomy; if bilateral, mineralocorticod antagonists

(Continued)

TABLE 6-3   Causes of Secondary Hypertension (Continued)

Cause	Clinical presentation	Diagnosis	Treatment
Pheochromocytoma (see Chapter 21)	Episodic headache, sweating, palpitations, tachycardia, tremor; HTN may be episodic or sustained (a few patients are normotensive); sometimes also associated with orthostatic hypotension; familial in some cases	Elevated urine and plasma levels of catecholamines or metanephrine before CT or MRI for localization; I-MIBG[123] scintigraphy sometimes necessary	Preoperative α- and β-blockade followed by surgical resection
Cushing disease and syndrome (see Chapter 21)	Uncommon; weight gain, truncal obesity, abdominal striae, skin atrophy, easy bruising, proximal muscle weakness, plethora, edema, psychological changes; if due to ACTH excess hyperpigmentation, hirsutism, amenorrhea, and acne may occur	Glucose intolerance, hypokalemia, metabolic alkalosis, and elevated urine or blood cortisol levels; dexamethasone suppression test; a 24-hour urinary cortisol virtually excludes the diagnosis; CT or MRI for localization	Generally surgical but medical treatment is occasionally used (e.g., adrenal enzyme inhibitors, cabergoline, and pasireotide)
Thyroid disease (see Chapter 21)	Uncommon; either hyper- or hypothyroidism may increase blood pressure; hyperthyroidism is characterized by sweating, tachycardia, weight loss, anxiety, tremor, and hyperreflexia; hypothyroidism is characterized by fatigue, cold intolerance, weight gain, goiter, and slowed reflexes	Thyroid function testing	Treatment of hyper- or hypothyroidism
Aortic coarctation	Fairly common cause in children but uncommonly first presents in adulthood; headache, cold feet, leg pain; lower BP in legs than arms; reduced or absent femoral pulse, delay in femoral compared with radial pulse, murmur (continuous systolic and diastolic) heard between the scapulae	Doppler echocardiography, CT, MRI	Surgical correction

CPAP, continuous positive airway pressure; CAD, coronary artery disease; PAD, peripheral arterial disease; CKD, chronic kidney disease; HF, heart failure; ACE, angiotensin-converting enzyme; ARB, angiotensin receptor blocker; MRA, magnetic resonance angiography; CTA, computed tomographic angiography; BUN, blood urea nitrogen; PRA, plasma renin activity; PAC, plasma aldosterone concentration; HTN, hypertension; MIBG, metaiodobenzylguanidine; ACTH, adrenocorticotropic hormone; BP, blood pressure.

- There is a high interpatient variability in response, with many patients responding well to one drug class but not to another.
- **The amount of BP reduction rather than the specific antihypertensive drug is the major determinant in reducing CV risk in hypertensive patients.**[25,26] However, this may not be the case with β-blockers and certain medication combinations.
- **In the general non-Black** (i.e., lacking specific overriding indications) population, initial medication management should include a **thiazide diuretic, calcium channel blocker (CCB), angiotensin-converting enzyme (ACE) inhibitor, or angiotensin receptor blocker (ARB).**[4]
- **In the general Black population** (i.e., lacking specific overriding indications), initial management should include a **thiazide diuretic or CCB.**[4,27,28]
- **β-Blockers should not be considered first-line therapy in patients without evidence-based indications** due to the lack of consistent data supporting an independent positive effect on CV morbidity and mortality and relatively less stroke protection compared to other first-line agents.[4,29–31]
- While the ALLHAT trial did demonstrate greater benefit of chlorthalidone (CTDN) in terms of HF, the JNC 8 did not conclude that this finding was compelling enough to recommend thiazide diuretic above the other first-line agents.[4,27]
- Many patients have **specific indications** for particular antihypertensive agents based on other comorbidities (Table 6-4).[3] Data regarding these indications are discussed in the appropriate sections below.
- A patient with mild HTN who is relatively unresponsive to one drug has an almost 50% likelihood of responding to a second drug, so trials of different agents are warranted before moving to combination therapy.[32]
- **Many patients will not reach treatment goal BP on one drug.**[3,4]
- The typical decrease in BP with a single agent is approximately 8 to 15 mm Hg systolic and 8 to 12 mm Hg diastolic.[33,34] Most patients with HTN, however, will eventually require two or more medications.[3,4]

TABLE 6-4	Indications for Individual Drug Classes						
Indication	Thiazide	BB	ACE-I	ARB	CCB	Aldo ANT	HDZ + NIT
General population	X		X	X	X		
Diabetes mellitus[a]	X		X[b]	X[b]	X		
Postmyocardial infarction		X	X[c]	X[c]		X[c]	
Heart failure	X[d]	X	X	X		X	X
Chronic kidney disease			X[e]	X[e]			
Atrial fibrillation rate control		X			X		
Blacks[a]	X				X		

[a]Combination therapy frequently required.
[b]First-choice agent according to the American Diabetes Association.
[c]In patients with left ventricular dysfunction.
[d]Loop rather than thiazide diuretic.
[e]Particularly for patients with albuminuria ≥30 mg/day (or albumin/creatinine ratio ≥30 mg/g).
ACE-I, angiotensin-converting enzyme inhibitor; Aldo ANT, aldosterone antagonist; ARB, angiotensin receptor blocker; BB, β-blocker; CCB, calcium channel blocker; HDZ, hydralazine; NIT, nitrate.
Data from Chobanian AV, Bakris GL, Black HR, et al. National High Blood Pressure Education Program Coordinating Committee on Prevention, Detection, Evaluation, and Treatment of High Blood Pressure: the JNC 7 report. *JAMA* 2003;289:2560–72.

- Combination therapy is appropriate if BP cannot be controlled with a single agent, in patients with stage 2 HTN, and in patients with specific indications for multiple agents (Table 6-4).
- Thiazide diuretics, CCBs, ACE inhibitors, and ARBs are all appropriate add-on agents.[4]
- Fixed-dose combination pills offer the advantage of convenience that may improve adherence but sometimes at a higher cost to the patient and with less flexibility in adjusting doses.

Specific Patient Populations

- **Diabetes**
  - ○ HTN occurs more frequently in diabetics compared with nondiabetics. These two conditions together significantly increase a patient's risk of developing both major CV events and microvascular disease.
  - ○ **The JNC 8 BP treatment goals are the same a nondiabetics (i.e., <140/90).**[4]
  - ○ **The American Diabetes Association (ADA) 2014 standards of care, however, recommend a goal of <140/80.**[35] An SBP of <130 is suggested for some patients (e.g., relatively young) if this can be attained without significant treatment burden.[35]
  - ○ The United Kingdom Prospective Diabetes Study (UKPDS) demonstrated a reduction in mortality (15%), MI (11%), and retinopathy/nephropathy (13%) for every 10 mm Hg reduction in SBP.[36]
  - ○ The JNC 8 recommendation regarding which particular drug to use/start in diabetics is the same as for nondiabetics, based on the lack of difference in CV outcomes.[4]
  - ○ The ADA specifically recommends that an **ACE inhibitor or an ARB** should be a component of antihypertensive treatment given their ability to retard loss of renal function and proteinuria independent of antihypertensive effects.[35,37-40]
  - ○ Most hypertensive diabetics will require more than one antihypertensive to achieve goal BP.
- **Ischemic heart disease**
  - ○ **β-Blockers reduce mortality following MI and should be initiated in all patients regardless of left ventricular (LV) function.** Immediate therapy should be avoided in acute MI patients with signs HF or risk factors for cardiogenic shock.[41-44]
  - ○ β-Blockers without intrinsic sympathomimetic activity are preferred; therefore, acebutolol and pindolol should not be used. When LV function is impaired (without evidence of unstable HF or shock), β-blockers with proven benefit in HF should be used (i.e., metoprolol, carvedilol, and bisoprolol).[41,42,44]
  - ○ ACE inhibitors also have mortality benefit in patients following an MI, **especially those with impaired LV function.**[41,42,45-48] An ARB may be substituted for patients intolerant to ACE inhibitors. Combined ACE inhibitor and ARB does not have further benefit and is associated with more adverse events. Perindopril has also been shown to decrease CV events in patients with stable CAD.[49]
  - ○ CCBs may be used if β-blockers are contraindicated or if additional BP or angina control is necessary. **A long-acting dihydropyridine is recommended** to limit the risk of heart block, bradycardia, and reflex tachycardia.
- **Heart failure**
  - ○ **ACE inhibitors, ARBs, β-blockers, aldosterone antagonists, and the combination of hydralazine and nitrates have all been shown to have mortality benefit in HF,** depending on disease severity.[50-58]
  - ○ Extended release metoprolol succinate, carvedilol, and bisoprolol all have proven benefit and are the preferred β-blockers.
  - ○ The addition or an ARB to ACE inhibitor therapy may be useful in some patients but patients should be monitored carefully for hyperkalemia, worsening renal function, and hypotension.[59,60] The concomitant use of an ACE inhibitor, ARB, and aldosterone antagonist is not recommended.

- ○ Loop diuretics constitute an important aspect of fluid management and are typically an essential part of the patient's regimen.
- ○ While CCBs may cause adverse effects due to their negative inotropic properties, long-acting dihydropyridines can provide additional BP control with less potential for myocardial depression than with verapamil and diltiazem.
- **Chronic kidney disease**
  - ○ **The JNC 8 BP goal for patients with CKD is the same as for the general population, <140/90.**[4]
  - ○ The Kidney Disease: Improving Global Outcomes (KDIGO) Working Group, however, recommends a more strict goal of <130/80 for patients with CKD not on dialysis and with albuminuria ≥30 mg/day (or albumin/creatinine ratio ≥30 mg/g or proteinuria ≥150 mg/day). Data most strongly support this goal for those with albuminuria ≥300 mg/day. The more lenient goal of <140/90 is recommended by KDIGO when albuminuria is <30 mg/day.[61]
  - ○ The National Kidney Foundation accepts these recommendations as reasonable but points out the lack of quality supporting data for the more stringent goals, particularly in those with moderate albuminuria (i.e., 30 to 300 mg/g).[62]
  - ○ KDIGO recommends that an **ACE inhibitor or an ARB** are first-line therapy in patients with albuminuria ≥30 mg/day (or albumin/creatinine ratio ≥30 mg/g), particularly in those with concurrent DM.[36-40,63-65] Again the data most strongly support this recommendation in those with albuminuria ≥300 mg/day.
  - ○ While adding an ARB to an ACE inhibitors reduces proteinuria more, data indicate that this may worsen outcome.[66,67]
- **Stroke**
  - ○ During the acute phase of an **ischemic stroke** (at least the first 24 hours), BP is often increased and is generally not treated unless it is severely elevated (>220/120 mm Hg) or there is other ongoing end-organ damage (e.g., myocardial ischemia, HF, dissection, acute kidney injury [AKI], encephalopathy).[68] An important exception is for patients who are to receive fibrinolytic therapy, in which case the BP should be lowered to <185/110 mm Hg and then to <180/105 mm Hg once it has been given. When to start or resume chronic antihypertensive therapy after an acute ischemic stroke is a matter of controversy; in most patients it is reasonable to initiate treatment after the first 24 hours.
  - ○ The acute management of BP in **intracerebral hemorrhage** is more complex and the BP can be extremely high in this circumstance. Guidelines recommend treatment for SBP >180 mm Hg (mean arterial pressure >130 mm Hg), with the aggressiveness of therapy and monitoring dependent on the degree of elevation and the concern for increased intracranial pressure.[69] With an acute subarachnoid hemorrhage antihypertensive treatment is very generally recommended to decrease SBP <160 mm Hg.[70]
  - ○ **Treatment of HTN to reduce the risk of recurrent stroke or TIA is clearly** indicated.[71-73] The PROGRESS trial demonstrated a reduction in recurrent stroke and all CV events in patients treated with perindopril and indapamide compared to placebo. The degree of reduction was dependent on the degree of BP lowering, which was most notable in the combined therapy patients.[74] Some patients had preexisting HTN and others did not. The same has been shown for indapamide alone.[72] A very large trial found no such difference with telmisartan versus placebo but the degree of achieved BP reduction was very small.[75] Whether the class of drug used is as or more important than the degree of BP lowering has yet to be clearly determined, particularly for combination therapy. Both the JNC 8 and the American Stroke Association (ASA) recommend initiating treatment in patients with a prior stroke or TIA for BP ≥140/90 mm Hg and for a goal BP of <140/90 mm Hg.[4,73]
- **Black patients**
  - ○ HTN is more common, is more severe, and has a higher morbidity in Blacks compared with non-Hispanic Whites.

○ Blacks have lower plasma renin levels, increased plasma volume, and higher peripheral vascular resistance (PVR) compared with non-Black patients.
○ Dietary sodium reduction may be more effective in this population with a greater decrease in BP compared with other demographic groups.[76,77]
○ **The JNC 8 does not make a specific BP target recommendations based solely on race and, therefore, treatment goals are the same as for non-Blacks.**
○ The 2010 International Society on Hypertension in Blacks (ISHIB) Consensus Statement recommends a goal of <135/85 for those with no evidence of end-organ damage, preclinical CVD, or overt CVD. A goal of <130/80 is recommended for Blacks with evidence of end-organ damage, preclinical CVD, or a history of CV events. In this context, end-organ damage was defined as albumin/creatinine ratio >200 mg/g, estimated glomerular filtration rate (eGFR) <60 mL/minute/1.73 m^2, or ECG or echocardiographic evidence of LVH. CV events were defined as HF, CAD, MI, PAD, stroke, TIA, or abdominal aortic aneurysm. Preclinical CVD was defined as metabolic syndrome, Framingham risk >20%, prediabetes, or DM.[28]
○ JNC 8 recommends either a **thiazide diuretic or CCB as first-line therapy** for Blacks, including those with DM.[4,27] ISHIB emphasizes the common necessity of combined therapy in Blacks.[28]
○ **While Blacks in general have less of a BP reduction with ACE inhibitors and ARBs, they can still be very effective, particularly when combined with a diuretic or dihydropyridine CCB.**[7,28] The ACE inhibitor and CCB (rather than thiazide diuretic) combination may be particularly effective at reducing CV outcomes.[78]

• **Older patients**
○ HTN becomes much more common with advancing age (>60), particularly isolated systolic HTN (i.e., SBP >140 and DBP <90). SBP may be a stronger predictor of CV events than DBP.
○ Data from clinical trials clearly support treating HTN in older patients.[21–24,79]
○ In elderly patients **starting with lower doses and titrating slowly** is, in general, reasonable advice. Care should be taken when increasing medications to avoid causing orthostatic hypotension and its symptoms. Following the standing BP may be helpful.[80]
○ When treating isolated systolic HTN it is generally agreed that there is no increased risk in lowering the DBP until it is <60.[7]
○ Thiazide diuretics, long-acting dihydropyridine CCBs, and ACE inhibitors/ARBs are all reasonable choices for initial therapy in older patients.[4]
○ The effectiveness of antihypertensive treatment in frail older patients is unknown.

Specific Drug Classes
• **Thiazide diuretics**
○ Thiazides commonly used for HTN include **hydrochlorothiazide (HCTZ), CTDN,** and indapamide. They are **a reasonable first choice for most patients.**[4]
○ Thiazides block sodium reabsorption at the distal convoluted tubule by inhibition of Na-Cl cotransporter, thereby decreasing plasma volume. Plasma volume, however, stabilizes after 2 to 3 weeks of therapy and partially returns to the pretreatment level. Therefore, the actual mechanism of sustained BP reduction is uncertain but may be due to a decrease in vascular resistance.
○ CTDN is thought to be 1.5 to 2 times more potent than HCTZ and has a much longer half-life.
○ They may be **particularly effective in Blacks and the elderly** who have a greater tendency to be sodium sensitive but are less effective in patients with renal insufficiency (eGFR <30 mL/minute/1.73 m^2). In the latter case, a loop diuretic may be more appropriate.
○ Multiple trials have shown thiazides to be effective in lowering BP, preventing initial and subsequent strokes, and reducing CV mortality.[21,27] These data are largely driven by the

use of CTDN in the ALLHAT trial, while the data supporting a reduction in CV events with HCTZ are minimal.[27]

○ **There is no randomized prospective trial data that specifically and directly compares the effectiveness of CTDN and HCTZ.** A large network meta-analysis indirectly compared the two drugs and found CTDN to be superior in preventing CV events, even when the achieved SBP reduction was the same.[81] Conversely, a large observational cohort did not find a difference in CV outcomes but did demonstrate a greater risk of hypokalemia with CTDN.[82]

○ The results of the ACCOMPLISH Trial indicate that the combination of HCTZ plus benazepril is inferior to amlodipine plus benazepril.[78] Given that many patients require combination therapy to achieve BP goals, these results could call into question the first-line drug of choice status of thiazides, particularly HCTZ, as CTDN was not studied in this trial.

○ Side effects include electrolyte abnormalities (hypokalemia, hypomagnesemia, hypercalcemia, and hyperuricemia), muscle cramps, dyslipidemia, and glucose intolerance. Electrolyte monitoring is warranted during initiation, dosage changes, and occasionally when on stable treatment.

• **Potassium-sparing diuretics**
  ○ **Spironolactone** and **eplerenone** inhibit the action of aldosterone by blocking the mineralocorticoid receptors in the cortical collecting ducts. Eplerenone is far more selective than spironolactone and does not have antiandrogenic or progestogenic effects. Amiloride and triamterene block the epithelial sodium channel and inhibit the reabsorption of sodium and secretion of potassium in the collecting ducts.
  ○ Spironolactone and eplerenone are **specifically indicated for patients with HF and reduced LV function after MI** to improve morbidity and mortality.[55,58,83]
  ○ Patients with **primary hyperaldosteronism** who refuse or are not candidates for surgery can be treated with potassium-sparing diuretics. Spironolactone and eplerenone have the advantage of fully blocking the systemic effects of aldosterone rather than counteracting its effect only in the collecting ducts.
  ○ Potassium-sparing diuretics are sometimes added to thiazides to offset the hypokalemic effect of the latter.
  ○ All potassium-sparing diuretics can cause hyperkalemia and monitoring of potassium and renal function is advisable, particularly in patients with DM and/or CKD. Spironolactone can cause gynecomastia, decreased libido, and impotence in men and mastodynia and amenorrhea in women.

• **Loop diuretics**
  ○ Loop diuretics inhibit sodium resorption by blocking the Na-K-Cl cotransporter in the ascending loop of Henle and include furosemide, bumetanide, torsemide, and ethacrynic acid. Ethacrynic acid does not contain a sulfa moiety and can be used in those with a sulfa allergy.
  ○ Short-acting loop diuretics should not generally be considered antihypertensive agents in patients without CKD.
  ○ **They are appropriate antihypertensives for patients with HTN and eGFR <30 mL/ minute/1.73 m²** because hypervolemia is often an important factor.
  ○ Side effects include electrolyte abnormalities (hypokalemia, hypomagnesemia, hypocalcemia, and hyperuricemia), ototoxicity (less common with oral rather than intravenous), and glucose intolerance.

• **ACE inhibitors**
  ○ Commonly used ACE inhibitors include benazepril, captopril, enalapril, fosinopril, lisinopril, perindopril, quinapril, ramipril, and trandolapril.
  ○ As the name clearly implies, these drugs inhibit ACE leading to a decreased conversion of angiotensin I to angiotensin II, which reduces vasoconstriction, reduces aldosterone secretion, promotes natriuresis, and increases vasodilatory bradykinins.

- ○ ACE inhibitors are **appropriate initial therapy in most patients.**[4]
- ○ ACE inhibitors are considered **first-line therapy in patients with HF or asymptomatic LV dysfunction, prior MI or high risk for CAD, DM, and CKD with moderate-to-severe albuminuria.**[36–38,45–47,51,63,65,84,85]
- ○ They work well in combination with other agents, particularly diuretics, due to the activation of the renin-angiotensin system (RAS). As noted above, however, the results of the ACCOMPLISH Trial indicate that the combination of benazepril plus HCTZ is inferior to benazepril plus amlodipine.[78] CTDN was not studied in this trial.
- ○ While adding an ARB to an ACE inhibitor further reduces proteinuria, data indicate that this may worsen outcome.[66,67]
- ○ ACE inhibitors are **absolutely contraindicated in pregnancy.**
- ○ Side effects include hyperkalemia, orthostatic hypotension, cough, angioedema, and worsening renal function. However, an increase in serum creatinine is expected in most patients and up to 30% is acceptable and not a reason to discontinue therapy.
- **ARBs**
  - ○ The ARBs include candesartan, irbesartan, losartan, olmesartan, telmisartan, and valsartan. These drugs directly block angiotensin II receptors resulting in vasodilation. They do not inhibit the breakdown of bradykinin and are much less likely to cause cough.
  - ○ **ARBs are appropriate as initial therapy in most patients and generally effective in the same clinical settings as an alternative to ACE inhibitors.**[39,40,48,56,57]
  - ○ ARBs **may be specifically beneficial in patients with LVH.**[31]
  - ○ While adding an ARB to an ACE inhibitor further reduces proteinuria, data indicate that combined therapy does not improve CV outcome and may worsen renal outcome.[66,67]
  - ○ ARBs are **absolutely contraindicated in pregnancy.**
  - ○ Side effects are similar to those of ACE inhibitors and include hypotension and a lower incidence of cough and angioedema.
- **Direct renin inhibitors**
  - ○ **Aliskiren** binds the active site of renin and inhibits the conversion of angiotensinogen to angiotensin I and subsequently dramatically reducing the levels of angiotensin II and aldosterone.
  - ○ Aliskiren is effective at lowering BP and has been studied as monotherapy and in combination with other drugs.[86–88]
  - ○ One study showed that the addition of aliskiren to losartan in patients with diabetic nephropathy may further reduce albuminuria.[89] A subsequent randomized controlled trial in a much larger but similar population was terminated early due to a trend toward more stroke, hypotension, hyperkalemia, and a lack of benefit on CV and renal outcomes.[90]
  - ○ At present, there are no long-term studies demonstrating a reduction in long-term hard CV or renal outcomes with aliskiren. It **should not be used as first-line therapy.**
  - ○ Side effects include hyperkalemia, decreased renal function, diarrhea, and cough.
- **Calcium channel blockers**
  - ○ CCBs selectively block the slow inward calcium channels in vascular smooth muscle causing arteriolar vasodilation.
  - ○ Long-acting dihydropyridine CCBs (e.g., amlodipine, felodipine, isradopine, nifedipine) are most commonly used for HTN while the nondihydropyridine CCBs (e.g., verapamil and diltiazem) are used for atrial fibrillation rate control and angina. CCBs are also indicated for coronary vasospasm or Raynaud phenomenon, and supraventricular arrhythmias.
  - ○ **CCBs are appropriate as an initial treatment of HTN in most patients.**[4,27]
  - ○ They may be particularly effective in older patients with isolated systolic HTN and Blacks.[3,27,28]

- As a class, CCBs have no significant effect on glucose tolerance, electrolytes, or lipid profiles and are not adversely affected by NSAIDs.
- Side effects include flushing, headache, dependent edema, gingival hyperplasia, and esophageal reflux.

- **β-Blockers:**
  - β-Blockers competitively inhibit the effects of catecholamines at β receptors to decrease heart rate and cardiac output. Individual drugs have variable selectivity for β_1 and β_2 receptors. β_1 receptors are located mainly in the heart and kidneys. β_2 receptors are found in the lungs, vascular smooth muscle (causing vasodilation), gastrointestinal (GI) tract, uterus, and skeletal muscle. Some β-blockers also have antagonistic effects on α_1 receptors. They also decrease plasma renin and release vasodilatory prostaglandins. The precise mechanism of sustained BP reduction, however, is uncertain.
  - The **nonselective β-blockers** antagonize both β_1 and β_2 receptors and include propranolol, timolol, and nadolol. There is some risk of bronchospasm in patients with chronic obstructive pulmonary disease (COPD) or reactive airway disease. There is a theoretical possibility of hypoglycemia and blunting of the adrenergic response to hypoglycemia.
  - **Cardioselective β-blockers** primarily act on β_1 receptors but lose some selectivity at higher doses. Examples include atenolol, bisoprolol, esmolol, and metoprolol. They seem to have less risk of inducing bronchospasm.
  - Some β-blockers are said to have intrinsic sympathomimetic activity including acebutolol and pindolol. They exert low-level agonist activity while simultaneously antagonizing the site. Acebutolol is β_1-selective and pindolol is nonselective. These drugs may be useful in patients with excessive bradycardia but do not have demonstrated benefit in patients post-MI.
  - The **mixed α- and β-blockers labetalol and carvedilol** have antagonist effects at both types of adrenergic receptors. Both have **vasodilating properties** through α_1-receptor blockade.
  - **Nebivolol** is a new vasodilating β-blocker with and additional unique mechanism of action—potentiating nitric oxide (NO).
  - The vasodilating β-blockers may be preferential to conventional nonselective β-blockers based on the latter being associated with inferior outcomes, an increased rate of stroke, and an increased risk of developing DM.[29] On the other hand, it is important to note that to date **there are no long-term outcome trials of vasodilating β-blockers used solely for the treatment of HTN.**
  - **β-Blockers are no longer considered appropriate first-line agents for patients without compelling indications** (e.g., MI or HF) due to the lack of data supporting an independent positive effect on morbidity and mortality.[4,29,30]
  - **β-Blockers reduce mortality following MI and should be initiated in all patients regardless of left ventricular (LV) function.** β-blockers without intrinsic sympathomimetic activity are preferred. When LV function is impaired (without evidence of unstable HF or shock), β-blockers with proven benefit in HF should be used (i.e., metoprolol, carvedilol, and bisoprolol).[41–43]
  - **β-blockers have been clearly shown to have mortality benefit in HF,** particularly metoprolol, carvedilol, and bisoprolol.[52–54]
  - β-blockers are also indicated for the treatment of tachyarrhythmias and angina.
  - Side effects of β-blockers include fatigue, nausea, dizziness, heart block (especially when used with CCBs), worsening of HF, dyslipidemia, erectile dysfunction, and bronchospasm. Abrupt withdrawal can precipitate angina and elevation of BP because of the increase in adrenergic tone with chronic β-blocker use.

- **α₁-Blockers:**
  - Prazosin, terazosin, and doxazosin block α_1 receptors on vascular smooth muscle cells, impairing catecholamine-induced vasoconstriction.

- ○ α_1-Blockers are less efficacious than thiazides, CCBs, and ACE inhibitors as monotherapy based on the ALLHAT and are **not recommended as first-line therapy.**[27]
- ○ They are characterized by a first-dose effect with a larger decrease in BP than subsequent doses making use before bedtime more appropriate than the morning.
- ○ They may decrease urinary symptoms in patients with prostate enlargement.
- ○ Side effects include orthostatic hypotension, GI distress, and drowsiness.
- **Centrally acting adrenergic agonists**
- ○ Clonidine and methyldopa stimulate α_2 receptors in the central nervous system leading to decreased peripheral sympathetic tone, PVR, heart rate, and cardiac output. Both are effective antihypertensives, but there are **no long-term outcome data** supporting either drug.
- ○ Clonidine can be quite useful for hypertensive urgencies. Refer to the Hypertension Urgencies and Emergencies section.
- ○ **Abrupt cessation can precipitate an acute withdrawal syndrome characterized by tachycardia, diaphoresis, and severe elevations in BP.**
- ○ Methyldopa is safe in pregnancy.
- ○ Side effects include bradycardia, sedation, orthostatic hypotension, depression, and sexual dysfunction. Methyldopa is associated with a lupus-like syndrome.
- **Other sympatholytic agents** such as reserpine, guanethidine, and guanadrel are no longer considered first- or second-line therapy because of their significant side effect profiles and the availability of more effective and much better-tolerated drugs.
- The so-called **direct-acting vasodilators** are hydralazine and minoxidil.
- ○ These agents hyperpolarize arteriolar smooth muscle by activating gated potassium channels to produce direct relaxation and, therefore, vasodilation. Hydralazine requires the presence of NO to be functional and minoxidil contains a NO moiety.
- ○ While these are potentially potent antihypertensive agents, **there are no randomized clinical trials demonstrating improvements in CV morbidity and mortality with either drug when used specifically for HTN.** Because of this, both are second-line therapy. Additionally, they have the potential for more frequent and significant side effects.
- ○ Hydralazine plus nitrate improves mortality in patients with HF compared to placebo.[50] Further evidence indicates that ACE inhibitor therapy is more beneficial than the combination of hydralazine and nitrate in HF patients.[91] In Blacks, the addition of hydralazine and nitrate to standard HF therapy (including RAS blockade and β-blockers) further improves mortality.[92] Whether these effects are ethnically specific is unresolved. **Care should be taken not to conflate these results with the use of hydralazine strictly as an antihypertensive. Additionally, oral nitrates are not appropriate for use as an ongoing BP-lowering agent.**
- ○ Both hydralazine and minoxidil may lead to reflex sympathetic hyperactivity and fluid retention that makes concomitant treatment with a diuretic and/or β-blocker desirable.
- ○ Side effects of hydralazine include headache, tachycardia, orthostatic hypotension, GI distress, and a lupus-like syndrome. Minoxidil can lead to weight gain, hirsutism, hypertrichosis, ECG abnormalities, and pericardial effusions.

Other Nonpharmacologic Therapy

- **Therapeutic lifestyle changes** described in Table 6-5 should be instituted in all patients with HTN and prehypertension.[3,7,19,20] These represent a critical component of both prevention and management of those on drug therapy.
- Therapeutic lifestyle changes may be employed as sole therapy for 6 to 12 months to manage stage 1 HTN in the absence of DM, end-organ damage, evidence of CVD, or multiple other risk factors.[3,7,19]

TABLE 6-5	Lifestyle Modifications to Prevent and Reduce Hypertension	
Modification	Recommendation	SBP reduction (range)
Weight reduction	Maintain normal body weight (body mass index 18.5–24.9 kg/m²)	1 mm Hg/1 kg or 3 mm Hg reduction with a loss of 5% of body weight
DASH dietary pattern	Consume a diet rich in fruits, vegetables, legumes, and low-fat dairy products with a reduced content of saturated and total fat	5–6 mm Hg
Mediterranean dietary pattern	No universal definition; consume a diet higher in fresh fruits, vegetables, whole grains, omega-3–rich fish, nuts; avoid red meat and higher-fat dairy products (e.g., butter); use olive oil; moderate red wine consumption	6–7 mm Hg
Sodium restriction	Reduce dietary sodium intake 1.5–2.4 g/day (3.75–6 g sodium chloride)	2–7 mm Hg
Exercise	Engage in regular moderate-to-vigorous aerobic physical activity such as brisk walking (3–4 sessions/week, about 40 minutes/session)	2–5 mm Hg
Reduce alcohol consumption	Limit consumption to ≤2 drinks (e.g., 24 oz beer, 10 oz wine, or 3 oz 80-proof whiskey) per day for most men and to ≤1 drink/day for women and lighter-weight persons	2–4 mm Hg

DASH, Dietary Approaches to Stop Hypertension.
Modified from Chobanian AV, Bakris GL, Black HR, et al. National High Blood Pressure Education Program Coordinating Committee on Prevention, Detection, Evaluation, and Treatment of High Blood Pressure: the JNC 7 report. *JAMA* 2003;289:2560–72.

- **Weight loss** results in a reduction of SBP on the order of 1 mm Hg/kg. Put another way, a 5% weight loss results in about a 3 mm Hg reduction in SBP.[93–96] Orlistat and sibutramine increase weight loss but the former my increase BP.[93]
- **Exercise:** Moderate- to vigorous-intensity aerobic activity 3 to 4 sessions/week, 40 minutes/session results in a 2 to 5 and 1 to 4 mm Hg reduction in SBP and DBP, respectively, independent of weight loss.[20]
- **Diet**
  - Reducing **sodium** levels decreases BP in some individuals but often enhances the antihypertensive effects of medications. Sodium intake should be restricted to 1.5 to 2.4 g/day (3.75 to 6 g sodium chloride). This degree of restriction may reduce SBP by 2 to 7 mm Hg.[20]
  - The Dietary Approaches to Stop Hypertension (DASH) diet and a Mediterranean diet pattern may be recommended.[20,97] The DASH diet consists of consuming a diet

rich in fruits, vegetables, legumes, and low-fat dairy products with a reduced content of saturated and total fat. Adding sodium limitation to the DASH diet augments BP reduction.[76]

  ○ There is no universal definition of the Mediterranean dietary pattern. In general, it entails consuming a diet higher in fresh fruits, vegetables, whole grains, omega-3–rich fish, nuts, and avoiding red meat and higher-fat dairy products (e.g., butter). Olive oil is the typical fat. It also often includes moderate red wine consumption.

• Cessation of **tobacco smoking** is advised for overall CV health but does not reduce basal BP.

• **Alcohol** intake should be limited to ≤2 drinks/day for men and ≤1 drink/day for women and smaller men. Restricting alcohol to these levels can reduce SBP by 2 to 4 mm Hg.[20] One drink is equivalent to 12 oz beer (350 mL), 5 oz wine (150 mL), or 1.5 oz 80-proof whiskey (45 mL).

• Although relieving stress may improve one's overall health, no studies have successfully demonstrated a link between stress reduction and a sustained reduction in BP.

SPECIAL CONSIDERATIONS

Resistant Hypertension

• Resistant HTN is defined as the **persistent elevation of BP above goal despite the concurrent use of antihypertensive agents from three different classes, including a diuretic.** This also includes BP that is adequately controlled on a four-drug regimen (i.e., controlled resistant HTN).[7,98] SBP is typically harder to control than DBP. Not surprisingly, patients with resistant HTN have worse CV outcomes.

• The term **refractory HTN** refers to those patients who remain uncontrolled despite all maximal medical therapy (prescribed and taken) and lifestyle modification.

• The exact prevalence of resistant HTN is unknown, but clinical trials and surveys suggest that it is a common phenomenon occurring in an estimated 20% to 30% of the population being treated for HTN.[98,99]

• Patient characteristics associated with resistant HTN include higher baseline BP, older age, LVH, CKD, DM, obesity, high sodium intake, female gender, and Black ethnicity.[98–100]

• Resistant HTN should be distinguished from so-called **pseudoresistance,** which may be due to nonadherence to therapy, poor BP measurement technique, white coat HTN, and submaximal/inappropriate medical management.

  ○ Patients should be queried carefully and often about **adherence.** Interventions to improve adherence should be carried out, for example, once-a-day regimens, combination pills, reducing cost, and minimizing troublesome side effects.

  ○ Improper **BP measurement technique** can lead to the false assumption of resistant HTN. Patients should sit quietly for several minutes after arrival before taking the BP and the proper size cuff must always be used. The physician is encouraged to confirm the BP measurements.

  ○ Twenty-four–hour ABPM or patient self-measurement may be necessary to determine which patients have **white coat HTN** (see the "Ambulatory Blood Pressure Monitoring" section). It is reasonable to suspect white coat HTN in patients who report symptoms of orthostasis and those with no evidence of common comorbidities or end-organ damage.

• Potentially modifiable factors that contribute to resistant HTN include obesity, high sodium intake, excess alcohol consumption, physical inactivity, and other drugs (e.g., NSAIDs, oral contraceptives, sympathomimetic compounds, glucocorticoids, cyclosporine, erythropoietin, and some herbal compounds). Lifestyle interventions to reduce weight, sodium, and alcohol and to increase activity should be strongly encouraged (see the "Other Nonpharmacologic Therapy" section).[98–100]

- **Secondary causes** of HTN (Table 6-3) are more common in patients with resistant HTN, particularly OSA, renal parenchymal disease, primary hyperaldosteronism, and renovascular disease. Screening should be based on clinical suspicion. These conditions are discussed in the "Secondary Hypertension" section.

- **Volume (and sodium) expansion** is generally considered to be an important contributing factor in most patients with resistant HTN. **Diuretic therapy should be maximized** (along with sodium intake restriction) and **CTDN is the preferred agent** rather than HCTZ.[81] In those with a eGFR <30 to 50 mL/minute/1.73 m^2, a loop diuretic is necessary—furosemide will need to be dosed at least bid.

- The preferred three-drug regimen is an ACE inhibitor (or ARB) plus a long-acting dihydropyridine CCB plus CTDN, all at maximal doses. β-Blockers should be used when there are specific indications.

- When a three-drug regimen (that includes a diuretic) does not achieve goal BP levels, a mineralocorticoid receptor antagonist is often recommended as the fourth agent. Data suggest that both **spironolactone** (12.5 to 50 mg daily) and **eplerenone** (50 mg daily to bid) can result in significant BP lowering in patients with resistant HTN without primary hyperaldosteronism and regardless of aldosterone level.[101–104] Patients should be monitored for hyperkalemia, particularly those with CKD and DM. Spironolactone, but not the more selective eplerenone, is also associated with gynecomastia and breast pain.

- When additional treatment is necessary, β-blockers, clonidine, hydralazine, and minoxidil are all potential options, but there are no randomized clinical trials to help determine which of these would be best and in what population of patients.

- When β-blockers are used, one of the newer vasodilating agents (i.e., labetalol, carvedilol, or nebivolol) may be preferable possibly due to greater BP lowering and more favorable metabolic effects compared to typical β-blockers.[105,106] There are no long-term outcome trials of vasodilating β-blockers used solely for the treatment of HTN. Also refer to the "Specific Drug Classes" section.

- The use of clonidine, hydralazine, and minoxidil in resistant HTN is largely empirical; all can lower BP but controlled trials demonstrating improved CV outcomes are lacking. Also refer to the "Specific Drug Classes" section.

- Combining two agents that inhibit the RAS (e.g., ACE inhibitor plus ARB or aliskiren) is not recommended due to the lack of improved outcomes and the possibility of more side effects.[66,67,89,90]

- Referral to a **hypertension specialist** is recommended, if BP cannot be controlled after 6 months of treatment or for specific secondary etiologies that may require assistance with diagnosis and treatment.[98]

Secondary Hypertension

- The large majority of patients who are hypertensive have primary HTN. Occasionally, secondary causes are identified, some of which can be cured and others specifically treated. It is possible to have secondary HTN on top of primary HTN.

- Generally speaking secondary HTN should be at least considered in the following situations:
  - Resistant HTN
  - Severe HTN in younger patients, particularly those with end-organ damage
  - Sudden elevations in previously controlled HTN and those who have experienced a hypertensive emergency (see the "Hypertensive Urgencies and Emergencies" section)
  - Persistent, otherwise unexplained, hypokalemia

- The more specific symptoms and signs of various causes of secondary HTN are presented in Table 6-3.

Obstructive Sleep Apnea

- OSA is a fairly common contributor to secondary HTN.[107,108]
- Risk factors for OSA include obesity, enlarged tonsils, macroglossia, and craniofacial abnormalities. Use of sedatives, narcotics, or alcohol can also increase the risk for OSA.
- Common complaints for patients with OSA include daytime sleepiness (including falling asleep with driving), not feeling refreshed upon awakening, awakening snorting or gasping, and poor concentration. Patients may report headaches upon awakening. The patient's bed partner may report witnessing apneic events. In addition, the bed partner may report disruption of their sleep due to the patient's loud snoring.
- The diagnosis is made by polysomnography with an apnea-hypopnea index >5. An index >30 is consistent with severe OSA. More severe OSA is more associated with HTN.
- Use of continuous positive airway pressure (CPAP) is associated with a reduction in BP but it is relatively modest, about –2/2 daytime and –4/2 nighttime.[109] Even this small reduction can be meaningful with regard to reducing CV events.

Renal Parenchymal Disease

- HTN is a major contributor to the development of CKD, but impaired renal function can also elevate BP resulting in a vicious cycle.
- Approximately 80% of patients with CKD have HTN characterized by a combination of sodium retention, activation of the RAS, enhanced sympathetic activity, and impaired endothelium-mediated vasodilation.
- Treatment should stress sodium restriction, use of diuretics, and the use of ACE inhibitors to reduce proteinuria and intraglomerular pressure.

Renovascular Disease

- Renal artery stenosis is an important correctable cause of HTN responsible for up to 10% of patients with severe HTN resistant to multiple medications. It can result from either fibromuscular disease (more common in the young and in women) or atheromatous disease (more common in the elderly with other CV risk factors).
- Critical stenosis of the renal artery leads to increased renin release from the ischemic kidney, which causes both volume expansion and increased PVR.
- Bilateral disease may present as a sudden decline in renal function after use of an ACE inhibitor or ARB. These agents should be avoided if bilateral disease is known.
- Fibromuscular dysplasia should be considered in young patients without family history.
- Commonly evaluated with duplex ultrasonography, magnetic resonance angiography, or computed tomography angiography.
- Angioplasty is typically done for fibromuscular disease. The choice of treatment for atherosclerotic disease can be quite challenging; both angioplasty with stenting and surgical revascularization are possible. Some patients will have an excellent BP response, some will have minimal effect, and others will have deterioration of renal function. Unilateral disease is more likely to benefit from revascularization.
- Medical treatment to control BP is indicated in all patients and ACE inhibitors or ARBs should be used if tolerated and the patient carefully monitored.

Primary Hyperaldosteronism

- Primary hyperaldosteronism is usually caused by a unilateral adrenal adenoma or bilateral adrenal hyperplasia, rarely adrenocortical carcinoma and familial syndromes.
- It can be difficult to distinguish based on clinical symptoms but should be considered in the presence of unexplained hypokalemia and metabolic alkalosis, especially if the patient is also on an ACE or ARB. However, about half of patients do not have hypokalemia.
- The initial screening test in appropriate patients is the plasma aldosterone concentration (PAC) to plasma renin activity (PRA) ratio. PAC is high and the PRA is very low,

increasing the ratio. If the ratio is <20, the diagnosis of primary hyperaldosteronism is excluded, whereas a ratio of >50 makes the diagnosis very likely. Confirmation is a salt suppression test (oral salt load ×3 days, followed by measurement of 24-hour urinary aldosterone). All drugs that interfere with the renin-angiotensin-aldosterone axis should be discontinued. Inappropriately high aldosterone excretion (>12 μg/day) with Na >200 mEq/day confirms the diagnosis.

- CT or MRI of the adrenal glands can help distinguish between the subtypes when the disease is confirmed. Adrenal vein sampling is sometimes necessary to determine laterality.
- Treatment includes surgical resection of a single adenoma or mineralocorticoid antagonists.

Pregnancy

- A complete discussion of HTN in pregnancy is beyond this scope of this book and will not be undertaken. Most of these patients will be cared for by an obstetrician or a maternal-fetal medicine subspecialist.
- Pregnancy-associated HTN may be preexisting primary HTN. Gestational HTN is defined as new onset BP ≥140/90 developing after 20 weeks' gestation. Preeclampsia is diagnosed when patients also have proteinuria or certain end-organ damage (e.g., thrombocytopenia, elevated creatinine, pulmonary edema, cerebral or visual symptoms, elevated transaminases). Preeclampsia may be superimposed on chronic primary HTN. Eclampsia is only diagnosed when a seizure has occurred. Severe gestational HTN is defined as BP ≥160/110.[110]
- The decision to treat HTN in pregnancy must be individualized and is based on multiple factors, including maternal condition, degree of BP elevation, the presence of end-organ damage, and fetal viability.
- Mild to moderate gestational HTN is generally followed carefully without medications.[110] Those with severe gestational HTN (≥160/110) may be treated with medications and are usually delivered preterm.
- Management of preeclampsia is more complex and may involve medical management and/or early delivery, sometimes before viability in those with severe preeclampsia.
- **Methyldopa** has proven safety and modest effectiveness. Other common and safe options include **labetalol** and long-acting **nifedipine. Hydralazine** is often used in the acute setting.
- ACE inhibitors and ARBs are contraindicated in pregnancy.

Hypertensive Urgencies and Emergencies

- **Hypertensive urgency,** also known as severe asymptomatic HTN, is BP usually ≥180/110 mm Hg and the **absence of end-organ damage.** There is, in fact, no absolute BP level above which an urgency can be declared for all patients. Patients with chronic severe elevations are a fairly low acute risk for poor outcomes. More rapid elevations are associated with increased risk.[7]
- **Hypertensive emergency** (crisis) is usually associated with a BP ≥180/120 mm Hg and is typified by the **presence of end-organ damage** (e.g., retinopathy, encephalopathy, cerebral hemorrhage, myocardial ischemia, HF, AKI, aortic dissection, microangiopathic hemolytic anemia, and preeclampsia).[7]
- Hypertensive encephalopathy signifies a loss of cerebrovascular autoregulation and the resultant neurologic manifestations (e.g., delirium, headache, visual disturbance, and seizures).
- The historic term malignant HTN referred to patients with papilledema, retinal exudates, and hemorrhages, and variable renal involvement, who, at the time, had a very poor prognosis because of the lack of effective treatments.
- Hypertensive urgencies and emergencies are usually due to primary HTN, but may be related to secondary causes of HTN, drugs, pregnancy, and central nervous system

disorders (e.g., head trauma). Medication nonadherence may be an important contributing factor in some patients.

- When evaluating patients with new (or apparently new) severe BP elevations, the physician should recheck the BP using the best possible technique. Repeating again after the patient has simply rested quietly for approximately a half hour can result in a significant decrease in BP to below a severe level.

- Patients should be carefully questioned about medications, adherence, use of drugs and/or elicit substances, and CV, pulmonary, neurologic, and renal symptoms. These areas should be examined and a funduscopic exam performed. The history and physical may rapidly uncover evidence of end-organ damage and in others laboratory testing may be necessary (e.g., renal function, urinalysis, ECG, CXR).

- **Hypertensive emergencies should be managed in the emergency department or in-patient setting.** Relatively prompt but modest reductions in BP (e.g., no more than 10% to 20% in the first hour) are indicated and can be achieved with various medications, including labetalol, nitroprusside, nitroglycerine, hydralazine, and fenoldopam. Management needs to individualized based on the nature of the emergency. The management of HTN in acute stroke is very briefly discussed above in the "Specific Patient Populations" section.

- Hypertensive urgencies are sometimes managed in the out-patient setting. Rapid BP lowering is generally not indicated. Patients on chronic antihypertensive therapy who have been nonadherent may be instructed to resume their medications. If the patient is felt to be at increased risk for acute complications due to the BP elevation, relatively fast-acting oral medications may be given to lower BP over a few hours. A reasonable short-term goal is approximately BP ≤160/100 mm Hg; however, there is no controlled trial data to support this or any other specific goal BP. What is clear is that **rapid reductions to a normal BP are unnecessary and can result in myocardial and cerebral ischemia.**

- Possible oral agents for reducing BP over a few hours include:[7]
  - Clonidine 0.1 to 0.2 mg PO.
  - Captopril 6.25 to 12.5 mg PO.
  - Labetalol 100 to 200 mg PO.
  - All can be repeated if necessary.
  - **Short-acting CCBs, particularly sublingual nifedipine, should not be used in typical medical patients** due to the risk of sudden drops in BP, reflex tachycardia, and myocardial ischemia.

- Patients with hypertensive urgency should be followed closely and started on an oral regimen appropriate for long-term management. If the patient has been nonadherent to a previously effective regimen, it should be resumed. If the patient is currently taking a regimen then it should be adjusted (e.g., doses maximized or additional agents added). And if the patient has not been previously prescribed antihypertensive treatment then medication should be started and it may be reasonable to start two medications.

REFERENCES

1. Lewington S, Clarke R, Qizilibash N, et al. Age-specific relevance of usual blood pressure to vascular mortality: a meta-analysis of individual data for one million adults in 61 prospective studies. *Lancet* 2002;360:1903–1913.

2. Centers for Disease Control and Prevention (CDC). Vital signs: awareness and treatment of uncontrolled hypertension among adults—United States, 2003–2010. *MMWR Morb Mortal Wkly Rep* 2012;61:703–709.

3. Chobanian AV, Bakris GL, Black HR, et al. National High Blood Pressure Education Program Coordinating Committee on Prevention, Detection, Evaluation,

and Treatment of High Blood Pressure: the JNC 7 report. *JAMA* 2003;289: 2560–2572.

4. James PA, Oparil S, Carter BL, et al. 2014 Evidence-based guideline for the management of high blood pressure in adults: report from the panel members appointed to the Eighth Joint National Committee (JNC 8). *JAMA* 2014;311:507–520.

5. Julius S, Nesbitt SD, Egan BM, et al.; Trial of Preventing Hypertension Study Investigators. Feasibility of treating prehypertension with an angiotensin-receptor blocker. *N Engl J Med* 2006;354:1685–1697.

6. Wolff T, Miller T. Evidence for the reaffirmation of the U.S. Preventive Services Task Force recommendation on screening for high blood pressure. *Ann Intern Med* 2007;147:787–791.

7. U.S. Department of Health and Human Services. National Institutes of Health. Nation Heart Lung, and Blood Institute. Complete Report. The Seventh Report of the Joint National Committee on Prevention, Detection, Evaluation, and Treatment of High Blood Pressure. NIH Publication No. 04–5230. Available at: http://www.nhlbi. nih.gov/health-pro/guidelines/current/hypertension-jnc-7/complete-report.htm. Last accessed 1/21/15.

8. Reeves RA. The rational clinical examinations. Does this patient have hypertension? How to measure blood pressure. *JAMA* 1995;273:1211–1218.

9. Dolan E, Stanton A, Hisjs L, et al. Superiority of ambulatory over clinic blood pressure measurement in predicting mortality: the Dublin outcome study. *Hypertension* 2005;46:156–161.

10. Pierdomenico SD, Cuccurullo F. Prognostic value of white-coat and masked hypertension diagnosed by ambulatory monitoring in initially untreated subjects: an updated meta analysis. *Am J Hypertens* 2011;24:52–58.

11. Pickering TG, Shimbo D, Haas D. Ambulatory blood pressure monitoring. *N Engl J Med* 2006;354:2368–2374.

12. Fagard RH, Cornelissen VA. Incidence of cardiovascular events in white-coat, masked and sustained hypertension versus true normotension: a meta-analysis. *J Hypertens* 2007;25:2193–2198.

13. Boggia J, Li Y, Thijs L, et al. Prognostic accuracy of day versus night ambulatory blood pressure: a cohort study. *Lancet* 2007;370:1219–1229.

14. Fan HQ, Li Y, Thijs L, et al. Prognostic value of isolated nocturnal hypertension on ambulatory measurement in 8711 individuals from 10 populations. *J Hypertens* 2010;28:2036–2045.

15. Pickering TG, Miller NH, Ogedegbe G, et al. Call to action on use and reimbursement for home blood pressure monitoring: executive summary. *Hypertension* 2008;52:1–9.

16. Gerstein HC, Mann JF, Zinman B, et al.; HOPE Study Investigators. Albuminuria and risk of cardiovascular events, death, and heart failure in diabetic and nondiabetic individuals. *JAMA* 2001;286:421–426.

17. Hillege HL, Fidler V, Diercks GF, et al.; Prevention of Renal and Vascular End Stage Diseased (PREVEND) Study Group. Urinary albumin excretion predicts cardiovascular and noncardiovascular mortality in general population. *Circulation* 2002;106:1777–1782.

18. Wachtell K, Ibsen H, Olsen MH, et al. Albuminuria and cardiovascular risk in hypertensive patients with left ventricular hypertrophy: the LIFE Study. *Ann Intern Med* 2003;139:901–906.

19. Elmer PJ, Obarzanek E, Vollmer WM, et al. Effects of comprehensive lifestyle modification on diet, weight, physical fitness, and blood pressure control: 18-month results of a randomized trial. *Ann Intern Med* 2006;144:485–495.

20. Eckel RH, Jakicic JM, Ard JD, et al. 2013 AHA/ACC guideline on lifestyle management to reduce cardiovascular risk. *Circulation* 2014;129:S76–S99.

21. SHEP Cooperative Research Group. Prevention of stroke by antihypertensive drug treatment in older persons with isolated systolic hypertension. Final results of the Systolic Hypertension in the Elderly Program (SHEP). *JAMA* 1991;265: 3255–3264.
22. Staessen JA, Fagard R, Thijs L, et al. Randomised double-blind comparison of placebo and active treatment for older patients with isolated systolic hypertension. The Systolic Hypertension in Europe (Syst-Eur) Trial Investigators. *Lancet* 1997;350:757–764.
23. Perry HM Jr, Davis BR, Price TR, et al. Effect of treating isolated systolic hypertension on the risk of developing various types and subtypes of stroke: the Systolic Hypertension in the Elderly Program (SHEP). *JAMA* 2000;284:465–471.
24. Beckett NS, Peters R, Fletcher AE, et al.; for the HYVET Study Group. Treatment of hypertension in patients 80 years of age or older. *N Engl J Med* 2008;358:1887–1898.
25. Turnbull F, Neal B, Ninomiya T, et al. Effects of different regimens to lower blood pressure on major cardiovascular events in older and younger adults: meta-analysis of randomised trials. *BMJ* 2008;336:1121–1123.
26. Law MR, Morris JK, Wald NJ. Use of blood pressure lowering drugs in the prevention of cardiovascular disease: meta-analysis of 147 randomised trials in the context of expectations from prospective epidemiological studies. *BMJ* 2009;338:b1665.
27. The ALLHAT Officers and Coordinators for the ALLHAT Collaborative Research Group. Major outcomes in high-risk hypertensive patients randomized to angiotensin-converting enzyme inhibitor or calcium channel blocker vs diuretic: The Antihypertensive and Lipid-Lowering Treatment to Prevent Heart Attack Trial (ALLHAT). *JAMA* 2002;288:2981–2997.
28. Flack JM, Sica DA, Bakris G, et al. Management of high blood pressure in blacks: an update of the International Society on Hypertension in Blacks consensus statement. *Hypertension* 2010;56:780–800.
29. Lindholm LH, Carlberg B, Samuelsson O. Should beta blockers remain first choice in the treatment of primary hypertension? A meta-analysis. *Lancet* 2005;366:1545–1553.
30. Wiysonge CS, Bradley HA, Volmink J, et al. Beta-blockers for hypertension. *Cochrane Database Syst Rev* 2012;(11):CD002003.
31. Dahlof B, Devereux RB, Kjeldsen SE, et al. Cardiovascular morbidity and mortality in the Losartan Intervention For Endpoint Reduction in Hypertension Study (LIFE): a randomised trial against atenolol. *Lancet* 2002;359:995–1003.
32. Materson BJ, Reda DJ, Preston RA, et al. Response to a second single antihypertensive agent used as monotherapy for hypertension after failure of the initial drug. Department of Veterans Affairs Cooperative Study Group on Antihypertensive Agents. *Arch Intern Med* 1995;155:1757–1762.
33. Materson BJ, Reda DJ, Cushman WC, et al. Single-drug therapy for hypertension in men. A comparison of six antihypertensive agents with placebo. The Department of Veterans Affairs Cooperative Study Group on Antihypertensive Agents. *N Engl J Med* 1993;328:914–921.
34. Neaton JD, Grimm RH Jr, Prineas RJ, et al. Treatment of Mild Hypertension Study. Final results Treatment of Mild Hypertension Study Research Group. *JAMA* 1993;270:713–724.
35. American Diabetes Association. Standards of medical care in diabetes—2014. *Diabetes Care* 2014;37:S14–S80.
36. UKPDS 39. Efficacy of atenolol and captopril in reducing risk of macrovascular and microvascular complications in type 2 diabetes: UKPDS 39. UK Prospective Diabetes Study Group. *BMJ* 1998;317:713–720.
37. Lewis EJ, Hunsicker LG, Bain RP, et al.; The Collaborative Study Group. The effect of angiotensin-converting enzyme inhibition on diabetic nephropathy. *N Engl J Med* 1993;329:1456–1462.

38. Laffel LM, McGill JB, Gans DJ; North American Microalbuminuria Study Group. The beneficial effect of angiotensin-converting enzyme inhibition with captopril on diabetic nephropathy in normotensive IDDM patients with microalbuminuria. *Am J Med* 1995;99:497–504.

39. Lewis EJ, Hunsicker LG, Clarke WR, et al.; for the Collaborative Study Group. Renoprotective effect of the angiotensin-receptor antagonist irbesartan in patients with nephropathy due to type 2 diabetes. *N Engl J Med* 2001;345:851–860.

40. Brenner BM, Cooper ME, de Zeeuw D, et al.; RENAAL Study Investigators. Effects of losartan on renal and cardiovascular outcomes in patients with type 2 diabetes and nephropathy. *N Engl J Med* 2001;345:861–869.

41. Amsterdam EA, Wenger NK, Brindis RG, et al. 2014 AHA/ACC guideline for the management of patients with non-ST-elevation acute coronary syndromes. *Circulation* 2014;130:e344–e426.

42. O'Gara PT, Kushner FG, Ascheim DD, et al. 2013 ACCF/AHA guideline for the management of ST-elevation myocardial infarction. *Circulation* 2013;127: e362–e425.

43. Freemantle N, Cleland J, Young P, et al. Beta blockade after myocardial infarction: systematic review and meta regression analysis. *BMJ* 1999;318:1730–1737.

44. The Capricorn Investigators. Effect of carvedilol on outcome after myocardial infarction in patients with left-ventricular dysfunction: The CAPRICORN randomised trial. *Lancet* 2001;357:1385–1390.

45. Pfeffer MA, Braunwald E, Moye LA, et al. Effect of captopril on mortality and morbidity in patients with left ventricular dysfunction after myocardial infarction. Results of the Survival and Ventricular Enlargement Trial. The SAVE Investigators. *N Engl J Med* 1992;327:669–677.

46. The Acute Infarction Ramipril Efficacy (AIRE) Study Investigators. Effect of ramipril on mortality and morbidity of survivors of acute myocardial infarction with clinical evidence of heart failure. *Lancet* 1993;342:821–828.

47. Køber L, Torp-Pedersen C, Carlsen JE, et al. A clinical trial of the angiotensin-converting-enzyme inhibitor trandolapril in patients with left ventricular dysfunction after myocardial infarction. Trandolapril Cardiac Evaluation (TRACE) Study Group. *N Engl J Med* 1995;333:1670–1676.

48. Pfeffer MA, McMurray JJ, Velazquez EF, et al. Valsartan, captopril, or both in myocardial infarction complicated by heart failure, left ventricular dysfunction, or both. *N Engl J Med* 2003;349:1893–1906.

49. The European Trial on Reduction of Cardiac Events with Perindopril in Stable Coronary Artery Disease Investigators. Efficacy of perindopril in reduction of cardiovascular events among patients with stable coronary artery disease: randomised, double-blind, placebo-controlled, multicentre trial (the EUROPA Study). *Lancet* 2003;362:782–788.

50. V-HeFT II, Cohn JN, Archibald DG, Ziesche S, et al. Effect of vasodilator therapy on mortality in chronic congestive heart failure. Results of a Veterans Administration Cooperative Study. *N Engl J Med* 1986;314:1547–1552.

51. The SOLVD Investigators. Effect of enalapril on survival in patients with reduced left ventricular ejection fractions and congestive heart failure. *N Engl J Med* 1991;325:293–302.

52. CIBIS Investigators and Committees. A randomized trial of beta-blockade in heart failure. The Cardiac Insufficiency Bisoprolol Study (CIBIS). *Circulation* 1994;90:1765–1773.

53. MERIT-HF Study Group. Effect of metoprolol CR/XL in chronic heart failure: Metoprolol CR/XL Randomised Intervention Trial in Congestive Heart Failure (MERIT-HF). *Lancet* 1999;353:2001–2007.

54. Packer M, Coats AJ, Fowler MB, et al. Effect of carvedilol on survival in severe chronic heart failure. *N Engl J Med* 2001;344:1651–1658.

55. Pitt B, Zannad F, Remme WJ, et al. The effect of spironolactone on morbidity and mortality in patients with severe heart failure. Randomized Aldactone Evaluation Study (RALES) Investigators. *N Engl J Med* 1999;341:709–717.

56. Cohn JN, Tognoni G. A randomized trial of the angiotensin-receptor blocker valsartan in chronic heart failure. The Valsartan Heart Failure Trial Investigators. *N Engl J Med* 2001;345:1667–1675.

57. Granger CB, McMurray JJ, Yusuf S, et al. Effects of candesartan in patients with chronic heart failure and reduced left-ventricular systolic function intolerant to angiotensin-converting-enzyme inhibitors: the CHARM-Alternative trial. *Lancet* 2003;362:772–776.

58. Zannad F, McMurray JJ, Krum H, et al.; EMPHASIS-HF Study Group. Eplerenone in patients with systolic heart failure and mild symptoms. *N Engl J Med* 2011;364:11–21.

59. McMurray JJ, Ostergren J, Swedberg K, et al. Effects of candesartan in patients with chronic heart failure and reduced left-ventricular systolic function taking angiotensin-converting-enzyme inhibitors: the CHARM-Added trial. *Lancet* 2003;362:767–771.

60. Phillips CO, Kashani A, Ko DK, et al. Adverse effects of combination angiotensin II receptor blockers plus angiotensin-converting enzyme inhibitors for left ventricular dysfunction: a quantitative review of data from randomized clinical trials. *Arch Intern Med* 2007;167:1930–1936.

61. Kidney Disease: Improving Global Outcomes (KDIGO) Blood Pressure Work Group. KDIGO clinical practice guideline for the management of blood pressure in chronic kidney disease. *Kidney Int Suppl* 2012;2:337–414.

62. Taler SJ, Agrawal R, Bakris GL, et al. KDOQI US commentary on the 2012 KDIGO clinical practice guideline for management of blood pressure in CKD. *Am J Kidney Dis* 2013;62:201–213.

63. Randomised placebo-controlled trial of effect of ramipril on decline in glomerular filtration rate and risk of terminal renal failure in proteinuric, non-diabetic nephropathy. The GISEN Group (Gruppo Italiano di Studi Epidemiologici in Nefrologia). *Lancet* 1997;349:1857–1863.

64. Wright JT Jr, Bakris G, Greene T, et al. Effect of blood pressure lowering and antihypertensive drug class on progression of hypertensive kidney disease: results from the AASK trial. *JAMA* 2002;288:2421–2431.

65. Fink AH, Ishani A, Taylor BC, et al. Screening for, monitoring, and treatment of chronic kidney disease stages 1 to 3: a systematic review for the U.S. Preventive Services Task Force and for an American College of Physicians Clinical Practice Guideline. *Ann Intern Med* 2012;156:570–581.

66. Mann JF, Schmieder RE, McQueen M, et al.; ONTARGET Investigators. Renal outcomes with telmisartan, ramipril, or both, in people at high vascular risk (the ONTARGET study): a multicentre, randomised, double-blind, controlled trial. *Lancet* 2008;372:547–553.

67. Yusuf S, Teo KK, Pogue J, et al.; ONTARGET Investigators. Telmisartan, ramipril, or both in patients at high risk for vascular events. *N Engl J Med* 2008;358:1547–1559.

68. Jauch EC, Saver JL, Adams HP Jr, et al. Guidelines for the early management of patients with acute ischemic stroke. *Stroke* 2013;44:870–947.

69. Morgenstern LB, Hemphill JC III, Anderson C, et al. Guidelines for the management of spontaneous intracerebral hemorrhage. *Stroke* 2010;41:2108–2129.

70. Connolly ES Jr, Rabinstein AA, Carhuapoma JR, et al. Guidelines for the management of aneurysmal subarachnoid hemorrhage. *Stroke* 2012;43:1711–1737.

71. Arima H, Chalmers J. PROGRESS: prevention of recurrent stroke. *J Clin Hypertens (Greenwich)* 2001;13:693–702.

72. Liu L, Wang Z, Gong L, et al. Blood pressure reduction for the secondary prevention of stroke: a Chinese trial and a systematic review of the literature. *Hypertens Res* 2009;32:1032–1040.

73. Kernan WN, Ovbiagele B, Black HR. Guidelines for the prevention of stroke in patients with stroke and transient ischemic attack. *Stroke* 2014;45:2160–2236.

74. PROGRESS Collaborative Group. Randomised trial of a perindopril-based blood-pressure-lowering regimen among 6,105 individuals with previous stroke or transient ischaemic attack. *Lancet* 2001;358:1033–1041.

75. Yusuf S, Diener HC, Sacco RL, et al. Telmisartan to prevent recurrent stroke and cardiovascular events. *N Engl J Med* 2008;359:1225–1237.

76. Sacks FM, Svetkey LP, Vollmer WM, et al. Effects on blood pressure of reduced dietary sodium and the Dietary Approaches to Stop Hypertension (DASH) diet. DASH-Sodium Collaborative Research Group. *N Engl J Med* 2001;344:3–10.

77. He FJ, Li J, Macgregor GA. Effect of longer term modest salt reduction on blood pressure: Cochrane systematic review and meta-analysis of randomised trials. *BMJ* 2013;346:f1325.

78. Jamerson K, Weber MA, Bakris GL, et al.; ACCOMPLISH Trial Investigators. Benazepril plus amlodipine or hydrochlorothiazide for hypertension in high-risk patients. *N Engl J Med* 2008;359:2417–2428.

79. MRC Working Party; Medical Research Council trial of treatment of hypertension in older adults: principal results. *BMJ* 1992;304:405–412.

80. Aronow WS, Fleg JL, Pepine CJ, et al. ACCF/AHA 2011 expert consensus document on hypertension in the elderly. *Circulation* 2011;123:2434–2506.

81. Roush GC, Holford TR, Guddati AK. Chlorthalidone compared with hydrochlorothiazide in reducing cardiovascular events: systematic review and network meta-analyses. *Hypertension* 2012;59:1110–1117.

82. Dhalla IA, Gomes T, Yao Z, et al. Chlorthalidone versus hydrochlorothiazide for the treatment of hypertension in older adults: a population-based cohort study. *Ann Intern Med* 2013;158:447–455.

83. Pitt B, Remme W, Zannad F, et al.; Eplerenone Post-Acute Myocardial Infarction Heart Failure Efficacy and Survival Study (EPHESUS) Investigators. Eplerenone, a selective aldosterone blocker, in patients with left ventricular dysfunction after myocardial infarction. *N Engl J Med* 2003;348:1309–1321.

84. Yusuf S, Sleight P, Pogue J, et al.; Heart Outcomes Prevention Evaluation (HOPE) Study Investigators. Effects of an angiotensin-converting enzyme inhibitor, ramipril, on cardiovascular events in high-risk patients. *N Engl J Med* 2000;342:145–153.

85. Pepine C, Handberg E, Cooper-DeHoff R, et al.; INVEST Investigators. A calcium antagonist vs a noncalcium antagonist hypertension treatment strategy for patients with coronary artery disease. The International Verapamil-Trandolapril Study (INVEST): a randomized controlled trial. *JAMA* 2003;290:2805–2816.

86. Grandman AH, Schmieder RE, Lins RL, et al. Aliskiren, a novel orally effective renin inhibitor, provides dose-dependent antihypertensive efficacy and placebo-like tolerability in hypertensive patients. *Circulation* 2005;111:1012–1018.

87. Schmieder RE, Philipp T, Guerediaga J, et al. Long-term antihypertensive efficacy and safety of the oral direct renin inhibitor aliskiren: a 12-month randomized, double-blind comparator trial with hydrochlorothiazide. *Circulation* 2009;119:417–425.

88. Brown MJ, McInnes GT, Papst CC, et al. Aliskiren and the calcium channel blocker amlodipine combination as an initial treatment strategy for hypertension control (ACCELERATE): a randomised, parallel-group trial. *Lancet* 2011;377:312–320.

89. Parving HH, Persson F, Lewsi JB, et al.; AVOID Study Investigators. Aliskiren combined with losartan in type 2 diabetes and nephropathy. *N Engl J Med* 2008;358:2433–2446.

90. Parving HH, Brenner BM, McMurray JJ, et al.; ALTITUDE Investigators. Cardiorenal end points in a trial of aliskiren for type 2 diabetes. *N Engl J Med* 2012;367:2204–2213.
91. Cohn JN, Johnson G, Ziesche S, et al. A comparison of enalapril with hydralazine-isosorbide dinitrate in the treatment of chronic congestive heart failure. *N Engl J Med* 1991;325:303–310.
92. Taylor AL, Ziesche S, Yancy C, et al.; A-HeFT Investigators. Combination of isosorbide dinitrate and hydralazine in blacks with heart failure. *N Engl J Med* 2004;351:2049–2057.
93. Horvath K, Jeitler K, Siering U, et al. Long-term effects of weight-reducing interventions in hypertensive patients: systematic review and meta-analysis. *Arch Intern Med* 2008;168:571–580.
94. Aucott L, Rothnie H, McIntyre L, et al. Long-term weight loss from lifestyle intervention benefits blood pressure?: a systematic review. *Hypertension* 2009;54:756–762.
95. Siebenhofer A, Jeitler K, Berghold A, et al. Long-term effects of weight-reducing diets in hypertensive patients. *Cochrane Database Syst Rev* 2011;(9):CD008274.
96. Jensen MD, Ryan DH, Apovian CM, et al. 2013 AHA/ACC/TOS guideline for the management of overweight and obesity in adults: a report of the American College of Cardiology/American Heart Association Task Force on Practice Guidelines and The Obesity Society. *Circulation* 2014;129:S102–S138.
97. Appel LJ, Moore TJ, Obarzanek E, et al. A clinical trial of the effects of dietary patterns on blood pressure. DASH Collaborative Research Group. *N Engl J Med* 1997;336:1117–1124.
98. Calhoun DA, Jones D, Textor S, et al. Resistant hypertension: diagnosis, evaluation, and treatment. A Scientific Statement from the American Heart Association Professional Education Committee of the Council for High Blood Pressure Research. *Circulation* 2008;117:e510–e526.
99. Vongpatanasin W. Resistant hypertension: a review of diagnosis and management. *JAMA* 2014;311:2216–2224.
100. Myat A, Redwood SR, Qureshi AC, et al. Resistant hypertension. *BMJ* 2012;345:e7473.
101. White WB, Carr AA, Krause S, et al. Assessment of the novel selective aldosterone blocker eplerenone using ambulatory and clinical blood pressure in patients with systemic hypertension. *Am J Cardiol* 2003;92:38–42.
102. Chapman N, Dobson J, Wilson S, et al.; ASCOT Investigators. Effect of spironolactone on blood pressure in subjects with resistant hypertension. *Hypertension* 2007;49:839–845.
103. Václavík J, Sedlák R, Plachy M, et al. Addition of spironolactone in patients with resistant arterial Hypertension (ASPIRANT): a randomized, double-blind, placebo-controlled trial. *Hypertension* 2011;57:1069–1075.
104. Oxlund CS, Henriksen JE, Tarnow L, et al. Low dose spironolactone reduces blood pressure in patients with resistant hypertension and type 2 diabetes mellitus: a double blind randomized clinical trial. *J Hypertens* 2013;31:2094–2102.
105. Gress TW, Nieto FJ, Shahar E, et al. Hypertension and antihypertensive therapy as risk factors for type 2 diabetes mellitus. Atherosclerosis Risk in Communities Study. *N Engl J Med* 2000;342:905–912.
106. Bakris GL, Fonseca V, Katholi RE, et al.; GEMINI Investigators. Metabolic effects of carvedilol vs metoprolol in patients with type 2 diabetes mellitus and hypertension: a randomized controlled trial. *JAMA* 2004;292:2227–2236.
107. Nieto FJ, Young TB, Lind BK, et al. Association of sleep-disordered breathing, sleep apnea, and hypertension in a large community-based study. Sleep Heart Health Study. *JAMA* 2000;283:1829–1836.

108. Marin JM, Agusti A, Villar I, et al. Association between treated and untreated obstructive sleep apnea and risk of hypertension. *JAMA* 2012;307:2169–2176.
109. Fava C, Dorigoni S, Dalle Vedove F, et al. Effect of CPAP on blood pressure in patients with OSA/hypopnea a systematic review and meta-analysis. *Chest* 2014;145:762–771.
110. American College of Obstetricians and Gynecologists. Task force on hypertension in pregnancy. Hypertension in pregnancy. *Obstet Gynecol* 2013;122:1122–1131.

Ischemic Heart Disease

Jayendrakumar S. Patel, Sandeep S. Sodhi,
Anuradha Godishala, and Mohammad A. Kizilbash

GENERAL PRINCIPLES

Epidemiology

- Ischemic heart disease (IHD) is the cause of 1 of every 6 deaths in the United States.[1]
- More than 1 million Americans experience a myocardial infarction (MI) each year.
- IHD does not always produce symptoms; 64% of women and 50% of men who die suddenly from IHD had no previous symptoms.
- After age 40, 49% of men and 32% of women will have an MI during the remainder of their lifetime.[1]

Risk Factors

- **Greater than 90% of patients experiencing acute coronary syndrome (ACS) will have at least one established coronary artery disease (CAD) risk factor.**[2]
- Traditionally, **major cardiovascular risk factors** have been defined as the following[3]:
  - Increased age
  - Diabetes (DM)
  - Hypertension (HTN)
  - Cigarette smoking
  - Elevated low-density lipoprotein (LDL) cholesterol
  - Low high-density lipoprotein (HDL) cholesterol
  - Family history of premature CAD, defined as first-degree male relative with an MI before age 55 or female relative before age 65
- **Risk equivalents for coronary heart disease**: Patients with known coronary heart disease (CHD) have a 20% or higher risk for a subsequent CHD event; similarly, some patients without established CHD may also be at high risk if they have[3,4]:
  - Diabetes mellitus (DM)
  - Peripheral arterial disease (PAD) or presence of an aortic aneurysm
  - Prior cerebrovascular accident (CVA) or transient ischemic attack (TIA)
  - Chronic kidney disease (CKD)
  - A high global risk score for CHD or cardiovascular disease (CVD)
- Other **less potent coronary heart disease risk factors**[5]:
  - Obesity, particularly central obesity
  - Physical inactivity
  - High-fat, high-cholesterol diet
  - Systemic autoimmune collagen vascular diseases
  - In women, history of preeclampsia or gestational diabetes
- **Novel cardiac risk factors**
  - **C-reactive protein** (CRP), as compared to other novel CVD risk factors, has gained more acceptance in its role in primary prevention. It is widely available, easily attained, and more often covered by health insurance carriers than other risk biomarkers or indirect measures of atherosclerosis, such as coronary calcium scoring.
    - CRP levels can be affected by various conditions (Table 7-1).[6]
    - CRP is a component of the Reynolds score, which is one of the available risk calculators for CVD events.

TABLE 7-1	Variables Associated with CRP Concentration

Increased levels of CRP	Decreased levels of CRP
Elevated blood pressure	Moderate alcohol consumption
Elevated body mass index	Increased activity/endurance exercise
Cigarette smoking	Weight loss
Metabolic syndrome/diabetes mellitus	Statin drug therapy
Low HDL/high triglycerides	Fibrate drug therapy
Estrogen/progesterone use	Niacin drug therapy
Chronic infections (e.g., gingivitis, bronchitis)	
Chronic inflammation (e.g., rheumatoid arthritis)	

CRP, C-reactive protein; HDL, high-density lipoprotein cholesterol.
Modified from Pearson TA, Mensah GA, Alexander RW, et al. Markers of inflammation and cardiovascular disease: application to clinical and public health practice. *Circulation* 2003;107:499–511.

- CRP has also been studied as part of a protocol to determine patient eligibility for statin therapy, which could supplement or supplant the traditional methods discussed such as the global risk score discussed in the Prevention section. Statin therapy can be considered in men older than 50 years and women older than 60 years with LDL <130 mg/dL and a CRP levels >2 mg/dL.[7]
- What is not yet known is whether similar patients with an LDL <130 mg/dL would benefit from statin therapy regardless of their CRP level.
- Although low levels of CRP are associated with lower rates of cardiovascular events, several studies have failed to demonstrate the incremental utility of CRP testing or have questioned the results of prior studies.[7–13]
- For patients with a high global risk score (GRS) or for use in secondary prevention efforts, CRP plays no current role.
  - **Other biomarkers**
    - Other biomarkers such as **homocysteine**, other **lipid parameters** (lipoproteins, apolipoproteins, particle size, and density), **fibrinogen, B-type natriuretic peptide, and genotyping** are not currently recommended for cardiovascular risk assessment in the asymptomatic individual.[14]
    - Urinalysis evaluation for microalbuminuria may be of benefit in risk assessment.
    - Lipoprotein-associated phospholipase A2 might be reasonable for cardiovascular risk assessment in intermediate-risk individuals.
- **Other medical conditions contributing to CVD risk**
  - A growing body of literature has suggested that **autoimmune conditions** such as rheumatoid arthritis and lupus are associated with higher rates of MI and other cardiovascular events.[15–17] This risk appears to be independent of hypercoagulable states that frequently accompany these disease processes, although chronic inflammation may play a pathogenic role. Paradoxically, chronic steroids and other immunosuppressive drugs may also increase the risk of CAD.
  - Infection with **human immunodeficiency virus** (HIV) may be associated with accelerated atherosclerosis, particularly when treatment includes medications such as protease inhibitors, which promote dyslipidemia and glucose intolerance.[18]
  - **Cocaine abuse may dramatically accelerate atherosclerosis in certain individuals**, particularly with chronic abuse. Both angina and MI may be precipitated acutely by cocaine-induced vasospasm, thrombosis, and increased myocardial demand from hyperadrenergic tone.[19]

Prevention

- **Treatment of cardiovascular risk factors has resulted in a 50% decrease in deaths from CHD over the past few decades.**[20] Despite impressive declines in mortality, CVD, which includes CHD, stroke/TIA, and PAD, remains the leading cause of death in men and women worldwide.[21]
- **The majority of known risk factors for CVD are modifiable by preventive measures, including lifestyle changes and adjunctive pharmacotherapy.** The INTERHEART study demonstrated that nine modifiable risk factors account for over 90% of the risk of an initial acute myocardial infarction.[22] Importantly, the presence of multiple risk factors confers at least additive risk.[23]
- **Assessment of risk in primary prevention should not be limited to risk for CHD but should also include risk for CVD events.** This is of particular concern in women who have a higher stroke burden than men.[5]
- A **GRS** can be calculated to determine the absolute risk of an atherosclerotic CVD (ASCVD) event over a specified time period, usually 10 years, based on the presence of major risk factors without known CHD or CHD risk equivalent. Risk calculators include the following:
  - The American Heart Association (AHA)/American College of Cardiology (ACC) atherosclerotic CVD (ASCVD) risk calculator based on the **Pooled Cohort Equations** and lifetime risk prediction tools (http://www.cardiosource.org/science-and-quality/practice-guidelines-and-quality-standards/2013-prevention-guideline-tools.aspx, last accessed December 23, 2014). These risk estimations were derived from large racially and geographically diverse cohort studies and predict so-called hard cardiovascular events, including stroke. The factors included are age, sex, race (non-Hispanic white vs. African American), systolic blood pressure, use of antihypertensive therapy, total and HDL cholesterol, diabetes, and smoking. **Formal estimation of 10-year ASCVD risk is recommended beginning at age 40 and should be repeated every 4 to 6 years in adults 40 to 79 years of age who are free from ASCVD.** Due to limitations of the data, calculated risks for Hispanics and Asian Americans may be overestimated.[14]
  - The Framingham Risk Score (FRS) for the prediction of CHD events (angina, MI, or coronary death) (http://cvdrisk.nhlbi.nih.gov/calculator.asp, last accessed December 23, 2014). The Framingham Study included only middle-aged Caucasian patients and assesses only the risk of developing CHD. The generalizability of the Framingham Risk Score to other populations remains questionable.
  - Other GRS include SCORE (Systematic Coronary Risk Evaluation) for CVD death, the Reynolds Risk Score for major CVD events, and the JBS3 (Joint British Societies) risk calculator for estimating both CVD risk and the impact of beneficial interventions (http://www.jbs3risk.com, last accessed December 23, 2014).
- Based on the GRS, patients are categorized as low or elevated risk for the development of ASCVD over the next 10 years.
  - **Low (<7.5%) ASCVD risk** patients generally do not need further testing or aggressive risk factor modification with pharmacotherapy, but therapeutic lifestyle interventions are strongly encouraged. Statin therapy may be considered in select patients 21 to 75 years of age (see Lipids below). In patients 20 to 59 years old, it may also be useful to calculate the 30-year or lifetime risk of ASCVD.[24]
  - **Elevated (≥7.5%) ASCVD** risk patients require intensive risk factor modification, typically through a combination of lifestyle changes and drug therapy, particularly statin medications. Further testing with labs, imaging, or ischemic evaluation is not routinely recommended, but may be indicated based on clinical context. **Frequent retesting to determine achievement of specific numeric treatment goals has been discouraged in favor of intermittent assessments of global risk.**

- **The concept of matching the intensity of risk factor management to the estimated risk of CVD is well established** and has resulted in an increased emphasis on the accuracy and reliability of risk assessment. The desire to improve existing risk estimation tools has stimulated interest in finding new risk markers for CVD. On the basis of current, albeit limited, evidence, several novel biomarkers have been identified that show promise for clinical utility. Assessment of one or more of the following may be considered when a risk-based treatment decision is uncertain even after formal risk estimation:
  - Family history of premature CVD (first-degree male relative <55 years or female relative <65 years) confers greater risk and supports revising risk assessment upward.
  - Coronary artery calcium (CAC) score by computed tomography. A score ≥300 Agatston units suggests higher risk.
  - Ankle-brachial index (ABI) ratios <0.9 or >1.3 imply the presence of peripheral vascular disease and thus elevate global CVD risk.
  - High-sensitivity C-reactive protein (hs-CRP) levels ≥2 mg/L have been associated with significantly higher rates of CVD events.
  - Carotid intima-media thickness (CIMT) assessed by ultrasound. CIMT is a measure of arterial wall thickness used to detect subclinical atherosclerosis. At this time, routine measurement of CIMT is not recommended since the added value in risk prediction is small and unlikely to be of clinical importance.[25]
- **Age**
  - The incidence of MI increases continuously with age, and >83% of people who die from CHD are in the geriatric population.[7]
  - In the FRS, age is the most heavily weighted risk factor; hence, a common critique is that it underestimates risk in younger individuals.
- **Lipids**
  - Lipid management is discussed in detail in Chapter 11.
  - **A fasting lipid profile is the preferred screening test and should be first obtained at age 21 and then reassessed every 4 to 6 years along with other traditional ASCVD risk factors** (i.e., age, sex, race, blood pressure, diabetes, and smoking).
  - Total cholesterol (TC), high-density lipoprotein (HDL), and triglyceride (TG) levels are measured directly. Very low-density lipoprotein (VLDL) level is estimated by dividing the triglyceride concentration by five.
  - LDL may be calculated from the following formula:

$$Total\ cholesterol = HDL + LDL + VLDL$$
$$LDL = TC - (HDL + TG/5)$$

  - This method is accurate only when triglyceride levels are <400 mg/dL.
  - Direct measurement of LDL is possible and necessary if triglycerides levels exceed this threshold.
  - HDL is the only nonatherogenic subtype of cholesterol, and elevated HDL levels are considered protective or a negative risk factor. Despite an inverse association between HDL levels and CVD risk, **therapies to raise HDL have failed to demonstrate improved outcomes.** This is consistent with recent trial data suggesting that low HDL is more likely a biomarker for CHD risk rather than causative of it.[26]
  - **Specific numeric therapeutic targets are no longer recommended** (e.g., LDL <100 mg/dL). Instead, the emphasis is on moderate- or high-intensity statin treatment in appropriate individuals. The four clear statin benefit groups are[24]
    - Patients ≥21 years old with LDL ≥190 mg/dL
    - Patients 40 to 75 years old with DM and LDL of 70 to 189 mg/dL
    - Patients 40 to 75 years old without clinical ASCVD or DM but with ≥7.5% 10-year risk of ASCVD (ACC/AHA Pooled Cohort Equations)
    - Patients with clinical ASCVD (secondary prevention)

- **Hypertension**
  - Blood pressure is directly related to the incidence of cardiovascular events, starting from a systolic BP of 115 mm Hg.[27] However, intensive blood pressure regimens with systolic goals <140/90 mm Hg have not been shown to reduce CVD risk in all populations, including diabetics and the elderly.[28]
  - The recently released report of the Eighth Joint National Committee (JNC 8) recommends a treatment goal of <140/90 for all patients, except those patients ≥60 years old without DM or CKD, for whom a goal of <150/90 is recommended.[29]
  - One notable exception is in those with systolic dysfunction where the aim is to achieve adequate doses of angiotensin-converting enzyme (ACE) inhibitors and β-blockers based on tolerability rather than blood pressure levels.
  - HTN management is discussed in further detail in Chapter 6.
- **Cigarette smoking**
  - Smoking is the leading cause of preventable death in the United States, and **tobacco cessation reduces the risk of cardiovascular events by 25% to 50%**.
  - Clinical studies have demonstrated the key role of physician counseling in facilitating an individual's interest and motivation for quitting.
  - Nicotine replacement may be helpful for some patients, but oral medications such as bupropion or varenicline may improve cessation rates.
  - Smoking cessation is discussed in Chapter 45.
  - Secondhand smoke also increases the risk of cardiovascular events and mortality.
- **Aerobic exercise**
  - The U.S. Department of Health and Human Services recommends goal activity levels of ≥150 minute/week of moderate intensity and/or ≥75 minute/week of vigorous-intensity exercise are recommended for both primary and secondary preventions of heart disease. Individual episodes of aerobic activity should be at least 10 minutes long and spread throughout the week.[30]
  - The ACC/AHA lifestyle management guidelines to reduce cardiovascular risk recommendations are very similar: three to four sessions per week, lasting on average 40 minutes per session, involving moderate- to vigorous-intensity physical activity.[31]
  - Exercise intensity should progress slowly over time. One method to assess intensity, in those not on AV nodal drugs, is to monitor heart rate.
  - Heavy exercise is considered more than 80% of the maximal predicted heart rate calculated as 220 minus age.
- **Diet**
  - Dietary modifications can have a powerful and beneficial effect on CVD. In general, a healthy diet emphasizes intake of vegetables, fruits, nuts, beans, high fiber grains, healthy fish at least twice a week (which may exclude tilapia); avoidance of trans fats; minimization of saturated fats in favor of monosaturated fats; and limits intake of red meat, sweets, and sugar-sweetened beverages. Total caloric intake should be appropriate for current weight, and calories should be restricted when necessary.[31]
  - Appropriate dietary plans to achieve these goals include the AHA Diet, the U.S. Department of Agriculture (USDA) Food Pattern, or the DASH (Dietary Approaches to Stop Hypertension) diet.[32–35]
  - Saturated fat intake should be <7% of total energy intake.
  - Fiber intake goal is 30 to 45 g/day.
  - 200 g/day of fruit and 200 g/day of vegetables should be consumed.
  - For those who already drink, alcohol should be limited to 1 drink/day (1 drink = 4 oz of wine or 12 oz of beer or 1 oz of spirits) in women and 1 to 2 drinks/day in men.
- **Obesity**
  - Obesity is the fastest growing cardiovascular risk factor. A calculated body mass index (BMI) >25 kg/m² is considered overweight, while >30 kg/m² is considered obese.

TABLE 7-2	American Heart Association Criteria for Metabolic Syndrome

Criteria (any three for diagnosis)	Men	Women
Elevated waist circumference[a]	≥102 cm (40 inches)	≥88 cm (35 inches)
Reduced high-density lipoprotein cholesterol	<40 mg/dL	<50 mg/dL
Elevated triglycerides	≥150 mg/dL or drug treatment for triglycerides	
Elevated blood pressure	Systolic ≥130 mm Hg or diastolic ≥85 mm Hg	
Elevated fasting glucose	≥100 mg/dL or drug treatment for glucose	

[a]Waist circumference measured horizontally at the iliac crest, at the end of normal expiration; lower cutoffs may be appropriate in Asian Americans (≥90 cm or ≥35 inches for men, ≥80 cm or ≥31 inches for women).
Modified fromGrundy SM, Cleeman JI, Daniels SR, et al. Diagnosis and management of the metabolic syndrome. *Curr Opin Cardiol* 2006;21:1–6.

Central obesity is defined as a waist circumference >40 inches for men and >35 inches for women.[36]
- Target BMI is between 18.5 and 25 kg/m^2, and initial weight loss goals should be 5% to 10% of total weight.
- **The metabolic syndrome** is correlated with obesity and associated with a higher risk for DM. The diagnostic criteria can be found in Table 7-2.[37]
- Metabolic syndrome was initially defined to identify patients with insulin resistance at risk for DM and CVD. However, it may not be a unique risk factor whose presence conveys a greater risk than the sum of its parts. Hence, its clinical utility is of uncertain significance. Treatment involves the same lifestyle changes recommended to all patients.[38]
- **Diabetes care in ischemic heart disease**
  - DM management is important, although intense control is no longer recommended, and it is imperative that therapy does not induce hypoglycemic episodes.[28]
  - Hemoglobin A1c goals of <7% may be considered in those with a short duration of DM and good life expectancy.
  - Hemoglobin A1c goals of 7% to 9% may be appropriate in older patients, those with end organ damage from DM, or prior hypoglycemic events.
  - **Rosiglitazone is contraindicated in patients with IHD/heart failure, although more recent evidence suggests the CVD concerns may have been unjustified.**

DIAGNOSIS

Clinical Presentation

History
- **The most common manifestation of CAD is angina,** which is generally described as a substernal pain or discomfort lasting minutes that is crushing, squeezing, pressure, suffocating, and/or heavy. Angina is not usually sharp or stabbing and does not typically change with respiration or position.[39]
- Some individuals may experience nausea, diaphoresis, epigastric discomfort, or dyspnea as the primary symptom of angina. Atypical symptoms are more common in women and the elderly.[39]

TABLE 7-3 Classification of Angina

Class	Onset of angina[a]
I	With strenuous activity
II	With moderate activity such as brisk walking or climbing stairs
III	With mild activity such as walking on level ground
IV	With minimal activity or at rest

[a]Unstable angina is generally considered class IV angina, or progression of classes II–III angina over the preceding 2 months.
Modified from Campeau L. Grading of angina pectoris. *Circulation* 1976;54:522–523.

- Symptoms can be precipitated by emotional or physical stress or illness.
- Symptoms may radiate into the arm, jaw, neck, or back and are frequently associated with a profound sense of discomfort or uneasiness.
- **Typical angina** has three features: (a) substernal chest discomfort of a characteristic quality and duration that is (b) provoked by stress or exertion, and (c) relieved by rest or nitroglycerin (NTG).[39]
  - Atypical angina has two of these three characteristics.
  - Noncardiac chest pain meets one or none of these characteristics.
- Of note, **diabetics may not experience chest discomfort** despite having significant CAD, and women and elderly patients often experience more atypical forms of chest discomfort.
- Since quality of angina varies significantly among individuals, the Canadian Cardiovascular Society has classified the amount of angina in terms of symptomatic limitations to performing daily activities (Table 7-3). This allows clinicians to titrate medical or surgical therapy to reduce anginal severity.[40]
- When evaluating patients in the ambulatory setting with symptoms suggestive of CHD, the **stability of the symptoms is key** in determining which patients need inpatient evaluation and which can be cared for in the ambulatory setting. Patients with angina should first be identified as having **stable or unstable angina**.
- Chronic stable angina is reproducibly precipitated in a predictable manner by exertion or emotional stress and relieved within 5 minutes by sublingual nitroglycerin or rest. To be considered stable, angina symptoms should be present and unchanged for 2 months or greater. These patients can be safely managed in the ambulatory setting.
- Patients with low-risk unstable angina are those with new-onset exertional angina or worsening existing exertional angina whose onset is between 2 weeks and 2 months of presentation with a normal exam, ECG, and cardiac markers. Other **low-risk features** include age <70 years, pain after exertion <20 minutes duration, lack of rest pain, and pain that is not rapidly worsening. Ambulatory management of these patients is possible, but treatment and testing should not be delayed and close follow-up should be assured.
- Patients with **symptoms suggestive of an ACS** or its complications (such as acute heart failure exacerbation) should be referred for prompt inpatient hospital evaluation and management.

Physical Examination
- Physical examination can help identify higher-risk CHD patients or noncardiac causes of chest pain (Table 7-4).
- Concerning physical exam findings include signs of heart failure (edema, rales, S3 heart sound), new or worsening mitral regurgitation murmur, hypotension, and tachycardia or bradycardia.
- Evidence of undiagnosed cardiac risk factors may be noted on examination (e.g., tendon xanthomas in hypercholesterolemia, abnormalities of pulse suggestive of PAD).

TABLE 7-4	Differential Diagnosis of Chest Pain

Cardiac	Noncardiac
Potentially dangerous	**Potentially dangerous**
Atherosclerotic coronary artery disease	Aortic dissection
Coronary stent thrombosis or in-stent restenosis	Pulmonary embolus
Hypertrophic cardiomyopathy	Esophageal rupture, Mallory-Weiss tear
Severe aortic stenosis	Peptic ulcer, cholecystitis, pancreatitis
Severe hypertension with subendocardial ischemia	Pneumonia
Arrhythmias	Pulmonary hypertension (usually with right ventricular strain)
Coronary vasospasm	Pneumothorax
Coronary artery aneurysm, dissection, fistula, embolus	Mediastinitis
Myocardial bridging	Supply-demand mismatch (e.g., tachycardia, severe anemia, hypoxia, thyrotoxicosis)
Anomalous coronary artery	
Usually not life threatening	**Usually not life threatening**
Mitral valve prolapse	Reflux, esophagitis, gastritis, esophageal spasm, biliary colic
Pericarditis	Costochondritis, chest wall trauma, musculoskeletal abnormality
Cardiac syndrome X (believed to represent microvascular dysfunction with widely patent coronaries)	Cervical or thoracic spine disease
	Pleurisy, pleuritis, bronchitis
	Herpes zoster

- Severe HTN alone may provoke coronary ischemia (hypertensive emergency). In patients with chest discomfort and elevated BP, rapid reduction of systolic BP by approximately one-third—generally in a monitored setting such as an emergency department—with gradual further reduction over the subsequent 48 hours is imperative.

Differential Diagnosis

- The differential diagnosis of chest pain is broad (Table 7-4). The diagnosis of obstructive CAD relies heavily on the history and ECG.
- **Ischemia from etiologies other than atherosclerotic CAD**
  - **Subendocardial ischemia related to myocardial strain** requires management of the underlying cause of strain (i.e., blood pressure control, β-blockers or calcium channel blockers [CCBs] for hypertrophic cardiomyopathy, valve replacement for aortic stenosis).
  - **Variant angina from coronary vasospasm** (an uncommon cause of angina, usually associated with ST-segment elevation on the ECG).
    - Treatment of spasm using CCBs and/or nitrates should be combined with interventions aimed at endothelial stabilization (e.g., tobacco cessation, aspirin therapy, weight loss and exercise, possibly ACE inhibitors). β-Blockers can worsen variant angina and should be avoided.
    - Provocation testing in the catheterization laboratory or 24-hour ECG monitoring to diagnose ST elevations may be necessary for definitive diagnosis.

○ Rarely, **myocardial bridging** (or certain congenital coronary artery anomalies) may also cause angina. This is best relieved by reducing inotropy and improving diastolic flow with β-blockers and possibly CCBs. Surgery for certain coronary anomalies may be necessary.

○ **Cocaine or other stimulants** may provoke ischemia via tachycardia, HTN, and vaso-constriction. Other than cessation of cocaine usage, management is similar to vasospasm, but β-blockers are generally avoided because of the risk of unopposed α-adrenergic stimulation. With acute intoxication, nitrates and benzodiazepines are the mainstay of treatment.

Diagnostic Testing

Laboratories

To identify precipitating causes of chest pain or assess risk, initial tests should include complete blood count, renal function and electrolytes, lipid panel fasting glucose, and an ECG.

Imaging

• Chest radiography may help identify aortopathies, structural heart disease/heart failure, or pulmonary/skeletal etiologies, which can cause chest discomfort.

• Echocardiography (echo) is indicated when chest symptoms or examination findings are potentially related to structural (e.g., valvular heart disease, hypertrophic cardiomyopathy, pericardial disease) or functional abnormalities (systolic or diastolic heart failure) with the heart. Echo may also be obtained in patients with prior MI or an abnormal ECG.

Diagnostic Procedures

Stress Testing

• **In patients without established IHD, determining the pretest probability of CAD is very important** in deciding which symptomatic patients should undergo stress testing to establish a diagnosis of CAD (Table 7-5).[39,41,42]

○ **Stress testing is most clinically useful in patients with symptoms and intermediate pretest probability of CAD** (test results will have the least false-positive and false-negative results). Stress testing in low pretest probability patients (<10% likelihood of CAD) will result in more false-positive tests.[39,43,44]

○ Patients with symptoms and high pretest probability of CAD, with severe stable angina (class III/IV despite appropriate medications), and with high-risk unstable angina (stress testing contraindicated) can proceed directly to cardiac catheterization.

TABLE 7-5	Pretest Probability of Coronary Artery Disease on Catheterization[a]						
	Asymptomatic		Nonanginal chest pain		Atypical/probable angina		Typical/definitive angina	
Age	Female	Male	Female	Male	Female	Male	Female	Male
30–39	<5	<5	2	4	12	34	26	76
40–49	<5	<10	3	13	22	51	55	87
50–59	<5	<10	7	20	31	65	73	93
60–69	<5	<5	14	27	51	72	86	94
	Very low <5%		**Low <10%**		**Intermediate 10%–90%**		**High >90%**	

[a]Based on data from Diamond and Forrester and the Coronary Artery Surgery Study.[42,43]
Modified from Fihn SD, Gardin JM, Abrams J, et al. 2012 ACCF/AHA/ACP/AATS/PCNA/SCAI/STS guideline for the diagnosis and management of patients with stable ischemic heart disease. *Circulation* 2012;129:e354–e471.

- Other situations where stress testing is indicated include the following:
  - Assessing change in angina pattern (low-risk unstable angina) in those with prior coronary revascularization on optimal medical therapy should be accompanied by cardiac imaging.
  - Assessing the functional significance of a coronary lesion noted at angiography should be considered with imaging.
  - Assessing for an ischemic etiology of a new diagnosis of left ventricular (LV) dysfunction in a patient without ischemic symptoms and not at high risk for CHD should be accompanied with cardiac imaging.
  - Assessing for an ischemic etiology/myocardial scar in the setting of ventricular tachycardia in a patient without ischemic symptoms and not at high risk for CHD should be accompanied with cardiac imaging.
  - Determining prognosis in patients with known symptomatic IHD or in those without known IHD but are at intermediate or higher likelihood of having CAD but invasive interventions are less desirable (with or without cardiac imaging).
  - To assess adequacy of medical therapy for symptomatic patients with CAD in whom ongoing symptoms may not be of ischemic origin.
  - Prior to starting cardiac rehabilitation, to assess ischemic burden after an ACS where revascularization was not performed, or in previously sedentary patients planning on embarking on vigorous exercise regimens or as part of an exercise prescription, especially in those at high risk for silent ischemia.
  - Preoperatively in some circumstances (see Chapter 2).
  - Although some guidelines suggest stress testing in some asymptomatic individuals (e.g., coronary calcium score >400 or airline pilots), we do not recommend stress testing in most asymptomatic individuals.
- Contraindications to exercise stress testing are listed in Table 7-6.[43]
- Generally, β-blockers, nondihydropyridine CCBs, and other antianginals (e.g., nitrates) should be held the day prior to stress testing to permit a normal heart rate/dilatory response in patients without established CAD. In patients with known CAD, these medications may be continued if adequacy of medical therapy is being tested.

TABLE 7-6	Contraindications to Exercise Testing
Absolute contraindications	**Relative contraindications**
Acute myocardial infarction within 2 days	Known left main coronary stenosis (not bypassed)
High-risk unstable angina	Moderate stenotic valvular heart disease
Uncontrolled symptomatic cardiac arrhythmias	Severe arterial hypertension (e.g., systolic blood pressure >200 mm Hg at rest)
Symptomatic severe aortic stenosis	Significant electrolyte abnormalities
Uncontrolled symptomatic heart failure	Uncontrolled tachyarrhythmia or bradyarrhythmia
Acute pulmonary embolus or pulmonary infarction	Significant obstruction of left ventricular outflow tract
Acute myocarditis or pericarditis	Mental or physical impairment precluding adequate exercise
Acute aortic dissection	High-degree atrioventricular block
Severe comorbidity limiting life expectancy and/or candidacy for revascularization	

Modified from Gibbons RJ, Balady GJ, Beasley JW, et al. ACC/AHA guidelines for exercise testing: executive summary. *Circulation* 1997;96:345–354.

Exercise Treadmill Testing
- Exercise treadmill testing (ETT) with or without cardiac imaging is the preferred method of stress testing and should always be attempted unless it is obvious that the patient cannot exercise or other contraindications to ETT are present.
  - ST elevation during stress testing localizes myocardial injury and suggests high-grade obstruction of an epicardial coronary artery. These patients are usually referred urgently for cardiac catheterization.
  - Inadequate heart rate response (<85% of the maximum predicted heart rate [MPHR]) can render the stress test nondiagnostic. Upsloping ECG changes may also result in an indeterminate test.
  - Downsloping or horizontal ST-segment depression is suggestive of ischemia although it does not necessarily localize the coronary lesion with accuracy.[45]
  - **A positive test is defined as ≥1 mm of ST depression in two contiguous ECG leads** 60 to 80 ms after the J-point when compared with the PR segment.
  - Apart from the ECG, the blood pressure response and heart rate response may be clinically useful. Hypertensive responses may require uptitration of blood pressure medications.
- Prognosis is directly related to exercise stress testing functional capacity, degree of exercise-induced angina, severity of ECG changes, and length of time for ECG changes to revert back to normal in recovery.
  - The **Duke treadmill score** incorporates several prognostic factors from exercise testing into a simple formula (Table 7-7).[46]
  - High-risk patients should be referred for coronary angiography, whereas intermediate-risk patients may be further stratified by either angiography or a repeat stress test with imaging to better assess ischemia.[39]

Pharmacologic Stress Testing.
- In patients unable to exercise or attain target heart rate, pharmacologic stress testing should be performed and is always accompanied by cardiac imaging.[39]

TABLE 7-7	Duke Treadmill Score[a] and Other Prognostic Factors during Exercise Stress Testing

High-risk findings
Duke treadmill score−11 or lower (suggests 5.25% annual CAD mortality)[a]
Systolic blood pressure reduction ≥10 mm Hg during exercise
Persistent ST-segment changes >5 minutes into recovery
Poor functional capacity (e.g., unable to progress beyond stage I of Bruce protocol, or <4 METs)
New ST depression >2 mm
New ST elevation >1 mm
Sustained ventricular tachycardia

Intermediate-risk findings
Duke treadmill score−10 to 4 (suggests 1.25% annual CAD mortality)[a]

Low-risk findings
Duke treadmill score ≥5 (suggests 0.25% annual CAD mortality)[a]
High exercise tolerance (i.e., >10 METs)

[a]Duke treadmill score = minutes of exercise on Bruce protocol − (5 × ST deviation in mm) − (4 × exercise angina score). Exercise angina score: 0 = no angina, 1 = angina during the test, 2 = angina causing test termination.
CAD, coronary artery disease; MET, metabolic equivalent.
Data from Mark DB, Shaw L, Harrell FE, et al. Prognostic value of a treadmill exercise score in outpatients with suspected coronary artery disease. *N Engl J Med* 1991;325:849–853.

- Pharmacologic stress tests involve redistribution of myocardial blood flow using vasodilators (adenosine or regadenoson) or adrenergic stimulation (dobutamine).
  - **Adenosine and regadenoson:** Adenosine can provoke bronchospasm in patients with severe reactive airway disease. Regadenoson is less likely to cause bronchospasm but should be avoided in these patients. Both agents are contraindicated in advanced AV block, sick sinus syndrome, and those taking oral dipyridamole. All caffeine products need to be withheld for 12 to 18 hours prior to use of these agents since caffeine can block the effect of the vasodilators. Aminophylline can be given to reverse the effects of adenosine or regadenoson.
  - **Dobutamine** may provoke arrhythmias or hypotension and should be avoided in patients with uncontrolled atrial fibrillation, known ventricular tachycardia, or known aortic dissection. β-Blockers can be given to reverse the effects of dobutamine.

Stress Tests with Imaging.

- Echocardiographic imaging, radionuclide myocardial perfusion imaging (MPI), or cardiovascular magnetic resonance (CMR) imaging can be used as imaging adjunct to stress testing and is recommended if the baseline ECG is abnormal (LV hypertrophy with secondary ST-segment changes, resting ST depression >1 mm, digoxin effects, left bundle branch block [LBBB], ventricular pacemaker beats, preexcitation) or in patients who cannot exercise to an adequate heart rate.[39]
- When LBBB or electronic ventricular pacing is present, exercise stress testing should be avoided in favor of a pharmacologic stress test to prevent a false-positive study due to septal abnormalities. In all other circumstances where stress testing is ordered, ETT with or without imaging is the stress test of choice.
- Sensitivity and specificity are improved with the addition of cardiac imaging as compared to ETT alone.
- High-risk findings during stress testing (Table 7-8) should prompt coronary angiography for prognostic assessment and potential revascularization in appropriate candidates.[39]
- Each stress imaging modality has its own advantages but similar sensitivities and specificities. In general, indications for stress echo and stress MPI are interchangeable; they are both currently preferred over stress CMR.
  - Stress echo allows assessment of both cardiac structure and function with higher specificity, lower cost, and no exposure to radiation, but acquisition and interpretation of stress images require expertise by a dedicated sonographer and echocardiographer. Dobutamine is the preferred pharmacologic agent in those who cannot undergo ETT.
  - Guidelines permit more liberal use of stress echo in patients with lower likelihood of CAD, as compared to stress MPI, even if they have a normal baseline ECG.
  - Stress radionuclide MPI has a high sensitivity for the detection of CAD and is less technically demanding. In patients with severe cardiomyopathies, stress images can be easier to interpret as compared to stress echo. False-negative studies in the presence of left main or triple vessel disease can occur due to balanced ischemia and should be considered when interpreting results. Exposure to nuclear isotopes that require specialized handling and licensing is a disadvantage of radionuclide MPI.
  - Stress CMR is currently limited to a few centers that have the necessary expertise to perform and interpret such studies. Advantages of CMR include the ability to look at cardiac structure/function without exposure to radiation. Additionally, viability of cardiac muscle and infiltrative diseases of the heart may also be assessed. Currently, stress CMR can only be performed as a pharmacologic stress test (vasodilator or dobutamine) and hence should generally not be considered in those who can exercise.

Coronary CT Angiography

- Coronary CT angiography (CCTA) noninvasively assesses coronary anatomy. CCTA is better suited to ruling out the presence of CAD (e.g., high negative predictive value in populations with lower pretest probability of CAD) and identifying congenital coronary anomalies.[47]

TABLE 7-8 Prognostic Markers from Stress Testing

High risk (>3% annual mortality or MI)
Severe resting LV systolic dysfunction (LVEF <35%) not easily explained by noncoronary causes
Resting perfusion abnormalities (≥10%) of the myocardium in the absence of a history or evidence of MI
Severe exercise-induced LV systolic dysfunction (↓ ≥10% with stress or <45% at peak exercise)
Stress-induced LV dilation
Exercise-induced ST elevation or VT/VF; ≥2 mm ST depression at low work load or during recovery
Stress-induced nuclear perfusion abnormalities (≥10%) or stress segmental scores indicative of multivessel abnormalities
Stress-induced wall motion abnormalities (>2 segments or 2 coronary territories)
Stress-induced wall motion abnormality at low heart rate (<120) or low-dose dobutamine (≤10 mg/kg/minute)

Intermediate risk (1%–3% annual mortality or MI)
Mild-to-moderate LV systolic dysfunction (LVEF 35%–49%) not easily explained by noncoronary causes
Resting perfusion abnormalities (5%–9.9%) of the myocardium in the absence of a history or evidence of MI
≥1 mm ST depression with symptoms on exertion
Stress-induced nuclear perfusion abnormalities (5%–9.9%) or stress segmental scores indicative of single-vessel disease without LV dilation
Small stress-induced wall motion abnormality (1–2 segments and 1 coronary territory)

Low risk (<1% annual mortality or MI)
Low-risk Duke treadmill score (≥5) or no new ST changes or no chest pain
Normal or small nuclear perfusion abnormality (<5%) in the absence of other high-risk features
No wall abnormalities with stress or no change in limited resting wall motion abnormalities

LV, left ventricle; LVEF, left ventricular ejection fraction; MI, myocardial infarction; VT, ventricular tachycardia; VF, ventricular fibrillation
Modified from Fihn SD, Gardin JM, Abrams J, et al. 2012 ACCF/AHA/ACP/AATS/PCNA/SCAI/STS guideline for the diagnosis and management of patients with stable ischemic heart disease. *Circulation* 2012;129:e354–e471.

- Since CCTA is not accompanied by stress testing, the physiologic significance of identified coronary lesions cannot be tested. Thus, an abnormal CCTA may lead to further testing, potentially increasing the cumulative radiation and iodinated contrast exposure. Another disadvantage occurs in patients with coronary stents (especially stents smaller than 3 mm) or significant coronary calcium where image reconstruction artifacts can make quantification of lesion severity less accurate.
- CCTA may be useful for those with persistent symptoms/multiple hospitalizations and inconclusive or normal stress testing results. CCTA can also be useful in assessing graft patency after coronary artery bypass grafting (CABG).
- **CCTA should not be used for screening asymptomatic patients to diagnose occult CAD**.
- CCTA can be considered a reasonable alternative for the assessment of CAD in symptomatic patients who cannot undergo ETT and are at low to intermediate likelihood risk of CAD.[47]

Coronary Angiography

- Diagnostic left heart catheterization is the gold standard for assessing the presence of CAD, defining coronary anatomy, lesion severity, and atherosclerotic burden. Cardiac catheterization can also assess LV systolic function and valvular function and can be used to obtain pressure measurements within the heart and vasculature.[39,48]
- In patients with suspected CAD and angina, coronary angiography is considered an appropriate test in the following scenarios[39,49]:
  - Angina with high-risk criteria by clinical assessment
  - Disabling angina (class III to IV) despite medical therapy
  - Angina with intermediate-risk stress test findings
  - High-risk stress test findings in patients with angina or without angina but stress testing suggests left main or triple vessel disease (Table 7-8)
  - Indeterminate stress test results despite high pretest probability of CAD
  - Angina or high likelihood of CAD in a patient with new LV systolic dysfunction
  - Survivors of sudden cardiac death (SCD) and life-threatening ventricular arrhythmias
  - Patients undergoing planned heart valve or other cardiac surgeries if CAD is possible
- Conventional angiography reliably identifies epicardial coronary lesions, but ancillary tools may be needed to determine the significance of some lesions. Interventional techniques such as fractional flow reserve or intravascular ultrasound can quantify the significance of a coronary stenosis by determining if the lesion is flow limiting or if there is greater plaque burden than visually noted.
- Complication rates from diagnostic catheterization are generally <1% to 2%, although higher risks are associated with increasing age, PAD, renal dysfunction, coagulopathy, and extremes of body weight. Mortality risk is approximately 0.1%.
- The transradial approach is an alternative strategy for catheterization as opposed to the more traditional femoral artery technique. The transradial approach is associated with a reduction in vascular access complications as well as lower bleeding rates. The transradial approach should always be considered in patients who cannot accept blood products based on religious or other objections.[50]

Treatment

- Patient education and adherence to lifestyle modification and medications is of paramount importance for the successful management of IHD. Clinicians must involve patients when formulating a treatment plan.
- Treatment is intended to reduce the risks of cardiovascular mortality and MI, while also reducing symptoms and improving quality of life.
- Outpatient therapies are directed toward increasing coronary blood flow, reducing myocardial oxygen demand, reducing thrombosis, preventing or reversing remodeling of ischemic or infarcted myocardium, and correcting any illness that may precipitate ischemia.

Medications

Antiplatelet Therapy

- Aspirin (ASA) therapy (75 to 100 mg) is the preferred antiplatelet therapy for primary prevention.[39,51] The risk-benefit ratio for ASA becomes more favorable as the GRS increases. Hence, bleeding risk and risk for CHD events needs to be weighed. Generally, ASA will be reserved for patients at high GRS. It should be noted that women tend to have higher rates of bleeding on ASA as compared to men.
- Antiplatelet therapy for established CAD consists of ASA and/or platelet P2Y12 receptor blockers (clopidogrel, prasugrel, and ticagrelor).
  - **Prasugrel** has a maintenance dose of 10 mg once daily. It is reserved for patients with ACS who undergo cardiac stenting only. It is contraindicated in patients with a prior TIA or stroke. It should be avoided in those ≥75 years of age or who weigh <60 kg.

- ○ **Ticagrelor** has a maintenance dose of 90 mg twice daily and is reserved for use in ACS whether stents were placed or not. It must not be used with ASA doses >100 mg. Compliance with twice daily dosing can be a problem.
- ○ **Clopidogrel** has a maintenance dose of 75 mg once a day. Only clopidogrel can be used in conjunction with warfarin and ASA due to a higher risk of bleeding with the other P2Y12 receptor blockers.
- **For patients beyond the first year post-ACS, lifelong single antiplatelet therapy with either aspirin (81 mg) or clopidogrel (in aspirin intolerant patients) is recommended.**
  - ○ ASA at 81 to 162/day reduces the risk of MI, stroke, and vascular death and reduces all-cause mortality in patients with known CAD.[39]
  - ○ **ASA doses of 162 to 325/day or greater are no more protective and are more gastrotoxic compared to lower doses.**[52]
  - ○ In surgical patients, aspirin should be continued during the pre- and postoperative period if feasible.
  - ○ Enteric coating may not be more protective against GI bleeding risk.[53]
  - ○ **Clopidogrel** may be substituted for patients with true aspirin allergy (e.g., anaphylaxis). Alternatively, aspirin desensitization may be pursued.
- **For patients within 1 year of ACS who did not undergo percutaneous coronary intervention (PCI) or CABG dual antiplatelet therapy [DAPT] with ASA (81 mg) and a platelet P2Y12 receptor blocker is recommended for up to 1 year.** Aspirin should be continued indefinitely. Either clopidogrel or ticagrelor may be used.
- **For patients within 1 year of ACS who underwent PCI with stenting or CABG, DAPT is recommended for a minimum of 1 year.**[54–57]
  - ○ In patients treated with stent placement, any platelet P2Y12 receptor blocker can be employed.
  - ○ In patients post-CABG, clopidogrel or ticagrelor may be used along with ASA.
- **For patients who underwent PCI with elective stenting (non-ACS indication):**
  - ○ All patients who receive a cardiac stent on an elective basis should preferably stay on ASA and clopidogrel for 1 year, especially if a drug-eluting stent (DES) was placed.[39]
  - ○ However, therapy beyond 1 month of combined clopidogrel and ASA therapy with bare metal stents (BMS) is less universally accepted and can be sufficient.
- **DAPT therapy after PCI with stent placement beyond the first year of therapy**[57]:
  - ○ Robust data on the routine use of DAPT beyond 1 year are lacking.
  - ○ It is reasonable to continue DAPT beyond 1 year for patients with higher risk for cardiac events (e.g., reduced LV function, complex PCI of bifurcating lesions or heavily calcified lesions, use of multiple stents or long areas of stenting), high-risk sites of stenting (e.g., left main, proximal left anterior descending [LAD]), or suboptimal stenting results in those who are not at high risk of bleeding.[39,47]
  - ○ Risk of late stent thrombosis (beyond 1 year) varies for different DES. Stent-specific data on late thrombosis should be considered and discussed with the patient when considering continuing or stopping platelet P2Y12 receptor blockers after 1 year. There is a lower rate of stent thrombosis associated with use of second-generation DES (everolimus- and zotarolimus-eluting stents) as compared to older DES types.
- **For patients who underwent PCI with stent placement who subsequently require nonemergent surgery (see Chapter 2):**
  - ○ **Nonemergent surgery should be delayed a minimum of 6 weeks after ACS, and DAPT therapy should not be interrupted within the first year.**
  - ○ If the cardiac stent was placed electively, ASA and clopidogrel therapy should be continued for a minimum of 4 weeks for BMS and 6 months for DES, after which ASA alone should be continued.

○ All platelet P2Y12 receptor blockers significantly increase bleeding complications during major surgery. Therefore, if therapy needs to be interrupted for surgery, P2Y12 receptor blockers should be withheld for 5 days for clopidogrel or ticagrelor and 7 days for prasugrel.

Antiischemic Therapy
β-Blockers

• β-Blockers (Table 7-9) have been shown to prevent reinfarction and improve survival. **They should be the first-line therapy for all patients with prior MI or LV systolic dysfunction** (<40%) in the absence of contraindications (hypotension, severe bradycardia or heart block, decompensated heart failure, Prinzmetal angina).[39]

• β-Blockers should be continued for 3 years in patients post-MI with normal LV function.

• No trials have shown an improvement in survival or reduction in the rate of MI for patients with stable IHD without a history of MI.

• In patients with LV systolic dysfunction, β-blocker therapy should be with carvedilol, metoprolol succinate, or bisoprolol, as these agents have been shown to reduce mortality.[39]

• Goal heart rate is generally 55 to 60 beats per minute with slow dose titration. The aim when treating stable angina is not to allow the exercise-induced heart rate to exceed 75% of the rate at which ischemia is experienced.

• Agents more selective for β1-receptors at low doses may cause fewer side effects related to β2-antagonism (e.g., bronchospasm).

TABLE 7-9 Commonly Used β-Blockers

Medication	Usual dosing regimen	Elimination half-life (hours)	Characteristics
Acebutolol	200–1,200 mg qd or divided bid	3–4 (metabolite 8–15)	β1 selective, ISA
Atenolol	25–100 mg qd	6–9	β1 selective, hydrophilic
Bisoprolol	2.5–20 mg qd	9–12	β1 selective
Carvedilol	3.125–50 mg bid	7–10	Combined α- and β-receptor antagonism
Carvedilol CR	10–80 mg qd	11	Combined α- and β-receptor antagonism
Labetalol	200–2,400 mg bid	6–8	Combined α- and β-receptor antagonism
Metoprolol tartrate	50–200 mg bid	3–4	β1 selective, lipophilic
Metoprolol succinate	25–200 mg qd	4–7	β1 selective, lipophilic
Nadolol	40–240 mg qd	14–24	Hydrophilic
Nebivolol	5–40 mg qd	12–19	β1 selective, nitric oxide–potentiating vasodilatory effect
Pindolol	5–20 mg bid or tid	3–4	ISA
Propranolol	10–80 mg qid	4–6	Lipophilic
Propranolol LA	60–320 qd	10	Lipophilic
Timolol	10–30 mg bid	3–4	Hydrophilic

CR, controlled release; ISA, intrinsic sympathomimetic activity.

Calcium Channel Blockers

- CCBs may reduce angina by inducing arteriolar vasodilation and reducing myocardial oxygen demand (Table 7-10). They may be added to β-blockers for patients with continued symptoms or used as second-line agents in individuals with contraindications to β-blockers.[39]
- CCBs, in conjunction with nitrates, are preferable when treating coronary vasospasm.
- Nondihydropyridines may be useful for suppressing atrial arrhythmias or atrioventricular conduction, but given their negative chronotropic and inotropic effects, these agents should be avoided in patients with LV systolic dysfunction.
- Short-acting nifedipine may cause reflex tachycardia, and any CCB may cause peripheral edema, constipation, headaches, or flushing.

Nitrates

- Nitroglycerin reduces preload (venodilation) and afterload (arterial dilation) in patients with angina and therefore improves both myocardial supply and demand as well as LV wall stress.
- Nitrates should be prescribed for anginal relief when β-blockers cannot be used or as add-on therapy to β-blockers.
- Headaches are common but benign and often treatable with acetaminophen. Hypotension may be precipitated in patients with intravascular depletion, severe aortic stenosis, hypertrophic cardiomyopathy, or concomitant therapy with phosphodiesterase-5-inhibitors (e.g., sildenafil, vardenafil, tadalafil).
- Sublingual nitroglycerin spray or tablets provide rapid relief for many individuals with stable angina, but prolonged discomfort after two to three doses should prompt immediate evaluation in an emergency department.
- Longer-acting nitrates (isosorbide dinitrate and mononitrate, transdermal nitroglycerin patch) may help avoid angina in chronic symptomatic CAD, but all forms require an 8- to 12-hour nitrate-free period to avoid tachyphylaxis.
- **These agents have never been demonstrated to improve long-term outcomes**, so nitrates should be prescribed for symptom relief in patients with inadequate responses or contraindications to β-blockers or CCBs.[39]
- As with CCBs, nitrates may help prevent or minimize angina from coronary vasospasm.

TABLE 7-10	Calcium Channel Blockers	
	Usual dosing regimen	Elimination half-life (hours)
Nondihydropyridines		
Diltiazem	30–120 mg tid or qid	3–5
Diltiazem CD	120–480 mg qd	5–8
Diltiazem LA	120–480 mg qd	6–9
Verapamil	80–120 mg tid or qid	3–7
Verapamil SR	120–480 mg qd	5–12
Dihydropyridines		
Amlodipine	2.5–10 mg qd	30–50
Felodipine	5–10 mg qd	9
Isradipine	2.5–5 mg bid	8
Isradipine SR	5–10 mg qd	8
Nicardipine	20–30 mg bid or tid	2–8
Nifedipine	10–30 mg tid or qid	2
Nifedipine SR	30–90 mg qd	7
Nisoldipine	10–40 mg qd or bid	7–12

CD, continuous duration; LA, long acting; SR, sustained release.

Ranolazine

Ranolazine is an anti-ischemic agent with unclear mechanism, which has been shown to reduce angina severity and frequency when added to β-blockers for chronic CAD. Reductions in clinical events have not been demonstrated conclusively to date.[39,58-60]

Other Medication Therapies
Angiotensin-Converting Enzyme Inhibitors

ACE inhibitors should be added for patients with IHD plus HTN, DM, LV systolic dysfunction (ejection fraction [EF] <40%), or mild-to-moderate renal dysfunction.[39] Angiotensin receptor blockers (ARBs) may be reasonable alternatives for patients with intolerance to ACE inhibitors (e.g., significant cough, angioedema).

Aldosterone Antagonists

Eplerenone, an aldosterone antagonist related to spironolactone, improves short- and long-term mortality and cardiovascular outcomes when given to patients with acute MI, LV systolic dysfunction (EF <40%), clinical HF or DM, and no other contraindication to aldosterone blockade (e.g., creatinine >2.5 mg/dL, hyperkalemia).[61-63] Therapy should be continued for 2 years after MI.

Statin Therapy

- **High-intensity statin therapy should be administered to all patients with CAD or CAD risk equivalents**. See Prevention above and Chapter 11, Dyslipidemia.[24]
- Patients with myalgias or other adverse effects on one particular statin should be tried on other statins. Other approaches include using lower doses of an initial statin and/or every-other-day dosing.
- High-dose, high-potency statins may modify plaque composition and reduce atherosclerotic progression over time but may be associated with a higher incidence of DM. Potential benefits regarding cardiovascular events very likely outweigh potential harm.[7,64-66]
- High-potency statins also have pleiotropic effects beyond lowering of LDL. Thus, all patients with CAD (prior CABG or PCI) should be treated with a statin at a moderate or higher dose irrespective of their baseline LDL.
- Adding niacin, fibrates, or omega-3 fish oil tablets to statin therapy has not shown any clear benefit beyond statin therapy alone. Alternative lipid-lowering agents can be considered in statin-intolerant patients.

Other Risk Reduction Therapy

- Influenza vaccine is recommended annually for patients with known CVD.[39]
- Discussion with patients about symptoms of depression and stress can help control angina. Treatment of major depressive disorder may be needed.
- Treatments not recommended for IHD include[39,49]:
  ○ Estrogen
  ○ Dipyridamole
  ○ Supplements with vitamins C, E, B_6, and B_{12}, beta carotene, garlic, coenzyme Q10, selenium, and chromium
  ○ Acupuncture
  ○ Chelation therapy

Other Nonpharmacologic Therapies

- Most patients may resume driving, sexual activity, commercial air travel, and return to work approximately 1 to 2 weeks after a myocardial infarction.
- Cardiac rehabilitation in a structured format has been shown to reduce long-term mortality after MI or coronary revascularization procedures by approximately 25%.[67]
- The initial goal is 50% to 60% of MPHR (estimated as 220 – age) for 10 to 30 minutes at least three times per week followed by a gradual escalation of exercise duration and heart rate to 75% to 85% of maximal predicted.[67]

- Warm-up and cool-down periods of 5 to 15 minutes are recommended.
- Elderly patients enjoy mortality and morbidity benefits equivalent to younger patients, and referral to cardiac rehabilitation is highly encouraged for this age group. Supervision and hemodynamic surveillance is recommended initially for this group.[68]
- Enhanced external counterpulsation (EECP) involves sequential inflations and deflations of cuffs on a subject's limbs, and for patients with refractory angina despite maximal medical and interventional therapy, symptoms may be improved after several weeks of daily therapy.[39,69–71]
- Spinal cord stimulation and transmyocardial revascularization can also be considered for those with refractory angina.[39]
- Persistent LV systolic dysfunction after MI (EF ≤35%), despite aggressive medication titration for at least 40 days, should prompt evaluation for an implantable defibrillator (potentially with cardiac resynchronization therapy [CRT] if the QRS is prolonged [LBBB ≥120 ms, non-LBBB QRS ≥150 ms]) in appropriate patients with mild-to-moderate HF symptoms and otherwise good 1-year prognosis.[72,73]
- Cardiac transplantation can be considered for individuals with medically or surgically refractory angina.

Surgical Management

Coronary Revascularization for Stable Ischemic Heart Disease

- In general, medical therapy with at least two, and preferably three, classes of antianginal agents should be attempted before medical therapy is considered a failure and coronary revascularization pursued.[48]
- **In patients with stable angina, medical therapy results in similar cardiovascular outcomes when compared to PCI except that PCI offers greater short- and long-term relief of anginal symptoms.** Patients should be aware, as part of the informed consent, that their risk for MI or death is not altered by PCI if the indication is stable angina.[39,48]
- **However, patients with certain coronary lesions have a survival advantage with revascularization as compared to medical therapy alone.**
- The choice between PCI and CABG surgery is dependent on the coronary anatomy, medical comorbidities, and patient preference.
- In general, patients with complex and diffuse disease do better with CABG, while PCI in select patients with the proper coronary anatomy can provide comparable results as CABG. Due to the extensive nature of CABG, patient comorbidities often necessitate PCI for revascularization.
- The decision regarding medical therapy alone, PCI, or CABG should consider whether both symptom and mortality benefits are sought or symptom relief alone is sufficient. PCI and CABG are both effective at symptom relief of angina.[39]
- Revascularization is shown to improve survival as compared to medical therapy alone in the following circumstances encountered in the outpatient setting:
  - CABG for >50 % left main disease or PCI if patient is ineligible for CABG and has left main anatomy suitable for PCI.
  - CABG or PCI in survivors of ischemia-mediated SCD.
  - CABG for three-vessel disease or disease in the proximal LAD and one other artery, two-vessel disease with extensive ischemia, and multivessel disease with an left ventricular ejection fraction (LVEF) of >35% when either reversible ischemia or viable myocardium is present.
- CABG carries a 1% to 3% mortality rate, 5% to 10% incidence of perioperative MI, and a small risk of perioperative stroke. The use of internal mammary artery grafts is associated with 90% graft patency at 10 years, compared with 40% to 50% for saphenous vein grafts. The long-term patency of a radial artery graft is 80% at 5 years. After 10 years of follow-up, 50% of patients develop recurrent angina or other adverse cardiac events related to late vein graft failure or progression of native CAD.[74–76]

FOLLOW-UP

- **Routine stress testing or angiography is not indicated after revascularization.**
  - ○ With the current DES and use of internal thoracic artery for bypass surgery, the pretest probability of restenosis is significantly lower than 10 to 20 years ago.[39]
  - ○ Although the practice is not universally accepted, stress testing may be considered for stable or asymptomatic patients in patients with known silent ischemia.
- In patients with recurrent symptoms following PCI, stress MPI is relatively inaccurate for the first 2 months after PCI, resulting in high rates of false-positive studies.[44]
- Above all else, modification of underlying risk factors is imperative because revascularization does not modify the progression of atherosclerosis. Future angina prevalence and ischemic burden is associated with progression of native CAD rather than with the type of revascularization performed.[76]

REFERENCES

1. Roger VL, Go A, Lloyd-Jones DM, et al. Heart disease and stroke statistics—2012 update. *Circulation* 2012;125:e2–e220.
2. Greenland P, Knoll M, Stamler J, et al. Major risk factors as antecedents of fatal and nonfatal coronary heart disease events. *JAMA* 2003;290:891–897.
3. Expert Panel on Detection, Evaluation, and Treatment of High Blood Cholesterol in Adults. Executive summary of the third report of the National Cholesterol Education Program. *JAMA* 2001;285:2486–2497.
4. Haffner SM, Lehto S, Ronnemaa T, et al. Mortality from coronary heart disease in subjects with type 2 diabetes and in nondiabetic subjects with and without prior myocardial infarction. *N Engl J Med* 1998;339:229–234.
5. Mosca L, Benjamin EJ, Berra K, et al. Effectiveness-based guidelines for the prevention of cardiovascular disease in women—2011 update. *J Am Coll Cardiol* 2011;57:1404–1423.
6. Pearson TA, Mensah GA, Alexander RW, et al. Markers of inflammation and cardiovascular disease: application to clinical and public health practice. *Circulation* 2003;107:499–511.
7. Ridker P, Danielson E, Fonseca F, et al. Rosuvastatin to prevent vascular events in men and women with elevated C-reactive protein. *N Engl J Med* 2008;359:2195–2207.
8. Naghavi M, Falk E, Hecht HS, et al. From vulnerable plaque to vulnerable patient—part III: executive summary of the Screening for Heart Attack Prevention and Education (SHAPE) task force report. *Am J Cardiol* 2006;98(suppl 1):2–15.
9. Elliott P, Chambers JC, Zhang W, et al. Genetic loci associated with C-reactive protein levels and risk of coronary heart disease. *JAMA* 2009;302:37–48.
10. Ridker PM, Cannon CP, Morrow D, et al. C-reactive protein levels and outcomes after statin therapy. *N Engl J Med* 2005;352:20–28.
11. de Lorgeril M, Salen P, Abramson J, et al. Cholesterol lowering, cardiovascular diseases, and the rosuvastatin-JUPITER controversy. A critical reappraisal. *Arch Intern Med* 2010;170:1032–1036.
12. Folsom AR, Chambless LE, Ballantyne CM, et al. An assessment of incremental coronary risk prediction using C-reactive protein and other novel risk markers: the Atherosclerosis Risk in Communities study. *Arch Intern Med* 2006;166:1368–1373.
13. Miller M, Zhan M, Havas S. High attributable risk of elevated C-reactive protein level to conventional coronary heart disease risk factors: the third National Health and Nutrition Examination Survey. *Arch Intern Med* 2005;165:2063–2068.
14. Goff DC, Lloyd-Jones DM, Bennett G, et al. 2013 ACC/AHA guideline on the assessment of cardiovascular risk. *Circulation* 2014;129:549–573.

15. Maradit-Kremers H, Gabriel SE. Epidemiology. In: St. Clair EW, Pisetsky DS, Haynes BF, eds. *Rheumatoid Arthritis*. Philadelphia, PA: Lippincott Williams & Wilkins; 2004:1–10.

16. Solomon DH, Karlson EW, Rimm EB, et al. Cardiovascular morbidity and mortality in women diagnosed with rheumatoid arthritis. *Circulation* 2003;107:1303–1307.

17. Urowitz MB, Ibañez D, Gladman DD. Atherosclerotic vascular events in a single large lupus cohort: prevalence and risk factors. *J Rheumatol* 2007;34:70–75.

18. Lai S, Lai H, Celentano DD, et al. Factors associated with accelerated atherosclerosis in HIV-1-infected persons treated with protease inhibitors. *AIDS Patient Care & STDS* 2003;17:211–219.

19. Lange RA, Hillis LD. Cardiovascular complications of cocaine use. *N Engl J Med* 2001;345:351–358.

20. Ford ES, Ajani UA, Croft JB, et al. Explaining the decrease in U.S. deaths from coronary disease, 1980–2000. *N Engl J Med* 2007;356:2388–2398.

21. Murray CJL, Lopez AD, eds. *The global burden of disease: A comprehensive assessment of mortality and disability from diseases, injuries, and risk factors in 1990 and projected to 2020*. Boston, MA: Harvard School of Public Health; 1996.

22. Yusuf S, Hawken S, Ounpuu S, et al. Effect of potentially modifiable risk factors associated with myocardial infarction in 52 countries (the INTERHEART study): case–control study. *Lancet* 2004;364:937–952.

23. Jackson R, Lawes CM, Bennett DA, et al. Treatment with drugs to lower blood pressure and blood cholesterol based on an individual's absolute cardiovascular risk. *Lancet* 2005;365:434–441.

24. Stone NJ, Robinson J, Lichtenstein AH, et al. 2013 ACC/AHA guideline on the treatment of blood cholesterol to reduce atherosclerotic cardiovascular risk in adults. *Circulation* 2014;129:S1–S45.

25. Den Ruijter HM, Peters SE, Anderson TJ, et al. Common carotid intima-media thickness measurements in cardiovascular risk prediction: a meta-analysis. *JAMA* 2012;308(8):796–803.

26. Voight BF, Peloso GM, Orho-Melander M, et al. Plasma HDL cholesterol and risk of myocardial infarction: a Mendelian randomization study. *Lancet* 2012;380:572–580.

27. Chobanian AV, Bakris GL, Black Her, et al. The seventh report of the joint national committee on prevention, detection, evaluation, and treatment of high blood pressure: the JNC 7 report. *JAMA* 2003;289:2560–2572.

28. Gerstein HC, Miller ME, Byington RP, et al.; The action to control cardiovascular risk in diabetes study group. Effects of intensive glucose lowering in type 2 diabetes. *N Engl J Med* 2008;358:2545–2559.

29. James OA, Oparil S, Carter BL, et al. 2014 evidence-based guideline for the management of high blood pressure in adults: report from the panel members appointed to the Eighth Joint National Committee (JNC 8). *JAMA* 2014;311:507–520.

30. U.S. Department of Health and Human Services. 2008 Physical Activity Guidelines for Americans. Available at: http://www.health.gov/paguidelines. Last accessed December 23, 2014.

31. Eckel RH, Jakicic JM, Ard JD, et al. 2013 AHA/ACC guideline on lifestyle management to reduce cardiovascular risk. *Circulation* 2014;129:S76–S99.

32. Lichtenstein AH, Appel LJ, Brands M, et al. Diet and lifestyle recommendations revision 2006. *Circulation* 2006;114:82–96.

33. U.S. Department of Health and Human Services. Dietary Guidelines for Americans, 2010. Available at: http://www.health.gov/dietaryguidelines/2010.asp. Last accessed December 23, 2014.

34. Svetkey LP, Simons-Morton D, Vollmer WM, et al. Effects of dietary patterns on blood pressure: subgroup analysis of the Dietary Approaches to Stop Hypertension (DASH) randomized clinical trial. *Arch Intern Med* 1999;159:285–293.

35. U.S. Department of Health and Human Services. Your guide to lowering your blood pressure with DASH. NIH Publication No. 06–5834, 2006. Available at: https://www.nhlbi.nih.gov/health/resources/heart/hbp-dash-introduction-html.htm. Last accessed December 23, 2014.

36. Jensen MD, Ryan DH, Apovian CM, et al. 2013 AHA/ACC/TOS guideline for the management of overweight and obesity in adults. *Circulation* 2014;129:S102–S138.

37. Grundy SM, Cleeman JI, Daniels SR, et al. Diagnosis and management of the metabolic syndrome. *Curr Opin Cardiol* 2006;21:1–6.

38. Kahn R, Buse J, Ferrannini E, et al. The metabolic syndrome: time for a critical appraisal. *Diabetes Care* 2005;28:2289–2304.

39. Fihn SD, Gardin JM, Abrams J, et al. 2012 ACCF/AHA/ACP/AATS/PCNA/SCAI/STS guideline for the diagnosis and management of patients with stable ischemic heart disease. *Circulation* 2012;129:e354–e471.

40. Campeau L. Grading of angina pectoris. *Circulation* 1976;54:522–523.

41. Diamond GA, Forrester JS. Analysis of probability as an aid in the clinical diagnosis of coronary artery disease. *N Engl J Med* 1979;300:1350–1358.

42. Chaitman BR, Bourassa MG, Davis K, et al. Angiographic prevalence of high-risk coronary artery disease in patient subsets (CASS). *Circulation* 1981;64:360–367.

43. Gibbons RJ, Balady GJ, Beasley JW, et al. ACC/AHA guidelines for exercise testing: executive summary. *Circulation* 1997;96:345–354.

44. Gibbons RJ, Balady GJ, Bricker JT, et al. ACC/AHA 2002 guideline update for exercise testing: summary article. *Circulation* 2002;106:1883–1892.

45. Mark DB, Hlatky MA, Lee KL, et al. Localizing coronary artery obstructions with the exercise treadmill test. *Ann Intern Med* 1987;106:53–55.

46. Mark DB, Shaw L, Harrell FE, et al. Prognostic value of a treadmill exercise score in outpatients with suspected coronary artery disease. *N Engl J Med* 1991;325:849–853.

47. Mark DB, Berman DS, Budoff MJ, et al. ACCF/ACR/AHA/NASCI/SAIP/SCAI/SCCT 2010 expert consensus document on coronary computed tomographic angiography. *Catheter Cardiovasc Interv* 2010;76:E1–E42.

48. Levine GN, Bates ER, Blankenship JC, et al. 2011 ACCF/AHA/SCAI Guideline for Percutaneous Coronary Intervention: executive summary. *Catheter Cardiovasc Interv* 2012;79:453–495.

49. Fihn SD, Blankenship JC, Alexander KP, et al. 2014 ACC/AHA/AATS/PCNA/SCAI/STS focused update of the guideline for the diagnosis and management of patients with stable ischemic heart disease. *Circulation* 2014;64:1929–1949.

50. Jolly SS, Niemela K, Xavier D, et al. Design and rationale of the radial versus femoral access for coronary intervention (RIVAL) trial: a randomized comparison of radial versus femoral access for coronary angiography or intervention in patients with acute coronary syndromes. *Am Heart J* 2011;161:254–260.

51. U.S. Preventive Services Task Force. Aspirin for the prevention of cardiovascular disease: U.S. Preventive Services Task Force recommendation statement. *Ann Intern Med* 2009;150:396–404.

52. Antithrombotic Trialists Collaborative. Collaborative meta-analysis of randomised trials of antiplatelet therapy for prevention of death, myocardial infarction, and stroke in high risk patients. *BMJ* 2002;324:71–86.

53. Kelly JP, Kaufman DW, Jurgelon JM, et al. Risk of aspirin-associated major upper-gastrointestinal bleeding with enteric-coated or buffered product. *Lancet* 1996;348:1413–1416.

54. Alonso-Coello P, Bellmunt S, McGorrian C, et al. Antithrombotic therapy in peripheral artery disease: antithrombotic therapy and prevention of thrombosis, 9th ed. *Chest* 2012;141:e669S–e690S.

55. Ho PM, Peterson ED, Wang L, et al. Incidence of death and acute myocardial infarction associated with stopping clopidogrel after acute coronary syndrome. *JAMA* 2008;299:532–539.
56. Vandvik PO, Lincoff AM, Gore JM, et al. Primary and secondary prevention of cardiovascular disease: antithrombotic therapy and prevention of thrombosis, 9th ed. *Chest* 2012;141:e637S–e668S.
57. Levine GN, Bates ER, Blankenship JC, et al. 2011 ACCF/AHA/SCAI guideline for percutaneous coronary intervention. *Circulation* 2011;124:e574–e651.
58. Stone PH, Gratsiansky NA, Blokhin A, et al. Antianginal efficacy of ranolazine when added to treatment with amlodipine: the ERICA (Efficacy of Ranolazine in Chronic Angina) trial. *J Am Coll Cardiol* 2006;48:566–575.
59. Chaitman BR, Pepine CJ, Parker JO, et al. Effects of ranolazine with atenolol, amlodipine, or diltiazem on exercise tolerance and angina frequency in patients with severe chronic angina: a randomized controlled trial. *JAMA* 2004;291:309–316.
60. Morrow DA, Scirica BM, Karwatowska-Prokopczuk E, et al. Effects of ranolazine on recurrent cardiovascular events in patients with non-ST-elevation acute coronary syndromes: the MERLIN-TIMI 36 randomized trial. *JAMA* 2007;297:1775–1783.
61. Pitt B, Remme W, Zannad F, et al. Eplerenone, a selective aldosterone blocker, in patients with left ventricular dysfunction after myocardial infarction. *N Engl J Med* 2003;348:1309–1321.
62. Pitt B, White H, Nicolau J, et al. Eplerenone reduces mortality 30 days after randomization following acute myocardial infarction in patients with left ventricular systolic dysfunction and heart failure. *J Am Coll Cardiol* 2005;46:425–431.
63. Zannad F, McMurray JJ, Krum H, et al. Eplerenone in patients with systolic heart failure and mild symptoms. *N Engl J Med* 2011;364:11–21.
64. Sattar N, Preiss D, Murray HM, et al. Statins and risk of incident diabetes: a collaborative meta-analysis of randomised statin trials. *Lancet* 2010;375:735–742.
65. Preiss D, Seshasai SR, Welsh P, et al. Risk of incident diabetes with intensive-dose compared with moderate-dose statin therapy: a meta-analysis. *JAMA* 2011;305:2556–2564.
66. Ridker PM, Pradhan A, MacFadyen JG, et al. Cardiovascular benefits and diabetes risks of statin therapy in primary prevention: an analysis from the JUPITER trial. *Lancet* 2012;380:365–371.
67. Suaya JA, Stason WB, Ades PA, et al. Cardiac rehabilitation and survival in older coronary patients. *J Am Coll Cardiol* 2009;54:25–33.
68. Lavie CJ, Milani RV, Littman AB. Benefits of cardiac rehabilitation and exercise training in secondary coronary prevention in the elderly. *J Am Coll Cardiol* 1993;22:678–683.
69. Arora RR, Chou TM, Jain D, et al. The multicenter study of enhanced external counterpulsation (MUST-EECP): effect of EECP on exercise-induced myocardial ischemia and anginal episodes. *J Am Coll Cardiol* 1999;33:1833–1840.
70. Soran O, Kennard ED, Kfoury AG, et al. Two-year clinical outcomes after enhanced external counterpulsation (EECP) therapy in patients with refractory angina pectoris and left ventricular dysfunction (report from The International EECP Patient Registry). *Am J Cardiol* 2006;97:17–20.
71. Cohn PF. Enhanced external counterpulsation for the treatment of angina pectoris. *Prog Cardiovasc Dis* 2006;49:88–97.
72. Tracy DM, Epstein AE, Darbar D, et al. 2012 ACCF/AHA/HRS focused update of the 2008 guidelines for device-based therapy of cardiac rhythm abnormalities. *Circulation* 2012;126:1784–1800.
73. Epstein AE, DiMarco JP, Ellnbogen KA, et al. ACC/AHA/HRS 2008 guidelines for device-based therapy of cardiac rhythm abnormalities. *Circulation* 2008;117:e350–e408.

74. Bourassa MG, Fisher LD, Campeau L, et al. Long-term fate of bypass grafts: the Coronary Artery Surgery Study (CASS) and Montreal Heart Institute experiences. *Circulation* 1985;72:V71–V78.
75. Post Coronary Artery Bypass Graft Trial Investigators. The effect of aggressive lowering of low-density lipoprotein cholesterol levels and low-dose anticoagulation on obstructive changes in saphenous-vein coronary-artery bypass grafts. *N Engl J Med* 1997;336:153–162.
76. Alderman EL, Kip KE, Whitlow PL, et al. Native coronary disease progression exceeds failed revascularization as cause of angina after five years in the Bypass Angioplasty Revascularization Investigation (BARI). *J Am Coll Cardiol* 2004;44:766–774.

Heart Failure and Cardiomyopathy

Sophia Airhart, Joel D. Schilling, and Michael W. Rich

Heart Failure

GENERAL PRINCIPLES

The primary goals of heart failure (HF) management in the outpatient setting are to improve patient symptoms, reduce mortality and hospitalizations, and delay disease progression. The role of the primary physician is to appropriately diagnose HF in at-risk or symptomatic individuals and to initiate management. Early referral to a cardiologist may also be appropriate in selected patients.

Definition

- **HF is a clinical syndrome** characterized by the inability of the heart to support the metabolic needs of the body while maintaining normal intracardiac filling pressures.
- The primary clinical manifestations of HF are symptoms and signs of increased fluid retention (e.g., pulmonary/peripheral edema, pleural effusions, ascites) and/or reduced cardiac output (e.g., fatigue, oliguria, hypotension).

Classification

- The classification of HF into disease stage and symptom class can help direct optimal patient management and assist in assessing prognosis.
- The New York Heart Association (NYHA) functional class is a standard tool for assessing the severity of patient symptoms.
  - **Class I:** No limitations of activity; no symptoms during ordinary activity
  - **Class II:** Mild limitation of activity; comfortable at rest and with mild exertion
  - **Class III:** Marked limitation of activity; comfortable at rest, but ordinary activity causes dyspnea and fatigue
  - **Class IV:** Unable to carry out any physical activity without symptoms; may have symptoms at rest
- The American College of Cardiology (ACC) staging is presented in Figure 8-1.[1]

Epidemiology

- HF afflicts more than 6 million people in the United States. At 40 years of age, the lifetime risk of developing HF for both men and women is one in five. HF incidence approaches 10 per 1,000 population after 65 years of age. Greater than 10% of deaths in the United States have HF mentioned on the death certificate.[2]
- Up to 30% of patients hospitalized with an HF exacerbation will be rehospitalized within the subsequent 3 months.[3]
- Mortality from HF ranges from 10% to 50% within 1 year of diagnosis depending on disease severity.[1,3]
- Up to 50% of patients who present with clinical HF have preserved left ventricular (LV) systolic function (EF $\geq$40%); this entity is known as **heart failure with preserved ejection fraction (HFPEF)**. Three-month mortality is similar in patients with preserved

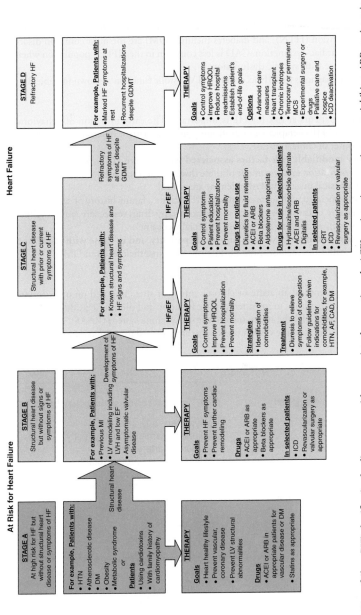

Figure 8-1 Heart failure (HF) classification by disease stage with appropriate therapeutic goals. ACEI, angiotensin-converting enzyme inhibitor; ARB, angiotensin receptor blocker; AF, atrial fibrillation; CAD, coronary artery disease; CRT, Cardiac resynchronization therapy; DM, diabetes mellitus; EF, ejection fraction; HTN, hypertension; ICD, implantable cardioverter-defibrillator; LV, left ventricular; LVH, left ventricular hypertrophy; MI, myocardial infarction; GDMT, guideline-directed medical therapy; HRQOL, health-related quality of life; MCS, mechanical circulatory support. Modified from: Yancy CW, Jessup M, Bozkurt B, et al. 2013 ACCF/AHA guideline for the management of heart failure: a report of the American College of Cardiology Foundation/American Heart Association Task Force on practice guidelines. *Circulation* 2013;128:e240–e327.

or reduced LV systolic function.[4] The mortality rate for HFPEF at 3 months following index hospitalization is approximately 10%, and the 5-year mortality is >50%.

Etiology

• The potential causes of HF are diverse. In the United States, coronary artery disease (CAD), hypertension (HTN), and diabetes mellitus (DM) are the most common disorders leading to cardiac dysfunction. CAD is less common in the HFPEF population when compared to those with systolic dysfunction.
• The differential diagnosis for HF according to LV systolic function is shown in Table 8-1.

Risk Factors

• Recognition of patients at risk for HF is important. The early initiation of behavioral interventions and HF therapies can significantly improve patient outcomes and delay or prevent the onset of clinical disease.
• **The primary modifiable risk factors associated with HF are HTN, DM, and CAD**; therefore, identification and treatment of these diseases and their risk factors (e.g., smoking, obesity, physical inactivity, dyslipidemia) are critical.
• Other factors associated with increased risk of HF include a family history of cardiomyopathy and exposure to cardiotoxins such as chemotherapy drugs (especially anthracyclines and trastuzumab), alcohol, or illicit drugs (especially cocaine).
• **HFPEF is more common in women, in elderly patients, and in those with HTN**, and common comorbidities include atrial fibrillation, renal insufficiency, and DM.[4]

Pathophysiology

• HF is the consequence of an acute or chronic injury or stress imposed on one or more cardiac structures that leads to impaired cardiac function and diminished cardiac reserve.
• During the course of HF, the renin-angiotensin-aldosterone system (RAAS), the sympathetic nervous system, and the vasopressin system are activated to maintain normal cardiac

TABLE 8-1	Causes of Heart Failure
HF with systolic dysfunction	**HF with preserved systolic function**
Coronary artery disease	Hypertension
Hypertension	Diabetic cardiomyopathy (early)
Myocarditis	Coronary artery disease
Viral	Hypertrophic cardiomyopathy
Autoimmune	Restrictive cardiomyopathy
Giant cell arteritis	Hypereosinophilic syndrome
Diabetic cardiomyopathy (late)	Amyloidosis
Familial/genetic cardiomyopathy	Hemochromatosis/iron overload
Toxin induced	Sarcoidosis
Chemotherapy (anthracyclines, trastuzumab)	Genetic
Cocaine	Constrictive pericarditis
Alcohol	Right HF (in the absence of left HF)
Postpartum cardiomyopathy	Pulmonary hypertension
Valvular cardiomyopathy	High-output HF
Tachycardia-induced cardiomyopathy	Hyperthyroidism
Congenital heart disease	Arteriovenous malformations
Idiopathic	Anemia
	Congenital heart disease

output and tissue perfusion. However, these initially adaptive neurohumoral pathways ultimately lead to further cardiac injury, fibrosis, and LV dilation. This process is known as **adverse myocardial remodeling**.

DIAGNOSIS

HF is a clinical diagnosis based on patient symptoms and physical findings consistent with cardiac dysfunction. Laboratory testing and echocardiography are also important tools to aid in the diagnosis and characterization of patients presenting with HF syndromes. HFPEF and HF with reduced ejection fraction (HFREF) cannot be reliably distinguished by history and physical examination alone.

Clinical Presentation

History
- **Shortness of breath,** including breathlessness during activity, at rest, or while sleeping (paroxysmal nocturnal dyspnea; PND). Patients often have difficulty breathing while lying flat and may need to elevate their upper body on pillows (orthopnea).
- **Swelling** in the feet, ankles, legs, or abdomen, which can be associated with weight gain. Patients may find that their shoes feel tight.
- Abdominal swelling, and decreased blood flow to the digestive system, can be associated with decreased appetite, nausea, or early satiety.
- Persistent coughing or wheezing, particularly coughing that produces white or pink-tinged mucous from fluid backup in the lungs.
- Generalized fatigue and memory loss and disorientation can also occur.
- The history should evaluate for **potential causes**:
  - **Ischemic heart disease:** chest pain, history of myocardial infarction (MI), presence of CAD risk factors
  - **Myocarditis:** recent viral illness, rheumatologic symptoms
  - **Genetic cardiomyopathy:** family history of HF or sudden death
  - **Toxic cardiomyopathy:** history of chemotherapy, alcohol or drug abuse
  - **Hypertensive cardiomyopathy:** history of HTN and inadequate blood pressure control
  - **Diabetic cardiomyopathy:** personal or family history of DM, obesity, polyuria
  - **Peripartum cardiomyopathy:** recent pregnancy
  - **Constrictive pericarditis:** history of chest irradiation or pericarditis
  - **Valvular heart disease:** history of a heart murmur, rheumatic fever
  - **Infectious endocarditis:** fever, chills, recent dental work, or other procedures
- **Define the patient's current functional status:**
  - How far can the patient walk before becoming short of breath?
  - How many flights of stairs can the patient climb?
  - Can the patient perform activities of daily living?
  - Compare functional status with previous visits to assess for change.
  - Determine the NYHA functional class.
- **Assess the patient's volume status**. Determine presence of PND, orthopnea, lower extremity (LE) edema, increased abdominal girth, and increased weight.
- **Determine adherence to diet and medications**:
  - Inquire about intake of salt and high sodium foods.
  - Ask about daily fluid intake.
  - Inquire about medication use, side effects, and reasons for nonadherence (if applicable).
  - Ask about use of any new medications (e.g., NSAIDs) or dietary supplements.

Physical Examination
- At each visit, heart rate, respiratory rate, blood pressure, and body weight should be reviewed to direct therapeutic changes.

- Another important function of the physical exam in an initial evaluation is to identify possible causes of HF (e.g., valvular disease, pericardial disease).
- Assessment of volume status on physical exam.
  - **Jugular venous distention (JVD):** Defined as jugular venous pulse >3 to 4 cm above the sternal notch with the patient at 45 degrees. JVD usually correlates with elevated left-sided intracardiac filling pressures unless pulmonary HTN, pericardial constriction, or severe tricuspid regurgitation is present.
  - **S3:** A low-frequency heart sound present following S2 that signifies impaired rapid, early diastolic filling of the LV. In patients with HF, this finding is specific but not sensitive for the presence of LV diastolic volume overload.
  - **Wet pulmonary crackles:** A sign of fluid accumulation in the alveolar air spaces. Present only in about 50% of HF patients with elevated intracardiac filling pressures due to pulmonary lymphatic compensation. Crackles, usually dry, can also be present in other forms of lung disease (e.g., pneumonia, pulmonary fibrosis).
  - **Hepatomegaly/ascites:** Reflects elevated central venous pressure (CVP) from right heart pressure or volume overload.
  - **LE pitting edema:** A late sign of fluid overload that is approximately 30% sensitive for diagnosing hypervolemia in HF patients; not a specific sign of HF as many other diseases can produce LE edema.
  - **Narrow pulse pressure (<30 mm Hg) and pulsus alternans:** Markers of significantly reduced cardiac stroke volume.

Diagnostic Testing

Laboratories
- Laboratory testing in HF can help in determining etiology but is more important for defining disease-modifying comorbidities such as DM, renal insufficiency, and anemia.
- The **initial lab evaluation for all patients** with newly diagnosed HF should include a complete blood cell count (CBC), basic metabolic panel (BMP), liver function tests, fasting lipid panel, fasting blood glucose, urinalysis (UA), and thyroid-stimulating hormone (TSH).
- In select patients with HF of unknown etiology, serum iron studies and tests for HIV and hepatitis C should also be considered.
- **B-type natriuretic peptide (BNP)** is released from myocytes in response to wall stress. A level >400 pg/mL is usually diagnostic of HF (in the absence of chronic kidney disease), whereas a level <100 pg/mL has a high negative predictive value for active HF. BNP levels have also been shown to correlate with the risk of future adverse events in HF patients. A BNP or N-terminal prohormone of brain natriuretic peptide (nt-proBNP) level is **most useful when the diagnosis of HF is uncertain;** levels may also be helpful for monitoring the clinical course and response to therapy and for assessing prognosis.

Electrocardiography
The 12-lead ECG is a useful point of care test to assess for evidence of myocardial ischemia or infarction, left ventricular hypertrophy (LVH), arrhythmias, and interventricular conduction delay (e.g., left bundle branch block [LBBB]).

Imaging
- The hallmarks of HF on **chest radiography** (CXR) are cardiomegaly, bilateral pulmonary infiltrates, and pleural effusions (R > L). In addition, the CXR evaluates for other potential causes of dyspnea such as pneumothorax, pneumonia, or chronic lung disease. Up to 50% of patients with chronic HF and elevated cardiac filling pressures have clear lung fields on CXR; therefore, this finding should not be used to exclude a diagnosis of HF.
- The **echocardiogram is a critical component in the evaluation and management of HF.**

- This imaging test provides information regarding LV and right ventricular (RV) systolic and diastolic function, LVH, valvular disease, pericardial disease, and pulmonary artery pressures.
- Diagnosis of HFPEF is usually based on echocardiographic criteria, mitral valve inflow, and tissue Doppler findings of normal LV systolic function with impaired diastolic function.
- Many aspects of HF disease management and prognosis are determined by the information obtained from the echocardiogram.

Diagnostic Procedures
- **All patients with unexplained HF should have an evaluation for ischemia.**
- Although not a standard test in the evaluation of HF, **myocardial perfusion imaging** (MPI) with thallium and sestamibi can be used in patients at lower risk for CAD to evaluate for ischemia. MPI may also be used to direct revascularization in patients with a known ischemic cardiomyopathy by identifying areas of ischemic but viable myocardium (i.e., hibernating myocardium).
- Similar to MPI, **exercise or dobutamine infusion can be combined with echocardiography** to assess exercise tolerance and/or identify active ischemia by detection of stress-induced wall motion abnormalities. A ramped dobutamine stress echo can also be used to assess myocardial viability in ischemic HF patients being evaluated for coronary bypass surgery.
- **Coronary angiography** is the gold standard for assessing occlusive coronary disease and should be considered unless the patient is a poor candidate (coagulopathy, renal failure, etc.) or the probability of CAD is very low.
- Newer imaging modalities may have a role in the initial assessment of HF. Both **CT and magnetic resonance angiography** could provide a noninvasive approach to evaluate for CAD in new-onset HF. Magnetic resonance imaging (MRI) also has potential value in identifying patients with myocarditis or other specific forms of cardiomyopathy (e.g., amyloidosis, sarcoidosis, arrhythmogenic right ventricular dysplasia [ARVD]). Additional studies are needed to define the role of these imaging techniques in HF.
- Routine **endomyocardial biopsy** for the evaluation of new-onset HF is not recommended. In most cases, the results are nondiagnostic and/or fail to impact management decisions. The use of endomyocardial biopsy can be considered in select patients in whom there is clinical suspicion for sarcoidosis, giant cell myocarditis, or amyloidosis.

TREATMENT

Chronic Heart Failure

- Numerous clinical trials have investigated pharmacologic therapy in chronic HF over the past 30 years. The results of these trials have led to the construction of detailed practice guidelines developed by the American College of Cardiology (ACC) and the American Heart Association (AHA) to help optimize outcomes in HF patients.[1]
- The **goals of treatment** are (1) to improve symptoms, maximize functional status, and improve quality of life; (2) to reduce mortality; (3) to minimize HF hospitalizations; and (4) to slow disease progression.
- Patients with ischemic or valvular cardiomyopathy should be evaluated for revascularization (via percutaneous intervention or surgery) and valve repair/replacement, respectively.
- The classification of HF patients into stages A to D can be used to direct the behavioral, pharmacologic, and device therapy that should be employed to reduce disease progression, hospitalizations, and mortality (Figure 8-1).[1] An overview of diuretic dosing in HF is presented in Table 8-2.[1]

TABLE 8-2	Dosing of Diuretics Commonly Used in Heart Failure		
Drug	Initial daily dose	Maximal total daily dose recommended	Duration of action
Loop diuretics			
Bumetanide	0.5–1 mg IV/PO qd or bid	10 mg	4–6 hours
Furosemide	20–40 mg IV/PO qd or bid	600 mg	6–8 hours
Torsemide	10–20 mg PO qd	200 mg	12–16 hours
Thiazide diuretics			
Chlorothiazide	250–500 mg PO qd or bid	1,000 mg	6–12 hours
Chlorthalidone	12.5–25 mg PO qd	50 mg	24–72 hours
Hydrochlorothiazide	25 mg qd	50 mg	6–12 hours
Indapamide	2.5 mg qd	5 mg	36 hours
Metolazone	2.5 mg qd	20 mg	12–24 hours
Potassium-sparing diuretics			
Amiloride	5 mg qd	20 mg	24 hours
Spironolactone	12.5–25 mg qd	25–50 mg	2–3 days
Triamterene	50–75 mg bid	200 mg	7–9 hours
Combination therapy			
Chlorothiazide	250–1,000 mg plus a loop diuretic		
Hydrochlorothiazide	25–100 mg plus a loop diuretic		
Metolazone	2.5–10 mg plus a loop diuretic		

Modified from Yancy CW, Jessup M, Bozkurt B, et al. 2013 ACCF/AHA guideline for the management of heart failure: a report of the American College of Cardiology Foundation/American Heart Association Task Force on practice guidelines. *Circulation* 2013;128:e240–e327.

- **The optimal treatment strategy for HFPEF remains undefined.** However, the following approaches are recommended:
  - Control blood pressure. Diuretics, angiotensin-converting enzyme (ACE) inhibitors, angiotensin receptor blockers (ARBs), calcium channel blockers (CCBs), and β-blockers are all reasonable agents to achieve this goal.
  - Control heart rate and use warfarin anticoagulation in patients with atrial fibrillation.
  - Use diuretics to treat congestive symptoms, being careful to avoid overdiuresis.
  - Treat underlying ischemia if present.

Medications
- The pharmacologic management of HFREF is detailed in Table 8-3.[5–24]
- HFREF is associated with a **two- to fourfold increased risk of thromboembolic events,** including stroke.
- To date, four randomized controlled trials have failed to show a difference in mortality between placebo versus aspirin versus warfarin in patients with EF <35%. A slight reduction in ischemic stroke has been observed with warfarin, but this is offset by an increased risk of CNS bleeding. The use of aspirin has been associated with increased hospitalization for HF.
- The general consensus is that patients with HFREF should not routinely receive antiplatelet or anticoagulant medications. However, those with atrial fibrillation, LV thrombus, or LV noncompaction should be treated with warfarin. If patients have CAD, aspirin is appropriate.
- In patients with HFREF, the risks and benefits of anticoagulation therapy must be carefully weighed on an individual basis.

TABLE 8-3 Pharmacologic Management of Heart Failure with Reduced Ejection Fraction

Agent	Practical use	Evidence	Additional information
Angiotensin-converting enzyme (ACE) inhibitors[5,6] *Decrease the conversion of angiotensin I to angiotensin II (a potent vasoconstrictor that promotes cardiac fibrosis, myocyte injury, and fluid retention)*	1. **ALL patients with systolic dysfunction (EF <40%) should receive ACE inhibitor therapy unless contraindicated** 2. Start at a low dose and titrate to levels shown to be effective in clinical trials; captopril has a short half-life and can be useful for initial titration in patients with borderline blood pressure or renal function • Captopril 6.25 mg tid → 50 mg tid • Enalapril 2.5 mg bid → 10–20 mg bid • Lisinopril 2.5–5 mg qd → 20–40 qd • Quinapril 5 mg bid → 20 mg bid • Ramipril 1.25–2.5 mg qd → 10 mg qd • Trandolapril 1 mg qd → 4 mg qd • Perindopril 2 mg qd → 8–16 mg qd	1. ACE inhibitor therapy improves survival in patients with: • Asymptomatic LV dysfunction • Moderate-to-severe HF • Post-MI LV dysfunction 2. ACE inhibitors reduce mortality by approximately 25% and have favorable effects on hospitalizations, exercise tolerance, and quality of life	Adverse reactions: • Cough (10%) • Angioedema (rare) • Hypotension • Hyperkalemia • Renal insufficiency • Teratogenic **Avoid NSAIDs** because they increase the risk of acute renal failure and hyperkalemia and antagonize the beneficial effects of ACE inhibitors **Check serum Cr and potassium levels within 2–4 weeks** of starting therapy or increasing the dose

(Continued)

TABLE 8-3 Pharmacologic Management of Heart Failure with Reduced Ejection Fraction (*Continued*)

Agent	Practical use	Evidence	Additional information
Angiotensin receptor blockers (ARB)[7–10] *Bind to and inhibit the type 1 angiotensin II receptor, causing effects similar to ACE inhibitors*	1. **Alternative to ACE inhibitor in patients intolerant to ACE inhibitor therapy** (because of cough or angioedema) 2. Initial and goal doses: • Valsartan 40 mg bid → 160 mg bid • Candesartan 4 mg qd → 32 mg qd 3. The addition of an ARB can be considered in **select** patients already receiving ACE inh bitor and β-blocker therapy who have persistent HF symptoms or recurrent hospitalizations	1. Improve survival in patients with: • Chronic HF • Post-MI LV 2. Reduce hospitalizations in patients with HF and preserved systolic function. 3. Combination therapy (ACE inhibitor + ARB) was investigated in subgroups of several trials and showed no benefit of combination therapy, but there was an increased incidence of hyperkalemia and hypotension; one trial demonstrated a 15% reduction in death or hospitalization with combination, whereas another showed benefit only in patients not receiving a β-blocker.	Adverse reactions: • Hypotension • Hyperkalemia • Renal insufficiency • Teratogenic Not associated with increased risk of cough Angioedema occurs less often than with ACE inhibitors **As with ACE inhibitor, check serum Cr and potassium levels within 2–4 weeks** of starting therapy or of dose increase

β-Blockers[11-16]
The chronic activation of β-adrenergic receptors in HF can lead to arrhythmias, myocyte apoptosis, and adverse LV remodeling

1. **ALL patients with chronic HF and LV systolic dysfunction should receive a β-blocker in the absence of contraindications**
2. Initiate once patients are clinically euvolemic and already on afterload-reducing medications
3. In patients already on β-blocker therapy who present with decompensated HF, the β-blocker should be continued at the same or slightly reduced dosage, discontinuation has been associated with worse outcomes
4. Initial and goal doses:
   - Carvedilol 3.125 bid → 25–50 mg bid
   - Carvedilol CR 10 mg qd → 80 mg qd
   - Metoprolol succinate 12.5–25 mg qd → 200 mg qd
   - Bisoprolol 1.25 mg qd → 5–10 mg qd

1. Improve survival and HF symptoms in patients with mild, moderate, or severe chronic HF and in the post-MI setting
2. Based on data from prospective, randomized trials; **carvedilol** ($β_1$-, $β_2$-, α-antagonist), or **metoprolol** succinate ($β_1$-antagonist), $β_1$-antagonist should be used for the treatment of chronic HF

Adverse reactions:
- Bradycardia
- Heart block
- Hypotension
- Fatigue
- Fluid retention
- Erectile dysfunction

β-Blockers are contraindicated in patients with severe decompensated HF, cardiogenic shock, marked bradycardia (HR<40–45 bpm), hypotension (systolic BP <90 mm Hg), or severe bronchospastic lung disease

In patients with reactive airway disease, β-blockers can worsen bronchospasm; however, this problem can be minimized by using $β_1$-selective agents (e.g., metoprolol succinate, bisoprolol)

(Continued)

TABLE 8-3 Pharmacologic Management of Heart Failure with Reduced Ejection Fraction (*Continued*)

Agent	Practical use	Evidence	Additional information
Aldosterone antagonists[17-19] *Inhibit aldosterone signaling and reduce cardiac fibrosis and adverse remodeling; weak diuretic*	1. **Recommended therapy for patients already on ACE inhibitor and β-blockers who have moderate-to-severe HF symptoms and/or frequent HF hospitalizations** 2. Strongly consider starting for patients with an EF of ≤40% after an acute MI 3. Initial and goal doses: • Spironolactone 12.5–25 mg qd → 25 mg qd • Eplerenone 25 mg qd → 25–50 mg qd • Start at a low dose in the elderly and in those with impaired renal function	1. Decreases mortality and HF hospitalizations by 30% in patients with NYHA class III to IV HF symptoms and EF of ≤30% 2. Associated with a 15% reduction in mortality over 1 year when added to standard therapy in patients with LV dysfunction following an MI 3. In patients with NYHA class II symptoms, EF of ≤30% CV death or first hospitalization for HF were reduced by 34%	Adverse reactions: • Hyperkalemia • Gynecomastia (only with spironolactone, in approximately 10%) **If the baseline potassium level is >5.0 mEq/L or the serum creatinine level is >2.5 mg/dL, then these agents should be avoided because of the risk of life-threatening hyperkalemia** **Potassium level should be checked within 1 week of starting therapy** and sooner if the patient has a potassium level of >4.5 mEq/L or a serum creatinine level of >1.5 mg/dL prior to initiating therapy

Digoxin[20,21]

Inhibits Na-K ATPase, which leads to an increase in intracellular calcium, thereby increasing cardiac contractility; reduces conduction through the AV node

1. Consider as adjunctive therapy for HF patients already on an ACE inhibitor and a β-blockers who have persistent HF symptoms, frequent hospitalizations, or chronic atrial fibrillation
2. Standard dose for HF is 0.125–0.25 mg daily; in patients with renal insufficiency, 0.125 mg three times per week is used
3. The use of a loading dose is not necessary for the management of HF
4. Goal digoxin level is 0.5–0.9 ng/mL
5. Discontinuation of digoxin can result in increased HF symptoms and hospitalizations

No survival benefit; however, digoxin has been associated with **reduced HF hospitalizations;** in post hoc analysis, digoxin levels <1 ng/mL were associated with more favorable outcomes

Digoxin toxicity can be life threatening and include:

1. Cardiac abnormalities (e.g., paroxysmal atrial tachycardia with block, accelerated junctional rhythm, bidirectional VT, atrial fibrillation with regular ventricular response; if severe, the patient can present with sustained VT or high-degree AV block
2. Gastrointestinal (e.g., nausea, vomiting, diarrhea)
3. Neurologic (e.g., lethargy, altered mental status, visual disturbances)

Beware of drug interactions; specifically, amiodarone, verapamil, flecainide, and quinidine, which may increase digoxin levels by up to 100%

Treatment of digoxin toxicity is dependent on the severity of the cardiac manifestations. Electrolyte disorders must be corrected (e.g., potassium and magnesium), and the use of temporary cardiac pacing, phenytoin, and/or digoxin-specific Fab fragments (Digibind) should be considered in select cases. Patients with life-threatening digoxin toxicity require hospitalization and close observation in a monitored setting

(Continued)

TABLE 8-3 Pharmacologic Management of Heart Failure with Reduced Ejection Fraction (*Continued*)

Agent	Practical use	Evidence	Additional information
Hydralazine/nitrates[22-24] *This vasodilator combination was the first pharmacologic therapy shown to modify the natural history and reduce mortality in patients with chronic HF*	1. **In African-American HF patients, hydralazine/nitrates are recommended if persistent HF symptoms are present *despite* use of ACE inhibitors and β-blockers** 2. Can be used as an **alternative vasodilator regimen for patients intolerant of ACE inhibitors/ARBs** (usually because of abnormal renal function or recurrent hyperkalemia) 3. Use as a fixed dose combination tablet or as individual components: • Combination pill (Bidil): 1 → 2 tablets (20 mg isosorbide dinitrate and 37.5 mg hydralazine) tid • Hydralazine 12.5–25 mg tid → 100 mg tid • Isosorbide mononitrate: 30 → 120 mg qd • Isosorbide dinitrate: 10 → 40 mg tid	1. Reduces mortality in patients with chronic HF 2. When compared with enalapril, ACE inhibitor therapy was associated with lower mortality, but other clinical outcomes were similar 3. There is an additive benefit of hydralazine/nitrate therapy in African-American patients with class III–IV HF symptoms who are already receiving an ACEI and β-blocker	Adverse reactions: • Headache • Hypotension • Orthostatic symptoms • Dose-related drug-induced lupus syndrome seen with hydralazine (rare) Erectile dysfunction agents (sildenafil and other phosphodiesterase inhibitors) must be avoided in patients taking nitrates to avoid profound hypotension Compliance can be a problem due to the frequent dosing and above side effects

Diuretics

Always use in conjunction with dietary sodium and fluid restriction. See Table 8-2 for dosing of the common diuretics. The dose used should be based on volume status, symptom severity, and renal function. The lowest dose necessary to maintain euvolemia should be used

1. Used for volume control
2. Hydrochlorothiazide and chlorthalidone are mild diuretics that are best suited for patients with mild HF and normal renal function
3. Loop diuretics are more potent and are frequently required in clinical HF
4. In patients with significant right-sided volume overload and a poor response to oral furosemide, the use of bumetanide or torsemide should be considered as these drugs have more reliable intestinal absorption
5. The addition of a thiazide diuretic to a loop diuretic can be a useful strategy to facilitate diuresis in patients refractory to loop diuretics

Despite their ability to relieve congestive HF symptoms, diuretics **have not been shown to alter the natural history of HF** and may be harmful in the long term because of their adverse renal and neurohormonal effects

Diuretic therapy activates the RAAS and the sympathetic nervous system, which can promote further adverse myocardial remodeling

Adverse reactions:
- Volume contraction (prerenal azotemia or hypotension)
- Electrolyte disorders (potassium, magnesium, sodium)
- Ototoxicity (seen rarely with high-dose furosemide)
- Allergic reaction to sulfa moiety
- Thiamine deficiency (seen with prolonged use of loop diuretics)

Diuretic therapy activates the RAAS and the sympathetic nervous system, which can promote further adverse myocardial remodeling

Electrolytes and renal function should be followed as the clinical situation dictates

AV, atrioventricular; Cr, creatinine; CV, cardiovascular; EF, ejection fraction; HF, heart failure; LV, left ventricle; MI, myocardial infarction; NYHA, New York Heart Association; RAAS, renin-angiotensin-aldosterone system; VT, ventricular tachycardia.

Other Nonpharmacologic Therapies

- The patient's **nonadherence** to medication regimen and diet is a major factor leading to worsened HF symptoms and increased hospitalizations. Therefore, patient education is vital to improve HF outcomes.
- A **low-salt diet** is necessary to avoid excessive fluid accumulation. In patients with mild-to-moderate HF, sodium intake should be restricted to 2 g/day. Avoidance of foods with high sodium content can help prevent decompensation.
- Patients also need to be educated about **fluid intake.** For most patients with HF, a 2 L/day maximum fluid intake is appropriate; however, in patients with more severe HF or when hyponatremia is present, more aggressive fluid restriction may be required.
- Patients should obtain (or be provided with) a home scale and maintain a record of **daily weights.** Increased weight of >2 to 3 pounds from baseline often indicates fluid retention and may warrant adjustment in diuretic dosage.
- **Exercise** in the form of low-impact aerobic activity is recommended for all HF patients in the absence of contraindications. Physical activity can prevent deconditioning and muscle atrophy, both of which worsen HF prognosis. Heavy weight lifting should be avoided.
- **Smoking cessation** should be emphasized in patients with current tobacco use; counseling and/or medications should be offered to patients interested in quitting.
- Patients with HF should have yearly **influenza vaccination** as well as the **pneumococcal pneumonia** vaccination to minimize the risk of pulmonary infections.
- **Implantable cardioverter-defibrillators** (ICDs):
  - Arrhythmic sudden cardiac death (SCD) accounts for about 50% of all HF-associated deaths.
  - ACE inhibitors, β-blockers, and aldosterone antagonists have all been associated with a reduction in SCD; however, despite these therapies, ICDs are associated with improved survival in selected chronic HF patients with reduced systolic function.
  - **All patients with an EF ≤35%, NYHA class II or III symptoms, and an estimated survival of >1 year should be considered for placement of an ICD for primary prevention of SCD.**
  - Patients with non-ischemic cardiomyopathy (NICM) should receive ACE inhibitors and β-blockers at optimal doses for at least 3 months prior to implanting an ICD, as many of these patients will have significant improvement in LV function with medical therapy.
  - Primary prevention ICD implantation should be delayed by at least 40 days following an acute MI or coronary revascularization.
  - **Evidence**
    - MADIT-I and MADIT-II established that ICDs reduce mortality by approximately 1% to 2% per year in selected patients with ischemic cardiomyopathy and an EF of ≤30%.[25]
    - Subsequently, the SCD-HeFT study evaluated patients with either ischemic or non-ischemic cardiomyopathy and an EF of ≤35% and found that an ICD improved survival in both patient groups.[26]
    - The DINAMIT study investigated the use of ICD therapy in patients with LV dysfunction within 40 days after acute MI and found no survival benefit with device implantation in this timeframe.[27]
    - Although effective at reducing ventricular ectopy, amiodarone has not been shown to reduce arrhythmic death in patients with HF who have reduced systolic function.
    - In general, implantation of a primary prevention ICD is not associated with improved survival during the first 12 to 18 months following insertion.[25,26]
  - **Adverse events**
    - Complications associated with ICD implantation include pneumothorax/hemothorax, cardiac rupture, bleeding at the generator site, pericarditis, and device infection, but the incidence of major complications is <5% among experienced operators.

- Inappropriate shocks occur in 10% to 25% of patients with ICDs, usually related to device sensing of a supraventricular tachycardia (most commonly atrial fibrillation). Device failure is another possible adverse event.
- Some patients report worse quality of life, especially after receiving an ICD shock.

- **Cardiac resynchronization therapy**
  - LBBB is present in 20% to 30% of patients with HF. Inter- and intraventricular dyssynchrony produced by LBBB can significantly reduce cardiac efficiency and increase mitral regurgitation.
  - Implanting an LV pacemaker lead transvenously via the coronary sinus or by a thoracotomy, in conjunction with an RV pacing lead (i.e., biventricular pacing), can improve ventricular synchrony.
  - Cardiac resynchronization therapy (CRT) may be considered for HF patients with an LVEF ≤35%, a QRS duration of >120 msec, and persistent NYHA class II to IV symptoms despite optimal medical therapy. The device can be implanted with or without ICD capabilities.
  - Patients with LBBB morphology and QRS duration ≥150 msec are most likely to benefit from CRT. Conversely, the value of CRT in patients without LBBB and QRS duration <150 msec is less certain.
  - **Evidence:** The two largest clinical trials evaluating the efficacy of CRT were COMPANION and CARE-HF.[28,29] Both studies demonstrated improved HF symptoms and fewer hospitalizations with CRT. CARE-HF also showed a significant 10% absolute risk reduction in mortality in patients receiving CRT (without ICD).
  - **Adverse events:** CRT devices are associated with the same procedural and infectious complications as described above for ICDs. Adverse events unique to CRT include diaphragmatic stimulation from the LV lead and a higher risk of pericardial tamponade from injury to the coronary sinus. Technical challenges or inadequate cardiac venous anatomy can preclude percutaneous placement of an LV lead. Such patients require a surgical approach for placement of the LV lead.

Advanced Chronic Heart Failure (Stage D)

- Definition: Severe HF symptoms (NYHA class IIIb or IV) and/or frequent hospitalizations for HF despite optimal medical therapy.
- Patients with end-stage HF represent about 5% of the total HF population; however, they have an extremely high mortality rate and are frequently hospitalized, mandating close medical attention.
- Potential candidates for heart transplantation and/or an LV assist device (LVAD) should be identified and referred to a HF specialist.
- Patients should be continued on ACE inhibitor/ARB, β-blockers, aldosterone antagonists, and digoxin as blood pressure and renal function allow.
- Congestive symptoms should be managed with diuretics; however, hypotension, renal dysfunction, and diuretic resistance are frequently encountered in these patients.
- Discussions regarding end-of-life care should occur between the patient and provider.

- **LVADs/Transplantation**
  - Advanced HF therapies such as heart transplantation or LVAD implantation should be considered for patients with advanced HF refractory to medical therapy who have few comorbidities. Cardiopulmonary exercise testing can also be useful to identify patients who might benefit from these treatments. A VO_2 max of <14 mL O_2/kg/minute is predictive of poor outcomes without advanced therapies.
  - The use of LVADs for permanent or destination therapy (DT) can be considered for advanced HF patients who are not transplant eligible, do not have other life-limiting organ dysfunction, and have a high risk of HF mortality within the next year (class I, level of evidence B, 2012).[30]

○ ACE inhibitors/ARBs, β-blockers, and aldosterone antagonists can reduce arrhythmias and decrease systemic afterload in LVAD patients and thus should be continued after device implant as renal function, potassium, and blood pressure allow.

○ **Evidence:** In the REMATCH trial, the HeartMate XVE (pulsatile pump) reduced mortality compared to medical therapy in patients with severe HF who were not eligible for cardiac transplantation (REMATCH).[31] More recently, the next-generation HeartMate II device (continuous-flow pump) was shown to be superior to the HeartMate XVE, with a 2-year survival rate free of disabling stroke and reoperation to replace the LVAD of 62% versus 7%, respectively.[32]

○ The most common outpatient **complications** observed in LVAD patients include infection, stroke/cardioembolic events, device thrombosis, gastrointestinal bleeding, ventricular arrhythmias, and recurrent HF (often right HF) with or without multiorgan failure.[33,34]

○ **Anticoagulation and antiplatelet therapy** is standard for LVAD patients due to the risk of in situ device thrombosis and stroke. The risk of stroke is approximately 10% per patient-year. Goal INR is typically 1.8 to 2.0; however, it is often individualized based on the risk of bleeding and/or thrombotic complications.

○ **Device-related infections** including pump, pump pocket, and driveline infections are serious and can progress to sepsis.

○ Device thrombosis is a life-threatening complication that can present as HF and/or hemolysis. The presence of dark urine mandates immediate further evaluation (CBC, UA, LDH, plasma-free hemoglobin, haptoglobin, bilirubin, echocardiogram). Device thrombosis requires urgent transplant or pump exchange.

○ Cryptogenic gastrointestinal bleeding is common in LVAD patients, occurring in about 25% of those on HeartMate II support. Close monitoring of INR and hemoglobin is important in the outpatient setting.

○ Ventricular arrhythmias remain problematic after LVAD implant. Although tolerated, patients often have palpitations, fatigue, and light-headedness. The use of β-blockers and antiarrhythmic agents can be effective. Most patients already have an ICD in place for prophylaxis although the value of ICDs in LVAD patients is unknown.

○ Right HF occurs in about 25% of patients who receive an LVAD leading to an excess of rehospitalizations and mortality. The optimal medical treatment is unknown, but changes in pump speed and/or the use of diuretics, pulmonary vasodilators, or inotropes can be considered.

• **Continuous intravenous inotropic therapy** can be used as a bridge to transplantation or for symptom palliation in patients who are not transplant or LVAD candidates. However, **chronic inotropes have been associated with increased mortality** and should therefore be initiated with caution.[35] The two inotropic agents currently in use are the β-adrenergic agonist dobutamine and the phosphodiesterase inhibitor milrinone. These medications should be initiated only in consultation with a HF specialist.

• The 1-year mortality for patients with NYHA class III to IV HF symptoms ranges from 50% to 90% depending on patient characteristics. In patients who are not candidates for transplantation or an LVAD, **palliative care and hospice** should be discussed as mechanisms to provide medical and emotional support during the end-of-life process. Discussions regarding turning off ICDs at the end of life should be undertaken to avoid unnecessary painful events.

Acute Decompensated Heart Failure in the Ambulatory Setting

• In contrast to chronic HF, the management of acute decompensated HF (ADHF) is based more on expert opinion than on clinical trial evidence.

• The **primary treatment goals** in acute HF syndromes are as follows: (1) to improve patient symptoms, (2) to identify and treat precipitating factors of decompensation, (3) to minimize cardiac and renal injury, and (4) to reduce hospitalization by managing selected cases of mild-to-moderate volume overload in the outpatient setting.

- **Identifying and treating potential triggers** of an HF exacerbation is critical to improving patient outcomes. The most common causes of decompensation in patients with established HF include the following:
  - Medication and dietary noncompliance
  - Arrhythmias (particularly atrial fibrillation or ventricular tachycardia (VT))
  - Ischemia
  - Uncontrolled HTN
  - Infections (e.g., pneumonia)
  - Substance abuse
  - Pulmonary embolism
- **Upstream management strategies**
  - Dependence on symptoms (orthopnea) and exam findings (pulmonary rales, peripheral edema, elevated JVP) alone has proven ineffective in averting ADHF hospitalizations. One strategy to improve the sensitivity of detecting early volume overload is through the use of **implantable hemodynamic sensors**.[36]
  - Several implantable sensors have been developed that monitor parameters such as intracardiac filling pressures or thoracic electrical impedance (a measure of lung fluid content).
  - These devices have the potential to reduce HF hospitalizations and improve outpatient medical therapy for HF. Early trials have suggested benefit, but definitive evidence requires further study.
- Patients should be considered for **hospital admission** if they have any of the following:
  - Severe symptoms or active myocardial ischemia
  - Uncontrolled or new-onset arrhythmias
  - Hypoxemia
  - Marked tachycardia or bradycardia
  - Worsening renal insufficiency (increased creatinine >0.5 to 1 mg/dL from baseline)
  - Suspected severe valve disease
  - Evidence of drug toxicity
- For mild HF exacerbations, further testing is not usually indicated. In moderate HF exacerbations, a BMP should be obtained to assess renal function and electrolyte levels.
- In select patients, a CXR, BNP, and/or CBC should be considered to assess HF severity and to evaluate for anemia or infection.
- If ischemia is suspected, an ECG and troponin level should be obtained.
- The treatment of HF exacerbations involves the use of diuretics and vasodilators.
- Table 8-4 provides a rational approach to the outpatient management of HF decompensation.

OUTCOME/PROGNOSIS

- There are many factors that can help determine prognosis in patients with HF. The following have been associated with worse outcomes in HF:
  - **Patient characteristics:** worse NYHA functional class, older age, inability to tolerate ACEI or β-blockers, male gender.
  - **HF etiology:** ischemic heart disease
  - **Lab data:** elevated blood urea nitrogen (BUN) and/or creatinine, hyponatremia, elevated BNP, elevated troponin, low hemoglobin
  - **Echocardiographic data:** lower EF, restrictive diastolic dysfunction, pulmonary HTN
  - **Hemodynamics:** chronically elevated pulmonary capillary wedge pressure pulmonary HTN

TABLE 8-4	Outpatient Management of Decompensated Heart Failure (HF)

Mild HF exacerbation	Moderate HF exacerbation
• Increase total diuretic dose by 50% and administer bid (e.g., 40 mg qd becomes 40 mg bid) for approximately 5–10 days. • Restrict Na to <2 g/day. • Continue ACEI or ARB and titrate if on low dose. • Continue β-blocker. • Monitor daily weights at home. • Target 1- to 2-pound weight loss per day. • Telephone follow-up in 3–5 days.	• Consider ordering BMP. • Increase loop diuretic dose by 50% and administer bid for approximately 7–10 days. • If inadequate response after 1–2 days, consider addition of metolazone at 2.5–5 mg/day. • Restrict Na to <2 g and fluid intake to <2 L. • Increase dose of ACEI/ARB if blood pressure and renal function allow and if not on target doses. • Monitor daily weights and blood pressure at home. • Target 2- to 3-pound weight loss per day. • Telephone follow-up in 3–5 days. • Office follow-up with BMP in 1 week.

ACEI, angiotensin-converting enzyme inhibitor; ARB, angiotensin receptor blockers; BMP, basic metabolic panel; Na, sodium.

- ○ **Patient comorbidities:** atrial fibrillation, renal insufficiency, chronic obstructive pulmonary disease (COPD), peripheral arterial disease, cognitive dysfunction
- ○ **Functional assessment:** decreased VO_2 max; decreased 6-minute walk distance
- • **The Seattle Heart Failure Model** uses several of the above factors to estimate patient survival and can be a useful tool to estimate prognosis in an individual patient. This tool can be accessed online at http://depts.washington.edu/shfm/ (last accessed April 30, 2014).

Hypertrophic Cardiomyopathy

GENERAL PRINCIPLES

- • Hypertrophic cardiomyopathy (HCM) is a genetic cardiomyopathy characterized by asymmetric septal hypertrophy associated with nondilated ventricular chambers, systolic anterior motion of the mitral valve, and variable degrees of LV outflow tract obstruction.
- • Systolic function is usually normal to hyperdynamic, but diastolic function is markedly abnormal.
- • Onset of symptoms in patients with HCM may be as early as the first decade of life, but up to 25% of patients with HCM are ≥65 years of age.
- • Many cases of HCM have a genetic component, with mutations in the myosin heavy-chain gene that follow an autosomal dominant transmission with variable phenotypic expression and penetrance. **Genetic counseling and family screening** are recommended for first-degree relatives at high risk for SCD because the disease is transmitted as an autosomal dominant trait.
- • HCM can be classified according to the presence or absence of LV outflow tract obstruction. LV outflow obstruction may occur at rest but is enhanced by factors that increase LV contractility or decrease ventricular volume.

DIAGNOSIS

- The clinical presentation can be highly variable. In severe cases, patients become symptomatic early in life, while in other cases, the cardiomyopathy is discovered as an incidental finding later in life.
- Sudden death is most common in children and young adults between the ages of 10 and 35 years and often occurs during periods of strenuous exertion.
- Bisferious carotid pulse may be present (in the presence of obstruction). Forceful double or triple apical impulse may be palpated.
- The characteristic coarse systolic outflow murmur localized along the left sternal border that is accentuated by maneuvers that decrease preload (e.g., standing, Valsalva maneuver).
- The ECG may show nonspecific findings, including left atrial enlargement, increased QRS voltage, conduction system disease, ST-T abnormalities, or atrial fibrillation.
- The clinical diagnosis of HCM is typically made with cardiac imaging. 2D echocardiography and Doppler flow studies can establish the presence of significant LV outflow gradient at rest or with provocation. Increasingly, cardiac magnetic resonance (CMR) imaging is indicated in patients with suspected HCM if echocardiography is inconclusive for diagnosis.
- Additional risk stratification can be pursued with 24- to 48-hour Holter monitoring and exercise testing.

TREATMENT

- Guidelines for management of HCM have been established by the American College of Cardiology Foundation and the American Heart Association.[37]
- Medical therapy can help alleviate symptoms and is directed toward controlling heart rate and reducing contractility. First-line agents are **β-blockers and nondihydropyridine CCBs**. The type 1 antiarrhythmic agent disopyramide can be added in patients with persistent symptoms.
- Oral diuretics can be helpful in patients with nonobstructive HCM or used cautiously in patients with obstructive HCM, when dyspnea or angina persists despite the use of β-blockers or verapamil or their combination. However, **overdiuresis can worsen outflow tract obstruction,** producing hypotension and increased symptoms.
- In patients with refractory symptoms and severe outflow tract obstruction, an alcohol septal ablation or surgical myomectomy can be considered.
- ICD implantation should be strongly considered in patients with syncope, VT, or a family history of SCD.
- **Surgical therapy** is useful in the treatment of symptoms but has not been shown to alter the natural history of HCM.
  - The most frequently used operative procedure involves septal myotomy-myectomy with or without mitral valve replacement (MVR).
  - Alcohol septal ablation, a catheter-based alternative to surgical myotomy-myectomy, appears to be equally effective at reducing obstruction and providing symptomatic relief compared with surgery.
  - Cardiac transplantation should be reserved for patients with end-stage HCM with symptomatic HF.[38]

Restrictive Cardiomyopathy

GENERAL PRINCIPLES

- Restrictive cardiomyopathy results from pathologic infiltration of the myocardium or several myocyte diastolic dysfunction.

- Myocardial infiltration results in abnormal diastolic ventricular filling and varying degrees of systolic dysfunction.
- Restrictive cardiomyopathy is **most commonly associated with amyloidosis or sarcoidosis**.
- Less common causes include glycogen storage diseases, hemochromatosis, endomyocardial fibrosis, hypereosinophilic syndromes, and genetic calcium handling diseases.

DIAGNOSIS

- Despite increased LV mass by echocardiography, the ECG is often characterized by low voltage.
- In restrictive cardiomyopathy, echocardiography with Doppler analysis may demonstrate thickened myocardium, an abnormal diastolic filling pattern, elevated intracardiac pressures, and either normal or abnormal systolic function.
- MRI may be helpful in suggesting a potential etiology for restrictive cardiomyopathy and in distinguishing this condition from constrictive pericarditis.
- Cardiac catheterization reveals elevated RV and LV filling pressures and a **classic dip-and-plateau pattern in the RV and LV pressure tracings.**
- RV **endomyocardial biopsy** may be diagnostic and should be considered in patients for whom a specific diagnosis has not been established.
- Restrictive cardiomyopathy and constrictive pericarditis have similar clinical presentations and hemodynamics, but differentiation is critical as surgical therapy may be effective for constriction.

TREATMENT

- Therapy targeted at amelioration of the underlying cause should be initiated.
- Cardiac hemochromatosis may respond to reduction of total body iron stores via phlebotomy or chelation therapy with deferoxamine or deferasirox.
- Cardiac sarcoidosis may respond to glucocorticoid therapy, but improved survival has not been established.
- There is currently no proven therapy for cardiac amyloidosis, but the efficacy of several agents is being evaluated.
- **Digoxin should be avoided** in patients with cardiac amyloidosis because of enhanced susceptibility to digoxin toxicity.

Constrictive Pericarditis

GENERAL PRINCIPLES

- Constrictive pericarditis may develop as a late complication of pericardial inflammation.
- The noncompliant pericardium causes impairment of ventricular filling and progressive elevation of venous pressure.
- Most cases are idiopathic, but pericarditis after cardiac surgery and mediastinal irradiation are common causes.
- Tuberculous pericarditis is a leading cause of constrictive pericarditis in some underdeveloped countries.
- Constrictive pericarditis may be difficult to distinguish from restrictive cardiomyopathy based on the history, physical examination, and hemodynamic findings.

DIAGNOSIS

- In contrast to cardiac tamponade, the clinical presentation of constrictive pericarditis is insidious, with gradual development of fatigue, exercise intolerance, and venous congestion.

- Physical exam findings include the following: JVD with **prominent X and Y descents**, inspiratory elevation of the jugular venous pressure (**Kussmaul sign**), peripheral edema, ascites, and a **pericardial knock** may be present during early diastole.
- Echocardiography may reveal pericardial thickening and diminished diastolic filling.
- CT scan or MRI demonstrates pericardial thickening and other features of constriction.
- Cardiac catheterization may be necessary to demonstrate **elevated and equalized diastolic pressures in all four cardiac chambers** as well as the more specific dynamic inspiratory changes associated with ventricular interdependence.

TREATMENT

- Definitive treatment requires complete pericardiectomy, which is accompanied by significant perioperative mortality (5% to 10%) but results in clinical improvement in 90% of patients.
- Patients who are minimally symptomatic can be managed with judicious sodium and fluid restriction and diuretic therapy but must be followed closely to detect hemodynamic deterioration.

Cardiac Tamponade

GENERAL PRINCIPLES

- Cardiac tamponade results from increased intrapericardial pressure due to fluid accumulation within the pericardial space.
- Pericarditis of any cause may lead to cardiac tamponade.
- Idiopathic (often presumed viral), malignancy, and end-stage renal disease are the most frequent causes.

DIAGNOSIS

- The diagnosis should be suspected in patients with elevated jugular venous pressure, hypotension, **pulsus paradoxus,** tachycardia, evidence of poor peripheral perfusion, and distant heart sounds.
- ECG often reveals a tachycardia with low voltage and electrical alternans.
- Echocardiography can confirm the diagnosis of pericardial effusion and demonstrate hemodynamic significance by right atrial and RV diastolic collapse, increased right-sided flows during inspiration, and respiratory variation of the transmitral flow.
- Right heart catheterization is rarely needed but may be helpful in determining the hemodynamic significance of a pericardial effusion, especially in patients with a subacute or chronic presentation. Hemodynamic findings of elevated, equalized diastolic pressures are present in patients with cardiac tamponade.

TREATMENT

- Treatment consists of drainage of the pericardial space via pericardiocentesis or surgical pericardiotomy. Urgent pericardiocentesis should be performed with echocardiographic guidance, if possible.
- **Diuretics, nitrates, and other preload-reducing agents are absolutely contraindicated for cardiac tamponade.**

REFERENCES

1. Yancy CW, Jessup M, Bozkurt B, et al. 2013 ACCF/AHA guideline for the management of heart failure: a report of the American College of Cardiology Foundation/American Heart Association Task Force on practice guidelines. *Circulation* 2013;128:e240–e327.

2. Go AS, Mozaffarian D, Roger VL, et al. Heart disease and stroke statistics–2013 update: a report from the American Heart Association. *Circulation* 2013;127:e6–e245.

3. Adams KF Jr, Fonarow GC, Emerman CL, et al. Characteristics and outcomes of patients hospitalized for heart failure in the United States: rationale, design, and preliminary observations from the first 100,000 cases in the Acute Decompensated Heart Failure National Registry (ADHERE). *Am Heart J* 2005;149:209–216.

4. Yancy CW, Lopatin M, Stevenson LW, et al. Clinical presentation, management, and in-hospital outcomes of patients admitted with acute decompensated heart failure with preserved systolic function: a report from the Acute Decompensated Heart Failure National Registry (ADHERE) database. *J Am Coll Cardiol* 2006;47:76–84.

5. Garg R, Yusuf S. Overview of randomized trials of angiotensin-converting enzyme inhibitors on mortality and morbidity in patients with heart failure. Collaborative Group on ACE inhibitor trials. *JAMA* 1995;273:1450–1456.

6. Reynolds G, Hall AS, Ball SG. What have the ACE-inhibitor trials in postmyocardial patients with left ventricular dysfunction taught us? *Eur J Clin Pharmacol* 1996;49 (Suppl 1):S35–S39.

7. Pfeffer MA, Swedberg K, Granger CB, et al. Effects of candesartan on mortality and morbidity in patients with chronic heart failure: the CHARM-Overall programme. *Lancet* 2003;362:759–766.

8. Cohn JN, Tognoni G. A randomized trial of the angiotensin-receptor blocker valsartan in chronic heart failure. *N Engl J Med* 2001;345:1667–1675.

9. Yusuf S, Pfeffer MA, Swedberg K, et al. Effects of candesartan in patients with chronic heart failure and preserved left-ventricular ejection fraction: the CHARM-Preserved trial. *Lancet* 2003;362:777–781.

10. McMurray JJ, Ostergren J, Swedberg CB, et al. Effects of candesartan in patients with chronic heart failure and reduced left-ventricular systolic function taking angiotensin-converting-enzyme inhibitors: the CHARM-Added trial. *Lancet* 2003;362:767–771.

11. MERIT-HF Study Group. Effect of metoprolol CR/XL in chronic heart failure: metoprolol CR/XL Randomised Intervention Trial in Congestive Heart Failure (MERIT-HF). *Lancet* 1999;353:2001–2007.

12. Packer M, Fowler MB, Roecker EB, et al. Effect of carvedilol on the morbidity of patients with severe chronic heart failure: results of the Carvedilol Prospective Randomized Cumulative Survival (COPERNICUS) study. *Circulation* 2002;106:2194–2199.

13. Packer M, Bristow MR, Cohn JN, et al. The effect of carvedilol on morbidity and mortality in patients with chronic heart failure. U.S. Carvedilol Heart Failure Study Group. *N Engl J Med* 1996;334:1349–1355.

14. McGavin JK, Keating GM. Bisoprolol: a review of its use in chronic heart failure. *Drugs* 2002;62:2677–2696.

15. Dargie HJ. Effect of carvedilol on outcome after myocardial infarction in patients with left-ventricular dysfunction: the CAPRICORN randomised trial. *Lancet* 2001;357: 1385–1390.

16. Torp-Pedersen C, Poole-Wilson PA, Swedberg K, et al. Effects of metoprolol and carvedilol on cause-specific mortality and morbidity in patients with chronic heart failure: COMET. *Am Heart J* 2005;149:370–376.

17. Pitt B, Zannad F, Remme WJ, et al. The effect of spironolactone on morbidity and mortality in patients with severe heart failure. Randomized Aldactone Evaluation Study Investigators. *N Engl J Med* 1999;341:709–717.

18. Pitt B, Remme WJ, Zannad F, et al. Eplerenone, a selective aldosterone blocker, in patients with left ventricular dysfunction after myocardial infarction. *N Engl J Med* 2003;348:1309–1321.

19. Zannad F, McMurray JJV, Krum H, et al. Eplerenone in patients with systolic heart failure and mild symptoms. *N Engl J Med* 2011;364:11–21.

20. The Digitalis Investigation Group. The effect of digoxin on mortality and morbidity in patients with heart failure. *N Engl J Med* 1997;336:525–533.

21. Ahmed A, Gambassi G, Weaver MT, et al. Effects of discontinuation of digoxin versus continuation at low serum digoxin concentrations in chronic heart failure. *Am J Cardiol* 2007;100:280–284.

22. Cohn JN, Archibald DG, Ziesche S, et al. Effect of vasodilator therapy on mortality in chronic congestive heart failure. Results of a Veterans Administration Cooperative Study. *N Engl J Med* 1986;314:1547–1552.

23. Cohn JN, Johnson G, Ziesche S, et al. A comparison of enalapril with hydralazine-isosorbide dinitrate in the treatment of chronic congestive heart failure. *N Engl J Med* 1991;325:303–310.

24. Taylor AL, Ziesche S, Yancy C, et al. Combination of isosorbide dinitrate and hydralazine in blacks with heart failure. *N Engl J Med* 2004;351:2049–2057.

25. Moss AJ. MADIT-I and MADIT-II. *J Cardiovasc Electrophysiol* 2003;14(Suppl 9):S96–S98.

26. Bardy GH, Lee KL, Mark DB, et al. Amiodarone or an implantable cardioverter-defibrillator for congestive heart failure. *N Engl J Med* 2005;352:225–237.

27. Hohnloser SH, Kuck KH, Dorian P, et al. Prophylactic use of an implantable cardioverter-defibrillator after acute myocardial infarction. *N Engl J Med* 2004;351:2481–2488.

28. Cleland JG, Daubert JC, Erdmann E, et al. The effect of cardiac resynchronization on morbidity and mortality in heart failure. *N Engl J Med* 2005;352:1539–1549.

29. Bristow MR, Saxon LA, Boehmer J, et al. Cardiac-resynchronization therapy with or without an implantable defibrillator in advanced chronic heart failure. *N Engl J Med* 2004;350:2140–2150.

30. Peura J, Colvin-Adams M, Francis GS, et al. Recommendations for the use of mechanical circulatory support: device strategies and patient selection: a scientific statement from the American Heart Association. *Circulation* 2012;126:2648–2667.

31. Rose EA, Gelijns AC, et al. Long-term mechanical left ventricular assistance for end-stage heart failure. *N Engl J Med* 2001;345:1435–1443.

32. Slaughter MS, Rogers JG, Milano CA, et al. Advanced heart failure treated with continuous-flow left ventricular assist device. *N Engl J Med* 2009;361:2241–2251.

33. Cowger J, Romano MA, Stulak J, et al. Left ventricular assist device management in patients chronically supported for advanced heart failure. *Curr Opin Cardiol* 2011;26:149–154.

34. Kirklin JK, Naftel DC, Kormos RL, et al. Second INTERMACS annual report: more than 1,000 primary left ventricular assist device implants. *J Heart Lung Transplant* 2010;29:1–10.

35. Abraham WT, Adams KF, Fonarow GC, et al. In-hospital mortality in patients with acute decompensated heart failure requiring intravenous vasoactive medications: an analysis from the Acute Decompensated Heart Failure National Registry (ADHERE). *J Am Coll Cardiol* 2005;46:57–64.

36. Merchant FM, Dec GW, Singh JP. Implantable sensors for heart failure. *Circ Arrhythm Electrophysiol* 2010;3:657–667.

37. Gersh BJ, Maron BJ, Bonow RO, et al. 2011 2011 ACCF/AHA guideline for the diagnosis and treatment of hypertrophic cardiomyopathy: a report of the American College of Cardiology Foundation/American Heart Association Task Force on Practice Guidelines. *Circulation* 2011;124:e783–e831.

38. Firoozi S, Elliot PM, Sharma S, et al. Septal myotomy-myectomy and transcoronary septal alcohol ablation in hypertrophic obstructive cardiomyopathy. A comparison of clinical, haemodynamic and exercise outcomes. *Eur Heart J* 2002;23:1617–1624.

Valvular Heart Disease
Jared G. Breyley and Brian R. Lindman

- Significant mitral or aortic valve disease is common and occurs in >10% of patients over 75 years old.
- History and physical examination play a prominent role in these patients as they often have physical findings long before the onset of symptoms.
- Primary care physicians are frequently the first doctors to recognize the physical findings in these patients. It is important to recognize cardiac murmurs that require further evaluation versus those that are benign flow murmurs (see Fig. 9-1).[1] It is also important to know when to refer these patients to cardiac specialists.
- The onset of symptoms (e.g., fatigue, increased dyspnea with exertion) in valvular heart disease is often quite insidious with a long period of asymptomatic progression in many patients.
- Advances in surgical and catheter-based techniques will provide additional, less invasive options for the treatment of severe valve disease.
- Determining whether and when to repair or replace a heart valve requires an integration of information about the severity of the valve disease, patient symptoms, and risk stratification.

Aortic Stenosis

GENERAL PRINCIPLES

- Aortic stenosis (AS) is usually present for many years before patients become symptomatic.
- There is a long latency with an excellent prognosis until chest pain, syncope, or heart failure develops.
- The operative mortality of isolated aortic valve replacement (AVR) is quite low in patients with isolated AS, normal left ventricular (LV) function, and relatively few comorbidities (<2% in experienced centers).[1]
- Treatment of high-risk and inoperable patients has been modified with the introduction of transcatheter aortic valve replacement (TAVR).

Pathophysiology

- AS results from an active valvular biology that leads to valve fibrosis and calcification; it occurs in 2% to 7% of patients >65 years of age.
- A bicuspid aortic valve occurs in 1% to 2% of the population and is associated with severe calcific AS at an earlier age (50s to 60s). It accounts for about 50% of valve replacements for AS.
- Maintenance of cardiac output in AS imposes a pressure overload on the LV, which leads to hypertrophic remodeling, diastolic dysfunction, increased myocardial oxygen demand, increased filling pressures, and eventually systolic dysfunction.

DIAGNOSIS

Clinical Presentation

History
- Generally, until the AS becomes severe, patients will not have symptoms directly attributable to the valve abnormality. Many patients with severe AS will be asymptomatic. Providers should be alert to the common scenario in which affected elderly patients subconsciously reduce activity and therefore report no symptoms.

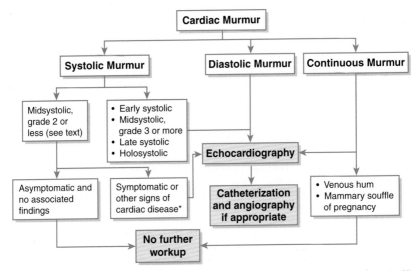

Figure 9-1 **Evaluation of heart murmurs.** (Modified from Bonow RO, Carabello BA, Chatterjee K, et al. 2008 Focused Update Incorporated Into the ACC/AHA 2006 Guidelines for the Management of Patients With Valvular Heart Disease. *J Am Coll Cardiol* 2008;52:e1–e142.)

- With the development of symptoms (e.g., angina, dizziness, syncope, heart failure), it is critical that these patients be seen and offered valve replacement expeditiously as the mean survival is 2 to 3 years for symptomatic severe AS.
- Risk factors for faster progression or a worse outcome include an elevated brain natriuretic peptide, abnormal exercise test, increased valve calcification, rapid increase in transvalvular gradient, higher transvalvular gradient, increased LV hypertrophic remodeling, diastolic dysfunction, and pulmonary hypertension.

Physical Examination
- The physical examination will reveal a harsh crescendo-decrescendo murmur heard over the aortic area and often radiating to the carotids.
- As the severity increases, the murmur peaks later and the aortic second sound (A_2) becomes softer.
- The carotid upstroke becomes weaker and is delayed as the significance of AS increases (*pulsus parvus et tardus*).

Diagnostic Testing
Electrocardiography
- Electrocardiogram often reveals LV hypertrophy with strain.

Imaging
- Echocardiography:
  - The development of quantitative Doppler echocardiography has revolutionized the care of these patients. The aortic valve area (AVA) and the peak jet across the valve can now be determined with accuracy (Table 9-1).
  - Any patient with a significant murmur (≥grade 3) in the aortic region should undergo echocardiography.

TABLE 9-1	Severity of Aortic Stenosis		
Indicator	Mild	Moderate	Severe
Valve area (cm²)	>1.5	1.0–1.5	<1.0
Jet velocity (m/s)	<3.0	3.0–4.0	>4.0
Mean gradient (mm Hg)	<25	25–40	>40

Modified from Bonow RO, Carabello BA, Chatterjee K, et al. 2008 Focused Update Incorporated Into the ACC/AHA 2006 Guidelines for the Management of Patients With Valvular Heart Disease. *J Am Coll Cardiol* 2008;52:e1–e142.

- ○ Exercise testing may be beneficial in asymptomatic patients to unmask symptoms and further risk-stratify patients.
- ○ Patients with an AVA <1 cm² but low gradients due to low flow and low ejection fraction (EF) benefit from a dobutamine echocardiogram to clarify the severity of the AS and assess for contractile reserve.
- Cardiac MRI: Detection of myocardial fibrosis by MRI has been associated with increased mortality in patients with AS and may be helpful in risk stratification.
- Cardiac catheterization: Because of the high prevalence of coronary disease in patients with AS, all patients with chest pain and/or planned AVR should undergo coronary angiography.

TREATMENT

Medications
- There is no medical therapy specifically targeting AS that has been shown to improve clinical outcomes.
- It is important to treat any associated cardiovascular comorbidities (hypertension, coronary artery disease, atrial fibrillation, and heart failure) with appropriate medical therapy.
- In particular, hypertension is quite common in patients with AS and often undertreated due to concerns about inducing hypotension. Inadequately treated hypertension adds an additional detrimental load on the LV beyond the valvular stenosis.

Surgical Management
- AVR is the definitive treatment for AS and improves survival and quality of life, even in very elderly patients (>80 years of age).
- AVR is indicated for symptomatic patients with severe AS, asymptomatic patients with an EF < 50%, or those with moderate or severe AS undergoing cardiac surgery for another reason.

Percutaneous Management
- TAVR is a rapidly evolving, less invasive therapeutic alternative to surgical AVR for patients with severe AS.
- Patients at high risk or ineligible for surgical AVR may be candidates for TAVR. They should be evaluated by a multidisciplinary heart team (cardiologist, cardiac surgeon) to determine the best management strategy.
- The PARTNER Trial showed that TAVR is noninferior to surgical AVR in high-risk patients and TAVR is superior to standard therapy in inoperable patients.[2]
- Additional trials to evaluate these techniques are underway as are ongoing device modifications.

MONITORING/FOLLOW-UP

- In patients with AS, the AVA decreases 0.1 cm^2/year on average, but there is significant variability from patient to patient in the rate of progression.
- Echocardiography is recommended every 3 years for mild AS, every 1 to 2 years for moderate AS, and at least yearly for severe AS.
- Patients with severe AS should be seen at least every 6 months to monitor clinically for the development of symptoms.

Aortic Regurgitation

GENERAL PRINCIPLES

Pathophysiology

- Mild aortic regurgitation (AR) is frequently documented by Doppler echocardiography, but severe AR requiring operative therapy is relatively uncommon.
- AR can result from intrinsic valve disease (e.g., bicuspid aortic valve, rheumatic heart disease, endocarditis, trauma, lupus, and other connective tissue disease).
- Dilatation of the aortic root can also cause severe AR (e.g., Marfan syndrome, aortic dissection, long-standing hypertension, ankylosing spondylitis, and syphilitic aortitis).
- Severe acute AR leads to marked increase in LV pressure since the LV is not compliant enough to accommodate the regurgitant volume. This may lead to pulmonary edema and/or cardiogenic shock.
- Since severe AR usually develops over years, the LV is allowed to dilate and accommodate the large regurgitant volume and maintain normal LV pressures. Over time, these compensatory mechanisms fail and the LV becomes markedly dilated, systolic function diminishes, and LV pressures increase.

DIAGNOSIS

Clinical Presentation

History
- Patients with acute severe AR are almost always symptomatic and often critically ill.
- Patients with chronic severe AR may be asymptomatic for years (compensated state) before developing symptoms, which are most commonly fatigue, dyspnea on exertion, palpitations, and heart failure.

Physical Examination
- Physical examination reveals bounding pulses, a wide pulse pressure, displaced PMI, and a diastolic decrescendo murmur often heard with the patient sitting up or bending forward.
- An Austin-Flint murmur can sometimes be heard at the apex as a low-pitch diastolic murmur due to regurgitant flow through the aortic valve that impedes opening of the anterior mitral valve leaflet and obstructs flow through the mitral valve.

Diagnostic Testing

Electrocardiography
- Electrocardiogram reveals LV hypertrophy and often left atrial enlargement.

Imaging
- Any patient with a diastolic murmur should undergo echocardiography.
- The echocardiogram should document the severity of AR, whether the valve is bicuspid, the size of the LV in systole and diastole, and the size of the aortic root.

• Transesophageal echo may be helpful to clarify whether there is a bicuspid valve and more accurately measure the dimension of the aorta.

TREATMENT

Medications
• Hypertension should be treated in patients with severe AR according to established guidelines.
• In the absence of hypertension, vasodilators may be considered as a chronic treatment for patients with symptomatic severe AR and reduced EF when surgery is not recommended or asymptomatic patients with severe AR and LV dilation with normal EF.
• Vasodilators may also be used in the acute setting in patients with severe HF symptoms as a bridge to AVR.

Surgical Management
• AVR is indicated for symptomatic patients with severe AR and for asymptomatic patients with EF <50% or severe LV dilatation (LV end-systolic dimension >50 to 55 mm; LV end-diastolic dimension >70 to 75 mm).
• Operative mortality is generally quite low and should be strongly considered even if the EF is markedly reduced.
• Concomitant surgery to repair/replace the aortic root is indicated in patients with an aortic root >4.5 to 5.0 cm with a bicuspid aortic valve or Marfan syndrome or >5.0 to 5.5 cm in the absence of those conditions. Operative therapy is also indicated for an increase of 0.5 cm/year in the aortic diameter.

MONITORING/FOLLOW-UP

• Patients with mild-to-moderate AR should be followed yearly with an echocardiogram performed every 2 to 3 years.
• Severe AR with normal LV function should be monitored clinically every 6 months with an echo usually once a year.
• Any change in symptoms warrants immediate evaluation.
• First-degree relatives of patients with Marfan syndrome or a bicuspid aortic valve should be screened with imaging.

Mitral Stenosis

GENERAL PRINCIPLES

Etiology
• Rheumatic heart disease is the most common cause of mitral stenosis (MS), particularly in young women. Mean age for severe MS is the fifth to sixth decades of life.
• With the decrease in rheumatic heart disease, the prevalence of MS has dropped dramatically in developed countries.
• Other causes of MS are rare (e.g., congenital) or less often progress to severe MS (e.g., mitral annular calcification).

Pathophysiology
• Leaflet and subvalvular thickening and calcification results in a decrease in the mitral valve orifice and the development of a diastolic transmitral pressure gradient.

- The transmitral pressure gradient depends on the severity of the obstruction (mitral valve area), flow across the valve (cardiac output), diastolic filling time (heart rate), and the presence of effective atrial contraction.
- Significant MS can lead to elevation of left atrial, pulmonary venous, and pulmonary artery pressures, which can lead to pulmonary vascular remodeling and right ventricular dysfunction.

DIAGNOSIS

Clinical Presentation
History
- The latency or delay between rheumatic fever and significant MS is typically decades; symptom onset can be insidious.
- In addition to dyspnea and/or fatigue, patients may present with cough and sometimes hemoptysis; symptoms of right heart failure may also occur.
- Symptoms may develop suddenly in the setting of fever, new-onset atrial arrhythmia, hyperthyroidism, or pregnancy due to an increased transvalvular gradient.
- Thirty to forty percent of patients with MS develop an atrial arrhythmia.

Physical Examination
- Physical examination reveals a loud S_1 and an opening snap in diastole followed by a mid-diastolic rumble heard best at the apex with the bell of a stethoscope with the patient in left lateral decubitus position.
- A right ventricular heave, loud P_2, and/or signs of right heart failure may also be present.

Diagnostic Testing
Electrocardiography
- Electrocardiogram often shows left atrial enlargement and right ventricular hypertrophy.

Imaging
- Echocardiography can frequently quantify the severity of MS (transvalvular gradient, valve area) and consequences of MS (elevated pulmonary pressures, MR, left atrial enlargement, right ventricular dysfunction).
- Stress echocardiography can be helpful in some cases to assess transmitral gradient and pulmonary artery pressures during exercise.
- If valvuloplasty is considered, transesophageal echocardiography should be performed to evaluate for any associated mitral regurgitation, left atrial clot, and significant calcification/tethering of the mitral valve and subvalvular apparatus.

TREATMENT

Medications
- Therapy is primarily aimed at rate control and prevention of thromboembolism.
- β-Blockers or nondihydropyridine calcium channel blockers (CCBs) tend to be more effective than digoxin for tachycardia associated with exertion.
- Anticoagulation is indicated for atrial arrhythmia (paroxysmal, persistent, or permanent), prior embolic event (even in sinus rhythm), and left atrial thrombus.
- Rhythm control strategies often fail in patients with significant MS.

Percutaneous Management
- Patients with moderate or severe MS with symptoms or associated pulmonary hypertension (at rest or with exercise) should be considered for percutaneous or surgical intervention.

- Patients with rheumatic MS are potentially candidates for percutaneous mitral balloon valvuloplasty (PMBV), whereas patients with calcific MS are not.
- Based on transesophageal echocardiography, patients with extensive calcification/fusion of the mitral leaflets and/or subvalvular apparatus, moderate or greater mitral regurgitation, or left atrial clot are not candidates for PMBV.
- PMBV is the procedure of choice in patients with rheumatic MS without these exclusions; these patients generally have an excellent result from PMBV that may last several years.

Surgical Management
- Those patients needing an intervention on their valve who are not candidates for PMBV should generally undergo valve replacement; valve repair is rarely an option for fibrotic, calcified valves.

MONITORING/FOLLOW-UP

- Asymptomatic patients with moderate to severe MS should be evaluated clinically every 6 months with an echo at least yearly or as clinically indicated.
- In asymptomatic patients, consideration should be given to performing periodic exercise stress tests to evaluate for exercise-induced pulmonary hypertension.
- Holter monitor should be considered in patients with palpitations to monitor for atrial arrhythmias.

Degenerative Mitral Regurgitation

GENERAL PRINCIPLES

Etiology
- Degenerative mitral valve disease refers to those processes that affect the mitral valve leading to regurgitation (myxomatous degeneration, mitral valve prolapse, rheumatic disease, and endocarditis).
- Mitral valve prolapse (MVP) occurs in 1% to 2% of the population and is characterized by prolapse of one or both mitral valve leaflets into the left atrium >2 mm in midsystole.

Pathophysiology
- In patients with acute severe MR (e.g., endocarditis, torn chordae), the sudden large-volume load from the ventricle into a noncompliant left atrium leads to increased pressures that are transmitted to the pulmonary vasculature, causing pulmonary congestion and edema. Forward cardiac output is reduced, and there is compensatory tachycardia to attempt to maintain forward flow.
- As the severity of chronic MR worsens over time, LV function can be maintained and the increased volume load accommodated at normal filling pressures by LV dilation and eccentric hypertrophy.
- As compensatory mechanisms fail, the LV and LA progressively dilate, LV dysfunction occurs, and atrial fibrillation and pulmonary hypertension can develop.

DIAGNOSIS

Clinical Presentation
History
- Patients with acute severe MR can present suddenly and be critically ill.

- Many patients with chronic severe MR are asymptomatic before they present with subtle dyspnea on exertion and fatigue.
- Patients may symptomatically decompensate with the development of atrial fibrillation.

Physical Examination
- Physical examination reveals a holosystolic murmur radiating to the axilla. Prolapse of the posterior and anterior leaflets may produce radiation of the murmur to the chest wall or back, respectively.
- A murmur may not be audible in the setting of acute severe MR, but does not rule out the diagnosis.

Diagnostic Testing
Electrocardiography
- Electrocardiogram may reveal left atrial enlargement and LV hypertrophy; in more end-stage cases, right ventricular hypertrophy may be present.

Imaging
- Chest radiography may reveal cardiomegaly, left atrial enlargement, and pulmonary vascular redistribution.
- Echocardiography:
  - Transthoracic echocardiography should be used to evaluate the severity of mitral regurgitation, mechanism of leak, LV dimensions and function, left atrial size, and pulmonary artery pressures. It is important to incorporate quantitative measurements of MR severity, particularly in those with moderate or severe MR.
  - Exercise stress evaluation with an echocardiogram should be considered to clarify whether symptoms are present in patients with severe MR and/or to evaluate for exercise-induced pulmonary hypertension.
  - Transesophageal echocardiogram should be performed to clarify the severity and mechanism of the MR and assess the feasibility of valve repair.

TREATMENT

Medications
- There are no medical therapies that have been demonstrated to improve clinical outcomes (e.g., delay the time to surgery) in patients with degenerative MR and normal LV function.
- Treat other cardiovascular comorbidities (e.g., hypertension and coronary artery disease) according to appropriate guidelines.
- Patients with severe acute MR may be bridged to definitive therapy (valve surgery) with vasodilators or a balloon pump to maximize forward flow and minimize pulmonary congestion.
- Patients with MVP with a history of TIAs should take ASA (75 to 325 mg), and those with palpitations should avoid/minimize the use of tobacco, alcohol, and caffeine as these may worsen symptoms.

Surgical Management
- Acute severe MR must be treated promptly with surgery.
- For chronic severe MR, surgery is indicated for symptoms or, in the absence of symptoms, when there is LV dilation (LV end-systolic dimension ≥ 4 cm) or EF $<60\%$. Surgery should also be considered in asymptomatic patients with the onset of an atrial arrhythmia and pulmonary hypertension (resting or exercise induced) or when the likelihood of successful valve repair is $>90\%$.

- Mitral valve repair is preferable to mitral valve replacement for degenerative mitral valve disease and should be performed by a high-volume valve repair surgeon.
- Patients with a concomitant atrial arrhythmia should be considered for a surgical maze procedure at the time of valve repair.

MONITORING/FOLLOW-UP

- Patients with severe MR should be monitored very closely for the onset of symptoms, LV dysfunction, LV dilation, atrial arrhythmia, or pulmonary hypertension.
- Echocardiography should be done every 1 to 2 years in patients with moderate MR and at least yearly in those with severe MR. Periodic assessment for exercise-induced pulmonary hypertension is also recommended.

Functional Mitral Regurgitation

GENERAL PRINCIPLES

- Functional MR may occur in patients with LV dysfunction and dilation. The regurgitation results from annular dilatation and papillary muscle displacement due to LV enlargement and remodeling, which causes tenting of the leaflets and inadequate coaptation.
- It may occur in the setting of nonischemic or ischemic dilated cardiomyopathy.
- Functional MR often leads to more severe regurgitation (MR begets MR) as the increased volume load leads to further adverse LV remodeling and dilation, more leaflet tenting, and more inadequate coaptation.

DIAGNOSIS

Clinical Presentation

- Patients have a history of LV dysfunction and often a history of myocardial infarction and/or heart failure preceding the development of MR.
- Patients with moderate to severe functional MR usually have an audible holosystolic murmur heard best at the apex radiating to the axilla; when LV dysfunction is severe, the murmur may be relatively soft.

Diagnostic Testing
Electrocardiography

- Electrocardiogram may reveal left atrial enlargement, LV enlargement, atrial arrhythmia, right ventricular hypertrophy, and/or pathologic Q waves depending on the severity and chronicity of disease and etiology of LV dysfunction.

Imaging

- Chest radiography may reveal cardiomegaly, left atrial enlargement, and pulmonary vascular redistribution.
- Transthoracic echocardiography should be used to evaluate the severity of mitral regurgitation, mechanism of leak, severity of leaflet tethering, LV dimensions and function, and pulmonary artery pressures. It is important to incorporate quantitative measurements of MR severity, particularly in those with moderate or severe MR.

TREATMENT

Medications

- Patients with functional MR have LV dysfunction, so treatment with all the medications indicated for LV dysfunction and heart failure is appropriate for these patients, including ACE inhibitors, β-blockers, aldosterone antagonists, diuretics, and cardiac resynchronization therapy.
- These therapies can lead to favorable reverse remodeling of the LV, which can reduce the severity of functional MR.

Surgical Management

- Whether and when to perform mitral valve surgery for patients with functional MR is controversial as there is conflicting evidence regarding the presence of any survival and/or quality-of-life benefit from surgical intervention.
- Unlike surgery for degenerative MR, it is not clear whether valve repair or replacement is preferable for functional MR.

Percutaneous Management

- A variety of devices are being developed and investigated as potentially less invasive alternatives to surgery for the reduction of functional MR.
- The mitral clip has been evaluated in the EVEREST Trial, and ongoing clinical trials are testing it in patients with functional MR who are at increased operative risk.

Endocarditis Prophylaxis

- In 2007, the American Heart Association (AHA) released its most recent guidelines regarding infective endocarditis (IE) prophylaxis; it contains major changes compared with prior guidelines.[3] There is a notable lack of data supporting the use of antibiotic prophylaxis in the setting of dental, gastrointestinal, and genitourinary procedures, and evidence of causation is circumstantial. The guidelines suggest that there be greater emphasis on oral health in individuals with high-risk cardiac conditions.
- The guidelines conclude that antibiotic prophylaxis is reasonable in a few clinical situations. Prophylaxis is now recommended only for patients undergoing certain dental procedures with cardiac conditions associated with the highest risk of adverse outcome (Table 9-2).

TABLE 9-2	Cardiac Conditions with the Highest Risk of Adverse Outcome from Infective Endocarditis

Prosthetic valve or prosthetic material used for valve repair
Previous infective endocarditis
Congenital heart disease (CHD)
Unrepaired cyanotic CHD, including palliative shunts and conduits
Completely repaired CHD with prosthetic material or device, whether placed by surgery or by catheter intervention, during the first 6 months after the procedure
Repaired CHD with residual defects at the site or adjacent to the site of a prosthetic patch or prosthetic device (which inhibit endothelialization)
Recipients of cardiac transplants who develop cardiac valvulopathy

Modified from Wilson W, Taubert KA, Gewitz M, et al. Prevention of infective endocarditis: guidelines from the American Heart Association. *Circulation* 2007;116:1736–1754.

TABLE 9-3 AHA Guidelines—Regimens for a Dental Procedure

		Regimen: single dose 30–60 minutes before the procedure	
Situation	Agent	Adults	Children
Oral	Amoxicillin	2 g	50 mg/kg
Unable to take oral medication	Ampicillin or	2 g IM or IV	50 mg/kg IM or IV
	Cefazolin or ceftriaxone	1 g IM or IV	50 mg/kg IM or IV
Allergic to penicillins or ampicillin, oral	Cephalexin[a,b] or	2 g	50 mg/kg
	Clindamycin or	600 mg	20 mg/kg
	Azithromycin or clarithromycin	500 mg	15 mg/kg
Allergic to penicillins or ampicillin and unable to take oral medication	Cefazolin or ceftriaxone[b] or	1 g IM or IV	50 mg/kg IM or IV
	Clindamycin	600 mg IM or IV	20 mg/kg IM or IV

[a]Or other first- or second-generation oral cephalosporin in equivalent adult or pediatric dosage.
[b]Cephalosporins should not be used in an individual with a history of anaphylaxis, angioedema, or urticaria with penicillins or ampicillin.
From Wilson W, Taubert KA, Gewitz M, et al. Prevention of infective endocarditis: guidelines from the American Heart Association. *Circulation* 2007;116:1736–1754; with permission.

- Only dental procedures that involve manipulation of the gingival tissue or the periapical region (i.e., near the roots) of teeth or perforation of the oral mucosa warrant prophylaxis. Tooth extractions and cleanings are included. In these instances, prophylactic antibiotics should be directed against viridans streptococci. The recommended regimens for dental procedures are shown in Table 9-3.[3]
- For procedures on infected skin, skin structures, or musculoskeletal tissue, it is reasonable that treatment of the infection itself should be active against staphylococci and β-hemolytic streptococci (e.g., antistaphylococcal penicillin or cephalosporin). For patients unable to tolerate penicillins or who are suspected or known to have an oxacillin-resistant *Staphylococcus aureus* (ORSA) infection, vancomycin or clindamycin may be used.

Anticoagulation

- Patients with mechanical prosthetic valves require long-term anticoagulation (Table 9-4).
- Long-term ASA is indicated for all heart valves.
- Patients with mechanical valves and atrial fibrillation or prior emboli should receive heparin as a bridge when warfarin is stopped for surgery.
- In general, warfarin is stopped for 72 hours prior to surgery and heparin is initiated when INR is <2.0. Low molecular weight heparin has been used as a bridge in small studies, but no large randomized studies have been performed, so no official recommendation has been made.

TABLE 9-4	Antithrombotic Therapy for Patients with Prosthetic Heart Valves			
Valve and duration	Aspirin (75–100 mg)	Warfarin (INR 2–3)	Warfarin (INR 2.5–3.5)	No warfarin
Mechanical				
AVR—low risk				
< 3 months	Class I	Class I	Class IIa	
> 3 months	Class I	Class I		
AVR—high risk	Class I		Class I	
MVR	Class I		Class I	
Biologic				
AVR—low risk				
< 3 months	Class I	Class IIa		Class IIb
> 3 months	Class I			Class IIa
AVR—high risk	Class I	Class I		
MVR—low risk				
< 3 months	Class I	Class IIa		
> 3 months	Class I			Class IIa
MVR—high risk	Class I	Class I		

From Godara H, Hirbe, A, Nassif M, et al., eds. *The Washington Manual of Medical Therapeutics*, 34th ed. Philadelphia, PA: Lippincott Williams & Wilkins; 2014, with permission.

REFERENCES

1. Bonow RO, Carabello BA, Chatterjee K, et al. 2008 Focused Update Incorporated Into the ACC/AHA 2006 Guidelines for the Management of Patients With Valvular Heart Disease. *J Am Coll Cardiol* 2008;52:e1–e142.
2. Leon MB, Smith CR, Mack M, et al. Transcatheter aortic-valve implantation for aortic stenosis in patients who cannot undergo surgery. *N Engl J Med* 2010;363:1597–1607.
3. Wilson W, Taubert KA, Gewitz M, et al. Prevention of infective endocarditis guidelines from the American Heart Association. *Circulation* 2007;116:1736–1754.

10 Arrhythmia and Syncope
Jason D. Meyers and Timothy W. Smith

GENERAL APPROACH TO ARRHYTHMIAS

- The primary care physician will frequently be the first to encounter or suspect an arrhythmia and will continue to care for the patient once the arrhythmia is diagnosed. This chapter focuses on arrhythmia diagnosis and management with an emphasis on issues arising in the primary care setting.
- The initial approach to any ongoing arrhythmia includes obtaining vital signs and a 12-lead electrocardiogram (ECG). If the patient is unstable (i.e., hypotensive, hypoxic, experiencing chest pain or dyspnea), immediate treatment according to ACLS (advanced cardiac life support) algorithms is necessary.
- Frequently, the clinician is faced with a patient whose symptoms are intermittent. If no ECG tracing from a previous event is available, an arrhythmia can be suspected but not definitively diagnosed. Efforts to confirm or detect the arrhythmia are a large part of the clinical approach.
- If an arrhythmia is suspected, a thorough history and physical exam should be performed.
- Symptoms of arrhythmias are frequently nonspecific and include palpitations, light-headedness, chest pain, presyncope/syncope, dyspnea, and a sense of anxiety. At the same time, many serious arrhythmias are frequently asymptomatic.
- The utility of the history and physical exam is to detect other signs of underlying cardiovascular disease. Fortunately, once an ECG or rhythm monitor recording of the arrhythmia is obtained, a diagnosis can often be made.
- In a few cases, such as preexcitation, the nature of the arrhythmia is evident on a baseline ECG. However, this is the exception, and often, other tools must be used to obtain a recording of the arrhythmia.

DIAGNOSTIC TOOLS

Several options are available for the diagnosis of arrhythmias and the correlation of arrhythmia with a patient's symptoms.

- **Holter monitor:** an ambulatory ECG monitor that records continuously for 24 or 48 hours. The entire time period is then reviewed for arrhythmias. This approach is useful only in patients with **daily symptoms.**
- **Event monitor or loop recorder:** an ambulatory ECG monitor that records continuously but saves data only when triggered, either by the patient in accordance with symptoms or by predefined criteria such as heart rate. Events are then transmitted via a transtelephonic system for interpretation. This is often the most cost-effective method of identifying arrhythmias and correlating them with symptoms.
- **Implantable event monitor:** for relatively rare events, an implantable device can be placed.

CLASSIFICATION

- The categorization of arrhythmias is complex and can include categories based on the underlying electrophysiologic mechanisms (reentry, triggered activity, enhanced automaticity), rate, site of origin, and ECG features.

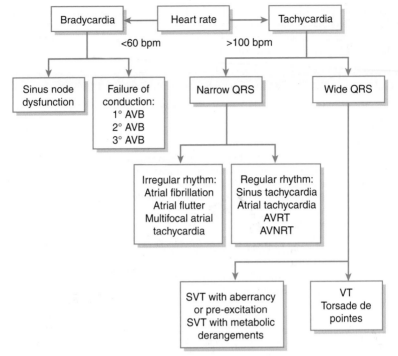

Figure 10-1 **Arrhythmia classification.** AVB, atrioventricular block; AVNRT, atrioventricular nodal reentrant tachycardia; AVRT, atrioventricular reentrant tachycardia; bpm, beats per minute; SVT, supraventricular tachycardia; VT, ventricular tachycardia.

- Although there are some inconsistencies, a practical taxonomy for arrhythmias is based on rate and prominent ECG features. Tachyarrhythmias are those with a rate >100 beats per minute (bpm), whereas bradyarrhythmias have a rate typically <50 bpm. The terms tachycardia and tachyarrhythmia or bradycardia and bradyarrhythmia are essentially synonymous and will be used interchangeably in this chapter.
- Figure 10-1 provides an overview of the traditional classification of arrhythmias.

TACHYARRHYTHMIAS

- Tachyarrhythmias exhibit a heart rate >100 bpm and can arise from either supraventricular or ventricular origins.
- Although the appropriate management is dictated by the origin and the mechanism (increased automaticity, reentry, or triggered activity), these details are often not immediately evident.
- For practical purposes, a distinction is often made between narrow-complex and wide-complex tachycardias (WCTs) on the basis of a QRS complex < or >120 ms.

NARROW-COMPLEX TACHYCARDIA

- Narrow-complex tachyarrhythmias invariably **originate above or at the atrioventricular (AV) node** with a resultant narrow QRS complex that reflects normal activation along the His-Purkinje system.

- Narrow-complex tachycardias are further divided based on the regularity of the rhythm.
- These arrhythmias include sinus tachycardia, atrial fibrillation (AF), atrial flutter, atrial tachycardias, and various reentrant arrhythmias (e.g., atrioventricular reentrant tachycardia [AVRT], atrioventricular nodal reentrant tachycardia [AVNRT]).

Initial Approach

- The first priority is to check the patient's vital signs and initiate the appropriate ACLS protocol if the patient is unstable.
- In the stable patient, obtain a 12-lead ECG. However, correct identification of the arrhythmia is often difficult with rapid heart rates.
- A helpful approach to tachyarrhythmias is to **promote vagal (parasympathetic) activity** with either carotid massage or administration of adenosine (Table 10-1). This serves to slow down AV nodal conduction, decreasing the rate and frequently allowing identification of the rhythm. In addition, reentrant rhythms that require the AV node for maintenance will be terminated by these maneuvers.
- **Carotid sinus massage**
  ○ In the absence of carotid bruits, apply circular pressure to one carotid sinus for 5 seconds.
  ○ Use caution in patients at risk for myocardial ischemia or cerebrovascular accident.
- **Adenosine** (Table 10-1)
  ○ Give 6-mg **rapid** IV push. Adenosine has a half-life of approximately 9 seconds, so the full dose must be pushed and flushed rapidly. A second dose of 12 mg can be used if the first dose has no effect.
  ○ Adenosine will cause complete heart block, although typically brief; appropriate resuscitation equipment and personnel should be available.
  ○ The patient should be warned that adenosine will cause a transient unpleasant feeling of presyncope.
  ○ Rarely, adenosine can cause severe bronchospasm and severe respiratory distress.

Sinus Tachycardia

GENERAL PRINCIPLES

- Although not an arrhythmia per se, it is important to consider sinus tachycardia when confronted with a rapid, narrow-complex tachycardia.
- Sinus tachycardia is almost invariably a response to an underlying condition such as fever, hypovolemia, pain, anemia, thyrotoxicosis, pulmonary disease, heart failure (HF), caffeine, illicit drug use/withdrawal, or anxiety.[1]
- In rare cases, however, the sinus tachycardia is genuinely inappropriate and may be due to a reentrant arrhythmia within the sinoatrial (SA) node.[2]

DIAGNOSIS

- Heart rate is typically 150 to 200 bpm. There is usually a slow increase and decrease in heart rate, not abrupt onset and termination.
- ECG will demonstrate P waves with a normal axis and morphology.
- Laboratory evaluation should include underlying causes such as anemia, thyrotoxicosis, and drug intoxication (either prescribed or illicit).

TREATMENT

- Treatment is focused on the underlying cause.[1]
- Treatment aimed solely at slowing the heart rate (e.g., β-blockers or calcium channel blockers [CCBs]) is **rarely appropriate** and should be pursued only if the underlying

TABLE 10-1 Antiarrhythmic Medications

Class	Mechanism	Indications	Side effects	Other comments
Class Ia	Decreases phase 0 repolarization and inhibits Na and K channels		Proarrhythmia, torsade de pointes	Prolongs QRS, QT, PR
Quinidine		AF atrial flutter, ventricular arrhythmias	Diarrhea, nausea, vomiting, rash, hypotension, fever, tinnitus, blurred vision, headache, thrombocytopenia, lupus-like syndrome	May enhance AV nodal conduction; increases digoxin level and warfarin effects; amiodarone increases quinidine levels; therapeutic range 2–6 mg/L
Procainamide		Ventricular arrhythmias (labeled); atrial arrhythmias (unlabeled)	Drug-induced SLE, GI symptoms, hypotension, rash, insomnia, hepatitis, myopathy, agranulocytosis, heart block/asystole	50%–85% develop ANA; 30%–50% develop SLE; adjust dose for renal dysfunction; therapeutic range 4–10 mg/L (NAPA <20 mg/L)
Disopyramide		Ventricular arrhythmias (labeled); atrial arrhythmias (unlabeled)	Anticholinergic effects, nausea, vomiting, hypotension, hypoglycemia, nervousness	Significant negative inotropic activity; adjust dosage in patients with renal insufficiency, hepatic disease, HF, and elderly; may enhance AV nodal conduction; therapeutic range 2–6 mg/L
Class Ib	Decreases phase 0 depolarization and slows down intracardiac conduction		CNS effects, seizures, coma, psychosis, tremor	No ECG changes
Lidocaine		Acute treatment of ventricular arrhythmias	Cardiac depression, bradycardia/asystole	Monitor levels for infusions for >24 hours Dependent on hepatic blood flow Therapeutic level 1.5–5 mg/L

(Continued)

TABLE 10-1 Antiarrhythmic Medications (Continued)

Class	Mechanism	Indications	Side effects	Other comments
Mexiletine		Ventricular arrhythmias	Nausea, vomiting, thrombocytopenia, AV block	Should be taken with food; reduce dosage in hepatic dysfunction, HF, and CrCl >10; therapeutic level 0.5–2 mg/L
Class Ic	Decreases phase 0 depolarization and markedly slows intracardiac conduction		Bradycardia, heart block, proarrhythmia	Avoid in patients with structural heart disease; prolongs PR and QRS
Flecainide		Paroxysmal AF and flutter; paroxysmal SVT (AVNRT); ventricular arrhythmia	Significant negative inotropy, blurry vision, headache, GI symptoms, neutropenia	Avoid in patients with HF; may increase defibrillation threshold; reduce dose in hepatic dysfunction, renal insufficiency, and HF; therapeutic level 0.2–1 mg/L
Propafenone		Ventricular arrhythmias (labeled); SVT (unlabeled)	Metallic/bitter taste, headache, GI upset, cholestatic jaundice	May worsen obstructive lung disease; reduce dose in hepatic dysfunction
Class II Metoprolol, carvedilol, atenolol, esmolol, and others	β-Adrenergic blockade	HTN; rate control in SVT; ventricular ectopy; angina/CAD	Bradycardia, bronchospasm in predisposed patients, fatigue, HF exacerbation, hypotension, sexual dysfunction, dizziness	Contraindications: bradycardia, heart block, cardiogenic shock, acute HF, severe bronchospastic lung disease; may blunt hypoglycemic symptoms
Class III Amiodarone	K channel inhibition Complex activity at multiple ion channels	Ventricular arrhythmias (labeled); atrial arrhythmias (unlabeled)	Proarrhythmia, torsade de pointes Hyper/hypothyroidism, chemical hepatitis, pulmonary fibrosis, bradycardia, heart block/bradycardia, skin photosensitivity	ECG effects: sinus bradycardia, PR, QRS, and QT prolongation

Dofetilide		Maintenance of sinus arrhythmia after cardioversion for AF	Can cause life-threatening ventricular arrhythmia	ECG effect: QTc prolongation; initiation of treatment requires 72 hours inpatient monitoring with QTc measurement after each dose; Only certified cardiologists can prescribe dofetilide
Sotalol	Combined β-blocker and K channel blocker	Ventricular arrhythmia (labeled); atrial fibrillation (unlabeled)	Proarrhythmia, including torsade de pointes	ECG effects: sinus bradycardia, QT and PR prolongation; reduce dose in renal dysfunction
Class IV				
Diltiazem	Calcium channel blockade	Rate control of atrial arrhythmias	Negative inotropy, headache, dizziness, edema, bradycardia, AV block, hypotension	
Verapamil		Rate control of atrial arrhythmia	Negative inotropy, constipation, hypotension, bradycardia, AV block	
Others				
Adenosine	Depression of AV conduction due to α_1-agonism	Conversion of reentrant SVT	Flushing, dyspnea, chest pressure, nausea, bronchospasm, heart block	May produce transient asystole
Digoxin	Increased AV node refractory period due to increased vagal tone	Rate control of AF, atrial flutter, or SVT	Bradycardia, AV block, anorexia, nausea, diarrhea, yellow-green halo around light, blurry vision, confusion, proarrhythmia	ECG effects: PR prolongation, ST depression; toxicity characterized by atrial arrhythmia in conjunction with heart block; toxicity possible at therapeutic levels; toxicity treated with electrolyte correction and use of Digibind; therapeutic levels 1–2 ng/mL

AF, atrial fibrillation; ANA, antinuclear antibody; AV, atrioventricular; AVB, atrioventricular block; AVNRT, atrioventricular nodal reentrant tachycardia; CAD, coronary artery disease; HF, heart failure; CNS, central nervous system; CrCl, creatinine clearance; GI, gastrointestinal; HTN, hypertension; K, potassium; NAPA, *n*-acetyl procainamide; SLE, systemic lupus erythematosus; SVT, supraventricular tachycardia.

cardiac disease (e.g., valvular disease, coronary artery disease [CAD], HF) results in intolerance of the elevated heart rate. The increased heart rate frequently represents a compensatory response, **which is necessary to maintain cardiac output**.
- It should be emphasized that an inappropriate sinus tachycardia is a rare condition and should be considered only after a rigorous exclusion of secondary causes of tachycardia.

Atrial Fibrillation

GENERAL PRINCIPLES

- AF is the most common sustained arrhythmia with an incidence of about 1% in the general population and about 10% in those >80.[1]
- It is most commonly associated with valvular disease, advanced age, hypertension, HF, CAD, and mechanical dilatation of the atria.[1,3]
- Hyperthyroidism is the most common noncardiac, treatable cause of AF.
- Frequently described as "lone" (i.e., occurring in the absence of other cardiac diseases), "first episode," "recurrent," "paroxysmal" (i.e., recurrent episodes that typically self-terminate), "persistent" (i.e., requiring electrical or chemical cardioversion), and "permanent" (i.e., cannot be converted to normal sinus rhythm).
- AF results in three distinct consequences.
  ○ The loss of AV synchrony with a resultant decrease in cardiac output due to the lack of the atrial contraction
  ○ **Increased thromboembolic risk** due to blood stasis in the noncontractile atrium
  ○ Decreased cardiac output and increased myocardial oxygen demand due to the increased ventricular rate
- The underlying electrical substrate for AF remains under investigation, although the role of the pulmonary veins as a site of initiation has led to new treatment options (see Treatment section below).

DIAGNOSIS

- ECG demonstrates chaotic atrial activity without evidence of P waves, although some coarse fibrillation waves may be evident in coarse AF (Fig. 10-2).
- Ventricular rate is typically 140 to 180 bpm but varies substantially depending on rapidity of AV nodal conduction.
- Laboratory evaluation should include tests of thyroid function.

TREATMENT

- Despite the intuitive appeal of treatment, which maintains sinus rhythm, several studies have shown that this strategy is unsuccessful at reducing the morbidity and mortality associated with AF, most likely reflecting the poor success rate of current therapies at maintaining sinus rhythm.[4-6] Therefore, current therapy focuses on addressing individually the adverse consequences of AF.

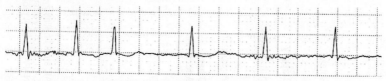

Figure 10-2 **Atrial fibrillation.** Note the irregular rhythm and lack of P waves.

- The two general treatment strategies are often referred to as "rate control," in which the AF rhythm is accepted, but the rate is controlled and "rhythm control," in which efforts are made to maintain sinus rhythm. As discussed below, **both strategies frequently require anticoagulation.**[6]

Control of Ventricular Rate

- Ventricular rate is controlled with medications that slow down AV nodal conduction.
- **β-Blockers and CCBs** are first-line agents for control of ventricular rate. Choice of specific agents is often determined by other indications or contraindications in a given patient.
- **Digoxin** can also provide control of resting ventricular rate, although it is less effective at reducing ventricular rate during exertion. In addition, digoxin is associated with more side effects than are other agents (Table 10-1). Its ideal use is in a patient with left ventricular (LV) dysfunction whose ventricular function also benefits from digoxin.
- In some cases, pharmacologic control of ventricular rate proves impossible. In these patients, invasive radio-frequency AV node ablation (resulting in complete heart block) with implantation of a permanent pacemaker is an option.

Maintenance of Sinus Rhythm

- Restoration and maintenance of sinus rhythm is a tempting goal but not always readily achievable. How aggressively sinus rhythm is pursued is dictated by the patient's overall cardiac function and the degree to which they can tolerate AF.
- Initial termination of AF is accomplished by synchronized direct current cardioversion (DCCV) with a success rate of ≥80%. DCCV requires sedation and hemodynamic monitoring and should be carried out in facility with emergency resuscitation and airway support available.
- Several medications may result in pharmacologic cardioversion, increase the success rate of DCCV, and improve maintenance of sinus rhythm once cardioversion is accomplished.[1]
- For patients with structural heart disease, preferred agents include amiodarone, sotalol, and dofetilide (Table 10-1).
- For patients without structural heart disease, preferred agents include amiodarone, flecainide, and propafenone (Table 10-1).
- Amiodarone (Table 10-1) is typically well tolerated but has several significant long-term side effects. It is, therefore, less favored for use in young patients who may require decades of therapy.[7]
- Initiation or adjustment of these medications frequently requires inpatient cardiac monitoring and should be performed in consultation with a cardiac electrophysiologist.

Atrial Fibrillation Ablation/Surgical Treatment Options

- New techniques of catheter-based AF ablation are becoming increasingly successful.
- Should noninvasive attempts to maintain sinus rhythm fail in a patient who does not tolerate AF well, invasive ablation techniques can be considered to restore the sinus rhythm.[6]
- Historically, the surgical Cox maze procedure was designed to eliminate AF by creating a pattern of scar lines in the atrium that interrupts the fibrillation. However, this technique is now more commonly performed in conjunction with other cardiac operations.
- Minimally invasive catheter-based techniques (such as electrical isolation of the pulmonary veins) may be a more suitable option for patients not requiring cardiac surgery with a success rate of 60% to 80% at experienced centers.
- The details of these techniques continue to undergo rapid development and are beyond the scope of this chapter.
- **Consultation with a cardiac electrophysiologist is warranted for any patient with poorly tolerated AF.**

Thromboembolic Risk

- Although, in theory, restoration of sinus rhythm obviates the need for anticoagulation, several studies have shown that **the risk of stroke from atrial thrombi is essentially unchanged by pharmacologic attempts to maintain sinus rhythm.**[4,5] However, given the risks of anticoagulation, attempts have been made to identify which patients are at high enough risk to justify warfarin therapy.
- Several different indices of thromboembolic risk have been developed. In general, patients with advanced age, HF, a history of stroke, diabetes, or hypertension are at greater risk of stroke in the context of AF.[4]
- It is essential to ensure the absence of left atrial thrombus **prior to** DCCV in any patient with AF lasting longer than 48 hours. This can be accomplished with transesophageal echocardiography with visualization of the left atrial appendage; transthoracic echocardiography is not adequate. Alternatively, the patient can be anticoagulated for a period of at least 3 to 4 weeks prior to cardioversion.[4]
- Importantly, **the risk of embolic events is highest in the several weeks following cardioversion, even if it is successful.** It is therefore essential to continue therapeutic anticoagulation for at least 4 weeks following cardioversion.
  - In recent years, a number of new agents have been approved for thromboembolism prevention in nonvalvular AF. The choice of a particular therapeutic anticoagulant should be tailored to each patient individually (see Chapter 14).
  - The role of transesophageal echocardiogram (TEE) to exclude thrombus prior to DCCV when therapeutically anticoagulated with an agent other than warfarin has not been well established.
- It should be emphasized that AF is typically a chronic/recurrent condition. The presumption is, therefore, that the patient requires permanent anticoagulation unless (a) a contraindication to anticoagulation exists or (b) the patient is clearly at low risk for embolic events.

AF and Preexcitation (Wolff-Parkinson-White Syndrome)

- AF in a patient with an AV bypass tract poses a special risk. In the normal heart, the maximal ventricular rate in AF is limited by the slow conduction of the AV node. When conduction occurs through a bypass tract, the ventricular rate can match the AF rate (400 to 700 bpm) resulting in degeneration into ventricular fibrillation (VF) and cardiovascular collapse.
- The ECG in preexcited AF is **characterized by an irregularly irregular rate with varying morphologies of a wide-complex QRS.**
- Treatment options include procainamide, amiodarone, or DCCV. **AV nodal blocking agents including adenosine, CCBs, β-blockers, and digoxin should be avoided** as they can cause acceleration of the bypass tract conduction. Expert consultation is required for definitive treatment and ablation of the bypass tract (Table 10-1).

Perioperative AF

- AF is common in the postoperative patient, especially after cardiac surgery and most specifically valvular surgery. Most episodes are self-limiting but in the interim pose **the same risks as any other episode of AF.** Because of the potential complications of anticoagulation, **prompt DCCV within the first 48 hours of AF is recommended.**
- Perioperative treatment with β-blockers has been shown to reduce the incidence of AF.[8]
- In addition, amiodarone (Table 10-1) is frequently used as either prophylactic **treatment or once the AF has occurred.**[8]
- The need for continued therapy should be reevaluated by a cardiologist several months after the operation.

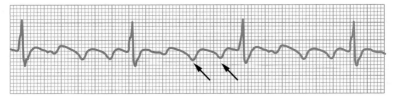

Figure 10-3 **Atrial flutter.** This is an example of 3:1 atrial flutter. Note sawtooth-shaped flutter waves (*arrows*).

Atrial Flutter

GENERAL PRINCIPLES

- Atrial flutter is sustained reentry within the atria, causing rapid fluttering of the atria.
- Although it is more electrically organized than AF, the atrial transport of blood is still less efficient than normal; flutter thus also has a risk of thromboembolism.
- Many of the same factors that predispose to AF are also related to atrial flutter. It is not uncommon for patients to have both rhythms and transition from one to the other.

DIAGNOSIS

- ECG demonstrates sawtooth flutter waves. In typical flutter, these sawtooth waves are most evident in the inferior leads (Fig. 10-3). Typical flutter waves have a negative vector in the inferior leads (II, III, aVF) while positive in the anterior precordium (V1, V2). In other forms of flutter, various appearances of the flutter waves are possible.
- Flutter waves are typically at a rate of 240 to 340 bpm; 300 bpm is classic.
- Ventricular rate is usually at a 2:1, 3:1, or 4:1 ratio with the atrial rate. Although the ventricular rate may be irregular due to variable conduction block, it is more typically regular with a fixed ratio to the atrial activity.

TREATMENT

- Medical treatment of atrial flutter is essentially identical to management of AF: control of ventricular rate, management of stroke risk with anticoagulation, and, when possible, maintenance of sinus rhythm.
- The stereotypical circuit in typical atrial flutter is readily amenable to catheter ablation techniques with a success rate of approximately 90%. However, a significant number of patients subsequently develop AF.[6]

Reentrant Supraventricular Tachycardia

GENERAL PRINCIPLES

- Although the term supraventricular tachycardia (SVT) would technically include all rhythms arising above the AV node, it is conventionally applied to a specific group of reentrant rhythms.[9,10]
- SVTs are divided into two main groups based on the anatomy of the reentrant circuit.
  - **AVNRT:** The entire reentrant circuit is contained in the AV node and the immediate surrounding tissue.
  - **AVRT:** The reentrant circuit includes atrial tissue, the AV node, ventricular tissue, and an accessory bypass tract.

- Common features of reentrant rhythms include one branch of the circuit with rapid conduction (and a long refractory period) and another branch with slow conduction (and a short refractory period). With this anatomy, an appropriately timed premature impulse can trigger the reentry and result in continuous cycling of electrical activity in this circuit.
- Different forms of AVRT and AVNRT are characterized by whether the antegrade impulse (forward, i.e., atrial to ventricular) occurs over the fast or slow pathway. The retrograde impulse (backward, i.e., ventricular to atrial) occurs over the other pathway.
- SVTs result in **retrograde P** waves as the retrograde signal stimulates the atrium. These rhythms can therefore be further divided into long RP in which the (retrograde) P wave occurs significantly after the QRS complex, reflecting retrograde conduction over a slow pathway, or short RP in which the (retrograde) P wave occurs rapidly after the QRS.
- AVRT and AVNRT typically occur in patients without other underlying cardiac diseases.

DIAGNOSIS

- Clinical presentations include palpitations, dyspnea, syncope, and angina/HF in patients with underlying cardiac disease.
- Accurate diagnosis of reentrant arrhythmias is frequently possible from the ECG.
- Reentrant rhythms typically have an abrupt onset and termination, in contrast to sinus tachycardia and AF, and exhibit heart rates in the range of 150 to 250 bpm.
- All reentrant SVTs exhibit retrograde P waves, which are negative in leads II, III, and aVF, reflecting activation of the atrium in a reverse, caudal-to-cranial direction.
- AVNRT represents approximately 70% of SVTs with AVRT constituting the remainder.[1]
- ECG features of common SVTs are summarized in Figure 10-4.
- **Typical AVNRT** (50% to 90% of AVNRTs): **Antegrade** conduction occurs over the **slow** pathway and retrograde conduction over the fast pathway. As a result, the retrograde P wave occurs within 100 ms of the QRS, making this a "short RP" rhythm. In fact, the

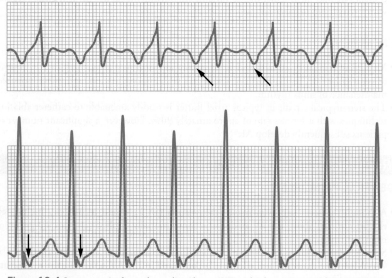

Figure 10-4 **Supraventricular tachycardia.** Above, SVT with a long RP interval; note inverted retrograde P waves in lead II (*arrows*). Below, SVT with a short RP interval; note inverted retrograde P waves in lead II (*arrows*).

RP interval is so brief that typically the P waves are obscured by the QRS or visible only as a pseudo-R in lead V1 or pseudo-S in lead II or III.

- **Atypical AVNRT: Antegrade** conduction occurs over the **fast** pathway and retrograde conduction over the slow pathway. As a result, the retrograde P wave is visible between the QRS complexes with a long RP interval.
- **Orthodromic AVRT** (95% of AVRTs): **Antegrade** conduction occurs via the **AV node** and **retrograde** conduction over the **accessory pathway**. Most commonly, the RP interval is short due to a fairly rapidly conducting accessory tract. However, a slowly conducting accessory tract is also possible and gives rise to a long RP tachycardia.
- **Antidromic AVRT**: This is a WCT but mentioned here for contrast with orthodromic AVRT. Antegrade conduction occurs over the accessory pathway with a resultant wide QRS complex.
- **AVNRT may be visualized as reentry within the AV node**. As a result, the tachycardia can continue regardless of events in the atria or ventricles, such as premature ventricular contractions (PVCs), premature atrial contractions (PACs), or bundle-branch block. In AVRT, the atrium and ventricle are part of the circuit. Atrial and ventricular events will therefore affect the tachycardia.
- **AVRT requires the existence of an accessory tract**. Accessory pathways may be "manifest," that is, visible as preexcited delta waves on the baseline ECG (Wolff-Parkinson-White pattern), or concealed, that is, lacking evidence of antegrade conduction but capable of retrograde conduction and therefore support of AVRT. A manifest pathway can result in either orthodromic or antidromic AVRT, whereas a concealed pathway is capable only of orthodromic AVRT.

TREATMENT

- The initial approach to a stable patient with a narrow-complex tachycardia is the use of vagal maneuvers such as the Valsalva maneuver or carotid sinus massage or the administration of adenosine, as discussed above (Table 10-1). This will usually result in the termination of the arrhythmia in the case of AVRT and AVNRT.
- Medical treatment consists of AV node blockade with β-blockers, CCBs, and digoxin (Table 10-1).
- DCCV usually terminates the arrhythmia and is required in unstable patients.
- The high success rate (>95%) of catheter ablation makes definitive invasive treatment of these rhythms equally first line with medical management.[9]

Atrial Tachycardia

- Atrial tachycardias encompass various intra-atrial arrhythmias, including intra-atrial reentry, automatic tachycardias, and triggered tachycardias.
- These rhythms are almost invariably associated with underlying cardiac disease, chronic obstructive pulmonary disease (COPD), electrolyte imbalances, or digoxin toxicity (Table 10-1).[1]
- ECG features of atrial tachycardia
  - P-wave axis and morphology are **different** from sinus rhythm.
  - Rhythm is typically regular.
  - QRS is usually identical to normal sinus rhythm.
  - An electrophysiology (EP) study is usually required to fully characterize the atrial arrhythmia.
- Medical treatment options are focused on treatment of the underlying abnormalities.
- For clinically significant atrial tachycardias, radiofrequency catheter ablation is often the treatment of choice.

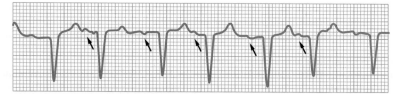

Figure 10-5 **Multifocal atrial tachycardia.** Note irregular rhythm and P wave with varying morphology and PR interval (*arrows*).

Multifocal Atrial Tachycardia

- Multifocal atrial tachycardia (MAT) is almost invariably associated with COPD or HF.[11]
- The underlying electrophysiologic mechanism likely involves increased automaticity or triggered activity.
- ECG features of MAT
  - Three or more different P-wave morphologies associated with different PR intervals (Fig. 10-5)
  - Atrial rate typically 100 to 130 bpm
- Treatment is focused on the underlying disease with little role for antiarrhythmic medications.
- In cases where treatment is necessary, CCBs and amiodarone (Table 10-1) have been shown to have some success.

WIDE-COMPLEX TACHYCARDIAS

- A WCT reflects activation that proceeds through the myocardium *without* use of the His-Purkinje system or does so in a slow and disorganized manner.
- As a result, the QRS is wide due to the slow propagation of the electrical signal. Only a few rhythms generate a wide QRS tachycardia:
  - A ventricular rhythm, that is, ventricular tachycardia (VT)
  - A supraventricular rhythm with aberrancy, that is, an intraventricular conduction delay such as left bundle branch block (LBBB) or right bundle branch block (RBBB)
  - A supraventricular rhythm with excitation through an accessory tract
  - Metabolic derangements (hyperkalemia or drug toxicity) resulting in a wide QRS

Initial Approach

- As with narrow-complex tachycardias, the first priority is evaluation of the patient's stability and application of ACLS protocols to the unstable patient.
- The immediate question that must be addressed when confronted with a WCT is whether the rhythm is ventricular in origin or supraventricular with aberrancy or preexcitation.
- Attention must also be paid to possible metabolic causes of a wide QRS complex, most importantly drug toxicity and hyperkalemia.
- The distinction between VT and SVT with aberrancy is challenging and is not always readily possible. However, several algorithms have been developed to distinguish these entities.[12]

Suggestive Features of Ventricular Tachycardia

- There are several suggestive features of VT.
  - An extreme rightward axis (–90 to 180 degree) suggests VT.
  - An initial R wave in aVR suggests VT.
  - Slight irregularity or irregularity at the onset of the rhythm suggests VT.

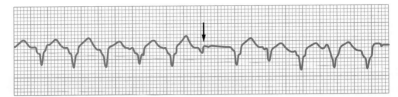

Figure 10-6 **Ventricular tachycardia.** Note fusion beat (*arrow*).

- ○ A QRS >140 ms in an RBBB-like tachycardia or a QRS >160 ms in an LBBB-like tachycardia suggests VT.
- ○ The presence of precordial concordance, that is, monomorphic QRS complexes, across the precordial leads that are either all entirely positive or all entirely negative suggests VT.
- ○ The presence of fusion beats (combination of a normal QRS and the ectopic beat) and capture beats (intermittent normal QRS complexes within the tachycardia) indicates AV dissociation and thus indicates VT (Fig. 10-6).
- In addition, several stepwise algorithms have been developed to distinguish VT from SVT in a WCT. The most commonly used criteria are those published by Brugada et al. and are summarized in Table 10-2.[13] At each step, either the rhythm is identified as VT or one proceeds to the next criterion.
- Although accurate, these criteria are frequently too cumbersome to be applied by those not readily familiar with them. The original Brugada criteria demonstrated a sensitivity of 99% and a specificity of 96.5%; however, further real-world studies demonstrated a sensitivity of 79% to 92% and a specificity of 44% to 56%.[14]
- A useful rule of thumb is that **any WCT is presumed to be VT until proven otherwise**. This assumption is justified by the fact that **up to 80% of WCT in the setting of heart disease is VT**.
- This approach is further reinforced by the fact that many of the pharmacologic treatments for SVT (adenosine and CCBs) have the potential to cause degeneration of VT to VF, whereas the treatments for VT (amiodarone and procainamide) are frequently effective

---

TABLE 10-2   Brugada Criteria for Wide-Complex Tachycardia

- Is there an RS in *any* precordial lead?
  - ○ If no, the rhythm is VT.
- If there is an RS in a precordial lead, measure the time from QRS onset to the nadir of the S wave.
  - ○ If >100 ms, the rhythm is VT.
- Is there evidence of AV dissociation? (e.g., P waves, fusion beats, capture beats)
  - ○ If so, the rhythm is VT.
- Examine the QRS morphology in V1, V2, and V6 for typical VT morphology:
  - ○ RBBB-like pattern (positive QRS polarity in V1 and V2):
    - - V1, V2: R or qR indicates VT.
  - ○ Other sources also include an RSR′ with R > R′ as indicative of VT.
    - - V6: rS (i.e., R wave smaller than S wave) indicates VT.
  - ○ LBBB-like pattern (negative QRS polarity in V1 and V2):
    - - V1, V2: broad initial R wave >40 ms indicates VT.

AV, atrioventricular; VT, ventricular tachycardia; LBBB, left bundle-branch block; RBBB, right bundle-branch block.
Modified from Brugada P, Brugada J, Mont L, et al. A new approach to the differential diagnosis of a regular tachycardia with a wide QRS complex. *Circulation* 1991;83:1649–1659.

and safe for SVT (Table 10-1). Therefore, use of VT treatments is preferred if the rhythm is unclear.

• **In summary, any WCT should be managed as VT.** Once the patient is stabilized, expert consultation is warranted to clarify the rhythm and future management.

Ventricular Arrhythmias

• Ventricular arrhythmias encompass a spectrum from single PVCs, couplets and triplets (two to three consecutive PVCs), to VT and VF.
• VT can be described as **sustained** (definitions vary but are typically defined as >30 seconds in duration or causing hemodynamic collapse requiring immediate cardioversion) or **non-sustained** (NSVT) (>3 beats but <30 seconds). The abbreviations SVT and NSVT refer to entirely different rhythms despite their similarity. Sustained VT is **not** abbreviated SVT.
• VT is described as **monomorphic** (in which all of the QRS complexes exhibit the same morphology) or **polymorphic**. Polymorphic VT is closer, both in mechanism and treatment, to VF than to monomorphic VT.
• Management of VT depends on the presence or absence of underlying cardiac disease.
• Reversible causes of VT should be evaluated including cocaine and digitalis intoxication, hypokalemia, hypomagnesemia, and acute ischemia.

VENTRICULAR ARRHYTHMIAS ASSOCIATED WITH STRUCTURAL HEART DISEASE

GENERAL PRINCIPLES

• VT can be associated with various underlying cardiac diseases, including ischemic cardiomyopathy; nonischemic cardiomyopathy; and infiltrative conditions including amyloidosis and sarcoidosis; either repaired or unrepaired congenital heart disease; and muscular dystrophies.
• Most studies have focused on ischemic and, more recently, nonischemic dilated cardiomyopathies. However, the general approach is applied to cardiomyopathies of other etiologies as well.

TREATMENT

• **Premature ventricular contractions**
  ○ PVCs in the context of structural heart disease are associated with an increased risk of sudden cardiac death (SCD).
  ○ However, pharmacologic suppression, although effective at reducing the incidence of PVCs, has failed to show a mortality benefit. In fact, **use of class I antiarrhythmics (Table 10-1) results in an increased mortality in the setting of ischemic heart disease**.[15,16]
  ○ In light of this, treatment of asymptomatic PVCs themselves is not warranted. Symptomatic PVCs may be treated with β-blockers, antiarrhythmic agents, and, in some circumstances, ablation.
• **Nonsustained VT**
  ○ NSVT in the context of structural heart disease is similarly associated with SCD. As with PVCs, pharmacologic therapy alone does not reduce the incidence of SCD.
  ○ For patients with at least moderately reduced ejection fraction (EF) (typically defined as ≤35%), an implantable cardiac defibrillator (ICD) is warranted for primary prevention, as discussed below, and the presence or absence of NSVT is largely immaterial.
• **Sustained VT**
  ○ Sustained VT requires immediate medical attention. In the unstable patient, termination of the rhythm requires immediate cardioversion.
  ○ In the stable patient, consideration can be given to pharmacologic termination with either amiodarone or lidocaine (Table 10-1).

- ○ Unless the rhythm is unequivocally the result of a transient and reversible cause, such as an electrolyte abnormality, ICD therapy is usually indicated.
- ○ Expert consultation is warranted for any sustained VT.
- **Polymorphic VT**
  - ○ In the context of ischemic heart disease, polymorphic VT has a worse prognosis than monomorphic VT. Management focuses on treatment of the underlying ischemic disease whenever possible.
  - ○ Other forms of polymorphic VT require different treatment and will be discussed below.
- **Long-term treatment options for VT**
  - ○ After acute termination of the VT, several long-term treatment options are available.
  - ○ **The first-line treatment is placement of an ICD**, which has been shown to reduce mortality when compared with pharmacologic therapy in multiple studies.[17–19]
  - ○ Although successful at reducing VT burden, **pharmacologic therapy has not been shown to reduce mortality from SCD**. As such, its role in treatment is limited to (a) patients with contraindications to ICD placement or (b) patients with an ICD with the intention of reducing the frequency of ICD shocks. First-line medications include amiodarone and sotalol (Table 10-1).
  - ○ In patients with persistent VT, catheter or surgical ablation procedures can be performed. These procedures are most successful in patients with a well-localized scar rather than a diffuse myocardial process.
  - ○ In extreme cases of refractory ventricular arrhythmias, cardiac transplantation can be considered.

VT ASSOCIATED WITH ACUTE MYOCARDIAL ISCHEMIA

- The significance of VT in the context of acute myocardial ischemia or infarction depends on the timing of the VT.
- Although VT shortly after acute myocardial infarction (AMI) is a poor prognostic sign with regard to in-hospital mortality, the long-term significance remains unclear. In contrast, late VT portends future malignant arrhythmias.
- One specific form of ischemic arrhythmia, which warrants special mention, is **accelerated idioventricular rhythm** (AIVR). This ventricular rhythm exhibits a wide QRS, a rate between 50 and 120 bpm, and is frequently associated with reperfusion, either spontaneous or medically accomplished. This is a benign rhythm that requires no treatment; there is no long-term prognostic significance of AIVR.

IDIOPATHIC VT NOT ASSOCIATED WITH STRUCTURAL HEART DISEASE

- A minority of ventricular arrhythmias are not associated with obvious structural heart disease, although as our understanding of these diseases progresses, it is frequently discovered that these patients have more subtle molecular or cellular derangements.
- Idiopathic VT is divided into monomorphic and polymorphic VT.
- Monomorphic VT, as found in conditions including repetitive monomorphic VT (RMVT), right ventricular outflow tract VT (RVOT VT), and idiopathic left ventricular VT, has a fairly benign prognosis. In contrast, polymorphic VT, as found in familial catecholaminergic VT, has a more malignant course. The details of these conditions are beyond the scope of this chapter, and any VT warrants referral to a cardiac electrophysiologist.

TORSADE DE POINTES

GENERAL PRINCIPLES

- **Torsade de pointes** (TdP) (twisting of the points) is a form of polymorphic VT that occurs in association with a baseline prolonged QT interval.

TABLE 10-3	Selected Medication Associated with QT Prolongation

Antiarrhythmic drugs
Quinidine
Procainamide
Disopyramide
Amiodarone
Sotalol
Dofetilide/ibutilide

Psychotropic drugs
Thioridazine
Phenothiazines
Tricyclic antidepressants
Haloperidol
Risperidone
Methadone

Antihistamines
Terfenadine
Astemizole

Antimicrobial drugs
Erythromycin
Clarithromycin
Telithromycin
Azithromycin

Other drugs
Cisapride
Domperidone
Droperidol
Ranolazine
HIV protease inhibitors
Organophosphate insecticides
Cocaine
Arsenic trioxide
Cesium chloride
Some Chinese herbs

- Congenital forms of TdP occur in the context of genetic long QT syndromes (discussed below).
- Most cases occur as the result of **acquired QT prolongation** due to medications, electrolyte abnormalities (hypokalemia, hypomagnesemia, and hypocalcemia), hypothyroidism, cerebrovascular events, ischemia, or severe HF.[20]
- In addition, **bradycardia** (which results in a relatively lengthened QT interval) can exacerbate TdP, although usually this occurs in the context of another precipitating factor.
- A substantial number of **medications** (summarized in Table 10-3 or available at www.qtdrugs.org) have been associated with QT prolongation, although not invariably with TdP.

DIAGNOSIS

- The ECG appearance of TdP consists of a WCT with a continuously changing axis, giving rise to an undulating appearance (Fig. 10-7).
- Further laboratory evaluation is focused on electrolyte levels, thyroid function, and myocardial ischemia.

TREATMENT

- Immediate DCCV is the treatment of choice for an unstable patient with TdP.
- Intravenous magnesium is frequently helpful in terminating stable TdP.
- Avoidance of QT-prolonging medications is crucial in these patients.

Ventricular Fibrillation

VF is a pulseless and **rapidly fatal rhythm without prompt defibrillation** and ACLS management.

WOLFF-PARKINSON-WHITE SYNDROME AND PREEXCITATION

GENERAL PRINCIPLES

- A wide variety of abnormal connections have been described that bypass the normal atria → AV node → bundle of His → Purkinje fiber pattern of excitation.

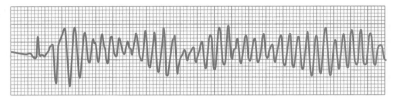

Figure 10-7 **Torsade de pointes.**

- The most common and clinically significant of such pathways are **Kent bundles**, which directly connect atrial and ventricular tissue and are responsible for the Wolff-Parkinson-White syndrome.
- Although other connections exist, their role in arrhythmias is more complex and the Kent bundles serve to illustrate this class of arrhythmias.[1]
- The clinical importance of these pathways is twofold. First, it provides the substrate for reentrant AVRT rhythms (see above). Second, by bypassing the slowed conduction of the AV node, it provides the potential for an atrial arrhythmia such as AF to be conducted to the ventricle at dangerously rapid rates.
- In general, preexcitation is not associated with other underlying cardiac diseases. In the absence of symptoms or a family history of SCD, the occurrence of malignant arrhythmias is rare.

DIAGNOSIS

- The Wolff-Parkinson-White pattern on ECG
  ○ A short PR interval of <120 ms
  ○ A wide QRS interval of >110 to 120 ms, frequently with a **slurred upstroke (delta wave)** in some leads
  ○ ST-T segment deviation opposite the QRS vector
- The Wolff-Parkinson-White syndrome consists of the above criteria on the baseline ECG in addition to an SVT (e.g., AVRT) **with symptoms**.

TREATMENT

- Acute management is typically required when the patient has developed a reentrant tachycardia or AF with a rapid ventricular response.
- Immediate DCCV is the treatment of choice in the **unstable patient**.
- **Use of AV nodal blocking agents** (adenosine, CCBs, and β-blockers) **should be avoided** in the case of preexcited AF since this can result in acceleration of the tachycardia via the accessory pathway (Table 10-1).
- IV procainamide or amiodarone (Table 10-1) can be used safely.
- **In patients without symptoms** and at low risk for SCD, treatment may not be necessary.
- Medical treatment options include amiodarone, sotalol, flecainide, or propafenone (Table 10-1).
- Radio-frequency ablation is 85% to 95% effective at eliminating the bypass tract.

Primary Prevention of Sudden Cardiac Death

- With the increased use of ICDs for the termination of potentially fatal ventricular arrhythmias, much attention has been devoted to identifying patients at the greatest risk for SCD.[21]
- The placement of an ICD in patients at high risk for SCD is termed primary prevention, in contrast to secondary prevention in patients who have already experienced either SCD or sustained VT/VF.

- The current ability to identify patients at highest risk for SCD remains limited, as only 30% of patients currently regarded as high risk (i.e., those who receive ICDs) ever experience an aborted arrest, and conversely, 50% of SCD occurs in patients not identified as high risk.[22]
- At this point in time, no screening of the general population is recommended for SCD risk factors beyond standard screening for cardiovascular health.
- Criteria for the placement of an ICD are summarized in Table 10-4. Briefly, placement of an ICD for primary prevention is warranted in patients with
  - Ischemic or nonischemic cardiomyopathy and EF ≤35% with clinical NYHA class II to III symptoms.
  - Ischemic cardiomyopathy and EF ≤40% with NSVT and inducible VT on EP study.

TABLE 10-4	Selected Indications for Automatic Implantable Cardiac Defibrillator Placement

Class I

Cardiac arrest due to VF or VT not due to a reversible cause

Spontaneous sustained VT in association with structural heart disease

LVEF ≤35% due to prior MI who are at least 40 days post-MI and are in NYHA functional class II or III

Nonischemic dilated cardiomyopathy (DCM) who have an LVEF ≤35% and who are in NYHA functional class II or III

Syncope of undetermined origin with hemodynamically significant sustained VT induced in EP study not amenable to drug therapy

Nonsustained VT with CAD, prior MI, LV dysfunction, and inducible VT/VF in EP study

Class IIa

ICD implantation is reasonable for patients with unexplained syncope, significant LV dysfunction, and nonischemic DCM

Familial and congenital conditions with a high risk of life-threatening ventricular arrhythmias, including hypertrophic cardiomyopathy, long QT syndrome, Brugada syndrome, and arrhythmogenic right ventricular dysplasia

Class IIb

Nonischemic heart disease who have an LVEF of ≤35% and who are in NYHA functional class I

Class III

Syncope of undetermined origin without inducible tachyarrhythmias and without structural heart disease

VF or VT resulting from arrhythmias amenable to surgical or catheter ablation

VT due to reversible causes, including AMI, electrolyte imbalance, drugs, or trauma

Significant psychiatric illness precluding reliable follow-up

Terminal illness with <6 months life expectancy

Class IV

Drug refractory HF patients who are not candidates for cardiac transplantation

CABG, coronary artery bypass graft; CAD, coronary artery disease; HF, congestive heart failure; EP, electrophysiology; LV, left ventricular; LVEF, left ventricular ejection fraction; MI, myocardial infarction; NYHA, New York Heart Association; VF, ventricular fibrillation; VT, ventricular tachycardia.
Class I: Evidence or general agreement that the treatment is useful and effective.
Class IIa: Conflicting evidence or divergence of opinion, with a weight of evidence favoring a benefit.
Class IIb: Conflicting evidence or divergence of opinion, with benefit less well established.
Class III: Evidence or general agreement that the treatment is not effective or is harmful.
Data from Epstein AE, DiMarco JP, Ellenbogen KA, et al. ACC/AHA/HRS 2008 guidelines for device-based therapy of cardiac rhythm abnormalities. *Circulation* 2008;117:e350–408.

BRADYARRHYTHMIAS

- A heart rate <60 bpm (or according to some, 50 bpm) constitutes bradycardia.
- A considerable variation in normal heart rate has been recorded among healthy patients. Of particular note, trained athletes frequently exhibit heart rates as low as 40 while at rest and can even include sinus pauses and AV nodal blocks. Similarly, heart rates decrease by approximately 24 bpm during sleep.[23]
- As a result of these considerations, **it is difficult to define a heart rate alone that warrants treatment.** Associated symptoms and the underlying mechanism of the bradycardia must be considered.
- Bradyarrhythmias may result in syncope, light-headedness, weakness, fatigue, dizziness, or HF symptoms.
- Broadly, pathologic bradyarrhythmias result from either a failure of impulse generation by the SA node or by a failure of impulse propagation (i.e., a conduction block).

Sinus Node Dysfunction

GENERAL PRINCIPLES

- **Sick sinus syndrome** is a broad term that encompasses various sinus node dysfunctions.
- One specific form of sick sinus syndrome is known as **tachycardia-bradycardia (or tachy-brady) syndrome.** This can take the form of almost any combination of tachyarrhythmia and bradyarrhythmia but frequently includes a prolonged sinus pause accompanying the termination of a tachyarrhythmia.
- Sick sinus syndrome can result from either intrinsic fibrosis of the sinus node or extrinsic causes including medications, hypothyroidism, hypothermia, increased intracranial pressure, electrolyte abnormalities, increased vagal tone, ischemia, and surgical trauma.

DIAGNOSIS

- Sick sinus syndrome can have a variety of ECG appearances, including inappropriate sinus bradycardia, sinus pauses, atrial tachyarrhythmias, and inappropriate heart rate responses to exercise.
- Laboratory testing should include thyroid function and electrolyte levels.

TREATMENT

- Reversible causes and offending medications should be addressed before considering pacemaker implantation. However, if a responsible medication (such as a β-blocker in a patient with CAD) is required, one can consider pacemaker implantation to permit continuation of the medication.
- Selected indications for pacemaker placement are summarized below in Table 10-5. They generally include bradycardias that are either of the following:
  ○ Likely to persist/recur and cause symptoms
  ○ Likely to progress to profound bradycardia or asystole

Conduction Abnormalities

GENERAL PRINCIPLES

- Normal cardiac conduction is initiated at the sinus node and spreads through the atrium to the AV node where it experiences a brief pause before continuing through the His-Purkinje system to activate the ventricular myocardium.

TABLE 10-5 Selected Indications for Permanent Pacemaker Placement

Class I
Bradycardia or AVB associated with symptoms
Third-degree AVB associated with:
   Documented asystole >3 seconds or escape rate <40 bpm
   Neuromuscular disease associated with AVB
Chronic bifascicular or trifascicular block associated with:
   Intermittent third-degree AVB
   Type II second-degree AVB
Congenital third-degree AVB

Class II
Asymptomatic third-degree AVB with escape rate >40 bpm
Asymptomatic second-degree type II AVB
Incidental finding of infra-His block on EP study

Class III
Sinus bradycardia or pauses not associated with symptoms
Asymptomatic first-degree AVB
Asymptomatic second-degree type I AVB
AV block expected to resolve

AVB, atrioventricular block; bpm, beats per minute; EP, electrophysiologic.
Class I: Evidence or general agreement that the treatment is useful and effective.
Class II: Conflicting evidence or divergence of opinion.
Class III: Evidence or general agreement that the treatment is not effective or is harmful.
Data from Epstein AE, DiMarco JP, Ellenbogen KA, et al. ACC/AHA/HRS 2008 Guidelines for device-based therapy of cardiac rhythm abnormalities. *Circulation* 2008;117:e350–e408.

- Defects in electrical conduction are described as atrioventricular block (AVB) and are categorized based on the behavior of conduction, which typically corresponds to the site/mechanism of the block.
- Causes of AV conduction block are similar to sinus node dysfunction and include fibrosis of the conduction system with age, medications, thyroid disease, infiltrative disease, increased vagal tone, ischemia, and surgical trauma.

DIAGNOSIS

- As with tachyarrhythmias, correlation of symptoms with bradycardia is important and may require the use of ambulatory monitoring. However, the bradyarrhythmia is frequently persistent and readily identified on the 12-lead ECG even at a time that the patient is asymptomatic or minimally symptomatic.
- Laboratory evaluation should include tests of thyroid function and electrolyte levels.
- The ECG features of AV blocks are summarized in Table 10-6.
- In addition, there are two special cases of AVB.
  - 2:1 AVB: Because of the absence of sequential conducted P waves, it is impossible to categorize 2:1 AV block as type 1 or type 2. The anatomic level (within the AV node or below the AV node) of the block must be inferred (e.g., if atropine or exercise results in enhanced AV nodal conduction and improvement in block, it is likely an intranodal block).
  - High-grade block: This term describes an AVB with multiple sequential nonconducted P waves. If the block is not associated with intense vagal activity, the anatomic level of the block is usually infranodal.

TABLE 10-6 Features of Conduction Abnormalities

Abnormality	ECG characteristics	Typical anatomic location of block	Example
First-degree AVB	PR interval >120 ms, but without failure of AV conduction (1:1 conduction)	Slowed conduction within the atrium and/or AV node	
Second-degree AVB, type I (Wenckebach block)	Intermittent failure of AV conduction (A:V > 1:1) Progressively increasing PR interval and (typically) shortening RR interval until a P wave fails to conduct PR interval after the blocked beat is shorter than previous PR interval	High AV node	Note that the nonconducted P wave (arrow) is superimposed on the T wave
Second-degree AVB, type II	Intermittent failure of conduction PR interval associated with conducted beats is constant (A:V > 1:1).	His-Purkinje system (infranodal)	
Third-degree AVB	AV dissociation	AV node	

AV, atrioventricular; AVB atrioventricular block.

TREATMENT

- Reversible causes and offending medications should be addressed before considering pacemaker implantation. However, if a responsible medication (such as a β-blocker in a patient with CAD) is required, one can consider pacemaker implantation to permit continuation of the medication.
- Indications for pacemaker placement are summarized in Table 10-5.[24]

CONGENITAL ARRHYTHMIAS

Management of congenital arrhythmias is a complex and rapidly evolving field. Any patient suspected of having a congenital arrhythmia syndrome requires evaluation by an experienced specialist.

Brugada Syndrome

- Brugada syndrome is due to **mutations in the sodium channel,** although the genetics of the disease are complex and incompletely understood.[25]
- Diagnostic criteria continue to evolve but include a typical ECG appearance of ST elevation in leads V1 to V3, an association with spontaneous VT/VF, and a familial pattern.
- Incidence is higher in men than in women and particularly prevalent among Asian males.
- Although pharmacologic therapy (usually amiodarone or quinidine, Table 10-1) can be considered, affected individuals usually require placement of an ICD for the prevention of SCD.

Long QT Syndrome

- To date, mutations in at least 13 genes that generate a congenital QT prolongation have been identified. Subtle differences in clinical features and ECG findings exist among some of these mutations.
- Patients can present with palpitations, syncope, SCD, and TdP.
- Management is complex and depends in part on the genotype of the affected individual. Referral to a cardiac electrophysiologist is warranted.[26]

Short QT Syndrome

- Short QT syndrome is a recently described genetic syndrome. To date, mutations in at least six different potassium and calcium channel genes have been associated with short QT syndrome.[27]
- Clinical features include a short QT interval (typically <330 ms when corrected for heart rate), a propensity for AF, and a risk of SCD.
- Patients with short QT syndrome have a high risk for sudden death, and ICD implantation is recommended as first-line therapy. Optimal medical management for this condition remains undefined.

Arrhythmogenic Right Ventricular Dysplasia/Cardiomyopathy

- Arrhythmogenic right ventricular dysplasia (ARVD) is characterized by a fibrofatty infiltrate of the right ventricle (RV), although the LV is sometimes involved, with a resultant thinning of the ventricular wall.[28]
- A subset of patients exhibit a familial pattern with mutations in genes involved in cell adhesion; however, mutations of other genes and at loci for which the gene is yet to be identified have also been associated with ARVD.
- Naxos disease is an autosomal recessive form of ARVD associated with palmoplantar keratosis and woolly hair.

- Clinical features of ARVD include arrhythmias (most commonly an RVOT VT), syncope, palpitations, and SCD. Despite the involvement of the RV, evidence of RV failure is relatively uncommon.
- Although sotalol and amiodarone may have role in suppressing the ventricular arrhythmias, only ICD placement is likely to reduce the risk of SCD (Table 10-1).

Familial Polymorphic Ventricular Tachycardia

- In contrast to TdP, familial polymorphic VT (also called catecholaminergic polymorphic VT) occurs in the absence of QT prolongation. Unlike the other forms of idiopathic VT, this condition is associated with a substantial risk of SCD.
- This syndrome occurs in the absence of apparent cardiac disease and typically manifests as syncope and sudden death; polymorphic VT and VF are most prominent during stress and physical exertion.
- Two genes have been implicated in this condition: the ryanodine receptor (with autosomal dominant transmission) and the calsequestrin 2 gene (with autosomal recessive transmission). Both proteins are involved in calcium handling by the sarcoplasmic reticulum.[29]
- Treatment includes β-blockers, given the catecholamine-induced nature of the arrhythmias. Even with medical treatment, the incidence of SCD is considerable and ICD placement is warranted when high-risk features (such as syncope) are present.

SYNCOPE

GENERAL PRINCIPLES

- Syncope and presyncope can result from a wide variety of mechanisms, including cardiac, neurologic, and metabolic. This section will focus only on the cardiac and, particularly, arrhythmic causes of syncope.
- Studies have estimated that approximately 15% of syncope cases result from arrhythmias. Further, it should be kept in mind that 30% to 50% of cases of syncope have no identifiable cause. Therefore, the diagnostic approach should **focus on the identification of high-risk predictors of future events rather than definitive diagnosis** of the episode in question.
- Cardiovascular causes of syncope include neurocardiogenic (also known as vasovagal syncope), valvular heart disease, hypertrophic cardiomyopathy, bradyarrhythmias, and tachyarrhythmias.
- Neurocardiogenic syncope is believed to result from a paradoxical bradycardic and/or hypotensive response to a catecholamine surge with resultant syncope.
- Although no findings in the history or physical exam are particularly sensitive or specific, **syncope resulting from cardiac arrhythmias tends to occur abruptly and with minimum prodromal symptoms, whereas neurocardiogenic syncope is frequently preceded by a feeling of flushing and light-headedness**.

DIAGNOSIS

- The cardiac evaluation of syncope should include echocardiography and a baseline ECG. Depending on the frequency of events, a Holter or event monitor can be considered to identify a causative arrhythmia.
- The role of tilt table testing is controversial. This diagnostic test is designed to elicit bradycardia and hypotension in response to persistent upright position after lying supine (on a tilting table with footstand) and thereby diagnose neurocardiogenic syncope. Sensitivity has been reported as high at 70%; however, 45% to 65% of normal individuals also exhibit a positive response to tilt table testing, markedly reducing the specificity of this test.[30] In addition, there is a small but distinct risk of cardiac arrest and death.

- The diagnosis of neurocardiogenic syncope can usually be made based on the history and exclusion of other causes without recourse to tilt table testing.

TREATMENT

- The management of symptomatic tachyarrhythmias and bradyarrhythmias is covered in the appropriate sections of this chapter.
- **Management of neurocardiogenic syncope can be difficult. Although placement of a pacemaker is tempting, the hypotensive response is frequently due to a vasodilatory effect and not a result of the bradycardia**. Therefore, patients often continue to have syncope despite control of the bradycardia. Only a subset of patients with a primarily bradycardic cause of their syncope are likely to benefit from a pacemaker.
- Behavioral modification plays an essential role in the control of neurocardiogenic syncope; patients are educated to avoid environmental triggers and volume depletion. Medications should be reviewed and vasodilatory medications eliminated.
- In selected patients, increased intake of salt and fluids can reduce both orthostatic and neurocardiogenic syncope.
- In general, **pharmacologic therapy has been found to be ineffective for neurocardiogenic syncope**.[31]
  - β-Blockers (some, such as acebutolol, with intrinsic sympathomimetic activity) have been used, though clinical trial data are conflicting.
  - Midodrine, an α-sympathomimetic drug, may inhibit vasodilation, but there is a risk of hypertension.
  - Some data support a role for selective serotonin reuptake inhibitors (SSRIs), such as paroxetine, and serotonin/norepinephrine reuptake inhibitors (SNRIs), such as venlafaxine.

IMPLANTABLE DEVICES FOR RHYTHM MANAGEMENT

With the increasing prevalence of both pacemakers and implanted defibrillators, it is important for the internist to be familiar with these devices.[32]

PACEMAKERS

- A pacemaker system consists of one or more electrical leads and a generator containing the battery and processor.
- Pacemaker systems may be either endocardial or epicardial. The more common endocardial system is placed by a percutaneous approach with the electrode leads in a subclavian vein and the generator placed in the subcutaneous pocket near the clavicle. The epicardial system is placed by a surgical approach with the electrodes on the epicardial surface and the generator located either in the upper abdomen or near the clavicle.
- The general principle of all pacemakers is to deliver stimuli that trigger a heartbeat in a pattern that most closely reproduces the normal cardiac activity.
- The full array of algorithms used by modern pacemakers is beyond the scope of this review. However, some general principles of pacemaker function (for pacemakers programmed in the dual/dual/dual [DDD] mode, the most common for patients not in AF) include the following:
  - If atrial activity is intact, the pacemaker will sense the atrial activity and deliver a ventricular stimulus (if necessary) in response to an atrial P wave.
  - If atrial activity is absent but the intrinsic conduction system is intact, the pacemaker will stimulate the atrium to generate a P wave, which is followed by conduction to the ventricle, generating a QRS complex. If the QRS does not occur within a programmed period of time, the pacemaker delivers a ventricular stimulus.

- If atrial activity is absent and the conduction system is not intact, the pacemaker will deliver stimuli to both the atrium and ventricle with a time delay that simulates the typical P wave and QRS timing.
- Pacemakers can be categorized by the number of leads.
  - **Dual chamber:** the most common configuration. Leads are placed in both the right atrium and the RV. This provides the greatest flexibility of pacemaker modes.
  - **Single chamber:** one lead in the RV. This design is used for patients in whom atrial pacing is not possible, such as permanent AF. Placement of a single atrial lead is an option in patients with an intact conduction system; the frequent progression of disease and subsequent requirement for a ventricular lead may make this an unappealing option.
  - **Biventricular:** In addition to the right atrial and right ventricular leads, a third lead is placed in a coronary vein (via the coronary sinus) to permit early activation of the left ventricle. This design is used in patients with severe HF and mechanical dyssynchrony. The selection of patients who will benefit from this device remains under investigation and is beyond the scope of this chapter. Current indications, however, are shown in Table 10-7.

TABLE 10-7 Selected Indications for Cardiac Resynchronization Therapy

Class I
CRT is indicated for patients who have LVEF ≤35%, sinus rhythm, LBBB with a QRS duration ≥150 ms, and NYHA class II, III, or ambulatory class IV symptoms on GDMT

Class IIa
CRT can be useful for patients who have LVEF ≤35%, sinus rhythm, LBBB with a QRS duration 120–149 ms, and NYHA class II, III, or ambulatory IV symptoms on GDMT
CRT can be useful for patients who have LVEF ≤35%, sinus rhythm, a non-LBBB pattern with a QRS duration ≥150 ms, and NYHA class III/ambulatory class IV symptoms on GDMT
CRT can be useful for patients on GDMT who have LVEF ≤35% and are undergoing new or replacement device placement with anticipated requirement for significant (>40%) ventricular pacing

Class IIb
CRT may be considered for patients who have LVEF ≤30%, ischemic etiology of heart failure, sinus rhythm, LBBB with a QRS duration of ≥150 ms, and NYHA class I symptoms on GDMT
CRT may be considered for patients who have LVEF ≤35%, sinus rhythm, a non-LBBB pattern with QRS duration 120–149 ms, and NYHA class III/ambulatory class IV on GDMT
CRT may be considered for patients who have LVEF ≤35%, sinus rhythm, a non-LBBB pattern with a QRS duration ≥150 ms, and NYHA class II symptoms on GDMT

Class III
CRT is not recommended for patients with NYHA class I or II symptoms and non-LBBB pattern with QRS duration <150 ms
CRT is not indicated for patients whose comorbidities and/or frailty limit survival with good functional capacity to <1 year

Class I: Evidence or general agreement that the treatment is useful and effective.
Class IIa: Conflicting evidence or divergence of opinion, with a weight of evidence favoring a benefit.
Class IIb: Conflicting evidence or divergence of opinion, with benefit less well established.
CRT, cardiac resynchronization therapy; GDMT, guideline-directed medical therapy; LBBB, left bundle branch block; LVEF, left ventricular ejection fraction; NYHA, New York Heart Association.
Data from Epstein AE, DiMarco JP, Ellenbogen KA, et al. ACC/AHA/HRS 2012 focused update of the 2008 guidelines for device-based therapy of cardiac rhythm abnormalities. *Circulation* 2012;126:1784–1800.

TABLE 10-8	Implanted Device Modes				
	First letter	**Second letter**	**Third letter**	**Fourth letter**	**Fifth letter**
Category	Chamber paced	Chamber sensed	Response to sensing	Programmability	Antitachycardia function
Letters	O = none; A = atrium; V = ventricle; D = dual (A + V)	O = none; A = atrium; V = ventricle; D = dual (A + V)	O = none; T = triggered; I = inhibited; D = dual (I + T)	O = none; P = simple programming; M = multiprogramming; C = communicating; R = rate-adaptive sensor	O = none; P = pacing; S = shock; D = dual (P and S)

- In addition to the lead configuration, pacemakers and defibrillators are described based on their mode. A five-letter code (although frequently only the first three or four letters are used) describes the sensing and pacing behavior of the device, as summarized in Table 10-8.
- Common modes of pacemakers
  - AAI or VVI: simple modes in which the pacemaker will sense and pace the atrium or ventricle at a given rate unless inhibited by intrinsic activity.
  - DDDR: a complex mode in which the pacemaker will sense and pace both the atrium and the ventricle in a pattern that attempts to recapitulate normal electrical activity. In addition, a sensor will increase the heart rate if physical activity is detected.
  - VOO: The pacemaker will deliver ventricular pacing a set rate without regard for endogenous activity. This mode has a theoretical risk of R-on-T-induced arrhythmia but is necessary during surgery or other procedures in which electrical interference could cause the pacemaker to fail to pace appropriately.

Pacemaker Management

- Patients with a pacemaker require regular follow-up with an electrophysiologist or cardiologist skilled in pacemaker management. However, the increased use of transtelephonic monitoring has reduced the need for office visits. More sophisticated home monitoring systems are also being introduced, most utilizing the Internet. Pacemaker batteries require replacement after approximately 3 to 7 years of use, depending on device details and the degree of pacemaker activity.
- Application of a strong magnet will convert any pacemaker to an asynchronous (VOO) mode as long as the magnet is in place over the device. In this mode, the pacemaker will deliver stimuli at a preset rate regardless of sensed cardiac (or extraneous) signals.

Pacemaker Complications and Malfunction

- **Device infection**
  - Device infection is a serious complication and may occur either shortly after implantation or because of seeding of the device at a later time.
  - The possibility of endocarditis and device infection must be considered in any patient with bacteremia or signs of local infection at the device site. Explantation of the device is frequently required for definitive treatment.
  - In the case of local infection, incision and drainage should be avoided because of the possibility of introducing infection to the device pocket. In general, patients with a possible device infection should be admitted to a facility with experience in this area.
- **Pacemaker syndrome**
  - In the setting of ventricular pacing, some patients experience a syndrome of neck/abdominal pulsations, palpitations, fatigue, dyspnea, and presyncope because of the lack of optimal AV synchrony and resulting decreased cardiac output and increased AV valvular regurgitation.
  - Avoiding ventricular-only pacing is the best approach to ameliorating symptoms.
- **Pacemaker-mediated tachycardia (PMT)**
  - Various reentrant arrhythmias may occur, which include the pacemaker as part of the circuit despite the use of programming features that minimize this complication. In this situation, application of a magnet to the pacemaker (see above) will interrupt the circuit and terminate the tachycardia.
  - Reprogramming may be necessary to prevent recurrences.
- **Failure to capture**
  - Obviously, failure of the pacemaker to stimulate cardiac contraction is a serious malfunction, especially in the pacemaker-dependent patient. In this situation, the first pri-

ority is to stabilize the patient with transcutaneous or temporary transvenous pacing if necessary.

○ Further evaluation includes consideration of electrolyte disturbances or AMI, both of which can increase the threshold for pacemaker capture. Interrogation of the device will then provide further information regarding device and lead function.

- **Failure to sense and oversensing**
  ○ Failure to sense intrinsic cardiac activity results in pacemaker-stimulated beats despite an adequate endogenous rhythm. This rarely presents an acute problem and can be evaluated with device interrogation and expert consultation.
  ○ More seriously, oversensing results when noncardiac signals (diaphragmatic or muscle potentials or environmental signals) are misinterpreted by the device as cardiac activity with a resulting suppression of pacemaker activity. In this case, application of a magnet to the device will result in asynchronous pacing until the problem can be further evaluated.

AUTOMATIC IMPLANTABLE CARDIAC DEFIBRILLATOR

- The role of the ICD (also sometimes referred to as automatic ICD) is to continuously monitor the cardiac rhythm and to terminate potentially lethal ventricular arrhythmias.[21]
- Two groups of patients are considered candidates for ICD placement. Patients who have experienced VT/VF and survived warrant ICD placement for secondary prevention of future events. In addition, prophylactic placement of ICDs for prevention of SCD in high-risk patients (primary prevention) has become the standard of care. However, accurate identification of high-risk patients continues to evolve.[24] The current guidelines are summarized in Table 10-3.
- As with pacemakers, both the more common endocardial and surgical epicardial systems can be placed.
- All ICDs have a basic backup pacing ability. For patients with indications for both a pacemaker and an ICD, a more comprehensive combination device that combines a full array of pacemaker and ICD functions is used.
- To terminate ventricular arrhythmias, ICDs use two techniques:
  ○ Antitachycardia pacing: a burst of pacing stimuli is delivered at a rate slightly faster than the tachycardia. Frequently, this will interrupt and terminate a reentrant rhythm.
  ○ Shock delivery: the device is capable of delivering a defibrillatory shock identical in function to external unsynchronized cardioversion.
- Complex and currently imperfect algorithms are used by the device to differentiate VT and VF from atrial arrhythmias. Heart rate remains the most important criterion for detection of ventricular arrhythmias. Inappropriate shocks due to atrial tachyarrhythmias are a risk of ICD therapy.

ICD Management

- Patients should be followed on a regular basis by the electrophysiologist who implanted or who monitors the device.
- As with pacemakers, remote follow-up is becoming more common, reducing the frequency of routine office visits.
- Discharge of the ICD is an uncomfortable and alarming experience for the patient. However, it should be remembered that this is the role of the device.
- A single shock does not necessarily require immediate evaluation; however, the patient should contact his or her cardiologist or electrophysiologist at the first opportunity.

Multiple shocks or shocks associated with symptoms such as syncope, chest pain, or shortness of breath warrant an immediate emergency department evaluation.

- **Magnet application**
  - Application of a strong magnet to the ICD activates a switch that **disables the antitachycardia functions** of the device; it has **no effect on the backup pacing function** (in contrast to the effect of a magnet on the pacemaker as discussed above).
  - This is used when the device is delivering shocks inappropriately. With the increased prevalence of devices and, consequently, device malfunction, any facility with ACLS equipment should have a magnet available for management of this situation.
  - Appropriate magnets can be obtained from the manufacturers of ICDs.

ICD Complications and Malfunction

- **Device Infection**: As with pacemakers, ICD infection is a serious problem and should be managed as discussed above.
- **Inappropriate defibrillator firing/shock**
  - The current algorithms used by the ICD to distinguish SVT from VT/VF are imperfect, sometimes resulting in inappropriate shocks for supraventricular rhythms. Inappropriate shocks may also result from extrinsic signals or noise, such as electrocautery or other electromagnetic interference (including that generated by arc welding).
  - Acute management of this situation includes ECG monitoring to determine the rhythm and application of a magnet if the shocks are inappropriate. Immediate availability of resuscitation personnel and equipment is necessary while the device is inactivated.
  - Expert consultation is required to address the reason for the inappropriate therapy.
- **Failure to treat VF/VT**: Episodes of VF/VT that are not treated by the device require expert consultation for possible reprogramming of the ICD. In the interim, the patient requires monitoring in a facility able to manage these rhythms.

Other Device Concerns

- **Perioperative management**
  - Several concerns arise with pacemaker or ICD function during an operation. Vibrations, pressure, and electrical signals from electrocautery can interfere with normal pacemaker function.
  - In general, reprogramming the pacemaker to a DOO/VOO mode and inactivation of the rate-responsive element will prevent these complications. After the procedure, the device should be interrogated to ensure that no damage occurred.
  - For thoracic operations, a chest radiograph should be performed to confirm that the lead position was not affected.
- **Magnetic resonance imaging (MRI) imaging**
  - **MRI imaging is contraindicated in patients with a pacemaker or ICD** because of the possibility of heating and torque forces on the device itself from the magnetic field as well as potential reprogramming of the device.
  - There is currently one MR conditional pacemaker system (leads and pulse generator) available. There are currently no approved MR conditional or MR safe ICDs. However, more MR conditional pacemakers and ICDs are likely to be approved within the next several years.
- **Radiation therapy**
  - Radiation therapy has minimal immediate effect on the device if the beam is not directed directly at or near the pulse generator; however, cumulative radiation doses can result in device damage and warrant regular device interrogation.

○ In addition, the shielding effect of the device may reduce the efficacy of the radiation treatment. Consultation with the patient's cardiologist and/or device manufacturer is desirable.

• **Cardioversion/defibrillation**
  ○ Application of external defibrillation or cardioversion may damage the device. The pads should be applied at a distance from the implanted device and proper device function confirmed once the patient is stabilized.
  ○ **This concern should not prevent the application of appropriate ACLS treatments to the unstable patient.**

• **Exposure to environmental electromagnetic radiation**
  ○ Electromagnetic interference (EMI) is ubiquitous in the modern world. Common sources include cell phones, antitheft devices, metal detectors, microwave ovens, and high-voltage power lines. However, **few cases of significant interference have been reported**.
  ○ Patients can limit the potential for interference by not carrying the cell phone in a pocket over the device and using the more distant ear during conversations and by not lingering in the field of antitheft or metal detectors.
  ○ **Modern microwave ovens are no longer considered a significant concern** (in contrast to early generation ovens).
  ○ Patients exposed to significant electrical signals from industrial equipment should consult their cardiologist.

• **Driving and physical activity**
  ○ Few clear guidelines have been published on the issue of physical activity; however, **avoidance of contact sports that risk device damage and competitive exertion in patients at risk for arrhythmias is reasonable**.
  ○ With regard to driving, physicians should be familiar with local statutes.
  ○ However, it is recommended that patients avoid driving until they are free of VT/VF and ICD shocks for a period of 6 months.

REFERENCES

1. Ellis K, Dresing T. Tachyarrhythmias. In: Griffin BP, Topol EJ, eds. *Manual of Cardiovascular Medicine*. Philadelphia, PA: Lippincott Williams & Wilkins; 2004:283–313.
2. Yusuf S, Camm AJ. The sinus tachycardias. *Nat Clin Pract Cardiovasc Med* 2005;2:44–52.
3. Falk RH. Atrial fibrillation. *N Engl J Med* 2001;344:1067–1078.
4. Lip GY, Tse HF. Management of atrial fibrillation. *Lancet* 2007;370:604–618.
5. Wyse DG, Waldo AL, DiMarco JP, et al. A comparison of rate control and rhythm control in patients with atrial fibrillation. *N Engl J Med* 2002;347:1825–1833.
6. Hall MC, Todd DM. Modern management of arrhythmias. *Postgrad Med J* 2006;82:117–125.
7. Zimetbaum P. Amiodarone for atrial fibrillation. *N Engl J Med* 2007;356:935–941.
8. Mayson SE, Greenspon AJ, Adams S, et al. The changing face of postoperative atrial fibrillation prevention: a review of current medical therapy. *Cardiol Rev* 2007;15:231–241.
9. Ganz LI, Friedman PL. Supraventricular tachycardia. *N Engl J Med* 1995;332:162–173.
10. Delacretaz E. Clinical practice. Supraventricular tachycardia. *N Engl J Med* 2006;354:1039–1051.
11. McCord J, Borzak S. Multifocal atrial tachycardia. *Chest* 1998;113:203–209.

12. Eckardt L, Breithardt G, Kirchhof P. Approach to wide complex tachycardias in patients without structural heart disease. *Heart* 2006;92:704–711.

13. Brugada P, Brugada J, Mont L, et al. A new approach to the differential diagnosis of a regular tachycardia with a wide QRS complex. *Circulation* 1991;83:1649–1659.

14. Isenhour JL, Craig S, Gibbs M, et al. Wide-complex tachycardia: continued evaluation of diagnostic criteria. *Acad Emerg Med* 2000;7:769–773.

15. Echt DS, Liebson PR, Mitchell LB, et al. Mortality and morbidity in patients receiving encainide, flecainide, or placebo. The Cardiac Arrhythmia Suppression trial. *N Engl J Med* 1991;324:781–788.

16. Waldo AL, Camm AJ, deRuyter H, et al. Effect of d-sotalol on mortality in patients with left ventricular dysfunction after recent and remote myocardial infarction. The SWORD Investigators. Survival with oral d-sotalol. *Lancet* 1996;348:7–12.

17. Bardy GH, Lee KL, Mark DB, et al. Amiodarone or an implantable cardioverter-defibrillator for congestive heart failure. *N Engl J Med* 2005;352:225–237.

18. Moss AJ, Zareba W, Hall WJ, et al. Prophylactic implantation of a defibrillator in patients with myocardial infarction and reduced ejection fraction. *N Engl J Med* 2002;346:877–883.

19. Moss AJ, Hall WJ, Cannom DS, et al. Improved survival with an implanted defibrillator in patients with coronary disease at high risk for ventricular arrhythmia. Multicenter Automatic Defibrillator Implantation Trial Investigators. *N Engl J Med* 1996;335:1933–1940.

20. Yap YG, Camm AJ. Drug induced QT prolongation and torsades de pointes. *Heart* 2003;89:1363–1372.

21. DiMarco JP. Implantable cardioverter-defibrillators. *N Engl J Med* 2003;349:1836–1847.

22. Zipes DP, Camm AJ, Borggrefe M, et al. ACC/AHA/ESC 2006 guidelines for management of patients with ventricular arrhythmias and the prevention of sudden cardiac death. *Circulation* 2006;114:e385–e484.

23. Mangrum JM, DiMarco JP. The evaluation and management of bradycardia. *N Engl J Med* 2000;342:703–709.

24. Epstein AE, DiMarco JP, Ellenbogen KA, et al. ACC/AHA/HRS 2008 guidelines for device-based therapy of cardiac rhythm abnormalities. *Circulation* 2008;117:e350–e408.

25. Rossenbacker T, Priori SG. The Brugada syndrome. *Curr Opin Cardiol* 2007;22:163–170.

26. Schwartz PJ. Management of long QT syndrome. *Nat Clin Pract Cardiovasc Med* 2005;2:346–351.

27. Abriel H, Zaklyazminskaya EV. Cardiac channelopathies: genetic and molecular mechanisms. *Gene* 2013;517:1–11.

28. Kies P, Bootsma M, Bax J, et al. Arrhythmogenic right ventricular dysplasia/cardiomyopathy: screening, diagnosis, and treatment. *Heart Rhythm* 2006;3:225–234.

29. Francis J, Sankar V, Nair VK, et al. Catecholaminergic polymorphic ventricular tachycardia. *Heart Rhythm* 2005;2:550–554.

30. Kapoor WN, Brant N. Evaluation of syncope by upright tilt testing with isoproterenol. A nonspecific test. *Ann Intern Med* 1992;116:358–363.

31. Chen LY, Shen WK. Neurocardiogenic syncope: latest pharmacological therapies. *Expert Opin Pharmacother* 2006;7:1151–1162.

32. Schoenfeld MH. Contemporary pacemaker and defibrillator device therapy: challenges confronting the general cardiologist. *Circulation* 2007;115:638–653.

11 Dyslipidemia

Clare E. Moynihan and Anne C. Goldberg

GENERAL PRINCIPLES

Lipids are sparingly soluble molecules that include cholesterol, fatty acids, and their derivatives. Plasma lipids are transported by lipoprotein particles composed of **apolipoproteins, phospholipids, free cholesterol, cholesterol esters,** and **triglycerides.** Human plasma lipoproteins are separated into **five major classes** based on density: chylomicrons (least dense), very-low-density lipoproteins (VLDLs), intermediate-density lipoproteins (IDLs), low-density lipoproteins (LDLs), and high-density lipoproteins (HDLs). A sixth class, lipoprotein (a), Lp(a), resembles LDL in lipid composition and has a density that overlaps that of LDLs and HDLs. Physical properties of plasma lipoproteins are summarized in Table 11-1.

Atherosclerosis and Lipoproteins

Nearly 90% of patients with coronary heart disease (CHD) have some form of dyslipidemia. Increased levels of LDL cholesterol, remnant lipoproteins, and Lp(a) as well as decreased levels of HDL cholesterol have all been associated with an increased risk of premature vascular disease.[1,2]

Clinical Dyslipoproteinemias

- Most dyslipidemias are multifactorial in etiology and reflect the effects of genetic influences coupled with diet, inactivity, smoking, alcohol use, and comorbid conditions such as obesity and diabetes mellitus (DM). Differential diagnosis of the major lipid abnormalities is summarized in Table 11-2. The major genetic dyslipoproteinemias are reviewed in Table 11-3.[3-5]
- Familial hypercholesterolemia and familial combined hyperlipidemia are disorders that contribute significantly to premature cardiovascular disease.
  - **Familial hypercholesterolemia** is an underdiagnosed, autosomal codominant condition with a prevalence of 1 in 200 to 1 in 500 people that causes elevated LDL cholesterol levels from birth.[6,7] It is associated with significantly increased risk of early cardiovascular disease when untreated.[8]
  - **Familial combined hyperlipidemia** has a prevalence of 1% to 2% and typically presents in adulthood, although obesity and high dietary fat and sugar intake have led to increased presentation in childhood and adolescence.[9]

Standards of Care for Hyperlipidemia

LDL cholesterol–lowering therapy, particularly with hydroxymethylglutaryl coenzyme A (HMG-CoA) reductase inhibitors (commonly referred to as statins), **lowers the risk of CHD-related death, morbidity, and revascularization procedures** in patients with (secondary prevention) or without (primary prevention) known CHD.[10-17] Prevention of atherosclerotic cardiovascular disease (ASCVD) is the primary goal of the 2013 American College of Cardiology (ACC)/American Heart Association (AHA) Guidelines. These guidelines address risk assessment, lifestyle modifications, evaluation and treatment of obesity, and evaluation and management of blood cholesterol.[18-21]

TABLE 11-1	Physical Properties of Plasma Lipoproteins[a]		
Lipoprotein	Lipid composition	Origin	Apolipoproteins
Chylomicrons	TG, 85%; chol, 3%	Intestine	A-I, A-IV; B-48; C-I, C-II, C-III; E
VLDL	TG, 55%; chol, 20%	Liver	B-100; C-I, C-II, C-III; E
IDL	TG, 25%; chol, 35%	Metabolic product of VLDL	B-100; C-I, C-II, C-III; E
LDL	TG, 5%; chol, 60%	Metabolic product of IDL	B-100
HDL	TG, 5%; chol, 20%	Liver, intestine	A-I, A-II; C-I, C-II, C-III; E
Lp(a)	TG, 5%; chol, 60%	Liver	B-100; Apo (a)

[a]Remainder of particle composition: protein and phospholipid.
Chol, cholesterol; HDL, high-density lipoprotein; IDL, intermediate-density lipoprotein; LDL, low-density lipoprotein; Lp(a), lipoprotein(a); TG, triglyceride; VLDL, very-low-density lipoprotein.

TABLE 11-2	Differential Diagnosis of Major Lipid Abnormalities	
Lipid abnormality	Primary disorders	Secondary disorders
Hypercholesterolemia	Polygenic, familial hypercholesterolemia, familial defective apo B-100	Hypothyroidism, nephrotic syndrome, anorexia nervosa
Hypertriglyceridemia	Lipoprotein lipase deficiency, apo C-II deficiency, familial hypertriglyceridemia, dysbetalipoproteinemia	Diabetes mellitus, obesity, metabolic syndrome, alcohol use, oral estrogen, renal failure, hypothyroidism, retinoids, lipodystrophies
Combined hyperlipidemia	Familial combined hyperlipidemia, dysbetalipoproteinemia	Diabetes mellitus, obesity, metabolic syndrome, hypothyroidism, nephrotic syndrome, hypothyroidism, lipodystrophies
Low HDL	Familial hypoalphalipoproteinemia, Tangier disease (ABCA1 mutations), apoA1 mutations, lecithin:cholesterol acyltransferase deficiency	Diabetes mellitus, obesity, metabolic syndrome, hypertriglyceridemia, smoking, anabolic steroids

HDL, high-density lipoprotein.

TABLE 11-3 Review of Major Genetic Dyslipoproteinemias

Type of genetic dyslipidemia	Typical lipid profile	Type of inheritance pattern	Phenotypic features	Other information
Familial hypercholesterol-emia (FH)[3]	• Increased total (>300 mg/dL) and LDL (>250 mg/dL) cholesterol • Homozygous form (rare) can have total cholesterol >600 mg/dL and LDL >550 mg/dL	Autosomal dominant (prevalence of 1 in 200–500 for het-erozygote form)	• Premature CAD • Tendon xanthomas • Xanthelasmata • Premature arcus corneae (full arc before age 40)	Mutations of the LDL receptor and of apolipoprotein B-100 and gain-of-function mutations of proprotein convertase/kexin subtype 9 (PCSK9) lead to impaired uptake and degradation of LDL.
Familial combined hyperlipidemia (FCH)	• High levels of VLDL, LDL, or both • LDL apo B-100 level >130 mg/dL	Autosomal dominant (prevalence of 1%–2%)	• Premature CAD • Patients do not develop tendon xanthomas	Genetic and meta-bolic defects are not established
Familial dysbetalipoproteinemia[5]	• Symmetric elevations of cholesterol and triglycerides (300–500 mg/dL) • Elevated VLDL to triglyceride ratio (>0.3)	Autosomal recessive	• Premature CAD • Tuberous or tuberoeruptive xanthomas • Planar xanthomas of the palmar creases are essentially pathognomonic.	ApoE mutation Many homozygotes are normolipidemic, and emergence of hyperlipidemia often requires a secondary metabolic factor such as diabetes mellitus, hypothyroidism, or obesity,

Familial hypertriglyceridemia (can result in chylomicronemia syndrome)	• Most patients have triglyceride levels in the range of 150–500 mg/dL. • Clinical manifestations may occur when triglyceride levels exceed 1,500 mg/dL.	Familial hypertriglyceridemia is an autosomal dominant disorder caused by overproduction of VLDL triglycerides and manifests in adults.	• Eruptive xanthomas • Lipemia retinalis • Pancreatitis • Hepatosplenomegaly	Patients may develop the chylomicronemia syndrome in the presence of secondary factors such as obesity, alcohol use, or diabetes.
Familial hyperchylomicronemia	Similar to familial hypertriglyceridemia	Onset before puberty indicates deficiency of lipoprotein lipase or apo C-II, both autosomal recessive.	Similar to familial hypertriglyceridemia	

CAD, coronary artery disease; LDL, low-density lipoprotein; VLDL, very-low-density lipoprotein.

DIAGNOSIS

Screening

- Screening for hypercholesterolemia should begin in **all adults aged 20 years or older.**[18]
- Screening is best performed with a lipid profile (total cholesterol, LDL cholesterol, HDL cholesterol, and triglycerides) obtained after a 12-hour fast.
- If a fasting lipid panel cannot be obtained, total and HDL cholesterol should be measured. Total cholesterol ≥220 mg/dL may indicate a genetic or secondary cause. A fasting lipid panel is required if total cholesterol is ≥220 mg/dL or triglycerides are ≥500 mg/dL.
- If the patient does not have an indication for LDL-lowering therapy, screening can be performed **every 4 to 6 years between ages 40 and 75.**[18]
- Patients hospitalized for an acute coronary syndrome or coronary revascularization should have a lipid panel obtained within 24 hours of admission if lipid levels are unknown.
- Individuals with hyperlipidemia should be evaluated for potential **secondary causes,** including hypothyroidism, DM, obstructive liver disease, chronic renal disease, nephrotic syndrome, or medications such as estrogens, progestins, anabolic steroids/androgens, corticosteroids, cyclosporine, retinoids, atypical antipsychotics, and antiretrovirals (particularly protease inhibitors).

Risk Assessment

- The 2013 guidelines identify four groups in whom the benefits of LDL-lowering therapy with HMG-CoA reductase inhibitors (statins) clearly outweigh the risks:[21]
  ○ Patients with **clinical ASCVD**
  ○ Patients with **LDL ≥190 mg/dL**
  ○ Patients with **DM aged 40 to 75 with LDL between 70 and 189 mg/dL**
  ○ Patients with a calculated **ASCVD risk ≥7.5%**
- For patients **without** clinical ASCVD or an LDL ≥190 mg/dL, the guidelines advise calculating a patient's risk for ASCVD based on age, sex, ethnicity, total and HDL cholesterol, systolic blood pressure (treated or untreated), presence of DM, and current smoking status.[18]
- The ACC/AHA risk calculator is available at http://my.americanheart.org/cvriskcalculator (last accessed December 22, 2014).
  ○ For patients of ethnicities other than African American or non-Hispanic White, risk could not be as well assessed. Use of the non-Hispanic White risk calculation is suggested, with the understanding that risk may be lower than calculated in East Asian Americans and Hispanic Americans and higher in American Indians and South Asians.
  ○ A 10-year risk should be calculated beginning at age 40 in patients without ASCVD or LDL ≥190 mg/dL.
  ○ Lifetime risk may be calculated in patients aged 20 through 39, and patients aged 40 through 59 with a 10-year risk under 7.5%, to inform decisions regarding lifestyle modification.

TREATMENT

- The 2013 guidelines recognize lifestyle factors, including diet and weight management as an important component of risk reduction for all patients.[19,20]
- Patients should be advised to adopt a diet that is high in fruits and vegetables, whole grains, fish, lean meat, low-fat dairy, legumes, and nuts, with lower intake of red meat, saturated and *trans* fats, sweets, and sugary beverages. Saturated fat should comprise no more than 5% to 6% of total calories (Table 11-4).[19]
- Physical activity, including aerobic and resistance exercise, is recommended in all patients.[19]

TABLE 11-4 Nutrient Composition of the Therapeutic Lifestyle Change (TLC) Diet

Nutrient	Recommended intake
Saturated fat[a]	<5% to 6% of total calories
Polyunsaturated fat	Up to 10% of total calories
Monounsaturated fat	Up to 20% of total calories
Total fat	25%–35% of total calories
Carbohydrate[b]	50%–60% of total calories
Fiber	20–30 g/day
Protein	Approximately 15% of total calories
Cholesterol	<200 mg/day
Total calories (energy)[c]	Balance energy intake and expenditure to maintain desirable body weight/prevent weight gain

[a]Trans fatty acids are another low-density lipoprotein (LDL)-raising fat that should be kept at a low intake.
[b]Carbohydrate should be derived predominantly from foods rich in complex carbohydrates, including grains (especially whole grains), fruits, and vegetables.
[c]Daily energy expenditure should include at least moderate physical activity (contributing approximately 200 Kcal/day).
Data from Eckel RH, Jakicic JM, Ard JD, et al. 2013 AHA/ACC guideline on lifestyle management to reduce cardiovascular risk: a report of the American College of Cardiology/American Heart Association Task Force on Practice Guidelines. *Circulation* 2014;129:S76–S99.

- For all obese patients (BMI ≥ 30), or overweight patients (BMI ≥ 25) who have additional risk factors, sustained weight loss of 3% to 5% or greater reduces ASCVD risk.[20]
- Consultation with a registered dietitian may be helpful to plan, start, and maintain a saturated fat–restricted and weight loss–promoting diet.
- Prior to the start of treatment, there should be a risk discussion between the patient and the clinician. Topics for discussion include the following:
  ○ Potential for ASCVD risk reduction benefits
  ○ Potential for adverse effects and drug–drug interactions
  ○ Heart-healthy lifestyle and management of other risk factors
  ○ Patient preferences

Clinical Atherosclerotic Cardiovascular Disease

- **Clinical ASCVD includes acute coronary syndromes, history of myocardial infarction, stable angina, arterial revascularization (coronary or otherwise), stroke, transient ischemic attack, or atherosclerotic peripheral arterial disease.**
- Secondary prevention is an indication for high-intensity statin therapy (Table 11-5), which has been shown to reduce events more than moderate-intensity statin therapy.
- If high-dose statin therapy is contraindicated or poorly tolerated, or there are significant risks to high-intensity therapy (including age >75 years), moderate-intensity therapy is an option.

LDL ≥ 190 mg/dL

- These individuals have elevated lifetime risk because of long-term exposure to very high LDL-C levels, and the risk calculator does not account for this.
- LDL-C should be reduced by at least 50%, primarily with high-intensity statin therapy (Table 11-5). If high-intensity therapy is not tolerated, maximum tolerated intensity should be used.
- Even high-intensity statin therapy may not be sufficient to reduce LDL-C by 50%, and nonstatin therapies are often required to achieve this goal.[22]

TABLE 11-5	Statin Therapy Regimens by Intensity

High intensity ($\downarrow$LDL $\geq$50%)	Medium intensity ($\downarrow$LDL 30%–50%)	Low intensity ($\downarrow$LDL <30%)
Atorvastatin 40–80 mg	Atorvastatin 10–20 mg	*Fluvastatin* 20–40 mg
Rosuvastatin 20–40 mg	Fluvastatin 40 mg bid–80 mg XL	Lovastatin 20 mg
	Lovastatin 40 mg	*Pitavastatin* 1 mg
	Pitavastatin 2–4 mg	Pravastatin 10–20 mg
	Pravastatin 40–80 mg	*Simvastatin* 10 mg
	Rosuvastatin 5–10 mg	
	Simvastatin 20–40 mg	

Italicized doses have not been studied in RCTs but achieve this level of LDL reduction in clinical use.
LDL, low-density lipoprotein; $\downarrow$, decreased.
Data from Stone NJ, Robinson JG, Lichtenstein AH, et al. 2013 ACC/AHA guideline on the treatment of blood cholesterol to reduce atherosclerotic cardiovascular risk in adults: a report of the American College of Cardiology/American Heart Association Task Force on Practice Guidelines. *Circulation* 2014;129:S1–S45.

- LDL apheresis is an optional therapy in patients with homozygous FH and those with severe heterozygous FH with insufficient response to medication. Lomitapide, a microsomal triglyceride transfer protein inhibitor, and mipomersen, an apolipoprotein B antisense oligonucleotide, are new medications indicated for the treatment of patients with homozygous FH.[7]
- As hyperlipidemia of this degree is often genetically determined, **discuss screening of other family members** (including children) to identify candidates for treatment. In addition, screen for and treat secondary causes of hyperlipidemia.[6]

Patients with Diabetes, Aged 40 to 75, LDL 70 to 189

- Using the AHA/ACC risk calculator, calculate the 10-year risk of an ASCVD event in these patients (categories, $\geq$7.5%, or $\leq$7.5%).
- **If the risk is $\geq$7.5%, consider high-intensity statin therapy** (Table 11-5).
- **Otherwise, these patients have an indication for moderate-intensity statin therapy**.

Patients without Diabetes, Aged 40 to 75, LDL 70 to 189

- Using the AHA/ACC risk calculator, calculate 10-year risk of an ASCVD event in these patients (categories, $\geq$7.5%, between 5.0% and 7.5%, and $\leq$5.0%).
- **A 10-year risk $\geq$7.5% is an indication for moderate- or high-intensity statin therapy**. The decision between moderate- and high-intensity therapy should be made with the patient based on anticipated, individualized risks and benefits.
- **A 10-year risk between 5% and 7.5% is reasonable for moderate-intensity statin therapy**.

Other Patient Populations

- Some patients not described above may still benefit from statin therapy—if the decision on treatment is unclear, the guidelines offer assessment of family history, high sensitivity C-reactive protein (hs-CRP), coronary artery calcium (CAC) score, or arterial-brachial index (ABI) as options to further define risk.[18,21]
  - A family history of premature ASCVD is defined as an event in a first-degree male relative before age 55 or in a first-degree female relative before age 65.
  - Higher risk is also indicated by an hs-CRP $\geq$2 mg/L; CAC $\geq$300 Agatston units or $\geq$75th percentile for age, sex, and ethnicity; or ABI $\leq$0.9.
  - The role of other biomarkers in risk assessment remains uncertain.

- ○ Depending on patient preference and assessment of risks and benefits, lower LDL-C levels can be considered for treatment (particularly LDL ≥160 mg/dL).
  - ○ **Patients with diabetes younger than 40 or older than 75 are reasonable candidates for statin therapy based on individual evaluation.**
- **Use of statin therapy should be individualized for patients older than 75.** In RCTs, patients older than 75 continued to have benefit from statin therapy, particularly for secondary prevention.[13,23] In addition, many ASCVD events occur in this age group, and patients without other comorbidities may benefit substantially from cardiovascular risk reduction.
- No official recommendation was made in the guidelines regarding initiation or continuation of statin therapy in patients on maintenance hemodialysis or with NYHA class II to IV ischemic systolic heart failure. Evidence from RCTs has not shown a benefit from statin therapy in these subpopulations.[21]

Hypertriglyceridemia

- Hypertriglyceridemia may be an **independent cardiovascular risk factor.**[24–26]
- Hypertriglyceridemia is often observed in the metabolic syndrome, and there are many potential etiologies for hypertriglyceridemia, including obesity, DM, renal insufficiency, genetic dyslipidemias, and therapy with oral estrogen, glucocorticoids, β-blockers, tamoxifen, cyclosporine, antiretrovirals, and retinoids.[27]
- The classification of serum triglyceride levels is as follows: Normal: <150 mg/dL. Borderline-high: 150 to 199 mg/dL. High: 200 to 499 mg/dL. Very high: ≥500 mg/dL.[26] The Endocrine Society has added two further categories: severe: 1,000 to 1,999 mg/dL (greatly increases the risk of pancreatitis) and very severe: ≥2,000 mg/dL.[9]
- Treatment of hypertriglyceridemia depends on the degree of severity.
  - ○ For patients with **very high triglyceride levels**, triglyceride reduction through a very-low-fat diet (≤15% of calories), exercise, weight loss, and drugs (fibrates, niacin, omega-3 fatty acids) is **the primary goal of therapy to prevent acute pancreatitis.**
  - ○ **When patients have a lesser degree of hypertriglyceridemia, controlling the LDL cholesterol level is the primary aim of initial therapy.** Lifestyle changes are indicated to lower triglyceride levels.[9]

Low HDL Cholesterol

- **Low HDL cholesterol is an independent ASCVD risk factor** that is identified as a non-LDL cholesterol risk and is included as a component of the ACC/AHA scoring algorithm.[18]
- Etiologies for low HDL cholesterol include genetic conditions, physical inactivity, obesity, insulin resistance, DM, hypertriglyceridemia, cigarette smoking, high (>60% calories) carbohydrate diets, and certain medications (β-blockers, anabolic steroids/androgens, progestins).
- Because therapeutic interventions for low HDL cholesterol are of limited efficacy, the guidelines recommend considering low HDL as a component of overall risk, rather than targeting low HDL as a specific therapeutic target.
- **There are no clinical trial data showing a benefit of pharmacologic methods of elevating HDL cholesterol.**

Starting and Monitoring Therapy

- Before starting therapy, guidelines recommend checking alanine aminotransferase (ALT), HgbA1c (if diabetes status is unknown), labs for secondary causes (if indicated), and creatine kinase (CK) if indicated.
- Evaluate for patient characteristics increasing the risk of adverse events from statins: impaired hepatic and renal function, history of statin intolerance, history of muscle

disorders, unexplained elevations of ALT >3× the upper limit of normal, drugs affecting statin metabolism, Asian ethnicity, and age >75 years.[21]

- A repeat fasting lipid panel is indicated 4 to 12 weeks after starting therapy to assess adherence, with reassessment every 3 to 12 months as indicated.
- In contrast to previous guidelines, **therapeutic targets are not recommended, as specific targets and a treat to target strategy have not been evaluated in RCTs**.
- In patients without the anticipated level of LDL reduction based on intensity of statin therapy (≥50% for high intensity, 30% to 50% for moderate intensity), assess adherence to therapy and lifestyle modifications, evaluate for intolerance, and consider secondary causes. After evaluation, if the therapeutic response is still insufficient on maximally tolerated statin therapy, it is reasonable to consider adding a nonstatin agent.
- CK should not be routinely checked in patients on statin therapy, but is reasonable to measure in patients with muscle symptoms.
- In 2012, the FDA stated that liver enzyme tests should be performed before starting statin therapy and only as clinically indicated thereafter. The FDA concluded that serious liver injury with statins is rare and unpredictable and that **routine monitoring of liver enzymes does not appear to be effective in detecting or preventing serious liver injury**.[28] Elevations of liver transaminases two to three times the upper limit of normal are dose dependent, may decrease on repeat even with continuation of statin therapy, and are reversible with discontinuation of the drug.

Treatment of Elevated Low-Density Lipoprotein Cholesterol

Statins

- Statins (Table 11-5) are the treatment of choice for elevated LDL cholesterol.[21,22,29]
- The lipid-lowering effect of statins appears within the first week of use and becomes stable after approximately 4 weeks of use.
- Common side effects (5% to 10% of patients) include gastrointestinal (GI) upset (e.g., abdominal pain, diarrhea, bloating, constipation) and muscle pain or weakness, which can occur without creatine kinase elevations. Other potential side effects include malaise, fatigue, headache, and rash.[29–31]
- **Myalgias are the most common cause of statin discontinuation** and are often dose dependent. They occur more often with increasing age and number of medications and decreasing renal function and body size.[31,32]
  - The AHA/ACC Guidelines recommend discontinuing statins in patients who develop muscle symptoms until they can be evaluated. For severe symptoms, evaluate for rhabdomyolysis.[21]
  - For mild-to-moderate symptoms, evaluate for conditions increasing the risk of muscle symptoms, including renal or hepatic impairment, hypothyroidism, vitamin D deficiency, rheumatologic disorders, and primary muscle disorders. Statin-induced myalgias are likely to resolve within 2 months of discontinuing the drug.
  - If symptoms resolve, the same or lower dose of the statin can be reintroduced.
  - If symptoms recur, use a low dose of a different statin and increase as tolerated.
  - If the cause of symptoms is determined to be unrelated, restart the original statin.
- **Statins have been associated with an increased incidence of DM, with the total benefit of statin use outweighing the potential adverse effects from an increase in blood sugar**.[33]
- Statins have very rarely been associated with reversible cognitive impairment and **have not been associated with irreversible or progressive dementia**.
- Because some of the statins undergo metabolism by the cytochrome P450 enzyme system, taking these statins in combination with other drugs metabolized by this enzyme system increases the risk of **rhabdomyolysis**.[29–31] Among these drugs are fibrates (greater risk with gemfibrozil), itraconazole, ketoconazole, erythromycin, clarithromycin, cyclosporine, nefazodone (no longer available in the United States or Canada), and protease inhibitors.[31]

- Statins may also interact with large quantities of grapefruit juice to increase the risk of myopathy, although the precise mechanism of this interaction is unclear.
- Simvastatin can increase the levels of warfarin and digoxin and has significant, dose-limiting interactions with amlodipine, amiodarone, dronedarone, verapamil, diltiazem, and ranolazine. Rosuvastatin may also increase warfarin levels.
- Since a number of drug interactions are possible depending on the statin and other medications being used, drug interaction programs and package inserts should be consulted.[34]
- The use of statins is contraindicated during pregnancy and lactation.

Bile Acid–Sequestrant Resins
- Currently available bile acid–sequestrant resins include the following:
  - **Cholestyramine**: 4 to 24 g PO/day in divided doses before meals
  - **Colestipol**: tablets, 2 to 16 g PO/day, and granules, 5 to 30 g PO/day in divided doses before meals
  - **Colesevelam**: 625 mg tablets; three tablets PO bid or six tablets PO daily (maximum 7 tablets daily) with food, or one packet of oral suspension daily
- Bile acid sequestrants typically lower LDL levels by 15% to 30% and thereby lower the incidence of CHD.[29,35]
- These agents should not be used as monotherapy in patients with triglyceride levels >250 mg/dL because they can raise triglyceride levels. They may be combined with nicotinic acid or statins.
- Common side effects of resins include constipation, abdominal pain, bloating, nausea, and flatulence.
- Bile acid sequestrants may decrease oral absorption of many other drugs, including warfarin, digoxin, thyroid hormone, thiazide diuretics, amiodarone, glipizide, and statins.
  - Colesevelam interacts with fewer drugs than do the older resins, but can affect the absorption of thyroxine.
  - Other medications should be given at least 1 hour before or 4 hours after resins.

Nicotinic Acid
- Niacin can lower LDL cholesterol levels by ≥15%, lower triglyceride levels by 20% to 50%, and raise HDL cholesterol levels by up to 35%.[24,36]
- Crystalline niacin is given 1 to 3 g PO/day in two to three divided doses with meals. Extended-release niacin is dosed at night, with a starting dose of 500 mg PO, and the dose may be titrated monthly in 500-mg increments to a maximum of 2,000 mg PO (administer dose with milk, applesauce, or crackers).
- Common side effects of niacin include flushing, pruritus, headache, nausea, and bloating. Other potential side effects include elevation of liver transaminases, hyperuricemia, and hyperglycemia.
  - Flushing may be decreased with the use of 325-mg aspirin 30 minutes before the first few doses.
  - Hepatotoxicity associated with niacin is partially dose dependent and appears to be more prevalent with over-the-counter time-release preparations.
- Avoid use of niacin in patients with gout, liver disease, active peptic ulcer disease, and uncontrolled DM.
  - Niacin can be used with care in patients with well-controlled DM (hemoglobin A_{1c} level ≤7%).
  - Serum transaminases, glucose, and uric acid levels should be monitored every 6 to 8 weeks during dose titration, then every 4 months.
- **The use of niacin in patients with well-controlled LDL cholesterol levels (with statins) has not been shown to be of benefit in clinical trials.**[37,38] Niacin can be useful as an additional agent in patients with severely elevated LDL cholesterol levels.

Ezetimibe

- Ezetimibe is currently the only available cholesterol absorption inhibitor. It appears to act at the brush border of the small intestine and inhibits cholesterol absorption.
- Ezetimibe may provide an additional 25% mean reduction in LDL when combined with a statin and provides an approximately 18% decrease in LDL when used as monotherapy.[39–42]
- The recommended dosing is 10 mg PO once daily. No dosage adjustment is required for renal insufficiency and mild hepatic impairment or in elderly patients. It is not recommended for use in patients with moderate-to-severe hepatic impairment.
- Side effects are infrequent and include GI symptoms (e.g., diarrhea, abdominal pain) and myalgias.
- In clinical trials, there was no excess of rhabdomyolysis or myopathy when compared with statin or placebo alone.
- Liver enzymes should be monitored when used in conjunction with fenofibrate and are not required in monotherapy or with a statin.
- Long-term clinical outcome trials of ezetimibe are ongoing. One clinical outcome trial showed decreased reduction of cardiovascular events with the combination of simvastatin and ezetimibe compared to placebo, in patients with chronic renal failure.[43] The effect on cardiovascular events of ezetimibe when added to a statin compared with statin alone has not been demonstrated.
- Ezetimibe is useful in patients with familial hypercholesterolemia who do not achieve adequate LDL cholesterol reductions with statin therapy alone.[44]

Treatment of Hypertriglyceridemia

Nonpharmacologic Treatment

- Nonpharmacologic treatments are important in the therapy of hypertriglyceridemia.
- Approaches include the following:
  - Changing oral estrogen replacement to transdermal estrogen
  - Decreasing alcohol intake
  - Encouraging weight loss and exercise
  - Controlling hyperglycemia in patients with DM
  - Avoiding simple sugars and very-high-carbohydrate diets[9,26]

Pharmacologic Treatment

- Pharmacologic treatment of severe hypertriglyceridemia consists of a fibric acid derivative (fibrates), niacin, or omega-3 fatty acids.
- Patients with severe hypertriglyceridemia should be treated with pharmacotherapy in addition to reduction of dietary fat, alcohol, and simple carbohydrates to decrease the risk of pancreatitis.
- Statins may be effective for patients with mild-to-moderate hypertriglyceridemia and concomitant LDL cholesterol elevation.[9,26,45]
- Fibric acid derivatives:
  - Currently available fibric acid derivatives include the following:
    - **Gemfibrozil**: 600 mg PO bid before meals
    - **Fenofibrate**: available in several forms, dosage typically 48 to 145 mg PO/day
  - Fibrates generally lower triglyceride levels by 30% to 50% and increase HDL cholesterol levels by 10% to 35%. They can lower LDL cholesterol levels by 5% to 25% in patients with normal triglyceride levels but may actually increase LDL cholesterol levels in patients with elevated triglyceride levels.[45,46]
  - Common side effects include dyspepsia, abdominal pain, cholelithiasis, rash, and pruritus.
  - Fibrates may potentiate the effects of warfarin.[29] Gemfibrozil given in conjunction with statins may increase the risk of rhabdomyolysis.[31,47–49]

- **Omega-3 fatty acids**
  - High doses of omega-3 fatty acids from fish oil can lower triglyceride levels.[50,51]
  - The active ingredients are eicosapentaenoic acid (EPA) and docosahexaenoic acid (DHA).
  - To lower triglyceride levels, 1 to 6 g of omega-3 fatty acids, either EPA alone or with DHA, are needed daily.
  - Main side effects are burping, bloating, and diarrhea.
  - Prescription forms of omega-3 fatty acids are available and are indicated for triglyceride levels >500 mg/dL. One preparation contains EPA and DHA; four tablets contain about 3.6 g of omega-3 acid ethyl esters and can lower triglyceride levels by 30% to 40%. Other preparations contain only EPA or contain unesterified EPA and DHA.
  - In practice, omega-3 fatty acids are being used as an adjunct to statin or other drugs in patients with moderately elevated triglyceride levels.
  - The combination of omega-3 fatty acids plus statin has the advantage of avoiding the risk of myopathy seen with the statin-fibrate combination.[52,53]

Treatment of Low High-Density Lipoprotein Cholesterol

- Low HDL cholesterol often occurs in the setting of hypertriglyceridemia and metabolic syndrome. Management of accompanying high LDL cholesterol, hypertriglyceridemia, and the metabolic syndrome may result in improvement of HDL cholesterol.[54]
- Nonpharmacologic therapies are the mainstay of treatment including **smoking cessation, exercise, and weight loss**.
- In addition, medications known to lower HDL levels, such as β-blockers (except carvedilol), progestins, and androgenic compounds, should be avoided.
- No clinical outcomes trials have shown a clear benefit to pharmacologic treatment for raising HDL cholesterol.

REFERENCES

1. Genest JJ, Martin-Munley SS, McNamara JR, et al. Familial lipoprotein disorders in patients with premature coronary artery disease. *Circulation* 1992;85:2025–2033.
2. Kugiyama K, Doi H, Motoyama T, et al. Association of remnant lipoprotein levels with impairment of endothelium-dependent vasomotor function in human coronary arteries. *Circulation* 1998;97:2519–2526.
3. Stone NJ, Levy RI, Fredrickson DS, et al. Coronary artery disease in 116 kindred with familial type ii hyperlipoproteinemia. *Circulation* 1974;49:476–488.
4. Innerarity TL, Mahley RW, Weisgraber KH, et al. Familial defective apolipoprotein B-100: a mutation of apolipoprotein B that causes hypercholesterolemia. *J Lipid Res* 1990;31:1337–1349.
5. Feussner G, Wagner A, Kohl B, et al. Clinical features of type III hyperlipoproteinemia: analysis of 64 patients. *Clin Investig* 1993;71:362–366.
6. Haase A, Goldberg AC. Identification of people with heterozygous familial hypercholesterolemia. *Curr Opin Lipidol* 2012;23:282–289.
7. Nordestgaard BG, Chapman MJ, Humphries SE, et al. Familial hypercholesterolaemia is underdiagnosed and undertreated in the general population: guidance for clinicians to prevent coronary heart disease: consensus statement of the European Atherosclerosis Society. *Eur Heart J* 2013;34:3478–3490a.
8. Goldberg AC, Hopkins PN, Toth PP, et al. Familial hypercholesterolemia: screening, diagnosis and management of pediatric and adult patients: clinical guidance from the National Lipid Association Expert Panel on Familial Hypercholesterolemia. *J Clin Lipidol* 2011;5:133–140.

9. Berglund L, Brunzell JD, Goldberg AC, et al. Evaluation and treatment of hypertriglyceridemia: an Endocrine Society clinical practice guideline. *J Clin Endocrinol Metab* 2012;97:2969–2989.

10. Randomised trial of cholesterol lowering in 4444 patients with coronary heart disease: the Scandinavian Simvastatin Survival Study (4S). *Lancet* 1994;344:1383–1389.

11. Sacks FM, Pfeffer MA, Moye LA, et al. The effect of pravastatin on coronary events after myocardial infarction in patients with average cholesterol levels. Cholesterol and Recurrent Events Trial investigators. *N Engl J Med* 1996;335:1001–1009.

12. Prevention of cardiovascular events and death with pravastatin in patients with coronary heart disease and a broad range of initial cholesterol levels. The Long-Term Intervention with Pravastatin in Ischaemic Disease (LIPID) Study Group. *N Engl J Med* 1998;339:1349–1357.

13. Heart Protection Study Collaborative Group. MRC/BHF Heart Protection Study of cholesterol lowering with simvastatin in 20,536 high-risk individuals: a randomised placebo-controlled trial. *Lancet* 2002;360:7–22.

14. Shepherd J, Cobbe SM, Ford I, et al. Prevention of coronary heart disease with pravastatin in men with hypercholesterolemia. West of Scotland Coronary Prevention Study Group. *N Engl J Med* 1995;333:1301–1307.

15. Downs JR, Clearfield M, Weis S, et al. Primary prevention of acute coronary events with lovastatin in men and women with average cholesterol levels: results of AFCAPS/TexCAPS. Air Force/Texas Coronary Atherosclerosis Prevention Study. *JAMA* 1998;279:1615–1622.

16. Sever PS, Dahlöf B, Poulter NR, et al. Prevention of coronary and stroke events with atorvastatin in hypertensive patients who have average or lower-than-average cholesterol concentrations, in the Anglo-Scandinavian Cardiac Outcomes Trial—Lipid Lowering Arm (ASCOT-LLA): a multicentre randomised controlled trial. *Lancet* 2003;361:1149–1158.

17. Colhoun HM, Betteridge DJ, Durrington PN, et al. Primary prevention of cardiovascular disease with atorvastatin in type 2 diabetes in the Collaborative Atorvastatin Diabetes Study (CARDS): multicentre randomised placebo-controlled trial. *Lancet* 2004;364:685–696.

18. Goff DC, Lloyd-Jones DM, Bennett G, et al. 2013 ACC/AHA guideline on the assessment of cardiovascular risk: a report of the American College of Cardiology/American Heart Association Task Force on Practice Guidelines. *Circulation* 2014;129:S49–S73.

19. Eckel RH, Jakicic JM, Ard JD, et al. 2013 AHA/ACC guideline on lifestyle management to reduce cardiovascular risk: a report of the American College of Cardiology/American Heart Association Task Force on Practice Guidelines. *Circulation* 2014;129:S76–S99.

20. Jensen MD, Ryan DH, Apovian CM, et al. 2013 AHA/ACC/TOS Guideline for the management of overweight and obesity in adults: a report of the American College of Cardiology/American Heart Association Task Force on Practice Guidelines and The Obesity Society. *Circulation* 2014;129:S102–S138.

21. Stone NJ, Robinson JG, Lichtenstein AH, et al. 2013 ACC/AHA guideline on the treatment of blood cholesterol to reduce atherosclerotic cardiovascular risk in adults: a report of the American College of Cardiology/American Heart Association Task Force on Practice Guidelines. *Circulation* 2014;129:S1–S45.

22. Robinson JG, Goldberg AC. Treatment of adults with familial hypercholesterolemia and evidence for treatment: recommendations from the National Lipid Association Expert Panel on Familial Hypercholesterolemia. *J Clin Lipidol* 2011;5:S18–S29.

23. Shepherd J, Blauw GJ, Murphy MB, et al. Pravastatin in elderly individuals at risk of vascular disease (PROSPER): a randomised controlled trial. *Lancet* 2002;360:1623–1630.

24. Sarwar N, Danesh J, Eiriksdottir G, et al. Triglycerides and the risk of coronary heart disease: 10,158 incident cases among 262,525 participants in 29 Western prospective studies. *Circulation* 2007;115:450–458.

25. Tirosh A, Rudich A, Shochat T, et al. Changes in triglyceride levels and risk for coronary heart disease in young men. *Ann Intern Med* 2007;147:377–385.

26. Miller M, Stone NJ, Ballantyne C, et al. Triglycerides and cardiovascular disease: a scientific statement from the American Heart Association. *Circulation* 2011;123:2292–2333.

27. International Diabetes Federation. IDF Worldwide Definition of the Metabolic Syndrome. Available at: http://www.idf.org/metabolic-syndrome. Last accessed December 22, 2014.

28. U.S. Food and Drug Administration. FDA Drug Safety Communication: Important safety label changes to cholesterol-lowering statin drugs. 2012. Available at: http://www.fda.gov/Drugs/DrugSafety/ucm293101.htm. Last accessed December 22, 2014.

29. Knopp RH. Drug treatment of lipid disorders. *N Engl J Med* 1999;341:498–511.

30. Chong PH. Lack of therapeutic interchangeability of HMG-CoA reductase inhibitors. *Ann Pharmacother* 2002;36:1907–1917.

31. Pasternak RC, Smith SC, Bairey-Merz CN, et al. ACC/AHA/NHLBI clinical advisory on the use and safety of statins. *Circulation* 2002;106:1024–1028.

32. Venero CV, Thompson PD. Managing statin myopathy. *Endocrinol Metab Clin North Am* 2009;38:121–136.

33. Sattar N, Preiss D, Murray HM, et al. Statins and risk of incident diabetes: a collaborative meta-analysis of randomised statin trials. *Lancet* 2010;375:735–742.

34. Kellick KA, Bottorff M, Toth PP. A clinician's guide to statin drug-drug interactions. *J Clin Lipidol* 2014;8:S30–S46.

35. The Lipid Research Clinics Coronary Primary Prevention Trial results. I. Reduction in incidence of coronary heart disease. *JAMA* 1984;251:351–364.

36. Illingworth DR, Stein EA, Mitchel YB, et al. Comparative effects of lovastatin and niacin in primary hypercholesterolemia. A prospective trial. *Arch Intern Med* 1994;154:1586–1595.

37. Boden WE, Probstfield JL, Anderson T, et al. Niacin in patients with low HDL cholesterol levels receiving intensive statin therapy. *N Engl J Med* 2011;365:2255–2267.

38. Group HC. HPS2-THRIVE randomized placebo-controlled trial in 25 673 high-risk patients of ER niacin/laropiprant: trial design, pre-specified muscle and liver outcomes, and reasons for stopping study treatment. *Eur Heart J* 2013;34:1279–1291.

39. Dujovne CA, Ettinger MP, McNeer JF, et al. Efficacy and safety of a potent new selective cholesterol absorption inhibitor, ezetimibe, in patients with primary hypercholesterolemia. *Am J Cardiol* 2002;90:1092–1097.

40. Knopp R. Effects of ezetimibe, a new cholesterol absorption inhibitor, on plasma lipids in patients with primary hypercholesterolemia. *Eur Heart J* 2003;24:729–741.

41. Gagné C, Bays HE, Weiss SR, et al. Efficacy and safety of ezetimibe added to ongoing statin therapy for treatment of patients with primary hypercholesterolemia. *Am J Cardiol* 2002;90:1084–1091.

42. Goldberg AC, Sapre A, Liu J, et al. Efficacy and safety of ezetimibe coadministered with simvastatin in patients with primary hypercholesterolemia: a randomized, double-blind, placebo-controlled trial. *Mayo Clin Proc* 2004;79:620–629.

43. Baigent C, Landray MJ, Reith C, et al. The effects of lowering LDL cholesterol with simvastatin plus ezetimibe in patients with chronic kidney disease (Study of Heart and Renal Protection): a randomised placebo-controlled trial. *Lancet* 2011;377:2181–2192.

44. Ito MK, McGowan MP, Moriarty PM. Management of familial hypercholesterolemias in adult patients: recommendations from the National Lipid Association Expert Panel on Familial Hypercholesterolemia. *J Clin Lipidol* 2011;5:S38–S45.

45. Brunzell JD. Clinical practice. Hypertriglyceridemia. *N Engl J Med* 2007;357:1009–1017.

46. Keech A, Simes RJ, Barter P, et al. Effects of long-term fenofibrate therapy on cardiovascular events in 9795 people with type 2 diabetes mellitus (the FIELD study): randomised controlled trial. *Lancet* 2005;366:1849–1861.

47. Rosenson RS. Current overview of statin-induced myopathy. *Am J Med* 2004;116:408–416.

48. Alsheikh-Ali AA, Kuvin JT, Karas RH. Risk of adverse events with fibrates. *Am J Cardiol* 2004;94:935–938.

49. Jones PH, Davidson MH. Reporting rate of rhabdomyolysis with fenofibrate + statin versus gemfibrozil + any statin. *Am J Cardiol* 2005;95:120–122.

50. Nestel PJ, Connor WE, Reardon MF, et al. Suppression by diets rich in fish oil of very low density lipoprotein production in man. *J Clin Invest* 1984;74:82–89.

51. Harris WS, Connor WE, Illingworth DR, et al. Effects of fish oil on VLDL triglyceride kinetics in humans. *J Lipid Res* 1990;31:1549–1558.

52. Maki KC, McKenney JM, Reeves MS, et al. Effects of adding prescription omega-3 acid ethyl esters to simvastatin (20 mg/day) on lipids and lipoprotein particles in men and women with mixed dyslipidemia. *Am J Cardiol* 2008;102:429–433.

53. Barter P, Ginsberg HN. Effectiveness of combined statin plus omega-3 fatty acid therapy for mixed dyslipidemia. *Am J Cardiol* 2008;102:1040–1045.

54. Ballantyne CM, Olsson AG, Cook TJ, et al. Influence of low high-density lipoprotein cholesterol and elevated triglyceride on coronary heart disease events and response to simvastatin therapy in 4S. *Circulation* 2001;104:3046–3051.

12

Disorders of Hemostasis

Tzu-Fei Wang, Charles S. Eby, and Ronald Jackups Jr.

GENERAL PRINCIPLES

- Normal hemostasis involves a complex sequence of interrelated reactions that lead to platelet aggregation (primary hemostasis) and activation of coagulation factors (secondary hemostasis) to produce a durable vascular seal.
- **Primary hemostasis** is an immediate but temporary response to vessel injury. Platelets and von Willebrand factor (vWF) interact to form a primary plug.
- **Secondary hemostasis** (coagulation) results in the formation of a fibrin clot (Fig. 12-1). Injury initiates coagulation by exposing extravascular tissue factor to blood, which initiates activation of factors VII, X, and prothrombin. The subsequent activation of other factors leads to the generation of thrombin, conversion of fibrinogen to fibrin, and formation of a durable clot.[1]

DIAGNOSIS

Clinical Presentation

History
- A detailed history can assess bleeding severity, congenital or acquired status, and primary or secondary hemostatic defects.
- Prolonged bleeding after dental extractions, circumcision, menstruation, labor and delivery, trauma, or surgery may suggest an underlying bleeding disorder.
- Strong family history may suggest an inherited bleeding disorder.

Physical Examination
- Primary hemostasis defects are suggested by mucosal bleeding and excessive bruising.
  - **Petechiae:** <2-mm foci of subcutaneous bleeding that do not blanch with pressure and typically present in areas subject to increased hydrostatic force: the lower legs and periorbital area (especially after coughing or vomiting)
  - **Ecchymoses:** >3-mm black-and-blue (or violaceous) patches due to rupture of small vessels from trauma
- Secondary hemostasis defects can produce hematomas (localized masses of clotted/unclotted blood), hemarthroses, or delayed bleeding after trauma or surgery.

Diagnostic Testing

Laboratories
The history and physical exam guide test selection: Initial studies should include platelet count, prothrombin time (PT), activated partial thromboplastin time (aPTT), and peripheral blood smear.

Primary Hemostasis Testing
- A **low platelet count** requires a review of a blood smear to rule out platelet clumping artifact (often due to the EDTA additive), giant platelets, and misclassification of other cells as platelets.
- The **bleeding time** (BT) measures time until bleeding cessation from a standardized skin incision, but it does not quantify the perioperative risk of bleeding.[2] While the BT is used to detect qualitative platelet defects, it is considered a poor test due to low accuracy and high interoperator variability. The platelet function analysis (PFA)-100 now replaces BT in most laboratories.

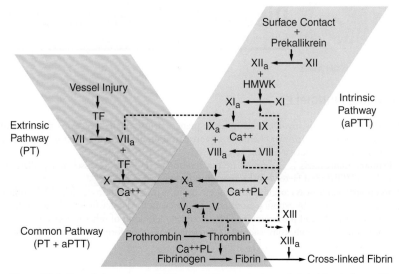

Figure 12-1 Coagulation cascade. *Solid arrows* indicate activation and *dashed lines* indicate additional substrates activated by factor VIIa or thrombin. aPTT, activated partial thromboplastin time; HMWK, high molecular weight kininogen; PL phospholipid; PT, prothrombin time; TF, tissue factor.

- The **PFA-100** instrument assesses vWF-dependent platelet activation in flowing citrated whole blood. Most patients with von Willebrand disease (vWD) and qualitative platelet disorders have prolonged closure times. Anemia (hematocrit <30%) and thrombocytopenia (platelet count of <100 × 10⁹/L) can cause artifactually prolonged closure times.
- **In vitro platelet aggregation** studies measure platelet secretion and aggregation in response to platelet agonists (e.g., adenosine diphosphate [ADP], collagen, arachidonic acid, and epinephrine), and they assist with the diagnosis of qualitative platelet disorders.
- Laboratory evaluation of vWD is discussed later in this chapter.

Secondary Hemostasis Testing

- **Prothrombin time (PT):** Measures time to form a fibrin clot after adding thromboplastin (tissue factor and phospholipid) and calcium to citrated plasma.
  - Sensitive to deficiencies of the **extrinsic pathway** (factor VII), **common pathway** (factors X and V and prothrombin), and **fibrinogen**.
  - Sensitive to anticoagulation therapy with **warfarin** and may also be prolonged with the use of direct thrombin inhibitors (DTIs) and factor Xa inhibitors.
  - Reporting a PT ratio as an international normalized ratio (INR) reduces interlaboratory variation for monitoring warfarin therapy.[3]
- **Activated partial thromboplastin time (aPTT):** Measures the time to form a fibrin clot after activation of citrated plasma by calcium, phospholipid, and negatively charged particles.
  - Sensitive to deficiencies of the **intrinsic pathway** (factors VIII, IX, and XI), **common pathway**, and **fibrinogen** and to clinically insignificant deficiencies of the **contact activators** (factor XII, prekallikrein, and high molecular weight kininogen).
  - Sensitive to anticoagulation therapy with **unfractionated heparin** and may also be prolonged with use of direct thrombin inhibitors (DTIs) and factor Xa inhibitors.
  - Although the aPTT may be prolonged with use of **low molecular weight heparin** (enoxaparin), monitoring of therapeutic anticoagulation should be performed with the **anti–factor Xa inhibitor** assay.

TABLE 12-1	Factor Deficiencies Causing Prolonged Prothrombin Time (PT) and/or Activated Partial Thromboplastin Time (aPTT) That Correct with 50:50 Mix

Abnormal assay	Suspected factor deficiencies
aPTT	XII, XI, IX, or VIII
PT	VII or multiple vitamin K–dependent factors
PT and aPTT	II, V, X, or fibrinogen

- **Thrombin time**: Measures time to form a fibrin clot after addition of thrombin to citrated plasma. Quantitative and qualitative deficiencies of fibrinogen, elevated fibrin degradation products, heparin, and DTIs may prolong the thrombin time.
- **Fibrinogen**: The addition of thrombin to dilute plasma and the measurement of a clotting time determine the effective functional concentration of fibrinogen. Conditions causing hypofibrinogenemia include decreased hepatic synthesis, massive hemorrhage, and disseminated intravascular coagulation (DIC).
- **D-dimers** result from plasmin digestion of fibrin. Elevated D-dimer concentrations occur in many disease states, including acute venous thromboembolism, DIC, trauma, and malignancy.
- **General workup of unexpected prolonged PT or aPTT** should include the following:
  - Consideration of preanalytic variables such as incomplete filling of sample tubes, heparin contamination (screen with thrombin time), high hematocrit (>55%), hemolysis, and lipemia.
  - A **mixing study** (performing PT or aPTT on the patient's plasma mixed 1:1 with normal pooled plasma) will differentiate factor deficiencies from inhibitors:
    - Correction of PT or aPTT to within reference range after mixing: simple deficiency of factor(s), depending on whether PT and/or aPTT is prolonged. Hemophilias, acquired deficiencies, and warfarin result in this pattern.
    - No or minimal correction: factor inhibitor, depending on whether PT and/or aPTT are prolonged. Autoantibodies and alloantibodies to factors result in this pattern, as do heparins, DTIs, and lupus anticoagulants.
  - **Common causes** of PT and aPTT prolongation (Table 12-1):
    - **PT and aPTT prolonged**: hypofibrinogenemia, common pathway factor (II, V, X) deficiencies, DIC, liver disease, dilutional coagulopathy, DTIs, factor Xa inhibitors, and superwarfarin (e.g., brodifacoum) toxicity
    - **PT only**: warfarin, vitamin K deficiency, liver disease, factor VII deficiency
    - **aPTT only**: Heparin, common hemophilias (factor VIII, IX, or XI deficiency)
    - Most common inhibitors that prolong the aPTT are factor VIII inhibitors (if bleeding is present) and lupus anticoagulants (if there is no history of bleeding)

PLATELET DISORDERS

Quantitative Platelet Disorders (Thrombocytopenia)

- Thrombocytopenia is defined as a platelet count of <140 to 150 × 10^9/L at most laboratories. In the absence of qualitative platelet defects or vascular damage, spontaneous bleeding often does not occur until the platelet count is <10 to 30 × 10^9/L.
- Thrombocytopenia occurs from decreased production, increased destruction, or sequestration of platelets (Table 12-2). Many infectious diseases are associated with thrombocytopenia through complex or poorly understood mechanisms.[4]

TABLE 12-2	Classification of Thrombocytopenia

Decreased platelet production
Marrow failure syndromes
  Congenital
  Acquired: aplastic anemia, paroxysmal
    nocturnal hemoglobinuria
Hematologic malignancies
Marrow infiltration
  Cancer
  Granuloma
Fibrosis
  Primary
  Secondary
Nutritional
  Vitamin B_{12} deficiency
  Folate deficiency
Physical damage
  Radiation
  Ethanol
  Chemotherapy

Increased splenic sequestration
Portal hypertension
Felty syndrome
Lysosomal storage disorders
Infiltrative hematologic malignancies
Extramedullary hematopoiesis

Increased platelet clearance
Immune-mediated mechanisms
Immune thrombocytopenia purpura
Thrombotic thrombocytopenia
  purpura
Posttransfusion purpura
Heparin-induced thrombocytopenia
Nonimmune mediated
Acute hemorrhage
DIC
Local consumption (e.g., aortic
  aneurysm)
HELLP syndrome

**Infections associated with
thrombocytopenia**
HIV
HHV-6
Ehrlichiosis
Rickettsia spp.
Malaria
Hepatitis C
Cytomegalovirus
Epstein-Barr virus
Helicobacter pylori
Escherichia coli O157:H7 (HUS)

DIC, disseminated intravascular coagulation; HELLP, Hemolysis (with microangiopathy), Elevated Liver enzymes, and Low Platelet count; HUS, hemolytic uremic syndrome.

Immune Thrombocytopenic Purpura

GENERAL PRINCIPLES

Immune thrombocytopenic purpura (ITP) is an acquired autoimmune disorder in which antiplatelet antibodies cause shortened platelet survival and suppress megakaryopoiesis, leading to thrombocytopenia and increased bleeding risk. ITP can be classified into primary (idiopathic) and secondary (associated with coexisting conditions, including systemic lupus erythematosus, antiphospholipid antibody syndrome, HIV, hepatitis C, *Helicobacter pylori*, and lymphoproliferative disorders).[4]

DIAGNOSIS

Clinical Presentation

• ITP typically presents as mild mucocutaneous bleeding and petechiae or thrombocytopenia discovered incidentally.

- Primary ITP often has the scenario of isolated thrombocytopenia in the absence of a likely underlying causative disease or medication.

Diagnostic Testing

- Laboratory tests do not confirm the presence of primary ITP, though they help to exclude some secondary causes.
- Serologic tests for antiplatelet antibodies do not help diagnose ITP because of poor sensitivity and low negative predictive value and should not be used routinely.[5]
- Bone marrow biopsy and aspirate studies are not necessary in patients with typical presentations of ITP, irrespective of age. However, if patients have other abnormalities identified in history, physical examination, or peripheral blood count, bone marrow biopsy may be needed to exclude other causes such as malignancy, especially in older patients (age >60 years) and patients who do not respond to standard ITP treatments.[6]
- All newly diagnosed adult ITP patients should be tested for HIV and HCV.

TREATMENT

- The decision to treat primary ITP depends upon the severity of thrombocytopenia and symptoms of bleeding.
- Management of secondary ITP includes treatment of the underlying disease and standard primary ITP therapy.
- **Initial therapy, when indicated, consists of glucocorticoids** (typically prednisone 1 mg/kg/day for 2 to 3 weeks then taper depending on the patient's responses and stability of platelet count).
- Steroid nonresponders or patients with active bleeding often also receive intravenous immunoglobulin (IVIG) (1 g/kg × 2 days) or anti–D immunoglobulin (WinRho) if Rh positive. Anti–D immunoglobulin is ineffective postsplenectomy.
- Approximately 80% of patients will respond to glucocorticoids initially with resolution of thrombocytopenia within 1 to 3 weeks.
- Steroid nonresponders and the 30% to 40% of patients who relapse during a steroid taper have chronic ITP. The therapeutic goals in refractory and relapsed ITP patients include a safe platelet count (>30 × 10^9/L) and minimization of treatment-related toxicities.
- **Treatment options for refractory or relapsed ITP**: The optimal sequence or choice of the following three treatment options has not been established and is usually determined by patient preference/conditions.
  - Splenectomy: **Two-thirds of patients with refractory ITP will obtain a durable complete response following splenectomy**. Administer pneumococcal, meningococcal, and *Haemophilus influenzae* type B vaccines at least 2 weeks before splenectomy.
  - Rituximab, an anti-CD20 monoclonal antibody, or much less commonly, other immunosuppressive agents such as cyclosporine, azathioprine, or androgen therapy with danazol.[6,7]
  - Thrombopoietin (TPO) receptor agonists:
    - Two small-molecule TPO receptor agonists are available for refractory ITP patients with increased bleeding risk. **Romiplostim** is given subcutaneously once weekly and **eltrombopag** orally once a day.
    - Both produce durable platelet count improvements in 80% to 90% of refractory ITP patients after 5 to 7 days.
    - Potential complications include transaminitis, thromboembolic events, and bone marrow fibrosis.[8]

Drug-Induced Thrombocytopenia

GENERAL PRINCIPLES

Drug-dependent immune thrombocytopenia results from drug-platelet interactions prompting antibody binding.[9] Medications that are commonly associated with thrombocytopenia are listed in Table 12-3.[10] An extensive list of medications with references can be found on the website of the University of Oklahoma Health Sciences (http://www.ouhsc.edu/platelets/DITP.html, last accessed January 2, 2015).

DIAGNOSIS

Key factors to diagnose drug-induced thrombocytopenia:

• Exposure of suspected drug(s) precede(s) thrombocytopenia.
• Normalization of platelet counts with discontinuation of suspected drug(s).

TABLE 12-3	Drugs Implicated in Immune Thrombocytopenia

Antibiotics
Cephalosporins
  Cefotetan
  Cephalothin
Gentamicin
Linezolid
Penicillins
  Penicillin
  Ampicillin
  Methicillin
Rifampin
Sulfonamides
Trimethoprim
Vancomycin

Anti-inflammatory drugs
Aspirin
Diclofenac
Ibuprofen
Indomethacin
Naproxen
Piroxicam
Sulindac
Tolmetin

Antihistamines
Chlorpheniramine
Cimetidine
Ranitidine

Antiarrhythmics
Amiodarone
Digoxin
Lidocaine
Procainamide
Quinidine

Anticoagulants
Heparin
Low molecular weight heparin

Platelet inhibitors
Abciximab
Eptifibatide
Tirofiban
Ticlopidine

Antihypertensives
α-Methyldopa
Acetazolamide
Captopril
Chlorothiazide
Furosemide
Hydrochlorothiazide
Spironolactone

Anticonvulsants
Carbamazepine
Phenytoin
Valproic acid

Other
Acetaminophen
Alemtuzumab
Cocaine
Fludarabine
Gold
Heroin
Iodinated contrast
Quinine
Sulfonylureas
Tricyclic antidepressants

- No other likely drugs present.
- No other more likely etiologies for thrombocytopenia.
- Thrombocytopenia recurs when patients are rechallenged with the same drug.

TREATMENT

- Discontinuation of the suspected offending agent(s) is the main therapy.
- Platelet transfusion for severe thrombocytopenia may decrease the risk of bleeding, but is discouraged for less severe thrombocytopenia without bleeding. IVIG, steroids, and plasmapheresis have uncertain benefits.

Thrombotic Thrombocytopenic Purpura

GENERAL PRINCIPLES

- The pathogenesis of thrombotic thrombocytopenic purpura (TTP) is the formation of disseminated platelet thrombi. Deficiency of the vWF-cleaving metalloprotease ADAMTS13 (most commonly autoantibody mediated) leads to elevated levels of abnormally large vWF multimers that spontaneously adhere to platelets and form occlusive vWF-platelet aggregates in the microcirculation and subsequent thrombotic microangiopathy (TMA).[11] Thrombocytopenia due to platelet consumption, microangiopathic hemolytic anemia (MAHA) due to platelet microthrombi, and organ ischemia are characteristic features.
- Sporadic (primary) TTP has an incidence of approximately 11.3 cases per 10^6 people and occurs more frequently in women and African Americans.[12]
- Secondary TTP refers to TMA associated with DIC, HIV, malignant hypertension, vasculitis, organ and stem cell transplant–related toxicity, adverse drug reactions, and, during pregnancy, preeclampsia/eclampsia and HELLP (Hemolytic anemia, Elevated Liver enzymes, Low Platelet count) syndrome.
- TMA may also be associated with certain drugs, including quinine, ticlopidine, calcineurin inhibitors (cyclosporine, tacrolimus), sirolimus, and chemotherapy agents such as gemcitabine and mitomycin C.

DIAGNOSIS

Clinical Presentation

- The classic **pentad** of TTP includes **consumptive thrombocytopenia, MAHA, fever, renal dysfunction, and fluctuating neurologic deficits,** but is only fully present in <30% of cases. The findings of thrombocytopenia and MAHA alone should raise suspicion for TTP.
- Patients with autosomal recessive inherited ADAMTS13 deficiencies have recurrent TTP (Upshaw-Schulman syndrome).

Diagnostic Testing

- **Schistocytes** and thrombocytopenia on peripheral blood smears are classical findings.
- Hemolysis workup is often positive including anemia, elevated reticulocyte count, low haptoglobin, elevated lactate dehydrogenase, and elevated indirect bilirubin.
- TTP is often associated with very low or undetectable ADAMTS13 enzyme activity and an ADAMTS13 inhibitory antibody. However, treatment should not be delayed for such testing, due to the urgency of the disease.

TREATMENT

- The mainstay of therapy is **plasma exchange** (PEX), requiring **emergent inpatient admission Glucocorticoids** (prednisone 1 mg/kg/day orally or methylprednisolone 1 g IV daily) are commonly initiated along with PEX. Treatment for refractory or relapsed TTP may include rituximab, cyclosporine, or vincristine.[13–16]
- Platelet transfusion in the absence of severe bleeding is relatively contraindicated because of the potential risk of additional microvascular occlusions.
- When TMA is suspected to be due to drugs, discontinuation of the offending agent is the preferred therapy. PEX is usually not effective.

Hemolytic-Uremic Syndrome

GENERAL PRINCIPLES

- The clinical **pentad** of TTP can also be found in hemolytic-uremic syndrome (HUS), but HUS is usually associated with higher incidence of renal dysfunction and lower incidence of neurologic manifestations.
- There are two types of HUS, typical and atypical.
  - **Typical HUS** (diarrhea associated) often follows acute infection with *Escherichia coli* (especially serotype O157:H7) or *Shigella dysenteriae* that produce Shiga-like toxins.
  - **Atypical HUS (aHUS)** has the clinical presentation of HUS without being preceded by the above-mentioned infections or diarrhea. Acquired and inherited defects in regulation of the alternative pathway of complement activation are frequently identified.[17]

DIAGNOSIS

Clinical Presentation

- Diarrhea (often bloody) and abdominal pain often precede typical HUS, and more pronounced renal dysfunction occurs.
- Familial atypical HUS often leads to chronic renal failure.

Diagnostic Testing

- Features of TMA and acute renal failure are usually present.
- In typical HUS, stool culture for *E. coli* O157 has a higher sensitivity than Shiga toxin assays.[18]
- ADAMTS13 activity is often normal or only mildly decreased (in contrast to TTP, which is associated with a very low ADAMTS13 activity).
- Workup for suspected aHUS should include molecular analysis of complement regulator factor H and I and MCP (membrane cofactor protein) genes as well as analysis for acquired inhibitors through reference laboratories.

TREATMENT

- Inpatient admission is recommended based on the severity of the presentation.
- Typical HUS:
  - Treatment is supportive care (e.g., hydration).
  - Antibiotics do not hasten recovery or minimize toxicity for HUS-associated infection.
  - **PEX is not recommended due to a demonstrated lack of benefit.**

- Atypical HUS:
  - PEX can provide some benefit, but is often less effective than for TTP.
  - Eculizumab, a monoclonal antibody against the complement protein C5, inhibits the complement-mediated renal injury.

Heparin-Induced Thrombocytopenia

GENERAL PRINCIPLES

- Heparin-induced thrombocytopenia (HIT) is an acquired hypercoagulable disorder caused by antibodies targeting heparin and platelet factor 4 (PF4) complexes, which can activate platelets, cause thrombocytopenia, and increase thrombin generation.[19]
- HIT typically presents with a decreased platelet count by at least 50% after exposure to unfractionated heparin (UFH) or (less likely) low molecular weight heparin (LMWH).
- The incidence of HIT varies with clinical setting, anticoagulant formulation, dose, duration of exposure, and previous exposure, ranging from 0.1% to 1% in medical and obstetric patients receiving prophylactic and therapeutic UFH to 1% to 5% in patients receiving prophylactic UFH after total hip or knee replacements or cardiothoracic surgery.[20]

DIAGNOSIS

Clinical Presentation

- Suspect HIT when thrombocytopenia occurs during heparin exposure by any route in the absence of other causes of thrombocytopenia and when platelet counts recover after cessation of heparin.
- HIT **usually develops between 5 and 14 days of heparin exposure** (typical-onset HIT). Exceptions include **delayed-onset HIT,** which occurs after stopping heparin, and **early-onset HIT,** which starts within the first 24 hours of heparin administration in patients with recent exposure to heparin.[20]
- Both venous and arterial thromboembolic complications occur due to activation of platelets. Thrombosis can precede, be concurrent with, or follow recognition of thrombocytopenia. Thrombi may occur at heparin injection sites as full-thickness skin infarctions, sometimes in the absence of thrombocytopenia. HIT **rarely causes severe thrombocytopenia ($<20 \times 10^9$/L) and bleeding**.

Diagnostic Testing

- A scoring system based on the "4Ts" improves diagnostic accuracy: thrombocytopenia, timing, thrombosis, and other explanations for thrombocytopenia (Table 12-4).[21] A 4 T score of 3 or below correlates with a low probability of HIT and high negative predictive value (0.998).[22] A HIT assay should **NOT** be ordered due to the high false-positive rate in this population.
- There are two main types of HIT assays:
  - **Serologic enzyme immunoassays** (PF4 EIA) to detect heparin-PF4 antibodies
  - **Functional assays**: platelet aggregometry or serotonin release assay to detect activation of control platelets in the presence of patient serum and heparin
- In comparison, serologic tests have higher sensitivity and serve as screening tests, whereas functional assays have higher specificity and may serve as confirmatory tests when the diagnosis is unclear.

TABLE 12-4 The 4Ts Scoring System[23]

Category	2 points	1 point	0 point
Thrombocytopenia	PLT count fall >50% and PLT nadir ≥20,000/mm³	PLT count fall 30%–50% or PLT nadir 10,000–19,000/mm³	PLT count fall <30% and PLT nadir <10,000/mm³
Timing of thrombocytopenia	Clear onset on days 5–10 or PLT fall ≤1 day (with prior heparin exposure within 30 days)	Suspected fall on days 5–10 but not clear, onset after day 10, or PLT fall ≤1 day (with prior heparin exposure 30–100 days ago)	PLT count fall ≤4 days without recent heparin exposure
Thrombosis or other sequelae	New confirmed thrombosis, skin necrosis, or acute systemic reactions after IV heparin	Progressive or recurrent thrombosis, nonnecrotizing skin lesions, or suspected thrombosis but not proven	None
Other causes of thrombocytopenia	None apparent	Possible	Definite

PLT, platelet.

TREATMENT

- When HIT is strongly suspected, begin treatment by **eliminating all heparin exposure**. Patients with thrombosis and those at high risk for thrombosis require alternative anticoagulation with a parenteral DTI, such as bivalirudin or argatroban (see Chapter 14). LMWH may cross-react with HIT antibodies and should not be used. **Do not treat with warfarin initially**, as it may exacerbate the prothrombic state of HIT via protein C depletion, resulting in skin necrosis or limb gangrene.
- Perform a lower extremity venous compression ultrasound since it often detects deep vein thrombosis in asymptomatic isolated HIT patients, and the presence of thrombosis mandates longer-duration anticoagulation.[19]
- Start warfarin only after the platelet count normalizes, and overlap with a DTI for 5 days. The recommended duration of anticoagulation therapy for HIT depends on the clinical scenario: For isolated HIT (without thrombosis), at least until the platelet count recovers, some experts advocate anticoagulation for 6 weeks after the normalization of platelet count; for HIT-associated thrombosis, typical thromboembolism therapy duration is recommended (see Chapter 14).

Posttransfusion Purpura

- Posttransfusion purpura (PTP) is a rare acquired autoimmune disorder in which **antiplatelet alloantibodies** cause shortened survival of transfused platelets and paradoxically of native platelets, leading to severe thrombocytopenia and increased bleeding risk.
- Thrombocytopenic purpura and bleeding typically occur **8 to 10 days after blood transfusion**. Due to the delay in presentation, its association to the preceding transfusion event is frequently missed.

- Testing for platelet antibodies may help to confirm the diagnosis, but treatment should not be delayed for testing. The most commonly identified antibody is anti–HPA-1a.
- **First-line therapy is IVIG** and is usually successful. Plasma exchange may be considered as second-line therapy if IVIG fails. Transfusion of HPA-1a–negative platelets may provide a better response in platelet counts during the thrombocytopenic phase. PTP is self-limiting, but may recur following future transfusions.

Gestational Thrombocytopenia

- Gestational thrombocytopenia is a benign and mild thrombocytopenia and occurs in 5% to 7% of otherwise uncomplicated pregnancies.
- Gestational thrombocytopenia occurs in the third trimester of pregnancy. The mother is asymptomatic, and thrombocytopenia spontaneously resolves after delivery. The fetus remains unaffected.
- Platelet counts should be no $<70 \times 10^9$/L. Lower platelet counts should prompt consideration of other causes and appropriate workup.
- Other important differential diagnoses of thrombocytopenia during pregnancy include ITP, preeclampsia, eclampsia, HELLP syndrome, TTP, and DIC.

Chemotherapy-Induced Thrombocytopenia

- Thrombocytopenia is a common temporary side effect of myelosuppressive chemotherapy.
- Treatment is supportive transfusion while patients receive chemotherapy.
- To prevent life-threatening hemorrhage, even in asymptomatic patients, prophylactic platelet transfusion is generally given for platelet count $<20 \times 10^9$/L in the outpatient setting and for platelet count $<10 \times 10^9$/L in the inpatient setting. Patients with bleeding or in need of procedures may require higher platelet counts (usually $>50 \times 10^9$/L but can vary depending on the severity of bleeding and the type of procedure).
- Frequently transfused patients may develop platelet refractoriness due to acquired HLA antibodies that rapidly clear transfused platelets. When suspected, a platelet count should be performed 15 to 60 minutes following transfusion to detect a poor platelet response (<20 to 30×10^9/L increment). Confirmation of refractoriness by identification of HLA antibodies may allow for the use of HLA-compatible or HLA-crossmatched platelet transfusions.

Thrombocytopenia Secondary to Liver Disease

Patients with cirrhosis often have thrombocytopenia due to multiple mechanisms:

- Splenic sequestration from splenomegaly
- Immune destruction by autoantibodies
- Bone marrow suppression from viruses (such as hepatitis C), toxins (such as alcohol), or medications (such as ribavirin or interferon)
- Decreased TPO production by the cirrhotic liver

Familial Thrombocytopenia

- Familial thrombocytopenia is uncommon and is often misdiagnosed as ITP.
- Patients usually present with an incidental finding of mild thrombocytopenia ($>100 \times 10^9$/L) without evidence of bleeding. Giant platelets may also be seen on peripheral smear (macrothrombocytopenia) that may not be counted by automated cell analyzers.
- A positive family history of thrombocytopenia is crucial to avoid misdiagnosis and exposure of patients to unnecessary ITP therapy.

Qualitative Platelet Disorders

GENERAL PRINCIPLES

- Qualitative platelet disorders should be suspected when patients present with **mucocutaneous bleeding and excessive bruising** in the setting of an adequate platelet count, normal PT and aPTT, and negative screening tests for vWD.
- Most platelet defects produce prolonged PFA-100 closure times. However, a high clinical suspicion of a disorder in a patient with normal test results should lead to in vitro platelet aggregation studies.
- **Inherited disorders of platelet function** include receptor defects, aberrant signal transduction, cyclooxygenase defects, secretory (e.g., storage pool disease) defects, and adhesion or aggregation defects. In vitro platelet aggregation studies can identify patterns of agonist responses consistent with a particular defect such as the rare autosomal recessive disorders of Bernard-Soulier syndrome (defect of platelet glycoprotein Ib/IX/V [vWF receptor]) and Glanzmann thrombasthenia (defect of glycoprotein IIb/IIIa [fibrinogen receptor]).
- **Acquired platelet defects** occur much more commonly than do hereditary platelet qualitative disorders.
  - **Conditions associated with acquired qualitative defects** include myeloproliferative diseases, myelodysplasia, acute leukemia, monoclonal gammopathy, metabolic disorders (e.g., uremia, liver failure), and exposure to cardiopulmonary bypass trauma.
  - **Drug-induced platelet dysfunction** occurs as a side effect of many drugs that include high-dose penicillin, aspirin and other nonsteroidal anti-inflammatory drugs (NSAIDs), and alcohol. Other drug classes, such as β-lactam antibiotics, β-blockers, calcium channel blockers, nitrates, antihistamines, psychotropic drugs, tricyclic antidepressants, and selective serotonin reuptake inhibitors, cause platelet dysfunction in vitro but rarely cause bleeding.
    - **Aspirin** irreversibly inhibits cyclooxygenase (COX)-1 and COX-2. Its effects can last for 7 to 10 days from last consumption of the medication.
    - Since **other NSAIDs** reversibly inhibit COX-1 and COX-2, their effects are shorter than aspirin. COX-2 inhibitors have minimal effects on platelets at therapeutic doses.
    - **Thienopyridines** (e.g., clopidogrel, prasugrel, ticlopidine) inhibit platelet aggregation by irreversibly blocking platelet ADP receptor P_2Y_{12}.
    - **Dipyridamole**, alone or in combination with aspirin, inhibits platelet function by increasing intracellular cyclic adenosine monophosphate.
    - **Abciximab, eptifibatide, and tirofiban** block glycoprotein IIb/IIIa–dependent platelet aggregation during management of acute coronary syndrome.

TREATMENT

- Transfusion of platelets is reserved for major bleeding episodes.
- Treatment of uremic platelet dysfunction includes the following:
  - Dialysis to improve uremia.
  - Increase of hematocrit to ≥30% by transfusion or erythropoietin.
  - Desmopressin (diamino-8-D-arginine vasopressin [DDAVP], 0.3 µg/kg IV) to stimulate release of vWF from endothelial cells.
  - Conjugated estrogens (0.6 mg/kg IV daily for 5 days) may improve platelet function for up to 2 weeks.
  - Platelet transfusions in actively bleeding patients, though transfused platelets can rapidly acquire the uremic defect.
- **Withhold antiplatelet agents for 7 to 10 days before elective invasive procedures.**

INHERITED COAGULATION DISORDERS

Hemophilia A

GENERAL PRINCIPLES

- Hemophilia A is an X-linked recessive coagulation disorder due to mutations in the gene encoding factor VIII. It affects approximately 1 in 5,000 live male births.
- Approximately 20% to 30% of cases occur in patients without a family history of hemophilia, reflecting the high rate of spontaneous germ line mutations in the factor VIII gene.[23]
- Factor VIII activity determines bleeding risk: severe (factor VIII level <1%), moderate (1% to 5%), and mild (5% to 40%).

DIAGNOSIS

Clinical Presentation

- The typical presentation involves patients with a history of recurrent bleeding, prolonged aPTT and normal PT, and possibly a positive family history of bleeding on the maternal side. Nearly all patients are male. Age at diagnosis may differ based on the severity of the disease.
- Patients with mild or moderate hemophilia may present with hemorrhage only when challenged by trauma or invasive procedures (dental extractions, surgery).
- Severe hemophiliacs present with spontaneous joint, muscle, and gastrointestinal (GI) bleeding. Spontaneous hemarthroses are particularly characteristic. Recurrent hemarthroses can lead to hemophilic arthropathy. Intracranial hemorrhage occurs in a few very severely affected patients in the perinatal period.

Diagnostic Testing

- PT and platelet count are normal.
- aPTT is prolonged but may be within the reference range in some mild hemophilics.
- Factor VIII activities are diagnostic (severe hemophilia, <1%; moderate, 1% to 5%; and mild, 5% to 40%).

TREATMENT

- The severity of factor VIII deficiency and the type of hemorrhage or expected surgery/invasive procedures determine intensity of therapy.
- In patients with mild-to-moderate hemophilia A and a minor bleeding episode, **DDAVP** (0.3 µg/kg IV or 300 µg intranasally dosed every 12 hours) typically increases factor VIII activity three- to fivefold and has a half-life of 8 to 12 hours. Tachyphylaxis typically occurs after several doses.[24]
- Patients with mild-to-moderate hemophilia A and major bleeding episodes or those with severe hemophilia A with any hemorrhage require **factor VIII replacement**.
  - Many hemophiliacs infuse **factor VIII concentrates** at home when needed. **Recombinant factor VIII concentrates** have become the first choice of agent, particularly for children who are initiated on factor VIII.
  - Plasma factor VIII activity level increases approximately 2% for every 1 IU/kg of factor VIII concentrate infused. Factor VIII must be dosed q12 hours given its half-life of 8 to 12 hours. The duration and intensity of factor replacement depend on the type of surgery/procedure and the target factor VIII activity. Measure factor VIII activity pre- and postinfusion initially to establish the patient's response to infusion.

○ Factor VIII concentrates dosed to a goal peak plasma activity of 30% to 50% typically stop minor hemorrhages. Major traumas and surgery require maintenance of factor VIII peak activities at >80% for extended periods.

○ Patients who have been treated with factor VIII concentrates should be evaluated for factor VIII inhibitors before an elective surgery or invasive procedure is performed (see section below on Complications of Therapy for Hemophilia).

Hemophilia B

• Hemophilia B is an X-linked recessive bleeding disorder secondary to mutations in the gene encoding factor IX. Hemophilia B affects approximately 1 in 30,000 male births.

• Hemophilia B is **clinically indistinguishable from hemophilia A**, except for deficient factor IX, rather than factor VIII, activities.

• **DDAVP cannot increase factor IX levels and is ineffective for hemophilia B patients**.

• Postinfusion peak targets, duration of replacement, and monitoring for treatment of hemophilia B–related bleeding episodes are similar to those provided for hemophilia A, with two differences: Plasma factor IX activity increases approximately 1% for every 1 IU/kg factor IX concentrate infused, and factor IX has a longer half-life of 18 to 24 hours, allowing for q24-hour dosing.

Complications of Therapy for Hemophilia

• **Alloantibodies to factor VIII and factor IX (i.e., inhibitors)** are among the most severe complications in response to factor replacement and can develop in up to 30% and 5% of severe hemophilia A and B patients, respectively. These alloantibodies **neutralize infused factor VIII or factor IX** and render them ineffective in correcting coagulopathy.

• Determination of the titer of a factor VIII or factor IX inhibitor predicts inhibitor behavior and guides therapy.

• **Treatments** for hemophiliacs with inhibitors include inpatient management of acute bleeding and eradication of inhibitors.

von Willebrand Disease

GENERAL PRINCIPLES

• vWD is **the most common inherited bleeding disorder**.

• vWD results from an inherited **quantitative or qualitative defect of von Willebrand factor (vWF)**. Most forms of vWD have an autosomal dominant inheritance with variable penetrance, although autosomal recessive forms (types 2N and 3) exist (Table 12-5).

• vWF circulates as multimers of variable size that facilitate adherence of platelets to injured vessel walls and stabilize factor VIII in plasma.

• Classification recognizes three main types of vWD (Table 12-5):[25]

○ **Type 1 vWD**, a qualitative deficiency of vWF antigen (vWF:Ag) and activity, accounts for 70% to 80% of cases.

○ **Type 2 vWD includes four subtypes**: 2A, selective loss of large multimers; 2B, loss of large and medium multimers due to increased affinity of vWF for platelet glycoprotein Ib; 2M, decreased platelet adhesion without loss of large multimers; and 2N, decreased binding affinity of vWF for factor VIII.

○ **Type 3 vWD** represents a virtually complete deficiency of vWF.[26]

TABLE 12-5 Hemostasis Test Patterns in von Willebrand Disease

	Type I	Type 2A	Type 2B	Type 2M	Type 2N	Type 3
PFA-100 closure time	↑/nl	↑	↑	↑	nl	↑
aPTT	↑/nl	↑/nl	nl/↑	nl/↑	↑	↑
vWF antigen	↓	↓/nl	↓/nl	↓/nl	Normal	Absent
vWF activity	↓	↓↓	↓↓	↓↓	Normal	Absent
Factor VIII:C	↓/nl	↓/nl	↓/nl	↓/nl	↓	↓↓
RIPA	N/A	Reduced	Enhanced	Reduced	Normal	Absent
Multimetric pattern	Normal	Missing large multimers	Missing large multimers	Normal	Normal	None detected
Inheritance	Dominant	Dominant	Dominant	Dominant	Recessive	Recessive

aPTT, activated partial thromboplastin time; factor VIII:c, procoagulant activity of factor VIII; nl, normal; PFA, platelet function analysis; RIPA, ristocetin-induced platelet aggregation; vWF, von Willebrand factor.

DIAGNOSIS

Clinical Presentation

- The characteristic clinical findings consist of mucocutaneous bleeding (epistaxis, menorrhagia, and GI bleeding) and easy bruising.
- Trauma, surgery, or dental extractions may result in life-threatening bleeding in severely affected individuals.
- Patients with mild vWD phenotypes may remain undiagnosed into adulthood.

Diagnostic Testing

- If personal and family bleeding histories support a reasonable pretest likelihood of an inherited primary hemostasis or bleeding disorder, **screening for vWD should begin with measurement of vWF antigen and activity and factor VIII activity** (Table 12-5).
  - **vWF:Ag** tests measure plasma concentrations of vWF by immunoassay. A deficiency of vWF:Ag detects type 1 and 3 vWD; low or normal levels may occur with type 2 forms.
  - **vWF:RCo** measures agglutination of normal platelets in the presence of patient plasma and ristocetin cofactor (RCo), which enhances the binding of vWF to glycoprotein Ib. Types 1, 3, 2A, 2B, and 2M can all cause decreased platelet agglutination.
  - **Factor VIII activity** may be reduced due to a quantitative deficiency of vWF (types 1 and 3) or vWF mutations that reduce factor VIII binding to vWF (type 2N).
- Suspect a quantitative vWF defect (type 1) with low vWF:Ag and RCo activity and a RCo/vWF:Ag ratio of >0.7.
- Suspect type 2 vWD when RCo/vWF:Ag activity has a ratio of <0.7. vWF multimer analysis by gel electrophoresis assesses for the presence (type 2M) or absence (types 2A and 2B) of large vWF multimers, and a ristocetin-induced platelet aggregation test (the patient's plasma and the patient's platelets incubated with ristocetin) distinguishes types 2A and 2M (attenuated) from type 2B (exaggerated) platelet aggregation responses.
- Type 2N appears clinically identical to mild forms of hemophilia A, except that it is inherited in an autosomal recessive pattern, and the half-life of infused factor VIII concentrates is much shorter.

TREATMENT

- DDVAP:
  - ◦ Minor bleeding in type 1 vWD usually responds to DDAVP.
  - ◦ DDAVP can induce variable responses in individual patients. Therefore, test dose administration to confirm clinically acceptable increments of vWF:Ag, vWF:RCo, and factor VIII is needed for all patients.
  - ◦ vWF:RCo activities of >50% control most hemorrhages.
  - ◦ DDAVP with or without the oral antifibrinolytic drug **aminocaproic acid** is recommended for inpatient minor invasive procedures.
  - ◦ DDAVP does not effectively treat some type 2A, 2M, and 2N vWD and all type 3vWD patients. Because of the risk of postinfusion thrombocytopenia, DDAVP is contraindicated in type 2B vWD.
- vWF concentrates: Severe bleeding and major surgery in vWD patients require **infusion of vWF concentrates** typically for 5 to 10 days.

ACQUIRED COAGULATION DISORDERS

Vitamin K Deficiency

- Hepatocytes require vitamin K to complete the synthesis of clotting factors II, VII, IX, and X and the natural anticoagulants protein C and protein S.
- **Vitamin K deficiency is usually caused by malabsorption states or poor dietary intake combined with antibiotic-associated loss of intestinal bacterial colonization.** Vitamin K deficiency is suspected when an at-risk patient has a prolonged PT that corrects after a 1:1 mix with normal pooled plasma.
- Vitamin K replacement is most commonly given orally or intravenously. With adequate replacement, PT should begin to normalize within 12 hours.
- FFP rapidly but temporarily (4 to 6 hours) corrects acquired coagulopathies secondary to vitamin K deficiency. **FFP should only be transfused to patients with active moderate-to-severe bleeding or an impending invasive surgical procedure.** Vitamin K is a safer method to manage prolonged PT in patients with no or mild bleeding.

Coagulopathy Due to Anticoagulant Therapy

Supratherapeutic concentrations of anticoagulants may exacerbate bleeding risk. Management, including reversal, is discussed in Chapter 14.

Liver Disease

- Liver disease can seriously impair hemostasis because the liver produces most of the coagulation factors with the exception of vWF.
- Hemostatic abnormalities associated with liver disease typically remain stable unless the liver's synthetic function rapidly worsens or the patient is not eating normally.
- Hemostatic complications of liver disease are hyperfibrinolysis, thrombocytopenia due to splenic sequestration, DIC, spontaneous bacterial peritonitis, GI hemorrhage, and cholestasis (which impairs vitamin K absorption).
- **Transfusion support should be reserved only for cases of moderate-to-severe bleeding or an impending invasive procedure in the setting of additional laboratory abnormalities:**
  - ◦ FFP for severe coagulopathy (PT or aPTT >1.5 times control is often used as a cutoff but is **not** evidence based)

○ Cryoprecipitate, given at a dose of 1.5 units/10 kg body weight, for severe hypofibrino-genemia (<100 mg/dL)
○ Platelet transfusion for moderate-to-severe thrombocytopenia

Disseminated Intravascular Coagulation

- DIC occurs in a variety of systemic illnesses, including sepsis, trauma, burns, shock, obstetric complications, and malignancies (notably acute promyelocytic leukemia).
- Exposure of tissue factor to the circulation generates excess thrombin and results in activa-tion and consumption of coagulation factors (including fibrinogen), regulators (protein C, protein S, and antithrombin), and platelets; formation of generalized microthrombi; and reactive fibrinolysis.
- Consequences of DIC include bleeding, organ dysfunction secondary to microvascular thrombi and ischemia, and, less commonly, large arterial and venous thrombosis.[27]
- Although no one test confirms a diagnosis of DIC, affected patients commonly have **prolonged PT and aPTT, thrombocytopenia, low fibrinogen, and a positive D-dimer**.
- DIC treatment consists of supportive care, correction of the underlying disorder if pos-sible, and administration of FFP, cryoprecipitate, and platelets as needed for hypofibrino-genemia and thrombocytopenia.

Acquired Inhibitors of Coagulation Factors

- Acquired inhibitors of coagulation factors may arise de novo (**autoantibodies**) or may develop in hemophiliacs (**alloantibodies**) following factor VIII or IX infusions.
- **The most common acquired inhibitor is directed against factor VIII**. Acquired factor VIII inhibitors most commonly occur in patients over 50 years old, during pregnancy, or postpartum or associated with malignancy or autoimmune diseases.
- Patients with coagulation factor inhibitors present with an abrupt onset of bleeding, pro-longed aPTT that does not correct after 1:1 mixing, markedly decreased factor activities, and a positive inhibitor titer (Bethesda titer).
- Bleeding complications in patients with factor VIII inhibitors (autoantibodies) are man-aged in the same manner as for hemophiliacs with alloantibodies to factor VIII (see above Inherited Bleeding Disorders section).
- Eradication of inhibitors consists of immunosuppression with cyclophosphamide, pred-nisone, rituximab, or vincristine.[28]

REFERENCES

1. Lippi G, Favaloro EJ, Franchini M, et al. Milestones and perspectives in coagulation and hemostasis. *Semin Thromb Hemost* 2009;35:9–22.
2. Gewirtz AS, Miller ML, Keys TF. The clinical usefulness of the preoperative bleeding time. *Arch Pathol Lab Med* 1996;120:353–356.
3. Kirkwood TB. Calibration of reference thromboplastins and standardisation of the pro-thrombin time ratio. *Thromb Haemost* 1983;49:238–244.
4. Cines DB, Bussel JB, Liebman HA, et al. The ITP syndrome: pathogenic and clinical diversity. *Blood* 2009;113:6511–6521.
5. Davoren A, Bussel J, Curtis BR, et al. Prospective evaluation of a new platelet glycopro-tein (GP)-specific assay (PakAuto) in the diagnosis of autoimmune thrombocytopenia (AITP). *Am J Hematol* 2005;78:193–197.
6. George JN, Woolf SH, Raskob GE, et al. Idiopathic thrombocytopenic purpura: a prac-tice guideline developed by explicit methods for the American Society of Hematology. *Blood* 1996;88:3–40.

7. Stasi R, Pagano A, Stipa E, et al. Rituximab chimeric anti-CD20 monoclonal antibody treatment for adults with chronic idiopathic thrombocytopenic purpura. *Blood* 2001;98:952–957.

8. Nurden AT, Viallard JF, Nurden P. New-generation drugs that stimulate platelet production in chronic immune thrombocytopenic purpura. *Lancet* 2009;373: 1562–1569.

9. Aster RH, Bougie DW. Drug-induced immune thrombocytopenia. *N Engl J Med* 2007;357:580–587.

10. Li X, Hunt L, Vesely SK. Drug-induced thrombocytopenia: an updated systematic review. *Ann Intern Med* 2005;142:474–475.

11. Furlan M, Robles R, Galbusera M, et al. von Willebrand factor-cleaving protease in thrombotic thrombocytopenic purpura and the hemolytic-uremic syndrome. *N Engl J Med* 1998;339:1578–1584.

12. Terrell DR, Williams LA, Vesely SK, et al. The incidence of thrombotic thrombocytopenic purpura-hemolytic uremic syndrome: all patients, idiopathic patients, and patients with severe ADAMTS-13 deficiency. *J Thromb Haemost* 2005;3:1432–1436.

13. Zheng X, Pallera AM, Goodnough LT, et al. Remission of chronic thrombotic thrombocytopenic purpura after treatment with cyclophosphamide and rituximab. *Ann Intern Med* 2003;138:105–108.

14. Bresin E, Gastoldi S, Daina E, et al. Rituximab as pre-emptive treatment in patients with thrombotic thrombocytopenic purpura and evidence of anti-ADAMTS13 autoantibodies. *Thromb Haemost* 2009;101:233–238.

15. Ferrara F, Annunziata M, Pollio F, et al. Vincristine as treatment for recurrent episodes of thrombotic thrombocytopenic purpura. *Ann Hematol* 2002;81:7–10.

16. George JN. How I treat patients with thrombotic thrombocytopenic purpura: 2010. *Blood* 2010;116:4060–4069.

17. Atkinson JP, Goodship TH. Complement factor H and the hemolytic uremic syndrome. *J Exp Med* 2007;204:1245–1248.

18. Tarr PI. Shiga toxin-associated hemolytic uremic syndrome and thrombotic thrombocytopenic purpura: distinct mechanisms of pathogenesis. *Kidney Int Suppl* 2009;112:S29–S32.

19. Cuker A, Cines DB. How I treat heparin-induced thrombocytopenia. *Blood* 2012;119:2209–2218.

20. Linkins LA, Dans AL, Moores LK, et al. American College of Chest Physicians. Treatment and prevention of heparin-induced thrombocytopenia: American College of Chest Physicians Evidence-Based Clinical Practice Guidelines (9th Edition). *Chest* 2012;141:495S–530S.

21. Lo GK, Juhl D, Warkentin TE, et al. Evaluation of pretest clinical score (4 T's) for the diagnosis of heparin-induced thrombocytopenia in two clinical settings. *J Thromb Haemost* 2006;4:759–765.

22. Cuker A, Gimotty PA, Crowther MA, et al. Predictive value of the 4Ts scoring system for heparin-induced thrombocytopenia: a systemic review and meta-analysis. *Blood* 2012;120:4160–4167.

23. Mannucci PM, Tuddenham EG. The hemophilias—from royal genes to gene therapy. *N Engl J Med* 2001;344:1773–1779.

24. Mannucci PM. Desmopressin (DDAVP) in the treatment of bleeding disorders: the first 20 years. *Blood* 1997;90:2515–2521.

25. Sadler JE, Budde U, Eikenboom JC, et al. Working Party on von Willebrand Disease Classification. Update on the pathophysiology and classification of von Willebrand disease: a report of the Subcommittee on von Willebrand Factor. *J Thromb Haemost* 2006;4:2103–1214.

26. Rodeghiero F, Castaman G, Tosetto A. How I treat von Willebrand disease. *Blood* 2009;114:1158–1165.
27. Levi M, Ten Cate H. Disseminated intravascular coagulation. *N Engl J Med* 1999;341:586–592.
28. Wiestner A, Cho HJ, Asch AS, et al. Rituximab in the treatment of acquired factor VIII inhibitors. *Blood* 2002;100:3426–3428.

13

Hematologic Diseases
Thomas Regenbogen and Morey A. Blinder

The internist often evaluates and manages hematologic disorders independently or in concert with a hematologist. This chapter seeks to guide the outpatient physician in the evaluation and management of common conditions. Disorders of coagulation and thrombocytopenia are covered in Chapter 12.

ANEMIA

GENERAL PRINCIPLES

- Anemia always reflects an underlying primary disease. An attempt should be made to diagnose the cause in every case.
- Anemia is defined as a decrease in circulating red blood cell mass: hemoglobin (Hgb) <12 g/dL or hematocrit (Hct) <36% in women and Hgb <14 g/dL or Hct <41% in men.
- Anemia may be classified into three etiologic groups: **blood loss (acute or chronic), decreased red cell production, and increased red cell destruction**.
- The morphologic classification has diagnostic utility for many presentations. The mean cellular volume (MCV) is used to classify anemia as **microcytic (<80 fL), normocytic (80 to 100 fL), and macrocytic (>100 fL)**.

DIAGNOSIS

Clinical Presentation

- Patients may be asymptomatic or have only minor complaints, especially with longer chronicity and slower decline in Hgb. Clinical findings will be present in most individuals at Hgb <7.0 g/dL.
- Symptoms and signs are generally due to tissue hypoxia. These include fatigue, pallor, dizziness, headaches, poor concentration, and weakness. Tachycardia and dyspnea on exertion are seen in severe anemia. High-output heart failure and shock may develop in the most severe cases.
- The history and physical examination in conjunction with basic laboratory data will either be diagnostic or narrow the differential diagnosis dramatically. As such, it is critical to address the following as part of the initial evaluation:
  - Gastrointestinal (GI) hemorrhage
  - Obstetric and menstrual history
  - Evidence of hemolysis or predisposition to hemolysis
  - Comorbidities such as gastrointestinal disease or resection, malabsorption, renal disease, rheumatologic disease, etc.
  - Comorbidities that may be exacerbated by anemia, such as cardiovascular disease
  - Personal or family history of anemia and prior treatments
  - Prescribed and over-the-counter medications, alcohol consumption, diet, ethnic background, and religious beliefs pertaining to blood transfusion
  - Clinical evidence of other cytopenias (e.g., infections or easy bruising)

Diagnostic Testing

- The evaluation should begin with a **complete blood count (CBC)** including red cell indices and **reticulocyte count**. Findings in the H&P help guide further evaluation. If iron deficiency is suspected, obtain an iron panel and ferritin level. If hemolysis is suspected, obtain a hepatic function panel, urinalysis, haptoglobin, and peripheral smear. Obtain serum vitamin B_{12} and serum folate levels with macrocytosis.
- The **relative reticulocyte count** measures the percentage of immature red cells in the blood. The absolute reticulocyte count (relative reticulocyte count multiplied by the red cell count) may be reported by some labs. The normal range for absolute reticulocyte count is 50,000 to 75,000 per µL.
  - The **reticulocyte index (RI)** = relative reticulocyte count × (patient Hct/normal Hct). RI is an indication of whether the bone marrow (BM) is responding appropriately based on the degree of anemia.
  - Individuals with normal erythrocyte proliferation will have an **RI >3%** to compensate for bleeding or hemolysis; however, an **RI <3%** with anemia indicates decreased production of erythrocytes (hypoproliferative anemia).
- A **BM biopsy** may be indicated in cases of normocytic anemia with a low reticulocyte count (e.g., to confirm iron deficiency in the setting of chronic disease states). It is also typically indicated in the evaluation of pancytopenia.

MICROCYTIC ANEMIA

Iron Deficiency Anemia

GENERAL PRINCIPLES

- **Iron deficiency** is the most common cause of anemia in the ambulatory setting.[1]
- GI bleeding is the most common etiology of iron deficiency in men and postmenopausal women in the developed world.
- Menstrual blood loss and pregnancy are common etiologies in premenopausal women; however, the clinician should not overlook GI bleeding in premenopausal women.
- The differential diagnosis of microcytic anemia includes iron deficiency, thalassemia, anemia of chronic inflammation (occasionally microcytic), sideroblastic, and occasionally myelodysplastic syndrome (MDS).
- Functional iron deficiency refers to adequate iron stores but inadequate mobilization for erythropoiesis, as is seen in patients with end-stage renal disease.

DIAGNOSIS

Clinical Presentation

History
- A careful history of both physiologic and abnormal hemorrhage must be obtained.
- Pica is an abnormal change in dietary habits (e.g., eating ice, clay, or starch) and is associated with iron deficiency anemia.
- Diseases of the stomach and proximal small intestine (e.g., *Helicobacter pylori* infection, achlorhydria, celiac disease, and bariatric surgery) often lead to impaired iron absorption.

Physical Examination
- The physical exam may be unremarkable as the classic signs are typically present only in severe iron deficiency.
- A digital rectal exam should be performed to examine for a mass and to test for occult blood.

Diagnostic Testing

- The MCV correlates with the degree of anemia; therefore, early mild iron deficiency may present as a normal or only slightly decreased MCV.
- Serum iron (SI) concentration is typically low, while total iron-binding capacity (TIBC) is typically elevated but can be low/normal with comorbid liver disease or inflammatory states. Transferrin increases linearly to approximately 400 mg/dL once patients are in negative iron balance, so that transferrin saturation (SI/TIBC) falls below 16% only when iron stores are exhausted. Pregnancy and oral contraceptive pills (OCP) use increase serum transferrin. Serum iron and TIBC have poor sensitivity and specificity for iron deficiency anemia.
- **Ferritin** is the primary storage form for iron in the reticuloendothelium and is the most accurate noninvasive marker of iron stores.
  - A ferritin level of <10 ng/mL in women or 20 ng/mL in men is a specific marker of low iron stores.
  - Ferritin is an acute-phase reactant, so normal levels may be seen in inflammatory states despite low iron stores. **A serum ferritin of >200 ng/mL generally excludes an iron deficiency.** However, in renal dialysis patients, a functional iron deficiency may be seen with a ferritin level of 500 to 1,200 ng/mL.[2]
- If the diagnosis of iron deficiency remains uncertain in the setting of normal renal function, a trial of oral iron repletion with repeat monitoring of Hgb/Hct 2 to 4 weeks after initiation is a reasonable diagnostic approach.
- A **BM aspiration** with special staining for iron is the definitive test for establishing iron deficiency but is rarely required due to improved serologic testing.

TREATMENT

- Evaluate and treat the underlying cause while treating the iron deficiency, if possible.
- If the anemia is severe (Hgb <7 g/dL) or if the patient is symptomatic with Hgb <10 g/dL, consider admission for transfusion and monitoring and to expedite evaluation if it is a new finding.[3]
- The majority of ambulatory patients may be treated with oral iron preparations (Table 13-1). We recommend **ferrous sulfate**, 325 mg PO, three times/day, 1 hour before meals and 2 hours from antacids. Each pill contains approximately 65 mg of elemental iron, of which 5 to 20 mg (about 10% to 30%) may be absorbed depending on patient-specific factors such as degree of anemia.
- In elderly adults, lower doses may be tolerated better yet equally effective over several months. Consider using 5- to 10-mL **iron sulfate elixir** in a quarter glass of orange juice before breakfast. Dental staining is a common adverse effect and may be avoided by using a straw.[4]
- Iron is best absorbed in the duodenum and proximal jejunum; therefore, delayed-release formulations will result in suboptimal absorption. Dosing with meals will also decrease absorption. A mildly acidic medium enhances absorption; thus, 250 mg of ascorbic acid may be given with the supplement.
- Common adverse effects are constipation, abdominal discomfort, or diarrhea. This is managed by decreasing frequency to BID, taking with meals, adding stool softeners, or reducing the elemental iron dose to <40 mg. A longer duration of therapy may be necessary.
- Serum ferritin should be monitored every 2 months during therapy, and normalization indicates repletion of iron stores. The Hgb/Hct typically increases after 1 to 2 weeks of therapy, but is variable depending on the cause of anemia and tolerability of treatment.
- If the underlying cause has resolved, therapy is discontinued once iron stores are replete. However, some patients will require long-term iron replacement.

TABLE 13-1   Pharmacologic Iron Supplementation

Generic name	Brand name[a]	Route	Common formulation[b]	Elemental iron[c]	Typical dose and schedule[d,e]	Generic (United States)	Notes
Ferrous sulfate	Feosol	PO	325 mg	65 mg	1 tab tid	Y	Start with qd dosing to improve tolerability.
	Feosol Elixir	PO	220 mg/5 mL	44 mg/5 mL	15 mL qd to bid	Y	1 tablespoon = 15 mL
Ferrous gluconate	Ferate	PO	325 mg	36 mg	1 tab tid	Y	
Ferrous fumarate	Ferrocite	PO	324 mg	106 mg	1 tab bid to tid	Y	
Polysaccharide-iron complex	Ferrex 150 / ProFe	PO	150 mg / 180 mg	150 mg / 180 mg	1 tab bid / 1 tab qd to bid	Y / Y	
Iron dextran	INFeD	IV/IM	2 mL	50 mg/mL	1,000 mg	N	Low molecular weight form (INFeD) is assoc. with fewer adverse events. Test dose required
Ferric gluconate	Ferrlecit	IV	5 mL	12.5 mg/mL	125 mg	Y	Newer preparations likely have a lower risk of anaphylactic reaction; however, a test dose is recommended in those with prior hypersensitivity to iron dextran or other medications.
Iron sucrose	Venofer	IV	2.5, 5, 10 mL	20 mg/mL	200–400 mg	N	
Ferumoxytol	Feraheme	IV	17 mL	30 mg/mL	517 mg	N	

[a]Brands are listed for reference but are not comprehensive; consult your local pharmacy or formulary for available brands and cost.
[b]Several dosage strengths may be available. For parenteral preparations, the common unit vial volume is shown.
[c]Always confirm elemental iron content when prescribing iron supplementation. Enteral absorption is typically 10%–30% of elemental iron.
[d]Dose iron based on the content of elemental iron. Typical enteral repletion dose is 150–300 mg elemental iron per day.
[e]Parenteral iron dosage should be calculated based on estimated iron deficiency, common single doses shown. See package insert for administration instructions.

- Occasionally, **intravenous iron** preparations may be required in the setting of bowel inflammation, rapid gastrointestinal transit, or malabsorption. In select severe cases, medication noncompliance is an indication for intravenous repletion. Treatment of anemia in the setting of CKD is discussed in Chapter 24.
- **Iron dextran** is commonly used, but newer formulations are available (Table 13-1):
  - The iron deficit may be calculated with a readily available formula; however, the typical requirement is 1,000 to 3,000 mg of elemental iron to replenish stores in the adult.
  - IV iron dextran therapy (INFeD, Dexferrum) can be complicated by serious side effects including **anaphylaxis**; therefore, an IV **test dose** of 25 mg in 50 mL of normal saline should be administered over 5 to 10 minutes. Methylprednisolone, diphenhydramine, and 1:1,000 epinephrine 1-mg ampule (for subcutaneous administration) should be immediately available at all times during the infusion.
  - Delayed reactions to IV iron, such as arthralgia, myalgia, fever, pruritus, and lymphadenopathy may be seen within 3 days of therapy and usually resolve spontaneously or with nonsteroidal anti-inflammatory drugs. Newer parenteral formulations are associated with fewer anaphylactic reactions; however, many clinicians recommend test doses, especially if the patient has had a reaction to dextran or has other drug allergies.[5]

REFERRAL

A referral to a hematologist is generally not required for treatment of iron deficiency unless the diagnosis is uncertain or there are complicating factors to standard treatment.

Thalassemia

GENERAL PRINCIPLES

- The **thalassemia syndromes** are autosomal recessive disorders characterized by reduced Hgb synthesis associated with mutations in the α- or β-chain of the molecule. They are among the most common genetic abnormalities.[6]
- **Beta-thalassemia** results in a decreased production of β-globin and an excess of α-globin, forming insoluble alpha tetramers, which are toxic to the cell.
- **Alpha-thalassemia** is due to deletion of one or more of the four α-globin genes leading to a β-globin gene excess, which is relatively less toxic.
- It is important to differentiate iron deficiency anemia from thalassemia.

Classification

- Beta-thalassemia:
  - **Thalassemia minor (trait)** occurs with one gene abnormality with variable amounts of β-chain underproduction. Patients are asymptomatic and present with microcytic, hypochromic erythrocytes and Hgb levels typically >10 g/dL.
  - **Thalassemia intermedia** occurs with dysfunction in both β-globin genes, characterized by a later clinical onset and milder anemia, which can require transfusions.
  - **Thalassemia major** (Cooley anemia) is caused by severe abnormalities of both genes and requires lifelong transfusion support unless the patient underwent successful stem cell transplantation in childhood.
- Alpha-thalassemia:
  - **Alpha-thalassemia minima** occurs with the deletion of one of four α-globin genes. Patients are not anemic and typically have normal MCV and Hgb electrophoresis.
  - **Alpha-thalassemia minor** clinically resembles beta-thalassemia minor; however, the Hgb electrophoresis pattern is normal.

○ **Hemoglobin H disease** is evident at birth and is characterized by moderate anemia predominantly due to chronic hemolysis, microcytosis, and 5% to 30% hemoglobin H. Oxidant drugs similar to those that exacerbate glucose-6-phosphate dehydrogenase deficiency should be avoided as they may increase hemolysis.

DIAGNOSIS

Clinical Presentation

History

• Mild thalassemia patients are typically asymptomatic and not transfusion dependent.
• Patients report a family or personal history of microcytic anemia not responsive to iron therapy.
• Patients with severe forms of thalassemia such as Cooley's anemia, many with thalassemia intermedia, and some with hemoglobin H may develop complications of chronic iron overload (e.g., cardiac, hepatic, or endocrine dysfunction).

Physical Examination

• Signs of hemolysis, including jaundice, hepatosplenomegaly, and leg ulcers, should be noted.
• Examine for signs of extramedullary hematopoiesis, (e.g., splenomegaly, mandibular enlargement, and other skeletal deformities).

Diagnostic Testing

• Typically thalassemia trait results in an MCV <75 fL but Hct >30%.
• Iron studies including serum ferritin level are obtained to initially evaluate microcytosis as well as periodically check for iron overload in patients with moderate-to-severe disease.
• Hemoglobin analysis by electrophoresis or high-pressure liquid chromatography establishes the diagnosis and severity of beta-thalassemia. Analysis will be normal in α-thalassemia because α chains are equally distributed among Hgb A, A2, and F.
  ○ Normally, Hgb A accounts for 96.5% to 98.5% of hemoglobin, Hgb A2 1.5% to 3.5%, and Hgb F <1.0%.
  ○ In β-thalassemia trait, Hgb A2 and F are increased. Low Hgb A fractions and elevated Hgb F are found in severe disease.
  ○ If α-thalassemia is suspected, α-globin gene deletion testing is confirmatory in the majority of cases.
  ○ Analysis may also reveal abnormal hemoglobin types, such as S, C, or M.
  ○ Ideally, the patient will not have had a blood transfusion in the 3 months before the test. Iron deficiency can falsely lower the Hgb A2 level.

TREATMENT

• Thalassemia trait requires no specific treatment. In patients with severe forms of the disease, red blood cell transfusions to maintain Hgb at 9 to 10 g/dL are needed to prevent the skeletal deformities that result from accelerated erythropoiesis.
• Transfusion-dependent anemia often results in iron overload. Chelation therapy with deferasirox 20 to 30 mg/kg PO daily is indicated to prevent hepatic, cardiac, and endocrine damage.[7] Chelation therapy should be continued with a target ferritin <1,000 mcg/L. Adverse effects of deferasirox include mild-to-moderate GI disturbances and skin rash.

Surgical Management

Splenectomy is indicated when there is a marked increase in transfusion requirements over the course of several months to a year. The benefit is typically transient, and splenectomy confers a higher risk of arterial and venous thrombosis as well as sepsis.

REFERRAL

Patients transitioning from pediatric care to adult care with moderate-to-severe forms of thalassemia should be referred to a hematologist.

PATIENT EDUCATION

- Educate patients that their condition may commonly be mistaken for iron deficiency and to avoid iron replacement therapy, unless the treating physician is aware they also have thalassemia.
- Patients should be offered genetic counseling.
- Patients may be directed to the Cooley's Anemia Foundation website, http:\\www.thalassemia.org (last accessed December 22, 2014).

MACROCYTIC ANEMIA

GENERAL PRINCIPLES

- May be an isolated abnormality or may accompany other cytopenias.
- The etiology can be determined in almost all cases with a thorough investigation.
- Elderly patients with vitamin B_{12} deficiency may present with subtle symptoms and a mild normocytic anemia.
- By definition, the MCV is >100 fL.
- An elevated MCV may be classified as megaloblastic, nonmegaloblastic, or false positive.
- Megaloblastic anemia is a term used to describe disorders of impaired DNA synthesis in hematopoietic cells that affect all proliferating cells.

Etiology

Megaloblastic

- **Folate deficiency** arises from a negative folate balance due to malnutrition, malabsorption, or increased requirement secondary to pregnancy or hemolytic anemia.
- Patients on long-term diets, alcoholics, elderly, and psychiatric patients are particularly at risk for nutritional folate deficiency.
- **Pregnancy and lactation** require higher (three- to fourfold) daily folate needs and are commonly associated with megaloblastic changes in maternal hematopoietic cells, leading to a dimorphic (combined folate and iron deficiency) anemia.
- Folate malabsorption may occur in celiac disease.
- **Drugs** that can interfere with folate absorption include ethanol, trimethoprim, pyrimethamine, diphenylhydantoin, barbiturates, and sulfasalazine.
- Patients who are undergoing dialysis require increased folate intake because of folate losses.
- Patients with hemolytic anemia, particularly sickle cell anemia, require increased folate for accelerated erythropoiesis and can present with aplastic crisis (rapidly falling erythrocyte counts) with folate deficiency.
- **Vitamin B_{12} deficiency** occurs insidiously over ≥3 years, due the relatively small daily B_{12} requirement (1 to 3 mcg) compared with larger total body stores (1 to 3 mg).
- In nonvegan adults, vitamin B_{12} deficiency is almost always due to malabsorption.[8]

- Causes of vitamin B_{12} deficiency include partial gastrectomy (up to 20% of patients within 8 years of surgery) or total gastrectomy and pernicious anemia (PA). Older patients with gastric atrophy may develop a vitamin B_{12} deficiency due to impaired absorption.
- PA occurs in individuals who are >40 years (mean age of onset is 60 years). Up to 30% of patients have a positive family history. PA is associated with other autoimmune disorders (Graves disease [30%], Hashimoto thyroiditis [11%], and Addison disease [5% to 10%]). Of patients with PA, 90% have antiparietal cell IgG antibodies and 60% have anti-intrinsic factor antibodies.
- Neurologic complications may occur even in the absence of anemia and may not fully resolve despite adequate treatment.

Nonmegaloblastic
- Reticulocytosis in response to peripheral red blood cell destruction or loss causes nonmegaloblastic macrocytic anemia given that reticulocytes are larger than mature red cells.
- Ethanol, medications (antiretrovirals, anticonvulsants, antifolates, chemotherapeutics, metformin, and cholestyramine), myelodysplasia, hypothyroidism, liver disease, hemolysis, hemorrhage, chronic obstructive pulmonary disease (COPD), and splenectomy account for most nonmegaloblastic macrocytosis.
- Cold agglutination, severe hyperglycemia, and marked leukocytosis may spuriously elevate the MCV.

DIAGNOSIS

Clinical Presentation
History
- Obtaining a targeted history to identify the abovementioned risk factors and causative agents is critical.
- Anemia may be the only overt sign of ethanol abuse and should prompt screening with a validated questionnaire.
- Folate-deficient patients present with sleep deprivation, fatigue, and manifestations of depression, irritability, or forgetfulness.
- When anemia due to vitamin B_{12} deficiency is clinically present, neurologic manifestations including peripheral neuropathy, paresthesias, lethargy, hypotonia, and seizures are also likely.

Physical Examination
- Physical examination may reveal poor nutrition, pigmentation of skin creases and nail beds, or glossitis.
- Jaundice or splenomegaly may indicate ineffective and extramedullary hematopoiesis.
- Vitamin B_{12} deficiency may cause decreased vibratory and positional sense, ataxia, paresthesias, confusion, and dementia.

Diagnostic Testing
- The initial workup includes CBC, reticulocyte index, peripheral smear, and vitamin B_{12} level.
- MCV >110 fL is more specific for megaloblastic anemia, but may be found in MDS as it reflects disordered hematopoiesis.
- The peripheral smear may show megaloblastic changes such as anisocytosis, poikilocytosis, and macroovalocytes; hypersegmented neutrophils (containing ≥ 5 nuclear lobes) are common. Dimorphic red cells indicate combined microcytic and macrocytic processes.
- If the peripheral smear is normal, consider adding thyroid and hepatic function panels to the initial laboratory work up.

- If the reticulocyte index is elevated, investigate for hemolysis.
- If the reticulocyte index is not elevated and
  - The vitamin B_{12} level is <100 pg/mL, there is vitamin B_{12} deficiency.
  - The vitamin B_{12} level is between 100 and 400 pg/mL, order serum methylmalonic acid (MMA) and homocysteine levels.
    - If the MMA is elevated, vitamin B_{12} deficiency is present.
    - If the MMA level is normal but homocysteine is elevated, folate deficiency is present.[9]
  - The vitamin B_{12} level is >400 pg/mL, check serum folate concentration. If folate is low, folate deficiency is present.
- BM biopsy may be necessary in the case of normal MMA, homocysteine, and folate levels to rule out an MDS.

TREATMENT

- Potassium monitoring and supplementation may be necessary when treatment is initiated to avoid complications of hypokalemia induced by enhanced hematopoiesis.
- Reticulocytosis should begin within 1 week of therapy, followed by a rising Hgb over 6 to 8 weeks.
- In one-third of patients, coexisting iron deficiency is present at diagnosis or develops during therapy and is a common cause for an incomplete response to repletion.[10]
- Folic acid, 1 mg PO daily, is given until the deficiency is corrected. High doses of folic acid (up to 5 mg PO daily) may be needed in patients with malabsorption syndromes.
- Vitamin B_{12} deficiency is corrected by administering **cyanocobalamin**. High-dose enteral replacement may be considered in highly motivated patients; however, the risk of relapse is higher than with parenteral therapy if treatment is discontinued prematurely.[11]
  - IM replacement is given daily for 1 week, then 1 mg/week for 4 weeks and then 1 mg/month for life. Monthly IM administration is approximately as cost-effective as enteral replacement.
  - Oral tablets or syrup, 50 to 1,000 mcg/day, may be given for maintenance indefinitely depending on the underlying cause.
  - Cyanocobalamin nasal spray (i.e., Nascobal) is approved for patients who have been repleted with intramuscular injections and have no nervous system involvement. It may be suitable for maintenance in those with malabsorption.
- Monitoring of red cell indices may confirm the diagnosis of vitamin B_{12} deficiency if there is a complete response.

MYELODYSPLASTIC SYNDROME

GENERAL PRINCIPLES

- **Myelodysplastic syndrome (MDS)** is a heterogeneous group of acquired, clonal disorders characterized by disordered hematopoiesis and potential transformation to acute myelogenous leukemia (AML) or pancytopenia.
- The natural history is variable, and mortality secondary to bone marrow failure is higher than with AML.[12]
- MDS should be strongly considered in the differential diagnosis of anemia in the elderly.

Classification

- There are several classifications; however, the most commonly used is the WHO, which lists the following subgroups based on cytopenia, percentage of bone marrow blasts, and cytogenetics:
  - Refractory anemia
  - Refractory anemia with ringed sideroblasts

○ Refractory anemia with excess blasts
○ 5q– syndrome
○ Chronic myelomonocytic leukemia[13]
• The International Prognostic Scoring System (IPSS) and its revision (IPSS-R) are most commonly used to stratify patients based on survival and risk of transformation to AML.[14]

Epidemiology

• The incidence of MDS increases from approximately 1:100,000 persons between 45 and 49 years old to 49.7 cases per 100,000 persons over the age of 85.[15] The vast majority of cases occur in individuals over the age of 60.
• Approximately 10% of anemia cases in the elderly are proven to be MDS, and it is the suspected diagnosis in as many as 16%.[16]

Risk Factors

• Most cases of MDS are idiopathic.
• Risk factors include some congenital diseases, ionizing radiation, prior chemotherapy, and exposure to benzene, which is commonly found in cigarette smoke.[15]

DIAGNOSIS

Clinical Presentation

• MDS may be asymptomatic and detected on laboratory analysis. Fatigue, easy bruising, or recurrent infections are common presenting complaints. Obtain a history of blood product transfusions and episodes of bleeding.
• Examining the skin may yield signs of thrombocytopenia and infection. Dermatosis (Sweet syndrome) or chloromas (dermal extramedullary leukemic cell accumulations) should prompt timely referral as they may signal malignant transformation.
• Scleral icterus may indicate hemolysis.

Diagnostic Testing

Laboratories
• CBC with reticulocyte count and peripheral smear. Anemia is usually present, and the MCV is typically elevated but may be normal or even low. The reticulocyte count is inappropriately low. Some patients present with leukopenia or thrombocytopenia or both. Rarely, thrombocytosis is present, and the hematologist may test for a JAK2 mutation. The peripheral smear may reveal dysplastic neutrophils, macrocytic erythrocytes, evidence of dysfunctional erythropoiesis, and normal platelets. The CBC may be initially repeated monthly to evaluate the progression of disease and less frequently thereafter.
• HIV serology, vitamin B_{12} profiles, serum folate, copper, ferritin, and iron studies are part of the routine initial evaluation of all patients. The hematologist may request HLA typing if the patient has had many transfusions or is a candidate for stem cell transplant.

Diagnostic Procedures
BM biopsy and aspirate are performed by the hematologist to diagnose and classify MDS.

TREATMENT

• **Supportive treatment**:
○ Scheduled or unscheduled transfusions of red blood cells or platelets.
○ Vaccinate for pneumococcal pneumonia, *Haemophilus influenzae* serotype b, seasonal influenza, and pertussis.
○ Providers should have an elevated index of suspicion for infections and pursue early treatment.

- **Chemotherapeutics**:
  - Treatment options include DNA hypomethylating agents (i.e., azacitidine), immuno-suppressants, and lenalidomide. Lenalidomide is approved for 5q– syndrome and has about a 50% chance of inducing transfusion independence.[17] The hematologist may also use granulocyte colony–stimulating factors. Younger patients with otherwise good health may benefit from higher-intensity regimens including stem cell transplant.
  - Referral to an academic center for clinical trial enrollment is encouraged, especially in those with refractory or recurrent disease.
- **Hematopoietic stem cell transplantation**:
  - This is the only treatment capable of cure and requires careful discussion between the patient, primary care physician, and hematologist. Comorbidities, goals of care, support structure, age of the patient, and the high morbidity and mortality of the procedure play important roles in this discussion.
  - Early referral to a tertiary center with a stem cell transplant program is ideal because the preliminary evaluation for transplant can be time consuming.
- **Treatment of the elderly**:
  - This group often has many comorbidities and poor prognostic indicators and may not be candidates for intensive therapy.
  - Trials of dose-reduced oral agents have found improved outcomes with a favorable toxicity profile in this demographic.[18]

REFERRAL

Referral to a hematologist once the diagnosis is suspected is recommended for definitive diagnosis, risk stratification, and treatment. If there are intermediate- or high-risk features, early referral for hematopoietic stem cell transplantation evaluation is appropriate.

PATIENT EDUCATION

Patients may be directed to the MDS Foundation, http:\\www.MDS-Foundation.org (last accessed December 22, 2014).

NORMOCYTIC ANEMIA

The causes of normocytic anemia include acute blood loss; malignancy (Chapter 35); BM infiltration; anemia of chronic disease (ACD), rheumatologic conditions, and chronic infection; and anemia of chronic renal insufficiency (Chapter 24).

Anemia of Chronic Disease

GENERAL PRINCIPLES

- Develops in patients with chronic inflammation due to malignancy, autoimmune disorders, and chronic infection.
- The etiology is multifactorial: defective iron mobilization due to increased levels of hepcidin, inflammatory cytokine-mediated suppression of erythropoiesis, and impaired endogenous erythropoietin (EPO) production.[19]
- Iron may inadequately mobilize in times of brisk of hematopoiesis in response to exogenous EPO.
- Anemia is thought to be a marker of the severity of the provocative disease.

DIAGNOSIS

- Measurement of serum hepcidin may become a diagnostic tool; however, this test is not yet widely available.[20]
- Mild-to-moderate normocytic, normochromic anemia is typical in ACD, but may be severe (Hgb <8 g/dL).
- Iron studies may reveal a low serum iron and low TIBC.
- Ferritin level <30 ng/dL indicates coexisting iron deficiency. If the ferritin is indeterminate, measuring soluble transferrin receptor (sTfR) can aid in identifying iron deficiency in the setting of ACD.

TREATMENT

- Treatment of the underlying disease process will improve ACD.
- Assess for iron deficiency and treat with intravenous iron. IV iron is preferred to enteral iron in ACD because of the poor enteral absorption during inflammatory states. Note that IV iron should not be given if active infection is suspected.
- Consider using an erythropoietin-stimulating agent (ESA) if the above strategies do not improve the anemia. Hgb should not be treated to levels >12 g/dL with ESA therapy due to the risk of cardiovascular events.[21]
- If there is a suboptimal (<1 g/dL) increase in hemoglobin 2 weeks after administration of ESA, reevaluate iron stores.
- Transfusion guidelines are patient specific:
  - Asymptomatic patients with Hgb <7 g/dL
  - Stable coronary artery disease with Hgb <8 g/dL
  - Symptomatic patients with Hgb <10 g/dL[3]

Aplastic Anemia

Aplastic anemia (AA) is an acquired immune-mediated disorder of hematopoietic stem cells, presenting in people of all ages as pancytopenia. Most cases are idiopathic in adults. AA must be differentiated from B_{12} deficiency, MDS, or other BM failure syndromes. Initial therapy is supportive, with early referral to a tertiary care center for immunosuppressive therapy and/or stem cell transplantation. Transfusions should be minimized and, when administered, should be leukodepleted and from nonfamily members. Patients with a history of AA are at an increased lifetime risk for developing paroxysmal nocturnal hemoglobinuria.[22]

Hemolytic Anemia

- Hemolytic anemia may be characterized as:
  - Acute or chronic
  - Immune versus non–immune mediated
  - Inherited or acquired
- The only abnormal laboratory values in acute hemolysis may be decreased Hgb and Hct. Internal hemorrhage can present with similar laboratory findings to hemolytic anemia.
- Maximal **reticulocyte** response occurs in 3 to 5 days. **Lactate dehydrogenase (LDH)** and **bilirubin** are increased in most patients reflecting an increase in red cell turnover. **Serum haptoglobin** is a sensitive early marker and is decreased by clearance of intravascular Hgb. The direct Coombs test (direct antibody test or DAT) identifies the presence of IgG or C3 bound to red cells; the indirect Coombs test indicates the presence of antibodies to red cells in the serum.

• Examination of the peripheral smear confirms hemolysis and may help identify the cause. Intravascular hemolysis may reveal **red cell fragmentation** (schistocytes, helmet cells), whereas **spherocytes** suggest extravascular, immune-mediated hemolysis. Polychromasia and nucleated erythrocytes can be seen with intense hemolysis and increased erythropoiesis.

Autoimmune Hemolytic Anemia

GENERAL PRINCIPLES

• **Autoimmune hemolytic anemia (AIHA)** is caused by antibodies to erythrocytes, leading to a shortened cell lifespan.
• **Warm-antibody AIHA** (WAIHA) is caused by IgG antibodies ± complement (C3) that react best at 37°C. It may be idiopathic or associated with an underlying malignancy (lymphoma, chronic lymphocytic leukemia [CLL], collagen vascular disorder) or drug induced.
• **Cold-antibody AIHA** (CAIHA or cold agglutinin disease) is less common than WAIHA and is caused by antibodies (usually IgM) and C3, which are most reactive with erythrocytes at lower temperatures. It may be chronic and associated with a B-cell neoplasm (lymphoma, CLL, Waldenström macroglobulinemia) or acute when caused by an infection (*Mycoplasma* spp., mononucleosis).

DIAGNOSIS

Clinical Presentation

• Mild cases of **WAIHA** may present with a stable anemia and reticulocytosis. In fulminant cases with an erythrocyte life span of <5 days, the anemia can be severe and the compensatory erythropoiesis inadequate. Patients may present with rapidly declining Hgb, fever, chest pain, and dyspnea. Jaundice, icterus, and dark urine reflect elevated indirect bilirubin from Hgb degradation.
• **CAIHA** may be characterized by severe acute hemolysis triggered by exposure to cold temperatures. Cyanosis can be seen in the extremities or other exposed areas. Chronic cold agglutinin disease is otherwise generally characterized by mild anemia with intermittent exacerbations.

Diagnostic Testing

• Laboratory evaluation of **WAIHA** shows a positive DAT for IgG, with 80% of patients also having antibodies detectable in the serum (positive indirect Coombs test). Plasma haptoglobin is decreased, LDH is increased, and the peripheral smear shows spherocytes.
• In **CAIHA**, IgM and C3 are present on the erythrocyte, but the DAT identifies only the presence of C3. IgG is negative on the DAT. The anemia is often mild and stable because serum complement inhibitors (C3 inactivator) limit complement activation on the erythrocyte membrane, which is temperature dependent.

TREATMENT

• Therapy for **WAIHA** is directed at identifying and treating any underlying cause.
• Steroid therapy (prednisone 1 to 2 mg/kg/day), splenectomy, and rituximab for patients with refractory disease are used to decrease the immune clearance of erythrocytes.
• Transfusion should not be delayed in situations of severe anemia or hemodynamic compromise. Fully typed and crossmatched red cells may be delayed due to the presence

of antibodies; therefore, O-negative blood should be given in emergent situations. Hemolysis of transfused red cells will occur at the same rate as the patient's own blood, but will not exacerbate the disease. The use of a blood warmer may be of marginal benefit.

- Cold avoidance and evaluation to identify underlying malignancy are important for **CAIHA**. Plasmapheresis may be helpful in the acute setting. Transfused blood must be prewarmed.
- Steroids and splenectomy are not effective in the treatment of IgM-mediated disease.[23]

Drug-Induced Hemolytic Anemia

- **Drug-induced hemolytic anemia** occurs by several mechanisms and is treated by identifying and withdrawing the causative agent. It presents similarly to WAIHA. The DAT may be positive or negative for IgG. It may also become negative soon after withdrawal of the offending agent.
- The role of steroids is not well defined, but they are often used due to diagnostic uncertainty. Common precipitants include cephalosporins (most commonly cefotetan and ceftriaxone), sulfamethoxazole/trimethoprim, dapsone, fluoroquinolones, NSAIDs, methyldopa, nitrofurantoin, and penicillin.

Microangiopathic Hemolytic Anemia

- Microangiopathic hemolytic anemia (MAHA) is a morphologic classification in which fragmented erythrocytes (schistocytes) are seen on peripheral blood smear.
- Processes that cause erythrocyte fragmentation and hemolysis include disseminated intravascular coagulation (DIC), thrombotic thrombocytopenic purpura (TTP), hemolytic-uremic syndrome (HUS), malignant hypertension, the preeclampsia/eclampsia syndromes, vasculitis, adenocarcinoma, and malfunctioning heart valves. DIC, TTP, and HUS are discussed in Chapter 12.

Sickle Cell Disease

GENERAL PRINCIPLES

- The sickle cell diseases are a group of hereditary Hgb disorders in which Hgb undergoes sickle shape transformation under conditions of deoxygenation.
- The most common are homozygous sickle cell anemia (Hgb SS) or other heterozygous conditions (Hgb SC, Hgb S-beta-thalassemia). Newborn screening programs for hemoglobinopathies now identify most patients in infancy.
- **Sickle cell trait** is present in 2.5 million people in the United States, occurring in 8% of African Americans.
- No abnormal hematologic findings are associated with sickle cell trait, which is a benign hereditary condition. Nevertheless, some risks have been reported. High-altitude hypoxia may lead to splenic infarction or cerebrovascular complications. Basic military training and competitive sports, particularly basketball and football, are associated with increased incidence of sudden death related to extreme exertion and dehydration.
- The National Institutes of Health provide useful guidelines for sickle cell disease (http://www.nhlbi.nih.gov/health-pro/guidelines/sickle-cell-disease-guidelines, last accessed December 22, 2014).[24]
- Sickle cell trait guidelines differ, but organizations such as the National Collegiate Athletic Association (NCAA) and military publish specific guidelines.

DIAGNOSIS

Clinical Presentation

- Clinical manifestations are variable but generally relate to complications from chronic hemolysis and/or vascular occlusion. Patients often have one syndrome that predominates.
  - **Vasoocclusive complications** include pain crises, avascular necrosis, priapism, and acute chest syndrome.
  - **Chronic hemolysis** complications include pulmonary hypertension, cholelithiasis, and leg ulcers.
  - Strokes, renal medullary infarctions, and priapism are complications of both forms.
- **Acute intermittent complications** account for much of the care provided to these patients and include the following:
  - **Acute painful episodes** (so-called sickle cell crisis):
    - Vasoocclusive pain crises are the most common manifestation of sickle cell disease. Pain is typically in the extremities, back, chest, and abdomen and lasts for 2 to 6 days. These crises may be idiopathic or precipitated by stress, dehydration, or infection.
    - Some patients with higher Hgb F levels have mild disease with few painful episodes and rarely require medical attention. Nevertheless, these patients are still at risk of all of the complications of the disease.
  - **Acute chest syndrome** occurs when hypoxia (<90% oxygen saturation) leads to increased intravascular sickling and irreversible occlusion of the microvasculature (predominantly pulmonary) circulation. Smokers and patients with lung pathology, such as pneumonia, are particularly at risk.[25]
  - **Aplastic crisis** presents with a sudden decrease in Hgb level. The RI is inappropriately low, reflecting suppression of erythropoiesis. The most common etiology in pediatric patients is infection with parvovirus B19. Folate deficiency should also be considered because of the chronic increased requirements for erythropoiesis.
  - **Cerebrovascular events**: stroke may occur at any age but is most common in children <10 years of age and is usually caused by large-vessel occlusion (i.e., middle cerebral artery).[26]
  - **Infections** in adults typically occur in tissues that are susceptible to vasoocclusive infarcts (bone, kidney, lung). *Staphylococcus* spp., *Salmonella* spp., and enteric organisms are the most common pathogens. Pneumonia is most likely to be caused by *Mycoplasma pneumoniae, Staphylococcus aureus,* or *Haemophilus influenzae* and must be distinguished from acute chest syndrome.
  - **Renal medullary infarction** results in chronic polyuria due to isosthenuria, leading to a chronic risk of dehydration.
  - **Renal tubular defects** caused by sickling in the anoxic hyperosmolar environment of the renal medulla may lead to isosthenuria and hematuria in both sickle cell trait and disease. These conditions predispose patients to dehydration, which increases the risk of vasoocclusive events.
  - **Cholelithiasis** is present in >80% of patients, primarily due to bilirubin stones.
  - **Avascular necrosis** (AVN) of the femoral heads occurs in up to 50% of patients and is a cause of severe pain in adults.
  - **Leg ulceration** occurring at the ankle is often chronic and recurring.
  - **Pregnancy** in a sickle cell patient should be considered high risk and is associated with increased spontaneous abortions or premature delivery, along with increased vasoocclusive crises.

Diagnostic Testing

- Hgb analysis by electrophoresis or high-pressure liquid chromatography is used to diagnose hemoglobinopathies and distinguishes homozygous sickle cell disease (Hgb SS) from other abnormal hemoglobin.
- The mean Hgb in Hgb SS disease is about 8 g/dL (range 5 to 10 g/dL). The MCV may be slightly elevated because of reticulocytosis but is low in Hgb S-β-thalassemia.
- Leukocytosis (10,000 to 20,000/mm³) and thrombocytosis (>450,000/mm³) are common due to enhanced stimulation of the marrow compartment and autosplenectomy.
- Peripheral smear shows sickle-shaped erythrocytes, target cells (particularly in Hgb SC and Hgb S-β-thalassemia), and Howell-Jolly bodies, indicative of functional asplenism.
- The degree of anemia and reticulocytosis is generally milder in Hgb SC disease.

TREATMENT

- Outpatient management of **acute painful episodes** consists of rehydration (oral fluids, 3 to 4 L/day), evaluation for and management of infections, analgesia, and, if needed, antipyretic and empiric antibiotic therapy.
  - ○ **Morphine** (0.3 to 0.6 mg/kg PO every 4 hours PRN) is the drug of choice for moderate-to-severe pain.
  - ○ Pain management is a complex problem that may require multidisciplinary approaches, including social services, psychiatric consultation, and pain service to optimize the use of opiate medications.
  - ○ Transfusion should only be used for severe symptomatic anemia in uncomplicated vaso-occlusive crises.
  - ○ **Indications for hospitalization** include inability to ingest adequate oral fluids, requirement for parenteral opioids or antibiotics, a declining Hgb level associated with inadequate erythropoiesis, or hypoxia.
  - ○ **Hydroxyurea** therapy (15 to 35 mg/kg PO daily) has been shown to increase levels of Hgb F and significantly decreases the frequency of vasoocclusive crises and acute chest syndrome in adults with sickle cell disease. It should be considered in most patients (nonpregnant) with Hgb SS or S β-thalassemia.[27]
- Individuals with suspected **acute chest syndrome** require immediate hospitalization and aggressive transfusion therapy, including red cell exchange. The presentation of acute chest syndrome is clinically indistinguishable from pneumonia; thus, empiric broad-spectrum antibiotics should be administered.
- **Priapism** is initially treated with hydration and analgesia. Persistent erections for >24 hours may require transfusion therapy or surgical drainage.
- **General prevention and maintenance** treatments include the following:
  - ○ **Dehydration and hypoxia** should be avoided because they may precipitate or exacerbate irreversible sickling.
  - ○ **Folic acid**, 1 mg PO daily, is generally administered to all patients with sickle cell disease because of chronic hemolysis.
  - ○ **Pneumococcal vaccine** is administered due to the risk of asplenism.
  - ○ **Ophthalmologic examinations** are recommended yearly for adults due to the high incidence of proliferative retinopathy leading to vitreous hemorrhage and retinal detachment.
  - ○ **Local and regional anesthesia** can be used without special precautions. Measures to avoid volume depletion, hypoxia, and hypernatremia are crucial.
  - ○ For **general anesthesia**, red blood cell transfusion to increase the Hgb concentration to 10 g/dL is strongly suggested and seems to be as effective as more aggressive regimens.[29]

COMPLICATIONS

- Patients with suspected **aplastic crisis** require hospitalization. Therapy includes folic acid, 5 mg/day, as well as red blood cell transfusions.
- **Cholelithiasis** may lead to acute cholecystitis or biliary colic. Acute cholecystitis should be treated medically with antibiotics, and cholecystectomy should be performed when the attack subsides. Elective cholecystectomy for asymptomatic gallstones is controversial; however, persistent abdominal complaints may suggest cholelithiasis as the cause.
- Treatment of AVN consists of local heat, analgesics, and avoidance of weight bearing. Hip and shoulder arthroplasty are usually effective in decreasing symptoms and improving function.
- In those with a history of stroke, the pediatric literature suggests transfusions to maintain the Hgb S concentration at <50% for at least 5 years to reduce the incidence of recurrent stroke.[30]
- **Leg ulcers** are treated with rest, leg elevation, and intensive local care. Referral to a wound care clinic or dermatologist is helpful.

Red Cell Enzyme Deficiencies

GENERAL PRINCIPLES

The most common hereditary enzyme deficiency is **glucose-6-phosphate dehydrogenase deficiency**, a sex-linked disorder that typically affects men. Erythrocytes that are deficient in this enzyme are more susceptible to hemolysis via oxidant stress, triggered by infections or drug exposure, leading to **chronic or episodic hemolysis**.

DIAGNOSIS

Clinical Presentation

- A mild form of the disease is seen in approximately 10% of African American men with anemia often precipitated by infection, fever, or medications such as sulfa, dapsone, antiretrovirals, and hydroxychloroquine.[31]
- A more severe form is the Mediterranean variant, in which hemolysis occurs when susceptible individuals ingest fava beans and present with fatigue, jaundice, and bilirubinuria.

Diagnostic Testing

- The peripheral smear classically shows bite cells.
- Diagnosis is made by demonstrating reduced levels of the enzyme. Because older senescent cells with lower enzyme levels hemolyze first during an acute hemolytic episode, a younger population of erythrocytes may result in a falsely elevated (normal) enzyme level; thus, the test should be repeated at least 6 weeks after the hemolytic event.

TREATMENT

Acute hemolytic episodes are largely intravascular and self-limited. Therapy is supportive and includes hydration and transfusion in addition to identifying and removing oxidant stresses such as drugs.

Polycythemia

GENERAL PRINCIPLES

- Polycythemia, defined as an abnormally elevated Hgb, Hct, or red cell mass, may be absolute or relative to plasma volume.
- It is most important to differentiate polycythemia vera (PV) from secondary and relative polycythemia because the treatment differs.[32]

DIAGNOSIS

Clinical Presentation

History
- Elicit either a history of lung disease or symptoms suggestive of such.
- Inquire about possible exposure to carbon monoxide, tobacco smoke, or high-altitude locations.
- Determine whether dehydration may be present such as with diuretic use.
- Symptoms suggestive of obstructive sleep apnea may be helpful in establishing the etiology.
- Testosterone replacement may increase the Hgb level by approximately 1 g/dL.

Physical Examination
- Examine for cyanosis, abnormal heart sounds suggestive of shunt, and lung sounds suggestive of obstructive disease.
- Splenomegaly is seen with PV and is typically not present in secondary or relative polycythemia.

Differential Diagnosis

Dehydration causes a relative polycythemia. Chronic hypoxemia, obstructive sleep apnea, and carbon monoxide poisoning may cause secondary polycythemia. PV is a myeloproliferative neoplasm (MPN).

Diagnostic Testing

- Repeat the CBC to confirm polycythemia.
- The next step is to rule out PV by checking **JAK2 V617F mutation** status and EPO level. JAK2 mutations are present in 94% of PV cases, and EPO may be low.[33] In cases of diagnostic uncertainty, red blood cell mass is used to differentiate absolute polycythemia from a relative reduction in plasma volume; however, this test is not widely available, and it will not differentiate PV from secondary polycythemia.
- Workup of secondary polycythemia is patient specific. Consider sleep study, echocardiogram, pulse oximetry, and carboxyhemoglobin.

TREATMENT

- PV may be initially treated with **phlebotomy** followed by maintenance therapy with continued phlebotomy or **hydroxyurea** to keep the Hct <45%.[34]
- **Aspirin** 81 mg daily reduces the high incidence of thrombotic events in PV.[35]
- Treatment of secondary polycythemia is dependent on the cause, and phlebotomy is rarely indicated. Aspirin is often used due to comorbid conditions but is not specifically indicated.

Thrombocytosis

GENERAL PRINCIPLES

- **Secondary thrombocytosis** may occur in response to recovery from bleeding or thrombocytopenia, postsplenectomy, iron deficiency, chronic infectious or inflammatory states, and malignancies.
- **Essential thrombocythemia** (ET) is a chronic MPN.
- Progression to myelofibrosis or acute myeloid leukemia occurs in a minority of ET patients.[36]
- Arterial thrombosis, including transient ischemic attacks and stroke, is common in ET. The risk of thrombosis increases with age, prior thrombosis, duration of disease, other comorbidities, and platelet count.[37]

DIAGNOSIS

Clinical Presentation

- Patients with secondary thrombocytosis generally do not have an increased risk of bleeding or thrombosis. However, patients postsplenectomy may have an increased risk of portal vein thrombosis. Platelet normalization occurs after improvement of the underlying disorder.
- ET may present asymptomatically with laboratory abnormalities or present with a thrombotic or hemorrhagic event.
- Erythromelalgia, due to microvascular occlusive platelet thrombi, presents as intense burning or throbbing of the extremities, typically involving the feet. Cold exposure usually relieves symptoms. Typical signs of erythromelalgia include erythema and warmth of affected digits.
- Approximately 50% of ET patients develop **mild splenomegaly**.

Diagnostic Testing

- The diagnosis of ET is currently based on the 2008 World Health Organization revised criteria.[13]
- The general practitioner can evaluate for a sustained platelet count of >450 × 10⁹/L, presence of **JAK2 V617F mutation**, and no cause for reactive thrombocytosis if the JAK2 mutation is absent.
- The hematologist may perform a BM aspirate and biopsy to evaluate for increased mature megakaryocytes and rule out myelofibrosis or other MPN.

TREATMENT

- Aspirin 81 mg daily is indicated unless there is history of significant hemorrhage.
- Platelet reduction therapy is indicated in patients >60 years old or with a prior thrombosis or hemorrhage, hypertension, diabetes, smoking, or hyperlipidemia. The majority of thrombotic complications occur at modest platelet count elevations. Treatment typically targets a platelet count of <400 × 10⁹/L. Platelet-lowering drugs include hydroxyurea, anagrelide, or interferon-α in pregnant patients or women in their childbearing years.[38] Hydroxyurea and anagrelide provide equivalent platelet count control, but anagrelide is associated with more adverse effects.[39]
- There is some evidence that **plateletpheresis** is beneficial in acute arterial thrombosis such as stroke or myocardial infarction.[40]

WHITE BLOOD CELL DISORDERS

Leukocytosis

GENERAL PRINCIPLES

- Leukocytosis is an elevation in the absolute WBC count (>10,000/mm^3).
- Neutrophilia is not often further evaluated until >20,000/mm^3.
- An elevated WBC count typically reflects the normal response of BM to an infectious or inflammatory process, steroid use, β-agonist or lithium therapy, splenectomy, stress, or smoking.
- Occasionally, leukocytosis is due to a primary BM abnormality in WBC production, maturation, or death (apoptosis) related to leukemia or MPN and can affect any cell in the leukocyte lineage.
- A WBC count >50,000/mm^3 may be termed a **leukemoid reaction** and must be interpreted in the clinical context with a high degree of suspicion for malignancy. Some infections such as *Clostridium difficile* colitis may evoke this type of response.
- Lymphocytosis is less common and is associated with viral infections, medication effect, or leukemia.
- Eosinophilia (>1,000/mm^3) has a limited differential. The most common cause worldwide is helminthic infections, while in developed nations, it is atopy. Other causes include malignancy, Addison disease, and collagen vascular disease.[41]

DIAGNOSIS

Clinical Presentation

History
- For mild neutrophilia, signs and symptoms of infection should be elicited. Cigarette smokers should be identified, and weight loss in this population may suggest malignancy. Recent corticosteroid use may produce a mild-to-moderate neutrophilia.
- Features of acute leukemia include bone pain, fatigue, night sweats, fever, or bleeding. Furthermore, neurologic deficiencies or cardiopulmonary distress are rare but suggestive of leukostasis secondary to leukemia.

Physical Examination
- Lymphocytosis secondary to CLL occasionally presents with splenomegaly and lymphadenopathy.
- Patients with chronic myelogenous leukemia (CML) present with leukocytosis and splenomegaly; they will rarely present with lymphadenopathy. The skin should be examined for chloromas.

Diagnostic Testing
- Repeat the CBC with differential and examine the peripheral smear.
- The presence of blasts on a peripheral smear is concerning for an acute leukemia and requires prompt evaluation. Acute leukemia may also have an associated elevation in LDH and uric acid due to rapid cell turnover.
- Unexplained lymphocytosis should also be assessed with peripheral flow cytometry and **BCR-abl molecular studies**.

TREATMENT

- Mild neutrophilia prompts a review of the patient's comorbidities and appropriate infectious disease workup. It often does not warrant evaluation by a hematologist. If there are

clinical features concerning for acute leukemia, such as circulating blasts or other cytopenias, contact a specialist directly or admit to a hospital as the acuity dictates.
• Chronic leukemias may be relatively asymptomatic and are typically evaluated and treated in an outpatient specialist setting.

Leukopenia

• Leukopenia is an abnormally low WBC count (<3,500 cells/mm^3) and may occur in response to infection, inflammation, malignancy, or vitamin deficiencies.
• Drug-induced neutropenia due to chemotherapeutic or immunosuppressive drugs is usually dose dependent.
• Idiosyncratic leukopenia may be caused by a broad range of medications and should be suspected when developing shortly after starting a new agent. Common classes are antiepileptics, antibiotics, NSAIDs, and some antipsychotics.[42]
• Severe neutropenia (absolute neutrophil count [ANC] <500/mm^3) increases the risk of a life-threatening bacterial infection. Neutropenic fever requires emergent evaluation, admission, panculture, and empiric broad-spectrum antibiotics.
• Unexplained pancytopenia with symptoms concerning for leukemia warrants immediate specialist evaluation.
• Chronic benign neutropenia is common in African Americans and is not clinically significant as their response to infection is normal.
• HIV infection may cause lymphopenia, while most other viral infections cause lymphocytosis.
• Growth factor support, such as G-CSF, should be considered in patients with chronic neutropenia and ongoing infections. An agent commonly used in the outpatient setting is filgrastim 5 mcg/kg (typically either 240 mcg or 480 mcg per dose) injected subcutaneously.

Monoclonal Gammopathies

An elevated total protein may be polyclonal or monoclonal. Common reasons for polyclonal gammopathy are chronic infection, inflammation, or liver disease. Monoclonal gammopathies are discussed individually below.

Monoclonal Gammopathy of Unknown Significance

• Monoclonal gammopathy of unknown significance (MGUS) refers to the presence of a monoclonal protein (M protein) totaling <3 g/dL in the absence of related organ failure (e.g., anemia, hypercalcemia, renal insufficiency, lytic bone lesions) or known underlying lymphoproliferative disorder.
• The incidence of MGUS increases with age; 3% of persons >50 years of age are affected, and people of African descent are twice as likely as Caucasians to have MGUS.
• Initial laboratory data should include CBC; basic metabolic panel including serum calcium, urinalysis, serum protein electrophoresis and immunofixation; and serum free light-chain assay. Normal urinalysis does not rule out proteinuria; thus, 24-hour urine collection for protein electrophoresis and immunofixation is needed to detect and quantify immunoglobulin light chains.
• A skeletal survey is important to document the absence of bone lesions. Advanced imaging and/or biopsy may be necessary to characterize suspicious lesions.
• MGUS evolves into a more serious lymphoproliferative malignancy at a rate of about 1% per year. Non-IgG MGUS may progress to multiple myeloma. IgM MGUS may transform to Waldenström macroglobulinemia or chronic lymphocytic leukemia.

- Three risk factors for progression have been identified: non-IgG gammapathy (IgM or IgA), abnormal serum free light-chain ratio (κ/λ ratio), and initial gammapathy concentration of >1.5 g/dL each increase the risk of progressing, and the presence of all three confers the highest risk of 58% at 20 years.[43]
- Referral is indicated for BM biopsy in patients at moderate to high risk of disease progression. Patients with MGUS should be monitored with CBC, electrolytes, renal function and serum protein electrophoresis (SPEP) every 6 to 12 months indefinitely due to the risk of malignant transformation.

Multiple Myeloma

- Multiple myeloma (MM) is a lymphoproliferative disorder that may present with unexpected skeletal fracture (long bone or vertebral body), renal failure (due to light chain proteinuria), cytopenia, hypercalcemia, or a combination of these. Fatigue and anemia may be the only presenting features particularly in older patients. A subset with hypogammaglobulinemia will present with recurrent bacterial infection such as pneumococcal pneumonia.
- The diagnosis is usually established by a BM examination with the presence of plasma cells >30% in the marrow or biopsy proven plasmacytoma.
- Initial treatment of hypercalcemia includes intravenous fluids and a bisphosphonate such as zoledronic acid 4 mg IV.
- Treatment of MM is rapidly changing and has become quite effective in controlling the disease. Care should be coordinated with a specialist and may include corticosteroids in combination with chemotherapy (melphalan, thalidomide, lenalidomide, or bortezomib). Palliative radiotherapy may be indicated for bone lesions, and orthopedic surgery may be necessary for impending fracture. The role of stem cell transplant is evolving as chemotherapy becomes more effective. Currently, it provides modest survival benefit and is typically indicated in those with poor-risk features.[44]
- The Multiple Myeloma Research Foundation website (http://www.themmrf.org, last accessed December 22, 2014) is an excellent online resource for clinicians and patients.

Amyloidosis

- Primary (amyloid light chain [AL]) amyloidosis is an infiltrative disorder due to monoclonal light-chain deposition in various tissues most often involving the kidney (renal failure, nephrotic syndrome), heart (nonischemic cardiomyopathy), peripheral nervous system (neuropathy), and GI tract/liver (macroglossia, diarrhea, nausea, vomiting). Unexplained findings in any of these organ systems should prompt evaluation for amyloidosis.[45]
- An M protein discovered by serum or urine protein electrophoresis or serum free light-chain assay is found in >95% of patients with AL amyloidosis. Biopsy of an affected organ, BM, or fat pad may also be helpful.
- Treatment options include chemotherapeutics similar to those used in MM; thus, specialty consultation is recommended.

THE BONE MARROW BIOPSY

Patients referred to a hematologist often undergo this procedure as part of the initial diagnostic workup and occasionally require repeated examinations. Patients may have preconceived ideas about this so it is helpful to counsel your patient since it is often not as painful as expected. Patients may experience localized pain that resolves over a few days. It has been shown that <1% of procedures are associated with an adverse event.[46] Of these, bleeding is the most common while infection is extremely unlikely. The provider may indicate a preference in terms of systemic anticoagulation management periprocedurally.

COUNSELING THE POTENTIAL STEM CELL DONOR

Unfortunately, misconceptions regarding stem cell donation and transplant have hindered enrollment. Counter to images of surgeons "scraping the bone marrow," the patient does not routinely undergo a surgical procedure for either donation or transplant of stem cells. Stem cell donation involves a SQ injection of G-CSF followed a few days later by a pheresis procedure. This has been shown to be safe with no long-term adverse effects.[47] Stem cell transplant is by intravenous infusion following bone marrow ablative therapy with chemotherapeutics and sometimes total body irradiation. All transplant recipients require central venous access.

REFERENCES

1. Fiebach NH, Barker LR, Burton JR, et al., eds. *Principles of Ambulatory Medicine*, 7th ed. Philadelphia, PA: Lippincott Williams & Wilkins; 2007:819–835.
2. Coyne DW, Kapoian T, Suki W, et al. Ferric gluconate is highly efficacious in anemic hemodialysis patients with high serum ferritin and low transferring saturation: results of the Dialysis Patients' Response to IV Iron with Elevated Ferritin (DRIVE) study. *J Am Soc Nephrol* 2007;18:975–984.
3. Carson JL, Grossman BJ, Kleinman S, et al. Red blood cell transfusion: a clinical practice guideline from the AABB. *Ann Intern Med* 2012;157:49–58.
4. Rimon E, Kagansky N, Kagansky M, et al. Are we giving too much iron? Low dose iron therapy is effective in octogenarians. *Am J Med* 2005;118:1142–1147.
5. Faich G, Strobos J. Sodium ferric gluconate complex in sucrose: safer intravenous iron therapy than iron dextrans. *Am J Kidney Dis* 1999;33:464–470.
6. Marengo-Rowe AJ. The thalassemias and related disorders. *Proc (Bayl Univ Med Cent)* 2007;20:27–31.
7. Meerpohl JJ, Antes G, Rücker G, et al. Deferasirox for managing iron overload in people with thalassaemia. *Cochrane Database Syst Rev* 2012;2:CD007476.
8. Stabler SP. Vitamin B_{12} deficiency. *N Engl J Med* 2013;368:149–160.
9. Kaferle J, Strzoda CE. Evaluation of macrocytosis. *Am Fam Physician* 2009;79:203–208.
10. Carmel R, Weiner JM, Johnson CS. Iron deficiency occurs frequently in patients with pernicious anemia. *JAMA* 1987;257:1081–1083.
11. Carmel R. How I treat cobalamin (vitamin B_{12}) deficiency. *Blood* 2008;112:2214–2221.
12. McQuilten ZK, Polizzotto MN, Wood EM, et al. Myelodysplastic syndrome incidence, transfusion dependence, health care use, and complications: an Australian population-based study 1998 to 2009. *Transfusion* 2014;54:2705-2715.
13. Vardiman JW, Thiele J, Arber DA, et al. The 2008 revision of the World Health Organization (WHO) classification of myeloid neoplasms and acute leukemia: rationale and important changes. *Blood* 2009;114:937–951.
14. Greenberg PL, Tuechler H, Schanz J, et al. Revised international prognostic scoring system for myelodysplastic syndromes. *Blood* 2012;120:2454–2465.
15. Ma X. Epidemiology of myelodysplastic syndromes. *Am J Med* 2012;125:S2–S5.
16. Shrier SL, Pang WW. Anemia in the elderly. *Curr Opin Hematol* 2012;19:133–140.
17. Fenaux P, Giagounidis A, Selleslag D, et al. A randomized phase 3 study of lenalidomide versus placebo in RBC transfusion-dependent patients with low-/intermediate-1-risk myelodysplastic syndromes with del5q. *Blood* 2011;118:3765–3776.
18. Lubbert M, Suciu S, Baila L, et al. Low-dose decitabine versus best supportive care in elderly patients with intermediate- or high-risk myelodysplastic syndrome (MDS) ineligible for intensive chemotherapy: final results of the randomized phase III study

of the European Organization for Research and Treatment of Cancer Leukemia Group and the German MDS Study Group. *J Clin Oncol* 2011;29:1987–1996.

19. Weiss G, Goodnough LT. Anemia of chronic disease. *N Engl J Med* 2005;352:1011–1023.

20. Ganz T, Nemeth E. Hepcidin and iron homeostasis. *Biochim Biophys Acta* 2012; 1823:1434–1443.

21. Fishbane S, Besarab A. Mechanism of increased mortality risk with erythropoietin treatment to higher hemoglobin targets. *Clin J Am Soc Nephrol* 2007;2:1274–1282.

22. Young NS, Maciejerski J. The pathophysiology of acquired aplastic anemia. *N Engl J Med* 1997;336:1365–1372.

23. Lechner K, Jäger U. How I treat autoimmune hemolytic anemias in adults. *Blood* 2010;116:1831–1838.

24. National Institutes of Health, Division of Blood Diseases and Resources. National Heart, Lung, and Blood Institute. *The Management of Sickle Cell Disease.* Washington, DC: National Institutes of Health; 2002. NIH Publication No. 02–2117.

25. Cohen RT, DeBaun MR, Blinder MA, et al. Smoking is associated with an increased risk of acute chest syndrome and pain among adults with sickle cell disease. *Blood* 2010;115:3852–3854.

26. Switzer JA, Hess DC, Nichols FT, et al. Pathophysiology and treatment of stroke in sickle-cell disease: present and future. *Lancet Neurol* 2006;5:501–512.

27. Brawley OW, Cornelius LJ, Edwards LR, et al. NIH consensus development statement on hydroxyurea treatment for sickle cell disease. *NIH Consens State Sci Statements* 2008;25:1–30.

28. Falletta JM, Woods GM, Verter JI, et al. Discontinuing penicillin prophylaxis in children with sickle cell anemia. Prophylactic Penicillin Study II. *J Pediatr* 1995;127:685–690.

29. Vichinsky EP, Haberkern CM, Neumayr L, et al. A comparison of conservative and aggressive transfusion regimens in the perioperative management of sickle cell disease. The Preoperative Transfusion in Sickle Cell Disease Study Group. *N Engl J Med* 1995;333:206–213.

30. Riddington C, Wang W. Blood transfusion for preventing primary and secondary stroke in people with sickle cell disease. *Cochrane Database Syst Rev* 2013;1:CD003146.

31. Youngster I, Arcavi L, Schechmaster R, et al. Medications and glucose-6-phosphate dehydrogenase deficiency: an evidence-based review. *Drug Saf* 2010;33:713–726.

32. Tefferi A. Polycythemia vera and essential thrombocythemia: 2012 update on diagnosis, risk stratification, and management. *Am J Hematol* 2012;87:285–293.

33. Rapado I, Albizua E, Ayala R, et al. Validity test study of JAK2 V617F and allele burden quantification in the diagnosis of myeloproliferative diseases. *Ann Hematol* 2008;87:741–749.

34. Marchioli R, Finazzi G, Specchia G, et al. Cardiovascular events and intensity of treatment in polycythemia vera. *N Engl J Med* 2013;368:22–33.

35. Landolfi R, Marchioli R, Kutti J, et al.; European Collaboration on Low-Dose Aspirin in Polycythemia Vera Investigators. Efficacy and safety of low-dose aspirin in polycythemia vera. *N Engl J Med* 2004;350:114–124.

36. Harrison CN. Essential thrombocythemia: challenges and evidence-based management. *Br J Haematol* 2005;130:153–165.

37. Harrison CN, Gale RE, Machin SJ, et al. A large proportion of patients with a diagnosis of essential thrombocythemia do not have a clonal disorder and may be at lower risk of thrombotic complications. *Blood* 1999;93:417–424.

38. Storen EC, Tefferi A. Long-term use of anagrelide in young patients with essential thrombocythemia. *Blood* 2001;97:863–866.

39. Harrison CN, Campbell PJ, Buck G, et al.; United Kingdom Medical Research Council Primary Thrombocythemia 1 Study. Hydroxyurea compared with anagrelide in high-risk essential thrombocythemia. *N Engl J Med* 2005;353:33–45.

40. Griest A. The role of blood component removal in essential and reactive thrombocytosis. *Ther Apher* 2002;6:36–44.

41. Rothenberg ME. Eosinophilia. *N Engl J Med* 1998;338:1592–1600.

42. Andersohn F, Konzen C, Garbe E. Systematic review: agranulocytosis induced by non-chemotherapy drugs. *Ann Intern Med* 2007;146:657–665.

43. Rajkumar SV, Kyle RA, Therneau TM, et al. Serum free light chain ratio is an independent risk factor for progression in monoclonal gammopathy of undetermined significance. *Blood* 2005;106:812–817.

44. Eshaghian S, Berenson JR. Multiple myeloma: improved outcomes with new therapeutic approaches. *Curr Opin Support Palliat Care* 2012;6:330–336.

45. Merlini G, Seldin DC, Gertz MA. Amyloidosis: pathogenesis and new therapeutic options. *J Clin Oncol* 2011;29:1924–1933.

46. Bain BJ. Bone marrow biopsy morbidity and mortality. *Br J Haematol* 2003;121: 949–951.

47. Moalic V. Mobilization and collection of peripheral blood stem cells in healthy donors: risks, adverse events and follow-up. *Pathol Biol (Paris)* 2013;61:70–74.

14

Venous Thromboembolism and Anticoagulant Therapy
Roger D. Yusen and Brian F. Gage

GENERAL PRINCIPLES

Definitions
- **Venous thromboembolism (VTE)** consists of the spectrum of disease defined by the presence of **deep vein thrombosis (DVT)** or **pulmonary embolism (PE)**.
- PE arises from DVT or intracardiac clots that embolize to the pulmonary arterial system.
- **Massive PE** often refers to PE associated with systemic hypotension despite resuscitative measures (e.g., hydration, vasopressors), while **submassive PE** may refer to nonmassive PE that has associated significant cardiac dysfunction (e.g., right heart strain on echo). Alternatively, some definitions of massive and submassive PE depend on clot burden, while others depend on prognosis.

Anatomy
- The anatomic location of DVT and PE may affect prognosis and treatment recommendations.
- DVTs can be classified as **deep** or **superficial** and as **proximal** or **distal.**
  - To emphasize its deep vein location, the term **femoral vein** replaced the term **superficial femoral vein.**
  - **Lower extremity proximal** DVTs occur in or superior to the popliteal vein (or the confluence of tibial and peroneal veins), whereas **distal lower extremity** DVTs occur inferior to the popliteal vein.
  - **Upper extremity proximal** DVTs occur in the axillary vein or more centrally, whereas **distal upper extremity** DVTs occur in the brachial vein or more peripherally.
- Location in the pulmonary arterial system characterizes **PEs** as **central** (main pulmonary artery, lobar, or segmental) or **distal** (subsegmental or smaller pulmonary artery branches).

Etiology/Pathophysiology
- Blood vessel damage or other events may produce a series of reactions that involve proteins, called clotting factors (identified by Roman numerals), and cause thromboses.
- Solidification of normally fluid blood into a dense aggregation of blood cells that is entangled within long fibrinous chains of molecules (fibrin) leads to a thrombosis.
- Acquired or genetic coagulation abnormalities can lead to thrombosis formation.
- Symptomatic DVTs most commonly develop in the lower limbs.
- Untreated DVTs may propagate proximally. **Without treatment, half of patients with proximal lower extremity DVT develop PE.**
- DVTs in the proximal lower extremities and pelvis produce most PEs.
- DVTs that occur in upper extremities, often secondary to an indwelling catheter, may also cause PE.
- DVT may occur concomitantly with **superficial thrombophlebitis**, which is seen in association with varicose veins, trauma, infection, and hypercoagulable disorders.

Risk Factors/Associated Conditions

- VTE has an increased incidence with conditions of blood **stasis, hypercoagulability, and venous endothelial injury.** Acute illnesses that lead to prolonged **immobilization** (trauma, surgery, and other major medical illnesses) also predispose to development of VTE.
- **Hypercoagulable states** may have an inherited or acquired etiology.
  - ○ **Acquired hypercoagulable states** may arise secondary to malignancy, nephrotic syndrome, obesity, pregnancy, and certain medications (e.g., estrogen, thalidomide, erythropoietin). Both **heparin-induced thrombocytopenia** (see Heparin-Induced Thrombocytopenia in Chapter 12) and the **antiphospholipid antibody (APA) syndrome** (see Chapter 33) can cause arterial or venous thrombi.
  - ○ **Inherited thrombophilic disorders** have a higher likelihood of occurring in the setting of a history of spontaneous VTE at a young age (<50 years), recurrent VTE, VTE in first-degree relatives, thrombosis in unusual anatomic locations, and recurrent fetal loss.[1]
  - ○ **Inherited risk factors for VTE** include genetic polymorphisms/mutations; deficiencies of the natural anticoagulants **protein C, protein S,** and **antithrombin; dysfibrinogenemia;** and **hyperhomocysteinemia.**
    - ▪ **Common mutations** that increase the risk of thrombosis affect the factor V gene (e.g., R506Q mutation) or the prothrombin (factor II) gene (e.g., G20210A mutation). For example, the factor V Leiden mutation can lead to resistance to the degrading properties of activated protein C, and this activated protein C resistance allows factor V to remain active longer.
    - ▪ **Homocystinuria** can cause arterial and venous thromboembolic events that often begin in childhood. Deficiency of cystathionine-β-synthase causes homocystinuria, though milder homocysteine elevations more commonly arise from an interaction between genetic mutations that affect enzymes involved in homocysteine metabolism and acquired factors such as inadequate folate consumption.[1] The diagnostic criterion for homocystinuria consists of an elevated fasting plasma homocysteine level.
- **Unusual spontaneous venous thromboses,** such as cavernous sinus thrombosis, mesenteric vein thrombosis, or portal vein thrombosis, may be the initial presentation of paroxysmal nocturnal hemoglobinuria (PNH) or myeloproliferative disorders.
- **Spontaneous (idiopathic) thrombosis,** despite the absence of an inherited thrombophilia and detectable autoantibodies, predisposes patients to future thromboses.[1]
- **Antiphospholipid antibody (APA) syndrome** may cause thrombosis, and the diagnosis requires the presence of at least one clinical and one laboratory criteria.[2]
  - ○ **Clinical criteria** consist of (a) the occurrence of arterial or venous **thrombosis** in any tissue or organ and (b) **pregnancy morbidities** (unexplained late fetal death; premature birth complicated by eclampsia, preeclampsia, or placental insufficiency; and at least three unexplained consecutive spontaneous abortions).
  - ○ **Laboratory criteria** consist of persistent (at least 12 weeks apart) detection of autoantibodies (lupus anticoagulant [LA], anticardiolipin antibody, and β_2-glycoprotein-1 antibodies) that react with negatively charged phospholipids.
  - ○ The APA syndrome may include other features, such as thrombocytopenia, valvular heart disease, livedo reticularis, neurologic manifestations, and nephropathy.

Prevention

VTE prevention, by identifying patients at high risk and instituting prophylactic measures, remains the ideal strategy for reducing its morbidity and mortality.

DIAGNOSIS

Clinical Presentation

- **DVT** may produce **pain and edema** in an affected extremity.
  - DVT has neither sensitive nor specific symptoms and signs. However, pretest assessment of the probability of a DVT provides useful information when combined with the results of compression ultrasound or a D-dimer test, or both, in determining whether to exclude or accept the diagnosis of DVT or perform additional imaging studies.[3]
- **Superficial thrombophlebitis** presents as a tender, warm, erythematous, and often palpable thrombosed vein. Accompanying DVT may produce additional symptoms and signs.
- **PE** has neither sensitive nor specific symptoms and signs.
  - PE may produce **shortness of breath, pleuritic chest pain,** shoulder or back pain, **hemoptysis, presyncope, syncope, tachycardia,** pleural rub, hypoxemia, hypotension, and right-sided heart failure.[4]
  - Validated **clinical risk factors** for a PE in outpatients who present to an emergency department include signs and symptoms of DVT, high suspicion of PE by the clinician, tachycardia, immobility in the past 4 weeks, history of VTE, active cancer, and hemoptysis.[5]
- **Clinical suspicion of DVT or PE should lead to objective testing**.

Differential Diagnosis

- The differential diagnosis for **unilateral lower extremity** symptoms and signs of **DVT**, such as swelling and pain, includes Baker cyst, hematoma, venous insufficiency, postphlebitic syndrome, lymphedema, sarcoma, arterial aneurysm, myositis, cellulitis, rupture of the medial head of the gastrocnemius, and abscess.
- **Symmetric bilateral lower extremity edema** often suggests the presence of heart, renal, or liver failure or a low albumin level.
- Additional diseases to consider in association with **lower extremity pain** include musculoskeletal and arteriovascular disorders.
- The **differential diagnosis of symptoms and signs of PE** includes dissecting aortic aneurysm, myocardial ischemia, heart failure, pneumonia, acute bronchitis, bronchocarcinoma, pericardial or pleural disease, and costochondritis. Other causes of pulmonary arterial occlusion, including in situ thrombi (e.g., sickle cell disease), marrow fat embolism, amniotic fluid embolism, pulmonary artery sarcoma, and fibrosing mediastinitis, mimic signs and symptoms of PE.

Diagnostic Testing

Laboratories
D-Dimer

- D-dimers, cross-linked fibrin degradation products, may increase with VTE, though other acute conditions (e.g., surgery) also elevate levels.
- Assays used to measure D-dimers differ in accuracy and thresholds for a positive test.
- D-dimer testing for DVT or PE has a low positive predictive value and specificity; **patients with an elevated D-dimer require further evaluation**.
- A sensitive quantitative D-dimer assay has a negative predictive value high enough to exclude a DVT in conjunction with a low (objectively defined) clinical probability and/or a negative noninvasive test.[6,7]
- A negative D-dimer in combination with a low pretest probability based on an objective scoring tool can exclude almost all PEs.[8]
- In the setting of a moderate-to-high clinical pretest probability (e.g., patients with cancer), a negative D-dimer does not have sufficient negative predictive value for excluding the presence of DVT or PE.[9]

Hypercoagulability Testing

- Most patients with VTE do not need hypercoagulability testing; selected individuals who have an idiopathic VTE and a high likelihood of having an inherited thrombophilic disorder (See Risk Factors section) typically undergo testing.
- Signs and symptoms of the **APA syndrome** should lead to laboratory evaluation.
  - Serologic tests (e.g., IgG and IgM β_2-glycoprotein-1 antibodies and IgG and IgM cardiolipin antibodies) or clotting assays (e.g., LA) detect APAs; performing both serologic and clotting assays improves sensitivity.
  - LAs may prolong the aPTT or PT/INR, but do not predispose to bleeding.
- To assess for PNH in the setting of unusual spontaneous venous thromboses, perform flow cytometry to detect missing antigens on red cells or leukocytes.

Imaging

DVT-Specific Testing

- Initial diagnostic testing for symptomatic acute DVT should consist of a **noninvasive test,** typically **venous compression ultrasound** (**US**; called **duplex examination** when performed with Doppler testing).[10]
  - Compression US has low sensitivity for detecting **calf DVT** and also may fail to visualize parts of the deep femoral vein, the pelvic veins, and the more central upper extremity venous system.
  - The presence of an **old DVT** on compression US may make new DVT harder to detect.
  - Noninvasive testing has a low sensitivity in **asymptomatic** patients.
  - **Simplified compression US** limited to only the common femoral vein in the groin and the popliteal vein (down to the trifurcation of the calf veins) has lower sensitivity than does a complete proximal lower extremity venous examination.
  - **Serial US testing** can improve the diagnostic yield. If a patient with a clinically suspected lower extremity DVT has a negative US of good quality, one can withhold anticoagulant therapy and repeat testing 3 to 14 days later.
  - Lower extremity venous compression US provides useful information in a patient with a suspected PE who has a nondiagnostic ventilation/perfusion (V/Q) or chest CT scan or when the clinician has a high suspicion of PE in the setting of a normal or low probability V/Q or a negative chest CT result. Detection of a proximal DVT may serve as a surrogate marker for PE, and this scenario often does not require further imaging.
- **Venography,** the gold standard technique for diagnosing DVT, has mostly been replaced by venous compression US because venography requires placement of an IV catheter, administration of iodinated contrast, and exposure to radiation. Contraindications to venography include renal dysfunction and dye allergy.
- MRI has good sensitivity for acute, symptomatic proximal DVT, but US is typically a much more practical test.
- **CT venography** testing for DVT may be done in conjunction with a contrast-enhanced PE protocol chest CT.[11] CT venography allows for visualization of the veins in the abdomen, pelvis, and proximal lower extremities, though the additional radiation burden raises concern, and lower extremity US is preferred.

PE-Specific Testing

- **Nondefinitive tests** such as ECG (e.g., sinus tachycardia; right-sided strain pattern, with characteristic S wave in lead I, Q wave in lead III, and T wave inversion in lead III; right bundle branch block), troponin and brain natriuretic peptide (BNP) levels, arterial blood gas, and chest radiography (CXR) help determine the pretest probability, focus the differential diagnosis, and assess cardiopulmonary reserve, but they do not diagnose or exclude PE.
- A negative **D-dimer** test adequately rules out PE in patients with a low clinical suspicion of PE, but patients with a moderate or high clinical suspicion should undergo imaging.

- **Contrast-enhanced spiral (helical) chest CT**
  - PE protocol chest CT requires IV administration of iodinated contrast and exposure to radiation.
  - Contraindications to PE protocol CT may include renal dysfunction and dye allergy.
  - **Multidetector CT** has better sensitivity than single-detector CT for evaluating patients with suspected PE.
  - Used according to standardized protocols in conjunction with expert interpretation, spiral CT has good accuracy for detection of large (proximal) PEs, but it has lower sensitivity for detecting small (distal) emboli.[12]
  - The **strategy combining D-dimer and chest CT** is as safe as the strategy using D-dimer followed by venous compression ultrasonography of the lower extremity and chest CT for the exclusion of PE.[13]
  - **Clinical suspicion discordant with the objective test finding** (e.g., high clinical suspicion with a negative CT scan or low clinical suspicion with a positive CT scan) **should lead to further testing**.
  - Advantages of CT scan over V/Q scan include more diagnostic results (positive or negative), with fewer indeterminate or inadequate studies, and the detection of alternative diagnoses, such as dissecting aortic aneurysm, pneumonia, and malignancy.[11]
- **V/Q scanning**
  - V/Q scanning requires administration of radioactive material (via both inhaled and IV routes).
  - V/Q scans may be classified as **normal, nondiagnostic** (i.e., very low probability, low probability, intermediate probability), or **high probability** for PE.
  - **V/Q scanning often produces a nondiagnostic result in the setting of an abnormal CXR.**
  - Use of clinical suspicion improves the accuracy of V/Q scanning; in patients with normal- or high-probability V/Q scans and matching pretest clinical suspicion, V/Q testing has a negative and positive predictive value of 96%.[14]
  - A low probability V/Q scan result combined with a low clinical suspicion of PE excludes most PE.[14]
- **MR angiography**
  - MR angiography requires IV administration of a nonionic contrast agent (e.g., gadolinium).
  - MR angiography is suboptimal for the evaluation of suspected acute PE; spiral chest CT is the preferred imaging.[15]
- **Pulmonary angiography**
  - Angiography is rarely performed for the evaluation of suspected PE because it requires placement of a pulmonary artery catheter, infusion of IV contrast, and exposure to radiation.
  - Similar to venography and PE protocol CT scanning, contraindications to angiography may include renal dysfunction and dye allergy.
- **Echocardiography** can assess cardiopulmonary reserve, evaluate for cardiac dysfunction, assess for intracardiac thrombus or clot in transit, and look for other diagnoses.

Prognostic Testing
- Several clinical factors are associated with worse prognosis of acute PE: hypoxemia, hypotension, tachycardia, acute RV strain, advanced age, cancer, chronic cardiopulmonary disease, and increased clot burden.[16]
- **Laboratory tests** such as **BNP** and **troponin** have prognostic value, though they do not rule in or rule out PE.[17]
- Combinations of **risk scores** (e.g., PE severity index [PESI], simplified PESI [sPESI], and Geneva) and diagnostic tests (e.g., troponin, BNP, echocardiography, and lower extremity venous compression US) assist with prognostication of patients with PE.[18,19]

Additional Testing

The search for an associated occult malignancy in patients with VTE should include a thorough history and physical, routine blood work, standard screening tests done according to recommended schedules (e.g., colonoscopy, mammography, Pap smear), and specific cancer screening tests indicated for distinct populations (e.g., low-dose chest CT to search for lung cancer in older patients with a significant smoking history).

TREATMENT

- **VTE therapy** should aim to prevent recurrence and extension of VTE, consequences of VTE (e.g., postphlebitic syndrome [pain, edema, and ulceration], pulmonary arterial hypertension [**PAH**], and death), and complications of therapy (e.g., bleeding and heparin-induced thrombocytopenia).
- Clinicians should perform standard baseline laboratory tests (i.e., complete blood cell count, metabolic profile, PT/INR, and aPTT) before starting anticoagulants.
- Clinicians should review each patient's medication list for drugs that could cause bleeding, clotting, or anticoagulant drug interactions.

Medications

- Unless a contraindication exists, the **initial treatment of VTE should consist of anticoagulation,** with unfractionated heparin (**UFH**), low molecular weight heparin (**LMWH**), pentasaccharide (fondaparinux), or a new oral anticoagulant **(Table 14-1).**
- IV UFH is usually reserved for inpatient treatment of VTE.
- SC LMWH, fondaparinux, or UFH and oral anticoagulants facilitate outpatient therapy, though SC drugs require the necessary training and resources for successful injection.
- Warfarin or other coumarins should not be used without initially overlapping with a more rapid acting anticoagulant.
- In general, the **oral factor Xa and factor IIa inhibitors** have similar efficacy and mortality risks when compared to traditional VTE therapy. However, the studies excluded

TABLE 14-1	Initial Treatment of Venous Thromboembolism
Drug	**Dosage**
UFH[a]	IV Heparin nomogram
	333 U/kg SC, followed by a fixed dose of 250 U/kg q12 hours
	Adjusted dose SC
Enoxaparin	1 mg/kg SC q12 hours or 1.5 mg/kg SC q24 hours
Tinzaparin	175 IU/kg SC daily
Dalteparin[a]	200 IU/kg SC daily for month 1, followed by 150 IU/kg SC
Fondaparinux	5 mg SC daily for weight <50 kg,
	7.5 mg SC daily for weight 50–100 kg,
	10 mg SC daily for weight >100 kg
Apixaban	10 mg PO bid for 7 days, and then 5 mg PO bid
Rivaroxaban	15 mg PO bid for 21 days, and then 20 mg PO daily
Dabigatran	150 mg PO bid after LMWH SC or UFH IV for 5–11 days

[a]Not an FDA-approved indication.
IU, anti-Xa units; for enoxaparin, 1 mg = 100 anti-Xa units.
Caution with the use of fondaparinux, tinzaparin, dalteparin, or enoxaparin for pregnancy, morbid obesity, or end-stage renal disease (CrCl <30 mL/minute); anti-Xa level monitoring is recommended in these settings.

patients that used drugs that may affect factor Xa and IIa inhibitor metabolism or elimination. Though rarely needed, the inability to reverse oral factor Xa and factor IIa inhibitors in the event of major or life-threatening bleeding raises additional concerns. Warfarin and other coumarins have a lower price and longer half-lives than the oral factor Xa and factor IIa inhibitors.

Unfractionated Heparin

- **UFH** comes from porcine intestinal mucosa, and it mainly works indirectly by catalyzing the inactivation of thrombin and factor Xa by antithrombin.
- At usual doses, UFH prolongs the thrombin time and aPTT and has a small effect on the PT/INR.
- Because the anticoagulant effects of UFH normalize within hours of discontinuation and **protamine sulfate** reverses it even faster, UFH is the anticoagulant of choice for patients with increased risk of bleeding.
- Abnormal renal function does not typically affect UFH dosing.
- For **therapeutic anticoagulation,** UFH is usually administered IV with a bolus followed by continuous infusion, but this is almost exclusively done in the inpatient setting.
- **Treatment doses of UFH may be administered SC**, initial dose of 333 U/kg SC, followed by a fixed unmonitored dose of 250 U/kg every 12 hours.[20] However, this regimen requires large-dose injections and is used infrequently.
- **Monitored and adjusted SC UFH** may be used to treat VTE, but this is not commonly done since many easier and potentially better alternatives exist. In addition, the therapeutic range (approximately 60 to 90 seconds) for aPTT is not standardized.

Low Molecular Weight Heparin

- **LMWHs** are produced by chemical or enzymatic cleavage of UFH, and they have a similar mechanism of action as UFH.
- Since LMWHs inactivate factor Xa to a greater extent than they do to thrombin (factor IIa), LWMHs minimally prolong the aPTT.
- Extensive clinical trials have confirmed the efficacy and safety of weight-based SC LMWH for the treatment of VTE.
- **Factor Xa monitoring is not recommended**, except in special circumstances where dose adjustments may be necessary, such as renal dysfunction, morbid obesity, cachexia, and pregnancy. Peak factor Xa levels, measured 4 hours after an SC dose, should be 0.6 to 1 IU/mL for q12-hour dosing and 1 to 2 IU/mL for q24-hour dosing.[21]
- Different LMWH preparations have different dosing recommendations **(Table 14-1)**.
- **Given the renal clearance of LMWHs, they are generally avoided in patients undergoing dialysis**.
- **Patients with a CrCl of 15 to 30 mL/minute** require dose adjustments (e.g., enoxaparin 1 mg/kg once daily instead of twice daily).
- **Patients with cancer** may have reduced recurrent VTE when treated long-term with LMWH rather than warfarin (or other coumarins). For example, subcutaneous dalteparin at dose of 200 IU/kg daily for 1 month, followed by a daily dose of 150 IU/kg, has been used successfully in patients with VTE and cancer.[22]
- **Protamine only partially reverses LMWH**.

Fondaparinux

- Fondaparinux, a **synthetic pentasaccharide that is structurally similar to a region of the heparin molecule, binds antithrombin** and functions as a selective indirect inhibitor of factor Xa.
- Because fondaparinux inhibits factor Xa and does not inhibit thrombin, it does not significantly prolong the aPTT.
- Large clinical trials have confirmed the efficacy and safety of weight-based subcutaneously dosed fondaparinux for the treatment of VTE.[23,24]

- Similar to the LMWHs, fondaparinux does not require **factor Xa monitoring,** except for patients with significant renal dysfunction.
- The recommended dose for VTE therapy ranges from 5 to 10 mg SC daily, depending on weight **(Table 14-1)**.[23,24]

Oral Direct Xa Inhibitors
- As compared to warfarin, the oral direct (i.e., do not require antithrombin) factor Xa inhibitors **rivaroxaban** and **apixaban** have a faster onset, shorter half-life, wider therapeutic window, and more predictable pharmacokinetics.
- In general, the features of the oral direct factor Xa inhibitors allow for fixed dosing without INR monitoring, though they may increase the INR and aPTT in a nonlinear fashion.
- Since both rivaroxaban and apixaban are **substrates of cytochrome P450 (CYP) 3A4,** strong inhibitors (e.g., clarithromycin) and inducers (e.g., St. John's wort) alter plasma concentrations.

Rivaroxaban
- The dose of oral **rivaroxaban** for acute VTE is 15 mg twice daily × 3 weeks, then 20 mg daily. **Therapy can be started at the time of diagnosis, without concomitant use of UFH or LMWH**. Therapy can also begin after transition from initial treatment with a parenteral agent (e.g., IV UFH).
- Rivaroxaban has similar efficacy and safety compared to therapy with subcutaneous enoxaparin and an oral vitamin K antagonist.[25,26]
- After 6 to 12 months of standard VTE treatment, continued treatment with rivaroxaban 20 mg PO daily compared to placebo for 6 to 12 additional months decreased the annual risk of symptomatic VTE recurrence by 82%, with a modest increase in hemorrhage.[25]
- Rivaroxaban's **predominant renal elimination** led to exclusion of patients with estimated CrCl <30 mL/minute from VTE treatment trials.
- Rivaroxaban is a substrate of the efflux transporter **P-glycoprotein** (Pgp), so concurrent use with drugs that interact with Pgp may lead to greater (e.g., amiodarone) or lesser (e.g., St. John's wort) rivaroxaban exposure.

Apixaban
- **Apixaban** has recently been approved by the FDA for VTE treatment (10 mg PO bid × 7 days, then 5 mg PO bid).
- Apixaban has similar efficacy to standard enoxaparin/warfarin therapy, but causes less bleeding.[27]
- After 6 to 12 months of standard VTE treatment, extended-duration treatment (12-month duration) with apixaban at a dose of either 5 mg or 2.5 mg twice daily decreased the annual risk of symptomatic VTE recurrence by about 80%, with a minimal increase in hemorrhage.[28]
- Apixaban has **limited renal elimination** but treatment trials excluded patients with an estimated CrCl <25 mL/minute.

Oral Direct Thrombin Inhibitors
Dabigatran
- Compared with warfarin, dabigatran has a more rapid onset, shorter half-life, wider therapeutic window, and more predictable pharmacokinetics.
- In general, dabigatran's features allow for oral anticoagulant therapy with fixed dosing without INR monitoring, though dabigatran may increase the INR, aPTT, and thrombin time in a nonlinear fashion.
- Compared with warfarin, studies suggest that dabigatran has a lower risk of intracranial (but not gastrointestinal) hemorrhage but a higher risk of myocardial infarction.[29–31]
- Dabigatran does not have FDA approval for VTE treatment in the United States, though it has approval in other countries (150 mg PO bid after LMWH or UFH for 5 to 11 days).

- After 6 to 18 months of standard VTE treatment, continued treatment with dabigatran (150 mg PO bid) compared to placebo for 6 additional months decreased the risk of VTE recurrence by 92%, with a modest increase in hemorrhage.[30]
- Dabigatran's **highly predominant renal elimination** led to exclusion of patients with estimated CrCl <30 mL/minute from dabigatran trials.
- Dabigatran is not a substrate, inhibitor, or inducer of CYP3A4. However, dabigatran is a substrate of the **efflux transporter Pgp**, and concurrent use with drugs that interact with Pgp leads to greater (e.g., dronedarone or amiodarone) or lesser (e.g., St. John's wort) dabigatran exposure.

Warfarin

- The oral anticoagulant warfarin **inhibits reduction of vitamin K to its active form** and leads to depletion of the vitamin K–dependent clotting factors II, VII, IX, and X and proteins C, S, and Z (see Fig. 12-1).
- Although warfarin has good oral absorption, it requires 4 to 5 days to achieve full anticoagulant effect.
  - The initial INR rise primarily reflects warfarin-related depletion of factor VII; the depletion of factor II takes several days due to its relatively long half-life.
  - Because of the warfarin-related rapid depletion of the anticoagulant protein C and a slower onset of its anticoagulant effect, patients may develop increased hypercoagulability during the first few days of warfarin therapy if warfarin is not combined with a parenteral anticoagulant.[32]
- The **starting dose** of warfarin depends upon factors such as age, size, concomitant drug use, and polymorphisms.[33] The starting dose ranges from approximately 3 mg in older or petite patients to 10 mg in young, robust outpatients. Patients with polymorphisms in genes for CYP2C9 or vitamin K epoxide reductase (VKORC1) may benefit from cautious low-dose warfarin initiation.[34]
- For most indications, such as VTE, warfarin has a **target INR of 2.5 and a therapeutic range** of 2 to 3, though patients with **mitral mechanical heart valves** should receive a higher level of anticoagulation (e.g., INR target range, 2.5 to 3.5). See Table 14-2.
- **Treatment of DVT/PE with warfarin requires overlap therapy with a faster acting anticoagulant** (UFH, LMWH, pentasaccharide, or rivaroxaban) **for at least 4.5 days and until patients achieve an INR of at least 2.0 for 2 days.**[35,36]
- **Warfarin nomogram dosing** has more success than does nonstandardized dosing.
- **INR monitoring** should occur frequently during the first month of therapy (e.g., twice weekly for 1 to 2 weeks, then weekly for 2 weeks, and then less frequently). Typical dose adjustments after the first few weeks of therapy change the weekly dose by 10% to 25%.

TABLE 14-2	**Anticoagulation with Artificial Heart Valves**	
Material	**Type/location**	**INR target**
Tissue	Aortic	ASA 325 mg lifelong; warfarin is an option for the initial 3–6 months.
	Mitral	INR 2.5 for 3 months, then ASA 325 mg lifelong
Mechanical[a]	St. Jude aortic	2.5 + low-dose ASA
	St. Jude mitral	3 + low-dose ASA
	Caged ball/caged disc	3 + lose-dose ASA

[a]Add ASA for any caged valve, known or suspected coronary artery disease, h/o prior stroke, or mitral valve repair.
ASA, acetylsalicylic acid; INR, international normalized ratio.

Subsequent dose adjustments should be smaller, with no dose adjustments needed for INRs that are in the therapeutic range (2 to 3).

○ Patients receiving a stable warfarin dose often have INR monitoring monthly. However, patients with labile INRs should have more frequent monitoring (e.g., weekly). Selected, stable patients can have INRs monitored every 6 to 12 weeks.[37]

○ The addition or discontinuation of **medications that affect warfarin**, especially antifungal agents or sulfa antibiotics, should trigger more frequent INR monitoring and may require dose adjustments of >25%.

○ In eligible patients, **home monitoring on point-of-care devices** can decrease adverse events.[38]

○ Compliant patients who have unacceptable INR lability, or those with LA and an elevated baseline INR, may benefit from long-term anticoagulation with an agent other than warfarin.

Other Treatments

• Select patients may benefit from **thrombolytic therapy**, catheter embolectomy, and emergency surgical thrombectomy, but these are inpatient issues.[35,36]

• **Inferior vena cava (IVC) filters** are used for acute VTE when there are **absolute contraindications to anticoagulation** (e.g., active bleeding, severe thrombocytopenia, or urgent surgery) or **recurrent PE despite therapeutic anticoagulation**.

○ Although prophylactic IVC filters in anticoagulated patients with acute DVT/PE reduce the risk of recurrent PE, a reduction in overall mortality has not been demonstrated, and they increase DVT recurrence.[39,40]

○ Relative indications for IVC filters include primary or metastatic CNS cancer or limited cardiopulmonary reserve after a PE.

○ Patients who had an IVC filter placed because of a temporary contraindication to anticoagulation should receive standard-duration anticoagulation when safe (to reduce the risk of filter-related thromboses and recurrent VTE).[35,36]

○ Several types of removable IVC filters exist and can provide a temporary barrier against emboli from the lower extremities, but filter removal requires a second procedure.

• **Leg elevation** reduces edema associated with DVT.

• **Ambulation** is encouraged for patients with DVT, especially after improvement of pain and edema, though strenuous lower extremity activity should initially be avoided.

• **Fitted graduated compression stockings** help to reduce the high incidence of postphlebitic syndrome in patients with lower extremity DVT.

• **Superficial vein thrombosis (SVT)**

○ **Oral NSAIDs** and **warm compresses** can relieve discomfort.

○ For **infusion thrombophlebitis** (superficial thrombophlebitis associated with a peripheral IV), anticoagulant therapy generally is not used.[35]

○ For patients with **spontaneous SVT**, treatment with low-dose LMWH (e.g., enoxaparin 40 mg SQ qd) for 8 to 12 days or fondaparinux 2.5 mg PO qd for 45 days may lower the short-term incidence of additional thrombosis.[36,41]

○ **Extensive SVT** can be treated with a prophylactic dose of fondaparinux for about 6 weeks.[35,36]

○ **Recurrent SVT** may be treated with anticoagulation.

○ **Surgical therapy** (with ligation of the saphenofemoral junction or stripping of thrombosed superficial veins) of SVT appears to be associated with higher rates of VTE than treatment with anticoagulants.[35,36]

• **Catheter-associated upper extremity DVT** does not necessarily require catheter removal if it is functional.[35]

Duration of Anticoagulation

• **Duration of anticoagulation** depends on patient preferences and values and the risk of recurrent VTE off anticoagulant therapy versus the added risk of bleeding complications from continued anticoagulation.[35,36]

- Patients with a **first episode of VTE provoked by surgical or nonsurgical transient risk factors** have a low risk of recurrence (<6%/year) after completing 3 months of anticoagulation.[35,36]
- Three months of anticoagulant therapy is also sufficient for patients with a **first episode of idiopathic VTE** associated with other transient risk factors, such as prolonged travel, minor injury, or oral contraceptive pills/hormone replacement therapy that has been stopped.[35,36]
- For patients with **unprovoked proximal lower extremity DVT or PE**, at least 3 months of anticoagulation should be prescribed.[35,36] Longer (extended) duration of anticoagulant therapy with warfarin (target INR of 2 to 3 or 1.5 to 2), apixaban (either 5 or 2.5 mg, twice daily), rivaroxaban (20 mg PO q day), or dabigatran (150 mg PO bid) reduces the relative risk of recurrent VTE, but it increases the risk of bleeding.[28,30]
- Patients with **cancer and VTE** should receive anticoagulation for more than 3 months and possibly until cancer resolution or development of a contraindication.[35,36]
- For patients with **a first VTE and one inherited hypercoagulable risk factor**, duration of anticoagulation depends on the type **of thrombophilia.**[36]
  - **Heterozygous factor V Leiden** and **heterozygous prothrombin 20210A** do not necessitate long-term therapy because they increase the odds of VTE recurrence modestly (approximately 1.5-fold).[42]
  - **Deficiency of protein S, protein C, or antithrombin** carries a high risk of recurrence, which necessitates long-term anticoagulation.[42]
- Patients with a **first VTE and antiphospholipid antibodies or two inherited risk factors** should receive a longer course of anticoagulation (e.g., 12 months), and indefinite therapy should be considered.
- Patients with **isolated calf DVT** or **upper extremity DVT** should typically receive standard-duration (e.g., 3 months) anticoagulation.[35,36]
- Patients with **recurrent idiopathic VTE** should receive extended-duration (more than 3 months) anticoagulation, possibly indefinitely, unless a contraindication develops, or patient preferences dictate otherwise.[35,36]
- Patients with a history of VTE, especially those with ongoing risk factors, should possibly receive temporary prophylactic anticoagulation during periods of increased VTE risk (e.g., prolonged air travel).[36]
- After completing the course of anticoagulant therapy, aspirin (e.g., 81 mg) use should be strongly considered to decrease the risk of recurrent VTE and acute coronary syndrome.[43]

SPECIAL CONSIDERATIONS

- **Outpatient VTE therapy**
  - Patients selected for **outpatient DVT therapy** should have no other indications for hospitalization (i.e., other problems or complications of VTE), adequate cardiopulmonary reserve, adequate instruction and understanding of the signs of bleeding and VTE recurrence, access to a telephone, ability to receive the anticoagulant, and adequate outpatient follow-up.[44]
  - Patients selected for outpatient PE therapy should have a low-risk classification and should meet eligibility criteria similar to those used for outpatient DVT therapy.[45]
  - **Pregnant** women with VTE (and without artificial heart valves) may undergo **long-term anticoagulation with SC LMWH, fondaparinux, or UFH,** and those who receive LMWH or fondaparinux should undergo factor Xa level monitoring.[46]
  - **Pregnant** women with VTE should **avoid warfarin and the oral thrombin and factor Xa inhibitors. Warfarin is contraindicated in the first trimester of pregnancy** because of its **teratogenicity,** and it is often avoided later in pregnancy because of the risk of fetal bleeding, but it is safe for infants of nursing mothers.

- For **failure of oral warfarin or other vitamin K antagonists**, with confirmed new VTE despite consistently therapeutic INRs, consider prescribing a different anticoagulant.

COMPLICATIONS/RISK MANAGEMENT

Bleeding

- **Major bleeding** occurs in 2% to 3% of patients who receive short-term anticoagulant therapy for VTE. The risk of intracranial hemorrhage is probably lower with oral thrombin and factor Xa inhibitors than with vitamin K antagonists. Antiplatelet agents used concomitantly with any anticoagulant nearly double the risk of bleeding.
- **Major bleeding in a patient with an acute VTE should lead to the discontinuation of anticoagulation.**[35,36]
- **Asymptomatic INR elevation on warfarin**
  - Asymptomatic minor INR elevations of >3.4 and <5 should be managed by holding or reducing warfarin dose until the INR falls to a safe level and then resuming warfarin at a lower dose.
  - Moderate (INR $\geq$5 but <9) elevation of the INR in asymptomatic patients should be treated by holding one or more warfarin doses. Treatment with oral vitamin K_1 1 to 5 mg probably does not reduce the risk of hemorrhage in this setting (as compared with warfarin cessation alone) but lowers the INR (Table 14-3).[47]
  - Severe (INR >9) elevation of the INR should be treated with vitamin K (e.g., oral vitamin K_1 2 to 10 mg) unless the INR is likely to be spurious (Table 14-3).[48]
- **General approach to bleeding with anticoagulants**
  - Stop the anticoagulant and other drugs (e.g., antiplatelet agents) that may exacerbate bleeding.
  - Provide supportive interventions (e.g., IV fluid, compression of bleeding site, surgery).
  - Check coagulation tests to see effect of the drug on board, follow CBC, and check CMP.
  - Red blood cell transfusion for anemia and platelet transfusion for patients on antiplatelet agents as needed.
- Anticoagulant-specific approaches may also be necessary.
- **Bleeding with warfarin (Table 14-3)**[49]:
  - **Prothrombin complex concentrate** (PCC), or **fresh frozen plasma** (FFP) if PCC not available, should be given to treat major bleeding associated with warfarin therapy.[50,51]
  - **Vitamin K** (e.g., 10 mg) by slow IV infusion should be given for serious hemorrhages caused by a high INR. Because of the long half-life of warfarin (approximately 36 hours, depending on CYP2C9 genotype), vitamin K should be repeated every 8 to 12 hours to prevent INR rebound.
- **Bleeding with UFH**
  - Stopping UFH usually restores hemostasis within a few hours.
  - With moderate-to-severe bleeding, give **FFP**.
  - For patients receiving UFH who develop major bleeding or have an UFH overdose, UFH can be completely reversed by infusion of **protamine sulfate** in situations where the potential benefits outweigh the risks (e.g., intracranial bleed, epidural hematoma, and retinal bleed).
  - After IV administration, UFH serum concentrations decline rapidly because of a short half-life, so only the UFH administered in the last 2 to 3 hours needs to be reversed with **protamine sulfate**.
  - **Approximately 1-mg protamine sulfate IV neutralizes 100 U of UFH**, up to a maximum dose of 250 mg.
- **Bleeding with LMWH**
  - With moderate-to-severe bleeding, give **FFP**.
  - **For major bleeding associated with LWMH**, protamine sulfate has less efficacy compared with its effect on UFH since it neutralizes only approximately 60% of LMWH.[52]

TABLE 14-3 Treatment of Elevated INR >5

Bleeding	INR	Action
None	5–9	Stop the anticoagulant; consider stopping other drugs (e.g., antiplatelet agents) that may exacerbate bleeding. Evaluate for food and drug interactions and for dosing or laboratory errors. Repeat INR in 1–4 days. If INR rising or at high risk for bleeding, give vitamin K 1–2.5 mg PO.
None	>9	Stop the anticoagulant and other drugs (e.g., antiplatelet agents) that may exacerbate bleeding. Evaluate for food and drug interactions and for dosing or laboratory errors. Repeat INR in 12–24 hours and in 48 hours. Vitamin K 2–10 mg PO; repeat vitamin K as needed.
Minor	Any	Stop the anticoagulant and other drugs (e.g., antiplatelet agents) that may exacerbate bleeding. Vitamin K 1–5 mg PO or IVPB INR q8–24 hours; repeat vitamin K as needed. If bleeding not controlled in 24 hours, treat as major bleeding.
Major	Any	Stop the anticoagulant and other drugs (e.g., antiplatelet agents) that may exacerbate bleeding. Provide supportive interventions (e.g., IV fluid, compression of bleeding site, surgery). PRBC transfusion for anemia, and PLT transfusion for severe thrombocytopenia or patients on antiplatelet agents, as needed Vitamin K 10 mg IV over 10–20 minutes If INR <4 (but elevated), then either 3-factor or 4-factor PCC should be given to the patient with major bleeding. For example, 35–39 IU/kg of a 3-factor PCC[60] If INR >4, then a 4-factor PCC will better replete factor VII.[61] The dose of PCC depends on the INR and formulation. For example, 35 IU/kg Kcentra (up to 3,500 IU) is recommended for an INR of 4–6. FFP (2–3 U) should be used when PCC is not available. Repeat INR in 6–12 hours, and continue vitamin K and PCC (or FFP) until INR remains normal AND bleeding has stopped.

FFP, fresh frozen plasma; INR, international normalized ratio; PCC, prothrombin complex concentrate; PLT, platelets; PRBC, packed red blood cells.

- **Bleeding with fondaparinux**
  - With moderate-to-severe bleeding, give **FFP**.
  - **For patients with very serious bleeding receiving fondaparinux,** give concentrated factor VIIa (up to 90 mcg/kg) and tranexamic acid (1-mg IV), but these agents can cause serious thrombosis.[53]
- **Bleeding with oral direct thrombin inhibitor (dabigatran)**[54]
  - An increase in the thrombin time (and INR and aPTT) may indicate dabigatran ingestion, but the coagulation tests do not indicate the degree of anticoagulation.
  - Determine amount consumed and timing of the last dose. Consider activated charcoal within 2 hours of last dose.

- ○ Consider dialysis for severe bleeding or overdose (especially with renal failure).
- ○ Consider using PCC for severe bleeding (limited data).
- **Bleeding with oral factor Xa antagonists**[54]
  - ○ An increase in the INR or aPTT may indicate a factor Xa antagonist ingestion, though the coagulation tests do not indicate the degree of anticoagulation.
  - ○ Consider using PCC for severe bleeding (limited data).

Other Complications

- **Occult gastrointestinal or genitourinary bleeding** is a relative and not absolute contraindication to anticoagulation, though its presence warrants investigation.
- **Warfarin-induced skin necrosis,** associated with rapid depletion of protein C, may occur during initiation of warfarin therapy.[32] Necrosis occurs most often in areas with a high percentage of adipose tissue, such as breast tissue, and it can be life threatening. Therapeutic anticoagulation with an immediate-acting anticoagulant (UFH, LMWH, etc.) and/or avoidance of loading doses of warfarin may prevent warfarin-induced skin necrosis.
- If possible, **anticoagulants should be avoided in patients about to undergo neuraxial procedures** (lumbar puncture, epidural/spinal anesthesia, and epidural catheter removal) because of the risk of development of **epidural hematomas and subsequent spinal cord compression** and paralysis.[55]
- **Osteoporosis** may occur with long-term heparin or warfarin use.[56]

Perioperative Management of Anticoagulants

- **Minor elective procedures** (including uncomplicated dental extractions, skin biopsies, placement of pacemakers, and cataract extraction) **can be done without cessation of anticoagulant therapy.**[57]
- Perioperative management of anticoagulation requires coordination with the surgeon (see Chapter 2).
- **Invasive procedures** typically benefit from discontinuation of anticoagulant therapy.
  - ○ **Warfarin**
    - Cessation for 5 days results in an INR ≤1.4 in most patients. However, patients taking >3 mg/day may require 6 days until the INR declines ≤1.4. If an INR of around 1.7 is acceptable for the procedure, the warfarin dose can be halved for 4 days preoperatively.[58]
    - To minimize time without therapeutic anticoagulation, UFH or LMWH or fondaparinux SC **bridging preprocedure therapy** can be initiated when the INR becomes subtherapeutic (e.g., 3 days after the last warfarin dose). In pregnant women with a mechanical heart valve, IV UFH appears safer than LMWH or fondaparinux.
    - After the procedure, resume warfarin (with or without UFH and LMW heparin, depending on the risks of bleeding and thrombosis).
  - ○ **UFH, LMWH, and fondaparinux.** Depending on the half-life of the anticoagulant, renal function (for LMWH and fondaparinux), and dosing frequency, stopping UFH for 6 hours, LMWH for 12 to 24 hours, and fondaparinux for 12 to 48 hours before an invasive procedure is usually adequate.
  - ○ **Oral direct thrombin inhibitor (dabigatran)**
    - Cessation of the oral direct thrombin inhibitor dabigatran for 24 to 48 hours should allow for invasive procedures in patients with normal bleeding risk whose Cr clearance is >50 mL/minute. With high bleeding risk or lower Cr clearance, 2 to 5 days of cessation may be necessary.[59]
    - Temporary interruption of dabigatran can cause stroke in patients who have atrial fibrillation.

- **Oral direct factor Xa inhibitors (rivaroxaban or apixaban)**
  - Cessation for 24 hours should allow for invasive procedures in patients whose Cr clearance >30 mL/minute.
  - With lower Cr clearance, rivaroxaban's half-life is prolonged and 2-day cessation is necessary.[59]

FOLLOW-UP

- In the case of a suspicious clinical presentation, **testing for intrinsic hypercoagulable risk factors** of the coagulation cascade ideally should wait until the patient is in stable health.[1] Hypercoagulable testing is not recommended for most patients with VTE.
  - **LA** testing can be done in the acute setting. A positive LA test result should be rechecked for persistent positivity at a later date.
  - Genetic testing for the **prothrombin gene mutation and factor V Leiden** can be done at any time.
  - Testing for **protein C, protein S, and antithrombin** deficiency or low activity can occur before initiating anticoagulation, but an acute thrombosis can depress their levels. Some anticoagulants may also affect these protein levels. Because proteins C and S are vitamin K dependent, levels should not be assessed during warfarin therapy.
- For patients with suspected lower extremity DVT, an initial negative compression ultrasound, and no satisfactory alternative explanation, serial compression ultrasonography in 3 to 14 days improves the diagnostic yield.
- If patient preferences or contraindications lead to the withholding of anticoagulant therapy for **calf DVT,** we recommend further evaluation with **a repeat compression ultrasonography** to assess for proximal extension, which would mandate therapy.
- Testing for PE in patients with DVT and testing for DVT in patients with PE will produce many positive findings, but such test results rarely affect therapy. However, baseline results may provide comparison data for patients who return with symptoms of VTE, though studies have not determined the cost-effectiveness of this practice.
- Prolongation of anticoagulation in patients with residual thrombosis on **compression ultrasonography at the end of standard duration anticoagulation** for proximal DVT reduces VTE recurrence but can cause hemorrhage.[60]
- Repeated **elevation of D-dimer at the end of standard duration anticoagulation** for a first episode of unprovoked VTE is associated with an increased risk of recurrence, though limited data exist regarding extension of anticoagulation duration based on D-dimer test results.[61]

REFERENCES

1. Seligsohn U, Lubetsky A. Genetic susceptibility to venous thrombosis. *N Engl J Med* 2001;344:1222–1231.
2. Miyakis S, Lockshin MD, Atsumi T, et al. International consensus statement on an update of the classification criteria for definite antiphospholipid syndrome (APS). *J Thromb Haemost* 2006;4:295–306.
3. Wells PS, Anderson DR, Bormanis J, et al. Value of assessment of pretest probability of deep-vein thrombosis in clinical management. *Lancet* 1997;350:1795–1798.
4. Stein PD, Beemath A, Matta F, et al. Clinical characteristics of patients with acute pulmonary embolism: data from PIOPED II. *Am J Med* 2007;120:871–879.
5. Wells PS, Anderson DR, Rodger M, et al. Excluding pulmonary embolism at the bedside without diagnostic imaging: management of patients with suspected pulmonary embolism presenting to the emergency department by using a simple clinical model and D-dimer. *Ann Intern Med* 2001;135:98–107.

6. Stein PD, Hull RD, Patel KC, et al. D-dimer for the exclusion of acute venous thrombosis and pulmonary embolism: a systematic review. *Ann Intern Med* 2004;140:589–602.

7. Wells PS, Owen C, Doucette S, et al. Does this patient have deep vein thrombosis? *JAMA* 2006;295:199–207.

8. Douma RA, Mos IC, Erkens PM, et al. Performance of 4 clinical decision rules in the diagnostic management of acute pulmonary embolism: a prospective cohort study. *Ann Intern Med* 2011;154:709–718.

9. Lee AY, Julian JA, Levine MN, et al. Clinical utility of a rapid whole-blood D-dimer assay in patients with cancer who present with suspected acute deep venous thrombosis. *Ann Intern Med* 1999;131:417–423.

10. Tapson VF, Carroll BA, Davidson BL, et al. The diagnostic approach to acute venous thromboembolism. Clinical practice guideline. American Thoracic Society. *Am J Respir Crit Care Med* 1999;160:1043–1066.

11. Stein PD, Fowler SE, Goodman LR, et al.; PIOPED II Investigators. Multidetector computed tomography for acute pulmonary embolism. *N Engl J Med* 2006;354:2317–2327.

12. Brotman DJ. Computed tomography for pulmonary embolism. *N Engl J Med* 2006;355:955.

13. Righini M, Le Gal G, Aujesky D, et al. Diagnosis of pulmonary embolism by multidetector CT alone or combined with venous ultrasonography of the leg: a randomised non-inferiority trial. *Lancet* 2008;371:1343–1352.

14. The PIOPED Investigators. Value of the ventilation/perfusion scan in acute pulmonary embolism. Results of the prospective investigation of pulmonary embolism diagnosis (PIOPED). *JAMA* 1990;263:2753–2759.

15. Stein PD, Chenevert TL, Fowler SE, et al. Gadolinium-enhanced magnetic resonance angiography for pulmonary embolism: a multicenter prospective study (PIOPED III). *Ann Intern Med* 2010;152:434–443.

16. Jiménez D, Aujesky D, Díaz G, et al. Prognostic significance of deep vein thrombosis in patients presenting with acute symptomatic pulmonary embolism. *Am J Respir Crit Care Med* 2010;181:983–991.

17. Lega JC, Lacasse Y, Lakhal L, et al. Natriuretic peptides and troponins in pulmonary embolism: a meta-analysis. *Thorax* 2009;64:869–875.

18. Jiménez D, Aujesky D, Moores L, et al. Combinations of prognostic tools for identification of high-risk normotensive patients with acute symptomatic pulmonary embolism. *Thorax* 2011;66:75–81.

19. Jiménez D, Aujesky D, Yusen RD. Risk stratification of normotensive patients with acute symptomatic pulmonary embolism. *Br J Haematol* 2010;151:415–424.

20. Kearon C, Ginsberg JS, Julian JA, et al.; Fixed-Dose Heparin (FIDO) Investigators. Comparison of fixed-dose weight-adjusted unfractionated heparin and low-molecular-weight heparin for acute treatment of venous thromboembolism. *JAMA* 2006;296:935–942.

21. Hirsh J, Lee AY. How we diagnose and treat deep vein thrombosis. *Blood* 2002;99:3102–3110.

22. Lee AY, Levine MN, Baker RI, et al. Low-molecular-weight heparin versus a coumarin for the prevention of recurrent venous thromboembolism in patients with cancer. *N Engl J Med* 2003;349:146–153.

23. Büller HR, Davidson BL, Decousus H, et al.; Matisse Investigators. Subcutaneous fondaparinux versus intravenous unfractionated heparin in the initial treatment of pulmonary embolism. *N Engl J Med* 2003;349:695–702.

24. Büller HR, Davidson BL, Decousus H, et al.; Matisse Investigators. Fondaparinux or enoxaparin for the initial treatment of symptomatic deep venous thrombosis: a randomized trial. *Ann Intern Med* 2004;140:867–873.

25. EINSTEIN Investigators; Bauersachs R, Berkowitz SD, et al. Oral rivaroxaban for symptomatic venous thromboembolism. *N Engl J Med* 2010;363:2499–2510.

26. EINSTEIN–PE Investigators, Büller HR, Prins MH, et al. Oral rivaroxaban for the treatment of symptomatic pulmonary embolism. *N Engl J Med* 2012;366:1287–1297.
27. Agnelli G, Buller HR, Cohen A, et al. Oral apixaban for the treatment of acute venous thromboembolism. *N Engl J Med* 2013;369:799–808.
28. Agnelli G, Buller HR, Cohen AN, et al. Apixaban for extended treatment of venous thromboembolism. *N Engl J Med* 2013;368:699–708.
29. Schulman S, Kearon C, Kakkar AK, et al. Dabigatran versus warfarin in the treatment of acute venous thromboembolism. *N Engl J Med* 2009;361:2342–2352.
30. Schulman S, Kearon C, Kakkar AK, et al. Extended use of dabigatran, warfarin, or placebo in venous thromboembolism. *N Engl J Med* 2013;368:709–718.
31. Larsen TB, Rasmussen LH, Skjøth F, et al. Efficacy and safety of dabigatran etexilate and warfarin in "real-world" patients with atrial fibrillation: a prospective nationwide cohort study. *J Am Coll Cardiol* 2013;61:2264–2273.
32. Sallah S, Thomas DP, Roberts HR. Warfarin and heparin-induced skin necrosis and the purple toe syndrome: infrequent complications of anticoagulant treatment. *Thromb Haemost* 1997;78:785–790.
33. Washington University in St. Louis. Warfarin Dosing. Last accessed December 22, 2014. http://www.warfarindosing.org/Source/Home.aspx
34. Crowther MA, Harrison L, Hirsh J. Reply: warfarin: less may be better. *Ann Intern Med* 1997;127:333.
35. Kearon C, Akl EA, Comerota AJ, et al. Antithrombotic therapy for VTE disease: antithrombotic therapy and prevention of thrombosis, 9th ed: American College of Chest Physicians Evidence-Based Clinical Practice Guidelines. *Chest* 2012;141:e419S–e494S.
36. Nicolaides A, Hull RD, Fareed J. Prevention and treatment of venous thromboembolism: international consensus statement (guidelines according to scientific evidence). *Clin Appl Thromb Hemost* 2013;19:116–231.
37. Schulman S, Parpia S, Stewart C, et al. Warfarin dose assessment every 4 weeks versus every 12 weeks in patients with stable international normalized ratios: a randomized trial. *Ann Intern Med* 2011;155:653–659.
38. Matchar DB, Jacobson A, Dolor R, et al. Effect of home testing of international normalized ratio on clinical events. *N Engl J Med* 2010;363:1608–1620.
39. Decousus H, Leizorovicz A, Parent F, et al. A clinical trial of vena caval filters in the prevention of pulmonary embolism in patients with proximal deep-vein thrombosis. Prévention du Risque d'Embolie Pulmonaire par Interruption Cave Study Group. *N Engl J Med* 1998;338:409–415.
40. PREPIC Study Group. Eight-year follow-up of patients with permanent vena cava filters in the prevention of pulmonary embolism: the PREPIC (Prevention du Risque d'Embolie Pulmonaire par Interruption Cave) randomized study. *Circulation* 2005;112:416–422.
41. Superficial Thrombophlebitis Treated By Enoxaparin Study Group. A pilot randomized double-blind comparison of a low-molecular-weight heparin, a nonsteroidal anti-inflammatory agent, and placebo in the treatment of superficial vein thrombosis. *Arch Intern Med* 2003;163:1657–1663.
42. Segal JB, Brotman DJ, Necochea AJ, et al. Predictive value of factor V Leiden and prothrombin G20210A in adults with venous thromboembolism and in family members of those with a mutation: a systematic review. *JAMA* 2009;301:2472–2485.
43. Brighton TA, Eikelboom JW, Mann K, et al. Low-dose aspirin for preventing recurrent venous thromboembolism. *N Engl J Med* 2012;367:1979–1987.
44. Yusen RD, Haraden BM, Gage BF, et al. Criteria for outpatient management of proximal lower extremity deep venous thrombosis. *Chest* 1999;115:972–979.
45. Aujesky D, Roy PM, Verschuren F, et al. Outpatient versus inpatient treatment for patients with acute pulmonary embolism: an international, open-label, randomised, non-inferiority trial. *Lancet* 2011;378:41–48.

46. Bates SM, Greer IA, Middeldorp S, et al. VTE, thrombophilia, antithrombotic therapy, and pregnancy: antithrombotic therapy and prevention of thrombosis, 9th ed: American College of Chest Physicians Evidence-Based Clinical Practice Guidelines. *Chest* 2012;141:e691S–e736S.

47. Crowther MA, Ageno W, Garcia D, et al. Oral vitamin K versus placebo to correct excessive anticoagulation in patients receiving warfarin: a randomized trial. *Ann Intern Med* 2009;150:293–300.

48. Gunther KE, Conway G, Leibach L, et al. Low-dose oral vitamin K is safe and effective for outpatient management of patients with an INR >10. *Thromb Res* 2004;113:205–209.

49. Gage BF, Yan Y, Milligan PE, et al. Clinical classification schemes for predicting hemorrhage: results from the National Registry of Atrial Fibrillation (NRAF). *Am Heart J* 2006;151:713–719.

50. Imberti D, Barillari G, Biasioli C, et al. Emergency reversal of anticoagulation with a three-factor prothrombin complex concentrate in patients with intracranial haemorrhage. *Blood Transfus* 2011;9:148–155.

51. Makris M, Van Veen JJ. Three or four factor prothrombin complex concentrate for emergency anticoagulation reversal? *Blood Transfus* 2011;9:117–119.

52. van Veen JJ, Maclean RM, Hampton KK, et al. Protamine reversal of low molecular weight heparin: clinically effective? *Blood Coagul Fibrinolysis* 2011;22:565–570.

53. Bijsterveld NR, Moons AH, Boekholdt SM, et al. Ability of recombinant factor VIIa to reverse the anticoagulant effect of the pentasaccharide fondaparinux in healthy volunteers. *Circulation* 2002;106:2550–2554.

54. Siegal DM, Crowther MA. Acute management of bleeding in patients on novel oral anticoagulants. *Eur Heart J* 2013;34:489–498.

55. Horlocker TT, Wedel DJ, Benzon H, et al. Regional anesthesia in the anticoagulated patient: defining the risks (the second ASRA Consensus Conference on Neuraxial Anesthesia and Anticoagulation). *Reg Anesth Pain Med* 2003;28:72–197.

56. Gage BF, Birman-Deych E, Radford MJ, et al. Risk of osteoporotic fracture in elderly patients taking warfarin: results from the National Registry of Atrial Fibrillation 2. *Arch Intern Med* 2006;166:241–246.

57. Birnie DH, Healey JS, Wells GA, et al. Pacemaker or defibrillator surgery without interruption of anticoagulation. *N Engl J Med* 2013;368:2084–2093.

58. Marietta M, Bertesi M, Simoni L, et al. A simple and safe nomogram for the management of oral anticoagulation prior to minor surgery. *Clin Lab Haematol* 2003;25:127–130.

59. Levy JH, Faraoni D, Spring JL, et al. Managing new oral anticoagulants in the perioperative and intensive care unit setting. *Anesthesiology* 2013;118:1466–1474.

60. Prandoni P, Prins MH, Lensing AW, et al.; AESOPUS Investigators. Residual thrombosis on ultrasonography to guide the duration of anticoagulation in patients with deep venous thrombosis: a randomized trial. *Ann Intern Med* 2009;150:577–585.

61. Cosmi B, Legnani C, Tosetto A, et al. Usefulness of repeated D-dimer testing after stopping anticoagulation for a first episode of unprovoked venous thromboembolism: the PROLONG II prospective study. *Blood* 2010;115:481–488.

15

Common Pulmonary Complaints

Adam Anderson, Peter G. Tuteur, and Adrian Shifren

INTRODUCTION

- Respiratory functions:
  - Ventilation: the movement of gas in and out of the lung structure
    - Minute ventilation (V_E): volume of gas exhaled per minute
    - Alveolar ventilation (V_A): the volume of gas ventilating perfused alveolae per minute
  - Gas exchange: the exchange of O_2 and CO_2 at the alveolar level
- Nonrespiratory functions:
  - Acid-base balance: change in V_A is inversely related to $PaCO_2$. Change in $PaCO_2$ is inversely related to the effect on blood pH.
  - Synthesis, activation, and inactivation of biologically active molecules.
  - Hemostatic function.
  - Lung defense mechanisms.
- When the ventilatory (airways) and the respiratory (alveoli and adjacent vascular structures) structures are altered by disease, function is impaired, and symptoms develop. Most pulmonary symptoms are included in the following categories:
  - Dyspnea (shortness of breath), exercise intolerance, breathlessness, and smothering
  - Cough
  - Expectoration (sputum, blood)
  - Wheezing (also consider stridor)
  - Chest pain (discomfort, ache, tenderness)

THE FOCUSED PULMONARY PHYSICAL EXAMINATION

- Examination should begin with observation of the general appearance of the patient, including respiratory rate, accessory muscle use, and ability to speak in full sentences. If any of these is acutely abnormal, more urgent evaluation is required.
- Examination of the thorax allows observation of breathing depth, regularity, and symmetry. Palpation of the chest wall can identify a focal or diffuse area of tenderness directing the examiner to consider diagnoses such as costochondritis, unexpected rib fracture, or even pleurisy.
- Percussion over the thorax can assist in narrowing the differential. Hyperresonance is expected in the setting of pneumothorax or significant bullous disease, while dullness is seen with pleural effusions or pneumonia.
- Auscultation should be performed, listening to both phases of ventilation, inspiration and expiration, during both tidal volume (relaxed) breathing and forceful expiration preceded by a deep inspiration.
- If cough regularly develops following deep inspiration, an interstitial pulmonary process becomes an important consideration in the differential diagnosis.
- Extrathoracic sites can then be examined looking for sinus tenderness, abnormal airway anatomy including potentially obstructing posterior pharyngeal tissue, tracheostomy site (open or healed), goiter, and conjunctivitis as seen in sarcoidosis or Sjögren syndrome.[1,2]

Auscultated Pulmonary Sounds

- Adventitious (added) sounds are crackles or wheezes.
- When **wheezing** (continuous musical sounds) is heard during tidal volume breathing or forceful expiration, airway narrowing is present.
- **Crackles** (rales) are intermittent sounds typically occurring during inspiration and are most meaningfully evaluated following a deep forceful expiration. These sounds might be considered "pulmonary opening snaps" produced when previously collapsed lung structures (airways or alveoli) open during the inspiratory phase. Awareness of the timing is critical for determining an appropriate differential diagnosis.
  - Crackles heard early in inspiration represent openings of previously collapsed larger airways as occurs in cystic fibrosis, bronchiectasis, and chronic bronchitis.
  - Crackles heard late in inspiration represent openings of previously collapsed distal structures such as alveoli or terminal bronchioles often abnormal in interstitial pulmonary processes or bronchiolitis obliterans.
- Coarse crackles (gurgles) are produced when fluid (mucus, blood) is present in the airways and gas moves through them. This can be confirmed by demonstrating change in location or character following forceful cough.

Dyspnea

GENERAL PRINCIPLES

- Shortness of breath or dyspnea (the subjective sensation of breathlessness) is a highly nonspecific symptom occurring in most primary pulmonary, cardiac, and some musculoskeletal disorders. An organized approach is essential.[3]
- Pulmonary diseases:
  - **Chest wall deformities**, such as kyphoscoliosis, may result in dyspnea because of mechanical reduction of lung volumes, diminished respiratory compliance, and mechanical respiratory muscle disadvantage.
  - **Increased abdominal girth**, as seen in morbid obesity and massive ascites, will worsen diaphragm dynamics resulting in dyspnea.
  - **Neuromuscular diseases**, such as myasthenia gravis or amyotrophic lateral sclerosis, often lead to dyspnea due to muscular weakness. Later in life, respiratory difficulties may develop in polio survivors, particularly those who had respiratory paralysis during their acute illness.
  - **Pleural effusions** and **pneumothorax** frequently have dyspnea as a primary symptom.
  - **Alveolar processes** such as bacterial pneumonia, pulmonary alveolar proteinosis, and sarcoidosis should be considered.
  - **Interstitial lung diseases** encompass several unique entities, but all may result in dyspnea and progressive pulmonary disability (see Chapter 17).
  - **Asthma** causes episodic or waxing and waning dyspnea.
  - **Chronic obstructive pulmonary disease** (COPD) is a common cause of dyspnea.
  - Upper airway flow may be affected by **tracheal stenosis** and may occur as a result of tracheal injury from prior intubation or from inflammation due to granulomatosis with polyangiitis (GPA) or relapsing polychondritis.
  - **External compression** of the airways may result from malignancies, goiter, or fibrosing mediastinitis.
  - **Vocal cord dysfunction** may result in symptoms that can be difficult to distinguish from those of asthma. Clues include central wheezing, which occurs on inspiration and expiration, and aphonia.
- Cardiovascular and miscellaneous causes
  - Acute cardiac dyspnea is often related to **pulmonary edema** either secondary to heart failure or as a result of myocardial infarction.
  - **Valvular disease**, specifically left-sided diseases including critical aortic stenosis and mitral stenosis, can lead to dyspnea.

○ **Constrictive pericarditis** may result in exertional dyspnea and peripheral edema.
○ **Pulmonary hypertension** will initially cause dyspnea on exertion but may be secondary to a separate process that can also cause dyspnea (e.g., interstitial lung disease).
○ **Acute pulmonary embolism (PE)** may present with a myriad of symptoms, dyspnea being a hallmark feature. **Chronic PE** may result in pulmonary hypertension.
○ Severe **anemia** may cause marked dyspnea likely from reduced oxygen-carrying capacity or high-output cardiac state. Similarly, **methemoglobinemia** and **carboxyhemoglobinemia** may result in decreased oxygen-carrying capacity.
○ **Deconditioning** may play a larger role in dyspneic patients than is often identified. Unfortunately, as patients develop dyspnea on exertion, they may adopt a more sedentary lifestyle that further worsens their exercise capacity.
○ **Anxiety** disorders may have dyspnea as a subjective complaint with limited objective evidence of physiologic impairment.

DIAGNOSIS

Clinical Presentation
History
• Assess the degree of disability; inquire whether dyspnea is present at rest or only with activity and if it is constant or episodic.
• Screen for angina, edema, orthopnea, or paroxysmal nocturnal dyspnea to uncover a cardiovascular etiology.
• Elicit and quantify the patient's smoking history, and record a thorough occupational exposure history.
• Table 15-1 provides additional characteristics that can aid in the differential diagnosis.

Physical Examination
• Elevated pulse and respiratory rate are nonspecific but suggest organic disease.
• Posture (leaning forward with the arms tripoding), accessory muscle use, and pursed-lip breathing suggest COPD.
• Examine for nasal polyps and purulent nasal discharge.
• Signs of current or past ear or nasal cartilage inflammation may suggest tracheal involvement from relapsing polychondritis or GPA.

TABLE 15-1	Characteristics of Shortness of Breath
Character	**Potential causes**
Increases when supine	• Phrenic nerve (diaphragmatic) dysfunction • Left ventricular dysfunction
Increases with exercise	• Ventilatory limitation: COPD, asthma, bronchiectasis, cystic fibrosis • Respiratory limitation: pulmonary embolism, pulmonary hypertension, left-to-right shunt • Cardiac dysfunction • Neuromuscular weakness • Interstitial pulmonary process
Sudden vs. slow onset	• Acute disease vs. chronic disease
Episodic	• Asthma, GERD, sinusitis, aspiration, bronchiectasis, exacerbation of chronic bronchitis
At altitude	• Impairment of oxygen gas exchange
Breathlessness associated with immersion—hot tub, swimming pool, bath tub	• Anemia • Altitude-associated pulmonary edema • Cardiac dysfunction • Diaphragmatic dysfunction

Diagnostic Testing

Imaging

- **Plain chest radiography**:
  - Posteroanterior and lateral chest radiographs (CXRs) should be one of the initial diagnostic evaluations.
  - Attention should be paid to the presence of cardiomegaly, effusions, edema, and lung volume size.
  - Location of lung involvement is also helpful for diagnosis:
    - Lower lobe involvement is characteristic of idiopathic pulmonary fibrosis, rheumatologic disease, and asbestosis.
    - Mid- and upper-lung zone development is associated with granulomatous diseases and silicosis.
  - **Computed tomography (CT):**
    - Detects approximately 10% of cases of interstitial lung disease not visible on CXR.
    - High-resolution CT (HRCT) may provide additional diagnostic clues and detect disease before it is clinically apparent.
    - When performed with contrast, it may reveal thromboembolic disease.
  - **Echocardiography** can reveal evidence of left ventricular dysfunction, valvular disease, and pericardial disease and can screen for pulmonary hypertension.

TREATMENT

- When possible, therapy should be directed by diagnosis.
- In general, supplemental oxygen should be adjusted to keep SpO_2 ≥89% both at rest and with exertion.
- For those with chronic dyspnea and exercise intolerance, pulmonary rehabilitation may reduce symptoms and optimize functional status.[4]

Cough

GENERAL PRINCIPLES

- Cough is the sudden exhalation of lung gas mixture; chronic cough is one that lasts for at least 8 weeks.
- The first response to the initiation of a cough reflex is deep inhalation followed by glottic closure and then maximum forceful expiratory maneuver with glottic opening. This may or may not be associated with the expectoration of phlegm, sputum (mucoid or purulent), or blood.
- Cough may be initiated by afferent stimulation of the upper airways structures such as the posterior pharynx, response to an inhaled irritant by larger airways, activation of stretch receptors of the alveolar wall, or stimulation of the diaphragm from either above or below.
- Identifying the etiology of cough is often a significant challenge.
- When the etiology is not immediately obvious, causes to consider include cough variant asthma, sinusitis or rhinitis with upper airway irritation, gastroesophageal reflux disease (GERD), nonbacterial (fungal) endobronchial infection, and interstitial pulmonary processes.[5–9]
- A differential diagnosis is presented in Table 15-2.

DIAGNOSIS

Clinical Presentation

History

- Recognition of the type and amount of expectoration often leads to a specific diagnosis.
- Nonproductive cough implies either a chronic irritating factor or an interstitial process potentially as simple as a viral pneumonitis or as complex as inflammation and/or scarring of the alveolar walls.

TABLE 15-2 Causes of Cough

Site of cough initiation	Potential associated conditions
Upper extrathoracic airways	
Posterior pharynx	• Sinusitis, tumor, allergic or nonallergic rhinitis
Epiglottis	• Epiglottitis (with sore throat)
Vocal cords	• Polyps, voice abuse
Trachea	• Aspiration, GERD
	• Status post tracheostomy
	• Compression of trachea
Large airways	
Intrathoracic trachea	• Stricture
Large named bronchi	• Bronchitis, bronchiectasis, cystic fibrosis, asthma
Alveolar walls	Interstitial pulmonary processes:
	• Uremia
	• Alveolar proteinosis
	• Radiation
	• Oxygen toxicity
	• Viral infection
	• Sarcoidosis
	• Hemosiderosis
	• Malignancy
	• Idiopathic
	• Tuberculosis
	• Fungal infection
	• Amyloid
	• Collagen vascular disease
	• Eosinophilic granuloma
	• Drugs or dust
Diaphragm	• Pleural effusion
	• Subpleural pulmonary infection/infarction
	• Subdiaphragmatic process (abscess, peritonitis)

- When mucus production is reported, an inflammatory process (acute or chronic) is likely present and may be associated with infection.
- Mucus production may not always be reported because of the social stigmata related to spitting.

Physical Examination
- Examine the ears for otitis, which is a rare cause of cough.
- Examine the nose for evidence of mucopurulent secretions, sinus tenderness, boggy turbinates, or polyps, all of which suggest upper airway irritation and perhaps a predisposition to asthma.
- Postnasal drip may also cause a cobblestone appearance of the tonsillar pillars/posterior pharynx.
- The throat should also be examined for signs of bulbar neurologic dysfunction.

Diagnostic Testing
- A **CXR** is a reasonable initial evaluation if the history and physical do not provide an adequate diagnosis. If it is abnormal, focus on directed evaluation of the abnormality.

If it is normal, obtaining sputum cytology, microbiologic stains, and cultures is neither warranted nor cost-effective.

- Imaging of the paranasal sinuses by **CT scan** is superior to conventional imaging. Sensitivity is probably very good, but specificity is uncertain.
- **Pulmonary function tests** (PFTs) should be obtained if the prior workup is otherwise negative and symptoms do not resolve.

TREATMENT

- When possible, therapy should be directed by diagnosis.
- Antitussive medications including menthol, benzonatate, dextromethorphan, and codeine for refractory cases can be trialed for symptomatic relief.[10–12]
- In extreme cases, nebulized lidocaine may be employed.

Upper Airway Cough Syndrome (Postnasal Drip)

- Intranasal glucocorticoids are the most effective therapy for allergic rhinitis and are also effective for several types of nonallergic rhinitis including vasomotor rhinitis.
- Other therapies for rhinitis include oral antihistamines (first generation are preferred because of their anticholinergic effects), intranasal azelastine, and intranasal ipratropium bromide.[13]
- If therapy is unsuccessful in relieving symptoms in 2 weeks, consider obtaining a sinus CT scan.

Postviral Bronchial Hyperreactivity

- Tends to be resistant to therapy but fortunately is self-limited.
- Ipratropium bromide is more effective than placebo in reducing cough in this entity.[14]
- Evidence for efficacy of inhaled steroids and oral steroids is weaker, but they can be given if cough persists despite ipratropium use.
- Resistant cough should be treated with antitussives and reassurance.

Angiotensin-Converting Enzyme Inhibitors

- Angiotensin-converting enzyme (ACE) inhibitors mediate cough via accumulation of bradykinin.[15]
- Discontinuing ACE inhibitors often results in relief of symptoms in less than a week, and virtually all patients are better in 4 weeks.
- Changing the ACE inhibitor is unlikely to be effective as this is a class effect; however, alternatives such as angiotensin receptor blockers (ARBs) can often be used.

Hemoptysis

GENERAL PRINCIPLES

- Defined as coughing up blood from a pulmonary source.
- On occasion, hemoptysis is confused with hematemesis or the expectoration of blood from a nasal or pharyngeal source.
- Blood originates from the bronchial circulation in most cases but has a pulmonary arterial source in pulmonary arteriovenous malformations, Rasmussen aneurysms in tuberculous cavities, and the diffuse alveolar hemorrhage syndromes of autoimmune origin.
- Hemoptysis is an infrequent complaint for those who seek primary care but is of great concern to the patient. When present in small amounts, the greatest concern is usually **lung cancer**. When there is a large amount, the event itself is frightening to the patient and the physician.

- Certain conditions are typically associated with hemoptysis: pneumonia, carcinoma of the lung, necrotizing pneumonitis, tuberculosis, acute and chronic bronchitis, hereditary hemorrhagic telangiectasia (Osler-Weber-Rendu syndrome), bronchiectasis, and cystic fibrosis.
- Of note, hemoptysis associated with anticoagulation therapy or hypocoagulable disease states usually develops only when there is an underlying pulmonary pathology.

DIAGNOSIS

Clinical Presentation

History
- Obtain an estimate of the volume of hemoptysis. If the history suggests acute hemoptysis of ≥60 mL, refer the patient immediately to a hospital emergency department.
- Although differentiating massive versus nonmassive hemoptysis is controversial, 200 mL/day or 100 mL/hour can be used.[16] Others define massive hemoptysis as that resulting in hemodynamic instability or gas exchange abnormalities.[17]
- Inquire about the appearance of the sputum.
  - Frothy pink sputum suggests heart failure or mitral stenosis.
  - Purulent sputum with fevers and chills suggests pneumonia.
  - Chronic production of sputum with streaks of blood suggests bronchitis.
  - Chronic large-volume purulent sputum punctated by episodes of frank blood suggests bronchiectasis.
- Chest pain may accompany pulmonary embolism, lung cancer involving the parietal pleura, and pneumonia.
- Determine the smoking history, and obtain an occupational history, specifically addressing asbestos exposure as a risk factor for lung cancer.

Physical Examination
- Fever suggests an infectious cause.
- Examine the nasopharynx carefully to rule out an upper airway source of bleeding.
- Halitosis may accompany a lung abscess.
- Lymphadenopathy can be found in either malignancy or infection.
- Auscultate the chest for signs of consolidation (pneumonia), a pleural rub (pulmonary infarction, pneumonia), or a localized wheeze (bronchial obstruction by a neoplasm).
- Synovitis and rash may suggest vasculitis.
- Telangiectasia on face, lips, tongue, and fingers may indicate hereditary hemorrhagic telangiectasia with coexistent pulmonary involvement.

Diagnostic Testing

Laboratories
- Obtain a complete blood cell count, prothrombin time, and partial thromboplastin time.
- Examine the urine for microscopic hematuria and red cell casts that may suggest a vasculitic pulmonary-renal syndrome, and obtain a serum creatinine.
- Evaluate sputum with a gram stain, acid-fast stain, culture, and cytologic examination.
- In cases in which pulmonary vasculitis is a consideration, obtain antinuclear antibodies and antineutrophil cytoplasmic antibodies.

Imaging
- The CXR can localize an infiltrate or mass. Volume loss or atelectasis suggests bronchial obstruction. Pulmonary cavitation may occur with a lung abscess, tuberculosis, or necrosing cancer.

- High-resolution CT without contrast is the best method for a diagnosis of bronchiectasis. It is also excellent for the diagnosis of aspergilloma and may detect a broncholith. High-resolution chest CT with contrast is the test of choice for evaluating potential arteriovenous malformations.[18]

Diagnostic Procedures
- Fiberoptic bronchoscopy should be strongly considered in all patients with an abnormal CXR and hemoptysis. The diagnostic sensitivity varies from study to study depending on the population evaluated, but is at best localizing or diagnostic in approximately half of cases.[19]
- Identification of the bleeding site is three times more likely if bronchoscopy is done within 48 hours.[20]
- In the setting of massive hemoptysis, bronchoscopy is primarily performed to ensure airway patency, to maintain ventilation, and to perform endobronchial blockade to spare the opposite lung.

TREATMENT

- The treatment of small-volume hemoptysis is directed at the underlying disease process.
- Hemoptysis that is associated with chronic bronchitis and bronchiectasis should be treated with antibiotics and antitussives.
- Massive hemoptysis can be lethal and generally demands aggressive evaluation and treatment.[21,22]

Noncardiac Chest Pain

GENERAL PRINCIPLES

- Noncardiac chest pain is pain due to causes other than heart disease. Often referred to as atypical chest pain, it is generally used to include all chest pain that is not caused by coronary artery disease.
- Noncardiac chest discomfort is quite common in ambulatory practice. Its greatest importance lies in the concern it causes to patients and physicians alike that significant heart disease underlies the symptom.
- This discussion assumes that the presence of coronary disease has been evaluated and ruled out. The remaining common causes involve the chest wall, pleura, and esophagus. Diseases of the gallbladder, pancreas, large and small bowel, and psychiatric disorders account for much of the remainder.[23]
- **Chest wall disorders**:
  ○ Musculoskeletal pain is more common than neurogenic pain.
  ○ Costochondral and chondrosternal pain is frequently the result of exercise, injury, or inflammation.
  ○ Rib fracture may occur from direct trauma.
  ○ Intercostal or pectoral muscle strain may result from exercise.
  ○ Nerve pain may be a result of preeruption herpes zoster or postviral or idiopathic neuritis.
- **Pleural disorders**:
  ○ Viral pleuritis may follow coxsackie B infection.
  ○ Pneumonia is often accompanied by pleural inflammation and sometimes pain.
  ○ Systemic lupus erythematosus is often complicated by pleural involvement producing pain.
  ○ Pulmonary infarction occurs in a minority of cases of pulmonary embolism but is often accompanied by pain.
  ○ Gastrointestinal causes of pleural effusions, with or without pain, include pancreatitis and esophageal rupture.

DIAGNOSIS

Clinical Presentation

History
- If one is notified of acute severe pain by phone, refer the patient to an emergency department for initial evaluation of coronary artery disease, aortic dissection, and pulmonary embolism, any of which may be rapidly fatal; office evaluation is not appropriate.
- **Musculoskeletal** pain is of widely varying duration, from a few seconds to days. The patient may notice that it hurts to touch or is worse with movements involving the trunk and arms.
- **Neurologic** pain is less likely to be increased by thoracic movement, but neck, arm, and shoulder movement may worsen nerve root irritation or thoracic outlet compression.
- **Pleuritic** pain is typically sharp and aggravated by inspiration and cough, but less so by movement. An exception is the pleural pain component that may accompany pericarditis.
- **Esophageal** pain is classically improved or relieved with antacids or H_2 blockers, and the duration is typically longer than that caused by angina. However, it may be dull or heavy rather than burning with radiation to the neck or arm.
- **Gallbladder** pain is usually of acute onset, associated with nausea and vomiting, and felt in the right upper quadrant or epigastrium with radiation to the right shoulder.
- **Pancreatitis** usually presents with severe epigastric pain with radiation to the back, nausea, and vomiting.

Physical Examination
- Many ambulatory patients with noncardiac chest pain look well.
- Tachycardia may accompany any of the acute illnesses and is characteristic of pulmonary embolism and infarction.
- Palpate the chest wall for tenderness. Although characteristic of musculoskeletal pain, it may also be present in empyema, pleurodynia, and rarely pulmonary infarction.
- Percuss and auscultate for dullness or hyperresonance; the former may herald pleural effusion or consolidation, the latter pneumothorax.
- Palpate the abdomen for right upper quadrant tenderness and a Murphy sign.
- Inspect the skin for the characteristic vesicular eruption of herpes zoster.
- Examine the cervical and thoracic spine for any signs of tenderness, and determine if pain is worsened by cervical spine motion or vertical compression.

Diagnostic Testing
- Although patients may need no further evaluation given their presentation, obtaining a normal ECG may be worth its cost in providing the patient and physician with reassurance.
- If chest wall tenderness follows trauma or is accompanied by systemic symptoms, plain radiography of the ribs may show evidence of fracture or malignancy.
- Pain that is radicular and unremitting may warrant magnetic resonance imaging (MRI) of the cervical or thoracic spine.
- If the symptoms suggest pleuropulmonary infection, obtain a CXR.
- Nonpleuritic pain without an obvious cause should prompt evaluation for a gastrointestinal source.

TREATMENT

Treatment is directed at the specific diagnosis that is responsible for the chest pain. Musculoskeletal pain is frequently controlled with nonsteroidal anti-inflammatory medications, which may also be helpful for nonspecific neuritis.

Pulmonary Function Tests

GENERAL PRINCIPLES

- Further evaluation of the above symptoms and signs is aided by objective assessment of pulmonary function.
- A detailed description of pulmonary function testing is beyond the scope of this chapter.
- PFTs neither provide a specific diagnosis nor determine disability. They simply quantify the degree of impairment of ventilation and gas exchange.
- In general, these measurements are performed at rest but can also be performed under the stress of exercise often uncovering more subtle impairment.
- In the pulmonary function laboratory, one can also assess ventilatory muscle function and determine the potential therapeutic effect of aerosolized bronchodilator medication and supplemental oxygen.
- The various PFTs available may be categorized as follows[24]:
  - Spirometry: forced vital capacity (FVC), forced expiratory volume in 1 second (FEV_1), the ratio of FEV_1 to FVC, and peak expiratory flow (PEF)
  - Lung volumes: total lung capacity (TLC), residual volume (RV), functional residual capacity (FRC), and expiratory reserve volume (ERV)
  - Diffusing capacity of the lung for carbon monoxide (DLCO)
  - Arterial blood gas analysis (ABG)
  - Six-minute walk/oxygen assessment
  - Cardiopulmonary exercise study
  - Bronchoprovocative testing (methacholine challenge)[25]

INTERPRETATION

- Many pulmonary function studies are effort dependent; therefore, the first step of PFT interpretation is to assess the validity of the measured values.[26–28]
- Specifically, one asks, did the technician/patient interaction result in maximum patient effort? The general definition of validity is that the two best attempts are within 5%.
- When this is not the case, all may not be lost because the best test still represents a minimum level of the patient's function, albeit less than the true maximum value.
- Figure 15-1 and Table 15-3 discuss the interpretation of PFTs.[27,28]

PREDICTED VALUES

- Predicted values are based on age, gender, height, and race.[29]
- Normal range is generally considered to be 80% to 120% of the mean predicted value.[30]
- Measured values are compared with the predicted range aiding the interpretive process.

ORDERING APPROPRIATE TESTS

- It is not medically appropriate to simply order "pulmonary function tests." Specific test designation is required. To do so most successfully, one must clearly keep in mind the clinical question prompting an order for pulmonary function studies.
- Spirometry alone may be appropriate to screen for impairment of ventilatory function but insufficient for a patient with advanced disease whose care may require information regarding the severity of an obstructive abnormality, the acute effect of bronchodilator administration, the presence or absence of air trapping, or the need for supplemental oxygen.
- When a restrictive ventilatory defect is considered, a TLC measurement is required for confirmation.

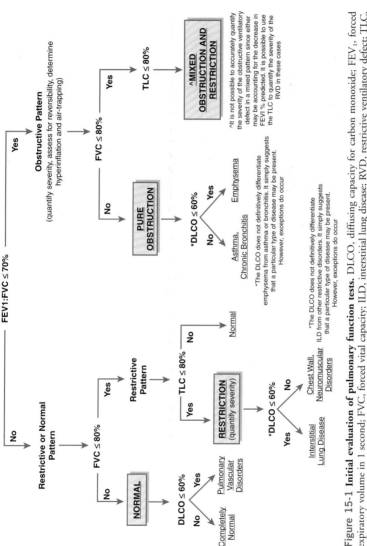

Figure 15-1 Initial evaluation of pulmonary function tests. DLCO, diffusing capacity for carbon monoxide; FEV$_1$, forced expiratory volume in 1 second; FVC, forced vital capacity; ILD, interstitial lung disease; RVD, restrictive ventilatory defect; TLC, total lung capacity. Data from: Pellegrino R, Viegi G, Brusasco V, et al. Interpretive strategies for lung function tests. *Eur Respir J* 2005;26:948–968 and Al-Ashkar F, Mehta R, Mazzone PJ. Interpreting pulmonary function tests: recognize the pattern and the diagnosis will follow. *Cleve Clin J Med* 2003;70:886–881.

TABLE 15-3 Pulmonary Function Test Interpretation

Type of physiologic abnormality	Criteria	Qualitative interpretation
Obstructive ventilatory defect	FEV_1/FEV <70% Decreased FEV_1	FEV_1 ≥70% = **mild** ventilatory defect FEV_1 60%–69% = **moderate** ventilatory defect FEV_1 50%–59% = **moderately severe** ventilatory defect FEV_1 35%–49% = **severe** ventilatory defect ≤34% = **very severe** ventilatory defect
Bronchial reactivity	Increased airways resistance (Raw) Decreased conductance (Gaw) Increased FEV_1 after administration of aerosolized bronchodilator Methacholine challenge test	>12% **and** 200 mL increase from baseline >20% FEV_1 fall at a concentration of methacholine ≤8 mg/mL
Restrictive ventilatory defect	TLC <80% (plethysmography) TLC <80% (dilution)	FEV_1 ≥70% = **mild** ventilatory defect FEV_1 60%–69% = **moderate** ventilatory defect FEV_1 50%–59% = **moderately severe** ventilatory defect FEV_1 35%–49% = **severe** ventilatory defect ≤34% = **very severe** ventilatory defect Dilution technique for measurement of TLC is less specific than plethysmography because of underestimation in the face of obstruction
Combined obstructive and restrictive ventilatory defects	Decreased FEV_1 and FEV_1/FEV and TLC	Discount assigned severity of obstructive ventilatory defect in face of restrictive ventilatory defect
Ventilatory muscle function	Supine spirometry MIP MEP MVV	Diaphragmatic dysfunction is suggested by >20% fall of FEV_1 and FVC in the supine position as compared to similar measurements taken sitting or standing Global muscle dysfunction is suggested by proportionately low MVV (MVV = FEV_1 × 40) and decreased MIP and MEP

FEV_1, forced expiratory volume in 1 second; FVC, forced vital capacity; MEP, maximum expiratory pressure; MIP, maximum inspiratory pressure; MVV, maximum voluntary ventilation; TLC, total lung capacity.

TABLE 15-4	Radiographic Studies for Pulmonary Complaints

Study	Radiation dose[31]	Use/indication
Standard PA and lateral CXR	0.1 mSv[a]	Screening, following longitudinal changes
CT of chest without contrast	7 mSv	Excellent for detailing parenchymal processes
CT of chest with contrast	7 mSv	Excellent for detailing parenchymal process and its relation to vascular structures
CT of chest with pulmonary embolism protocol	15 mSv	Most sensitive test for identifying pulmonary embolism
High-resolution CT of chest	7 mSv	Best for defining interstitial process
MRI chest	None	Assessment of foci of activity: inflammation and malignancy
Ventilation/perfusion scan	2.5 mSv	Less specific and sensitive alternative to PE protocol CT to identify pulmonary embolism

[a]As a reference, the annual background radiation dose from radioactive material occurring naturally in the environment and from cosmic radiation is approximately 3 mSv.
mSv, millisievert; CT, computed tomography; CXR, chest radiography; PA, posteroanterior; PE, pulmonary embolism.

RADIOGRAPHIC STUDIES

A detailed discussion of radiographic studies is not within the scope of this work. Table 15-4 should serve as a guideline for the usefulness of available studies.[31]

REFERENCES

1. Maitre B, Similowski T, Derenne JP. Physical examination of the adult patient with respiratory diseases: inspection and palpation. *Eur Respir J* 1995;8:1584–1593.
2. Kritek P, Choi A. Approach to the patient with disease of the respiratory system. In: Longo DL, Fauci AS, Kasper DL, et al., eds. *Harrison's Principles of Internal Medicine*, 18th ed. New York, NY: McGraw-Hill; 2012, Chapter 251.
3. Parshall MB, Schwartzstein RM, Adams L, et al. An official American Thoracic Society statement: update on the mechanisms, assessment, and management of dyspnea. *Am J Respir Crit Care Med* 2012;185:435–452.
4. Nici L, Donner C, Wouters E, et al. American Thoracic Society/European Respiratory Society statement on pulmonary rehabilitation. *Am J Respir Crit Care Med* 2006;173:1390–1413.
5. Irwin RS, Baumann MH, Bolser DC, et al. Diagnosis and management of cough executive summary: ACCP evidence-based clinical practice guidelines. *Chest* 2006;129:1S–23S.
6. Chung KF, Pavord ID. Prevalence, pathogenesis, and causes of chronic cough. *Lancet* 2008;371:1364–1374.
7. Pratter MR. Overview of common causes of chronic cough: ACCP evidence-based clinical practice guideline. *Chest* 2006;129:59S–62S.
8. Irwin RS. Chronic cough due to gastroesophageal reflux disease: ACCP evidence-based clinical practice guideline. *Chest* 2006;129:80S–94S.

9. Dicpinigaitis PV. Chronic cough due to asthma: ACCP evidence-based clinical practice guideline. *Chest* 2006;129:75S–79S.
10. Bolster DC. Cough suppressant and pharmacologic protussive therapy: ACCP evidence-based clinical practice guideline. *Chest* 2006;129:238S–249S.
11. Pratter MR, Brightling CE, Boulet LP, et al. An empiric integrative approach to the management of cough: ACCP evidence-based clinical practice guideline. *Chest* 2006;129:222S–231S.
12. Pavord ID, Chung KF. Management of chronic cough. *Lancet* 2008;371:1375–1384.
13. Spencer CM, Faulds D, Peters DH. Cetirizine. A reappraisal of its pharmacological properties and therapeutic use in selected allergic disorders. *Drugs* 1993;46:1055–1080.
14. Braman SS. Postinfectious cough: ACCP evidence-based clinical practice guideline. *Chest* 2006;129:138S–146S.
15. Dicpinigaitis PV. Angiotensin-converting enzyme inhibitor-induced cough: ACCP evidence-based clinical practice guidelines. *Chest* 2006;129:169S–173S.
16. Bidwell JB, Pachner RW. Hemoptysis: diagnosis and management. *Am Fam Physician* 2005;72:1253–1260.
17. Ibrahim WH, Massive haemoptysis: the definition should be revised. *Eur Respir J* 2008;32:1131–1132.
18. McGuinness G, Beacher JR, Harkin TJ, et al. Hemoptysis: prospective high-resolution CT/bronchoscopic correlation. *Chest* 1994;105:1155–1162.
19. O'Neil KM, Lazarus AA. Hemoptysis. Indications for bronchoscopy. *Arch Intern Med* 1991;151:171–174.
20. McCalley SW. Clinical efficacy of early and delayed fiberoptic bronchoscopy in patients with hemoptysis. *Am Rev Respir Dis* 1982;125:269–270.
21. Jean-Baptiste E. Clinical assessment and management of massive hemoptysis. *Crit Care Med* 2001;28:1642–1647.
22. Karmy-Jones R, Cuschieri J, Vallieres E. Role of bronchoscopy in massive hemoptysis. *Chest Surg Clin N Am* 2001;11:873–906.
23. Cayley WE. Diagnosing the cause of chest pain. *Am Fam Physician* 2005;72:2012–2021.
24. Miller MR, Hankinson J, Brusasco V, et al. Standardization of spirometry. *Eur Respir J* 2005;26:319–338.
25. American Thoracic Society. Guidelines for methacholine and exercise challenge testing—1999. ATS statement. *Am J Respir Crit Care Med* 2000;161:309–329.
26. Barreiro TJ, Perillo I. An approach to interpreting spirometry. *Am Fam Physician* 2004;69:1107–1114.
27. Pellegrino R, Viegi G, Brusasco V, et al. Interpretative strategies for lung function tests. *Eur Respir J* 2005;26:948–968.
28. Al-Ashkar F, Mehra R, Mazzone PJ. Interpreting pulmonary function tests: recognize the pattern, and the diagnosis will follow. *Cleve Clin J Med* 2003;70:866–881.
29. Hankinson JL, Odencrantz JR, Fedan KB. Spirometric reference values from a sample of the general U.S. population. *Am J Respir Crit Care Med* 1999;159:179–187.
30. Hardie JA, Buist AS, Vollmer WM, et al. Risk of over-diagnosis of COPD in asymptomatic elderly never-smokers. *Eur Respir J* 2002;20:1117–1122.
31. Mettler F, Huda W, Yoshizumi T, et al. Effective doses in radiology and diagnostic nuclear medicine. *Radiology* 2008;248:254–263.

16 Chronic Obstructive Pulmonary Disease and Asthma

Kiran Sarikonda, Ajay Sheshadri, Mario Castro, and
Jeffrey J. Atkinson

Chronic Obstructive Pulmonary Disease

GENERAL PRINCIPLES

Definition

Chronic obstructive pulmonary disease (COPD) is "a common preventable and treatable disease state characterized by persistent airflow limitation that is usually progressive and associated with enhanced chronic inflammatory response to noxious particles or gases."[1]

Classification

COPD is a complex disease in which patients may have components of chronic bronchitis, emphysema, and airway hyperreactivity:

- **Chronic bronchitis** is defined as cough, productive of at least two tablespoons of sputum, for at least 3 months in 2 consecutive years.
- **Emphysema** is a pathologic definition referring to permanent enlargement of the airspaces distal to the terminal bronchioles, accompanied by destruction of their walls and without obvious fibrosis.
- **Airway hyperreactivity** is an enhanced constrictive response of airway smooth muscle resulting in increased obstruction; typically due to an external stimulus like antigens, chemicals, or infections. Although asthmatics that smoke can develop COPD, many nonasthmatic individuals with COPD demonstrate at least occasional airway hyperreactivity after fixed airflow obstruction has been established. **Asthma** differs from COPD in that the airflow limitation is largely reversible, although some patients with asthma develop poorly reversible airflow limitation over time. Asthma is a different disease entity with regard to pathogenesis, and therapeutic response and will be addressed separately.

Epidemiology

- COPD is currently the fourth leading cause of morbidity and mortality in the United States and is projected to be the third leading cause by 2020.[2]
- Women have exceeded men in mortality attributed to COPD since 2010.
- Approximately 4% to 6% of adult white males and 1% to 3% of adult white females have COPD. It is estimated that 20 million adults in the United States have COPD, the majority of whom do not carry a physician diagnosis of COPD.
- The predominant risk factor for COPD in the United States and other industrialized countries is cigarette smoking, but additional other environmental and likely genetic factors contribute to disease development (Table 16-1). Biomass fuels utilized for cooking in closed spaces may be a more important risk factor worldwide.

TABLE 16-1	Risk Factors for Chronic Obstructive Pulmonary Disease (COPD)

Major COPD risk factors	Comments
Cigarette smoking	15%–20% of smokers develop airflow obstruction Smoking results in accelerated age-related lung decline (80–100 mL/year compared to 20–30 mL/year in nonsmokers)
α_1-Antitrypsin deficiency	Significant early lung disease usually develops only in smokers, but occupational exposures may also contribute
	Panacinar emphysema or lower lobe predominant disease in young individuals should increase suspicion, but typical upper lobe predominant disease is common
	Bronchiectasis with mild emphysema can be seen
Air pollution	May interfere with lung development and increase susceptibility but also increases exacerbation risk
	Particulates more important than photochemical pollutants
Occupational exposures	Dust (organic and inorganic), fumes, and gases
	Gold miners, farmers, grain handlers, cement workers, cotton workers, plastic manufacturing, construction, and utility work

DIAGNOSIS

Clinical Presentation
- COPD is an insidious disease, with dyspnea being the predominant presenting symptom. However, dyspnea typically does not develop until the FEV_1 (forced expiratory volume in 1 second) is ≤60% of predicted.
- The etiology of the dyspnea is multifactorial and includes the following:
  - Expiratory airflow obstruction with air trapping[3]
  - Hyperinflation that reduces diaphragm efficiency and results in abnormalities of chest wall and respiratory muscle function
  - Mucus hypersecretion
  - Bronchoconstriction
  - Maldistribution of ventilation, resulting in ventilation-perfusion mismatching
  - Physical deconditioning
  - Nutritional abnormalities and weight loss

History
- Important symptoms of COPD include the following: dyspnea, chronic cough, sputum production, chest tightness, and wheezing (occasionally).
- Exacerbations of combinations of these symptoms, requiring antibiotic therapy or even hospitalization.
- Symptoms of weight loss, recurrent hemoptysis, or hoarseness should precipitate a thorough search for concurrent malignancy.

Physical Examination
- Signs on physical examination are often present only with more advanced disease and include the following: wheezing, prolonged expiration, barrel-shaped chest (hyperinflation), pursed lip breathing, accessory muscle use, and peripheral edema from cor pulmonale.

- Clubbing is not a physical exam finding that occurs in COPD and should prompt a search for additional or alternative etiologies.

Diagnostic Testing

Laboratories
- α_1-Antitrypsin levels should be checked in patients with the following problems[4]:
  - Premature onset of COPD or significant impairment before the age of 50
  - Predominance of basilar emphysema
  - A family history of α_1-antitrypsin deficiency or early-onset emphysema
  - Chronic bronchitis with airflow obstruction in a patient who never smoked
  - Unexplained bronchiectasis or cirrhosis
- Genetic phenotyping should be performed if the α_1-antitrypsin level is low.

Imaging
- Imaging studies, such as chest radiographs (CXR), are not sufficient to exclude lung cancer and offer little additional prognostic or therapeutic information.
- Routine chest computed tomography (CT) scanning is not indicated in the care of patients with COPD. However, annual low-dose CT protocols do detect early cancer, despite a high false-positive rate, and confer a survival advantage that is similar to routine mammography.[5] These protocols are now indicated in smokers over 50 years old with a >30-pack-year history and within 15 years of the last cigarette. It is not known if coexistent COPD results in a greater survival advantage with screening, but given the increased lung cancer risk in individuals with COPD, routine screening in patients outside the guideline population will require future study.

Diagnostic Procedures
- The crucial step in the diagnosis and ongoing assessment of obstructive lung disease is formal **pulmonary function testing** (PFT).
- Spirometry is the only reliable means for diagnosing COPD and, importantly, also classifies the severity of the disease.[6]
- The sine qua non for making the diagnosis of obstructive lung disease is a reduced ratio of the FEV_1 to the forced vital capacity (FVC).
- The grading of COPD severity by PFTs is presented in Table 16-2.
- A comprehensive pulmonary assessment often includes other testing of pulmonary function (Table 16-3). As disease severity increases, an oxygen evaluation becomes important.

TABLE 16-2 Grading the Severity of COPD

Severity of COPD	Postbronchodilator FEV_1/FVC ratio	FEV_1 (% predicted)
Mild	<0.7	>80
Moderate	<0.7	50–80
Severe	<0.7	30–50
Very severe	<0.7	<30

COPD, chronic obstructive pulmonary disease; FEV_1, forced expiratory volume in 1 second; FVC, forced vital capacity.
Data from Rabe KF, Hurd S, Anzueto A, et al. Global strategy for the diagnosis, management, and prevention of chronic obstructive pulmonary disease: GOLD executive summary. *Am J Respir Crit Care Med* 2007;176:532–555.

TABLE 16-3	Pulmonary Function Testing in COPD

Test	Comments
Spirometry both pre- and postbronchodilator	Useful to make the diagnosis Able to grade disease severity Useful to follow patients serially A significant response to bronchodilator (FEV_1 increase by >12% and 200 mL) is more suggestive of reactive airway disease
Lung volumes by body plethysmography, helium dilution, or nitrogen washout	Useful to detect air trapping (elevated residual volume) and hyperinflation (elevated total lung capacity)
DLCO	Tends to be very low in emphysema, less severely decreased with chronic bronchitis
Arterial blood gases	Should be performed with moderate or severe impairment to assess for resting hypoxemia and detect hypercapnia
Oxygen evaluation (6-minute walk test)	Useful to detect oxyhemoglobin desaturation with exercise Provides an assessment of resting and exertional oxygen needs Quantifies the distance the patient can walk

COPD, chronic obstructive pulmonary disease; FEV_1, forced expiratory volume in 1 second; DLCO, diffusing capacity of the lung for carbon monoxide.

TREATMENT

- An overview of the general management of COPD is given in Figure 16-1.[6,7] Each component of this management plan will be discussed in detail below.
- General consideration should be given to comorbidities as most patients with COPD have a higher frequency of cardiac disease, osteoporosis, gastroesophageal reflux, depression, and lung cancer.
- Death from cardiac disease or lung cancer is more common than directly from COPD.
- Individuals with COPD benefit from cardiac treatments, such as β-blockers, even with severe disease.

Medications

Short-Acting Bronchodilators
- Metered-dose inhalers (MDIs) that contain a β_2-agonist, an anticholinergic agent, or both can result in improvement of airflow obstruction and hyperinflation and therefore less dyspnea. Commonly used inhalers for COPD are detailed in Table 16-4.
- These agents are the mainstay of symptomatic therapy in COPD, and patients can use two to four puffs every 4 to 6 hours.[8] Regular use of short-acting bronchodilators does not preserve lung function or alter mortality.[9]
- Combination therapy with both anticholinergic agents and β_2-agonists is appropriate in patients with more severe disease.[10]
- Proper MDI technique should be verified at outpatient visits, and if patients have difficulty, a spacer device may prove beneficial. Nebulized agents may also be used in patients unable to acquire proper technique.

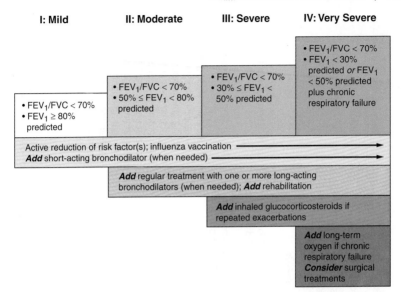

I: Mild **II: Moderate** **III: Severe** **IV: Very Severe**

Figure 16-1 **Therapy at each stage of COPD, the GOLD guidelines.** COPD, chronic obstructive pulmonary disease; FEV_1, forced expiratory volume in 1 second; FVC, forced vital capacity. (Modified from Rabe KF, Hurd S, Anzueto A, et al. Global strategy for the diagnosis, management, and prevention of chronic obstructive pulmonary disease: GOLD executive summary. *Am J Respir Crit Care Med* 2007;176:532–555, with permission.)

- Frequent MDI use can lead to failure of patients to recognize an MDI containing no active medication, as propellant quantity exceeds active drug. Patients need to be counseled; presence of propellant does not ensure active drug is also present.

Long-Acting Bronchodilators
- Current guidelines endorse the regular use of long-acting agents to improve symptoms and quality of life. Reduction in exacerbations of COPD has been demonstrated for several of these medications.[6,11,12] Multiple formulations are available (Table 16-4).
- The long-acting β_2-agonists (LABAs, Table 16-4) produce bronchodilation for 12 hours or more, potentially reducing nocturnal symptoms. Whether agents acting >12 hours offer greater efficacy, compliance, or simply convenience has not been addressed.
- Long-acting antimuscarinic (anticholinergic) agents (LAMA, Table 16-4) can improve airflow over a 24-hour period.
  - A large trial compared LAMA with LABA therapy in predominantly GOLD 2 and 3 diseases and demonstrated a slight therapeutic advantage of anticholinergics. However, this trial and several large anticholinergic trials have excluded subjects with higher-risk cardiac disease.[12]
  - Increased potential cardiac risk with anticholinergic agent use in clinical practice may outweigh the marginal benefit in subjects with advanced coronary disease.
- Many patients with significant dyspnea are managed with combinations of short-acting and long-acting bronchodilators. Use of both LABA and LAMA medications simultaneously likely has an additive symptomatic effect, but whether this also results in further exacerbation reduction is not known. Symptomatic dyspnea relief with simultaneous therapy is an option for some patients but may be cost prohibitive.

TABLE 16-4   Commonly Used Inhalers in COPD and Cystic Fibrosis

Drug name	Trade names	Formulation	Adult dose	Comments
Albuterol	Proventil-HFA Ventolin-HFA ProAir HFA Proventil Ventolin AccuNeb	MDI: 90 μg/spray NEB: 2.5 mg/3 mL	2 puffs INH q4–6 hour prn 2.5 mg NEB q4–6 hour prn	Short-acting β2-agonist
Levalbuterol	Xopenex-HFA Xopenex	HFA: 45 μg/puff NEB: 0.31, 0.63, or 1.25 mg/3 mL	1–2 puffs INH q4–6 hour prn 0.63 mg NEB q6–8 hour prn	Short-acting β2-agonist
Ipratropium bromide	Atrovent HFA Atrovent	MDI: 17 μg/spray NEB: 500 μg/2.5 mL	2 puffs INH q4–6 hour prn 500 μg q4-6 hour prn	Short-acting anticholinergic
Albuterol/ipratropium bromide	Combivent	MDI: 120/21 μg/spray	1–2 puffs INH q6 hour	Combination short-acting β2-agonist and short-acting anticholinergic
Salmeterol	Serevent	DPI: 50 μg/blister	1 INH q12 hour	Long-acting β2-agonist
Formoterol	Foradil	DPI: 12 μg/INH	1 INH q12 hour	Long-acting β2-agonist
Arcapta neohaler	Indacerol	DPI: 75 μg/capsule	1 capsule q day	Long-acting β2-agonist
Arformoterol tartrate	Brovana	NEB: 15 μg/2 mL	1 NEB q12 hour	Long-acting β2-agonist
Tiotropium	Spiriva	DPI: 18 μg	1 INH q24 hour	Long-acting anticholinergic
Aclidinum	Tudorza Pressair	DPI: 400 μg	1 INH q12 hour	Long-acting anticholinergic
Fluticasone /Salmeterol	Advair	DPI: 100 μg/50 μg 250 μg/50 μg 500 μg/50 μg	1 INH q12 hour	Combination of an inhaled corticosteroid and a long-acting β2-agonist
Budesonide/Formotorol	Symbicort	DPI: 160 μg/4.5 μg		

COPD, chronic obstructive pulmonary disease; DPI, dry powder inhaler; HFA, hydrofluoroalkane; INH, inhalation; MDI, metered-dose inhaler; NEB, nebulizer; solution or nebulized.

Inhaled Corticosteroids

- Inhaled corticosteroids (ICS) combined with LABAs have a role in reducing exacerbation frequency of patients with more than one exacerbation per year and GOLD 3+ disease.[11]
- There is an increased risk of pneumonia, so caution should be taken to utilize these medications in combination with LABAs and for the outcome of exacerbation reduction and not symptomatic relief alone.
- ICS as a monotherapy do not confer the same level of benefit. Use as part of a combined inhaler (Table 16-4) is preferred to improve compliance.
- Oral thrush is a common side effect, and mouth rinse or using medication prior to brushing teeth typically prevents this complication.

Macrolides

- One randomized placebo-controlled trial that included subjects with greater than one annual exacerbation and GOLD 2+ COPD demonstrated a significant reduction in COPD exacerbations.[13]
- Subset analysis may suggest that current smokers and older subjects received less benefit.
- Thought should be given to the possibility of atypical mycobacterial disease before chronic therapy is initiated, as later eradication is complicated if the mycobacteria develop resistance to macrolide antibiotics.
- Higher than expected levels of hearing loss were observed in the trial and likely warrant audiometry testing in older patients selected for chronic use.

Phosphodiesterase-4 (PDE4) Inhibitors

- Currently, one PDE4 inhibitor is available for use in COPD (Table 16-4).
- This medication has the narrow indication of reduction of exacerbation frequency in GOLD 3+ subjects with chronic bronchitis.[14]
- Similar to macrolides, the benefit in current smokers is less clear.
- GI distress is relatively common with this class of medications and may be a relative contraindication in patients with low BMI at the outset.

Methylxanthines

- Theophylline use has declined steadily due to its potential toxicity; however, this long-acting oral bronchodilator can be used as add-on therapy in patients who are still dyspneic despite maximal inhaled bronchodilator use.[15]
- Theophylline has multiple drug interactions, and drug levels need to be monitored routinely and whenever potentially interacting medications are added to a patient's regimen. Therapeutic range is between 6 and 12 mg/L.
- Common side effects include anxiety, tremor, nausea, and vomiting.
- Toxicity is manifested as tachyarrhythmias and seizures.

Oral Corticosteroids

- ICS are used in COPD, but the use of chronic oral corticosteroids has less supportive clinical evidence.
- A brief trial of oral corticosteroids may benefit as many as 30% of patients with COPD with wheezing, frequent exacerbations, or severe impairment. An objective improvement in FEV_1 should be evident to justify maintenance therapy with an oral steroid. Doses in the range of 40 mg/day for 1 to 2 weeks are generally initiated and then tapered off as soon as possible.
- Chronic use of oral steroids is discouraged because of the systemic side effects including osteoporosis, hyperglycemia, risk of peptic ulcer disease, immunosuppression, and cataracts.

Replacement Therapy

- Augmentation therapy with α_1-antitrypsin is available and is indicated in patients with α_1-antitrypsin deficiency and obstructive lung disease who have quit smoking.[16]
- Hepatitis vaccination should be performed prior to starting therapy.
- The efficacy of this therapy has been supported by radiographic measurement of emphysema progression but not rate of change in FEV_1.
- The therapy is very expensive and is given intravenously at weekly or monthly intervals to achieve trough levels equivalent to a heterozygote (80 mg/dL).

Other Nonpharmacologic Therapy

- **Oxygen therapy** has been shown to reduce mortality in hypoxemic patients with COPD and also improve physical and mental function.[17,18]
- Arterial blood gases (ABGs) should be obtained to document whether hypoxemia is present when breathing room air in individuals with more severe disease. Pulse oximetry can be used for oxygen titration after an arterial oxyhemoglobin saturation is obtained. It should be noted that in current smokers lower oxygen saturation can be present as carboxyhemoglobin levels can reach >10% but do not result in reduced noninvasive saturation measurements.
- The **indications for oxygen therapy** as derived from the Nocturnal Oxygen Therapy Trial Group (NOTT) are as follows[17]:
  - PaO_2 < 55 mm Hg or SpO_2 < 88% at rest
  - PaO_2 < 56 to 59 mm Hg or SpO_2 < 89% if there is P pulmonale, cor pulmonale, or hematocrit >55%
  - With exercise if accompanied by desaturation to levels listed above
  - With sleep if accompanied by desaturation to levels listed above
- Desaturation is common during sleep in patients with COPD, so formal overnight oximetry with oxygen titration may be helpful. If this is not available, patients are generally told to increase their resting oxygen setting by 1 L during sleep.
- Many patients develop worsening hypoxemia during acute exacerbations of COPD. These supplemental requirements may decrease after treatment of the exacerbation, so a follow-up oxygen evaluation should be performed 1 to 3 months later.
- Prescriptions for oxygen should specify the oxygen dose (L/minute) for rest, exercise, and sleep as well as the delivery system.
- There are three main forms of **oxygen delivery** for patients:
  - **Oxygen concentrators:** These are large devices, which are normally placed in the patient's home for home use. Patients need an additional portable mode of delivery, which is discussed below. Concentrators require power, and the portable tanks also function as a reserve if power failures occur.
  - **Compressed gas:** A portable form of therapy that can occasionally be difficult to carry or push around because of the size and weight of the gas canisters.
  - **Liquid oxygen:** This is the most expensive but most mobile form of therapy for patients. A large reservoir is typically present at home with refillable smaller portable tanks. Therefore, no concentrator pairing is need with liquid.
- The oxygen is normally delivered to the patient via a continuous-flow, dual-prong nasal cannula.
- Patients with COPD rarely require very high concentrations of oxygen, as **the predominant cause of hypoxemia is ventilation-perfusion mismatch.** However, higher requirements necessitate the use of a reservoir system like an Oxymizer device.
- Demand pulse systems that deliver oxygen only during inspiration are also available and can extend tank life for individuals with higher flow requirements.

Surgical Management

- **Bullectomy** can be performed in patients with dyspnea in whom a bulla or bullae occupy at least 50% of a hemithorax and compress the normal lung.

- **Lung volume reduction surgery** (LVRS) can have excellent spirometric and functional outcomes in highly selected patients with severe emphysema (FEV_1 <35%) and apical target areas, which consist of poorly functioning and volume-occupying lung, which can be surgically resected.[19] Individuals with low diffusing capacities and therefore little residual functioning compressed lung do not achieve improvement with LVRS and, in fact, have increased mortality.
- **Lung transplantation** can be performed in patients who have severe obstruction (FEV_1 <25%), hypercapnia, pulmonary hypertension, and marked limitation of activities of daily living (ADLs), but who are young without significant comorbidities.[20]

Lifestyle/Risk Modification

Smoking Cessation

- The beneficial effect of smoking cessation is well demonstrated by the Lung Health Study.[9] Subjects with COPD who continued to smoke experience higher yearly declines in lung function than sustained quitters.
- The Framingham offspring cohort has given additional data on smoking cessation, as cessation after 40 years had less of an impact in normalizing annual decline.[21] This cohort included lung function in young women, demonstrating early smoking may also cause harm via suppressing maximal lung function.
- It is well recognized that in addition to rate of decline, continued smoking also increases the risk of subsequent exacerbations and symptom severity, such as sputum production. Therefore, smoking cessation has the potential to preserve lung function, reduce symptoms, and decrease morbidity and mortality.
- Nicotine addiction causes a state of dependence; therefore, effective smoking cessation requires a multidisciplinary approach that includes consideration of pharmacologic treatment of addiction.[22] Smoking cessation is discussed in detail in Chapter 45.

Pulmonary Rehabilitation

- Dyspnea significantly impairs quality of life in COPD; pulmonary rehabilitation comprises a multidimensional continuum of services aimed at improving functional status both physically and psychologically. Rehabilitation programs can reduce exacerbation frequencies and significantly improve quality of life and ability to perform ADLs.[23] Insurance benefits are important to evaluate as coverage can vary significantly.
- Any patient with moderate COPD should be considered for referral to a comprehensive pulmonary rehabilitation program, particularly those with persistent dyspnea on maximal pharmacologic therapy, frequent exacerbations and hospital admissions, and impaired functional status and quality of life.
- These programs consist of the following[24]:
  - Nutrition and psychosocial support and counseling
  - Graded exercise programs to enhance functionality
    - Typically, sessions are three times a week with a goal of 30 minutes of continuous aerobic activity. Patients are exercised on tracks, treadmills, and bicycles and also perform arm ergometry and light weight lifting to promote upper body strength. Attention is also paid to increasing flexibility.
    - Patients are monitored with pulse oximetry, and oxygen is titrated during the exercise program. The workload is gradually increased until patients reach 80% of their maximum heart rate or breathlessness.
    - Often, coverage is for a single initiation period with continued lifelong exercise to be performed by the patient independently. Reinitiation of previous independent exercise often relies on the discharging physician after hospitalizations for COPD exacerbations.
- Oxygen assessments and potentially noninvasive cardiac stress testing should be performed prior to initiation of a rehabilitation program in patients at risk for significant coronary artery disease.

TABLE 16-5	The Medical Research Council (MRC) Dyspnea Scale

Grade	Degree of breathlessness related to activity
1	Not troubled by breathlessness except on strenuous exercise
2	Short of breath when hurrying or walking up a slight hill
3	Walks slower than contemporaries on level ground because of breathlessness or has to stop for breath when walking at own pace
4	Stops for breath after walking about 100 m or after a few minutes on level ground
5	Too breathless to leave the house or breathless when dressing or undressing

Adapted from Fletcher CM, Elmes PC, Fairbairn MB, et al. The significance of respiratory symptoms and the diagnosis of chronic bronchitis in a working population. *BMJ* 1959;2:257–266.

Patient Education
It is important that patients understand the nature, chronicity, treatment options, and prognosis of COPD. Educational materials are available from the American Lung Association (http://www.lung.org, last accessed January 20, 2015).

Health Maintenance
Yearly influenza vaccination is recommended for all patients, as well as a pneumococcal vaccine every 5 years. Yearly CT screening is indicated in the previously discussed high-risk population.

OUTCOMES/PROGNOSIS

- The **BODE index** is a multidimensional grading system to provide a better assessment of mortality risk and includes parameters that can be obtained at routine outpatient visits[25]:
  - **B**ody mass index (BMI)
  - FEV_1 (**o**bstruction)
  - **D**yspnea, graded by the Medical Research Council dyspnea scale (Table 16-5)
  - **E**xercise tolerance (6-minute walk distance)
- The highest possible score is 10 points, with lower scores indicating a lower risk of death (Table 16-6).

TABLE 16-6	The BODE Index

Variable	Point on BODE index			
	0	1	2	3
FEV_1 (% predicted)	≥65	50–64	36–49	≤35
6-Minute walk distance (m)	≥350	250–349	150–249	≤149
MRC dyspnea scale	0–1	2	3	4
BMI	>21	≤21		

BMI, body mass index; FEV_1, forced expiratory volume in 1 second; MRC, Medical Research Council.
Adapted from Celli BR, Cote CG, Marin JM, et al. The body-mass index, airflow obstruction, dyspnea, and exercise capacity index in chronic obstructive pulmonary disease. *N Engl J Med* 2004;350:1005–1012.

Acute Exacerbations of COPD

GENERAL PRINCIPLES

- Acute exacerbations are a common occurrence in patients with COPD and tend to occur more frequently in those patients who continue to smoke.
- These episodes are characterized by a change in the patient's baseline dyspnea, cough and/ or sputum production beyond day-to-day variability, and sufficient to warrant a change in management.
- Exacerbations are often precipitated by viral or bacterial respiratory infections but can be precipitated by other noxious stimuli like air pollution. Exacerbations account for a significant portion of the costs of managing COPD due to frequent physician visits, hospitalization, and time away from work.[26]

DIAGNOSIS

- Patients who are experiencing exacerbations often have worsening of their hypoxemia and hypercapnia during these episodes; evaluation is indicated to identify patients who may require hospitalization.
- Evaluation should focus on the severity of the dyspnea; the patients' ability to sleep, eat, and care for themselves; and underlying comorbidities.
- Physical exam findings of altered mental status, hemodynamic abnormalities, increased accessory muscle use, and significant comorbidities should prompt hospitalization.
- A CXR should also be performed in these patients.

TREATMENT

- Management, whether pursued as an outpatient or as an inpatient, consists of maximizing bronchodilator therapy, corticosteroids (oral prednisone at a dose of 40 mg/day for 7 to 10 days), and antibiotics if there is evidence of purulent sputum.[27]
- The antibiotic chosen can be narrow spectrum to cover *Haemophilus influenzae, Moraxella* spp., or *Streptococcus pneumoniae* in patients who do not have recent nosocomial risk factors. Reasonable choices include azithromycin, amoxicillin-clavulanate, an oral second-generation cephalosporin, or moxifloxacin.
- Gram-negative organisms (including *Pseudomonas aeruginosa*) are not unusual in patients with severe COPD, comorbid illnesses, and recurrent exacerbations, so coverage should be broadened in patients with these risk factors. For outpatients, ciprofloxacin or levofloxacin is acceptable. For inpatients, more aggressive treatment is warranted, such as piperacillin-tazobactam, cefepime, or levofloxacin.

Asthma

GENERAL PRINCIPLES

- Asthma is a chronic inflammatory disorder of the airways characterized by airway hyperresponsiveness and variable airflow obstruction in response to a wide variety of stimuli that is at least partially reversible either spontaneously or with treatment.[28]
- Many cell types play a role in the inflammation, in particular, mast cells, eosinophils, and Th2 lymphocytes.
- In susceptible individuals, this inflammation causes paroxysms of wheezing, chest tightness, dyspnea, and cough.

• Asthma is a chronic disease with episodic acute exacerbations that are interspersed with symptom-free periods.
• Exacerbations are characterized by a progressive increase in asthma symptoms that can last minutes to hours. They are triggered by viral infections, allergens, and occupational exposures and occur when airway reactivity is increased and lung function becomes unstable.

Classification

• Asthma severity should be classified based on both level of impairment (symptoms, activity limitation, lung function, and rescue medication use) and risk (exacerbations, lung function decline, medication side effects). At the initial evaluation, this assessment will determine level of severity in patients not on controller medications (Table 16-7). The level of severity is based upon the most severe category in which any feature appears. On subsequent visits or if the patient is on a controller medication, this assessment is based on the lowest step of therapy to maintain clinical control (Table 16-8).
• Patients who have had two or more exacerbations requiring systemic corticosteroids in the past year may be considered in the same category as those who have persistent asthma, regardless of level of impairment.

Epidemiology

• In the United States, asthma is the leading cause of chronic illness among children (20% to 30%).
• The prevalence of asthma and asthma-related mortality had been increasing from 1980 to the mid-1990s, but since the 2000s, mortality has decreased.[29]
• African Americans are more likely than whites to be hospitalized and have a higher rate of mortality due to asthma.

TABLE 16-7	Classification of Asthma Severity on Initial Assessment			
	Intermittent	Mild persistent	Moderate persistent	Severe persistent
Daytime symptoms	≤2 days/week	≥2 days/week but not daily	Daily	Throughout the day
Nighttime symptoms	≤2×/month	3–4×/month	≥1×/week but not nightly	Nightly
Activity limitations	None	Minor	Some	Extreme
Reliever medicine use	≤2 days/week	≥2 days/week but not daily	Daily	Several times per day
FEV₁ or PEF	≥80%	≥80%	60%–80%	<60%
Exacerbations	0–1×/year	≥2×/year	≥2×/year	≥2×/year
Management	Step 1	Step 2	Step 3 And consider short-course OCS	Step 4 or 5 And consider short-course OCS

OCS, oral corticosteroids; FEV_1, forced expiratory volume over 1 second; PEF, peak expiratory flow.
GINA Report, Global Strategy for Asthma Management and Prevention, 2011—www.ginasthma.org and National Asthma Education and Prevention Program-Expert Panel Report 3, 2007—http://www.nhlbi.nih.gov/guidelines/asthma/asthgdln.pdf

TABLE 16-8	Assessment of Asthma Control		
	Well controlled	Not well controlled	Very poorly controlled
Daytime symptoms	≤2 days/week	>2 days/week	Throughout the day
Nighttime symptoms	≤2x/month	1–3x/week	≥4x/week
Activity limitations	None	Some	Extreme
Reliever medicine use	≤2x/week	>2x/week	Frequent
FEV₁ or PEF	≥80%	60%–80%	≤60%
Validated questionnaire	ACT ≥20 ACQ <0.75	ACT 16–19 ACQ >1.5	ACT ≤15
Exacerbations	0–1/year	≥2x/year	≥2x/year
Management	Maintain at lowest step possible	Step up one step	Step up one to two steps and consider short-course OCS
Follow-up	1–6 months	2–6 weeks	2 weeks

FEV_1, forced expiratory volume over 1 second; PEF, peak expiratory flow; ACT, Asthma Control Test; ACQ, Asthma Control Questionnaire; OCS, oral corticosteroids.

Pathophysiology

Asthma is characterized by airway obstruction, hyperinflation, and airflow limitation resulting from multiple processes:

- Acute and chronic airway inflammation characterized by infiltration of the airway wall, mucosa, and lumen by activated eosinophils, mast cells, macrophages, and T lymphocytes
- Bronchial smooth muscle contraction resulting from mediators released by a variety of cell types including inflammatory, local neural, and epithelial cells
- Epithelial damage manifested by denudation and desquamation of the epithelium leading to mucous plugs that obstruct the airway
- Airway remodeling characterized by the following findings:
  - Subepithelial fibrosis, specifically thickening of the lamina reticularis from collagen deposition
  - Smooth muscle hypertrophy and hyperplasia
  - Goblet cell and submucosal gland hypertrophy and hyperplasia resulting in mucus hypersecretion
  - Airway angiogenesis
  - Airway wall thickening due to edema and cellular infiltration

DIAGNOSIS

Clinical Presentation

History

- The patient's medical history is of critical importance in establishing the diagnosis of asthma and also identifying characteristic triggers for exacerbations of the patient's symptoms. Asthma may have its onset in infancy through adulthood, and the symptoms may be intermittent or persistent.[30] Asthma is less likely to be the sole cause of respiratory symptoms in patients presenting for the first time after 50 years of age or who have >20-pack-year history of smoking.

- The history at the initial visit and all subsequent visits should focus on the following features:
  - Presence of cough, which can occasionally be productive of yellow sputum and classically is worse at night or in the early morning[31]
  - Presence of wheezing
  - Shortness of breath
  - A feeling of chest tightness
  - Nocturnal awakenings
  - A history of episodic symptoms and/or seasonal variation
  - Triggers of asthma: exercise, allergen exposure (mold, pollen, dust mites, pet dander, cockroaches), changes in weather, and occupational allergens and irritants such as perfumes, cleaners, or detergents
  - Symptoms suggestive of gastroesophageal reflux disease
  - History of sinusitis/allergic rhinitis and postnasal drip
  - History of missed work/school days
  - Prior history of hospitalization and intubation
  - Presence of tobacco abuse
  - History of aspirin sensitivity
  - Personal or family history of atopy
  - Prior therapeutic response to asthma medications

Physical Examination
- Wheezing and prolonged expiratory phase can be noted, but a normal lung examination does not exclude asthma.
- Signs of atopy, such as eczema, rhinitis (pale, boggy nasal mucous membranes), or nasal polyps often coexist with asthma.
- Patients with more severe airflow obstruction may exhibit tachypnea or accessory muscle use but may not have any wheezing due to poor air movement and can ultimately develop a pulsus paradoxus.

Differential Diagnosis

Other conditions may present with wheezing and need to be considered, especially in patients with refractory asthma. Many of the conditions in Table 16-9 can be differentiated from asthma by the absence of reversibility with bronchodilators, review of the flow volume loop, and consideration of the onset and temporal course of the symptoms.

Diagnostic Testing

- Routine laboratory tests are not indicated for the diagnosis of asthma, but a complete blood count with differential may reveal eosinophilia in some patients. Serum IgE level should be checked in patients with difficult to control asthma to evaluate for allergic bronchopulmonary aspergillosis and use of anti-IgE therapy.
- Allergy skin testing and in vitro testing for allergen specific IgE can be useful in management of asthma, to provide guidance for environmental modification.
- CXR and/or CT of the chest are not routinely indicated and are performed only if a complicating pulmonary process such as pneumonia or pneumothorax is suspected or to rule out other causes of respiratory symptoms in patients being evaluated for asthma.
- An objective measurement of airflow obstruction with PFTs is essential to the diagnosis of asthma.
- In patients with asthma, **PFTs** demonstrate an obstructive pattern, the hallmark of which is a decrease in expiratory flow rates:
  - A reduction in FEV_1 and a proportionally smaller reduction in the FVC occurs. This produces a decreased FEV_1/FVC ratio (generally <0.7). With mild obstructive disease

TABLE 16-9 Common Mimics of Asthma

Upper airway obstruction
- Tumor
- Epiglottitis
- Vocal cord dysfunction
- Obstructive sleep apnea

Lower airway disease
- Allergic bronchopulmonary aspergillosis
- Alpha-1-antitrypsin deficiency
- Chronic obstructive pulmonary disease
- Bronchiectasis
- Cystic Fibrosis
- Bronchiolitis obliterans
- Tracheobronchomalacia

Localized airway obstruction
- Endobronchial foreign body
- Endobronchial tumor (carcinoid)

Other
- Congestive heart failure
- Churg-Strauss syndrome
- Hypersensitivity pneumonitis
- Eosinophilic pneumonia
- Gastroesophageal reflux disease
- Chronic sinusitis
- Hyperventilation with panic attacks
- Dysfunctional breathlessness

that involves only the small airways, the FEV_1/FVC ratio may be normal, with the only abnormality being a decrease in airflow at midlung volumes (forced expiratory flow 25% to 75%).
- ○ The clinical diagnosis of asthma is supported by an obstructive pattern that improves after bronchodilator therapy. Improvement is defined as an increase in FEV_1 of >12% and 200 mL after two to four puffs of a short-acting bronchodilator. Most patients will not demonstrate reversibility at each assessment.
- ○ In patients with chronic, severe asthma, the airflow obstruction may no longer be completely reversible. In these patients, the most effective way to establish the maximal degree of airway reversibility is to repeat PFTs after a course of oral corticosteroids (usually 40 mg/day for 10 to 14 days).
- **Lack of demonstrable obstruction or reactivity does not rule out a diagnosis of asthma.** If spirometry is normal, bronchoprovocation testing with methacholine or mannitol may identify patients with airway hyperresponsiveness.[32] This test is not specific for asthma; however, a negative test makes the diagnosis less likely.
- **Measurement of peak expiratory flow rate** (PEFR), with handheld peak flow meters, can be a useful indicator of airflow obstruction and is helpful in outpatient management of the disease.[33]
- ○ The clinician should be aware of the limitations of PEFR measurement. PEFR is very effort and technique dependent.
- ○ Reduced peak flows are not synonymous with obstruction, and complete PFT is needed to distinguish an obstructive from restrictive abnormality.

○ **Thus, PEFR monitoring is best used in patients in whom the diagnosis of asthma has already been established.** Patients can identify their personal bests and can be educated on the appropriate management when their PEFR starts decreasing.

TREATMENT

- The current NIH/NHLBI guidelines updated in 2007 are a very useful resource for clinicians to guide asthma management[28] (Tables 16-7, 16-8, and 16-10).
- The major goals of asthma therapy are to avoid impairment and to minimize risk.
  ○ Freedom from symptoms (including nocturnal symptoms)
  ○ No limitation of daily activities including exercise
  ○ Optimization of lung function
  ○ Minimize acute exacerbations and emergency visits
  ○ Minimize medication side effects and tailor medications to individual patient profiles
- To attain these goals, periodic patient visits are necessary; patient and caregiver education is critical to prevent clinical deterioration. Visits should be an opportunity to assess for symptoms, medication usage, especially short-acting bronchodilators, obtain an objective assessment of lung function, and to educate the patient on appropriate self-management.
- Medical management involves chronic management and a plan for acute exacerbations (**asthma action plan**). Most often it includes the daily use of an anti-inflammatory medication (long-term control medications) and as-needed use of a short-acting bronchodilator (quick-relief medications).
- The stepwise approach to increasing severity of asthma provides general guidelines to assist clinical decision making, and clinicians should tailor medications to the needs of individual patients.
  ○ When initiating therapy for a patient not already on controller medicine, one should assess patient's severity and assign the patient to the highest level in which any one feature has occurred over the previous 2 to 4 weeks (Table 16-7).
  ○ Assessment of control on subsequent visits is used to modify therapy when following patients already on controller medication (Table 16-8).

Medications

- The goal of the stepwise approach is to gain control of symptoms as quickly as possible. Either start with aggressive therapy (e.g., add a course of oral steroids or a higher dose of inhaled steroids to the therapy) or start at the step that corresponds to the patient's initial severity and step up treatment, if necessary.
- At the same time, level of control varies over time, and consequently, medication requirements vary as well, so therapy should be reviewed every 3 months to check whether stepwise reduction is possible.
- Medications commonly used for asthma are detailed in Table 16-11.
- **Inadequate control is indicated by increased use of short-acting β_2-agonists.**
- Patients with exercise-induced bronchospasm should take two to four puffs of an inhaled β_2-agonist 10 to 30 minutes before exercise.
- **Inhaled corticosteroids** (ICS) are the agents of choice for patients with persistent asthma.[28] Dosing is based on the severity and control of asthma. Systemic corticosteroid absorption can occur with high-dose ICS, and thus, high-dose ICS should be reserved for patients with severe disease or for those who otherwise require oral corticosteroids.
- **Long-acting bronchodilators** (LABA) **should not be used as monotherapy in persistent asthma.**[34] However, when used with ICS, salmeterol and formoterol have consistently been shown to improve lung function, both day and nighttime symptoms, reduce exacerbations, and minimize the required dose of ICS.
- **Leukotriene-modifying agents** (montelukast, zafirlukast, and zileuton) can be used as add-on therapy in patients with persistent asthma to improve asthma control and

TABLE 16-10	Stepwise Approach for Managing Asthma in Adults
Step 6	Daily Medications: • Inhaled corticosteroid (high dose) **AND** • Long-acting inhaled β_2-agonist **AND** • Oral corticosteroid **AND** consider: Omalizumab for patients who have allergies
Step 5	Daily medications: • Inhaled corticosteroid (high dose) **AND** • Long-acting inhaled β_2-agonist **AND** consider: Omalizumab for patients who have allergies
Step 4	Daily medications: • Inhaled corticosteroid (medium dose) **AND** • Long-acting inhaled β_2-agonist Alternatives: Inhaled corticosteroid (medium dose) plus either leukotriene modifier or theophylline
Step 3	Daily medication: • Inhaled corticosteroid (medium dose) **OR** • Inhaled corticosteroid (low dose) **AND** • Long-acting inhaled β_2-agonist Alternatives: Inhaled steroid (low dose) plus either leukotriene modifier or theophylline
Step 2	Daily medication: • Inhaled corticosteroid (low dose) is preferred Alternatives: Nedocromil, cromolyn, leukotriene modifier, or sustained-release theophylline
Step 1	Short-acting bronchodilator as needed
All patients	**Quick relief** with a short-acting bronchodilator: inhaled β_2-agonist (2–4 puffs) as needed for symptoms

Modified from National Asthma Education and Prevention Program Expert Panel Report 3 (EPR3): Guidelines for the Diagnosis and Management of Asthma. Full Report 2007. National Institutes of Health, National Heart, Lung, and Blood Institute, Publication No. 08-4051, 2007.

potentially reduce the dose of inhaled corticosteroid.[35] However, in comparison to ICS + LABA, they are not as effective in improving asthma outcomes.

• **Omalizumab,** a monoclonal anti-IgE antibody, has been shown to reduce asthma exacerbations and improve asthma control symptoms in poorly controlled, moderate-to-severe persistent allergic asthma.[36] Potential candidates for omalizumab must have allergy testing to document sensitization to a perennial allergen. The therapy is expensive, and the drug is dosed based on patient weight and baseline IgE levels.

Other Nonpharmacologic Therapies
Bronchial thermoplasty is a novel therapy for severe asthma in which a specialized radiofrequency catheter is introduced through a bronchoscope to deliver thermal energy to airways in order to reduce smooth muscle mass surrounding the airways. Though asthma symptoms may worsen immediately after the procedure, long-term asthma-related quality of life and health care utilization have been shown to improve with bronchial thermoplasty.[37]

TABLE 16-11 Medications Commonly Used for Asthma

Drug name	Trade names	Formulation	Adult dose
Short-acting β₂-agonists			
Albuterol	Proventil Ventolin Proventil HFA Ventolin HFA AccuNeb ProAir HFA Generic	MDI: 90 µg/spray NEB: 2.5 mg/3 mL	2 INH q4–6 hours prn 2.5 mg NEB q4–6 hours prn
Levalbuterol	Xopenex Xopenex-HFA	HFA: 45 µg/puff NEB: 0.31, 0.63 or 1.25 mg/3 mL	1–2 INH q4–6 hours prn 0.63 mg NEB q6–8 hours prn
Pirbuterol	Maxair	MDI: 200 µg/INH	1–2 INH q4–6 hours prn
Long-acting β₂-agonists			
Salmeterol	Serevent	DPI: 50 µg/blister	1 INH q12 hours
Formoterol	Foradil	DPI: 12 µg/capsule	1 INH q 12 hours
Combination inhaled corticosteroid with a long-acting β₂-agonist			
Fluticasone propionate/salmeterol	Advair Advair HFA	DPI: 100/50, 250/50, 500/50 µg/INH HFA: 45/21, 115/21, 230/21 µg/INH	DPI: 1 INH q12 hours HFA: 2 INH q12 hours
Budesonide/formoterol fumarate dihydrate	Symbicort	Inhalation aerosol: 80/4.5 µg/INH 160/4.5 µg/INH	2 INH q12 hours

Drug name	Formulation	Low dose	Medium dose	High dose
Inhaled corticosteroids (comparative daily dosages)				
Beclomethasone dipropionate	MDI: 40 µg/spray 80 µg/spray	160–480 µg daily 40 µg: 4–12 INH 80 µg: 2–6 INH	480–800 µg daily 40 µg: 12–20 INH 80 µg: 6–10 INH	>800 µg daily 40 µg: >20 INH 80 µg: >10 INH
Budesonide	DPI: 180 µg/spray	180–360 µg daily 1–2 INH	360–540 µg daily 2–3 INH	>540 µg daily >3 INH

Drug	Formulation			
Flunisolide	MDI: 250 µg/spray	500–1,000 µg daily 2–4 INH	1,000–2,000 µg daily 4–8 INH	>2,000 µg daily >8 INH
Fluticasone	MDI: 44 µg/spray 110 µg/spray 220 µg/spray	88–264 µg daily 44 µg: 2–6 INH 110 µg: 2 INH	264–660 µg daily	>660 µg daily 110 µg: > 6 INH 220 µg: > 3 INH
Triamcinolone acetonide	MDI: 100 µg/spray	400–1,000 µg daily 4–10 INH	1,000–2,000 µg daily 10–20 INH	> 2,000 µg daily > 20 INH

Drug	Formulation	Adult dose	Comments
Leukotriene modifiers			
Montelukast (Singulair)	10-mg tablets	10 mg PO daily	Blocks leukotriene D$_4$
Zafirlukast (Accolate)	10-mg tablets 20-mg tablets	20 mg PO q12 hours	Food decreases bioavailability Take 1 hour before or 2 hours after meals
Zileuton (Zyflo)	600-mg tablets	600 mg PO q6 hours	Monitor ALT levels Inhibits 5-lipoxygenase
Other agents **Theophylline** Bronkodyl Uniphyl Elixophyllin Slo-Bid Slo-Phyllin Theo-24 Theo-Dur Theolair	Multiple including liquid, capsules, sustained-release tablets	300–600 mg/day divided bid to tid	Multiple drug interactions Narrow therapeutic index Follow levels frequently (goal levels of 5–15 µg/mL) Phosphodiesterase inhibitor
Cromolyn (Intal)	MDI: 800 µg/ spray	2 INH qid	One dose prior to exercise or allergen exposure provides prophylaxis for 1 hour
Nedocromil (Tilade)	MDI: 1.75 mg/ spray	2 INH qid	One dose prior to exercise or allergen exposure provides prophylaxis for 1 hour

MDI, metered-dose inhaler; HFA, hydrofluoroalkane; NEB, nebulizer solution or nebulized; DPI, dry powder inhaler; INH, inhalation.

SPECIAL CONSIDERATIONS

- During **pregnancy,** patients should have more frequent follow-up as the severity often changes and requires medication adjustment. There is more potential risk to the fetus with poorly controlled asthma compared to asthma medication exposure, most of which are generally considered safe.[38]
- **Occupational asthma** requires a detailed history of occupational exposure to a sensitizing agent, lack of asthma symptoms prior to exposure, and a documented relationship between symptoms and the workplace. Beyond standard asthma medical treatment, exposure avoidance is crucial.
- **Acute exacerbations of asthma are common.**
  - Patients experiencing severe asthma exacerbations (PEF or FEV_1 <40%) should receive systemic corticosteroids.
  - Oxygen should be administered to keep the oxygen saturation >90%.
  - The response to initial treatment (60 to 90 minutes, three treatments every 20 minutes with a short-acting bronchodilator) can be a better predictor of the need for hospitalization than the severity of an exacerbation.
  - A low threshold for hospital admission is appropriate for patients who do not respond to initial therapy, have history of recent hospitalization, or have a previous life-threatening exacerbation.
  - In addition, presence of a pulsus paradoxus >12 mm Hg, hypoxemia, and normocapnia despite tachypnea or hypercapnia ($PaCO_2$ >42 mm Hg) should trigger hospital admission.
  - The management of the hospitalized patient with an asthma exacerbation will not be discussed here, except to highlight the need for patient education prior to discharge, a written patient action plan, PEFR meter use reinforcement, and planning for outpatient follow-up.[39]

PATIENT EDUCATION

- One of the primary intents of **asthma education** is to develop a partnership with the patient and family.
- Information about asthma should be provided including
  - Chronicity of the disease and common triggers of exacerbations
  - Role of short-acting β_2-agonists and long-term controllers
  - Importance of communication
- Teach and discuss inhaler and spacer techniques.
- Discuss environmental control measures.
- Address misconceptions, fears, and financial concerns.
- **Develop an action plan for exacerbations.**

Cystic Fibrosis

GENERAL PRINCIPLES

Epidemiology

- Cystic fibrosis (CF) is the most common lethal genetic disease in Caucasians, with an incidence of 1 in 2,500 live births.[40]
- Although it is less common in non-Caucasians, the diagnosis needs to be considered in patients of diverse backgrounds.
- The diagnosis of CF is typically made during childhood, and most states implemented newborn screening programs by 2008, but historically, **8% of patients are diagnosed during adolescence or adulthood.**
- The median survival has been extended to approximately 37 years, and within the next 5 to 10 years, it is expected that over half of CF patients will be adults.

Pathophysiology

- CF is an autosomal recessive disorder that is caused by mutations of the cystic fibrosis transmembrane conductance regulator (CFTR) protein, located on chromosome 7.[41] CFTR protein normally regulates and participates in the transport of electrolytes across epithelial cell membranes.[42]
- There is considerable phenotypic variation in disease expression with the greatest modifier being the specific genetic mutation. More than 1,500 CFTR domain mutations have been identified and can result in defective protein synthesis, processing, regulation, and activity.
- The primary clinical manifestations of the disease are related to **abnormal electrolyte transport in exocrine organs** resulting in thickened secretions.
- The abnormal airway secretions in patients with CF predispose them to chronic infection and chronic colonization with organisms such as *S. aureus* and mucoid strains of gram-negative organisms such as *P. aeruginosa*. The chronic infection results in chronic airway inflammation and ultimately bronchiectasis.

DIAGNOSIS

- The diagnosis of CF in previously undiagnosed adults is based on clinical and family history in combination with persistently elevated concentrations of sweat chloride (the main laboratory confirmation used) or genetic confirmation revealing two known disease-causing CF mutations.[43]
- Atypical patients may lack classic symptoms and signs or have normal to indeterminant sweat tests. Although genotyping may assist in the diagnosis, it alone cannot establish or rule out the diagnosis of CF. Evidence of functional changes must be present.
- Although often overlooked, in males with an indeterminant diagnostic workup a testicular ultrasound demonstrating the presence of bilateral vas deferens can rule out cystic fibrosis, as the formation of a normal vas deferens is most sensitive to CFTR dysfunction.
- Newborn screening has identified a new subgroup of patients who do not have disease but have an abnormal sweat test or genetic testing showing a mutation that could cause CFTR-related organ dysfunction.[44] Although these patients will carry a diagnosis of CFTR-related metabolic syndrome (CRMS), whether this will represent a milder spectrum of disease in adults or merely a laboratory entity is not known.

Clinical Presentation

Pulmonary Manifestations

- Pulmonary symptoms lead to the consideration of the diagnosis of CF in 50% of cases.
- Symptoms typically include cough and purulent sputum production with dyspnea ensuing as the disease progresses. **Almost all patients eventually develop chronic sinopulmonary disease, bronchiectasis, and obstructive lung disease.**
- Acute pulmonary exacerbations, characterized by cough, increased sputum volume and purulence, malaise, and weight loss, typically in the absence of fevers, may lead to significant deterioration and subsequent hospitalization.
- Endobronchial infection occurs early in life, and the flora tends to change with time.[45]
  - *S. aureus* and *H. influenza* tend to be found in younger patients, and in older individuals, it is replaced by mucoid strains of *P. aeruginosa*.
  - Recurrent isolation of unusual gram-negative organisms like *Burkholderia* spp. or nontuberculous mycobacteria are more common in CF patients but often require special specimen processing due to *P. aeruginosa* overgrowth.
- Additional respiratory problems include episodes of hemoptysis, pneumothorax, and allergic bronchopulmonary aspergillosis.[46,47]

Extrapulmonary Manifestations

- Extrapulmonary manifestations of CF include **exocrine pancreatic insufficiency,** seen in 90% of patients, resulting in fat malabsorption; deficiency of fat-soluble vitamins A, D, E, and K; and malnutrition.
- CF involvement of the gastrointestinal (GI) tract causes considerable problems including steatorrhea, constipation, impaction, distal ileal obstruction syndrome, volvulus, intussusception, rectal prolapse, and increased risk of GI cancers.
- CF also affects the endocrine pancreas causing diabetes mellitus and pancreatitis. Significant hepatobiliary complications include the development of cirrhosis with portal hypertension, cholelithiasis, and cholecystitis.
- Male patients with CF tend to be infertile due to an absence of the vas deferens, whereas female patients may have fertility problems due to amenorrhea and abnormally thick cervical mucus production.[48]
- Many individuals with CF suffer from growth retardation, osteopenia, and osteoporosis related to nutritional deficiencies.[49]
- A CF-associated arthropathy as well as leukocytoclastic vasculitis with lower extremity palpable purpura can develop and may coincide with exacerbations.
- Digital clubbing appears in childhood in virtually all patients with significant bronchiectasis.

Differential Diagnosis

- All adult patients with unexplained **bronchiectasis** should be considered as possible cases of undiagnosed CF and should have sweat testing performed.[50]
- **Primary ciliary dyskinesia** or **immunoglobulin deficiency** may lead to bronchiectasis, sinusitis, and infertility, but few GI symptoms and no sweat electrolyte abnormalities are present.
- Men with **Young syndrome** have bronchiectasis, sinusitis, and azoospermia, but the respiratory disease is usually mild, and GI symptoms or sweat manifestations are not present.
- **Shwachman syndrome,** consisting of pancreatic insufficiency and cyclic neutropenia, may also lead to lung disease, but sweat chloride concentrations are normal, and the neutropenia is distinguishing.
- Idiopathic bronchiectasis with or without nontuberculous mycobacterial infection can present similarly to milder CF mutations but needs to be differentiated as treatments are not identical.

Diagnostic Testing

Skin Sweat Testing

- Standardized quantitative pilocarpine iontophoresis remains the gold standard for the diagnosis of CF and is best performed at a laboratory with experience.
- A sweat chloride concentration of >60 mmol/L is consistent with the diagnosis of CF.[50]
- The diagnosis should be made only if there is an elevated sweat chloride concentration on two separate occasions in a patient with a typical phenotype or with a history of CF in a sibling.
- Borderline sweat test results (40 to 60 mmol/L sweat chloride) or nondiagnostic test results in the setting of high clinical suspicion should also lead to repeat sweat testing, nasal potential difference testing, testicular ultrasound, or genetic testing.[51]
- Abnormal sweat chloride concentrations are rarely detected in non-CF patients (e.g., significant malnutrition, Addison disease, or untreated hypothyroidism).

Genetic Testing

- Genetic tests have detected >1,200 CF mutations on chromosome 7. The most common CFTR mutation in patients is ΔF508.
- Most commercially available probes are quite sensitive but test for only a minority of the known CF mutations, although they are able to identify >90% of the abnormal CF genes in Ashkenazi Jews.
- For patients to have clinical disease, two of the recessive genes must be abnormal. Care should be taken in interpreting the presence of mutations and polymorphisms in the

absence of symptoms. Identified abnormalities do not always result in disease as they may be on the same allele or simply do not alter protein function or localization. The Clinical and Functional Translation of CFTR website (www.cftr2.org, last accessed January 21, 2015) is a good resource for information related to clinical phenotype of genetic variants.

Nasal Potential Difference

Nasal potential difference measurements can be performed at experienced centers and are able to detect the abnormal epithelial chloride secretion that is typical of CF.[51]

Other Tests

- **CXR** may show hyperinflation and upper lobe predominant bronchiectasis.
- **PFTs** typically show expiratory airflow obstruction with air trapping and hyperinflation. Impairments of gas exchange also occur and can progress to hypoxemia and hypercapnia.
- **Sputum cultures** typically identify *P. aeruginosa* and *S. aureus*, or both. Most laboratories require labeling specimens as a CF patient so plating on special media occurs.
- Testing for **malabsorption** is often not formally performed, because clinical evidence of steatorrhea, low fat-soluble vitamin levels (A, D, and E), and a prolonged prothrombin time (vitamin K) as well as a clear response to pancreatic enzyme treatment are usually considered sufficient for diagnosing exocrine insufficiency.
- Testing for sinusitis or infertility, especially obstructive azoospermia in males, would also be supportive of the diagnosis of CF.

TREATMENT

- The goals of CF therapy include maintenance of a normal nutritional status, improving quality of life, decreasing the number of exacerbations, and decreasing mortality.[52] The major focus of therapy is on clearance of airway secretions and controlling infections.
- Care at a comprehensive CF core center is recommended. These centers are designed to address the multiple organ system involvement typical of the disease and are typically staffed by pulmonary specialists who lead teams of nurses, nutritionists, and social workers to help the patients live with a chronic illness.
- Specialty consultation with gastroenterologists, endocrinologists, and occasionally interventional radiologists may be required during the course of care of each individual patient.

Medications

- Refer to Tables 16-4 and 16-12 for an overview of pharmacologic therapies for CF.
- **Bronchodilators** such as β_2-agonists (Table 16-4) are used to treat the reversible components of airflow obstruction and help facilitate mucus clearance. Many patients with CF have acute improvements in FEV_1 as well as symptomatic improvement with bronchodilators.[53] Anticholinergics have not been demonstrated to provide benefit in CF.
- **Recombinant human deoxyribonuclease** ("DNase," dornase alfa) digests extracellular DNA, decreasing the viscoelasticity of the sputum.
  - Dornase alfa improves pulmonary function and decreases the incidence of respiratory tract infections that require parenteral antibiotics.[54]
  - The recommended dose of dornase alfa is 2.5 mg/day inhaled using a jet nebulizer.
  - Adverse effects may include pharyngitis, laryngitis, rash, chest pain, and conjunctivitis.
- **Hypertonic saline,** inhaled twice to four times a day, can be used as an additional regimen in patients already using bronchodilators and dornase alfa. Clinical trials have shown improved mucus clearance, small improvements in lung function, and fewer exacerbations requiring antibiotic therapy.[55] Four milliliters of a 7% saline is used and should be preceded by an inhaled bronchodilator to offset the bronchospasm that can occur from this therapy. This is a relatively time-consuming therapy and must utilize a sterile endotoxin-free solution, which may not be covered by prescription plans.

TABLE 16-12 Additional Medications Commonly Used for Cystic Fibrosis

Drug	Formulation	Adult dose	Comments
Dornase alfa (Pulmozyme)	NEB: 2.5 mg/ 2.5 mL ampule	Daily	Typically after nebulized bronchodilator
Hypertonic saline (7% HyperSal)	NEB: 4 mL	BID	Can have initial bronchospastic reaction
Tobramycin Inhaled Solution (TOBI)	NEB: 300 mg/ 5 mL ampule	BID : alternating 28 days on and off cycles	Typically after bronchodilator Pulmozyme and any airway clearance
Aztreonam inhaled (Cayston)	NEB: 75 mg reconstituted in 1 mL diluent	TID : alternating 28 days on and off cycles	Same as for tobramycin solution, requires Altera Nebulizer
Azithromycin (Zithromax)	500 mg PO	Q M, W, F	Taken chronically in pseudomonas infected patients
Ivacaftor (Kalydeco)	150 mg PO	BID	Only for patients with a known G551D mutation. Very expensive

- **Antibiotic therapy** forms an integral component of the care of patients with CF. The airways become infected in most patients with CF, and the typical pathogens in adulthood include *P. aeruginosa* and *S. aureus*.
  - **Sputum cultures** provide the clinician with an idea which antibiotics are effective against the colonizers/pathogens during acute exacerbations. However, antibiotic therapy should never be withheld due to lack of in vitro efficacy given treatment with IV antibiotics was equally successful when regimens utilized two antibiotics of different classes despite lack of in vitro susceptibility.
  - Routine sputum cultures are also useful in identifying new infecting organisms, which can impact treatment, isolation procedures, and outcomes in patients with CF, including the following: *P. aeruginosa* in previously negative patients, *Burkholderia cepacia*, *Achromobacter xylosoxidans*, *Stenotrophomonas maltophilia*, *Aspergillus* spp., methicillin-resistant *S. aureus* (MRSA), and nontuberculous mycobacteria (*Mycobacterium avium complex* or *Mycobacterium abscessus*).
  - **Aerosolized antibiotics** are frequently used in patients with CF. Inhaling aerosolized tobramycin (300 mg nebulized bid for 28 days on, alternating with 28 days off) using an appropriate nebulizer and compressor improves pulmonary function, decreases the density of *P. aeruginosa*, and decreases the risk of hospitalization.[56] Aztreonam lysinate (75 mg tid on alternating 28-day cycles) demonstrated similar benefits to tobramycin solution despite enrollment of a more aggressively treated cohort.[57]
  - **Macrolide antibiotic therapy** with azithromycin (500 mg, PO), used chronically three times per week in patients without concurrent nontuberculous mycobacterial infection, has been shown to improve lung function and reduce exacerbations in individuals with chronic *P. aeruginosa*.[58]
- **Systemic glucocorticoids** are indicated only for refractory lung disease that has demonstrated subjective (less dyspnea) and objective (decreased airflow obstruction, improved exercise tolerance, or both) benefit during a trial period. Short courses of glucocorticoid therapy may be helpful to some patients, but long-term therapy should be avoided to minimize the side

effects, which include glucose intolerance, osteopenia, and growth retardation. There is very little data to support the use of ICS in patients with CF, unless they have concomitant asthma.

- **Pancreatic enzyme supplementation** should be instituted after pancreatic insufficiency, and malabsorption have been demonstrated. Enzyme dose is titrated to achieve one to two semisolid stools per day. Enzymes are taken immediately before meals and snacks.
  - Dosing of pancreatic enzymes should be initiated at 500 units lipase/kg/meal and should not exceed 2,500 units lipase/kg/meal.
  - High doses (>6,000 units lipase/kg/meal) may be associated with chronic intestinal strictures.
- **Pancreatic endocrine dysfunction,** specifically diabetes mellitus, is best treated with meal carbohydrate-based insulin as the typical diabetic dietary restrictions are liberalized (high-calorie diet with unrestricted fat) to encourage appropriate growth and weight maintenance. Occasionally, mild or early disease responds to metformin.
- **Constipation or distal intestinal obstruction** can be life threatening, but surgical intervention can frequently be prevented by a combination of treatments similar to preparation for a colonoscopy. Frequently, chronic use of **polyethylene glycol** laxatives is necessary to prevent recurrence.
- **Vitamin supplementation** is recommended, especially the fat-soluble vitamins that are not well absorbed in the setting of pancreatic insufficiency. Vitamins A, D, E, and K should all be supplemented orally on a regular basis. Iron deficiency anemia requires iron supplementation and occasionally intravenous replacement in refractory cases.
- Osteopenia should be aggressively treated.
- Sinus regimens including nasal irrigation limit sinusitis, but symptomatic chronic sinus symptoms are common even in adults with mild pulmonary disease.
- **Vaccinations** including a yearly influenza vaccine and a pneumococcal vaccine every 5 years are recommended.

Other Nonpharmacologic Treatment

- **Mucus mobilization/airway clearance** can be accomplished using various airway clearance techniques, including postural drainage with chest percussion and vibration, with or without mechanical devices (flutter valves, high-frequency chest oscillation vests, and low and high positive expiratory pressure devices), and breathing and coughing exercises.[59]
- **Pulmonary rehabilitation** and exercise is recommended as it improves secretion mobilization and functional status.
- **Oxygen therapy** is indicated in patients with CF, based on the same criteria as in patients with COPD. Rest and exercise oxygen assessments should be performed as clinically indicated. Although there will likely never be a trial confirming enhanced survival, the presence of secondary pulmonary hypertension at the time of transplant evaluation of many CF patients suggests benefits similar to COPD should occur.

Surgical Management

- Most patients with CF die from pulmonary disease, and **lung transplantation** may be an option.
- An FEV_1 <20% of the predicted normal value, alveolar gas exchange abnormalities (resting hypoxemia or hypercapnia), evidence of pulmonary hypertension, or increased frequency or severity of pulmonary exacerbations should lead to consideration of lung transplantation as a treatment option.[60]
- Bilateral transplantation is always performed due to chronic endobronchial infection.
- Survival rates of 40% to 60% at 5 years are standard.

SPECIAL CONSIDERATIONS

- **Acute exacerbations of CF pulmonary disease** are marked by dyspnea, increasing cough, increased mucus production, worsening of spirometry, but rarely fevers.[61]

○ Mild exacerbations can be treated with **oral antibiotics.** Typical drugs for staphylococcal species include cephalexin, dicloxacillin, trimethoprim-sulfamethoxazole, or doxycycline. Most patients infected with *P. aeruginosa* will require ciprofloxacin (750 mg bid). Typical treatment intervals are 2 to 3 weeks with reassessment to ensure adequate clinical and spirometric improvement.

○ Many patients with exacerbations will eventually require initiation of **IV antibiotics.** Choice of these agents is dictated by the sputum sensitivities, if available. Combination therapy with a semisynthetic penicillin, a third- or fourth-generation cephalosporin, a carbapenem or a quinolone, and an aminoglycoside is the typical therapy recommended during acute exacerbations.[62]

○ The presence of MRSA on sputum culture testing often necessitates addition of vancomycin or linezolid.

○ Treatment is typically 2 weeks and can be completed outside of the hospital.

○ Drug dosing tends to be higher due to altered pharmacokinetics probably due to more rapid metabolism of larger charged molecules in CF patients.

○ Once-daily IV tobramycin dosing is as effective and simpler than multiple daily-dose regimens but still requires monitoring of peak and trough levels given toxicity.[63] Patients need to be monitored chronically for side effects, including ototoxicity given frequency of use in a disease with recurrent exacerbations.

○ Home IV antibiotic therapy is common, administered through a peripherally inserted central catheter (PICC) line, subclavian Hohn catheter, or an established Port-A-Cath.

○ Initial hospitalization is recommended to allow access to comprehensive therapy and diagnostic testing as well as establishment of appropriate dosing and monitoring of the aminoglycoside.

- ***B. cepacia complex*:** Acquisition of this organism is associated with accelerated decline of lung function and shortened survival in patients with CF. In addition, colonization with this organism is a contraindication to lung transplantation at some centers because of the resistance patterns of this pathogen.[64] Patients colonized by *Burkholderia* spp. should be kept separated from other patients with CF (different clinic days, different floors in the hospital).

- **Allergic bronchopulmonary aspergillosis** can occur in patients with CF.[47]

- **Nontuberculous mycobacteria,** normally *Mycobacterium avium-intracellulare* (MAI) and rarely *M. abscessus,* can infect patients with CF. Treatment decisions depend on symptoms, radiographic appearance, and pulmonary function. In general, the same therapies are required as in patients with non-CF bronchiectasis.

- **Hemoptysis** in CF is common, especially small amounts of blood during pulmonary exacerbations. Massive hemoptysis is usually treated with IV antibiotics, airway control and ventilatory support if needed, and radiographic embolization of the bronchial arteries feeding the site of hemoptysis. Embolization may need to be repeated because of the extensive bronchial collaterals seen with CF. Limited pulmonary resection is a last resort.[46]

- **Pneumothorax** in patients with CF tends to occur as lung function worsens. Treatment consists of chest tube drainage. For persistent air leaks, pleurodesis may be required.[46]

- Women with CF who become pregnant normally tolerate the pregnant state well as long as their lung function is not severely impaired with associated pulmonary hypertension.[65] Close monitoring of lung function and glycemic control is needed.

MONITORING/FOLLOW-UP

- Spirometry is the best objective measurement of lung function in CF, and routine spirometric monitoring is recommended. A significant decline in spirometry, even in the absence of increased symptoms, mandates intensification of therapy.
- Sputum cultures and sensitivity testing should also be sent from outpatient visits.
- A1C monitoring of diabetic patients is advised.
- Yearly vitamin levels (vitamins A, E) as well as bone densitometry are recommended.

REFERENCES

1. Celli BR, MacNee W. Standards for the diagnosis and treatment of patients with COPD: a summary of the ATS/ERS position paper. *Eur Respir J* 2004;23: 932–946.
2. Raherison C, Girodet PO. Epidemiology of COPD. *Eur Respir Rev* 2009;18:213–221.
3. Hogg JC, Chu F, Utokaparch S, et al. The nature of small-airway obstruction in chronic obstructive pulmonary disease. *N Engl J Med* 2004;350:2645–2653.
4. Stoller JK, Aboussouan LS. Alpha1-antitrypsin deficiency. *Lancet* 2005;365:2225–2236.
5. Aberle DR, Adams AM, Berg CD, et al. Reduced lung-cancer mortality with low-dose computed tomographic screening. *N Engl J Med* 2011;365:395–409.
6. Vestbo J, Hurd SS, Agusti AG, et al. Global strategy for the diagnosis, management and prevention of chronic obstructive pulmonary disease: GOLD executive summary. *Am J Respir Crit Care Med* 2013;187(4):347–365.
7. Rabe KF, Hurd S, Anzueto A, et al. Global strategy for the diagnosis, management, and prevention of chronic obstructive pulmonary disease: GOLD executive summary. *Am J Respir Crit Care Med* 2007;176:532–555.
8. Ram FS, Sestini P. Regular inhaled short acting beta2 agonists for the management of stable chronic obstructive pulmonary disease: Cochrane systematic review and meta-analysis. *Thorax* 2003;58:580–584.
9. Anthonisen NR, Connett JE, Kiley JP, et al. Effects of smoking intervention and the use of an inhaled anticholinergic bronchodilator on the rate of decline of FEV1. The Lung Health Study. *JAMA* 1994;272:1497–1505.
10. COMBIVENT Inhalation Aerosol Study Group. In chronic obstructive pulmonary disease, a combination of ipratropium and albuterol is more effective than either agent alone. An 85-day multicenter trial. *Chest* 1994;105:1411–1419.
11. Calverley PM, Anderson JA, Celli B, et al. Salmeterol and fluticasone propionate and survival in chronic obstructive pulmonary disease. *N Engl J Med* 2007;356:775–789.
12. Vogelmeier C, Hederer B, Glaab T, et al. Tiotropium versus salmeterol for the prevention of exacerbations of COPD. *N Engl J Med* 2011;364:1093–1103.
13. Albert RK, Connett J, Bailey WC, et al. Azithromycin for prevention of exacerbations of COPD. *N Engl J Med* 2011;365:689–698.
14. Wedzicha JA, Rabe KF, Martinez FJ, et al. Efficacy of roflumilast in the chronic obstructive pulmonary disease frequent exacerbator phenotype. *Chest* 2013;143:1302–1311.
15. Ram FS, Jardin JR, Atallah A, et al. Efficacy of theophylline in people with stable chronic obstructive pulmonary disease: a systematic review and meta-analysis. *Respir Med* 2005;99:135–144.
16. Stoller JK, Aboussouan LS. alpha1-Antitrypsin deficiency. 5: intravenous augmentation therapy: current understanding. *Thorax* 2004;59:708–712.
17. Nocturnal Oxygen Therapy Trial Group. Continuous or nocturnal oxygen therapy in hypoxemic chronic obstructive lung disease: a clinical trial. *Ann Intern Med* 1980; 93:391–398.
18. Crockett AJ, Cranston JM, Moss JR, et al. Domiciliary oxygen for chronic obstructive pulmonary disease. *Cochrane Database Syst Rev* 2005;(4):CD001744.
19. Fishman A, Martinez F, Naunheim K, et al. A randomized trial comparing lung-volume-reduction surgery with medical therapy for severe emphysema. *N Engl J Med* 2003;348:2059–2073.
20. Thabut G, Ravaud P, Christie JD, et al. Determinants of the survival benefit of lung transplantation in patients with chronic obstructive pulmonary disease. *Am J Respir Crit Care Med* 2008;177:1156–1163.
21. Kohansal R, Martinez-Camblor P, Agusti A, et al. The natural history of chronic airflow obstruction revisited: an analysis of the Framingham offspring cohort. *Am J Respir Crit Care Med* 2009;180:3–10.

22. Treating tobacco use and dependence: 2008 update U.S. Public Health Service Clinical Practice Guideline executive summary. *Respir Care* 2008;53:1217–1222.

23. Parshall MB, Schwartzstein RM, Adams L, et al. An official American Thoracic Society statement: update on the mechanisms, assessment, and management of dyspnea. *Am J Respir Crit Care Med* 2012;185:435–452.

24. American Thoracic Society. Pulmonary rehabilitation-1999. *Am J Respir Crit Care Med* 1999;159:1666–1682.

25. Celli BR, Cote CG, Marin JM, et al. The body-mass index, airflow obstruction, dyspnea, and exercise capacity index in chronic obstructive pulmonary disease. *N Engl J Med* 2004;350:1005–1012.

26. Connors AF Jr, Dawson NV, Thomas C, et al. Outcomes following acute exacerbation of severe chronic obstructive lung disease. The SUPPORT investigators (Study to Understand Prognoses and Preferences for Outcomes and Risks of Treatments). *Am J Respir Crit Care Med* 1996;154:959–967.

27. Niewoehner DE, Erbland ML, Deupree RH, et al. Effect of systemic glucocorticoids on exacerbations of chronic obstructive pulmonary disease. Department of Veterans Affairs Cooperative Study Group. *N Engl J Med* 1999;340:1941–1947.

28. National Asthma Education and Prevention Program. *Expert Panel Report 3 (EPR-3): Guidelines for the Diagnosis and Management of Asthma. Full Report 2007.* Bethesda, MD: National Institutes of Health, National Heart, Lung, and Blood Institute, Publication No. 08-4051; 2007. Available at: http://www.nhlbi.nih.gov/guidelines/asthma/index.htm (last accessed February 21, 2014).

29. Moorman JE, Rudd RA, Johnson CA, et al. National surveillance for asthma—United States, 1980–2004. *MMWR Surveill Summ* 2007;56(8):1–54.

30. Yunginger JW, Reed CE, O'Connell EJ, et al. A community-based study of the epidemiology of asthma. Incidence rates, 1964–1983. *Am Rev Respir Dis* 1992;146:888–894.

31. Irwin RS, Curley FJ, French CL. Chronic cough: the spectrum and frequency of causes, key components of the diagnostic evaluation, and outcome of specific therapy. *Am Rev Respir Dis* 1990;141:640–647.

32. Crapo RO, Casaburi R, Coates AL, et al. Guidelines for methacholine and exercise challenge testing-1999. *Am J Respir Crit Care Med* 2000;161:309–329.

33. Cowie RL, Revitt SG, Underwood MF, Field SK. The effect of a peak flow-based action plan in the prevention of exacerbations of asthma. *Chest* 1997;112:1534–1538.

34. Nelson HS, Weiss ST, Bleecker ER, et al. The salmeterol multicenter asthma research trial: a comparison of usual pharmacotherapy for asthma or usual pharmacotherapy plus salmeterol. *Chest* 2006;129:15–26.

35. Phipatanakul W, Greene C, Downes SJ, et al. Montelukast improves asthma control in asthmatic children maintained on inhaled corticosteroids. *Ann Allergy Asthma Immunol* 2003;91:49–54.

36. Soler M, Matz J, Townley R, et al. The anti-IgE antibody omalizumab reduces exacerbations and steroid requirement in allergic asthmatics. *Eur Respir J* 2001;18:254–261.

37. Castro M, Rubin AS, Laviolette M, et al. Effectiveness and safety of bronchial thermoplasty in the treatment of severe asthma: a multicenter, randomized, double-blind, sham-controlled clinical trial. *Am J Respir Crit Care Med* 2010;181(2):116–124.

38. Källén B, Rydhstroem H, Aberg A. Congenital malformations after the use of inhaled budesonide in early pregnancy. *Obstet Gynecol* 1999;93:392–395.

39. Rodrigo GJ, Rodrigo C, Hall JB. Acute asthma in adults: a review. *Chest* 2004;125:1081–1102.

40. Cohen-Cymberknoh M, Shoseyov D, Kerem E. Managing cystic fibrosis: strategies that increase life expectancy and improve quality of life. *Am J Respir Crit Care Med* 2011;183:1463–1471.

41. Rommens JM, Iannuzzi MC, Kerem B, et al. Identification of the cystic fibrosis gene: chromosome walking and jumping. *Science* 1989;245:1059–1065.
42. Denning GM, Ostedgaard LS, Cheng SH, et al. Localization of cystic fibrosis transmembrane conductance regulator in chloride secretory epithelia. *J Clin Invest* 1992;89:339–349.
43. Stern RC. The diagnosis of cystic fibrosis. *N Engl J Med* 1997;336:487–491.
44. Wagener JS, Zemanick ET, Sontag MK. Newborn screening for cystic fibrosis. *Curr Opin Pediatr* 2012;24:329–335.
45. Conrad D, Haynes M, Salamon P, et al. Cystic fibrosis therapy: a community ecology perspective. *Am J Respir Cell Mol Biol* 2013;48:150–156.
46. Flume PA, Mogayzel PJ Jr, Robinson KA, et al. Cystic fibrosis pulmonary guidelines: pulmonary complications: hemoptysis and pneumothorax. *Am J Respir Crit Care Med* 2010;182:298–306.
47. Stevens DA, Moss RB, Kurup VP, et al. Allergic bronchopulmonary aspergillosis in cystic fibrosis—state of the art: Cystic Fibrosis Foundation Consensus Conference. *Clin Infect Dis* 2003;37(suppl 3):S225–S264.
48. Dodge JA. Male fertility in cystic fibrosis. *Lancet* 1995;346:587–588.
49. Haworth CS, Selby PL, Webb AK, et al. Low bone mineral density in adults with cystic fibrosis. *Thorax* 1999;54:961–967.
50. Davis PB, Del Rio S, Muntz JA, et al. Sweat chloride concentration in adults with pulmonary diseases. *Am Rev Respir Dis* 1983;128:34–37.
51. Alton EW, Currie D, Logan-Sinclair R, et al. Nasal potential difference: a clinical diagnostic test for cystic fibrosis. *Eur Respir J* 1990;3:922–926.
52. Flume PA, O'Sullivan BP, Robinson KA, et al. Cystic fibrosis pulmonary guidelines: chronic medications for maintenance of lung health. *Am J Respir Crit Care Med* 2007;176:957–969.
53. Cropp GJ. Effectiveness of bronchodilators in cystic fibrosis. *Am J Med* 1996;100:19S–29S.
54. Fuchs HJ, Borowitz DS, Christiansen DH, et al. Effect of aerosolized recombinant human DNase on exacerbations of respiratory symptoms and on pulmonary function in patients with cystic fibrosis. The Pulmozyme Study Group. *N Engl J Med* 1994;331:637–642.
55. Elkins MR, Robinson M, Rose BR, et al. A controlled trial of long-term inhaled hypertonic saline in patients with cystic fibrosis. *N Engl J Med* 2006;354:229–240.
56. Ramsey BW, Pepe MS, Quan JM, et al. Intermittent administration of inhaled tobramycin in patients with cystic fibrosis. Cystic Fibrosis Inhaled Tobramycin Study Group. *N Engl J Med* 1999;340:23–30.
57. McCoy KS, Quittner AL, Oermann CM, et al. Inhaled aztreonam lysine for chronic airway *Pseudomonas aeruginosa* in cystic fibrosis. *Am J Respir Crit Care Med* 2008;178:921–928.
58. Saiman L, Marshall BC, Mayer-Hamblett N, et al. Azithromycin in patients with cystic fibrosis chronically infected with *Pseudomonas aeruginosa*: a randomized controlled trial. *JAMA* 2003;290:1749–1756.
59. Flume PA, Robinson KA, O'Sullivan BP, et al. Cystic fibrosis pulmonary guidelines: airway clearance therapies. *Respir Care* 2009;54:522–537.
60. Kreider M, Kotloff RM. Selection of candidates for lung transplantation. *Proc Am Thorac Soc* 2009;6:20–27.
61. Flume PA, Mogayzel PJ Jr, Robinson KA, et al. Cystic fibrosis pulmonary guidelines: treatment of pulmonary exacerbations. *Am J Respir Crit Care Med* 2009;180:802–808.
62. Zobell JT, Waters CD, Young DC, et al. Optimization of anti-pseudomonal antibiotics for cystic fibrosis pulmonary exacerbations: II. Cephalosporins and penicillins. *Pediatr Pulmonol* 2013;48:107–122.

63. Smyth A, Tan KH, Hyman-Taylor P, et al. Once versus three-times daily regimens of tobramycin treatment for pulmonary exacerbations of cystic fibrosis—the TOPIC study: a randomised controlled trial. *Lancet* 2005;365:573–578.

64. Chaparro C, Maurer J, Gutierrez C, et al. Infection with Burkholderia cepacia in cystic fibrosis: outcome following lung transplantation. *Am J Respir Crit Care Med* 2001;163:43–48.

65. Goss CH, Rubenfeld GD, Otto K, et al. The effect of pregnancy on survival in women with cystic fibrosis. *Chest* 2003;124:1460–1468.

Anthony Boyer and Murali M. Chakinala

Interstitial Lung Disease

GENERAL PRINCIPLES

- Interstitial lung diseases (ILDs), also known as diffuse parenchymal lung diseases, are a heterogeneous group of disorders characterized by infiltration of cellular and noncellular material into the lung parenchyma.
- The role of the primary care physician is to recognize the presentation of an ILD, start the initial workup, know when to involve the pulmonary specialist, and be aware of the disease course and treatment options.
- There are >100 distinct types of ILDs, yet no universal classification system exists; however, they can be categorized on the basis of etiology and presentation (Table 17-1).[1]
- The prevalence of ILDs is estimated to be 80.9 per 100,000 in males and 67.2 per 100,000 in females.[2] Idiopathic pulmonary fibrosis (IPF) is the most common form, accounting for 25% to 35% of cases.[1] Sarcoidosis and connective tissue disease (CTD)-related ILDs are the next most prevalent.
- Mechanisms of these diseases are not well understood, but many suspect injury to the alveolar epithelium that causes inflammation and an abnormal host response that ultimately leads to fibrosis. Collagen deposition causes stiff lungs with poor distensibility, resulting in a restrictive ventilatory pattern and impaired gas exchange. ILDs not only affect the interstitial compartment of the lungs but also involve the alveoli, microvasculature, and small airways.
- Pulmonary hypertension may be a late complication in the disease course.

DIAGNOSIS

Clinical Presentation

A general approach to the diagnosis of ILD is presented in Figure 17-1.[3]

History
- History is an extremely important component of the evaluation of ILDs.
- Demographics can be helpful (e.g., lymphangioleiomyomatosis [LAM] is most common in young women). Age of onset of disease is highly variable. IPF typically presents in the seventh decade or later, while CTD-related ILD often presents in the third to fifth decade.
- The temporal course of symptoms should be noted. For example, acute interstitial pneumonia (AIP), cryptogenic organizing pneumonia (COP), acute eosinophilic pneumonia (AEP), and alveolar hemorrhage syndromes develop quite rapidly (days to weeks), whereas IPF, nonspecific interstitial pneumonitis (NSIP), hypersensitivity pneumonitis (HP), and sarcoidosis have a more insidious onset (months to years).

TABLE 17-1	Classification Scheme for the Interstitial Lung Diseases (ILDs)
Category	**Disease**
Idiopathic interstitial pneumonias	Acute interstitial pneumonitis (AIP)/diffuse alveolar damage (DAD)
	Idiopathic pulmonary fibrosis (IPF)/usual interstitial pneumonia (UIP)
	Nonspecific interstitial pneumonitis (NSIP)
	Cryptogenic organizing pneumonitis (COP)
	Respiratory bronchiolitis-interstitial lung disease (RB-ILD)
	Desquamative interstitial pneumonia (DIP)
	Lymphocytic interstitial pneumonia (LIP)
Occupational/ environmental	Hypersensitivity pneumonitis (HP)
	Pneumoconiosis
	Heavy metal disease (e.g., cobalt)
	Berylliosis
	Asbestosis
	Silicosis
	Noxious gas/fumes/vapors
Immune related	Connective tissue disease related: systemic lupus erythematosus, rheumatoid arthritis, scleroderma/systemic sclerosis, antisynthetase syndrome, polymyositis, and dermatomyositis
	Vasculitis—granulomatosis with polyangiitis (GPA, formerly Wegener granulomatosis), Churg-Strauss, microscopic polyangiitis
	Goodpasture disease
Eosinophilic interstitial lung disease	Acute eosinophilic pneumonia (AEP)
	Chronic eosinophilic pneumonia (CEP)
Treatment related	Drugs (see http:\\www.pneumotox.com)—amiodarone, nitrofurantoin, methotrexate
	Chemotherapy—bleomycin, busulfan, BCNU
	Radiation induced
Malignancy	Lymphangitic carcinomatosis
	Bronchoalveolar cell carcinoma
	Amyloidosis
Others	Sarcoidosis
	Lymphangioleiomyomatosis (LAM)
	Pulmonary alveolar proteinosis (PAP)
	Pulmonary Langerhans cell histiocytosis (PLCH)
	Neurofibromatosis

- **The most common presenting symptom is dyspnea on exertion.** Cough is also common. Nonpulmonary symptoms, such as dysphagia, Raynaud phenomenon, myalgias, and arthralgias, point toward an underlying CTD.
- Active smoking is associated with respiratory bronchiolitis-ILD (RB-ILD), desquamative interstitial pneumonia (DIP), and pulmonary Langerhans cell histiocytosis (PLCH).
- Occupational and environmental exposures can reveal disorders such as HP and pneumoconiosis.

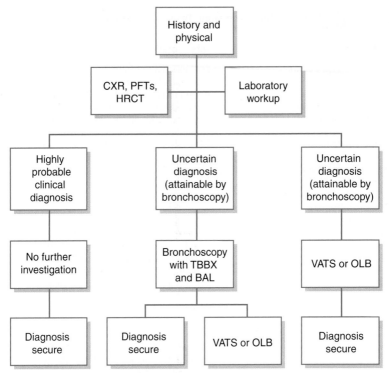

Figure 17-1 Approach to diagnosing interstitial lung diseases. (BAL, bronchoalveolar lavage; CXR, plain chest radiography; HRCT, high-resolution computed tomography; OLB, open lung biopsy; PFTs, pulmonary function tests; TBBX, transbronchial biopsy; VATS, video-assisted thoracoscopic surgery). (Modified from British Thoracic Society. The diagnosis, assessment and treatment of diffuse parenchymal lung disease in adults. *Thorax* 1999;54:S1–S28.)

- Medication history (e.g., amiodarone) or treatment with chemotherapy agents and radiation may reveal an underlying cause.
- Family history may also be important (e.g., familial form of IPF).

Physical Examination
- The hallmark feature of ILD is **auscultatory crackles**; IPF is associated with fine crackles that mimic Velcro ripping apart.
- Clubbing of the nails is an important clue in the diagnosis of IPF.
- Systemic findings of fever, joint pains, and rashes are more indicative of an associated CTD or sarcoidosis.
- Findings of a CTD, including cutaneous telangiectasias, sclerodactyly, arthritis, myositis, and joint deformities, may be present on examination.
- Advanced cases can exhibit findings of pulmonary hypertension and cor pulmonale.

Diagnostic Testing
Laboratory Tests
Laboratory tests should be interpreted in the appropriate clinical setting (Table 17-2).[4] Angiotensin-converting enzyme level for sarcoidosis is generally not useful due to its low sensitivity and specificity.

TABLE 17-2   Helpful Blood and Urine Tests to Evaluate ILDs

Laboratory test	Interpretation
Complete blood count	Eosinophilia may support eosinophilic pneumonia or a drug-related ILD. Anemia may support alveolar hemorrhage.
Creatine kinase, aldolase, anti-Jo1 antibody	Elevated levels support polymyositis or dermatomyositis in patients with muscle pain.
Urinary sediment	RBC casts or dysmorphic RBCs may suggest a systemic vasculitis.
Antinuclear antibody, rheumatoid factor, antiribonucleic protein antibody, anticentromere antibody, antitopoisomerase antibody	Elevated results *may* support a CTD-related ILD.
cANCA, p-ANCA	Positive cANCA followed by the detection of antiproteinase-3 antibody supports GPA. Positive p-ANCA followed by the detection of antimyeloperoxidase antibody supports microscopic polyangiitis or Churg-Strauss syndrome.
Antiglomerular basement membrane antibody	A positive result in a patient with alveolar hemorrhage is a diagnostic for Goodpasture disease.
Hypersensitivity pneumonitis serum precipitins	Results should be interpreted on the basis of clinical context. Sensitivity and specificity are variable.

cANCA, cytoplasmic antineutrophilic cytoplasmic antibody; CTD, connective tissue disease; ILD, interstitial lung disease; p-ANCA, perinuclear antineutrophilic cytoplasmic antibody; RBC, red blood cell.
Data from Reynolds H, Matthay R. Diffuse interstitial and alveolar lung diseases. In: George RB, Light RW, Matthay MA, et al. eds. *Chest Medicine: Essentials of Pulmonary and Critical Care Medicine.* Philadelphia, PA: Lippincott Williams & Wilkins; 2006:262–313.

Imaging
- **Plain chest radiography** can be helpful in revealing an ILD but not typically diagnostic. CXR can be normal in up to 10% of patients with clinically significant ILDs.[4] Radiographic patterns that may be associated with ILDs include the following[1,5]:
  - Small lung volumes: IPF and CTD related
  - Preserved or large lung volumes: ILDs associated with airway involvement such as HP, LAM, PLCH, combined pulmonary fibrosis and emphysema (CPFE), and neurofibromatosis-associated ILD
  - Upper lobe predominance: sarcoidosis, silicosis, and PLCH
  - Lower lobe predominance: IPF and asbestosis
  - Peripheral zone predominance: COP and chronic eosinophilic pneumonia (CEP)
  - Migratory infiltrates: COP, HP, and eosinophilic pneumonia
- High-resolution computed tomography (HRCT) is the most helpful radiographic test to evaluate ILDs and will also help guide location for lung biopsy and possible mediastinal lymph node sampling. Patterns on HRCT that may be associated with ILDs include the following[1,4]:
  - Reticular lines with honeycombing and traction bronchiectasis: IPF, CTD related, asbestosis, and sarcoidosis

- Nodules: pneumoconiosis, malignancy, rheumatoid arthritis (RA), granulomatosis with polyangiitis (GPA, formerly Wegener granulomatosis), HP, and sarcoidosis (nodular pattern particularly along bronchovascular bundles is common in sarcoidosis)
  - Cystic disease: LAM and PLCH
  - Honeycombing: IPF, asbestosis, CTD related, chronic HP
  - Ground-glass opacities: alveolar hemorrhage, HP, AIP, drug-induced diseases, pulmonary alveolar proteinosis (PAP), NSIP
  - Multifocal consolidation: COP or secondary bronchiolitis obliterans organizing pneumonia (BOOP)
  - Hilar/mediastinal lymphadenopathy: sarcoidosis, berylliosis, silicosis
  - Crazy paving: PAP

Diagnostic Procedures
- **Pulmonary function tests** (PFTs) should include spirometry, lung volumes, diffusion capacity, and exercise oximetry as well as an arterial blood gas in certain circumstances.
  - PFTs classically show a **restrictive ventilatory defect**: low total lung capacity, low vital capacity, low forced expiratory volume in 1 second (FEV_1), and low forced vital capacity (FVC) but normal or high FEV_1/FVC.[5]
  - Preserved lung volumes in the setting of ILD should raise suspicion for HP, PLCH, LAM, or CPFE.
  - An obstructive ventilatory defect in the setting of ILD could indicate sarcoidosis, HP, PLCH, or LAM due to concomitant airway involvement.
  - Abnormal gas exchange is often evident with a low diffusion capacity for carbon monoxide (DL_{CO}) and **hypoxemia, particularly with exercise**. Elevated DL_{CO} is consistent with alveolar hemorrhage.
- **Lung biopsy** can provide a firm histopathologic diagnosis allowing a clinician to more accurately predict prognosis, assess disease activity, and exclude neoplastic or infectious processes that may mimic an ILD.
  - In IPF, a biopsy is not always required as the aforementioned clinical and radiographic criteria can accurately predict the diagnosis in >90% of cases (Table 17-3).[6]
  - There are three routes for lung biopsies: transbronchial lung biopsy via **bronchoscopy**, wedge biopsy via **open thoracotomy** or open lung biopsy, and biopsy via **video-assisted thoracoscopic surgery (VATS)**.[2] ILD pathology is frequently inhomogeneous. Thus, large specimens typically >2 cm in diameter from more than one lobe of the lung are ideal.
  - There are six idiopathic interstitial pneumonias classified on the basis of histopathology (Table 17-4).[2,6]

Differential Diagnosis
- **IPF** is histologically identical to UIP, but with no known inciting agent. It typically affects patients >50 years of age and men much more commonly than women. Diagnosis of IPF can be made without a surgical lung biopsy (Table 17-3).[6] Distinguishing IPF from fibrosing NSIP may be very difficult.

TABLE 17-3	**Criteria for Diagnosis of IPF**

- Exclusion of known causes of ILDs (e.g., drugs, exposures, CTDs)
- Presence of UIP pattern on HRCT in patients not subjected to surgical lung biopsy
- Specific combinations of HRCT and surgical lung biopsy pattern in patients subjected to surgical lung biopsy

ILD, interstitial lung disease; CTD, connective tissue disease; UIP, usual interstitial pneumonia; HRCT, high-resolution computed tomography.

TABLE 17-4	Summary of Features of the Idiopathic Interstitial Pneumonias					
	IPF	**NSIP**	**DIP and RB-ILD**	**COP/BOOP**	**AIP**	**LIP**
Duration	Chronic (>12 months)	Subacute to chronic (months to years)	Subacute (weeks to months)	Subacute (<3 months)	Abrupt (1–2 weeks)	Chronic (>12 months)
HRCT findings	Peripheral, subpleural, basal predominance; Reticular opacities; Architectural distortion; Traction bronchiectasis; Honeycombing; Minimal "ground-glass"; Temporally heterogeneous with areas of end-stage honeycombing and adjacent unaffected areas	Peripheral, subpleural, basal, symmetric; Ground-glass attenuation/consolidation; Lower lobe volume loss; Occasional subpleural sparing	DIP: diffuse ground-glass opacities in the middle and lower lungs; RB-ILD: bronchial wall thickening; centrilobular nodules; patchy ground-glass opacities	Subpleural or peribronchial; Patchy consolidation; Nodules	Diffuse and bilateral; Ground-glass opacities often with lobular sparing	Diffuse; Centrilobular nodules; Ground-glass attenuation; Septal and bronchovascular thickening; Thin-walled cysts
Treatment	Poor response to corticosteroids or cytotoxic agents	Corticosteroids and steroid-sparing agents	**Smoking cessation**; effectiveness of corticosteroids unknown	Corticosteroids	Effectiveness of corticosteroids unknown	Corticosteroids
Prognosis	5-year mortality = 80%; median survival 2–3 years after diagnosis	Cellular NSIP: 5-year mortality <10% (median survival >10 years); Fibrotic NSIP: 5-year mortality = 10% (median survival 6–8 years)	DIP: 5-year mortality <5%; RB-ILD: no deaths reported	5-year mortality <5% (deaths are rare)	60% mortality in <6 months	Limited data

AIP, acute interstitial pneumonia; BOOP, bronchiolitis organizing pneumonia; COP, cryptogenic organizing pneumonia; DIP, desquamative interstitial pneumonia; HRCT, high-resolution computed tomography; IPF, idiopathic pulmonary fibrosis; LIP, lymphocytic interstitial pneumonia; NSIP, nonspecific interstitial pneumonitis; RB-ILD, respiratory bronchiolitis-interstitial lung disease.
Data from King TE. Clinical advances in the diagnosis and therapy of the interstitial lung diseases. *Am J Respir Crit Care Med* 2005;172:268–279.

- **NSIP** is a pattern of lung response to a variety of injuries. Diseases associated with NSIP include CTD such as scleroderma, rheumatoid arthritis, and polymyositis-dermatomyositis. Presentation is similar to IPF although NSIP may be a more subacute presentation, and patients may have signs and symptoms of a CTD. CXR is similar to other idiopathic interstitial pneumonias, and HRCT characteristically shows ground-glass opacities with varying degrees of fibrosis. There are **three histologic subgroups**: cellular (Group I), mixed cellular and fibrosis (Group II), and fibrosis (Group III).

- **COP is defined histologically by BOOP**, which encompasses collagenous granulation tissue in the lumens of small airways and alveolar ducts with surrounding alveolar chronic inflammation. It classically presents like pneumonia, but the patient fails to respond to antibiotics. BOOP may be caused by drugs, inhalational exposures, or infection. COP can be diagnosed only if known causes of BOOP are excluded. CXR and HRCT show patchy peripheral infiltrates that may be migratory. The diagnosis can usually be made by transbronchial biopsy.

- **Sarcoidosis** is the second most common ILD. Infectious granulomatous disease should be ruled out before initiating therapy. HRCT typically reveals nodular infiltrates in a lymphatic distribution with an **upper and midlung predominance**. Mediastinal and bilateral hilar lymphadenopathy is common.

- **HP** is also known as **extrinsic allergic alveolitis**. Inflammation is caused by repeated inhalation of an inciting agent in a sensitized host. Presentation can be acute, subacute, or chronic depending on the type and level of exposure to the offending agent. Common forms of HP include bird-fancier's disease, farmer's lung disease, and hot tub lung, but dozens of others have been reported. HRCT is variable and includes centrilobular nodules, ground-glass opacities, or extensive honeycombing.

- **GPA** is a **necrotizing granulomatous vasculitis** of the upper and lower respiratory tract and can cause a rapidly progressive glomerulonephritis. Presentations include sinusitis, epistaxis, ulcers, hemoptysis, and dyspnea. Specificity of **cytoplasmic antineutrophilic cytoplasmic antibody (cANCA)** testing is 99% but requires confirmation with positive antibody to proteinase 3. Sensitivity ranges from 30% to 60%. There is a strong correlation between cANCA and disease activity.[4] Radiographic features are variable but include heterogeneous pulmonary infiltrates and pulmonary nodules. Pathologic specimens include the presence of inflammatory masses with necrotic areas and granulomatous vasculitis.

- There are a variety of **eosinophilic lung diseases** including acute and chronic eosinophilic pneumonia (AEP and CEP, respectively), allergic bronchopulmonary aspergillosis, Churg-Strauss syndrome, and idiopathic hypereosinophilic syndrome. AEP typically has an acute, severe presentation characterized by diffuse infiltrates. CEP is a slow, progressive disease that may have severe pulmonary and systemic symptoms. Radiographic findings commonly show peripheral pulmonary infiltrates that can cross fissures. Bronchoalveolar lavage (BAL) eosinophils should be >25%, and peripheral eosinophilia is typical.

- **PAP** is characterized by the accumulation of periodic acid-Schiff–positive, lipid-rich proteinaceous material in the alveolar spaces. **Granulocyte macrophage colony–stimulating factor (GM-CSF) mutations** or acquired inactivating antibodies play a critical role in the pathogenesis. Disease onset is typically gradual. CXR shows a diffuse alveolar filling process. HRCT shows diffuse ground-glass opacities in a pattern referred to as crazy paving. BAL demonstrates thick milky effluent due to a large amount of proteinaceous material.

- **LAM** is a rare cystic disease, which causes progressive airflow obstruction in young women. Pneumothoraces are common. HRCT shows numerous uniform thin-walled cysts.

- **PLCH** is a disease that features activation and proliferation of Langerhans cells. **Greater than 90% of cases occur in smokers.**[4] Symptoms of cough and dyspnea typically occur insidiously. CXR shows diffuse micronodular infiltrates. HRCT shows numerous irregular cysts and centrilobular nodules.

TREATMENT

- The most recent international guidelines do not find evidence to support any pharmacologic therapy for IPF, including corticosteroid monotherapy.[6] A recent trial noted increased mortality and morbidity with combination prednisone, azathioprine, and *N*-acetylcysteine.[7] The role of alternative pharmacologic agents, such as acetylcysteine (as monotherapy) or pirfenidone, has yet to be fully elucidated.[6] Early referral for lung transplantation is advised, if no contraindications exist.
- **NSIP**, especially when exhibiting predominantly cellular pathology, responds to immunosuppressive therapy and has a significantly better prognosis than IPF.[8]
- **COP** tends to be steroid responsive but has a high rate of relapse (up to 50%).[4]
- First-line treatment for **sarcoidosis** is steroids, typically 0.5 mg/kg/day, but when and in whom to initiate therapy is still controversial. Generally, steroids for chronic ILD are not initiated unless significant pulmonary symptoms exist and fail to remit after an extended period of time (e.g., 6 to 12 months). Extrapulmonary disease (ophthalmologic, cardiac, and CNS) usually requires treatment. Steroid-sparing agents such as methotrexate, imuran, and leflunomide can be considered in patients unable to wean from high-dose steroids. Tumor necrosis factor-alpha (TNF-α) inhibitors can be considered in refractory disease.[9]
- **HP** treatment includes removal of the offending exposure. Steroids can be used if very symptomatic.
- The mainstay of treatment for **GPA** was oral cyclophosphamide plus corticosteroids; however, recent evidence suggests that rituximab with corticosteroids is as effective at inducing remission in severe disease. Untreated disease follows a rapidly fatal course.[4,10]
- **AEP** often responds to corticosteroids. **CEP** is also responsive to corticosteroids but may relapse in approximately 50% of patients.
- Spontaneous recovery from **PAP** occurs in >25% of patients. Corticosteroids have no clear benefit.[4] Subcutaneous GM-CSF has shown some benefit. In patients with severe respiratory failure, repetitive whole-lung lavage with saline is necessary.
- **LAM** treatment options include antiestrogen agents, oophorectomy, and sirolimus.[11]
- Smoking cessation is beneficial for **PLCH**. Corticosteroid therapy early in the disease may be helpful.

Pulmonary Hypertension

GENERAL PRINCIPLES

- Pulmonary hypertension (PH) is frequently encountered during the evaluation of respiratory or cardiac conditions.
- While mild PH (i.e., PASP <50 or mean PAP <30) can occur in the setting of acute conditions (e.g., pulmonary embolism, pulmonary edema, acute respiratory distress syndrome), chronic PH should prompt an evaluation to determine its origins and guide therapy.
- Internists and primary care physicians should be aware of basic pulmonary physiology, the differential diagnosis of PH, and how to evaluate the condition in order to identify which patients need therapeutic intervention.
- PH is defined as **mean PAP ≥25 mm Hg at rest.**

TABLE 17-5	2008 Dana Point Clinical Classification of Pulmonary Hypertension (PH)

Group I: Pulmonary arterial hypertension (PAH)
Idiopathic (IPAH)
Heritable
    BMPR2
    ALK-1, endoglin (with or without hereditary hemorrhagic telangiectasia)
    Unknown
Drugs and toxins induced
Associated with (APAH)
    Pulmonary arterial hypertension
    HIV infection
    Portal hypertension
    Congenital heart disease
    Schistosomiasis
    Chronic hemolytic anemia
Persistent pulmonary hypertension of the newborn

Group I: Pulmonary venoocclusive disease and/or pulmonary capillary hemangiomatosis

Group II: Pulmonary hypertension due to left heart disease
Systolic dysfunction
Diastolic dysfunction
Valvular disease

Group III: Pulmonary hypertension due to lung disease and/or hypoxia
Chronic obstructive lung disease
Interstitial lung disease
Other pulmonary diseases with mixed restrictive and obstructive pattern
Sleep-disordered breathing
Alveolar hypoventilation disorders
Chronic exposure to high altitude
Developmental abnormalities

Group IV: Chronic thromboembolic pulmonary hypertension (CTEPH)

Group V: PH with unclear and/or multifactorial mechanisms
Hematologic disorders: myeloproliferative disorders, splenectomy
Systemic disorders: sarcoidosis, PLCH, LAM, neurofibromatosis, vasculitis
Metabolic disorders: glycogen storage disease, Gaucher disease, thyroid disorders
Others: tumoral obstruction, fibrosing mediastinitis, chronic renal failure on dialysis

BMPR-2, bone morphogenic protein receptor, type 2; ALK-1, activin receptor-like kinase 1 gene; PLCH, pulmonary Langerhans cell histiocytosis; LAM, lymphangioleiomyomatosis. Data from Galie N, Hoeper MM, Humbert M, et al. Guidelines for the diagnosis and treatment of pulmonary hypertension: the Task Force for the Diagnosis and Treatment of Pulmonary Hypertension of the European Society of Cardiology (ESC) and the European Respiratory Society (ERS), endorsed by the International Society of Heart and Lung Transplantation (ISHLT). *Eur Heart J* 2009;30:2493–2537.

- There are five main groups of PH delineated in the 2008 Dana Point clinical classification scheme (Table 17-5).[12,13] Mechanisms leading to PH differ among categories:
  - **Group I** encompasses conditions distinguished by **severe vascular remodeling**.
  - **Group II** patients develop pulmonary venous hypertension from elevated downstream pressures in the left side of the heart.

- ○ **Group III** patients encounter lung destruction as a result of underlying lung disease and/or vascular remodeling due to chronic hypoxemia.
- ○ **Group IV** disease results from progressive obliteration of vasculature due to embolization of foreign material.
- ○ **Group V** conditions have variable mechanisms for developing PH, including vasculature compression, lung destruction, or vascular remodeling.
- **Pulmonary arterial hypertension (PAH)** is a category of diseases that share pathobiology resulting from **vasoconstriction, endothelial and smooth cell proliferation**, and **in situ thrombosis**.
  - ○ Prevalence of PAH is estimated to be 15 to 26 cases per million adults.[14,15]
  - ○ PAH is defined as elevated pulmonary artery pressures in the setting of normal LV filling pressures (i.e., PAOP ≤15 mm Hg).
  - ○ Notable for severely elevated pulmonary artery pressures that can ultimately result in right ventricular failure.
  - ○ Most common types are idiopathic PAH and PAH associated with collagen vascular diseases, particularly progressive systemic sclerosis or scleroderma.
- **Pulmonary venous hypertension** is the most frequently encountered type of PH in western countries, while PH associated with lung disease and/or hypoxemia is second most common.
- **The leading cause of death in patients with PAH is right heart failure**.

DIAGNOSIS

Clinical Presentation

- The core problem in PH is the deranged relationship between the flow of blood (i.e., the cardiac output) through the pulmonary vasculature and the pressures generated.
- Initially, pulmonary pressures rise as the peripheral vascular resistance (PVR) is climbing, but most patients will be asymptomatic as the right ventricle (RV) compensates through hypertrophy. Patients eventually become symptomatic from the inability to augment cardiac output during periods of exertion.
- Common complaints are **dyspnea** and **diminished exercise tolerance**.
- Patients may also report **palpitations** during activity, which is the self-perception of tachycardia required to meet cardiac output demands.
- **Hoarseness** can also be encountered because of left recurrent laryngeal nerve compression by the enlarging pulmonary artery (i.e., Ortner syndrome).
- As the condition progresses with additional increase in the PVR and RV afterload, peak cardiac output declines further until even resting cardiac output is depressed. **Fatigue** and **syncope** herald overt right heart failure exhibited by **lower extremity edema**, ascites, and early satiety/right upper quadrant pain from hepatic congestion.
- Ultimately, dilation of the RV and displacement of interventricular septum encroach upon the LV leading to impaired LV filling and precipitous decline in cardiac output.

Diagnostic Testing

- The objectives for the evaluation of chronic PH are to delineate the type of PH, identify contributory factors, and assess severity.
- PH should be considered in the following situations:
  - ○ Unexplained dyspnea or diminished exercise tolerance
  - ○ Dyspnea and/or hypoxemia out of proportion to other pulmonary physiologic measures
  - ○ Isolated right heart failure
  - ○ Risk factors for PAH (e.g., kindred with familial PAH, systemic sclerosis)
  - ○ Suggestive ECG findings: right axis deviation, right atrial enlargement (P wave taller than 2.5 mm in inferior leads), and right ventricular hypertrophy (prominent R wave

in V_1/V_2 or prominent S wave in V_5/V_6), right ventricular strain (ST-T–segment depression and T-wave inversions in the right precordial leads or a pattern of S wave in I with Q-wave and T-wave inversion in III)

○ Prominent central pulmonary arteries on CXR
- An algorithm for evaluating PH is outlined in Figure 17-2. The evaluation can be done concurrently if echocardiography confirms the suspicion of PH.
- Patients with severe PH, which is considered discordant to the degree of underlying cardiac or pulmonary conditions, require evaluation to exclude additional causes of PH.

Right Heart Catheterization

Before beginning vasodilator therapy for PAH (or Group I PH), right heart catheterization should be done to
- Confirm elevated pulmonary artery and right heart pressures
- Exclude left heart disease
- Screen for missed left-to-right shunts
- Infer prognosis based on the magnitude of right atrial pressure (RAP) elevation and cardiac index depression[16]

Vasodilator Challenge

- Perform an acute vasodilator challenge in PAH patients who are not in extreme right heart failure. Avoid if mean RAP >20 mm Hg or cardiac index <1.5 L/minute/m².
- Vasodilators of choice include inhaled nitric oxide, IV epoprostenol, and IV adenosine.
- A significant response is a **decline in mean PAP ≥10 mm Hg to a concluding mean PAP ≤40 mm Hg with stable or improved cardiac output.**[17]
- A significant vasodilator response in PAH is rare but, if present, identifies a subgroup of patients who may respond to long-term calcium channel blockers and confers a better prognosis.

Functional Assessment

- **Before beginning therapy for PAH, patients should have a baseline functional assessment** performed to assist with longitudinal monitoring.
- The World Health Organization functional classification is detailed in Table 17-6.[18] Prognosis is considerably worse for patients in functional class III or IV than for patients in functional class I or II.
- **6-minute walk test** (6 MW): distance covered during a 6-minute walk has correlated with functional class and survival in idiopathic PAH patients.[19]

TREATMENT

Treatment approach in PAH depends on the specific diagnosis, as mechanisms of PAH vary widely across categories (Table 17-5).[12,13]

Treatment of Group I PAH

General Therapies
- Avoid vasoconstrictive substances: over-the-counter decongestants, nicotine, and cocaine.
- Avoid strong Valsalva maneuvers that can induce syncope: heavy lifting or straining during micturition or defecation.
- Avoid excessive dietary salt intake (2 to 3 g/day).
- Routine vaccinations against influenza and *Streptococcus pneumoniae*.
- Avoid pregnancy because of historically high maternal mortality.
- Minimize exposure to high altitudes (>5,000 feet), including airline travel.
- In patients with right-to-left shunts (e.g., large patent foramen ovale or atrial septal defects), use filters on IVs to prevent inadvertent systemic air embolism.

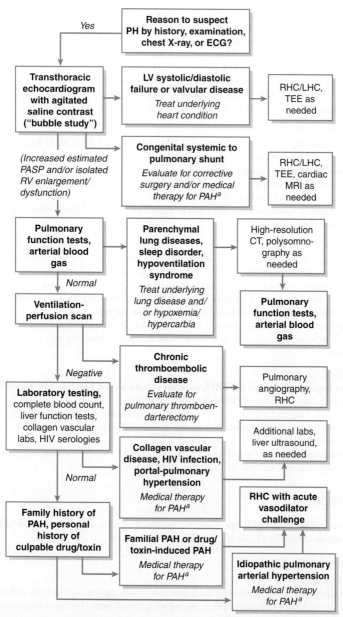

Figure 17-2 Diagnostic algorithm for the evaluation of pulmonary hypertension. Patients with unexplained pulmonary hypertension or pressures that are discordantly high for the presumed underlying cause should be considered for RHC. [a]Prior to medical therapy, patients should complete right heart catheterization and baseline functional assessments. (CT, computed tomography; ECG, electrocardiogram; LHC, left heart catheterization; LV, left ventricle; PAH, pulmonary artery hypertension; PASP, pulmonary artery systolic pressure; PH, pulmonary hypertension; RHC, right heart catheterization; RV, right ventricle; TEE, transesophageal echocardiogram).

TABLE 17-6	World Health Organization Functional Classification Scheme
Class I:	No limitation of physical activity Ordinary physical activity does not cause undue dyspnea or fatigue, chest pain, or near syncope
Class II:	Slight limitation of physical activity Ordinary physical activity causes undue dyspnea or fatigue, chest pain, or near syncope
Class III:	Marked limitation of physical activity Less than ordinary physical activity causes undue dyspnea or fatigue, chest pain, or near syncope
Class IV:	Inability to perform any physical activity without symptoms Dyspnea and/or fatigue may be present at rest, and discomfort is increased by any physical activity

Modified from *Diseases of the Heart and Blood Vessels: Nomenclature and Criteria for Diagnosis of the Heart and Great Blood Vessels*, 6th ed. New York: New York Heart Association/Little Brown; 1964.

Conventional Therapies
- **Diuretics** are used to control excess volume and minimize RV encroachment on LV.
- **Long-term oxygen therapy** is indicated to maintain SaO_2 >90% at all times, unless a right-to-left intracardiac shunt is present.
- **Warfarin** is recommended for patients without contraindications to chronic anticoagulation. Recommendation is stronger for idiopathic PAH patients.[20] Caution must be exercised in patients with systemic sclerosis, cirrhosis/portal hypertension, and certain patients with congenital systemic-to-pulmonary shunts because of unique bleeding tendencies.
- **Digoxin** has weak inotropic effects on the RV but can also assist with management of tachyarrhythmias.

Pulmonary Vasomodulators
- **Calcium channel blockers** are beneficial for only a very small minority of patients with PAH and **should not be used without confirming vasoresponsiveness with an acute vasodilator challenge** (see above).[20] Titrate to maximum tolerated dose over several weeks with close monitoring for side effects, such as fatigue, hypotension, and edema.
- Three classes of specific pulmonary vasomodulators, **endothelin receptor antagonists, phosphodiesterase-5 inhibitors, and prostacyclin analogues** (i.e., prostanoids), are detailed in Table 17-7.
- Initial choice of PAH-specific therapy should be individualized to severity of condition, based on predictors of prognosis (Fig. 17-3).[21]
  - Poor predictors (bolded factors are considered especially significant): **scleroderma PAH**, portopulmonary hypertension, familial PAH, men >60, renal insufficiency, B-type natriuretic peptide (BNP) >180, PVR >32 Wood units (even much lower PVR values confer poor prognosis), **RAP >20**, DL_{CO} ≤32%, **pericardial effusion**, systolic blood pressure <110, resting HR > 92, **WHO functional class IV**, and 6 MW distance <165 m.
  - Favorable predictors: NYHA (or WHO) functional class I, 6 MW distance >440 meters, BNP <50, and DL_{CO} ≥80%.
- The more advanced a patient's condition, the more likely they are to need continuous prostanoid infusion.
- Combining agents from different classes can be considered if treatment response to a single agent is suboptimal.[20]

TABLE 17-7 Available PAH-Specific Therapies

Drug Class	Drug	Route	Dose	Toxicity/adverse effects
Endothelin receptor antagonists (ERAs)	Bosentan	PO	125 mg bid	Hepatotoxicity, teratogenicity, edema
	Ambrisentan	PO	5–10 mg daily	Teratogenicity, edema
Phosphodiesterase-5 inhibitor	Sildenafil	PO	20 mg tid	Headache, hypotension, dyspepsia, myalgia
	Tadalafil	PO	40 mg daily	Headache, hypotension, dyspepsia, myalgia
Prostanoids	Iloprost	Inhaled	2.5–5 mg 6–9x/day	Headache, cough, syncope
	Treprostinil	SQ, IV	Continuous infusion with variable dose	Extremity pain, headache, diarrhea, site pain (SQ), catheter complications (IV)
		Inhaled	9 puffs (54 mcg) qid	Headache, flushing, cough, throat pain
	Epoprostenol	IV	Continuous infusion with variable dose	Catheter complications, jaw pain, diarrhea, headache, extremity pain, skin flushing, rash

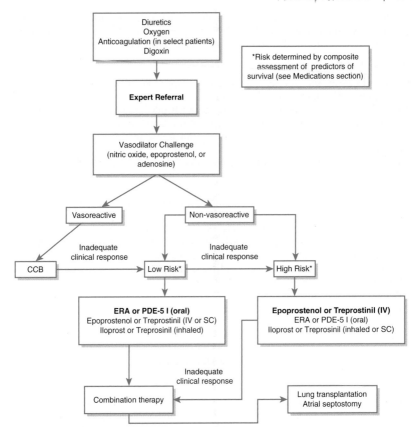

Figure 17-3 **PAH treatment algorithm.** Only patients with acute vasodilator responses (see PH treatment section) should receive CCB. Typical first-line therapy for "low-" and "high"-risk patients is listed first in the respective boxes. (CCB, calcium channel blocker; ERA endothelin receptor antagonist; PDE-5 I, phosphodiesterase-5 inhibitor).

- Due to the complexity of some therapies, an individual's comorbid conditions, cognitive abilities, and psychosocial makeup must also be heavily factored.

Interventional Therapies
- **Atrial septostomy** is a percutaneously created right-to-left shunt in the interatrial septum. It is indicated for severe, medically refractory right heart failure. It results in a net increase in oxygen delivery through augmentation of cardiac output, in spite of lower oxygen saturations.
- There are percutaneous and surgical options for **closure of systemic-to-pulmonary shunts**, depending on the type and size of defect. Determination requires calculation of net direction of shunting. Generally, shunts can be closed if the ratio of pulmonary blood flow to systemic blood flow (Q_p/Q_s) >1.5, pulmonary resistance to systemic resistance (PVR/SVR) <0.3, and the PVR index is <6 (Wood units × m²).[22,23]
- **Lung transplantation** is indicated for advanced functional class PAH patients on maximal medical therapy.[24] Bilateral lung transplantation is favored if there are no significant cardiac defects. Heart-lung transplantation is required for patients with complex defects,

including ventricular septal defects. The right ventricle recovers systolic function within the first few months of surgery. Thirty-day and 1-year survival is lower for the PAH group, but long-term results (median 4.5 years) are comparable to other transplanted groups.[25]

Treatment of Group II

- Group II patients should receive appropriate therapy to lower left-sided filling pressures and optimize LV function in order to minimize passive PH.
- Therapeutic choices depend on the underlying left-sided problem and are beyond the scope of this chapter. General treatment recommendations include diuretics to remove excess fluid, antihypertensive agents, rate control agents, inotropes, and interventional treatments.[26,27]
- **There is no proven role for pulmonary vasomodulators in Group II PH**.

Treatment of Group III

- Group III patients need therapy to minimize deleterious effects of lung disease on PH.
- Bronchodilators are used for the management of airway disease.
- Immunomodulatory therapy as indicated for specific interstitial disease.
- **Long-term oxygen therapy is essential if SaO_2 is $\leq 89\%$ or PaO_2 is ≤ 59**. Patients should be tested at rest and during exercise. Patients not meeting criteria during daytime should be evaluated while sleeping; supplemental oxygen is indicated if SaO_2 is $\leq 88\%$ or PaO_2 is ≤ 55, especially when polycythemia is present.
- Patients with sleep-disordered breathing (e.g., obstructive sleep apnea) can develop mild PH and should receive appropriate treatment, most commonly noninvasive positive pressure ventilation (NIPPV).
- Patients with alveolar hypoventilation syndromes (e.g., central hypoventilation, chest wall diseases) can develop severe chronic PH and should be treated with NIPPV.
- **There is no proven role for pulmonary vasomodulators**.

Treatment of Groups IV and V

- Group IV patients need careful evaluation to determine extent and location of vascular occlusions, which are most commonly venous thromboemboli. Patients who have significant proximal vessel involvement (e.g., at least at the segmental vessel level) should be offered pulmonary thromboendarterectomy.[24]
- Management of group V patients depends on the specific condition and the mechanism of PH.

REFERENCES

1. Ryu JH, Daniels CE, Hartman TE, et al. Diagnosis of interstitial lung diseases. *Mayo Clin Proc* 2007;82:976–986.
2. King TE. Clinical advances in the diagnosis and therapy of the interstitial lung diseases. *Am J Respir Crit Care Med* 2005;172:268–279.
3. The diagnosis, assessment and treatment of diffuse parenchymal lung disease in adults. Introduction. *Thorax* 1999;54(suppl 1):S1–S14.
4. Reynolds H, Matthay R. Diffuse interstitial and alveolar lung diseases. In: George RB, Light RW, Matthay MA, et al. eds. *Chest Medicine: Essentials of Pulmonary and Critical Care Medicine*. Philadelphia, PA: Lippincott Williams & Wilkins; 2006:262–313.
5. Raghu G, Brown KK. Interstitial lung disease: clinical evaluation and keys to an accurate diagnosis. *Clin Chest Med* 2004;25:409–419.
6. Raghu G, Collard HR, Egan JJ, et al. An official ATS/ERS/JRS/ALAT statement: idiopathic pulmonary fibrosis: evidence-based guidelines for diagnosis and management. *Am J Respir Crit Care Med* 2011;183:788–824.

7. Raghu G, Anstrom KJ, et al. Idiopathic Pulmonary Fibrosis Clinical Research Network. Prednisone, azathioprine, and N-acetylcysteine for pulmonary fibrosis. *N Engl J Med* 2012;366:1968–1977.

8. Kim DS, Collard HR, King TE. Classification and natural history of the idiopathic interstitial pneumonias. *Proc Am Thorac Soc* 2006;3:285–292.

9. Baughman RP, Culver DA, Judson MA. A concise review of pulmonary sarcoidosis. *Am J Respir Crit Care Med* 2011;183:573–581.

10. Stone JH, Merkel PA, Spiera R, et al. Rituximab versus cyclophosphamide for ANCA-associated vasculitis. *N Engl J Med* 2010;363:221–232.

11. McCormack FX, Inoue Y, Moss J, et al. Efficacy and safety of sirolimus in lymphangioleiomyomatosis. *N Engl J Med* 2011;364:1595–1606.

12. Galie N, Hoeper MM, Humbert M, et al. Guidelines for the diagnosis and treatment of pulmonary hypertension: the Task Force for the Diagnosis and Treatment of Pulmonary Hypertension of the European Society of Cardiology (ESC) and the European Respiratory Society (ERS), endorsed by the International Society of Heart and Lung Transplantation (ISHLT). *Eur Heart J* 2009;30:2493–2537.

13. Simonneau G, Robbins IM, Beghetti M, et al. Updated clinical classification of pulmonary hypertension. *J Am Coll Cardiol* 2009;54:S43–S54.

14. Humbert M, Sitbon O, Chaouat A, et al. Pulmonary arterial hypertension in France: results from a national registry. *Am J Respir Crit Care Med* 2006;173:1023–1030.

15. Peacock AJ, Murphy NF, McMurray JJ, et al. An epidemiological study of pulmonary arterial hypertension. *Eur Respir J* 2007;30:104–109.

16. D'Alonzo GE, Barst RJ, Ayres SM, et al. Survival in patients with primary pulmonary hypertension. Results from a national prospective registry. *Ann Intern Med* 1991;115:343–349.

17. Badesch DB, Abman SH, Ahearn GS, et al. Medical therapy for pulmonary arterial hypertension: ACCP evidence-based clinical practice guidelines. *Chest* 2004;126:35S–62S.

18. Rubin LJ. Diagnosis and management of pulmonary arterial hypertension: ACCP evidence-based clinical practice guidelines. *Chest* 2004;126:7S–10S.

19. Miyamoto S, Nagaya N, Satoh T, et al. Clinical correlates and prognostic significance of six-minute walk test in patients with primary pulmonary hypertension. Comparison with cardiopulmonary exercise testing. *Am J Respir Crit Care Med* 2000;161:487–492.

20. Barst RJ, Gibbs JS, Ghofrani HA, et al. Updated evidence-based treatment algorithm in pulmonary arterial hypertension. *J Am Coll Cardiol* 2009;54:S78–S84.

21. Benza RL, Gomberg-Maitland M, Miller DP, et al. The REVEAL Registry risk score calculator in patients newly diagnosed with pulmonary arterial hypertension. *Chest* 2012;141:354–362.

22. Duffels MG, Engelfriet PM, Berger RM, et al. Pulmonary arterial hypertension in congenital heart disease: an epidemiologic perspective from a Dutch registry. *Int J Cardiol* 2007;120:198–204.

23. Steele PM, Fuster V, Cohen M, et al. Isolated atrial septal defect with pulmonary vascular obstructive disease—long-term follow-up and prediction of outcome after surgical correction. *Circulation* 1987;76:1037–1042.

24. Keogh AM, Mayer E, Benza RL, et al. Interventional and surgical modalities of treatment in pulmonary hypertension. *J Am Coll Cardiol* 2009;54:S67–S77.

25. Christie JD, Edwards LB, Kucheryavaya AY, et al. The Registry of the International Society for Heart and Lung Transplantation: 29th adult lung and heart-lung transplant report-2012. *J Heart Lung Transplant* 2012;31:1073–1086.

26. Jessup M, Abraham WT, Casey DE, et al. 2009 focused update: ACCF/AHA Guidelines for the Diagnosis and Management of Heart Failure in Adults: a report of the American College of Cardiology Foundation/American Heart Association Task Force on Practice

Guidelines: developed in collaboration with the International Society for Heart and Lung Transplantation. *Circulation* 2009;119:1977–2016.

27. Dickstein K, Cohen-Solal A, Filippatos G, et al. ESC Guidelines for the diagnosis and treatment of acute and chronic heart failure 2008: the Task Force for the Diagnosis and Treatment of Acute and Chronic Heart Failure 2008 of the European Society of Cardiology. Developed in collaboration with the Heart Failure Association of the ESC (HFA) and endorsed by the European Society of Intensive Care Medicine (ESICM). *Eur Heart J* 2008;29:2388–2442.

18 Sleep Disorders

Tonya Russell

Obstructive Sleep Apnea

GENERAL PRINCIPLES

Definition

- Obstructive sleep apnea (OSA) is a condition in which there is cessation or decreased airflow during sleep due to upper airway narrowing or obstruction despite ongoing respiratory effort.
- Apneas are complete cessation of airflow.
- Hypopneas are diminished airflow (<70% of baseline) associated with a 4% oxygen desaturation.
- Respiratory effort–related arousals (RERAs) are a change in airflow that does not meet criteria for apnea or hypopnea, but are associated with an arousal.
- All respiratory events (e.g., apneas and hypopneas) must last at least 10 seconds.
- The apnea-hypopnea index (AHI) represents the number of apneas and hypopneas per hour of sleep.
- The respiratory disturbance index (RDI) represents the number of apneas, hypopneas, and RERAs per hour of sleep.

Classification

- An AHI of <5 in adults is normal.
- An AHI of 5 to 14 in adults is mild sleep apnea.
- An AHI of 15 to 29 in adults is moderate sleep apnea.
- An AHI of >30 in adults is severe sleep apnea.

Epidemiology

- The prevalence of OSA, as defined by an AHI >5 events per hour, is estimated to be 24% of men and 9% of women.
- The prevalence of obstructive sleep apnea-hypopnea syndrome (OSAHS), as defined by an AHI >5 in association with daytime sleepiness, is 4% of men and 2% of women.[1]

Pathophysiology

- Obstructive apneas and hypopneas result from excessive soft tissue or structural abnormalities of the upper airway resulting in cessation of breathing (apneas) or decreased airflow (hypopneas) during sleep.
- Obstructive events can be associated with snoring, arousals from sleep, and oxygen desaturations.

Risk Factors

- Risk factors for OSA include obesity, enlarged tonsils, macroglossia, and craniofacial abnormalities.
- Use of sedatives, narcotics, or alcohol can also increase the risk for OSA.
- Medical conditions that can contribute to decreased muscle tone, weight gain, or craniofacial abnormalities such as hypothyroidism or acromegaly can also increase the risk of OSA.

Prevention

- Weight loss may help to prevent OSA.
- Avoidance of sedatives, narcotics, and alcohol can be of benefit.
- Treatment of underlying medical conditions that may be contributing to OSA is of benefit.

Associated Conditions

- Patients with OSA are more likely to be hypersomnolent.
- Patients with OSA have an increased risk of motor vehicle collisions.[2,3]
- OSAHS increases the risk for hypertension, with the risk increasing as the severity of OSA increases.[4,5] Treatment of OSA can improve the control of hypertension, but it may take several weeks before the effects are seen.[6–9]
- Patients with severe untreated OSA (AHI >30) have a higher risk of fatal and nonfatal cardiovascular events when compared with healthy controls and patients with severe OSAHS treated with continuous positive airway pressure (CPAP).[10] There was no difference in other cardiovascular risk factors between the untreated and the CPAP-treated severe OSAHS groups.
- There is increased risk of congestive heart failure in patients with OSA.[11]
- OSA is associated with an adjusted hazard ratio of 1.97 for risk of stroke or death from any cause.[12]
- Studies have demonstrated impaired glucose tolerance and increased insulin resistance in patients with OSA even when controlled for obesity.[13,14] Treatment of OSA with CPAP has been shown to improve glycemic control.[15]

DIAGNOSIS

Clinical Presentation

History

- Common complaints for patients with OSA include daytime sleepiness (including falling asleep while driving), not feeling refreshed upon awakening, awakening snorting or gasping, and poor concentration. Patients may report headaches upon awakening.
- The patient's bed partner may report witnessing apneic events. In addition, the bed partner may report disruption of his or her sleep due to the patient's loud snoring.

Physical Examination

- The physical exam should note the patient's weight and body mass index.
- Neck circumference should be measured. Neck circumference >17 inches in men and >16 inches in women is associated with increased risk of OSA.
- Inspection of the oropharynx should be performed to assess Mallampati class and for macroglossia and enlarged tonsils.

Diagnostic Criteria

Sleep apnea is diagnosed when the AHI is >5 on either an in-lab polysomnogram or at-home unattended (no technician) ambulatory study.

Differential Diagnosis

- Central sleep apnea is a different type of sleep-disordered breathing in which there is cessation of airflow and no respiratory effort.
- Other causes of daytime sleepiness such as restless legs syndrome (RLS), periodic limb movements, sleep deprivation, narcolepsy, or idiopathic hypersomnia should be considered.

Diagnostic Testing

- The gold standard for diagnosing OSA is with an in-lab overnight polysomnogram.
  - Typically, the monitoring includes electroencephalogram, electrooculogram, and electromyogram leads for sleep staging.
  - In addition, respiratory effort is monitored by thoracic and abdominal belts, as well as airflow via thermistor and pressure transducer.
  - Electrocardiogram and oxygen saturations are recorded, and in situations in which hypoventilation is a concern, transcutaneous carbon dioxide levels may be monitored.
  - In-lab polysomnogram studies are often performed as split studies. Per the American Academy of Sleep Medicine recommendations, if a patient has an AHI >40 events per hour during the first 2 hours of sleep, a CPAP titration can be started during the same study.[16]
- Portable polysomnographic monitoring devices can be used to diagnose OSA.
  - Portable devices typically monitor airflow, respiratory effort, pulse oximetry, and snoring. However, data regarding body position and sleep state are often not obtained.
  - If a portable study is negative and there is still a clinical suspicion for OSA, an in-lab polysomnogram should be pursued.
  - Portable devices should not be used in patients in whom there is concern for other sleep-related conditions such as obesity hypoventilation syndrome, central sleep apnea, narcolepsy, or periodic limb movements. In addition, they should not be used in patients with severe cardiac or pulmonary disease.

TREATMENT

Medications

- Modafinil is a stimulant medication approved for use in patients with continued daytime sleepiness despite adequate therapy of OSAHS with CPAP and no other obvious cause for sleepiness.[17]
- Weight reduction should be encouraged in obese patients.
- Treatment of underlying endocrine disorders, such as hypothyroidism and acromegaly, should be pursued.

Other Nonpharmacologic Therapies

- CPAP is the standard therapy for OSA. It is typically initiated for home use after a CPAP titration has been performed in a sleep center. During titrations, CPAP is increased to relieve snoring as well as obstructive apneas and hypopneas.
- Autotitrating positive airway pressure (APAP) devices are available. These machines titrate through a range of pressures on the basis of algorithms within the device to determine snoring and changes in airflow. Several studies have shown that APAP is as effective as CPAP in treating OSA.
  - In patients who require a wide range of pressures to resolve their OSA and have trouble tolerating higher pressures during the entire night (e.g., a patient who requires lower pressures in the lateral position or during non–rapid eye movement sleep and higher pressures in the supine position or during rapid eye movement sleep), APAP may be a more tolerable option.
  - APAP is not a good option for patients with significant comorbid conditions.[18]
- Patients who have difficulty tolerating CPAP may prefer bilevel positive airway pressure devices.
- Potential side effects and barriers to use of CPAP, as well as potential remedies, are outlined in Table 18-1.
- Oral appliances can be used to treat OSA. Overall, the success rate is approximately 50%, although patients with more severe OSA are less likely to respond.

TABLE 18-1 Complications Related to CPAP and Potential Remedies

Complication	Remedy
Excessive nasal dryness/epistaxis	Use humidifier
Excessive nasal congestion	Decrease humidity; nasal steroids
Mouth dryness	Use humidifier; full face mask
Eye dryness	Ensure good mask fit to limit air leaks
Claustrophobia	Use lower profile masks such as nasal pillows
Aerophagia	Lowest possible therapeutic pressure; APAP
Frequent mask leaks	Refit with new mask; shave facial hair
Skin breakdown	Proper mask fit to prevent excessive tightening of head gear

APAP, autotitrating positive airway pressure; CPAP, continuous positive airway pressure.

- ○ Complications from oral appliances include temporomandibular joint pain, tooth and gum irritation, and occlusal changes, although most complications are temporary.
- ○ Oral appliances should be fitted by practitioners specializing in dental sleep medicine.
- ○ Patients being considered for oral appliances for snoring or OSA should undergo evaluation with overnight polysomnogram before starting therapy. If OSA is present on the baseline study, a repeat polysomnogram should be performed with the appliance in place to document resolution of the OSA.[19]
- Nasal expiratory positive airway pressure devices are small resistance valves that insert into the nostrils. The resistance generated by exhaling through the valve creates a positive pressure in the upper airway. These devices are best used in patients with milder OSA or those who cannot tolerate CPAP. A polysomnogram should be performed with the devices in place to ensure the adequacy of therapy.

Surgical Management

- Patients who want to consider surgery for OSA should be evaluated by an otolaryngologist to determine whether the area of upper airway obstruction is amenable to surgery.
- Tracheotomy can be curative for OSA, as the area of upper airway obstruction is bypassed.
- Uvulopalatopharyngoplasty is a common surgery performed for OSA. Response to surgery varies from 40% to 60% depending upon how surgical success is defined. Patients with higher AHIs are less likely to respond. Complications can include voice changes, foreign body sensation, and nasal reflux.[20]
- Laser-assisted uvulopalatoplasty differs from uvulopalatopharyngoplasty in that the tonsils and pharyngeal pillars are not excised. Currently, the recommendations for use of laser-assisted uvulopalatoplasty are only in primary snoring, not OSA.[21]
- Patients being considered for surgical treatment for snoring or OSA should undergo evaluation with overnight polysomnogram prior to surgery. If OSA is present on the baseline study, a postsurgical polysomnogram should be performed to document resolution of the OSA.[22]
- OSA may improve with weight loss following bariatric surgery.

Lifestyle/Risk Modification

- Weight loss should be encouraged.
- Patients should limit alcohol, sedatives, and narcotics.
- Driving precautions should be discussed with patients.

Insomnia

GENERAL PRINCIPLES

- Insomnia is the inability to initiate or maintain sleep.
- While approximately one-third of the general population has experienced insomnia at some point, of those patients with severe insomnia, approximately 80% have reported symptoms for more than a year.[23]
- See Table 18-2 for causes of insomnia and associated characteristics.
- Risk factors for insomnia depend upon the underlying cause, but can include depression, anxiety, acute life stressors, stimulant use, withdrawal from sedating drugs, or poor sleep hygiene.
- Following good sleep hygiene techniques can prevent insomnia. Good sleep hygiene consists of activities such as maintaining a regular sleep schedule, avoiding stimulants (caffeine and nicotine) close to bedtime, and avoiding reading or watching TV in bed. Treatment of conditions such as depression and anxiety may also help to prevent insomnia.
- Insomnia may be triggered by depression and anxiety. However, insomnia may also worsen depression and anxiety.
- Patients with insomnia may exhibit increased irritability, difficulty concentrating, and complaints of somatic pain.

DIAGNOSIS

Clinical Presentation

- Patients report difficulty with initiating and/or maintaining sleep.
- Patients may report racing thoughts that prevent them from sleeping.
- Often, patients are fatigued, but not overtly sleepy during the day.
- Elicit any history of use of medications or drugs that can contribute to insomnia or confounding medical conditions such as chronic pain, RLS, depression, or anxiety.
- In addition, the history should be directed to evaluate the patient's sleep schedule and to assess for poor sleep hygiene.
- There are no specific physical exam findings for insomnia.

TABLE 18-2	Causes of Insomnia and Associated Characteristics
Cause	**Characteristic**
Restless legs syndrome	Uncomfortable sensation in legs interfering with ability to fall asleep
Pain	Any underlying condition associated with chronic pain
Mental disorder	Underlying depression or anxiety
Adjustment insomnia	Associated with acute stressor
Inadequate sleep hygiene	Poor sleep habits, for example, irregular sleep times; excessive caffeine, nicotine, or alcohol use; using the bedroom for non–sleep-related activities
Psychophysiologic insomnia	Increased arousal, frequent inability to "turn off thoughts"
Idiopathic insomnia	Occurring since childhood
Drug or substance abuse	Chronic use of pain medicines, stimulants, alcohol, or sedative-hypnotics
Circadian rhythm disturbance	Advanced or delayed sleep phase

Diagnostic Criteria

- In general, a patient should complain of difficulty initiating and/or maintaining sleep that is associated with perceived limitation in daytime functioning such as fatigue, poor concentration, or irritability. There should be adequate opportunity for sleep.
- More specific criteria depend upon the cause of the insomnia.

Differential Diagnosis

Patients with paradoxical insomnia or sleep state misperception feel they suffer from insomnia. However, objective testing such as polysomnogram or actigraphy demonstrates normal sleep time and pattern. Often, their daytime impairment is less severe than patients with insomnia.

Diagnostic Testing

- If there is clinical concern, a polysomnogram can be performed to rule out other causes of poor sleep maintenance, such as periodic limb movements or sleep-disordered breathing.
- Actigraphy can be used to confirm reported sleep patterns and sleep times.
- Urine drug screen can be used to screen for use of illicit drugs that may trigger insomnia.

TREATMENT

Medications

- Over-the-counter medications are frequently used by patients to treat insomnia. Table 18-3 lists common over-the-counter medications and their potential side effects. There are no strong data to support the efficacy of these agents.[24]
- The prescription medications that are approved for treatment of insomnia are the benzodiazepine receptor agonists and the melatonin receptor agonists. Of these, eszopiclone (nonbenzodiazepine hypnotic) and ramelteon (melatonin agonist) are the only ones FDA approved for long-term use. The benzodiazepine receptor agonists are considered controlled substances, whereas the melatonin receptor agonists are not.[24]
- Frequently, sedating antidepressants are also prescribed for insomnia in off-label use, although data supporting their use are lacking. Table 18-4 outlines the prescription medications for insomnia as well as some of the potential side effects.[24]
- Treatment of underlying medical or psychiatric conditions potentially contributing to insomnia should be instituted.

TABLE 18-3	Over-the-Counter Medications for Insomnia and Their Side Effects	
Medication	**Dosage**	**Side effects**
Antihistamine (diphenhydramine)	25–75 mg	Hangover effect, dizziness, anticholinergic effects (dry mouth, urinary retention, delirium)
Melatonin	0.3–5 mg	Fatigue, headache, drowsiness, possible vasoconstriction
Valerian root	1.5–3 g of herb or root 400–900 mg of aqueous extract	Dizziness, headache, excitability, hepatic toxicity (in combination products)
Alcohol	Self-dosing	Impaired cognition and motor skills, anterograde amnesia; although initially sedating, as alcohol is metabolized it can cause fragmentation of sleep

TABLE 18-4 Prescription Medications Used for Insomnia

Medication	Class	Dosage	Half-life	Side effects
Temazepam	Benzodiazepine	7.5–30 mg	11 hours	Hangover effect, anterograde amnesia, rebound insomnia, withdrawal symptoms
Eszopiclone	Nonbenzodiazepine	1–3 mg	6 hours	Hangover effect, headache, dizziness, possible impaired memory at peak concentrations
Zolpidem		5–10 mg	4 hours	
Zolpidem extended release		6.25–12.5 mg	4 hours	
Zaleplon		5–10 mg	1 hour	
Ramelteon	Melatonin receptor agonist	8 mg	1–3 hours	Dizziness, headache, fatigue, somnolence
Trazodone	Antidepressant	50–100 mg	6–12 hours	Headache, somnolence, rebound insomnia, priapism
Amitriptyline	Tricyclic antidepressant	25–100 mg	10–26 hours	Somnolence, dizziness, dry mouth, arrhythmias
Mirtazapine	Antidepressant	7.5–45 mg	20–40 hours	Somnolence, dry mouth, increased weight

TABLE 18-5	Components of Cognitive-Behavioral Therapy for Insomnia
Component	**Description**
Sleep hygiene education	Avoiding excessive caffeine, alcohol, nicotine; optimizing sleeping environment
Stimulus control	Consistent wake-up time, out of bed during prolonged awakenings, reserving the bedroom for sleeping, avoiding napping
Sleep restriction	Minimize the amount of time spent in bed not sleeping
Imagery	Form a relaxing image that helps prevent intrusive thoughts from interfering with sleep
Muscle relaxation	Progressive relaxation of muscle groups to relieve muscle tension

Other Nonpharmacologic Therapies

- Cognitive-behavioral therapy (CBT) encompasses a wide variety of techniques aimed at breaking the cycle of insomnia.[25] Table 18-5 describes various components of CBT for insomnia.
- CBT has been shown to be beneficial in improving the nighttime and daytime symptoms associated with insomnia.[26–28]

Lifestyle/Risk Modification

- Patients should be encouraged to keep a regular sleep schedule with a consistent bedtime and waking time.
- Patients should avoid the use of stimulants such as caffeine and nicotine.
- Patients should modify their sleeping environment to minimize environmental disturbances.
- Patients should avoid activities such as watching TV or reading in bed.

Restless Legs Syndrome

GENERAL PRINCIPLES

- RLS consists of an uncomfortable sensation in the extremities (most commonly the legs), which is worse in the evening and nighttime, but can occur during the day in sedentary situations, and is temporarily relieved by movement.
- Prevalence of RLS is estimated to be between 2.5% and 15% of the population. In some patients with RLS, there is a hereditary link.[29]
- The severity of symptoms can be highly variable.
- The role of dopamine in RLS has been most strongly supported by the improvement of symptoms with dopamine agonists.[30]
- Iron is necessary for the rate-limiting step in dopamine synthesis. Therefore, low iron levels may decrease dopamine synthesis.[31] Ferritin levels <50 μg/L have been associated with increased severity of RLS. Iron supplementation is recommended in the setting of RLS when ferritin is <50 μg/L.[32]
- RLS can be associated with other underlying conditions such as pregnancy, uremia, and anemia.
- Pharmacologic agents such as caffeine, nicotine, alcohol, dopamine antagonists, diphenhydramine, serotonin reuptake inhibitors, and tricyclic antidepressants may worsen RLS.[33] Avoiding pharmacologic agents associated with RLS may help prevent symptoms.

DIAGNOSIS

Clinical Presentation

- Patients will report an uncomfortable sensation in the legs, which can sometimes involve the arms. Typically, the sensation is bilateral. If a patient reports mainly unilateral symptoms, consideration should be given to the possibility of a spinal cord lesion.
- The sensations should have a circadian rhythm to them in that they are worse in the late evening and earlier part of the night. However, some patients experience symptoms during the day when in prolonged sedentary situations.
- The sensations are typically temporarily relieved by movement, but return upon cessation of the movement.
- There are no specific physical exam findings for RLS.

Diagnostic Criteria

- RLS is a clinical diagnosis in which the four essential criteria, as outlined in Table 18-6, are met.[34]
- Periodic limb movements are frequently seen on the polysomnograms of patients with RLS, although a polysomnogram is not required to make the diagnosis of RLS.
- RLS is a clinical diagnosis. However, a polysomnogram can be performed if the presence of periodic limb movements would change therapy.
- A ferritin should be checked to evaluate if iron supplementation may be beneficial.

Differential Diagnosis

Musculoskeletal pain, neuropathy, leg cramps, and sleep starts are in the differential diagnosis for RLS.

TREATMENT

- An oral iron supplement can be prescribed if the ferritin is <50 ng/mL.
- Dopamine agonists (pramipexole and ropinirole) are the initial therapy in patients with RLS that require treatment and have a normal ferritin. These medications should be initiated at the lowest dose and titrated every 5 to 7 days until relief of symptoms or maximal dose is reached.[33]
- Gabapentin at a starting dose of 600 mg and titrated up to 2,400 mg as needed can also be used to treat RLS symptoms without significant side effects.[35]
- Benzodiazepines and opioids can also be effective in treating RLS symptoms.
- Caffeine should be limited as it can worsen RLS symptoms.
- Avoidance of medications that can trigger RLS (such as serotonin reuptake inhibitors) should be attempted.

TABLE 18-6	Clinical Criteria for Restless Legs Syndrome

Urge to move legs associated with an uncomfortable sensation in legs.
The urge to move legs or the uncomfortable sensation is worsened during periods of inactivity.
Movement temporarily improves or relieves the urge to move or uncomfortable sensation in the legs.
Symptoms are worse in the evening.

Data from Allen RP, Picchietti D, Hening WA, et al. Restless legs syndrome: diagnostic criteria, special considerations, and epidemiology. A report from the restless legs syndrome diagnosis and epidemiology workshop at the National Institutes of Health. *Sleep Med* 2003;4:101–119.

REFERENCES

1. Young T, Palta M, Dempsey J, et al. The occurrence of sleep-disordered breathing among middle-aged adults. *N Engl J Med* 1993;328:1230–1235.
2. Young T, Blustein J, Finn L, et al. Sleep-disordered breathing and motor vehicle accidents in a population-based sample of employed adults. *Sleep* 1997;20:608–613.
3. Terán-Santos J, Jiménez-Gómez A, Cordero-Guevara J, et al. The association between sleep apnea and the risk of traffic accidents. *N Engl J Med* 1999;340:847–851.
4. Nieto FJ, Young T, Lind BK, et al. Association of sleep-disordered breathing, sleep apnea, and hypertension in a large community-based study. *JAMA* 2000;282:1829–1836.
5. Peppard PE, Young T, Palta M, et al. Prospective study of the association between sleep-disordered breathing and hypertension. *N Engl J Med* 2000;342:1378–1384.
6. Becker HF, Jerrentrup A, Ploch T, et al. Effect of nasal continuous positive airway pressure treatment on blood pressure in patients with obstructive sleep apnea. *Circulation* 2003;107:68–73.
7. Logan AG, Tkacova R, Perlikowski SM, et al. Refractory hypertension and sleep apnoea: effect of CPAP on blood pressure and baroreflex. *Eur Respir J* 2003;21:241–247.
8. Robinson GV, Smith DM, Langford BA, et al. Continuous positive airway pressure does not reduce blood pressure in nonsleepy hypertensive OSA patients. *Eur Respir J* 2006;27:1229–1235.
9. Campos-Rodriguez F, Grilo-Reina A, Perez-Ronchel J, et al. Effect of continuous positive airway pressure on ambulatory BP in patients with sleep apnea and hypertension: a placebo-controlled trial. *Chest* 2006;129:1459–1467.
10. Marin JM, Carrizo SJ, Vicente E, et al. Long-term cardiovascular outcomes in men with obstructive sleep apnoea-hypopnoea with or without treatment with continuous positive airway pressure: an observational study. *Lancet* 2005;365:1046–1053.
11. Shahar E, Whitney C, Redline S, et al. Sleep-disordered breathing and cardiovascular disease: cross-sectional results of the Sleep Heart Health Study. *Am J Respir Crit Care Med* 2001;163:19–25.
12. Yaggi HK, Concato J, Kernan WN, et al. Obstructive sleep apnea as a risk factor for stroke and death. *N Engl J Med* 2005;353:2034–2041.
13. Ip MSM, Lam B, Ng MTM, et al. Obstructive sleep apnea is independently associated with insulin resistance. *Am J Respir Crit Care Med* 2002;165:670–676.
14. Punjabi NM, Shahar E, Redline S, et al. Sleep-disordered breathing, glucose intolerance, and insulin resistance: the Sleep Heart Health Study. *Am J Epidemiol* 2004;160:521–530.
15. Babu AR, Herdegen J, Fogelfeld L, et al. Type 2 diabetes, glycemic control, and continuous positive airway pressure in obstructive sleep apnea. *Arch Intern Med* 2005;165:447–452.
16. Kushida CA, Littner MR, Morgenthaler T, et al. Practice parameters for the indications for polysomnography and related procedures: an update for 2005. *Sleep* 2005;28:499–521.
17. Morgenthaler TI, Kapen S, Lee-Chiong T, et al. Practice parameters for the medical therapy of obstructive sleep apnea. *Sleep* 2006;29:1031–1035.
18. Berry RB, Parish JM, Hartse KM. The use of auto-titrating continuous positive airway pressure for treatment of adult obstructive sleep apnea. *Sleep* 2002;25:148–173.
19. Ferguson KA, Cartwright R, Rogers R, et al. Oral appliances for snoring and obstructive sleep apnea: a review. *Sleep* 2006;29:244–262.
20. Sher AE, Schechtman KB, Piccirillo JF. The efficacy of surgical modifications of the upper airway in adults with obstructive sleep apnea syndrome. *Sleep* 1996;19:156–177.
21. Littner M, Kushida CA, Hartse K, et al. Practice parameters for the use of laser-assisted uvulopalatoplasty: an update for 2000. *Sleep* 2001;24:603–619.

22. Thorpy M, Chesson A, Derderian S, et al. Practice parameters for the treatment of obstructive sleep apnea in adults: the efficacy of surgical modifications of the upper airway. *Sleep* 1996;19:152–155.

23. Sateia MJ, Doghramji K, Hauri PJ, et al. Evaluation of chronic insomnia. *Sleep* 2000; 23:243–308.

24. Morin AK, Jarvis CI, Lynch AM. Therapeutic options for sleep-maintenance and sleep-onset insomnia. *Pharmacotherapy* 2007;27:89–110.

25. Morgenthaler TI, Kramer M, Alessi C, et al. Practice parameters for the psychological and behavioral treatment of insomnia: an update. An American Academy of Sleep Medicine report. *Sleep* 2006;29:1415–1419.

26. Harvey AG, Sharpley AL, Ree MJ, et al. An open trial of cognitive therapy for chronic insomnia. *Behav Res Ther* 2007;45:2491–2501.

27. Edinger JD, Wohlgemuth WK, Radtke RA, et al. Cognitive behavioral therapy for treatment of chronic primary insomnia—a randomized controlled trial. *JAMA* 2001;285:1856–1864.

28. Morin CM, Bootzin RR, Buysse DJ, et al. Psychological and behavioral treatment of insomnia: update of recent evidence (1998–2004). *Sleep* 2006;29:1398–1414.

29. Masood A, Phillips B. Epidemiology of restless legs syndrome. In: Chokroverty S, Hening W, Walters A, eds. *Sleep and Movement Disorders*. Philadelphia, PA: Elsevier Science; 2003:316–321.

30. Henning WA, Allen RP, Earley CJ, et al. An update on the dopaminergic treatment of restless legs syndrome and periodic limb movement disorder. *Sleep* 2004;27:560–583.

31. Allen RP, Earley CJ. Dopamine and iron in the restless legs syndrome. In: Chokroverty S, Hening W, Walters A, eds. *Sleep and Movement Disorders*. Philadelphia, PA: Elsevier Science; 2003:333–340.

32. Sun ER, Chen CA, Ho G, et al. Iron and the restless legs syndrome. *Sleep* 1998; 21:381–387.

33. Hening WA. Current guidelines and standards of practice for restless legs syndrome. *Am J Med* 2007;120:S22–S27.

34. Allen RP, Picchietti D, Hening WA, et al. Restless legs syndrome: diagnostic criteria, special considerations, and epidemiology. A report from the restless legs syndrome diagnosis and epidemiology workshop at the National Institutes of Health. *Sleep Med* 2003;4:101–119.

35. Garcia-Borreguero D, Larrosa O, de la Llave Y, et al. Treatment of restless legs syndrome with gabapentin: a double-blind, crossover study. *Neurology* 2002;59:1573–1579.

19 | Pleural Effusion and Solitary Pulmonary Nodule
Alexander Chen

Pleural Effusion

GENERAL PRINCIPLES

- A pleural effusion is the abnormal accumulation of fluid in the pleural space. The pleural space normally contains only a small amount of fluid that is not radiographically apparent.
- Effusions are categorized into two types: transudates and exudates. This differentiation is defined by laboratory testing and identifies effusions secondary to diseases that do not directly damage the pleural surfaces (transudates) versus diseases that do directly damage the pleural surfaces (exudates). This designation is important since the management of the two types of effusions is distinctly different.
  - **Transudative pleural effusions** result from alteration of hydrostatic and oncotic factors that increase the formation or decrease the absorption of pleural fluid (e.g., increased mean capillary pressure [heart failure] or decreased oncotic pressure [cirrhosis or nephrotic syndrome]).
  - **Exudative pleural effusions** occur when damage or disruption of the normal pleural membranes or vasculature (e.g., tumor involvement of the pleural space, infection, inflammatory conditions, or trauma) leads to increased capillary permeability or decreased lymphatic drainage.
- When transudative effusions are identified, the underlying systemic disease should also be identified (heart failure [HF], liver disease, kidney disease) and treatment should be directed toward the primary disorder.
- Exudative effusions frequently indicate a process (malignancy, infection, etc.) that directly injures the pleura and deserves further investigation and therapy, typically focused on the pleural space.
- Pleural effusions occur in a wide variety of disease states; however, **90% of pleural effusions are the result of only five diseases**: HF (36%), pneumonia (22%), malignancy (14%), pulmonary embolism (PE) (11%), and viral disease (7%).[1]

DIAGNOSIS

Clinical Presentation

- The underlying cause of the effusion typically dictates the symptoms, although patients may be asymptomatic. Pleural inflammation, abnormal pulmonary mechanics, and worsened alveolar gas exchange produce symptoms and signs of disease.
- Inflammation of the parietal pleura leads to pain in locally involved areas (intercostal) or referred distributions (e.g., shoulder pain from phrenic nerve).
- Dyspnea is frequent and may be present out of proportion to the size of the effusion. Cough can occur.
- Clinical signs of pleural effusion include chest pain, dyspnea, and cough, though these are neither sensitive nor specific for diagnosing a pleural effusion.
- Unfortunately, a definitive diagnosis based upon pleural fluid analysis is possible in less than half of all effusions. Therefore, it is important to define the clinical setting of a pleural effusion with a thorough history and physical examination to aid in diagnosis.

- Obtain a detailed history with review of systems to identify symptoms of HF, underlying malignancy, PE, myocardial infarction, surgery or trauma, connective tissue diseases, or other underlying or recent infections.
- Social history focused on smoking history and possible TB exposures.
- Family history focused on malignancy, heart disease, and connective tissue diseases.
- Signs of a pleural effusion on physical exam include asymmetric chest wall expansion, dullness to percussion, diminished breath sounds, and the presence of a pleural rub.

Diagnostic Testing

Imaging

- Prior to any invasive diagnostic or therapeutic procedure, the patient should undergo imaging to confirm the presence, character, and size of the effusion.
- Pleural effusions are often initially detected by **plain chest radiography** (CXR).
  - Effusions are seen as blunting of the costophrenic angle or opacification of the base of the hemithorax without loss of volume of the hemithorax (which would suggest atelectasis) or presence of air bronchograms (which would suggest pneumonia).
  - CXR can also detect masses or infiltrates that may give clues to an etiology.
  - Decubitus chest films are frequently obtained to demonstrate that at least a portion of the fluid is not loculated and therefore, amenable to thoracentesis (see Table 19-1 and Figure 19-1).
- **Computed tomography** (CT) with contrast given by PE protocol is recommended if PE is suspected.
  - CT without contrast is adequate for the evaluation of pleural effusion if PE is clinically less likely.
  - CT can be used to further define masses, lymphadenopathy, or other abnormal findings on chest radiography.
  - CT with contrast given by standard protocol (in which the images are timed such that the contrast bolus is in the systemic vasculature) helps differentiate pleural fluid from lung masses and atelectatic lung; it also serves to identify and define the extent of pleural fluid thickening and pleural nodularity.
- **Ultrasound** is one of the best modalities to assess for pleural fluid loculations.
  - It provides real-time guidance for pleural procedures and can reduce both the complications and failure rate of thoracentesis.
  - Ultrasound of the pleural space may be used to characterize pleural fluid as well as pleural space anatomy (e.g., presence of septations and adhesions).
  - Ultrasound of the pleural space may guide management for pleural drainage procedures, as in tube thoracostomy versus thoracentesis for loculated pleural effusions and surgical versus medical management for complex septated pleural effusions.

Diagnostic Procedures

Thoracentesis

- Once a pleural effusion has been identified, the clinician must decide whether to sample the pleural fluid for either diagnostic or therapeutic benefit or both. Table 19-1 shows indications for thoracentesis, while Figure 19-1 is a schematic for the evaluation of an unknown effusion.
- If a patient has significant symptoms of dyspnea, cough, pain, or a supplemental oxygen requirement, a therapeutic thoracentesis is warranted.

TABLE 19-1	Indications for Thoracentesis

1. Pleural effusion of unknown etiology
2. Fever in setting of long-standing pleural effusion
3. Air-fluid level in the pleural space
4. Rapid change in size of effusion
5. Concern that empyema is developing

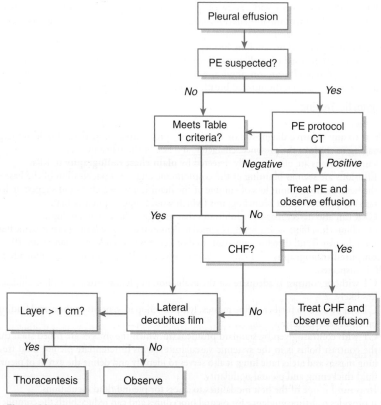

Figure 19-1 Evaluation of the unknown pleural effusion. CHF, congestive heart failure; CT, computed tomography; PE, pulmonary embolism.

- Thoracentesis can be performed safely, in the absence of disorders of hemostasis, on effusions that demonstrate a **>10 mm on a lateral decubitus film**.
- Loculated effusions can be localized with ultrasonography or CT scan.
- The most common serious complications of thoracentesis are pneumothorax, bleeding, and introduction of infection into the pleural space.
- Proper technique and sonographic guidance minimize the risk of complications.
- **Pleural fluid appearance** may be helpful in diagnostic and therapeutic considerations.
  - Red-tinged or serosanguineous pleural effusions indicate the presence of blood. This is either due to the procedure (and therefore should clear with continued aspiration) or from the primary disorder (commonly malignancy, PE, or trauma).
  - The presence of gross blood should lead to the measurement of a pleural fluid hematocrit. Hemothorax is defined as a pleural fluid blood hematocrit ratio of more than 0.5, and chest tube drainage should be implemented.
  - Malodorous fluid or frank pus is consistent with an empyema, and tube thoracostomy should occur immediately.
  - Turbid or milky fluid should prompt evaluation for chylothorax.
- The most important aspect of pleural fluid analysis is the laboratory evaluation, allowing the **designation of a pleural effusion as either transudate or exudate** using Light criteria (Table 19-2) or Heffner criteria (Table 19-3).[1-3] Of note, in patients who have an exudative effusion by chemical criteria, but high clinical suspicion for heart, liver, or

TABLE 19-2 Light Criteria for Definition of an Exudate

An exudate is defined by meeting any one or more of the following criteria:

1. Serum to effusion protein ratio of >0.5
2. Serum to effusion LDH ratio of >0.6
3. Effusion LDH >200 IU/dL or >2/3 of the upper value of normal for serum LDH

A transudate is defined when none of these three parameters are met.

kidney disease, then a serum to pleural fluid albumin gradient should be checked. A gradient of >1.2 g/dL suggests that the pleural fluid is likely due to congestive heart failure (CHF), liver, or kidney disease.[4]

- The most frequently used criteria for defining pleural fluid as either exudate or transudate is Light criteria.[1] These criteria have a 97.9% sensitivity for detecting an exudative effusion.[5] At the time of thoracentesis, a simultaneous measurement of serum lactate dehydrogenase (LDH) and protein must be sampled to properly use the criteria.
- Heffner criteria have a similar sensitivity to Light criteria (98.4%) and do not require simultaneous blood work for interpretation.[3]
- High cell counts are more typically seen in exudative effusions; however, this is not a component of Light criteria.
  - A high **neutrophil count** is suggestive of an infectious process, especially bacterial, and should prompt consideration of an empyema.[6]
  - **Eosinophilia** (>10% of total nucleated cell count) is suggestive of air or blood in the pleural space.[7] If neither of these is present, consideration should be given to fungal or parasitic infection, drug-induced disease, PE, asbestos-related disease, and Churg-Strauss syndrome.[8]
  - **Lymphocytosis** (>50% of the total nucleated cell count) is suggestive of malignancy or tuberculosis.[6]
  - **Mesothelial cells**, when present, argue against the diagnosis of tuberculosis.
  - **Plasma cells** in abundance suggest multiple myeloma.
- **Routine stains** should be obtained to quickly determine if an effusion is infected and to direct antibiotic therapy if indicated (Table 19-4). Staining for acid-fast bacilli and culture for tuberculosis are performed when clinically indicated.
- A **glucose** concentration <60 mg/dL is probably due to tuberculosis, malignancy, rheumatoid arthritis, or a parapneumonic effusion.[9–11] For parapneumonic effusions, with a glucose <60 mg/dL, tube thoracostomy should be considered (Table 19-4).
- Pleural fluid with a **low pH** usually corresponds to a low glucose and a high LDH; otherwise, the low pH may be due to poor sample collection technique (proper pH testing on pleural fluid involves anaerobic collection in a heparinized syringe and stored on ice).
  - A pH of <7.3 is seen with empyema, tuberculosis, malignancy, collagen vascular disease, or esophageal rupture.
  - For parapneumonic effusions with a pH < 7.2, tube thoracostomy should be considered (Table 19-4).[8,12]

TABLE 19-3 Heffner Criteria for Definition of an Exudate

An exudate is defined by meeting any one or more of the following criteria:

1. Pleural fluid protein >2.9 g/dL
2. Pleural fluid LDH >0.45 times the upper limit of normal
3. Pleural fluid cholesterol >45 g/dL

A transudate is defined when none of these three parameters are met.

TABLE 19-4	Indication for Tube Thoracostomy in Parapneumonic Effusions

Radiographic
- Pleural fluid loculation
- Effusion filling more than half of hemithorax
- Air-fluid level present

Microbiologic
- Pus in pleural space
- Positive gram stain for microorganisms
- Positive pleural fluid cultures

Chemical
- Pleural fluid pH <7.2
- Pleural fluid glucose <60 mg/dL

- Cytology is positive in approximately 60% of malignant effusions.[13] Priming the fluid collection bag with unfractionated heparin may increase the yield. Of note, the volume of pleural fluid analyzed does not impact the yield of cytologic diagnosis.[14]
- An elevation in amylase suggests pancreatic disease, malignancy, or esophageal rupture but should not be routinely measured unless there is a clinical suspicion.[15] Malignancy and esophageal rupture have salivary amylase elevations and not pancreatic amylase elevations.
- Turbid or milky fluid should prompt an investigation for **chylothorax**. The fluid should be centrifuged. If the cloudiness clears, then the appearance was merely secondary to cells and debris. If the supernatant does not clear and instead remains turbid, then pleural lipids should be checked. Elevation of triglycerides (>110 mg/dL) suggests that a chylothorax is present,[2,8] usually due to a disruption of the thoracic duct from trauma, surgery, or malignancy (e.g., lymphoma). Chylomicrons in the pleural fluid will confirm this.

Other Diagnostic Procedures
- When there is clinical suspicion for a certain diagnosis, other invasive procedures may be useful.
- **Closed pleural biopsy** typically adds little to the diagnostic yield of thoracentesis, except in the diagnosis of tuberculosis. For tuberculous effusions, pleural fluid cultures alone are positive in only 20% to 25% of cases. However, the combination of pleural fluid studies and pleural biopsy (demonstrating granulomata or organisms) is 90% sensitive in establishing TB as the etiology of the effusion.
- **Diagnostic thoracoscopy** has largely replaced closed pleural biopsy. Thoracoscopy allows visually directed biopsies, thus increasing the diagnostic yield for malignancy, while maintaining the high diagnostic yield for TB.

Differential Diagnosis

- **Transudative pleural effusions** usually have low protein and LDH. The glucose level is usually similar to the serum level, and the pH is generally higher than blood pH. Most transudates are clear, straw colored, nonviscous, and odorless. White blood cell (WBC) count is usually <100 cells/HPF, and the RBC count is usually <10,000 cells/HPF. Transudates should lead to further evaluation of the heart, liver, and kidney with therapy directed accordingly.
- **Exudative pleural effusions** usually have high-protein or LDH values and meet one of Light criteria as described above. Diagnosis of the etiology of the pleural fluid should proceed with a careful history and physical followed by pleural fluid analysis. There is a broad differential for exudative pleural effusions, and once a diagnosis is determined, therapy should be directed toward the cause.

- ○ **Parapneumonic effusions** are exudates that develop secondary to pulmonary infections.
  - ▪ Patients with pneumonia and an effusion should undergo rapid diagnostic testing because an infected pleural space (empyema) needs to be treated without delay.
  - ▪ In an **uncomplicated parapneumonic effusion,** bacterial infection in the pleural space is presumed to be absent, pH > 7.2, and glucose >60 mg/dL.
  - ▪ In **complicated parapneumonic effusions,** bacterial invasion of the pleural space is assumed to be present, pH < 7.2, glucose <60 mg/dL, and/or Gram stain and/or culture positive. **Empyema** is any uncomplicated parapneumonic effusion that appears grossly purulent.
  - ▪ Complicated parapneumonic effusions and empyema should be managed with **chest tube drainage** when indicated based on the size, presence of loculations, gross appearance of the fluid, or biochemical analysis of the pleural fluid (Table 19-4).[12]
  - ▪ Antibiotics should be administered broadly and then narrowed as directed by culture data.
  - ▪ Multiple chest tubes are sometimes required to adequately drain the pleural space.
  - ▪ Failure to adequately and quickly drain the pleural space can lead to organization of the pleural fluid and formation of a thick pleural "rind," which may necessitate surgical removal (known as **decortication**).
- ○ Malignant pleural effusions arise from tumor involvement of the pleura or mediastinum. In addition, patients with cancer are at increased risk of pleural effusions from other secondary causes such as PE, postobstructive pneumonia, chylothorax, and drug and radiation reactions. It may be appropriate for some patients with stable effusions without significant symptoms to avoid further invasive procedures and observe only.

TREATMENT

- **Therapeutic thoracentesis** may improve patient comfort and relieve dyspnea.
  - ○ Repeated thoracenteses are reasonable if they achieve symptomatic relief and if fluid reaccumulation is slow.
  - ○ The incidence of reexpansion pulmonary edema is approximately 1% and is related to changes in pleural pressure more so than the absolute volume of pleural fluid that is removed.[16]
  - ○ Unfortunately, 95% of malignant effusions recur, and the median time to recurrence is <1 week.
- **Pleurodesis** is an effective procedure indicated for a recurrent pleural effusion in a patient whose symptoms were relieved with initial drainage but has rapid reaccumulation.
  - ○ Chemicals used for pleurodesis include talc, doxycycline or minocycline, and bleomycin (considered less effective and more expensive).
  - ○ Chemical sclerosant is instilled into the pleural space to promote fusion of the visceral and parietal pleura (pleurodesis).
  - ○ Systemic analgesics and lidocaine added to the sclerosing agent should be used to reduce the significant discomfort associated with this procedure.[17]
  - ○ If chest tube drainage remains high (>100 mL/day) >2 days after the initial pleurodesis, a second dose of sclerosing agent can be administered.
- **A chronic indwelling pleural catheter** (e.g., PleurX catheter) can provide good symptomatic control of an effusion via intermittent patient-controlled drainage.
  - ○ The PleurX catheter is better at controlling symptoms than doxycycline pleurodesis.[18]
  - ○ Furthermore, repeated drainage leads to pleurodesis in roughly 50% of patients, allowing the catheter to be removed.
  - ○ Chronic indwelling catheters can be used for palliation with trapped lung compared when chemical pleurodesis is ineffective due to incomplete apposition of the visceral and parietal pleura.
- **Pleurectomy or mechanical pleural abrasion** of the pleural lining can promote pleurodesis. This requires thoracotomy and should be reserved for patients with a good prognosis who have had ineffective pleurodesis by other means.

• Chemotherapy and mediastinal radiotherapy may control effusions in responsive tumors, such as lymphoma or small cell bronchogenic carcinoma.

Solitary Pulmonary Nodule

GENERAL PRINCIPLES

• The **solitary pulmonary nodule** (SPN) is defined as a ≤3 cm isolated, spherical, well-circumscribed lesion completely surrounded by aerated lung without associated atelectasis, hilar enlargement, or pleural effusion.[19,20]
• A lesion >3 cm is referred to as a **pulmonary mass,** and the probability of malignancy is much higher.[19,20] Some authorities also distinguish **subcentimeter nodules** as <8 to 10 mm, which are much less likely to be malignant.[19]
• The large majority of SPNs are discovered incidentally on plain CXR or chest CT obtained for other reasons.[19]
• The prevalence of SPNs is highly dependent on the characteristics of the population studied (e.g., age, smoking status) and the technique used (e.g., CXR or CT). It has been reported to range from 0.2% to 7% for CXRs and 8% to 51% for CT.[19,21–23] **Some SPNs detected on CXR will be false positives**.
• Importantly, **long-term survival is dramatically better after resection of a malignant SPN compared to that for advanced lung cancer.**
• **Screening high-risk patients with low-dose CT scans significantly decreases lung cancer–attributed mortality in this patient population.**[24]

TABLE 19-5	Partial Differential Diagnosis of the SPN
Neoplastic	**Infectious**
Malignant	Granulomatous
Primary lung cancer	Tuberculosis
Adenocarcinoma (including the	Nontuberculous mycobacteria
bronchoalveolar variant)	Histoplasmosis
Squamous cell	Coccidioidomycosis
Small cell	Cryptococcosis
Large cell	Aspergillosis
Carcinoid	Blastomycosis
Metastatic (e.g., breast, colorectal,	Round pneumonia
germ cell, head and neck,	Lung abscess/septic embolus
melanoma, prostate, renal cell)	Parasitic (e.g., ascariasis, dirofilariasis,
Lymphoma	echinococcosis, paragonimiasis)
Benign	
Hamartoma	**Other**
	Healed or nonspecific granulomas
Vascular	Nonspecific inflammation or fibrosis
AV malformation	Round atelectasis
Hemangioma	Bronchogenic cyst
Focal hemorrhage	Intrapulmonary lymph node
Pulmonary infarct	Lipoid pneumonia
	Pulmonary sequestration
Inflammatory	Amyloid
Sarcoidosis	
Granulomatosis with polyangiitis	
(formerly Wegener)	
Rheumatoid arthritis	

- The rate of malignancy in patients with SPNs varies greatly depending on study populations and methods of detection used. Characteristics that increase the risk of malignancy will be discussed below. Table 19-5 outlines a differential diagnosis for SPN.

DIAGNOSIS

Clinical Presentation

- The vast majority of patients with a SPN will be asymptomatic with regard to the nodule itself. Age, smoking status, history of extrathoracic cancer, and history of prior lung cancer are perhaps the most important historical features that increase the likelihood that an SPN is malignant.[19,20,25–28]
- Patients should also be asked about constitutional symptoms that may be due to malignancy or infection such as fever, chills, sweats, weight loss, anorexia, weakness, fatigue, and malaise.
- The physical examination is usually normal with regard to the SPN. Nonetheless, a careful pulmonary examination is indicated.

Diagnostic Testing

Chest Radiography

- CXR factors suggestive of malignancy are as follows[19,21,25,26,29]:
  - **Likelihood of malignancy increases rapidly with size**. Those <1 cm are not usually malignant, but **SPNs >2 cm often are malignant**.
  - **Upper lobe lesions**, particularly on the right, are more likely to be malignant.
  - **Irregular or spiculated margins** increase the likelihood of malignancy. Smooth margins are more likely to be benign, and scalloped margins have intermediate likelihood.
  - **Stippled and/or eccentric calcifications** are associated with malignancy. Laminated, central, and dense calcifications suggest a granuloma, while the "popcorn" pattern suggests hamartoma. Patients with obviously benign calcifications do not need to be evaluated further.
  - The **doubling time** for malignant SPNs is usually between 20 and 300 days, often <100 days. One doubling time equates to an approximately 30% increase in diameter. Based on these assumptions, most authorities agree that **SPNs that are stable in size for 2 years are less likely to be malignant. Because of the importance of growth rate, it is critical to compare with previous CXRs or CTs.** Slowly growing bronchoalveolar cancers are known to exist, and they may subsequently become more aggressive. This seems to be particularly true of lesions with a ground-glass appearance, and lengthier follow-up may be indicated in these cases.[30]
- The American College of Chest Physicians (ACCP) recommends that clinicians **estimate the pretest probability of malignancy before ordering further imaging studies or biopsy**.[19] When appropriate, this may be done qualitatively using all of the factors discussed above. Several prediction models have been developed.[25,31,32] The prediction model developed by Swensen et al.[33] has been validated but is no more accurate than expert clinician assessment. In this model, the independent predictors are age (OR 1.04 for each year), current or past smoking (OR 2.2), history of cancer diagnosed ≥5 years ago (OR 3.8) (patients with cancer <5 years ago were excluded); and nodule diameter (OR 1.14 for each mm), spiculation (OR 2.8), and upper lobe location (OR 2.2).[25]

Chest Computed Tomography

High-resolution chest CT is clearly more sensitive and specific for detection and characterization of SPNs. **The ACCP recommends that all patients with an indeterminate SPN on CXR have high-resolution CT of the chest performed**.[18] If there are any prior chest

CTs, these should be reviewed. In addition to the radiographic features discussed above, CT characteristics suggestive of malignancy include the following[19–21,29,34,35]:

- Vascular convergence.
- Dilated bronchus leading into the nodule.
- Pseudocavitation.
- Thick (>15 mm), irregular-walled cavitation.
- Dynamic contrast enhancement >15 Hounsfield units (HU).
- Fat attenuation (−40 to −120 HU) is strongly suggestive of hamartoma or lipoma. Some metastatic malignancies (e.g., liposarcoma or renal cell carcinoma) may occasionally contain fat.

Positron Emission Tomography
- Fluorodeoxyglucose positron emission tomography (^{18}**F-FDG PET**) may also be used to further characterize SPNs.[36] Reviews have estimated the sensitivity to be 87% to 96.8% and specificity 77.8% to 83%.[37] Sensitivity is less for subcentimeter (<8 to 10 mm) SPNs.
- It is important to recognize that false negatives can occur, and if clinical suspicion still exists, a biopsy should be strongly considered.
- **The ACCP recommends ^{18}F-FDG PET for patients with low-to-moderate pretest probability and an SPN >8 to 10 mm with indeterminate (i.e., not clearly benign) CT characteristics.**[19] In some centers, PET and CT can be combined in a single scan.

Further Evaluation
- Once the clinical and imaging characteristics are known, the choice of subsequent management can be a close call between risk and benefit. Alternatives include observation with serial radiographs, biopsy, and surgery. Each of these has advantages and disadvantages that depend greatly on the likelihood of malignancy.
- **Observation** is appropriate for those with a very low likelihood of malignancy (<5%). Reasonable follow-up consists of serial high-resolution CT scans at 3, 6, 12, and 24 months. Any sign of growth is presumptive evidence of malignancy. If the lesion is stable after 2 years, then the risk of malignancy is very low.[19]
- Observation with serial CT scans may also be appropriate for SPNs >8 to 10 mm:
  ○ With a low likelihood (<30% to 40%) of malignancy and a negative ^{18}F-FDG PET scan or dynamic contrast enhancement <15 HU
  ○ With a nondiagnostic biopsy and a negative ^{18}F-FDG PET scan
  ○ If the patient declines aggressive evaluation[19]
- **Biopsy** is recommended for SPNs >8 to 10 mm in patients who would be appropriate candidates for surgical cure when:
  ○ The clinical likelihood of malignancy and results of imaging studies are not in agreement (e.g., high clinical suspicion but a negative ^{18}F-FDG PET scan)
  ○ A specific treatment is available for a benign diagnosis (e.g., fungal infection)
  ○ The patient wants biopsy confirmation prior to committing to surgery (this may be most useful when the risks of surgery are high).[18]
- Usually, the preferred biopsy technique is **CT-guided transthoracic needle aspiration**, especially for more peripheral lesions. Sensitivity and specificity are variable and depend on multiple factors including lesion size, expertise of the radiologist, availability of an onsite cytopathologic examination, needle size, and number of needle passes.[19,21,29,34,38–40] The reported rate of pneumothorax is variable, ranging from approximately 12% to 44%. Most do not require chest tube placement. Factors associated with pneumothorax include increased lesion depth, smaller SPN size, emphysema, smaller needle-pleural angle, lateral biopsy site, and lesion site near a fissure.[19,41–46]

- **Bronchoscopic biopsy** may be a viable alternative in specific situations (e.g., central lesions, lesions adjacent to a bronchus, an air bronchogram is in the lesion) when there is available expertise.[19]
- Newer technology including **radial probe endobronchial ultrasound, electromagnetic navigation, and virtual bronchoscopy** may improve the diagnostic yield of bronchoscopy for peripheral nodules over conventional bronchoscopic methods.[47,48]
- **Surgical management** is recommended for indeterminate SPNs >8 to 10 mm in appropriate surgical candidates when the clinical likelihood is moderate to high, the ^{18}F-FDG PET is positive, and the patient prefers to undergo a definitive procedure.[18] There are typically two surgical options:
  - **Thoracotomy** is the most definitive approach particularly for more centrally located SPNs that are not accessible by other techniques.
  - **Video-assisted thoracoscopic surgery (VATS)** is a minimally invasive technique with a lower mortality rate. It is usually the preferred method for SPNs in the peripheral third of the lung.
- **Stereotactic body radiation therapy (SBRT)** is a nonsurgical approach to managing early-stage lung cancer using highly focused radiation for patients who are not surgical candidates and offers local control rates similar to those achieved with surgery in this patient population.

REFERENCES

1. Light RW, Macgregor MI, Luchsinger PC, et al. Pleural effusions: the diagnostic separation of transudates and exudates. *Ann Intern Med* 1972;77:507–513.
2. Light RW. *Pleural Diseases*, 5th ed. Philadelphia, PA: Lippincott Williams & Wilkins; 2007.
3. Heffner JE, Brown LK, Barbieri CA. Diagnostic value of tests the discriminate between exudative and transudative pleural effusions. Primary Study Investigators. *Chest* 1997;111:970–980.
4. Roth BJ, O'Meara TF, Cragun WH. The serum-effusion albumin gradient in the evaluation of pleural effusions. *Chest* 1990;98:546–549.
5. Romero S, Candela A, Martin D, et al. Evaluation of different criteria for the separation of pleural transudates from exudates. *Chest* 1993;104:399–404.
6. Light RW, Erozan YS, Ball WC Jr. Cells in pleural fluid. Their values in differential diagnosis. *Arch Intern Med* 1973;132:854–860.
7. Spriggs AI, Boddington MM. *The Cytology of Effusions: Pleural, Pericardial, and Peritoneal and of Cerebrospinal Fluid*, 2nd ed. New York: Grune & Stratton; 1968.
8. Light RW. Clinical practice. Pleural effusions. *N Engl J Med* 2002;346:1971–1977.
9. Balbir-Gurman A, Yigla M, Nahir AM, et al. Rheumatoid pleural effusion. *Semin Arthritis Rheum* 2006;35:368–373.
10. Rodriguez-Panadero F, Lopez Mejias J. Low glucose and pH levels in malignant pleural effusions. Diagnostic significance and prognostic value in respect to pleurodesis. *Am Rev Respir Dis* 1989;139:663–667.
11. Heffner JE, Brown LK, Barbieri C, et al. Pleural fluid chemical analysis in parapneumonic effusions. A meta-analysis. *Am J Respir Crit Care Med* 1995;151:1700–1708.
12. Colice GL, Curtis A, Deslauriers J, et al. Medical and surgical treatment of parapneumonic effusions: an evidence-based guideline. *Chest* 2000;118:1158–1171.
13. Prakash UB, Reiman HM. Comparison of needle biopsy with cytologic analysis for the evaluation of pleural effusion: analysis of 414 cases. *Mayo Clin Pro* 1985;60:158–164.
14. Sallich SM, Sallach, JA, Vazquez E, et al. Volume of pleural fluid required for diagnosis of pleural malignancy. *Chest* 2002;122:1913–1917.

15. Branca P, Rodriguez RM, Rogers JT, et al. Routine measurement of pleural fluid amylase is not indicated. *Arch Intern Med* 2001;161:228–232.

16. Feller-Kopman D, Berkowitz D, Boiselle P, et al. Large volume thoracentesis and the risk of re-expansion pulmonary edema. *Ann Thorac Surg* 2007;84:1656–1662.

17. Walker-Renard PB, Vaughn LM, Sahn SA. Chemical pleurodesis for malignant pleural effusions. *Ann Intern Med* 1994;120:56–64.

18. Putman JB, Light RW, Rodriguez RM, et al. A randomized comparison of indwelling pleural catheter and doxycycline pleurodesis in the management of malignant pleural effusion. *Cancer* 1999;86:1992–1999.

19. Gould MK, Fletcher, J, Iannettoni MD, et al. Evaluation of patients with pulmonary nodules: when is it lung cancer?: ACCP evidence-based clinical practice guidelines (2nd edition). *Chest* 2007;132:108S–130S.

20. Ost D, Fein AM, Feinsilver SH. Clinical practice. The solitary pulmonary nodule. *N Engl J Med* 2003;348:2535–2542.

21. Wahidi MM, Govert JA, Goudar RK, et al. Evidence for the treatment of patients with pulmonary nodules: when is it lung cancer?: ACCP evidence-based clinical practice guidelines (2nd edition). *Chest* 2007;132:94S–107S.

22. Henschke CI, McCauley DI, Yankelevitz DF, et al. Early Lung Cancer Action Project: overall design and findings from baseline screening. *Lancet* 1999;354:99–105.

23. Holin SN, Dwork RE, Glaser S, et al. Solitary pulmonary nodules found in a community-wide chest roentgenographic survey. *Am Rev Tuberc* 1959;79:427–439.

24. The National Lung Screening Trial Research Team. Reduced lung cancer mortality with low-dose computed tomographic screening. *N Engl J Med* 2011;365:395–409.

25. Swensen SJ, Silverstein MD, Ilstrup DM, et al. The probability of malignancy in solitary pulmonary nodules. Application to small radiologically indeterminate nodules. *Arch Intern Med* 1997;157:849–855.

26. Gould MK, Ananth L, Barnett PG. A clinical model to estimate the pretest probability of lung cancer in patient with solitary pulmonary nodules. *Chest* 2007;131:383–388.

27. Schultz EM, Sanders GD, Trotter PR, et al. Validation of two models to estimate the probability of malignancy in patients with solitary pulmonary nodules. *Thorax* 2008;63:335–341.

28. Mery CM, Pappas AN, Bueno R, et al. Relationship between a history of antecedent cancer and the probability of malignancy for a solitary pulmonary nodule. *Chest* 2004;125:2175–2181.

29. Winer-Muram HT. The solitary pulmonary nodule. *Radiology* 2006;239:34–49.

30. Aoki T, Nakata H, Watanabe H, et al. Evolution of peripheral lung adenocarcinomas: CT findings correlated with histology and tumor doubling time. *AJR Am J Roentgenol* 2000;174:763–768.

31. Gurney JW. Determining the likelihood of malignancy in solitary pulmonary nodules with Bayesian analysis. Part I. Theory. *Radiology* 1993;186:405–413.

32. Gurney JW, Lyddon DM, McKay JA. Determining the likelihood of malignancy in solitary pulmonary nodules with Bayesian analysis. Part II. Application. *Radiology* 1993;186:415–422.

33. Swensen SJ, Silverstein MD, Edell ES, et al. Solitary pulmonary nodules: clinical prediction model versus physicians. *Mayo Clin Proc* 1999;74:319–329.

34. Jeong YJ, Yi CA, Lee KS. Solitary pulmonary nodules: detection, characterization, and guidance for further diagnostic workup and treatment. *AJR Am J Roentgenol* 2007;188:57–68.

35. Swensen SJ, Viggiano RW, Midthun DE, et al. Lung nodule enhancement at CT: multicenter study. *Radiology* 2000;214:73–80.

36. Herder GJ, van Tinteren H, Golding RP, et al. Clinical prediction model to characterize pulmonary nodules: validation and added value of 18F-fluorodeoxyglucose positron emission tomography. *Chest* 2005;128:2490–2496.

37. Gould MK, Maclean CC, Kuschner WG, et al. Accuracy of positron emission tomography for diagnosis of pulmonary nodules and mass lesions: a meta-analysis. *JAMA* 2001;285:914–924.
38. Lacasse Y, Wong E, Guyatt GH, et al. Transthoracic needle aspiration biopsy for the diagnosis of localized pulmonary lesions: a meta-analysis. *Thorax* 1999;54:884–893.
39. Wallace MJ, Krishnamurthy S, Broemeling LD, et al. CT-guided percutaneous fine-needle aspiration biopsy of small (≤1-cm) pulmonary lesions. *Radiology* 2002;225:823–828.
40. Ohno Y, Hatabu H, Takenaka D, et al. CT-guided transthoracic needle aspiration biopsy of small (<20 mm) solitary pulmonary nodules. *AJR Am J Roentgenol* 2003;180:1665–1669.
41. Kazerooni EA, Lim FT, Mikhail A, et al. Risk of pneumothorax in CT-guided transthoracic needle aspiration biopsy of the lung. *Radiology* 1996;198:371–375.
42. Cox JE, Chiles C, McManus CM, et al. Transthoracic needle aspiration biopsy: variable that affect risk of pneumothorax. *Radiology* 1999;212:165–168.
43. Yeow KM, See LC, Lui KW, et al. Risk factors for pneumothorax and bleeding after CT-guided percutaneous coaxial cutting needle biopsy of lung lesions. *J Vasc Interv Radiol* 2001;12:1305–1312.
44. Ko JP, Shepard JO, Drucker EA, et al. Factors influencing pneumothorax rate at lung biopsy: are dwell time and angle of pleural puncture contributing factors? *Radiology* 2001;218:491–496.
45. Saji H, Nakamura H, Tsuchida T, et al. The incidence and the risk of pneumothorax and chest tube placement after percutaneous CT-guided lung biopsy: the angle of the needle trajectory is a novel predictor. *Chest* 2002;121:1521–1526.
46. Yeow KM, Su IH, Pan KT, et al. Risk factors of pneumothorax and bleeding: multivariate analysis of 660 CT-guided coaxial cutting needle lung biopsies. *Chest* 2004;126:748–754.
47. Eberhardt R, Anantham D, Herth F, et al. Electromagnetic navigation diagnostic bronchoscopy in peripheral lung lesions. *Chest* 2007;131:1800–1805.
48. Kurimoto N, Miyazawa T, Okimasa S, et al. Endobronchial ultrasonography using a guide sheath increases the ability to diagnose peripheral pulmonary lesions endoscopically. *Chest* 2004;126:959–965.

20 Diabetes Mellitus

Cynthia J. Herrick and Janet B. McGill

GENERAL PRINCIPLES

- Diabetes mellitus (DM) is characterized by hyperglycemia resulting from defects in insulin secretion, insulin action, or both.
- Chronic hyperglycemia is associated with long-term damage of various organs.
  - Microvascular complications, which are directly linked to hyperglycemia, include retinopathy, nephropathy, and neuropathy.
  - Persons with DM are at increased risk of macrovascular events, increased morbidity from these events, and increased cardiovascular mortality.
- DM is a chronic illness that requires multicomponent medical care focused on glycemic control, regulation of blood pressure, lipid-lowering therapy, and preventative care, including cancer screening. Patient education is a key component of treatment.
- Management of diabetic emergencies such as ketoacidosis and hyperosmolar syndrome will not be covered in this manual.

Classification

Type 1 Diabetes Mellitus

- Type 1 DM (T1DM) accounts for 5% to 10% of those with diabetes.[1]
- Both the incidence and prevalence of T1DM are increasing across all age groups.
- The pathogenesis of T1DM is cellular-mediated autoimmune destruction of the pancreatic β-cells, leading to near-total or absolute insulin deficiency.[2]
- T1DM has strong human leukocyte antigen (HLA) associations; and one or more autoantibodies (e.g., to glutamic acid decarboxylase, insulinoma-associated autoantigen 2, insulin, and zinc transporter 8) are present in 85% to 90% of individuals with recent-onset disease.[2]
- The onset of T1DM is usually in childhood or adolescence, but can occur at any age.
  - The rate of β-cell destruction is variable—generally more rapid in children and young adults, but slower in adults over the age of 30, sometimes taking years to progress to complete insulin deficiency.[2]
  - Latent autoimmune diabetes in adults (LADA) is characterized by the presence of autoantibodies, but slow and sometimes incomplete β-cell destruction. Up to 10% of patients with type 2 diabetes mellitus (T2DM) have one or more autoantibodies present, depending on the population studied.
- Patients with T1DM are **dependent on insulin for survival and are at risk for ketoacidosis if insulin treatment is interrupted.**
- Patients are typically not obese at the time of diagnosis, but the presence of obesity does not exclude the diagnosis.
- Persons with T1DM have an increased risk of other autoimmune diseases such as Graves disease, Hashimoto thyroiditis, Addison disease, celiac sprue, pernicious anemia, autoimmune hepatitis, vitiligo, alopecia, myasthenia gravis, and systemic diseases such as rheumatoid arthritis and systemic lupus erythematosis.[3]

Type 2 Diabetes Mellitus

- T2DM is the most common form of diabetes, accounting for up to 90% of all cases of DM, and is strongly associated with obesity.[1]
- The pathogenesis of T2DM is not completely understood, but is characterized by insulin resistance (in most cases) followed by progressive insulin deficiency.[4] Other abnormalities

include tonically elevated glucagon levels, impaired incretin secretion or action, and elevated free fatty acids and inflammatory markers.
- Most patients are obese or have an increased percentage of intra-abdominal fat, which can worsen insulin resistance.
- Treatment options for T2DM include several oral and injectable non–insulin therapies, which can be augmented or replaced by insulin as needed, depending on the degree of β-cell dysfunction.[4]
- **Ketoacidosis rarely occurs in these patients** but can arise in the setting of illness or infection, and occasionally as the result of so called glucose toxicity, which causes a functional impairment of beta cells.
- The risk of developing T2DM increases with age, obesity, and lack of physical activity.
- T2DM is typically preceded by conditions such as impaired fasting glucose (IFG) and impaired glucose tolerance (IGT) or in women with a prior history of gestational diabetes mellitus (GDM).[1]
- The risk of developing T2DM varies among racial and ethnic groups, and despite a strong genetic predisposition, the genetic defects are complex and not clearly defined.
- Mild hyperglycemia is asymptomatic, leading to delayed diagnosis in many cases.

Other Types of Diabetes Mellitus
- Monogenetic diabetes
  - Defects in over 20 different genes result in diabetes, often with distinct clinical characteristics.[5] Monogenic diabetes (MD) accounts for >1% of cases of diabetes with childhood onset.[5] Some forms of MD are diagnosed in adolescence or in young adults and were previously referred to as maturity-onset diabetes of the young (MODY).[6]
  - Most of the patients with MD have impaired insulin secretion with minimal or no defects in insulin action and are autosomal dominant.[7]
- Diseases of the exocrine pancreas
  - Trauma, pancreatectomy, and acquired illnesses such as pancreatitis, infection, and pancreatic carcinoma can result in insulin deficiency.
  - Inherited conditions such as cystic fibrosis and hemochromatosis will also damage β-cells and impair insulin secretion.
- Drug- or chemical-induced diabetes
  - Toxins and drugs such as intravenous pentamidine can permanently destroy pancreatic β-cells, while steroids and others cause β-cell dysfunction and/or insulin resistance.[8]
  - Patients receiving α-interferon have been reported to develop diabetes associated with islet cell antibodies.[9]
- Endocrine disorders such as Cushing disease and acromegaly result in the secretion of hormones that antagonize insulin action and can result in IGT or T2DM.
- Gestational diabetes mellitus
  - GDM complicates 3% to 10% of all pregnancies, depending on the population studied, and generally appears in the second or third trimester.[10]
  - Women with GDM are at higher risk for developing T2DM in the 5 to 10 years after delivery and should undergo more frequent screening.

Prevention
- T2DM is generally preceded by IGT, IFG, or both. Numerous interventions are effective in reducing progression to T2DM from these at-risk conditions.[1]
- Lifestyle intervention, including diet and exercise, is effective in all age groups studied.[11]
- Metformin can be used in those who are at risk for diabetes, especially if <60 years of age.[1,11]
- Other therapies have been tested, but are not recommended due to adverse safety profiles.

DIAGNOSIS

- Diabetes screening in asymptomatic individuals should follow these guidelines:
  - All adults who are overweight (body mass index [BMI] > 25 kg/m²) and have additional risk factors (Table 20-1).[1]
  - In the absence of the above criteria, testing for diabetes should begin at age 45 years.
  - If results are normal, testing should be repeated at least at 3-year intervals, with more frequent testing if clinically indicated.
- Upon diagnosis, the initial evaluation should include a complete medical history that addresses the following:
  - Classify the type of diabetes.
  - Identify the presence of diabetes-related complications.
  - Assess microvascular and macrovascular risk factors, including blood pressure and lipid profile.
  - Document ethnicity and family history of diabetes.
  - Form a comprehensive management plan targeting glycemic, lipid, cardiovascular, and nutritional goals.

Diagnostic Criteria

- Patients must meet ONE of the following criteria to be diagnosed with diabetes[1,12]:
  - **FPG (fasting plasma glucose) of ≥126 mg/dL** (7.0 mmol/L). Fasting is defined as no caloric intake for at least 8 hours. Confirmation with a second measurement is advised.
  - **Symptoms of hyperglycemia and a random plasma glucose of ≥200 mg/dL** (11.1 mmol/L). Classic symptoms of hyperglycemia include polyuria, polydipsia, and unexplained weight loss.
  - **OGTT (oral glucose tolerance test) 2-hour plasma glucose of ≥200 mg/dL** (11.1 mmol/L). The patient should receive a glucose load containing 75 g of anhydrous glucose dissolved in water.
  - **Hemoglobin A1C (A1C) ≥ 6.5%.**[12]
- Official diagnostic criteria differentiating the two types of diabetes are lacking. A history of diabetic ketoacidosis (DKA), low or absent C-peptide, and/or the presence of autoantibodies characterize T1DM. Mild hyperglycemia at presentation, a history of GDM, and/or obesity characterize T2DM.

TABLE 20-1	Risk Factors for Diabetes Mellitus

Physical inactivity
First-degree relative with diabetes
Members of a high-risk ethnic population (e.g., African American, Latino, Native American, Asian American, Pacific Islander)
Women who delivered a baby weighing >9 pound or were diagnosed with GDM
Hypertension (>140/90 mm Hg or on therapy for hypertension)
HDL cholesterol level >35 mg/dL (0.90 mmol/L) and/or a triglyceride level >250 mg/dL (2.82 mmol/L)
Women with polycystic ovarian syndrome
Impaired glucose tolerance or impaired fasting glucose on previous testing
Other clinical conditions associated with insulin resistance (e.g., severe obesity, acanthosis nigricans)
History of cerebrovascular disease

GDM, gestational diabetes mellitus; HDL, high-density lipoprotein.

TABLE 20-2 Assessing Risk for Gestational Diabetes

Very high risk	Low risk
Severe obesity	Age < 25 years
Prior history of GDM or delivery of large for gestational age infant	Weight normal before pregnancy
Presence of glycosuria	Member of an ethnic group with a low prevalence of diabetes
Diagnosis of PCOS	No known diabetes in first-degree relatives
Strong family history of type 2 diabetes	No history of abnormal glucose tolerance
	No history of poor obstetrical outcome

GDM, gestational diabetes mellitus; PCOS, polycystic ovarian syndrome.

- **Gestational diabetes**
  - Women should undergo risk assessment (Table 20-2) and be screened for undiagnosed T2DM at the first prenatal visit using standard diagnostic criteria.[12]
  - Women without a diagnosis of diabetes or positive diagnostic test in the first trimester should undergo a 2-hour, 75-g glucose OGTT at 24 to 28 weeks of gestation.[10]
  - Women with a history of GDM have a higher risk of developing T2DM, so screening for T2DM should occur at 6 to 12 weeks postpartum and every 3 years thereafter.

TREATMENT

- Patients should receive care from a physician-coordinated team including, but not limited to, physicians, certified diabetic nurse educators, dietitians, pharmacists, and mental health professionals with expertise in diabetes.
- All treatment plans should emphasize the role of the patient as an integral component of care with emphasis on self-management education.
- In developing a management plan, consideration should be given to the patient's age, school/work schedule, physical activity, eating patterns, social situation and personality, cultural factors, and other medical conditions.
- All treatment recommendations should be individualized and based on life expectancy, comorbidities, cognitive abilities, risk of hypoglycemia, and glucose-lowering effectiveness.[13]
- In T2DM, a number of modifiable environmental factors play a role in disease development. Interventions that target obesity, a sedentary lifestyle, and nutrition have been shown to have a beneficial effect on hyperglycemia, lowering A1C by 0.25% to 2.9%.[1]

Glycemic Goals

- Glycemic control should be assessed by both self-monitoring of capillary blood glucose (SMBG) and periodic A1C testing.[12]
- Data have shown that targeting the following goals for glycemic control is associated with the lowest risk of long-term complications for both T1DM and T2DM.[9,10]
  - **Preprandial capillary BG values between 90 and 130 mg/dL (3.9 to 7.2 mmol/L).**
  - **Postprandial capillary BG values ≤ 180 mg/dL (<10.0 mmol/L).**
  - **A1C targets should be individualized. Tight glycemic control (A1C < 6.5%) is appropriate for patients managed on non–hypoglycemia-inducing therapies, while less tight control (A1C < 7% to 7.5%) may be appropriate for higher-risk patients, including those with CV disease and T2DM patients treated with insulin. Hypoglycemia should be avoided in all patients.**

- Goals for nonpregnant adults should be individualized and may vary based on the following: duration of diabetes, age and life expectancy, comorbid conditions, known cardiovascular disease (CVD) or advanced microvascular complications, hypoglycemia unawareness, and individual patient considerations.

Self-Monitoring of Capillary Blood Glucose

- For patients using noninsulin, non–hypoglycemia-inducing therapy, SMBG should occur daily or less often. Surveillance with pre and postprandial blood glucose is informative, even if done infrequently.
- For patients using basal insulin only, SMBG is recommended twice daily.
- Patients treated with multiple daily insulin injections or insulin pump therapy should perform SMBG four or more times daily. Improved glucose control is observed with greater testing frequency in patients with T1DM.
- Physicians should review records of SMBG at every visit to titrate medical therapy.
- Frequent glucose monitoring and continuous glucose monitoring (CGM), used along with intensive insulin regimens, have been shown to be useful in the management of adults with T1DM, especially those with hypoglycemia unawareness and/or frequent hypoglycemic episodes.[12]

Hemoglobin A1C

- **A1C should be measured at least twice annually in patients who have met treatment goals without hypoglycemia.**
- **A1C should be measured quarterly in patients whose therapy has changed or who have not meet glycemic goals.**
- A1C testing does not replace examination of glucose meter downloads or SMBG records. Point-of-care testing for hemoglobin A1C allows for timely decisions on therapy changes.[14]
- Limitations of hemoglobin A1C testing
  ○ Inaccurate A1C values may result from the following factors: conditions that affect erythrocyte turnover, hemoglobin variants, and recent blood transfusions.
  ○ Does not provide a measure of glycemic variability or hypoglycemia.
- Other measures of chronic glycemia such as fructosamine are available, but are not widely utilized.

Hypoglycemia

- Hypoglycemia is a common occurrence in patients with T1DM or T2DM treated with insulin or insulin secretagogues.[15]
- **The preferred treatment of hypoglycemia is 15 to 20 g of glucose,** although any form of carbohydrate that contains glucose can be used.
- Fats should be avoided acutely because they can delay the acute glycemic response.[16]
- Patients should be instructed to recheck an SMBG level 10 to 15 minutes after treatment.
  ○ If SMBG shows continued hypoglycemia, the treatment should be repeated.
  ○ Once SMBG returns to normal, the individual should evaluate his or her risk of recurrence, and modify insulin doses or consume additional calories as needed.
  ○ Overtreatment of hypoglycemia can cause rebound hyperglycemia and increase the variability in glucose values.
- Severe hypoglycemia is defined as hypoglycemia that requires the assistance of another person and cannot be treated with oral carbohydrate due to patient confusion or unconsciousness.
- **Patients with a history of frequent mild hypoglycemia or one episode of severe hypoglycemia should be prescribed glucagon,** and caregivers or family members of these individuals should be instructed on proper administration.
- **Hypoglycemia unawareness** is characterized by repetitive hypoglycemia that results in a deficiency of the protective counterregulatory hormone and autonomic responses.[15]
- Individuals with hypoglycemia unawareness should have higher glycemic goals temporarily to partially reverse hypoglycemia unawareness and reduce the risk of future episodes.[15]

Medications

Oral Agents

- Therapy with one agent is recommended for those patients with an A1C < 7.5%. For those with an A1C 7.5% to 9%, two agents offer greater efficacy. Three agents may be needed if the A1C is >9%, or insulin can be considered. In general, additional medications are added to the background regimen of metformin, though changes are often made when insulin is started.[17]
- As disease progression occurs in T2DM, medications can be used in combinations to achieve glycemic targets.

Metformin

- Doses are 500, 750, 850, or 1,000 mg given 2 to 3 times per day, not to exceed 2,550 mg daily.
- The primary effect is to decrease hepatic glucose output and lower fasting glycemia.
- **Therapy with metformin as a single agent will lower A1C by approximately 1% to 1.5%.**[18]
- Metformin is well tolerated in about 80%, tolerated at lower than maximal doses in 10%, and not tolerated in about 10%.
- **Metformin is contraindicated in patients with serum creatinine >1.5 mg/dL in men and >1.4 mg/dL in women**. Reduced creatinine clearance increases the risk of lactic acidosis in persons taking metformin. Other risk factors for lactic acidosis in which metformin should be discontinued include hypovolemia, serious infection, tissue hypoxia, alcoholism, and severe cardiopulmonary disease.
- Recent studies suggest that metformin is safe at reduced doses until the eGFR falls below 30 mL/minute.[19]

Sulfonylureas

- Sulfonylureas (SUs) enhance endogenous insulin secretion, and they are similar to metformin in efficacy and **lower A1C by approximately 1% to 1.5%.**
- The **primary adverse effect is hypoglycemia,** which can be severe and prolonged, especially in elderly patients or those with liver or renal disease. Patients who are known to skip meals should not take an SU because of an increased risk of hypoglycemia.
- Glyburide (1.25 to 20 mg daily) is associated with the highest risk of hypoglycemia when compared to other SU and is no longer recommended as a first-line antidiabetic agent.
- Other second-generation SUs include **glimepiride** (1 to 8 mg once daily), **glipizide** (5 to 40 mg/day, >15 mg/day should be given in divided doses), **glipizide extended release** (5 to 20 mg once daily), gliclazide (starting 40 to 80 mg once daily to a maximum of 320 mg/day, doses >160 mg must be split bid), and gliclazide modified release (30 to 120 mg once daily). They are the preferred agents of this class of antidiabetic drugs. Gliclazide is not available in the US.
- Weight gain is common after initiation of therapy.
- Although the onset of the hypoglycemic effect is quite rapid with SUs, durability of the glucose-lowering effect is inferior to the use of a thiazolidinedione (TZD) or metformin when used as monotherapy.[20]

Glinides

- These drugs also stimulate endogenous insulin secretion but bind to a different site within the SU receptor.
- They have a shorter circulating half-life than SU and are administered more frequently.
  - Because of their short half-life, they are **less likely to cause prolonged hypoglycemia.**
  - Glinides are a good choice for patients who would otherwise tolerate a SU but who have experienced hypoglycemia because of variable meal times and/or skipped meals.
- The two currently available glinides are repaglinide and nateglinide.
- Repaglinide (0.5 to 4 mg ac/tid) is almost as effective as metformin or SU at **decreasing hemoglobin A1C level by 1.5%,** but nateglinide (60 to 120 mg ac/tid) is somewhat less potent.[21]
- The risk of weight gain is similar to that with most SUs.

α-Glucosidase Inhibitors

- α-Glucosidase inhibitors, acarbose (25 to 100 mg ac/tid), miglitol (25 to 100 mg ac/tid), and voglibose (0.2 to 0.3 mg ac/tid) decrease the digestion and absorption of polysaccharides in the small intestine.[22]
- These agents lower postprandial glucose without causing hypoglycemia and **lower A1C by 0.5% to 0.8%.**
- The most common side effects are bloating and flatulence.
- Long-term use of acarbose has been shown to reduce the risk of myocardial infarction.[23]

Thiazolidinediones

- TZDs are peroxisome proliferator–activated γ-receptor agonists.
- Only pioglitazone (15 to 45 mg daily) is currently available in the US.
- The primary mechanism of action of TZD is to increase the peripheral tissue sensitivity to insulin.
- **When used as monotherapy, they have been shown to lower the hemoglobin A1C level by 0.5% to 1.4% and have better durability of effect than metformin or SU.**[20]
- The most common side effects are weight gain and fluid retention. There is also a **twofold greater risk of congestive heart failure.**[24]
- Several **meta-analyses suggested an increase in risk for myocardial infarction** with rosiglitazone.[25] In randomized clinical trials, pioglitazone has been neutral or beneficial in patients with cardiovascular risk factors.[26]
- Other concerning effects of TZDs include an increase in fracture risk and lower bone mineral density, especially in postmenopausal women.[27] **Pioglitazone has been associated with an increased risk of bladder cancer.**[28]

Dipeptidyl Peptidase-4 Inhibitors

- The gut insulinotropic hormones, **incretins,** include glucagon-like peptide-1 (GLP-1) and glucose-dependent insulinotropic peptide (GIP).[29] Both hormones are rapidly degraded by the enzyme dipeptidyl peptidase-4 (DPP-4). DPP-4 inhibitors enhance the effects of GLP-1 and GIP, increasing glucose-mediated insulin secretion and suppressing glucagon secretion.[30]
- DPP-4 inhibitors **lower A1C by 0.6% to 0.9%.**[29]
- Currently, sitagliptin (25 to 100 mg once daily), saxagliptin (2.5 to 5 mg once daily), linagliptin (5 mg once daily) and alogliptin (6.25 to 25 mg once daily) are available in the US. Vildagliptin (50 mg bid or 50 mg once daily when used with a SU) is available in Europe and Asia. All but linagliptin require dosage reduction in moderate to severe renal impairment.
- They are very well tolerated and have few side effects.[30]
- DPP-4 inhibitors can be used with other oral therapies and with insulin but should not be used with GLP1 receptor agonists.

Sodium-Glucose Cotransporter 2 (SGLT2) Inhibitor

- The mechanism of action of the SGLT2 inhibitors is to inhibit glucose reabsorption in the proximal tubule of the kidney, causing loss of glucose in the urine.[31]
- Dapagliflozin (5 and 10 mg) and canagliflozin (100 and 300 mg) are available in the US. Both are contraindicated in moderate to severe renal dysfunction.
- The SGLT2 inhibitors **lower A1C by 0.7% to 1.2%** and can be safely used with other therapies.[32]
- The major side effects are genital yeast infections, which can occur in 10% to 20% of patients newly treated, and hypovolemia.

Colesevelam

- This bile acid sequestrant has glucose-lowering properties when given in full doses.
- A1C is reduced by 0.4% to 0.6%, along with lowering of low-density lipoprotein (LDL).

Bromocriptine Mesylate

- Bromocriptine lowers glucose by an unknown mechanism.
- The tablets are 0.8 mg, dosed 1.6 to 4.8 mg once daily.

- It may also help with sleep or circadian rhythm.
- Cannot be used in patients who are taking antipsychotic agents.

Noninsulin Injectable Agents
Amylin Agonists
- Pramlintide, a synthetic analogue of the β-cell hormone amylin, has been shown to slow gastric emptying, inhibit glucagon secretion, and decrease postprandial hyperglycemia.[33]
- Pramlintide is administered subcutaneously before meals.
- **The addition of pramlintide to insulin therapy can decrease the A1C by 0.5% to 0.7%.**
- The major side effects are gastrointestinal, predominantly nausea, which tends to improve over time. **Weight loss** is associated with treatment and may be secondary to gastrointestinal side effects.
- **Pramlintide is approved for use only as adjunctive therapy with insulin,** in patients with T1DM or T2DM taking premeal regular or rapid-acting analogues.

Glucagon-Like Peptide-1 Agonists
- GLP-1 is a peptide produced by the small intestine that has been shown to potentiate glucose-stimulated insulin secretion and reduce glucagon secretion from alpha cells.[34]
- **Exenatide,** a synthetic GLP-1 agonist, is available as a short-acting agent that is administered twice daily (5 or 10 mg) or in a once weekly formulation (2 mg).
- Liraglutide is administered once daily subcutaneously in doses of 0.6 to 1.8 mg.
- GLP-1 agonists **lower A1C by 0.5% to 1.6%.**
- Additional actions of GLP-1 agonists include suppressing glucagon secretion and slowing gastric emptying.[34]
- Gastrointestinal side effects, including nausea, vomiting, or diarrhea, are common but tend to resolve over time or with dose reduction.
- Weight loss of 1 to 5 kg is observed in patients taking GLP-1 agonist therapy.[35]
- Pancreatitis risk may increase with use of GLP agonists, but the magnitude is not defined and appears to be small. Also thyroid C-cell tumors were increased in rodents but not in humans.
- Both liraglutide and exenatide can be used with oral antidiabetes therapies except for DPP-4 inhibitors and are approved for use with insulin.

Insulin
- **Insulin remains the most effective medication in the treatment of hyperglycemia and should be considered for initial therapy when the A1C is >9%.**[17]
- Insulin is available as human insulin (regular or NPH) or as analogues (lispro, aspart, glulisine, detemir, and glargine). Insulins are generally grouped by their onset and duration of action into rapid acting (lispro, aspart, glulisine), short acting (human regular insulin), intermediate acting (human NPH), or long acting (detemir, glargine).
  - **Rapid-acting insulin** has an onset of about 1 hour, peak activity at about 2 hours, and duration of action of 4 hours.
  - **Short-acting insulin** (e.g., regular) has an onset of 1 to 2 hours, peak activity of 3 to 4 hours, and duration up to 6 hours.
  - **Intermediate-acting insulin** (e.g., NPH) has an onset of about 2 hours, peak at 6 to 8 hours, and duration of action of 12 to 16 hours.
  - **Long-acting insulins** have a nearly flat, peakless profile and duration of action of 16 to 20 hours (detemir) or 22 to 25 hours (glargine).
- **Basal insulin,** using either intermediate- or long-acting insulin, is often added to oral or GLP-1 therapy.
- Conventional insulin therapy describes the use of one or two injections per day of regular and NPH insulin, sometimes premixed, given in fixed amounts.
- **Intensive insulin therapy, also known as multiple daily injection (MDI) or basal-bolus therapy,** describes more complex regimens that utilize basal insulin with rapid-acting insulin three or more times daily to cover meals.

Type 1 Diabetes

- **The majority of patients with T1DM will be treated with intensive insulin therapy with MDI or an insulin pump.**
- Since the arrival of both rapid- and long-acting insulin analogs, intensive glucose control in patients with T1DM is less associated with prolonged hypoglycemia.[36]
- Both **insulin glargine and detemir** are long-acting insulin analogs that have very modest peaks of activity, making them **ideal to provide a continuous basal insulin** level in a T1DM patient.
  - Dosing for insulin glargine is typically once daily, but in certain cases, patients may require twice-daily dosing.
  - Dosing for insulin detemir is twice daily.
- The rapid-acting insulins available are **insulin lispro, aspart, and glulisine.**[37]
  - All have an onset of action within 5 to 15 minutes, peak action at 30 to 90 minutes, and a duration of action of 2 to 4 hours.
  - These agents **decrease postprandial hyperglycemia.**
  - They have been shown to reduce the frequency of hypoglycemia when compared with regular human insulin.
  - Rapid-acting insulin should be injected **immediately before meals,** and the doses can be rapidly adjusted to match the hyperglycemia and carbohydrate intake in most T1DM patients.
- Most newly diagnosed patients with T1DM can be **started on a total daily dose of 0.3 to 0.4 units of insulin/kg/day, although most will ultimately require 0.7 to 0.8 units/ kg/day.**
- MDI regimens should be designed in collaboration with an endocrinologist, diabetes educator, and nutritionist to clearly match the needs and lifestyle of the individual.
- As a general rule of thumb, **approximately half of the total daily dose should be given as a basal insulin, and the remainder is given as short- or rapid-acting insulin, divided before meals.**

Type 2 Diabetes

- T2DM patients with persistent hyperglycemia despite oral hypoglycemic therapy may require the addition of insulin to their regimen or the transition to an insulin-based regimen alone.
- Insulin suppresses hepatic glucose production, which may help to improve the effectiveness of the oral agents and keep the patient's overall hyperinsulinemia to a minimum.[38]
- Basal insulin, given once bedtime, is a common starting point for insulin therapy.
  - **A safe starting dose is typically 10 units or 0.2 units/kg.**
  - This dose should be titrated up to achieve an FPG level of 90 to 130 mg/dL.
  - If nocturnal or symptomatic hypoglycemia occurs in patients taking bedtime NPH, the dose should be decreased or the patient should be switched to insulin glargine.
- For most T2DM patients, adding basal insulin to a regimen of oral or GLP-1 hypoglycemic agents is adequate to achieve glycemic goals.
- For patients who no longer respond to oral agents, preprandial boluses are necessary. These patients should be transitioned to an insulin-based regimen with the guidance of an endocrinologist.
- Very insulin-resistant T2DM patients may require high doses of insulin. Humulin U-500 insulin can be helpful, but the therapy should be guided by an endocrinologist with the help of a diabetes educator.
- Treatment targets and regimens should be individualized to minimize the risk of hypoglycemia, avoid unnecessary complexity, and provide the safe use of pharmaceuticals in patients with declining renal, hepatic, cardiac, or cognitive function. Overzealous glucose lowering with a goal of normalization of glucose values has been associated with increased mortality in patients with T2DM and CV risk factors.[39]

Other Nonpharmacologic Therapies

- Individual psychological and social issues can impair a patient's ability to adhere to a diabetes treatment regimen.[16] Self-management is often limited by attitudes toward the illness, personal expectations, patient's mood and affect, quality of life, psychiatric history, and financial, social, and emotional resources.
- Indications for referral to a mental health specialist familiar with diabetes management include:
  - Noncompliance with medical regimen
  - Depression with the possibility of self-harm
  - Debilitating anxiety (alone or with depression)
  - Indications of an eating disorder
  - Cognitive functioning that significantly impairs judgment or self-care
- Adjusting treatment regimens to assess barriers to adherence may improve overall quality of care.

Surgical Management

Bariatric surgery may be considered for adults with BMI of >35 kg/m^2 and T2DM, if the diabetes is difficult to control with lifestyle and pharmacologic therapy.[40] Longer-term concerns of bariatric surgery include vitamin and mineral deficiencies, osteoporosis, and hypoglycemia from insulin hypersecretion, although the latter effect is rare.

Lifestyle/Risk Modification

Diet

- **All patients with diabetes and prediabetes should undergo medical nutrition counseling** under the guidance of a registered dietician.[41]
- In overweight and obese individuals, **modest weight loss** has been shown to reduce insulin resistance and improve glycemic control.[42]
  - Both low-carbohydrate and low-fat calorie-restricted diets may be effective up to 1 year.[43]
  - For patients on low-carbohydrate diets, monitor lipid profiles, renal function, and protein intake and adjust hypoglycemic therapy as needed.
- Macronutrient content and distribution should be individualized to achieve desired weight and to account for personal preferences, cultural influences, and the presence of other illnesses.
  - **Saturated fat intake should be <7% of total calories** and trans fat intake should be discouraged.
  - Monitoring carbohydrate intake through carbohydrate counting, exchanges, or estimation is a key strategy in achieving glycemic control.
  - **The recommended dietary allowance for digestible carbohydrate is 130 g/day.** This is based on the amount of glucose required for central nervous system function without additional reliance on glucose production from protein and fat stores.[41]
- Sweeteners and sugar alcohols:
  - FDA-recommended nonnutritive sweeteners are acesulfame potassium, aspartame, neotame, saccharin, and sucralose.
  - All have been shown to be safe for people with diabetes and women during pregnancy.
  - FDA-approved sugar alcohols are erythritol, isomalt, lactitol, maltitol, mannitol, sorbitol, xylitol, tagatose, and hydrogenated starch hydrolysates.
  - The use of sugar alcohols may cause diarrhea, especially in children.
- Adults with diabetes should **limit alcohol intake to <1 drink/day for women and <2 drinks/day for men.**
- Vitamins and supplements:
  - Routine supplementation with antioxidants (such as vitamins E and C and carotene) is not advised.

○ Data on routine chromium supplementation are not conclusive and are not currently recommended.
○ Many patients will require added soluble vitamins (B complex), vitamin D, and calcium. Replacement should be individualized.[44]

Activity
- Regular exercise can improve blood glucose, reduce cardiovascular risk, and assist with weight loss.
- Structured exercise regimens in patients with T2DM have been shown to decrease A1C levels independent of changes in BMI.[45]
- **Adults with diabetes should exercise for ≥150 minutes/week.**
- Prior to recommending a program of physical activity, physicians should assess risk factors for coronary artery disease (CAD). Dynamic screening of asymptomatic diabetic patients is not recommended, so providers should use their clinical judgment for each individual case.
- Carbohydrate intake and medication adjustments will need to be addressed to avoid hypoglycemia, especially in individuals taking insulin and/or insulin secretagogues.
- Vigorous aerobic or resistance exercise may be contraindicated in patients with severe nonproliferative or active proliferative retinopathy due to the risk of triggering vitreous hemorrhage or retinal detachment.[46]
- Non–weight-bearing activities such as swimming, bicycling, or arm exercises are typically better tolerated by patients with severe peripheral neuropathy.

SPECIAL CONSIDERATIONS

- Influenza and pneumonia are associated with higher mortality and morbidity in people with diabetes.
- Diabetic patients are at increased risk of the bacteremic form of pneumococcal infection and nosocomial bacteremia.[47]
- The Centers for Disease Control and Prevention's Advisory Committee on Immunization Practices recommends **influenza and pneumococcal vaccines for all individuals with diabetes.**[1]
  ○ Influenza vaccine should be administered yearly.
  ○ Pneumococcal polysaccharide vaccine should be administered to all diabetic patients >2 years of age. A one-time revaccination is recommended for individuals >65 years old previously immunized when they were <65 if the vaccine was administered >5 years ago. Other indications for repeat vaccination include nephrotic syndrome, chronic kidney disease, and immunocompromised states.
  ○ Hepatitis B vaccination is now recommended for persons with diabetes ages 19 to 59 and should be considered for adults ≥60.

COMPLICATIONS

Cardiovascular Disease
- CVD remains the biggest cause of morbidity and mortality in patients with diabetes.
- Diabetes is an independent risk factor for CVD, and patients with T2DM typically have concomitant risk factors such as HTN and hyperlipidemia.
- **In diabetic patients, aspirin is recommended for primary and secondary prevention of cardiovascular events.**[48]
- In previous clinical trials, variable doses have been used, from 75 to 325 mg/day.
- The United States Preventive Services Task Force (USPSTF) recommends aspirin use when 10-year CVD risk is ≥6% (Framingham score). It should be considered in men

>40 years of age, postmenopausal women, and younger patients with CVD risk factors, such as diabetes.[48]
- The use of clopidogrel in diabetic patients, who are aspirin intolerant or as adjunctive therapy with aspirin, demonstrated a decrease in secondary CVD events.[49]

Hypertension
- HTN in diabetic patients is a risk factor for both CVD and microvascular complications.
- The diagnostic cutoff for HTN is lower in diabetic patients because of the synergistic effect of high blood pressure and hyperglycemia on CVD. **HTN in a diabetic patient is defined as a blood pressure of >130/80 mm Hg.**
- Clinical trials have shown that there is a reduction in the incidence of CV events, stroke, and development of nephropathy when lower blood pressure targets are achieved.[50,51]
- There are no well-controlled trials of nonpharmacologic therapies for the treatment of HTN in patients with diabetes, but given their benefit in nondiabetic patients, the following can be recommended in conjunction with medical therapy:
  ○ Reduce sodium intake.
  ○ Reduce excess body weight.
  ○ Increase consumption of fruits, vegetables, and low-fat dairy products.
  ○ Avoid excessive alcohol consumption.
  ○ Increase activity levels.
- Pharmacologic therapies for lowering blood pressure should include medications that are effective in both controlling HTN and reducing cardiovascular events.
- **Inhibitors of the renin-angiotensin system are especially useful for the treatment of diabetic patients with HTN and should be considered first-line agents.**[51]
  ○ Angiotensin-converting enzyme (ACE) inhibitors and angiotensin receptor blockers (ARBs) have been shown to reduce CVD outcomes.
  ○ For patients with T2DM and significant nephropathy, ARBs were superior to calcium channel blockers in reducing heart failure.
- Most patients with HTN and diabetes will require multidrug therapy to reach treatment goals.
- During pregnancy, patients with diabetes should have a target blood pressure goal of systolic blood pressure 110 to 129 mm Hg and diastolic blood pressure 65 to 79 mm Hg.[52]
  ○ Treatment with ACE inhibitors and/or ARBs is contraindicated.
  ○ Antihypertensive drugs known to be safe in pregnancy include methyldopa, labetalol, diltiazem, clonidine, and prazosin.

Dyslipidemia
- Many clinical trials have shown benefits of pharmacologic lipid-lowering therapy in patients with T2DM, both for primary and secondary prevention.[53]
- While many patients with T2DM have metabolic syndrome characteristics of low HDL and high triglycerides, the initial treatment target remains LDL.
- Lifestyle intervention, including medical nutrition therapy, increased physical activity, weight loss, and smoking cessation, may allow some patients to reach lipid goals.
- Nutrition counseling should focus on reducing dietary saturated fat, cholesterol, and transunsaturated fat. Improved glycemic control can improve dyslipidemia in patients with very high triglycerides.
- **For most patients with diabetes, the primary goal of therapy is to lower LDL cholesterol level to a target goal of <100 mg/dL** (2.60 mmol/L).[54] Multiple studies have shown that statins are the drugs of choice for LDL cholesterol lowering.[54]
- **In high-risk patients with a history of acute coronary syndrome or cardiovascular events, therapy with high doses of statins to achieve LDL cholesterol level of <70 mg/dL may further reduce their risk of subsequent events.**[54] However, the newest guidelines from the American College of Cardiology and the American Heart Association

focus less on specific numeric goals and more so on the intensity of treatment. Diabetics should receive moderate- to high-intensity statin therapy (see Chapter 11).[55]

- If the HDL cholesterol level is <40 mg/dL, niacin can be used to raise the HDL cholesterol level, but there was no benefit on CV outcomes.
- The ADA and American College of Cardiology discussed the use of apolipoprotein B (apo B) in patients with diabetes in a 2008 consensus panel.[56]
  ○ For patients who are high risk for CAD and diabetes, in whom the LDL cholesterol goal would be <70 mg/dL, apo B should be measured. A target level is <80 mg/dL.
  ○ For patients on statins with an LDL goal of <100 mg/dL, the target for apo B should be <90 mg/dL.

Smoking Cessation
- Studies of patients with diabetes have shown a much higher risk of CVD and premature death in smokers.
- Smoking results in earlier development of microvascular complications.
- Physicians should routinely assess tobacco use and encourage cessation (Chapter 45).

Screening for Cardiovascular Disease
- Silent ischemia and sudden death are more common in patients with diabetes and have prompted attempts to identify those at risk for CV events. Using a risk factor–based approach may fail to identify patients with silent ischemia.[57]
- **Screening for asymptomatic CAD in patients with T2DM does not affect cardiac event rates or outcomes and is not recommended.**[58] Intensive medical therapy is equivalent to revascularization in diabetic patients.[59]
- Currently, the recommendation is to assess cardiovascular risk factors annually in all diabetic patients and to treat accordingly. The pertinent risk factors are as follows: dyslipidemia, HTN, smoking, family history of premature coronary disease, and presence of micro- or macroalbuminuria.

Nephropathy
- Diabetic nephropathy is the leading cause of end-stage renal disease (ESRD).
- Microalbuminuria, defined as albuminuria in the range of 30 to 299 mg/24 hours, is the earliest stage of diabetic nephropathy in both T1DM and T2DM.
  ○ Microalbuminuria may be CVD risk factor in addition to a renal risk factor.
  ○ Patients with proteinuria (>300 mg of albumin/day) have a more rapid decline of kidney function than those with microalbuminuria or no albumin in their urine.
  ○ Progressive kidney disease due to diabetes can occur in the absence of proteinuria.
- Intensive glycemic control can delay the onset of microalbuminuria as well as the progression from microalbuminuria to macroalbuminuria.[60]
- Treatment of blood pressure with an ACE inhibitor or ARB can reduce the progression of nephropathy.[61,62]
- Patients with progressive nephropathy despite optimal glycemic and blood pressure control and therapy with ACE inhibitor and/or ARBs should be referred for further evaluation by a nephrologist and should consider dietary protein restriction.
- **The preferred method for screening for microalbuminuria is a random spot collection of urine with a calculation of the albumin:creatinine ratio.**
  ○ Two out of three measurements within 3 to 6 months should be elevated prior to diagnosis of albuminuria.
  ○ Exercise, infection, fever, heart failure, hyperglycemia, and HTN may precipitate urinary albumin excretion over baseline values.
- **Serum creatinine should be measured at least yearly in patients with diabetes,** regardless of the degree of urine albumin excretion. Creatinine should be used to estimate glomerular filtrations rate and to determine the stage of chronic kidney disease.

Diabetic Retinopathy

- The prevalence of diabetic retinopathy correlates with the duration of diabetes and the level of glycemic control.[63]
- Diabetic retinopathy is the most common cause of blindness in middle-aged adults. Other eye disorders, such as glaucoma and cataracts, also occur at an earlier age and more frequently in diabetic patients.
- Intensive glycemic control has been shown to prevent or delay the progression of diabetic retinopathy.[64]
- Diabetic retinopathy is completely asymptomatic; therefore, regular dilated eye examinations are recommended to identify progressive disease that will benefit from intervention before vision is lost.[63]
- Retinopathy is estimated to take at least 5 years to develop after the onset of hyperglycemia.[63]
  - Patients with T1DM should have an initial comprehensive, dilated eye examination within 5 years after the onset of diabetes.
  - Patients with T2DM should have an initial comprehensive, dilated eye examination soon after diagnosis.
- Subsequent examinations for both T1DM and T2DM patients are repeated annually if there is no documented retinopathy. Examinations should occur more frequently if retinopathy is progressing or to determine effectiveness of treatment.

Neuropathy

Neurologic manifestations of diabetes include symmetric polyneuropathy, mononeuropathy, autonomic neuropathy, and motor neuropathy. The most prevalent are chronic sensorimotor diabetic polyneuropathy (DPN) and autonomic neuropathy.[65]

Peripheral Neuropathy

- Diabetic patients should be screened annually for DPN by measuring ankle reflexes, pinprick sensation, vibration perception (using a 128-Hz tuning fork), and checking for protective sensation with a 10-g monofilament test at the distal plantar aspect of both great toes and metatarsal joints.
- **Loss of monofilament perception and reduced vibration perception can predict the development of foot ulcers.**[65]
- The primary treatment of diabetic neuropathy is optimal glycemic control.
- Patients with painful DPN may benefit from pharmacologic treatment of their symptoms with tricyclic drugs or anticonvulsants.

Autonomic Neuropathy

- A careful history and physical examination are the most helpful tools in the diagnosis of autonomic neuropathy.
- Common clinical manifestations of autonomic neuropathy are presented in Table 20-3.

TABLE 20-3 Clinical Manifestations of Diabetic Autonomic Neuropathy

---

Resting tachycardia (>100)
Exercise intolerance
Orthostatic hypotension (a fall in systolic blood pressure > 20 mm Hg upon standing)
Constipation and/or gastroparesis
Erectile dysfunction
Hypoglycemic autonomic failure

TABLE 20-4	Risk Factors for Ulcers and Amputations

Previous amputation
Past foot ulcer history
Peripheral neuropathy
Foot deformity
Peripheral vascular disease
Vision impairment
Diabetic nephropathy (especially patients on dialysis)
Poor glycemic control
Cigarette smoking

- Gastroparesis should be suspected in individuals with erratic glucose control or with upper gastrointestinal symptoms without other identified cause. The treatment of gastroparesis symptoms may improve with dietary changes and prokinetic agents.
- Treatments for erectile dysfunction often involves phosphodiesterase type 5 inhibitors. More invasive therapies, such as intracorporeal or intraurethral prostaglandins, vacuum devices, or penile prostheses, are often required and should be comanaged with a professional specializing in erectile dysfunction.

Foot Care
- Major causes of morbidity and mortality in diabetic patients with neuropathy include foot ulceration and amputation.
- Risk factors for ulcers or amputations are shown in Table 20-4.
- **All diabetic patients should have a comprehensive foot examination yearly.**
- Physicians should document any history of previous foot ulceration or amputation, neuropathic or peripheral vascular symptoms, impaired vision, tobacco use, and foot care practices.
- Assessment should include the following: general inspection of skin integrity and musculoskeletal deformities, documentation of pedal pulses and history of claudication, and neurologic examination to identify loss of protective sensation using a 10-g monofilament.
- **A diagnostic ankle-brachial index (ABI) should be performed in any patient with symptoms of peripheral arterial disease.**[66] Screening ABI may be performed in patients >50 years of age. Screening ABI should be considered in patients <50 years of age who have other peripheral arterial disease risk factors (e.g., smoking, HTN, hyperlipidemia, or duration of diabetes >10 years).
- **Patients should be counseled on the importance of foot care, appropriate footwear, and the risk associated with impaired sensation.** Patients with loss of protective sensation should be instructed to visually inspect their feet daily.
- Nail care and debridement of calluses should be performed by a foot care specialist or health professional.
- Foot ulcers and wound care may require care by a podiatrist, orthopedic or vascular surgeon, or rehabilitation specialist experienced in the management of individuals with diabetes.

REFERENCES

1. American Diabetes Association. Diagnosis and classification of diabetes mellitus. *Diabetes Care* 2013;36:S67–S71.
2. Atkinson MA, Eisenbarth GS, Michaels AW. Type 1 diabetes. *Lancet* 2014;383:69–82.
3. Dittmar M, Kahaly GJ. Polyglandular autoimmune syndromes: immunogenetics and long-term follow-up. *J Clin Endocrinol Metab* 2003;88:2983–2992.

4. Butler AE, Janson J, Bonner-Weir S, et al. Beta-cell deficit and increased beta-cell apoptosis in humans with type 2 diabetes. *Diabetes* 2003;52:102–110.

5. Irgens HU, Molnes J, Johansson BB, et al. Prevalence of monogenic diabetes in the population-based Norwegian childhood diabetes registry. *Diabetologia* 2013;56:1512–1519.

6. Fajans SS, Bell GI, Bowden DW, et al. Maturity onset diabetes of the young (MODY). *Diabet Med* 1996;13:S90–S95.

7. Murphy R, Ellard S, Hattersley AT. Clinical implications of a molecular genetic classification of monogenic β-cell diabetes. *Nat Clin Pract Endocrinol Metab* 2008; 4:200–213.

8. Bouchard P, Sai P, Reach G, et al. Diabetes mellitus following pentamidine-induced hypoglycemia in humans. *Diabetes* 1982;31:40–45.

9. Fabris P, Betterle C, Floreani A, et al. Development of type 1 diabetes mellitus during interferon alfa therapy for chronic HCV hepatitis. *Lancet* 1992;340:548.

10. Metzger BE, Gabbe SG, Persson B, et al.; International Association of Diabetes and Pregnancy Study Groups Consensus Panel. International association of diabetes and pregnancy study groups recommendations on the diagnosis and classification of hyperglycemia in pregnancy. *Diabetes Care* 2010;33:676–682.

11. Knowler WC, Barrett-Connor E, Fowler SE, et al. Reduction in the incidence of type 2 diabetes with lifestyle intervention or metformin. *N Engl J Med* 2002;346:393–403.

12. American Diabetes Association. Diagnosis and classification of diabetes mellitus. *Diabetes Care* 2013;36:S11–S66.

13. Inzucchi Se, Bergenstal RM, Buse JB, et al. Management of hyperglycemia in type 2 diabetes: a patient-centered approach. Position statement of the American Diabetes Association (ADA) and the European Association for the Study of Diabetes (EASD). *Diabetologia* 2012;55:1577–1596.

14. Miller CD, Barnes CS, Phillips LS, et al. Rapid A1c availability improves clinical decision-making in an urban primary care clinic. *Diabetes Care* 2003;26:1158–1163.

15. Cryer PE, Davis SN, Shamoon H. Hypoglycemia in diabetes. *Diabetes Care* 2003; 26:1902–1912.

16. Young-Hyman D. Psychosocial factors affecting adherence, quality of life, and well-being: helping patients cope. In: Bode B, ed. *Medical Management of Type 1 Diabetes*, 4th ed. Alexandria, VA: American Diabetes Association; 2004:162–182.

17. Garber AJ, Abrahamson MJ, Barzilay JI, et al. American Association of Clinical Endocrinologists' comprehensive diabetes management algorithm 2013 consensus statement—executive summary. *Endocr Pract* 2013;19:536–557.

18. DeFronzo R, Goodman A. The Multicenter Metformin Study Group: efficacy of metformin in patients with non-insulin-dependent diabetes mellitus. *N Engl J Med* 1995;333:541–549.

19. Shaw JS, Wilmot RL, Kilpatrick ES. Establishing pragmatic estimated GFR thresholds to guide metformin prescribing. *Diabet Med* 2007;24:1160–1163.

20. Kahn SE, Haffner SM, Heise MA, et al. Glycemic durability of rosiglitazone, metformin, or glyburide monotherapy. *N Engl J Med* 2006;355:2427–2443.

21. Rosenstock J, Hassman DR, Madder RD, et al. Repaglinide versus nateglinide monotherapy: a randomized, multicenter study. *Diabetes Care* 2004;27:1265–1270.

22. Rosak C, Mertes G. Critical evaluation of the role of acarbose in the treatment of diabetes: patient considerations. *Diabetes Metab Syndr Obes* 2012;5:357–367.

23. Hanefeld M, Catagay M, Petrowitsch T, et al. Acarbose reduces the risk for myocardial infarction in type 2 diabetic patients: meta-analysis of seven long-term studies. *Eur Heart J* 2004;25:10–16.

24. Singh S, Loke YK, Furberg CD. Thiazolidinediones and heart failure: a teleoanalysis. *Diabetes Care* 2007;30:2248–2254.

25. Nissen SE, Wolski K. Effect of rosiglitazone on the risk of myocardial infarction and death from cardiovascular causes. *N Engl J Med* 2007;356:2457–2471.

26. Dormandy JA, Charbonnel B, Eckland DJA, et al. Secondary prevention of macrovascular events in patients with type 2 diabetes in the PROactive Study (PROspective pioglitAzone Clinical Trial in macroVascular Events): a randomized controlled trial. *Lancet* 2005;366:1279–1289.

27. Meier C, Kraenzlin ME, Bodmer M, et al. Use of thiazolidinediones and fracture risk. *Arch Intern Med* 2008;168:820–825.

28. Colmers IN, Bowker SL, Majumdar SR, et al. Use of thiazolidinediones and the risk of bladder cancer among people with type 2 diabetes: a meta-analysis. *CMAJ* 2012; 184:E675–E683.

29. Deacon CF. Dipeptidyl peptidase-4 inhibitors in the treatment of type 2 diabetes: a comparative review. *Diabetes Obes Metab* 2011;13:7–18.

30. Dalle S, Remy B, Gourdy P. Specific actions of GLP1 receptor agonists and DPP4 inhibitors for the treatment of pancreatic β-cell impairments in type 2 diabetes. *Cell Signal* 2013;25:570–579.

31. Chen LH, Leung PS. Inhibition of the sodium glucose co-transporter-2: its beneficial action and potential combination therapy for type 2 diabetes. *Diabetes Obes Metab* 2013;15:392–402.

32. Nisley SA, Kolanczyk DM, Walton AM. Canagliflozin, a new sodium-glucose cotransporter 2 inhibitor, in the treatment of diabetes. *Am J Health Syst Pharm* 2013;70:311–319.

33. Riddle M, Frias J, Zhang B, et al. Pramlintide improved glycemic control and reduced weight in patients with type 2 diabetes using basal insulin. *Diabetes Care* 2007;30:2794–2799.

34. Derosa G, Maffioli P. GLP-1 agonists exenatide and liraglutide; a review of their safety and efficacy. *Curr Clin Pharmacol* 2012;7:214–228.

35. Kendall DM, Riddle MC, Rosenstock J, et al. Effects of exenatide (exendin-4) on glycemic control and weight over 30 weeks in patients with type 2 diabetes treated with metformin and a sulfonylurea. *Diabetes Care* 2005;28:1083–1091.

36. Ratner RE, Hirsch IB, Neifing JL, et al. Less hypoglycemia with insulin glargine in intensive insulin therapy for type 1 diabetes. U.S. Study Group of Insulin Glargine in Type 1 Diabetes. *Diabetes Care* 2000;23:639–643.

37. Hirsch IB. Insulin analogues. *N Engl J Med* 2005;352:174–183.

38. Riddle MC, Rosenstock J, Gerich J. The treat-to-target trial: randomized addition of glargine or human NPH insulin to oral therapy of type 2 diabetic patients. *Diabetes Care* 2003;26:3080–3086.

39. Action to Control Cardiovascular Risk in Diabetes Study Group; Gerstein HC, Miller ME, Byington RP, et al. Effects of intensive glucose lowering in type 2 diabetes. *N Engl J Med* 2008;358:2545–2559.

40. Buchwald H, Estok R, Fahrbach K, et al. Weight and type 2 diabetes after bariatric surgery: systematic review and meta-analysis. *Am J Med* 2009;122:248–256.

41. Franz MJ, Bantle JP, Beebe CA, et al. Evidence-based nutrition principles and recommendations for the treatment and prevention of diabetes and related complications. *Diabetes Care* 2002;25:148–198.

42. Klein S, Sheard NF, Pi-Sunyer X, et al. Weight management through lifestyle modification for the prevention and management of type 2 diabetes: rationale and strategies: a statement of the American Diabetes Association, the North American Association for the Study of Obesity, and the American Society for Clinical Nutrition. *Diabetes Care* 2004;27:2067–2073.

43. Stern L, Iqbal N, Seshadri P, et al. The effects of low-carbohydrate versus conventional weight loss diets in severely obese adults: one-year follow-up of a randomized trial. *Ann Intern Med* 2004;140:778–785.

44. Rabbini N, Thornalley PJ. Emerging role of thiamine therapy for prevention and treatment of early-stage diabetic nephropathy. *Diabetes Obes Metab* 2011;13:577–583.

45. Boulé NG, Kenny GP, Haddad E, et al. Meta-analysis of the effect of structured exercise training on cardiorespiratory fitness in Type 2 diabetes mellitus. *Diabetologia* 2003; 46:1071–1081.

46. Aiello LP, Wong J, Cavallerano J, et al. Retinopathy. In: Ruderman N, Devlin JT, Kriska A, eds. *Handbook of Exercise in Diabetes*, 2nd ed. Alexandria, VA: American Diabetes Association; 2002:401–413.

47. Smith SA, Poland GA. Use of influenza and pneumococcal vaccines in people with diabetes. *Diabetes Care* 2000;23:95–108.

48. US Preventive Services Task Force. Aspirin for the primary prevention of cardiovascular events: recommendation and rationale. *Ann Intern Med* 2002;136:157–160.

49. Bhatt DL, Marso SP, Hirsch AT, et al. Amplified benefit of clopidogrel versus aspirin in patients with diabetes mellitus. *Am J Cardiol* 2002;90:625–628.

50. Tight blood pressure control and risk of macrovascular and microvascular complications in type 2 diabetes: UKPDS 38: UK Prospective Diabetes Study Group. *BMJ* 1998;317:703–713.

51. Bangalore S, Kumar S, Lobach I, et al. Blood pressure targets in subjects with type 2 diabetes mellitus/impaired fasting glucose: observations from traditional and Bayesian random-effects meta-analyses of randomized trials. *Circulation* 2011;123: 2799–2810.

52. Sibai BM. Treatment of hypertension in pregnant women. *N Engl J Med* 1996; 335:257–265.

53. Heart Protection Study Collaborative Group. MRC/BHF Heart Protection Study of cholesterol-lowering with simvastatin in 5963 people with diabetes: a randomised placebo-controlled trial. *Lancet* 2003;361:2005–2016.

54. Nissen SE, Tuzcu EM, Schoenhagen P, et al. Effect of intensive compared with moderate lipid-lowering therapy on progression of coronary atherosclerosis: a randomized controlled trial. *JAMA* 2004;291:1071–1080.

55. Stone NJ, Robinson J, Lichtenstein AH, et al. 2013 ACC/AHA guideline on the treatment of blood cholesterol to reduce atherosclerotic cardiovascular risk in adults: a report of the American College of Cardiology/American Heart Association Task Force on Practice Guidelines. *Circulation* 2014;63(25 Pt B):2889–2934.

56. Brunzell JD, Davidson M, Furberg CD, et al. Consensus statement from the American Diabetes Association and the American College of Cardiology Foundation. *Diabetes Care* 2008;31:811–822.

57. Scognamiglio R, Negut C, Ramondo A, et al. Detection of coronary artery disease in asymptomatic patients with type 2 diabetes mellitus. *J Am Coll Cardiol* 2006;47: 65–71.

58. Young LH, Wackers FJ, Chyun DA, et al. Cardiac outcomes after screening for asymptomatic coronary artery disease in patients with type 2 diabetes: the DIAD study: a randomized controlled trial. *JAMA* 2009;301:1547–1555.

59. Boden WE, O'Rourke RA, Teo KK, et al. Optimal medical therapy with or without PCI for stable coronary disease. *N Engl J Med* 2007;356:1503–1516.

60. Effect of intensive therapy on the development and progression of diabetic nephropathy in the Diabetes Control and Complications Trial: the Diabetes Control and Complications (DCCT) Research Group. *Kidney Int* 1995;47:1703–1720.

61. Lewis EJ, Hunsicker LG, Bain RP, et al. The effect of angiotensin-converting-enzyme inhibition on diabetic nephropathy. The Collaborative Study Group. *N Engl J Med* 1993;329:1456–1462.

62. Brenner BM, Cooper ME, de Zeeuw D, et al. Effects of losartan on renal and cardiovascular outcomes in patients with type 2 diabetes and nephropathy. *N Engl J Med* 2001;345:861–869.

63. Antonetti DA, Klein R, Gardner TW. Diabetic retinopathy. *N Engl J Med* 2012; 366:1227–1239.

64. The Diabetes Control and Complications Trial Research Group. The effect of intensive treatment of diabetes on the development and progression of long-term complications in insulin–dependent diabetes mellitus. *N Engl J Med* 1993;329:977–986.

65. Boulton AJ, Vinik AI, Arezzo JC, et al. Diabetic neuropathies: a statement by the American Diabetes Association. *Diabetes Care* 2005;28:956–962.

66. American Diabetes Association. Peripheral arterial disease in people with diabetes (Consensus Statement). *Diabetes Care* 2003;26:3333–3341.

21

Endocrine Diseases
William E. Clutter

EVALUATION OF THYROID FUNCTION

Thyroid-Stimulating Hormone

- **Plasma thyroid-stimulating hormone (TSH) assay is the initial test of choice in most patients with suspected thyroid disease.**
- TSH levels are elevated in even mild primary hypothyroidism and can be suppressed to <0.1 µU/mL in subclinical hyperthyroidism (i.e., thyroid hormone excess too mild to cause symptoms). **A normal TSH level excludes hyperthyroidism and primary hypothyroidism.**
- TSH levels usually are within the reference range in secondary hypothyroidism and are not useful for detection of this rare form of hypothyroidism.
- Abnormal TSH levels are not specific for clinically important thyroid disease, which should usually be **confirmed by plasma thyroid hormone measurement.**
- TSH is mildly elevated (up to 20 µU/mL) in some euthyroid patients with nonthyroidal illnesses and in subclinical hypothyroidism.
- TSH levels may be suppressed to <0.1 µU/mL in nonthyroidal illness, in subclinical hyperthyroidism, and during treatment with dopamine or high doses of glucocorticoids.
- TSH levels remain <0.1 µU/mL for some time after hyperthyroidism is corrected.

Free Thyroxine

- Measurement of free T_4 confirms the diagnosis of clinical hypothyroidism in patients with elevated plasma TSH and confirms the diagnosis and assesses the severity of hyperthyroidism when plasma TSH is <0.1 µU/mL.
- It is also used to diagnose secondary hypothyroidism and adjust thyroxine therapy in patients with pituitary disease.
- **Measurement of total plasma T_4 alone is not adequate,** because thyroxine-binding globulin (TBG) levels are altered in many circumstances.

Effect of Nonthyroidal Illness

- Many illnesses alter thyroid tests without causing true thyroid dysfunction. These changes must be recognized to avoid mistaken diagnosis and therapy.
- **The low T_3 syndrome occurs in many illnesses,** during starvation, and after trauma or surgery. Conversion of T_4 to T_3 is decreased, and plasma T_3 levels are low. It may be an adaptive response to illness, and thyroid hormone therapy is not beneficial.
- The low T_4 syndrome occurs in severe illness. It may be due to decreased TBG levels, inhibition of T_4 binding to TBG, or suppressed TSH secretion.
- TSH levels decrease early in severe illness, sometimes to <0.1 µU/mL. During recovery, they rise, sometimes to levels higher than the normal range (but rarely higher than 20 µU/mL).

Effects of Drugs

- Iodine-containing drugs (e.g., amiodarone, radiographic contrast media) may cause hyperthyroidism or hypothyroidism in susceptible patients.
- Many drugs alter thyroid function tests, especially plasma T_4, without causing true thyroid dysfunction (Table 21-1).
- In general, plasma TSH levels are a reliable guide to determining whether true hyperthyroidism or hypothyroidism is present.

TABLE 21-1	Effects of Drugs on Thyroid Function Tests
Effect	**Drug**
Decreased free and total T$_4$	
True hypothyroidism (TSH elevated)	Iodine (amiodarone, radiographic contrast)
	Lithium
Inhibition of TSH secretion	Glucocorticoids
	Dopamine
Multiple mechanisms (TSH normal)	Phenytoin
Decreased total T$_4$ only	
Decreased TBG (TSH normal)	Androgens
Inhibition of T$_4$ binding to TBG (TSH normal)	Furosemide (high doses)
Increased free and total T$_4$	
True hyperthyroidism (TSH <0.1 μU/mL)	Iodine (amiodarone, radiographic contrast)
Inhibited T$_4$–T$_3$ conversion (TSH normal)	Amiodarone
Increased free T$_4$ only	
Displacement of T$_4$ from TBG in vitro (TSH normal)	Heparin, low molecular weight heparin
Increased total T$_4$ only	
Increased TBG (TSH normal)	Estrogens, tamoxifen, raloxifene

T$_3$, triiodothyronine; T$_4$, thyroxine; TBG, thyroxine-binding globulin; TSH, thyroid-stimulating hormone.

Hypothyroidism

GENERAL PRINCIPLES

- Primary hypothyroidism (due to disease of the thyroid itself) accounts for >90% of cases.[1]
- Hypothyroidism is readily treatable and should be suspected in any patient with compatible symptoms, especially in the presence of a goiter or a history of radioactive iodine (RAI) therapy or thyroid surgery.
- **Chronic lymphocytic thyroiditis (Hashimoto disease) is the most common cause** and may be associated with Addison disease and other endocrine deficits. Its prevalence is greatest in women and increases with age.
- **Iatrogenic hypothyroidism** due to thyroidectomy and RAI therapy is also a common cause.
- Transient hypothyroidism occurs in **postpartum thyroiditis and subacute thyroiditis,** usually after a period of hyperthyroidism.
- **Drugs** that may cause hypothyroidism include iodine and iodine-containing drugs like amiodarone, lithium, α- and β-interferon, interleukin-2, thalidomide, sunitinib, and bexarotene.
- **Secondary hypothyroidism** due to TSH deficiency is uncommon but may occur in any disorder of the pituitary or hypothalamus. It rarely occurs without other evidence of pituitary disease.

DIAGNOSIS

Clinical Presentation

- Most symptoms of hypothyroidism are nonspecific and develop gradually. They include cold intolerance, fatigue, somnolence, poor memory, constipation, menorrhagia, myalgias, and hoarseness.
- Mild weight gain may occur, but **hypothyroidism does not cause obesity**.
- Signs include slow deep tendon reflex relaxation, bradycardia, facial and periorbital edema, dry skin, and nonpitting edema (myxedema).
- Rare manifestations include hypoventilation, pericardial or pleural effusions, deafness, and carpal tunnel syndrome.

Diagnostic Testing

- Laboratory findings may include hyponatremia and elevated plasma levels of cholesterol, triglycerides, and creatine kinase.
- The ECG may show low-voltage and T-wave abnormalities.
- **Thyroid imaging with ultrasound or radionuclide scan is not useful** in diagnosis of hypothyroidism.
- **In suspected primary hypothyroidism, TSH is the best initial diagnostic test.** A normal value excludes primary hypothyroidism, and a markedly elevated value (>20 µU/mL) confirms the diagnosis. If plasma TSH is elevated moderately (5 to 20 µU/mL), plasma free T_4 should be measured. A low free T_4 confirms clinical hypothyroidism.
- **A clearly normal free T_4 with an elevated plasma TSH indicates subclinical hypothyroidism,** in which thyroid function is impaired but increased secretion of TSH maintains plasma T_4 levels within the reference range. These patients may have nonspecific symptoms that are compatible with hypothyroidism as well as a mild increase in serum cholesterol and low-density lipoprotein cholesterol levels. **They develop clinical hypothyroidism at a rate of 2.5% per year.**
- **If secondary hypothyroidism is suspected because of evidence of pituitary disease, plasma free T_4 should be measured.** Plasma TSH levels are usually within the reference range in secondary hypothyroidism and cannot be used alone to make this diagnosis. **Patients with secondary hypothyroidism should be evaluated for other pituitary hormone deficits and for a mass lesion of the pituitary or hypothalamus.**
- In severe nonthyroidal illness, the diagnosis of hypothyroidism may be difficult. Plasma free T_4 measured by routine assays may be low. Plasma TSH is still the best initial diagnostic test. Marked elevation of plasma TSH (>20 µU/mL) establishes the diagnosis of primary hypothyroidism. A normal TSH value is strong evidence that the patient is euthyroid, except when there is evidence of pituitary or hypothalamic disease, in which case free T_4 should be measured. Moderate elevations of plasma TSH (<20 µU/mL) may occur in euthyroid patients with nonthyroidal illness and are not specific for hypothyroidism.

TREATMENT

Thyroid Hormone Replacement

- Levothyroxine (T_4) is the drug of choice.[1] The average replacement dose is 1.6 µg/kg PO qd, and most patients require doses between 75 and 150 µg qd. Young and middle-aged patients should be started on 100 µg daily. In otherwise healthy elderly patients, the initial dose should be 50 µg daily. Patients with heart disease should be started on 25 µg daily and monitored carefully for exacerbation of cardiac symptoms.
- The need for lifelong treatment should be emphasized.

- Thyroxine should be taken 30 minutes before a meal, since dietary fiber interferes with its absorption, and should not be taken with medications such as calcium or iron supplements that affect its absorption.

Follow-Up and Dose Adjustment

- In primary hypothyroidism, the goal of therapy is to **maintain plasma TSH within the normal range.** After 6 to 8 weeks, plasma TSH should be measured. The dose of T_4 then should be adjusted in 12- to 25-µg increments at intervals of 6 to 8 weeks until plasma TSH is normal. Thereafter, annual TSH measurement is adequate to monitor therapy.
- **Overtreatment,** indicated by a plasma TSH below the normal range, should be avoided, as it **increases the risk of osteoporosis and atrial fibrillation.**
- In secondary hypothyroidism, plasma TSH cannot be used to adjust therapy. The goal of therapy is to maintain plasma free T_4 near the middle of the reference range. The dose of T_4 should be adjusted at 6- to 8-week intervals until this goal is achieved. Thereafter, annual measurement of plasma free T_4 is adequate to monitor therapy.
- Coronary artery disease may be exacerbated by treatment of hypothyroidism. The dose should be increased slowly, with careful attention to worsening angina, heart failure, or arrhythmias.

Difficult-to-Control Hypothyroidism

- Difficulty in controlling hypothyroidism is most often due to poor compliance with therapy. Observed therapy may be necessary in some cases.
- Other causes of increasing T_4 requirements include the following:
  ○ Malabsorption due to intestinal disease
  ○ Drugs that interfere with T_4 absorption (e.g., calcium carbonate, ferrous sulfate, colesevelam, cholestyramine, sucralfate, aluminum hydroxide)
  ○ Other drug interactions that increase T_4 clearance (e.g., rifampin, carbamazepine, phenytoin, estrogen) or block conversion of T_4 to T_3 (amiodarone)
  ○ Pregnancy, in which T_4 requirement increases in the first trimester
  ○ Gradual failure of remaining endogenous thyroid function after treatment of hyperthyroidism

Subclinical Hypothyroidism

Subclinical hypothyroidism should be treated with T_4 if any of the following is present: symptoms compatible with hypothyroidism, goiter, hypercholesterolemia that warrants treatment, and plasma TSH >10 µU/mL.[2] Untreated patients should be monitored annually, and T_4 should be started if symptoms develop or serum TSH increases to >10 µU/mL.

Pregnancy

- Thyroxine dose increases by an average of 50% in the first half of pregnancy.[3] In women with primary hypothyroidism, plasma TSH should be measured as soon as pregnancy is confirmed and monthly thereafter through the second trimester.
- The thyroxine dose should be increased as needed to maintain plasma TSH within the lower half of the normal range. After delivery, the prepregnancy dose should be resumed.

Urgent Therapy

- Urgent therapy is rarely necessary for hypothyroidism.
- Most patients with hypothyroidism and concomitant illness can be treated in the usual manner; however, **hypothyroidism may impair survival in critical illness** by contributing to hypoventilation, hypotension, hypothermia, bradycardia, or hyponatremia. Such patients should be admitted to the hospital for therapy of hypothyroidism and the concomitant illness.

- Confirmatory tests should be obtained before thyroid hormone therapy is started in a severely ill patient, including serum TSH and free T_4.
- T_4, 50 to 100 μg IV, can be given every 6 to 8 hours for 24 hours, followed by 75 to 100 μg IV daily until oral intake is possible.
- **Such rapid correction is warranted only in extremely ill patients.**
- Vital signs and cardiac rhythm should be monitored carefully to detect early signs of exacerbation of heart disease.
- Hydrocortisone, 50 mg IV every 8 hours, usually is recommended during rapid treatment with thyroid hormone on the grounds that replacement of thyroid hormone may precipitate adrenal failure.

Hyperthyroidism

GENERAL PRINCIPLES

- Hyperthyroidism should be suspected in any patient with compatible symptoms, as it is a readily treatable disorder that may become highly debilitating.[4]
- **Graves disease** causes most cases of hyperthyroidism, especially in young patients. This autoimmune disorder may also cause two signs that are not found in other causes of hyperthyroidism: proptosis (exophthalmos) and pretibial myxedema.
- **Toxic multinodular goiter** (MNG) is a common cause in older patients.
- Unusual causes include iodine-induced hyperthyroidism, usually precipitated by drugs (e.g., amiodarone or radiographic contrast media), thyroid adenomas (which present as a single nodule), subacute thyroiditis (painful tender goiter with transient hyperthyroidism), painless thyroiditis (nontender goiter with transient hyperthyroidism, often postpartum), and surreptitious ingestion of thyroid hormone.
- TSH-induced hyperthyroidism is extremely rare.

DIAGNOSIS

Clinical Presentation

- Symptoms include heat intolerance, weight loss, weakness, palpitations, oligomenorrhea, and anxiety.
- Signs include brisk deep tendon reflexes, fine tremor, proximal weakness, stare, and eyelid lag.
- Cardiac abnormalities may be prominent, including sinus tachycardia, atrial fibrillation, and exacerbation of coronary artery disease or heart failure. In the elderly, hyperthyroidism may present with only atrial fibrillation, heart failure, weakness, or weight loss, and a high index of suspicion is needed to make the diagnosis.
- Presence of proptosis or pretibial myxedema indicates Graves disease (although many patients with Graves disease lack these signs).
- Palpation of the thyroid can determine whether a diffuse or nodular goiter is present; most hyperthyroid patients with a diffuse nontender goiter have Graves disease.
- History of recent pregnancy, neck pain, or iodine administration suggests causes other than Graves disease.
- The differential diagnosis is presented in Table 21-2.

Diagnostic Testing

- **Plasma TSH is the best initial diagnostic test.**
  - If plasma TSH is <0.1 μU/mL, plasma free T_4 should be measured to determine the severity of hyperthyroidism and as a baseline for therapy.
  - If plasma free T_4 is elevated, the diagnosis of clinical hyperthyroidism is established.

TABLE 21-2	Differential Diagnosis of Hyperthyroidism
Signs	**Diagnosis**
Diffuse, nontender goiter	Graves disease (rarely painless thyroiditis)
Multiple thyroid nodules	Toxic multinodular goiter
Single thyroid nodule	Thyroid adenoma
Tender painful goiter	Subacute thyroiditis
Normal thyroid gland	Graves disease (rarely painless thyroiditis or factitious hyperthyroidism)
Proptosis or pretibial myxedema	Graves disease

- ○ If plasma TSH is <0.1 μU/mL but free T_4 is normal, the patient may have clinical hyperthyroidism due to elevation of plasma T_3 alone; in this case, plasma T_3 should be measured. This combination of test results may also be due to suppression of TSH by nonthyroidal illness.
- **Subclinical hyperthyroidism** may lower TSH to <0.1 μU/mL, and therefore, suppression of TSH alone does not confirm that symptoms are due to hyperthyroidism. Subclinical hyperthyroidism is present when the plasma TSH is suppressed to <0.1 μU/mL, but the patient has no symptoms that are definitely caused by hyperthyroidism and plasma levels of T_4 and T_3 are normal.[5]
- In rare cases, 24-hour **RAI uptake** (RAIU) is needed to distinguish Graves disease or toxic MNG (in which RAIU is elevated) from postpartum thyroiditis, iodine-induced hyperthyroidism, or factitious hyperthyroidism (in which RAIU is very low).

TREATMENT

- Some forms of hyperthyroidism (subacute or postpartum thyroiditis) are transient and require only symptomatic therapy.
- Three methods are available for definitive therapy: RAI, thionamides, and subtotal thyroidectomy, none of which controls hyperthyroidism rapidly.
- During treatment, patients are followed by clinical evaluation and measurement of plasma free T_4. **Plasma TSH is useless in assessing the initial response to therapy,** as it remains suppressed until after the patient becomes euthyroid.
- Regardless of the therapy used, all patients with Graves disease require lifelong follow-up for recurrent hyperthyroidism or development of hypothyroidism.

Symptomatic Therapy

- β-Adrenergic antagonists are used to relieve such symptoms as palpitations, tremor, and anxiety until hyperthyroidism is controlled by definitive therapy or until transient forms of hyperthyroidism subside. The initial dose of atenolol, 25 to 50 mg daily, is adjusted to alleviate symptoms and tachycardia. β-Adrenergic antagonist therapy should be reduced gradually, then stopped as hyperthyroidism is controlled.
- Verapamil at an initial dose of 40 to 80 mg tid can be used to control tachycardia in patients with contraindications to β-adrenergic antagonists.

Thionamides

- Methimazole and propylthiouracil (PTU) **inhibit thyroid hormone synthesis.**[4] PTU also inhibits extrathyroidal conversion of T_4 to T_3. **These drugs have no permanent effect on thyroid function**. Because of a better safety profile, methimazole should be used rather than PTU except in specific situations.

- Once thyroid hormone stores are depleted (after several weeks to months), T$_4$ levels decrease.
- In the majority of patients with Graves disease, hyperthyroidism recurs within 6 months after therapy is stopped. Spontaneous remission of Graves disease occurs in approximately one-third of patients during thionamide therapy, and, in this minority, no other treatment may be needed. Remission is more likely to occur in mild, recent-onset hyperthyroidism and with a small goiter.
- Before starting therapy, patients must be warned of side effects and precautions. Usual starting doses are methimazole, 10 to 40 mg PO daily, or PTU, 100 to 200 mg PO tid; higher initial doses can be used in severe hyperthyroidism.
- Restoration of euthyroidism takes up to several months. Patients are evaluated at 4-week intervals with assessment of clinical findings and plasma free T$_4$. If plasma free T$_4$ levels do not fall after 4 to 8 weeks, the dose should be increased. Doses as high as methimazole, 60 mg PO daily, or PTU, 300 mg PO qid, may be required. Once the plasma free T$_4$ level falls to normal, the dose is adjusted to maintain plasma free T$_4$ within the normal range.
- No consensus exists on the optimal duration of therapy, but periods of 6 months to 2 years are used most commonly. Regardless of the duration of therapy, patients must be monitored carefully for recurrence of hyperthyroidism after the drug is stopped.
- Side effects are most likely to occur within the first few months of therapy.
  ○ Minor side effects include rash, urticaria, fever, arthralgias, and transient leukopenia. **Agranulocytosis** occurs in 0.3% of patients who are treated with thionamides. Other life-threatening side effects include **hepatitis, vasculitis, and drug-induced lupus erythematosus**. Complications usually resolve if the drug is stopped promptly.
  ○ Patients must be warned to stop the drug immediately if jaundice or symptoms suggestive of agranulocytosis (e.g., fever, chills, sore throat) develop and to contact their physician promptly for evaluation.
  ○ Routine monitoring of the white blood cell count is not useful for detecting agranulocytosis, which develops suddenly.
  ○ Methimazole has been associated with congenital abnormalities and should not be used in early pregnancy or in women attempting pregnancy.

Radioactive Iodine Therapy

- A single dose permanently controls hyperthyroidism in about 90% of patients, and further doses can be given if necessary.[4] Usually, 24-hour RAIU is measured and used to calculate the dose.
- A pregnancy test is done immediately before therapy in potentially fertile women, since RAI is contraindicated in pregnancy.
- Thionamides interfere with RAI therapy and should be stopped 3 days before treatment. If iodine treatment has been given, it should be stopped at least 2 weeks before RAI therapy.
- Most patients with Graves disease are treated with 10 to 12 mCi, although treatment of toxic MNG requires higher doses.
- Several months are usually needed to restore euthyroidism. Patients are evaluated at 4- to 6-week intervals, with assessment of clinical findings and plasma free T$_4$. If thyroid function stabilizes within the normal range, the interval between follow-up visits is increased gradually to annual intervals.
- T$_4$ therapy is started if hypothyroidism develops, indicated by a low or low-normal FT$_4$. TSH may remain suppressed for several weeks after hypothyroidism develops and is not a reliable indicator in early hypothyroidism.
- If symptomatic hyperthyroidism persists after 6 months, RAI treatment is repeated.
- Side effects:
  ○ **Hypothyroidism occurs in most patients within the first year** and continues to develop at a rate of approximately 3% per year thereafter.

- ○ A slight rise in plasma T_4 may occur in the first 2 weeks after therapy, owing to release of stored hormone. This is clinically important only in patients with severe cardiac disease, which may worsen as a result. Such patients should be treated with thionamides to restore euthyroidism and to deplete stored hormone before treatment with RAI.
- ○ No convincing evidence has been found that RAI has a clinically important effect on the course of Graves eye disease.
- ○ RAI does not increase the risk of malignancy.
- ○ There is no increase in congenital abnormalities in the offspring of women who conceive after RAI therapy.

Subtotal Thyroidectomy

- This procedure provides long-term control of hyperthyroidism in most patients.[4]
- **Surgery may trigger a perioperative exacerbation of hyperthyroidism,** and patients should be prepared for surgery by one of two methods.
  - ○ A thionamide is given until the patient is nearly euthyroid. Supersaturated potassium iodide (SSKI), 40 to 80 mg (1 to 2 drops) PO bid, is then added, and surgery is scheduled 1 to 2 weeks later. Both drugs are stopped postoperatively.
  - ○ Atenolol, 50 to 100 mg daily, and SSKI, 1 to 2 drops PO bid, are started 1 to 2 weeks before surgery is scheduled. The dose of atenolol is increased, if necessary, to reduce the resting heart rate below 90 beats/minute. Atenolol, but not SSKI, is continued for 5 to 7 days after surgery.
- Patients should be evaluated 4 to 6 weeks after surgery, with assessment of clinical findings and plasma free T_4 and TSH. If thyroid function is normal, the patient is seen at 3 and 6 months and then annually. If hypothyroidism develops, T_4 therapy is started. Hyperthyroidism persists or recurs in 3% to 7% of patients.
- **Complications of thyroidectomy include hypothyroidism in 30% to 50% of patients and hypoparathyroidism in 3%.** Rare complications include permanent vocal cord paralysis due to recurrent laryngeal nerve injury and perioperative death. The complication rate appears to depend on the experience of the surgeon.

Choice of Definitive Therapy

- **In Graves disease, RAI therapy is the treatment of choice for almost all patients.** It is simple, is highly effective and causes no life-threatening complications.
- RAI cannot be used in pregnancy. **PTU should be used to treat hyperthyroidism in the first trimester of pregnancy, with consideration of then changing to methimazole.** Thionamides provide long-term control of hyperthyroidism in fewer than one-half of patients and carry a small risk of life-threatening side effects.
- Thyroidectomy should be used only in patients who refuse RAI therapy and who relapse or develop side effects with thionamide therapy.

Other Causes of Hyperthyroidism

- Toxic MNG and toxic adenoma should be treated with RAI (except in pregnancy).
- Transient forms of hyperthyroidism due to thyroiditis should be treated symptomatically with atenolol.
- Iodine-induced hyperthyroidism is treated with methimazole and atenolol.
- Although treatment of some patients with amiodarone-induced hyperthyroidism with glucocorticoids has been advocated, nearly all patients with amiodarone-induced hyperthyroidism respond well to methimazole.[6]
- **Subclinical hyperthyroidism increases the risk of atrial fibrillation in the elderly and predisposes to osteoporosis in postmenopausal women and should be treated in these groups of patients.**[5] Asymptomatic young patients can be observed for spontaneous remission or worsening hyperthyroidism that warrants therapy.

Urgent Therapy

- Urgent therapy is warranted when hyperthyroidism exacerbates heart failure or coronary artery disease and in rare patients with severe hyperthyroidism complicated by fever and delirium. Such patients should be admitted to the hospital for therapy.
- PTU, 300 mg PO every 6 hours, should be started immediately.
- Iodide (SSKI, 1 to 2 drops PO every 12 hours) should be started 2 hours after the first dose of PTU to inhibit thyroid hormone secretion rapidly.
- Propranolol, 40 mg PO every 6 hours (or an equivalent dose of a parenteral β-adrenergic antagonist), should be given to patients with angina or myocardial infarction, and the dose should be adjusted to prevent tachycardia. Propranolol may benefit some patients with heart failure and marked tachycardia but can further impair left ventricular function. In patients with clinical heart failure, it should be given only with careful monitoring of left ventricular function.
- Plasma free T_4 is measured every 4 to 6 days, and treatment with iodine is discontinued when free T_4 approaches the normal range.
- RAI therapy should be scheduled 2 weeks after iodine is stopped.

Hyperthyroidism in Pregnancy

- **RAI is contraindicated in pregnancy,** and therefore patients **should be treated with PTU,** with consideration of changing to methimazole after the first trimester.[3] The dose should be adjusted to maintain the plasma free T_4 near the upper limit of the normal range to avoid fetal hypothyroidism. The dose required often decreases in the later stages of pregnancy.
- Atenolol, 25 to 50 mg PO daily, can be used to relieve symptoms while awaiting the effects of PTU.
- The fetus and neonate should be monitored carefully for hyperthyroidism.

Euthyroid Goiter

- The diagnosis of euthyroid goiter is based on palpation of the thyroid and on evaluation of thyroid function. If the thyroid is enlarged, the examiner should determine whether the enlargement is diffuse or multinodular or whether a single nodule is present. **All three forms of euthyroid goiter are common, especially in women.**
- Imaging studies, such as thyroid scans or ultrasonography, provide no useful additional information about goiters that are diffuse or multinodular by palpation and should not be performed in these patients. Furthermore, **30% to 50% of people have nonpalpable thyroid nodules that are detectable by ultrasound. These nodules rarely have any clinical importance,** but their incidental discovery may lead to unnecessary diagnostic testing and treatment.[7]
- Almost all euthyroid **diffuse goiters** in the United States are due to chronic lymphocytic thyroiditis (Hashimoto thyroiditis). As Hashimoto disease may also cause hypothyroidism, plasma **TSH should be measured even in patients who are clinically euthyroid.** Small diffuse goiters usually are asymptomatic, and therapy is seldom required. The patient should be monitored regularly for the development of hypothyroidism.
- MNG is common in older patients, especially women. Most patients are asymptomatic and require no treatment. In a few patients, hyperthyroidism (toxic MNG) develops.
  - In rare patients, the gland compresses the trachea or esophagus, causing dyspnea or dysphagia, and treatment is required. Thyroxine treatment has little or no effect on the size of MNGs and is not indicated. RAI therapy reduces gland size and relieves symptoms in most patients.[8] Subtotal thyroidectomy can also be used to relieve compressive symptoms.
  - The risk of malignancy in MNG is low and is comparable to the frequency of incidental thyroid carcinoma in clinically normal glands. Evaluation for thyroid carcinoma with needle biopsy is warranted only if one nodule is disproportionately enlarged.

Single Thyroid Nodules

- **Single thyroid nodules are usually benign, but about 5% are thyroid carcinomas.**[9]
- Clinical findings that increase the likelihood of carcinoma include the presence of cervical lymphadenopathy, a history of radiation to the head or neck in childhood, and a family history of medullary thyroid carcinoma or multiple endocrine neoplasia syndromes type 2A or 2B. A hard fixed nodule, recent nodule growth, or hoarseness due to vocal cord paralysis also suggests malignancy. However, **most patients with thyroid carcinomas have none of these risk factors,** and nearly all palpable single thyroid nodules should be evaluated with needle aspiration biopsy. Patients with thyroid carcinoma should be managed in consultation with an endocrinologist.
- Nodules with benign cytology should be reevaluated periodically by palpation and biopsied again if they enlarge.
- T_4 therapy has little or no effect on the size of single thyroid nodules and is not indicated.
- **Imaging studies cannot distinguish benign from malignant nodules and are not necessary for the evaluation of a palpable thyroid nodule.**
- The management of nonpalpable thyroid nodules discovered incidentally by ultrasound is controversial.[7]

Adrenal Failure

GENERAL PRINCIPLES

- Adrenal failure may be due to disease of the adrenal glands (primary adrenal failure, Addison disease), with deficiency of cortisol and aldosterone and elevated plasma adrenocorticotropic hormone (ACTH) or due to ACTH deficiency caused by disorders of the pituitary or hypothalamus (secondary adrenal failure) with deficiency of cortisol alone.
- Findings in adrenal failure are nonspecific and, without a high index of suspicion, the diagnosis of this potentially lethal but readily treatable disease is easily missed.
- Adrenal failure should be suspected in patients with hypotension (including orthostatic hypotension), persistent nausea, weight loss, hyponatremia, or hyperkalemia.
- Primary adrenal failure:
  - ○ Often due to autoimmune adrenalitis, which may be associated with other endocrine deficits (e.g., hypothyroidism).
  - ○ Infections of the adrenal gland such as tuberculosis and histoplasmosis may cause adrenal failure.
  - ○ Hemorrhagic adrenal infarction may occur in the postoperative period, in coagulation disorders and hypercoagulable states, and in sepsis (i.e., Waterhouse-Friderichsen syndrome). Adrenal hemorrhage often causes abdominal or flank pain and fever; CT scan of the abdomen reveals high-density bilateral adrenal masses.
  - ○ Adrenoleukodystrophy causes adrenal failure in young males.
  - ○ In patients with AIDS, adrenal failure may develop because of disseminated cytomegalovirus, mycobacterial or fungal infection, or adrenal lymphoma, or treatment with ketoconazole, which inhibits steroid hormone synthesis.
- **Secondary adrenal failure is most often due to glucocorticoid therapy;** ACTH suppression may persist for a year after therapy is stopped. Any disorder of the pituitary or hypothalamus can cause ACTH deficiency, but usually other evidence of these disorders can be seen.

DIAGNOSIS

Clinical Presentation

- Symptoms include anorexia, nausea, vomiting, weight loss, weakness, and fatigue.
- Orthostatic hypotension and hyponatremia are common.

- Usually symptoms are chronic, but shock that is fatal unless treated promptly may develop suddenly. Often, this adrenal crisis is triggered by illness, injury, or surgery.
- Hyperpigmentation (due to marked ACTH excess), hyperkalemia, and volume depletion (due to aldosterone deficiency) occur only in primary adrenal failure.

Diagnostic Testing

- **The short cosyntropin stimulation test is used for diagnosis.**
  - Cosyntropin, 250 μg, is given IV or IM, and plasma cortisol is measured 30 minutes later. The normal response is a stimulated plasma cortisol >20 μg/dL.
  - This test detects primary and secondary adrenal failure, except within a few weeks of onset of pituitary dysfunction (e.g., shortly after pituitary surgery).
- The distinction between primary and secondary adrenal failure usually is clear.
  - Hyperkalemia, hyperpigmentation, or other autoimmune endocrine deficits indicate primary adrenal failure, whereas deficits of other pituitary hormones, symptoms of a pituitary mass (e.g., headache, visual field loss), or known pituitary or hypothalamic disease indicate secondary adrenal failure.
  - If the cause is unclear, the plasma ACTH level distinguishes primary adrenal failure (in which it is markedly elevated) from secondary adrenal failure.
  - Evidence of adrenal enlargement or calcification on abdominal CT indicates that the cause is infection or hemorrhage.
  - Patients with secondary adrenal failure should be tested for other pituitary hormone deficiencies and should be evaluated for a pituitary or hypothalamic tumor.

TREATMENT

Adrenal Crisis

- **Adrenal crisis with hypotension must be treated immediately.** These patients should be admitted to the hospital for therapy and be evaluated for an underlying illness that precipitated the crisis.
- If the diagnosis of adrenal failure is known, hydrocortisone, 100 mg IV every 8 hours, should be given, and 0.9% saline with 5% dextrose should be infused rapidly until hypotension is corrected.
  - The dose of hydrocortisone is decreased gradually over several days as symptoms and precipitating illness resolve and then is changed to oral maintenance therapy.
  - Mineralocorticoid replacement is not needed until the dose of hydrocortisone is <100 mg/day.
- If the diagnosis of adrenal failure has not been established, a single dose of dexamethasone, 10 mg IV, should be given, and a rapid infusion of 0.9% saline with 5% dextrose should be started.
  - A cosyntropin stimulation test should be performed.
  - Dexamethasone is used because it does not interfere with subsequent measurements of cortisol.
  - After the 30-minute plasma cortisol measurement, hydrocortisone, 100 mg IV every 8 hours, should be given until the test result is known.

Outpatient Maintenance Therapy

- **All patients with adrenal failure require cortisol replacement with prednisone.** Most patients with primary adrenal failure also require replacement of aldosterone with fludrocortisone.
- Prednisone, 5 mg PO every morning, should be started.
  - Patients should initially be evaluated every 1 to 2 months.
  - The dose of prednisone is adjusted to eliminate symptoms and signs of cortisol deficiency or excess, with most patients requiring between 4 mg every morning to as much as 5 mg every morning and 2.5 mg every evening.

- ○ The goal of therapy is the lowest dose of prednisone that relieves symptoms, to avoid the possibility of producing signs of Cushing syndrome.
  - ○ Eventually, annual follow-up is adequate **unless an acute illness develops.**
  - ○ Concomitant therapy with rifampin, phenytoin, or phenobarbital accelerates glucocorticoid metabolism and increases the dose requirement.
- During illness, injury, or the perioperative period, the dose of glucocorticoid must be increased.
  - ○ **For minor illnesses,** the patient should double the dose of prednisone for 3 days. If the illness resolves, maintenance dose is resumed. **Vomiting requires immediate medical attention,** with IV glucocorticoid therapy and IV fluid. Patients can be given a 4-mg vial of dexamethasone, to be self-administered IM for vomiting or severe illness if medical care is not immediately available.
  - ○ **For severe illness** or injury, hydrocortisone, 50 mg IV every 8 hours, should be given, with the dose tapered as severity of illness wanes. The same regimen is used in patients who are undergoing surgery, with the first dose of hydrocortisone given preoperatively. Usually, the dose can be reduced to maintenance therapy 2 to 3 days after uncomplicated surgery.
- In primary adrenal failure, **fludrocortisone**, 0.1 mg PO qd, should be given. During follow-up visits, supine and standing blood pressure and serum potassium should be monitored.
- The dose of fludrocortisone is adjusted to maintain blood pressure and serum potassium within the normal range; the usual dose is 0.05 to 0.2 mg PO qd.
- Patients should be educated in management of their disease, including adjustment of prednisone dose during illness. They should wear a medical identification tag or bracelet.

Cushing Syndrome

GENERAL PRINCIPLES

- Cushing syndrome (the clinical effects of increased glucocorticoid hormone) is **most often iatrogenic** due to therapy with glucocorticoid drugs.
- ACTH-secreting pituitary microadenomas (Cushing disease) account for approximately 80% of cases of endogenous Cushing syndrome. Adrenal tumors and ectopic ACTH secretion account for the remainder.

DIAGNOSIS

Clinical Presentation

- Clinical features include truncal obesity, rounded face, fat deposits in the supraclavicular fossae and over the posterior neck, hypertension, hirsutism, amenorrhea, and depression.
- More specific findings include thin skin, easy bruising, reddish striae, proximal muscle weakness, and osteoporosis.
- Diabetes mellitus develops in some patients.
- Hyperpigmentation or hypokalemic alkalosis suggests Cushing syndrome because of ectopic ACTH secretion.

Diagnostic Testing

- The diagnosis is based on increased cortisol excretion, lack of normal feedback inhibition of ACTH and cortisol secretion, or loss of the normal diurnal rhythm of cortisol secretion.[10]
- **Overnight dexamethasone suppression test can be done as a screening test.** 1-mg dexamethasone given PO at 11:00 PM; plasma cortisol measured at 8:00 AM the next day;

normal plasma cortisol level <2 µg/dL. Salivary cortisol may be measured at home during the nadir of normal plasma cortisol at 11:00 PM.

- If the overnight dexamethasone suppression test or 11 PM salivary cortisol is abnormal, 24-hour urine cortisol should be measured. **Twenty-four–hour urine cortisol** measurement can also be done as a screening test. **A normal value virtually excludes the diagnosis.**
- If the 24-hour urine cortisol is more than four times the upper limit of the reference range in a patient with compatible symptoms, the diagnosis of Cushing syndrome is established.
- In patients with milder elevations of urine cortisol, a **low-dose dexamethasone suppression test** should be performed. Dexamethasone, 0.5 mg PO every 6 hours, is given for 48 hours, starting at 8:00 AM. Urine cortisol is measured during the last 24 hours, and plasma cortisol is measured 6 hours after the last dose of dexamethasone. Failure to suppress plasma cortisol to <2 µg/dL and urine cortisol to less than the normal reference range is diagnostic of Cushing syndrome.
- Testing should not be done during severe illness or depression, which may cause false-positive results.
- Phenytoin therapy also causes false-positive dexamethasone suppression test results by accelerating metabolism of dexamethasone.
- **Random plasma cortisol levels are not useful for diagnosis,** because the wide range of normal values overlaps that of Cushing syndrome.
- After the diagnosis of Cushing syndrome is made, tests to determine the cause should be done in consultation with an endocrinologist.

TREATMENT

The treatment of hypercortisolism is dependent on its cause, and a complete discussion of management is beyond the scope of this chapter. Stopping exogenous glucocorticoids when possible is clearly indicated. Other treatments usually require the assistance of an endocrinologist or neurosurgeon.

Incidental Adrenal Nodules

GENERAL PRINCIPLES

Adrenal nodules are a common incidental finding on abdominal imaging studies. **Most incidentally discovered nodules are benign adrenocortical tumors** that do not secrete excess hormone, but the differential diagnosis includes adrenal adenomas that cause Cushing syndrome or primary hyperaldosteronism, pheochromocytoma, adrenocortical carcinoma, and metastatic cancer.[11]

DIAGNOSIS

Clinical Presentation
The patient should be evaluated for symptoms and signs of Cushing syndrome. Hypertension suggests the possibility of primary hyperaldosteronism or pheochromocytoma. Episodes of headache, palpitations, and sweating suggest pheochromocytoma. Hirsutism suggests the possibility of an adrenocortical carcinoma.

Diagnostic Testing
- The imaging characteristics of the nodule may suggest a diagnosis (e.g., benign adrenocortical nodule) but are not specific enough to obviate further evaluation.
- Patients who have potentially resectable cancer elsewhere and in whom an adrenal metastasis must be excluded may require positron emission tomography.

- In other patients, the diagnostic issue is whether a syndrome of hormone excess or an adrenocortical carcinoma is present.
- Plasma potassium, fractionated metanephrines, and dehydroepiandrosterone sulfate should be measured, and an overnight dexamethasone suppression test should be performed.
- Patients with hypertension and hypokalemia should be evaluated for primary hyperaldosteronism by measuring the ratio of plasma aldosterone (in ng/dL) to plasma renin activity (in ng/mL/hour) in a single blood sample.
  ○ This sample can be obtained from an ambulatory patient without special preparation.
  ○ If the ratio is <20, the diagnosis of primary hyperaldosteronism is excluded, whereas a ratio of >50 makes the diagnosis very likely.
  ○ Patients with an intermediate ratio should be further evaluated in consultation with an endocrinologist.
- An abnormal overnight dexamethasone suppression test should be evaluated further (see Cushing Syndrome).
- Elevation of plasma dehydroepiandrosterone sulfate or a large nodule suggests adrenocortical carcinoma.

TREATMENT

- If there is clinical or biochemical evidence of a pheochromocytoma, the nodule should be resected after appropriate α-adrenergic blockade with phenoxybenzamine.
- Most incidental nodules are <4 cm in diameter, do not produce excess hormone, and do not require therapy. One repeat imaging procedure 3 to 6 months later is recommended to ensure that the nodule is not enlarging rapidly (which would suggest an adrenal carcinoma).
- A policy of resecting all nodules >4 cm in diameter appropriately treats the great majority of adrenal carcinomas while minimizing the number of benign nodules removed unnecessarily.

Hypercalcemia

GENERAL PRINCIPLES

- Approximately 50% of serum calcium is ionized (free), and the remainder is complexed, primarily to albumin. Changes in serum albumin alter total calcium concentration without affecting the clinically relevant ionized calcium level, and if serum albumin is abnormal, clinical decisions should be based on **albumin-corrected or ionized calcium levels.**
- Parathyroid hormone (PTH) increases serum calcium by stimulating bone resorption, increasing renal calcium reabsorption, and promoting renal conversion of vitamin D to its active metabolite calcitriol (1,25-dihydroxyvitamin D [$1,25(OH)_2D$]). Serum calcium regulates PTH secretion by a negative feedback mechanism; hypercalcemia suppresses PTH release.
- Vitamin D is converted by the liver to 25-hydroxyvitamin D [25(OH)D], which in turn is converted by the kidney to $1,25(OH)_2D$. The latter metabolite increases serum calcium by promoting intestinal calcium absorption and plays a role in bone formation and resorption.
- Other factors that raise serum calcium include PTH-related peptide, which acts on PTH receptors, and some cytokines produced by plasma cells and lymphocytes.
- The major causes of hypercalcemia are listed in Table 21-3. >95% of cases are due to primary hyperparathyroidism or malignancy.
- **Primary hyperparathyroidism:**
  ○ Causes most cases of mild hypercalcemia in ambulatory patients.
  ○ It is a common disorder, especially in elderly women. **Approximately 85% of cases are due to an adenoma of a single gland,** 15% to enlargement of all four glands, and 1% to parathyroid carcinoma.

TABLE 21-3	Major Causes of Hypercalcemia

Common
    Primary hyperparathyroidism
    Malignancy
Uncommon
    Sarcoidosis, other granulomatous diseases
    Drugs (vitamin D toxicity, calcium carbonate, lithium)
    Hyperthyroidism

- Familial syndromes that include primary hyperparathyroidism (e.g., the multiple endocrine neoplasia syndromes) cause enlargement of all four glands.
- **Malignancy** causes most severe, symptomatic hypercalcemia. Common causes of malignant hypercalcemia include the following:
- Breast carcinoma (which is usually metastatic to bone when hypercalcemia occurs).
- Squamous carcinoma of the lung, head and neck, or esophagus (which may produce humoral hypercalcemia without extensive bone metastases).
- Multiple myeloma.
- **Most malignant hypercalcemia is due to secretion of PTH-related peptide by the tumor,** except for myeloma, in which hypercalcemia is mediated by cytokines.
- Other causes of hypercalcemia are uncommon and are almost always suggested by the history or physical examination.[12]
- Thiazide diuretics cause persistent hypercalcemia only in patients with increased bone turnover, for example, due to mild primary hyperparathyroidism.
- Sarcoidosis and other granulomatous disorders may cause hypercalcemia by excessive synthesis of $1,25(OH)_2D$.
- Familial benign hypercalciuric hypercalcemia is a rare autosomal dominant disorder that causes asymptomatic hypercalcemia from birth. It is due to a genetic defect in the calcium-sensing receptor on parathyroid cells and should be suspected if there is a family history of asymptomatic hypercalcemia.

DIAGNOSIS

Clinical Presentation
- **Most symptoms of hypercalcemia are present only if serum calcium is above 12 mg/dL.**
- In the majority of patients, mild, asymptomatic hypercalcemia is found incidentally.
- Severe symptomatic hypercalcemia is usually due to malignancy and the cancer is almost always clinically apparent.
- The history and physical examination should focus on duration of hypercalcemia (if >6 months without obvious cause, primary hyperparathyroidism is almost certain), history of renal stones, symptoms and signs of malignancy, evidence for any of the unusual causes of hypercalcemia (e.g., calcium supplements, vitamin D, or lithium), and family history of hypercalcemia or other components of multiple endocrine neoplasia syndromes.
- Mild hypercalcemia causes polyuria. Polyuria combined with nausea and vomiting may cause marked dehydration, which impairs calcium excretion and may cause rapidly worsening hypercalcemia.
- Severe hypercalcemia may cause renal failure, and chronic hypercalcemia may cause nephrolithiasis (not seen in hypercalcemia of malignancy).

- Gastrointestinal symptoms include anorexia, nausea, vomiting, and constipation.
- Neurologic findings of severe hypercalcemia include weakness, fatigue, confusion, stupor, and coma.
- Decreased bone density (and rarely a specific bone disorder, osteitis fibrosa) can result from chronic hyperparathyroidism.

Diagnostic Testing

- Mildly elevated serum calcium levels should be repeated with serum albumin to allow for correction, and ionized calcium should be measured to determine whether hypercalcemia is actually present.
- The serum intact PTH level should be measured.
  - If serum PTH is elevated in a patient with hypercalcemia, the diagnosis of primary hyperparathyroidism is confirmed.
  - Intact PTH is suppressed to below the reference range or to the lower part of the reference range in all other causes of hypercalcemia except familial benign hypercalcemia.
  - If the PTH level is suppressed, evaluation for other causes of hypercalcemia should be directed by clinical findings and may include a chest radiography, bone scan, and serum and urine protein electrophoresis.
- Vitamin D intoxication can be confirmed by measurement of elevated serum levels of 25(OH)D. The diagnosis of sarcoidosis as the cause of hypercalcemia is supported by elevated serum levels of 1,25(OH)$_2$D.
- In rare cases in which the diagnosis remains unclear, measurement of serum levels of PTH-related peptide may help confirm or exclude malignancy.
- ECG manifestations include a shortened QT interval.

TREATMENT

- Patients with symptoms of hypercalcemia or serum calcium levels >13 mg/dL should be admitted to the hospital for evaluation and therapy. Treatment of severe hypercalcemia includes measures that increase calcium excretion and decrease resorption of calcium from bone. The purpose is to relieve symptoms, while the cause of hypercalcemia is found and treated.
- Severely hypercalcemic patients are almost always dehydrated, and the first step in therapy is **extracellular fluid (ECF) volume repletion** with 0.9% saline to restore the glomerular filtration rate and promote calcium excretion. At least 3 to 4 L should be given in the first 24 hours, and a positive fluid balance of at least 2 L should be achieved.
- After ECF volume is restored, infusion of 0.9% saline (100 to 200 mL/hour) promotes calcium excretion. Serum electrolytes, calcium, and magnesium should be measured every 6 to 12 hours. **Furosemide adds little** to the effect of saline diuresis and may prevent adequate restoration of ECF volume. It should not be given unless clinical evidence of heart failure develops.

Zoledronic Acid

- Zoledronic acid is a bisphosphonate that inhibits bone resorption and should be used if symptoms persist or the serum calcium continues to be >12 mg/dL after initial volume repletion.
- A dose of 4 mg in 100 mL 0.9% saline is infused over 15 minutes.
- Serum calcium should be measured daily.
- Hypercalcemia abates gradually over several days and remains suppressed for 1 to 2 weeks.
- Treatment can be repeated when hypercalcemia recurs.
- Side effects include asymptomatic hypocalcemia, hypomagnesemia, hypophosphatemia, and transient low-grade fever.

Glucocorticoids

- **Steroids are effective in hypercalcemia due to myeloma, sarcoidosis, and vitamin D intoxication.**
- The initial dose is prednisone, 20 to 50 mg PO bid or its equivalent.
- It may take 5 to 10 days for serum calcium to fall.
- After serum calcium stabilizes, the dose should be gradually reduced to the minimum needed to control symptoms of hypercalcemia.

Management of Primary Hyperparathyroidism

- The most effective therapy for primary hyperparathyroidisim is parathyroidectomy.
- However, in the asymptomatic majority of patients, surgery may not be indicated. The natural history of asymptomatic hyperparathyroidism is not fully known, but in many patients, the disorder has a benign course, with little change in clinical findings or serum calcium for years. The major concern in these patients is the possibility of progressive loss of bone mass and increased risk of fracture. Deterioration of renal function is also possible but unlikely in the absence of nephrolithiasis. Currently, it is impossible to predict the patients in whom problems will develop.
- **Indications for parathyroidectomy** include the following:[13]
  - Symptoms due to hypercalcemia
  - Nephrolithiasis
  - Hip or spine bone mass by dual-energy radiography >2.5 standard deviations below the gender-specific mean peak bone mass (a T score < –2.5)
  - Serum calcium >1 mg/dL above the upper end of the reference range
  - Age <50 years
  - Infeasibility of long-term follow-up
- Surgery is a reasonable choice in otherwise healthy patients even if they do not meet these criteria, because experienced surgeons have a success rate of 90% to 95% with low perioperative morbidity and correction of hyperparathyroidism is followed by an increase in bone mass and a decrease in the risk of fracture.
- Preoperative localization of an adenoma by sestamibi scan may permit a limited neck dissection, which further decreases the risk of complications.
- Asymptomatic patients who do not meet criteria for parathyroidectomy or who refuse surgery can be followed by assessing clinical status, serum calcium and creatinine levels, and bone mass at 1- to 2-year intervals.[13] Surgery should be recommended if any of the above criteria develop or if there is progressive decline in bone mass or renal function.

Hyperprolactinemia

GENERAL PRINCIPLES

- The major causes of hyperprolactinemia are presented in Table 21-4.[14]
- In women, the most common causes of pathologic hyperprolactinemia are prolactin-secreting pituitary microadenoma (i.e., an adenoma with a diameter of <1 cm) and idiopathic hyperprolactinemia.
- In men, the most common cause is prolactin-secreting macroadenoma.
- Hypothalamic or pituitary lesions that cause deficiency of other pituitary hormones often cause hyperprolactinemia by compressing the pituitary stalk.
- In women, hyperprolactinemia causes amenorrhea or irregular menses and infertility. Only one-half of these women have **galactorrhea.** Prolonged estrogen deficiency increases the risk of osteoporosis.
- In men, hyperprolactinemia causes androgen deficiency and infertility but not gynecomastia. Mass effects of a large pituitary tumor (e.g., headaches, visual field loss) and hypopituitarism are common in men with hyperprolactinemia.

TABLE 21-4	Major Causes of Hyperprolactinemia

Pregnancy and lactation
Prolactin-secreting pituitary adenoma (prolactinoma)
Idiopathic hyperprolactinemia
Drugs:
   Dopamine antagonists (phenothiazines, haloperidol, atypical antipsychotics, metoclopramide)
   Others (verapamil, cimetidine, some antidepressants)
Interference with synthesis or transport of hypothalamic dopamine:
   Hypothalamic lesions
   Nonfunctioning pituitary macroadenomas
Primary hypothyroidism
Chronic renal failure

DIAGNOSIS

- The history and physical should include symptoms and signs of prolactin excess, pituitary mass effect, and hypothyroidism. A careful medication history should be obtained.
- Hyperprolactinemia is common in young women, and plasma prolactin should be measured in women with amenorrhea, whether or not galactorrhea is present. Mild elevations should be confirmed by repeat measurements. Laboratory evaluation should include plasma TSH and a pregnancy test.
- **Prolactin levels >200 ng/mL occur only in prolactinomas,** and levels between 100 and 200 ng/mL strongly suggest this diagnosis.
- **Levels <100 ng/mL may be due to any cause except prolactin-secreting macroadenoma,** and such levels in a patient with a large pituitary mass indicate that it is not a prolactinoma.
- Testing for hypopituitarism is needed only in patients with a macroadenoma or hypothalamic lesion and should include measurement of plasma free T_4, a cosyntropin stimulation test (see *Adrenal Failure* section, above), and measurement of plasma testosterone in men.
- Magnetic resonance imaging (MRI) of the pituitary should be performed in most cases, as nonfunctional pituitary or hypothalamic tumors may present with mild hyperprolactinemia.

TREATMENT

Microadenomas and Idiopathic Hyperprolactinemia

- Most patients are treated because of infertility or to prevent estrogen deficiency and osteoporosis.[14]
- Some women may be observed without therapy by periodic follow-up of prolactin levels and symptoms. In most patients, hyperprolactinemia does not worsen and prolactin levels sometimes return to normal. **Enlargement of microadenomas is rare.**
- Dopamine agonists suppress plasma prolactin and restore normal menses and fertility in most women.
  - Initial doses are **bromocriptine,** 1.25 to 2.5 mg PO at bedtime with a snack, or **cabergoline,** 0.25 mg PO twice per week.
  - Doses are adjusted by measurement of plasma prolactin at 2- to 4-week intervals to the lowest dose that suppresses prolactin to the normal range. Maximally effective doses are 2.5 mg bromocriptine tid and 1.5 mg cabergoline twice per week.

○ Initially, patients should use barrier contraception, as fertility may be restored quickly.

○ Side effects include nausea and orthostatic hypotension, which can be minimized by increasing the dose gradually and usually resolve with continued therapy. Side effects are less severe with cabergoline.

• Women who want to become pregnant should be managed in consultation with an endocrinologist.

• Women who do not want to become pregnant should be followed with clinical evaluation and plasma prolactin every 6 to 12 months.

○ Every 2 years, plasma prolactin should be measured after bromocriptine has been withdrawn for several weeks to determine whether the drug still is needed.

○ Follow-up imaging studies are not warranted unless prolactin levels increase substantially.

○ Transsphenoidal resection of prolactin-secreting microadenomas is used only in the rare patients who do not respond to or cannot tolerate bromocriptine. Prolactin levels usually return to normal, but up to one-half of patients relapse.

Prolactin-Secreting Macroadenomas

• **These tumors should be treated with a dopamine agonist,** which usually suppresses prolactin levels to normal, reduces tumor size, and improves or corrects abnormal visual fields in about 90% of cases.[14]

• The dose is adjusted as described as above, except that if mass effects are present, the dose should be increased to maximally effective levels over a period of several weeks.

• Visual field tests, if initially abnormal, should be repeated 4 to 6 weeks after therapy is started. Pituitary imaging should be repeated 3 to 4 months after initiation of therapy. The full effect on tumor size may take >6 months. If tumor shrinkage and correction of visual abnormalities are satisfactory, therapy can be continued indefinitely, with periodic monitoring of plasma prolactin.

• Further imaging is generally not warranted unless prolactin levels rise despite therapy.

• **Transsphenoidal surgery is indicated to relieve mass effects and to prevent further tumor growth** if the tumor does not shrink or if visual field abnormalities persist during dopamine agonist therapy. However, the likelihood of surgical cure of a prolactin-secreting macroadenoma is low, and most patients require further therapy with a dopamine agonist.

• Women with prolactin-secreting macroadenomas should not become pregnant unless the tumor has been resected surgically or has decreased markedly in size on dopamine agonist therapy, as the risk of symptomatic enlargement during pregnancy is 15% to 35%. Contraception is essential during dopamine agonist treatment.

Male Hypogonadism

GENERAL PRINCIPLES

• The testes have two distinct but related roles:
  ○ Secretion of testosterone (the major androgen) by the Leydig cells, which produce and maintain sexual characteristics
  ○ Production of spermatozoa by the seminiferous tubules, a process that requires high local concentrations of testosterone

• The testes are regulated by the pituitary gland, which secretes the gonadotropins, luteinizing hormone (LH), and follicle-stimulating hormone (FSH). Gonadotropin secretion is regulated by the hypothalamus via secretion of LH-releasing hormone and by negative feedback by gonadal hormones.

TABLE 21-5	Major Causes of Androgen Deficiency

Testicular disorders
    Klinefelter syndrome
    Orchitis (mumps, other viruses)
    Trauma
    Drug (including alcohol)
    Autoimmune testicular failure
Hypothalamic pituitary dysfunction
    Congenital luteinizing hormone–releasing hormone deficiency (Kallmann
      syndrome)
    Hyperprolactinemia
    Cushing syndrome
    Other pituitary or hypothalamic disorders
    Chronic illness
Combined defects
    Hepatic cirrhosis
    Chronic renal failure

- Hypogonadism due to disease of the testes results in diminished feedback on the pituitary and increased secretion of gonadotropins. If hypogonadism is due to disorders of the pituitary or hypothalamus, serum gonadotropin levels are within or below the reference range.
- Male hypogonadism may present with androgen deficiency or infertility because of oligospermia (low sperm count). Androgen deficiency is always associated with infertility, but oligospermia often occurs in men with normal testosterone levels.

Etiology

- Male hypogonadism may be due to disorders of the testes or due to dysfunction of the pituitary or hypothalamus (Table 21-5). Cirrhosis and chronic renal failure also impair gonadotropin secretion and testicular function.
- **Testicular disorders**
  - **Klinefelter syndrome** (47, XXY karyotype) occurs in approximately 1 in 1,000 male births. Seminiferous tubules fail to develop normally, and because of this, the testes are small and firm with no spermatogenesis. The degree of androgen deficiency ranges from mild to severe. Klinefelter syndrome usually presents as delayed puberty or persistent gynecomastia after puberty.
  - **Viral orchitis** in adults, most often due to mumps, can cause testicular atrophy. It usually causes infertility alone, but androgen deficiency occurs in severe cases.
  - **Alcohol** causes testicular dysfunction directly and indirectly via hepatic cirrhosis.
  - **Drugs** that impair androgen synthesis or action include ketoconazole, cimetidine, and spironolactone.
  - Infertility without androgen deficiency is usually **idiopathic** but may be due to milder forms of the disorders that cause androgen deficiency or due to cryptorchidism that was not corrected early in childhood.
  - Azoospermia (complete absence of sperm in the ejaculate) with normal testosterone levels may be due to obstruction or absence of the vas deferens.
- **Hypothalamic-pituitary dysfunction**
  - Any disorder of the hypothalamus or pituitary may cause androgen deficiency alone or combined with other pituitary hormone deficiencies.
  - **Hyperprolactinemia** in men is usually due to a prolactin-secreting pituitary macroadenoma.

○ **Kallmann syndrome** (congenital deficiency of LH-releasing hormone) presents as failure of puberty. Other pituitary hormones are usually intact. Most patients have anosmia (lack of sense of smell).

DIAGNOSIS

Clinical Presentation

- The history should include the age at onset of puberty, libido, potency and frequency of intercourse, frequency of shaving, testicular injury or infection, past fertility, medications, and chronic illnesses.
- Physical signs may include testicular atrophy (testes <15 mL in volume or <4 cm in greatest diameter), decreased facial and body hair, gynecomastia, and lack of sense of smell.
- Impotence (erectile dysfunction) with a normal libido is usually due to neurologic or vascular disorders or drugs rather than due to androgen deficiency.

Diagnostic Testing

- Androgen deficiency is confirmed by measurement of plasma **testosterone**.[15] If testosterone is low, plasma **LH** should be measured.
  - ○ Low testosterone levels should be confirmed with repeat testing in the morning.
  - ○ An elevated LH indicates a testicular cause of androgen deficiency.
  - ○ If LH is not elevated, hypothalamic or pituitary dysfunction is responsible, and serum **prolactin** should be measured, secretion of other pituitary hormones should be assessed, and the pituitary and the hypothalamus should be imaged.
- Men with infertility but normal serum testosterone levels should be evaluated by semen analysis.
  - ○ The most important characteristic is sperm concentration, with the normal range considered to be >20 million/mL.
  - ○ Interpretation is complicated by variability of the sperm count in normal men.
  - ○ Oligospermia should be confirmed by at least two semen analyses.

TREATMENT

- Androgen deficiency can be treated by injected or topical testosterone.[15] Treatment is appropriate only for those with repeatedly and clearly low testosterone levels and symptoms of hypogonadism.
  - ○ **Testosterone ester** (testosterone enanthate or cypionate) can be given at a dose of 150 to 250 mg IM every 2 weeks. In most men, a dose of 200 mg is satisfactory.
  - ○ **Testosterone gel** can be applied topically. The starting dose is 5 g once daily.
  - ○ Side effects of androgens include acne, gynecomastia, erythrocytosis, benign prostatic hypertrophy, progression of prostate cancer, and cardiovascular disease.
  - ○ Men older than age 50 years should undergo appropriate screening for prostate cancer.
  - ○ Patients should be followed at 6- to 12-month intervals, with assessment of their clinical response.
  - ○ Measurement of serum testosterone is necessary only if there is an inadequate clinical response to therapy.
- Infertility due to testicular disorders such as idiopathic oligospermia is correctable only by assisted reproduction techniques.
  - ○ Patients with azoospermia and normal levels of testosterone and gonadotropins should be evaluated for obstruction of the vas deferens in consultation with a urologist.
  - ○ Patients with hypogonadism due to pituitary or hypothalamic disorders who desire fertility should be referred to an endocrinologist for treatment.

Hirsutism

GENERAL PRINCIPLES

- Hirsutism is the male pattern growth of dark terminal hair in a woman.[16] It is a common complaint and may indicate **androgen excess**. However, there is a broad range of hair growth in normal women, and many patients with hirsutism have no evidence of androgen excess.
- Even slight increases in androgen production can cause noticeable hair growth in women. More severe androgen excess causes **virilization** (including deepening of the voice and male pattern baldness).
- The major issue in evaluating hirsutism is to exclude the possibility that a woman is one of the small minority with a serious cause (such as Cushing syndrome or an ovarian or adrenal tumor).
- Androgen excess can originate from the ovaries or adrenals. Exogenous androgens can also cause hirsutism.
- **By far, the most common cause is the polycystic ovary syndrome,** which includes hirsutism, infertility, and amenorrhea or irregular menses that are not due to another identifiable disorder.
  - Hirsutism and menstrual irregularity usually begin at puberty.
  - A wide range of abnormality is found in this syndrome, from mild hirsutism alone (sometimes called idiopathic hirsutism) to amenorrhea with enlarged ovaries.
  - These women are **resistant to insulin,** and the resulting high insulin levels play a role in stimulating ovarian androgen production.
- Rare ovarian tumors may produce hirsutism. Adrenal causes of hirsutism include Cushing disease, congenital adrenal hyperplasia, and, rarely, adrenal carcinoma.

DIAGNOSIS

- The history should include the age at onset of hirsutism, symptoms of virilization, any abnormality of menses, and fertility.
- The physical examination should include the extent of hair growth, signs of Cushing syndrome or virilization, and palpation for ovarian enlargement. Signs of virilization like frontal and temporal balding, laryngeal enlargement and deepening of the voice, increased muscle mass, and clitoral enlargement are common features of virilization and suggest a serious underlying cause.
- **Serum total and free testosterone should be measured.**[16]
- Testing for Cushing syndrome should be performed if there are any symptoms or signs to suggest this disorder.
- Multiple ovarian cysts are a common finding in women with normal menses and no hirsutism; ultrasound of the ovaries should not be performed unless an ovarian tumor is suspected.
- Almost all patients with no evidence of virilization and mild elevation of free testosterone have a disorder that falls within the spectrum of polycystic ovary syndrome. They can be treated for this without further evaluation.
- Patients with evidence of virilization or with serum total testosterone levels >200 ng/dL may have an ovarian or adrenal tumor and should be further evaluated in consultation with an endocrinologist.

TREATMENT

- Patients with mild hirsutism may not require medical therapy if cosmetic measures such as plucking or shaving produce a satisfactory result.
- The response of hair growth to drug therapy is slow and often incomplete.

- **Oral contraceptives** suppress ovarian androgen production and may improve hirsutism.
- In women with the polycystic ovary syndrome, drugs that improve insulin resistance may reduce androgen production and improve menstrual abnormalities and fertility.[16]
  - **Metformin,** 500 to 1,000 mg bid, can be used in patients with normal renal function.[16] It should be started at a dose of 500 mg daily, and the dose gradually increased over a several-week period.
  - Side effects include diarrhea, nausea, and abdominal cramps.
  - Patients should be followed at 6-month intervals, with assessment of hair growth, menstrual regularity, and serum-free testosterone.
- **Spironolactone,** 25 to 100 mg bid, is an androgen and aldosterone antagonist that can reduce excess hair growth.[16]
  - Side effects include irregular menses, nausea, and hyperkalemia.
  - It should not be used in patients with renal dysfunction since they are more prone to hyperkalemia. It should not be used by women desiring fertility, and women must use contraception.
  - Combination therapy with an oral contraceptive may be more effective and allows regular menses.
  - Patients should be followed at 6-month intervals, with assessment of hair growth, menstrual regularity, and serum potassium.

REFERENCES

1. Garber JH, Cobin RH, Gharib H, et al. Clinical practice guidelines for hypothyroidism in adults: cosponsored by the American Association of Clinical Endocrinologists and the American Thyroid Association. *Thyroid* 2012;22:1200–1235.
2. Surks MI, Ortiz E, Daniels GH, et al. Subclinical thyroid disease: scientific review and guidelines for diagnosis and management. *JAMA* 2004;291:228–238.
3. De Groot L, Abalovich M, Alexander EK, et al. Management of thyroid dysfunction during pregnancy and postpartum: an Endocrine Society clinical practice guideline. *J Clin Endocrinol Metab* 2012;97:2543–2565.
4. Bahn RS, Burch HB, Cooper DS. Hyperthyroidism and other causes of thyrotoxicosis: management guidelines of the American Thyroid Association and American Association of Clinical Endocrinologists. *Thyroid* 2011;21:593–646.
5. Cooper DS. Approach to the patient with subclinical hyperthyroidism. *J Clin Endocrinol Metab* 2007;92:3–9.
6. Osman F, Franklyn JA, Sheppard MC, et al. Successful treatment of amiodarone-induced thyrotoxicosis. *Circulation* 2002;105:1275–1277.
7. Topliss D. Thyroid incidentaloma: the ignorant in pursuit of the impalpable. *Clin Endocrinol (Oxf)* 2004;60:18–20.
8. Weetman AP. Radioiodine treatment for benign thyroid diseases. *Clin Endocrinol (Oxf)* 2007;66:757–764.
9. Cooper DS, Doherty GM, Haugen BR, et al. Revised American Thyroid Association management guidelines for patients with thyroid nodules and differentiated thyroid cancer. *Thyroid* 2009;19:1167–1214.
10. Nieman LK, Biller BMK, Findling JW, et al. The diagnosis of Cushing's syndrome: an endocrine society clinical practice guideline. *J Clin Endocrinol Metab* 2008;93:1526–1540.
11. Young WF Jr. Clinical practice. The incidentally discovered adrenal mass. *N Engl J Med* 2007;356:601–610.
12. Jacobs TP, Bilezikian JP. Clinical review: rare causes of hypercalcemia. *J Clin Endocrinol Metab* 2005;90:6316–6322.

13. Bilezikian JP, Khan AA, Potts JT. Guidelines for the management of asymptomatic primary hyperparathyroidism: summary statement from the third international workshop. *J Clin Endocrinol Metab* 2009;94:335–339.

14. Melmed S, Casanueva FF, Hoffman AR. Diagnosis and treatment of hyperprolactinemia: an Endocrine Society clinical practice guideline. *J Clin Endocrinol Metab* 2011;96:273–288.

15. Bhasin S, Cunningham GR, Hayes FJ. Testosterone therapy in men with androgen deficiency syndromes: an Endocrine Society clinical practice guideline. *J Clin Endocrinol Metab* 2010;95:2536–2559.

16. Martin KA, Chang RJ, Ehrmann DA. Evaluation and treatment of hirsutism in premenopausal women: an Endocrine Society clinical practice guideline. *J Clin Endocrinol Metab* 2008;93:1105–1120.

22

Nutrition and Obesity
Melissa Sum and Shelby Sullivan

General Nutritional Considerations

DEFINITIONS

- **Macronutrients**: provide energy and consist of protein, carbohydrate, and fat.
- **Micronutrients**: do not provide energy and consist of vitamins and minerals.
- **Essential nutrients**: nutrients not synthesized by the body and therefore completely supplied by the diet.
- **Malnutrition**: may refer to a state of overnutrition or undernutrition. For the purposes of this chapter, will be referred to a state of undernutrition.
- **Obesity**: results from macronutrient overnutrition though obese patients may have micronutrient deficiencies.
- **Body mass index** (BMI) = weight (kg)/height^2 (m^2):
  - Underweight: BMI <18.5 kg/m^2
  - Normal weight: BMI 18.5 to 25.0 kg/m^2
  - Overweight: BMI >25 kg/m^2
  - Obesity: BMI >30 kg/m^2
  - Morbid obesity: BMI >40 kg/m^2
- A BMI outside of the normal range is associated with increased morbidity for most patients.
- Special populations may have a high BMI, but normal body fat such as athletic men or women with more muscle mass than the general population; or a normal BMI, but high body fat such as an elderly person with less muscle mass than the general population.

Dietary Guidelines

Dietary Reference Intakes

- Estimates of daily nutrient intakes that can be used for planning and assessing diets for healthy individuals.
- Consist of four reference intakes: estimated average requirement (EAR), recommended dietary allowance (RDA), tolerable upper limit (UL), and adequate intake (AI).
- Current dietary reference intakes (DRIs) can be found on the US Department of Agriculture (USDA) website.[1]
- EAR: estimated daily intake of essential nutrients adequate to meet the nutritional needs of 50% of the individuals in a specific age and gender group.
- RDA:
  - Estimated daily intake of essential nutrients adequate to meet the nutritional needs of practically all (97% to 98%) individuals in a specific age and gender group.
  - 2 standard deviations above the EAR.
  - If the EAR for a given nutrient cannot be established through sufficient scientific data, the RDA for that nutrient cannot be established. When the RDA cannot be established, the AI is used instead.
- UL: The daily upper limit of intake of essential nutrients safe for most individuals. Data are lacking for many nutrients, and therefore lack of an UL does not mean that one does not exist.

- AI: The AI is used as a goal for the nutrient intake of individuals and is based on observed or experimental calculations. When sufficient data are not available to estimate an average requirement, an AI is set.

USDA Dietary Guidelines for Americans

- Developed by the USDA and the Department of Health and Human Services and revised every 5 years, most recently in 2010.
- Generally encourage Americans to eat fewer calories, to be more active, and to make wiser food choices.
- Guidelines note populations with special needs in the executive summary.
- Guidelines are the basis of the food guide plate.
- The **USDA food guide plate** was first released in 2011 (see Fig. 22-1). It replaced the previously used food guide pyramid that had been criticized for its lack of translatability to most Americans' dining habits. The USDA food guide plate emphasizes the following[2]:
  - ○ **Proportionality**: shown by the division of the plate into the four nearly comparable-sized components of fruits, vegetables, protein, and grains to suggest how much food a person should choose from each group. It encourages people to make half their plate fruits and vegetables.
  - ○ **Moderation**: represented by the division of one plate into quarters.
  - ○ **Variety**: symbolized by the five colors representing the four food groups on the plate and the dairy product next to it.
- The USDA website (www.choosemyplate.gov [last accessed 1/5/15]) contains links to SuperTracker, which helps patients plan, analyze, and track their diet and physical activity to identify ways to improve. It also contains a feature that allows patients to set personal calorie goals.

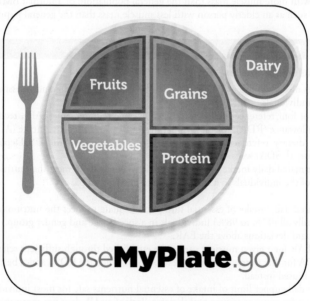

Figure 22-1 **United States Department of Agriculture MyPlate.** (From http://www.choosemyplate.gov [last accessed 1/5/15])

Calculating Energy Requirements

• Total energy expenditure = basal metabolic rate (BMR) + the energy expenditure of activity + the thermic effect of food.
• The thermic effect of food is a small percentage of total energy expenditure and is largely ignored when energy requirements are estimated.
• **Harris-Benedict equations** estimate BMR on the basis of gender, height, age, and weight:
  ○ Male: BMR (kcal) = 66.5 + (13.8 × weight in kg) + (5 × height in cm) − (6.8 × age in years).
  ○ Female: BMR (kcal) = 655 + (9.6 × weight in kg) + (1.9 × height in cm) − (4.7 × age in years).
• Energy needs are then calculated by multiplying BMR by an activity factor between 0.8 and 1.8 that adjusts for the stress of various medical conditions and for the level of activity.
• Table 22-1 can be used for an easy reference to determine energy requirements.

Macronutrients

Protein

• Components of protein include essential and nonessential amino acids. Essential amino acids are histidine, isoleucine, leucine, lysine, methionine/cystine, phenylalanine/tyrosine, threonine, tryptophan, and valine.
• Types of protein:
  ○ Complete proteins contain all essential amino acids and are derived from animal sources and select plant sources such as soy, quinoa, spirulina, buckwheat, hemp seed, and amaranth.
  ○ Incomplete proteins do not contain all essential amino acids.
• Sources of protein include meat, dairy products other than cream and butter, and plant products such as grains, legumes, and vegetables.
• Plant proteins can be ingested in combination so that their amino acid patterns become complementary. Vegans can meet requirements when grains, legumes, and leafy greens are combined.
• The RDA for protein intake in young healthy adults of both sexes is 0.8 g/kg body weight/day. **The average American's daily protein intake far exceeds the RDA**.
• Protein requirements increase during growth, pregnancy, lactation, and rehabilitation.

Carbohydrates

• Carbohydrates are composed of saccharide units.
• Types of carbohydrates:
  ○ Complex carbohydrates: polysaccharides, starch, which is digestible, and fiber, which is indigestible.
  ○ Sugars: monosaccharides (glucose, fructose), disaccharides (sucrose, lactose, maltose), or oligosaccharides; sucrose and lactose are the primary dietary sugars.
• Carbohydrates typically comprise 45% to 65% total daily calories.

TABLE 22-1	Energy Requirements Based on BMI
BMI	**Energy requirements (kcal/kg/day)**
<15	36–45
15–19	31–35
20–29	26–30
≥30	15–25

BMI, body mass index.

- **Fiber**:
  - Fiber is found in all plant sources (whole grains, legumes, and prunes are very good sources) and is commercially available in sources such as psyllium (e.g., Metamucil) and methylcellulose (e.g., Citrucel).
  - Fiber intake for males is 30 to 38 g/day and for females is 21 to 29 g/day.
  - **Most Americans do not consume the recommended amount of fiber** and may benefit from supplementation.
  - **Soluble fiber** is soluble in water and fermentable by intestinal bacteria. Pectin, gum, mucilages, and some hemicelluloses are considered soluble fibers. Benefits of soluble fiber include the following:
    - Delayed gastric emptying, slowed intestinal transit, and decreased glucose absorption with benefits in obese patients
    - Improvement in glycemic control in diabetic patients
    - A decrease in luminal wall tension (pain and cramps) and diarrhea in irritable bowel syndrome
    - Binding of fatty acids, cholesterol, and bile acids leading to lower serum lipid levels and atherosclerosis prevention
  - Insoluble fiber is insoluble in water and not fermented by intestinal bacteria. Cellulose, lignin, and some hemicelluloses are considered insoluble fibers. Sources of insoluble fiber include certain plant sources (whole grains, flax seed, and certain vegetables such as celery, potato skin, and green beans). Benefits of insoluble fiber include the following:
    - Increased intestinal transit and increased fecal bulk, resulting in a laxative effect
    - May reduce the rates of diverticulosis and colonic neoplasms

Fat
- Components of fat include glycerol backbone with three fatty acid chains. Fats are categorized by the following:
  - Fatty acid chain length: short-chain, medium-chain, and long-chain fatty acids.
  - Degree of hydrogen saturation of the fatty acid chains: polyunsaturated (multiple unsaturated sites), monounsaturated (a single unsaturated site), and saturated (completely saturated).
  - Ability of the body to synthesize the fat: essential or nonessential. Essential fatty acids are omega-3 α-linolenic acid and omega-6 linolenic acid. All other fatty acids are nonessential.
- **Increasing saturation is associated with increasing risk of coronary artery disease**. Unsaturated fatty acids may be hydrogenated to form trans fats.
- Polyunsaturated fats are divided into *n–6* and *n–3* fatty acids according to their molecular structure. A high ratio of *n–6* fatty acid to *n–3* fatty acid intake may be atherogenic.
- Fat should comprise no more than 35% of total daily calories, and saturated fat should comprise no more than 7% of total daily calories.
- **Trans fats** are made by hydrogenating vegetable oils, which solidifies the oils and increases the shelf life and flavor of the foods that contain them. They contribute to increased blood low-density lipoprotein (LDL) cholesterol, decreased blood high-density lipoprotein (HDL) cholesterol, and coronary artery disease. Trans fat should comprise no more than 1% of total daily calories.
- Monounsaturated fats (when substituted for saturated fat) have beneficial effects on the cholesterol profile decreasing LDL and triglyceride levels while increasing HDL.

Cholesterol
- Dietary fats and cholesterol are packaged into lipoproteins for delivery to the tissues.
- The classification of lipoproteins can be found in Chapter 11.
- LDL, very–low-density lipoprotein (VLDL), intermediate-density lipoprotein (IDL), and chylomicrons carry cholesterol to the tissues with LDL carrying 70% of serum cholesterol.
- HDL returns cholesterol from the tissues to the liver and carries 20% to 30% of serum cholesterol. HDL levels are inversely correlated with the risk of heart disease.

TABLE 22-2 Dietary Sources of Fats

Type of fat	Food source	Atherogenicity
Saturated fats	Dairy and meat products	High
Monounsaturated fats	Olive and canola oils, avocado, nuts	Low
Polyunsaturated fats (*n–6*)	Margarines, vegetable oils	High
Polyunsaturated fats (*n–3*)	Seed oils (linseed, rapeseed, soya, and walnut oils)	Low
	Nuts, green leafy vegetables	
	Fatty fish (tuna, salmon, sardines, mackerel, herring) and fish oils	
Trans fats	Vegetable shortening, margarine, cookies, and snack foods	High
Cholesterol	Egg yolks, dairy and meat products	High

- Reduced saturated fat, trans fat, and cholesterol intake; weight loss; and dietary adjuncts such as soluble fiber, plant sterols and stanols, and soy protein may decrease LDL cholesterol levels.
- Aerobic exercise, weight loss through decreasing caloric intake, smoking cessation, omega-3 fatty acid intake, increased soluble fiber intake, and drinking one to two servings of alcohol daily have been associated with increased HDL levels.[3]
- Cholesterol intake should be <300 mg/day (Table 22-2).

Alcohol
- Alcohol is structurally similar to carbohydrates.
- Each gram of ethanol yields 7 kcal and can be a significant source of empty calories.
- The alcohol contents in one 1.5-oz shot of hard liquor, one 12-oz beer, and one 5-oz glass of wine are roughly equivalent. One serving of an alcoholic beverage provides 14 to 20 g ethanol (100 to 140 calories) plus additional calories found in additives such as cream, sodas, or fruit juices.
- Ethanol is known to increase HDL in serum; thus, moderate ethanol use may convey a cardioprotective effect.
- Alcohol interferes with thiamine absorption and formation of its active metabolite.

Macronutrient Substitutes
- Artificial sweeteners and sugar substitutes provide sweetness with a reduction in calories. Five artificial sweeteners have been approved by the U.S. Food and Drug Administration (FDA): saccharin, aspartame, acesulfame, sucralose, and neotame (Table 22-3).
- The fat replacement olestra is a mixture of hexa-, hepta-, and octaesters of sucrose with long-chain fatty acids.
  - Olestra imparts taste indistinguishable from fat yet is too large to be absorbed.
  - It is currently found primarily in snack foods such as chips.
  - Side effects include cramping, flatulence, and diarrhea from fat malabsorption. Poor absorption of fat-soluble vitamins may occur because they are excreted with olestra.

Micronutrients
- Vitamins are essential organic compounds that are required to maintain growth, metabolism, and overall health. Vitamins are either fat soluble (vitamins A, D, E, and K) or water soluble (all other vitamins) (Table 22-4).

TABLE 22-3 Current Artificial Sweeteners

Chemical name	Trade name	Year of approval (limited/full)	Sweetness[a]	Health concerns	Heat stable?
Saccharin	Sweet 'N Low	Available before creation of the FDA	300×	Bladder cancer FDA required a warning label until 2001 when research showed that the urine precipitate found in laboratory animals was not found in humans. Still banned or restricted in certain countries	Yes
Aspartame	NutraSweet Equal Canderel	1981/1996	200×	Brain cancer Must be avoided by patients with phenylketonuria because phenylalanine is a metabolite of aspartame	No
Acesulfame K	Sunett Sweet One	1988/2003	200×	None to date	Yes
Sucralose	Splenda	1998/1999	600×	None to date	Yes
Neotame	None	2002/2002	7,000–13,000×	None to date	Intermediate

[a]As compared to sucrose.
FDA, Food and Drug Administration.

TABLE 22-4 Water- and Fat-Soluble Vitamins

Vitamin	Function	Source	Deficiency	Toxicity
A	Visual pigments Cell differentiation Gene regulation	Liver, fish Yellow-orange vegetables and fruits Green leafy vegetables	Night blindness Hyperkeratotic skin Xerophthalmia/blindness	Dermatitis Increased intracrania pressure Bone pain/hypercalcemia Liver fibrosis Birth defects in pregnancy
D	Calcium homeostasis Bone metabolism	Fortified milk Herring, salmon, sardines, liver	Osteomalacia	Hypercalcification of bone Kidney stones Soft tissue calcification Hypercalcemia
E	Membrane antioxidant	Vegetable oils Wheat germ, rice bran Nuts, seeds	Neuropathy Myopathy	Bleeding
K	Clotting Calcium metabolism	Green leafy vegetables Olive and soybean oils	Coagulopathy	Interferes with warfarin
C	Biosynthesis of collagen and carnitine Metabolism of drugs and steroids	Citrus fruits Green vegetables	Bleeding dyscrasia Scurvy (poor wound healing, bleeding diathesis)	Hemolytic anemia with IV Osmotic diarrhea False-positive FOBT Oxalate and UA kidney stones (hypothetical) Increased Fe absorption in patients with Fe overload
B_1 (thiamine)	Coenzyme for oxidative decarboxylations of 2-keto acids and transketolations	Brewers' yeast Meats (especially pork) Sunflower seeds, wheat germ, nuts, legumes Enriched grain products	Beriberi: High-output CHF (wet) Peripheral neuropathy (dry) Wernicke encephalopathy	Excessive IV or IM: Convulsion Cardiac arrhythmias Anaphylactic shock

(Continued)

TABLE 22-4 Water- and Fat-Soluble Vitamins (Continued)

Vitamin	Function	Source	Deficiency	Toxicity
B$_2$ (Riboflavin)	Coenzyme in redox reactions of fatty acids and the TCA cycle	Liver, meats Brewers' yeast Dairy products and eggs Fortified cereals Broccoli, spinach, mushrooms	Cheilosis Glossitis Angular stomatitis Corneal vascularization Anemia Personality changes	None
B$_3$ (niacin)	Precursor of NAD and NADP, which are important in redox reactions	Meat, poultry, fish Dairy products and eggs Fortified cereals Fortified flour Corn, potato Noncitrus fruits and juices	Pellagra: Diarrhea Dermatitis Confusion or dementia	Histamine-induced exacerbations of asthma and PUD Liver toxicity Elevated serum uric acid Glucose intolerance
B$_6$ (pyridoxine)	Coenzyme in amino acid metabolism Heme and neuro-transmitter synthesis	Liver Oatmeal Bananas Chicken Potatoes	Dermatitis Glossitis Peripheral neuropathy Convulsions Anemia	Sensory neuropathy
B$_{12}$ (cobalamin)	Coenzyme in metabolism of propionate, amino acids, and single-carbon fragments	Wheat germ, rice Clams, oysters, crab, tuna Liver, beef	Personality changes Megaloblastic anemia Depression Neuropathy Psychosis Glossitis	None

Folic acid	Coenzyme in single-carbon metabolism	Fortified cereals Brewers' yeast Legumes Leafy green vegetables Citrus fruit and juices Meat, poultry, fish	Megaloblastic anemia Diarrhea Fatigue Depression Confusion Glossitis	None May correct the bone marrow effects of B_{12} deficiency without correcting its neurologic manifestations
Biotin	Coenzyme for carboxylations Important in gluconeogenesis and fatty acid synthesis	Cereals Egg yolks (whites contain avidin, which binds biotin plus reduces bioavailability) Liver, soy Brewers' yeast Nuts, legumes	Anorexia Paresthesias Depression/hallucinations Dermatitis, hair loss	None
Pantothenic acid	Coenzyme for fatty acid metabolism	Meat, liver, fish, poultry Milk products and egg yolks Legumes Whole grain cereals Brewers' yeast	Paresthesias Ataxia Muscle cramps Depression Hypoglycemia	None
Choline	Precursor for acetylcholine and phospholipids	Soybeans Milk products and egg yolks Peanuts Whole grain cereals Potatoes, tomatoes Bananas and oranges	Fatty liver Elevated transaminases	Hypotension Cholinergic diaphoresis Diarrhea Salivation

CHF, congestive heart failure; FOBT, fecal occult blood testing; NAD, nicotinamide adenine dinucleotide; NADP, nicotinamide adenine dinucleotide phosphate; PUD, peptic ulcer disease; TCA, tricarboxylic acid; UA, uric acid.

- Dietary minerals are inorganic compounds that do not supply energy (Table 22-5). They are important in regulating metabolism, tissue catabolism, and anabolism, including
  - Cellular regulation and fluid balance
  - Coenzymes and cofactors
  - Bone and tooth formation

DRUG-NUTRIENT INTERACTIONS

- Food can enhance or impede medication effects.
- Medication can influence food and nutrient intake, absorption, metabolism, and excretion.
- It is beyond the scope of this chapter to list all possible interactions; however, some common interactions may be found in Table 22-6.

DIETARY SUPPLEMENTS

- Products (other than tobacco) intended to supplement the diet that contain one or more of the following ingredients: a vitamin; a mineral; an herb or other botanical; an amino acid; a dietary substance used to supplement a diet by increasing the total daily intake; or a concentrate, metabolite, constituent, extract, or combination of these ingredients (Table 22-7).
- Americans spend billions of dollars annually on supplements.
- **Supplements do not require FDA approval** and therefore vary greatly in strength, potency, and purity. Some products may contain no active ingredient. Contamination with pesticides, drugs, or heavy metals may occur, and it is the burden of the FDA to show that a product is not safe.
- Supplements may interact with other dietary supplements or prescription medications.
- Nonspecific side effects such as gastrointestinal (GI) distress, headache, allergic reactions, and medication interactions have been described for all supplements. Long-term effects of supplementation are not known.
- Some common complementary and alternative medicine dietary supplements are listed in Table 22-8.

Overnutrition and Obesity

GENERAL PRINCIPLES

- Overnutrition is the excess of one or more nutrients; it occurs when nutrient intake exceeds nutrient expenditure. Although macronutrients may be consumed in excess, micronutrient intake may be inadequate.
- Excess of vitamins and minerals can occur due to dietary supplements, complementary/alternative treatments, and some fad diets.
- Overweight is defined by BMI >25 kg/m^2 and obesity BMI >30 kg/m^2.
- Greater than 60% of Americans are overweight, >30% are obese, and approximately 5% are morbidly obese, and these rates have doubled in the past 20 years.[1]
- Obesity is associated with many comorbidities, including diabetes mellitus, hypertension, hyperlipidemia, atherosclerosis, gout, cardiovascular disease, and sleep apnea.

DIAGNOSIS

Clinical Presentation
History
- Obtain a general medical history including a careful diet history, thorough family history, and evaluation for medical and psychiatric comorbidities.

TABLE 22-5	Minerals			
Mineral	Function	Source	Deficiency	Toxicity
Calcium	Component of bones and teeth Signal transduction Muscle contraction Clotting	Dairy products Sardines, clams, oysters Turnips, mustard greens Legumes Broccoli	Rickets Osteoporosis Tetany	Milk-alkali syndrome Kidney stones Impaired iron absorption
Phosphorus	Component of bones and teeth, cell membranes, phospholipids, ATP	Meat, poultry, fish Eggs Dairy products Legumes	Rickets Rhabdomyolysis Paresthesia/ataxia Hemolysis Acidosis	Hypocalcemia Tetany
Magnesium	Component of bones Role in nerve conduction Protein synthesis Enzyme activation	Nuts, grains, chocolate Nuts, legumes Grains, corn Peas, carrots Seafood Brown rice	Depression Muscle weakness Tetany Convulsions Growth failure	Osmotic diarrhea Flushing Double vision Slurred speech Weakness, paralysis Cardiopulmonary failure
Potassium	Water and electrolyte balance Cell membrane transfer	Fruits Potato Beans Wheat bran Dairy products Eggs	Weakness Apathy Cardiac arrhythmias Paralysis	Cardiac arrhythmia Cardiac arrest

(Continued)

TABLE 22-5	Minerals (*Continued*)			
Mineral	**Function**	**Source**	**Deficiency**	**Toxicity**
Iron	Oxygen transport	Organ meats, clams, oysters Molasses Nuts, legumes, seeds Leafy green vegetables Enriched grains and cereals	Microcytic anemia Listlessness and fatigue Impaired cognitive development	GI distress Hemochromatosis
Zinc	Cofactor in metabolism Protein synthesis Collagen formation Alcohol detoxification Taste and smell	Oysters Wheat germ Beef, liver, poultry Whole grains	Growth retardation Abnormal taste and smell Changes in skin, hair, and nails	GI distress Anemia from copper deficiency (competitive absorption) Pulmonary fibrosis
Copper	Utilization of iron stores Lipid, collagen, pigment, and neurotransmitter synthesis	Liver, meat, fish Shellfish Whole grains Legumes Eggs	Anemia Growth retardation Skin/hair abnormalities Mental deterioration	GI distress Mental deterioration Hemolytic anemia Liver failure Renal dysfunction
Selenium	Protects against free radicals	Grains Meats, poultry, fish Dairy products	Osteopenia Myopathy Cardiomyopathy	Nausea and vomiting Neuropathy Dermatitis
Chromium	Regulation of blood glucose	Mushrooms, prunes, asparagus Organ meats Whole grains and cereals	Glucose intolerance Lipid abnormalities	Renal failure Dermatitis Pulmonary cancer

	Function	Food Sources	Deficiency	Toxicity
Iodine	Thyroid hormone synthesis	Iodized table salt Saltwater seafood Sunflower seeds Mushrooms Liver, eggs	Goiter Hypothyroidism	Thyroid dysfunction Acneiform rash
Manganese	Brain and bone function Collagen	Wheat bran Legumes Nuts Lettuce, blueberries, pineapple	Impaired growth Skeletal abnormalities Impaired CNS function	Neurotoxicity Parkinsonian-like symptoms Pneumoconiosis
Molybdenum fluoride	Metabolism of purines and pyrimidines Maintenance of teeth and bones	Seafood, poultry, meat Soybeans, lentils Buckwheat Oats, rice bread Fluorinated drinking water Fish, meat Legumes Grains	Neurologic abnormalities Dental caries Bone disorders	Fetal abnormalities Chronic toxicity: bone, kidney, nerve, and muscle dysfunction Mottled teeth Acute toxicity: acidosis, cardiac arrhythmias, death

ATP, adenosine triphosphate; CNS, central nervous system; GI, gastrointestinal.

TABLE 22-6 Important Food/Nutrient and Medication Interactions

Food/Nutrient	Medication	Interaction
Grapefruit juice	Carbamazepine Calcium channel blockers Cyclosporin Saquinavir Astemizole Statins Cisapride Buspirone Clomipramine Benzodiazepines Tacrolimus	Increases medication concentrations Mediated by suppression of the P-450 enzyme CYP3A4 Effect lasts 24 hours Drugs with high presystemic metabolism are affected the most
Tyramine-containing foods: aged cheese, overripe fruit, spoiled foods, fermented/dry salami or sausage, soy sauce, marmite-concentrated yeast extract, sauerkraut, fava and broad beans, banana peel, tap beer	Monoamine oxidase inhibitors Furazolidone Isoniazid Procarbazine	Leads to hypertensive crisis Mediated by release of norepinephrine by culprit foods and monoamine oxidase inhibitors Suggested upper limit of tyramine is 6 mg/day
Potassium supplements	Spironolactone Triamterene Amiloride	Can cause hyperkalemia

Vitamin K–rich foods: dark leafy green vegetables, soybean, canola, cottonseed, olive oils	Warfarin Phenindione	Suppresses warfarin effect Intake permitted but should be consistent
Vitamin B_6	Hydralazine Isoniazid Chloramphenicol Cycloserine	Inhibits absorption of vitamin B_6
Fat-soluble vitamins	Cholestyramine Colestipol Mineral oil	Inhibits absorption of fat-soluble vitamins
Folic acid	Sulfasalazine Phenytoin Primidone Colestipol Cholestyramine Methotrexate Pyrimethamine Nitrofurantoin Trimethoprim	Inhibits absorption of folic acid
Vitamin B_{12}	Histamine-2 receptor antagonists Proton pump inhibitors Chloramphenicol Cycloserine	Inhibits absorption of vitamin B_{12}

TABLE 22-7 Common Dietary Supplements

Functional food	Structure function	Natural sources (all may be found in dietary supplements)	Potential benefits	Grade of evidence for benefit[a]	Potential side effects
Creatine	Nitrogenous organic acid Involved in the transfer of phosphate to ADP Provides energy for muscle activity	Synthesized by the body Food sources (meat, milk, and fish)	Improved athletic performance Hyperlipidemia Cardiac diseases Muscular and neuromuscular diseases	C C C C	Asthma exacerbation Liver and kidney toxicity Muscle breakdown Electrolyte imbalances Altered glycemic control Stroke Decreased function of vitamins A, D, E, and K
Coenzyme Q10	Benzoquinone Cofactor in electron transport Antioxidant	Food sources (fish, fish oils, nuts, meats)	Hypertension Neurodegenerative and muscular diseases Cardiac diseases Mitochondrial diseases Cancer Migraines HIV Kidney failure Diabetes	C B C C C C C D	Organ damage during exercise Liver toxicity Thyroid dysfunction Platelet dysfunction Hypoglycemia
Glucosamine	Amino sugar Component of cartilage	Synthesized by the body	Osteoarthritis Venous insufficiency Inflammatory bowel disease Rheumatoid arthritis	A[b] C C C	Allergic potential in those with shellfish allergies Hypertension Palpitations Cataracts Bleeding Altered glycemic control

Supplement	Properties	Sources	Uses	Evidence	Adverse effects
Chondroitin	Glycosaminoglycan Component of cartilage	Cartilage	Osteoarthritis	A[b]	Hair loss
			Ophthalmologic uses	B	Breathing difficulties
					Hypertension
			Coronary disease	C	Asthma exacerbation
			Psoriasis	C	Bleeding
			Interstitial cystitis	C	Edema
					Bone marrow suppression
Lipoic acid	Antioxidant Cofactor in glucose metabolism	Synthesized by the body Food sources (organ meats, beef, yeast, broccoli, spinach)	Neuropathy	B	Malodorous urine
			Glucose utilization	c	Hypoglycemia
			Neurodegenerative disorders	c	Biotin deficiency
Omega-3 fatty acids: α-linolenic acid eicosapentaenoic acid docosahexaenoic acid	Polyunsaturated fatty acid with a carbon-carbon double bond in the ω-3 position Anti-inflammatory	Food sources: Wild-caught oily fish (salmon, herring, mackerel, anchovies, sardines) Flaxseed Mussels and clams Eggs from free-range chickens Kiwifruit Walnuts	Secondary prevention of CV disease	A	Hemorrhagic risk at high doses
			Hypertension	A	Impairment of glycemic control in diabetics
			Hypertriglyceridemia	A	Immunosuppression
			Primary prevention of CV disease	B	Increase in LDL cholesterol in some patients
			Protection from cyclosporine toxicity	B	
			Varicose veins	C	
			ADHD	C	
			Developmental and learning problems	C	
			Arthritis	C	

(Continued)

TABLE 22-7 Common Dietary Supplements (*Continued*)

Functional food	Structure function	Natural sources (all may be found in dietary supplements)	Potential benefits	Grade of evidence for benefit[a]	Potential side effects
Probiotics: *Lactobacillus* spp. *Bifidobacterium* spp.	Beneficial bacteria or yeasts Reconstitute the gut flora after disruption caused by stressors such as antibiotics, toxins, or disease preventing harmful bacteria from taking over.	Food sources: Dairy products Probiotic fortified foods	Chronic pouchitis Antibiotic-associated diarrhea	B C	None

[a]National Institutes of Health grade of evidence for benefit.
A: Strong scientific evidence for this use
B: Good scientific evidence for this use
C: Unclear scientific evidence for this use
D: Fair scientific evidence against this use
E: Strong scientific evidence against this use
[b]The most recent grade of evidence for glucosamine and chondroitin in osteoarthritis was assigned before publication of the GAIT trial. Clegg DO, Reda DJ, Klein MA, et al. Glucosamine, chondroitin sulfate, and the two in combination for painful knee osteoarthritis. *N Engl J Med* 2006;354:795–808.
[c]NIH evidence grading unavailable at this time.
ADHD, attention deficit hyperactivity disorder; ADP, adenosine diphosphate; LDL, low-density lipoprotein.

TABLE 22-8 Popular Herbal and Botanical Dietary Supplements

Name	Common names	Reported indications for use	Adverse side effects
Echinacea purpurea E. angustifolia E. pallida	American or purple coneflower	Colds, flu, or other infections, wound care	No toxic effects
Valeriana officinalis	Valerian, all-heal, garden heliotrope	Insomnia, anxiety, headaches, depression	Headaches, dizziness, fatigue
Tanacetum parthenium	Feverfew, bachelor's buttons, featherfew	Fevers, headaches, stomachaches, toothaches, insect bites, infertility, menstrual and childbirth problems, migraines, rheumatoid arthritis, psoriasis, allergies, asthma, tinnitus, nausea, dizziness	Aphthous ulcers, mucosal irritation, loss of taste, rebound headaches, anxiety, joint pain, uterine contractions, and miscarriage
Ginkgo biloba	Gingko, fossil tree, maidenhair tree, Japanese silver apricot, kew tree, yinhsing	Asthma, bronchitis, tinnitus, dementia, claudication, sexual dysfunction, multiple sclerosis	Headache, dizziness Increased bleeding risk, seizures, or death if uncooked seeds are consumed
Hypericum perforatum	St. John's wort, goat weed, Klamath weed, hypericum	Depression, anxiety, sleep disorders	Photosensitivity, anxiety, dry mouth, dizziness, headache, sexual dysfunction, many drug interactions
Serenoa repens	Saw palmetto, cabbage palm, American dwarf palm tree	Benign prostatic hypertrophy, hormone imbalances, bladder disorders, decreased sex drive, pelvic pain, hair loss	Decreased sex drive, breast tenderness

(Continued)

TABLE 22-8 Popular Herbal and Botanical Dietary Supplements (*Continued*)

Name	Common names	Reported indications for use	Adverse side effects
Piper methysticum	Kava kava, awa, kava pepper	Anxiety, insomnia, menopausal symptoms	Liver failure, dystonia, many drug interactions, drowsiness, yellow skin
Panax ginseng	Asian ginseng, ginseng	Recovery from illness, energy enhancement, erectile dysfunction, hepatitis C, menopausal symptoms, hypertension, diabetes	Headaches, insomnia, breast tenderness, menstrual irregularities, hypertension, hypoglycemia
Cimicifuga racemosa	Black cohosh, black snake root, macrotys, bugbane, bugwort, rattle root, rattle weed	Rheumatism, menopausal symptoms, menstrual irregularities, labor induction, premenstrual syndrome	Headaches, weight disturbances, possible link to hepatitis, may be unsafe for pregnant women and women with a history of breast cancer
Ephedra ≥40 species	Chinese Ephedra, Ma Huang	Increased energy, weight loss	Stroke, myocardial infarction, sudden death, hypertension, insomnia, anxiety, psychosis, worsening of kidney disease, diabetes
Pausinystalia yohimbe	Yohimbe bark, yohimbine	Aphrodisiac, erectile dysfunction	Hypertension, insomnia, palpitations, anxiety, headache, drug interactions (MAOIs, SSRIs, TCAs), kidney failure

MAOIs, monoamine oxidase inhibitors; SSRIs, serotonin reuptake inhibitors; TCAs, tricyclic antidepressants.

- When obesity is present, the evaluating physician should consider factors that affect intake and ability to perform physical exercise, and remember that obese patients may have micronutrient deficiencies.
  - What quantity and type of foods are being consumed?
  - What type of lifestyle does the patient lead?
  - Is there evidence for secondary causes of obesity including genetic syndromes, hypothyroidism, insulinoma, or Cushing syndrome?

Physical Examination
- Distribution of body fat can be evaluated via waist to hip ratio although this is not routinely done in many offices and has significant operator variability.
- Comorbid conditions include insulin resistance, male hypogonadism, polycystic ovarian syndrome, cardiovascular disease, obstructive sleep apnea, gallstone disease, osteoarthritis, as well as component of bones and teeth and reproductive cancers.

Diagnostic Testing

Laboratory assessment in the obese patient should aim to assess comorbidities and rule out secondary causes, if suspected. At minimum, laboratory assessment should include a fasting lipid panel and fasting blood glucose in addition to blood pressure monitoring.

TREATMENT

Lifestyle changes (diet and exercise) are the cornerstones of weight loss, though medications and bariatric surgery can be considered when diet and exercise fail in certain populations. Treatment decisions must take into account each patient's readiness for change (motivation, stress levels, time availability) and barriers to change.

Medications

- Indications for medical therapy include:
  - BMI >30 kg/m^2 or BMI >27 kg/m^2 with concomitant obesity-related risk factors or diseases
  - Unable to achieve weight loss goal despite therapeutic lifestyle changes
  - No contraindications to use
- Weight loss medications are meant to be used as an **adjunct to and not as a substitute for therapeutic lifestyle changes**.
- They should be discontinued if the patient has not responded within 1 to 2 months.
- The use of such a medication should be considered long term (if not lifelong) in patients who respond, as patients will regain weight quickly if the drug is stopped.
- Medications approved for short-term use (phentermine, diethylpropion, benzphetamine, phendimetrazine) are not typically used because of their limitations on duration of use and addictive properties and will not be discussed further here.

Orlistat
- Orlistat works by inhibiting pancreatic lipase and reduces the absorption of fat by 30% at recommended doses.
- Studies have shown that patients who take orlistat and make therapeutic lifestyle changes will lose about 4% more weight than patients making therapeutic lifestyle changes alone.[4]
- Contraindicated in patients with malabsorption syndromes.
- Side effects include diarrhea, bowel incontinence, flatulence, and oily spotting.
- Interferes with absorption of fat-soluble vitamins, and a multivitamin should be taken to prevent deficiency.
- Costs approximately $2,600 per year of treatment at recommended doses.

- A half-strength over-the-counter version of orlistat is available under the trade name Alli.
  - It inhibits fat absorption by 25% as compared with 30% for full-strength orlistat.
  - Side effects are the same as for full-strength orlistat and are still significant despite the reduced dose.
  - Costs approximately $500 to $700 per year.

Lorcaserin
- Lorcaserin was approved by the FDA in June 2012.
- It selectively activates 5-HT$_2$C receptors and thought to centrally act to increase satiety by acting on anorexigenic proopiomelanocortin neurons in the hypothalamus.
- Studies have shown that patients who take lorcaserin and make therapeutic lifestyle changes lose ≥5% of their body weight compared to patients making therapeutic lifestyle changes alone, and lorcaserin also helps manage the weight loss for up to 2 years.[5-8]
- Contraindicated in pregnant patients.
- Side effects include headache, upper respiratory infections, nasopharyngitis, dizziness, nausea, vomiting, and diarrhea.

Phentermine/topiramate
- This combination was approved by the FDA in July 2012.
- Phentermine is a sympathomimetic substance that is thought to suppress appetite by releasing norepinephrine in the hypothalamus, resulting in increased serum leptin levels.
- Topiramate is thought to suppress appetite by augmenting GABA channels.
- Studies have shown phentermine/topiramate to increase the number of patients able to achieve and maintain >5% and >10% weight loss over placebo.[9-11]
- It is contraindicated in patients who are pregnant and with hyperthyroidism, glaucoma, or patients or have been on monoamine oxidase inhibitors within the previous 14 days.
- Side effects include constipation, dizziness, paraesthesia, and dry mouth.

Surgical Management
- Bariatric surgery is used as an adjunct to and not as a substitute for therapeutic lifestyle changes.
- Indications:
  - BMI >40 kg/m^2 or BMI 35 to 40 kg/m^2 with life-threatening cardiopulmonary disease, severe diabetes, or lifestyle impairment
  - Failure to achieve weight loss with other treatment modalities
- Contraindications:
  - History of medical noncompliance
  - Psychiatric illness
  - High risk of death during the procedure
- Requires involvement of a team of medical, surgical, psychiatric, and nutrition experts.
- Most common current techniques include laparoscopic adjustable gastric banding and Roux-en-Y gastric bypass; less common techniques include biliopancreatic diversion and biliopancreatic diversion with duodenal switch.
- Patients should be aware of multiple complications and risks associated with the procedure. Complication rates are lower at centers with more experience.

Lifestyle/Risk Modification
- **Decreasing caloric intake**
  - Set small goals and start with one or two small changes that the patient agrees to.
  - Recommend substitutions (e.g., baked potato instead of french fries).
  - Encourage more low-calorie foods at meals and for snacks.
  - Recommend eating regular meals.
  - Do not deny patients their favorite foods, but stress the importance of portion control.
  - Discuss triggers to eating.
  - Consider referral to a nutritionist/dietician.

- **Increasing physical activity**
  - Helps sustain weight loss.[12]
  - Activity should be recorded in an activity diary.
  - Encourage 30 to 60 minutes of moderate physical activity on most days of the week.
  - Encourage activities that your patient enjoys.
  - Incorporate exercise into daily activities (e.g., walking to do nearby errands, ride your bike to work, walk the dog, take the stairs instead of the elevator).

Undernutrition

GENERAL PRINCIPLES

- Undernutrition is a deficiency of one or more nutrients and occurs when nutrient availability fails to meet metabolic requirements. It may result from inadequate nutrient intake, malabsorption, increased metabolic demands, ineffective substrate use, or any combination of these.
- The overall incidence of undernutrition in the US is not well defined but in hospitalized patients may be as high as 40% on admission, with those most undernourished risking further weight loss during the hospital course.[13]
- Undernutrition results in loss of skeletal and cardiac muscle function, impairment of immune function, apathy, depression, and prolonged hospital stays. Death can occur when weight falls to two-thirds of ideal body weight.[14]
- Risk factors for undernutrition include advanced age, chronic medical illnesses, drug-nutrient interactions, low socioeconomic status, and social isolation.

DIAGNOSIS

Clinical Presentation

History
- Obtain a complete diet history.
  - Ask open-ended questions and be nonjudgmental.
  - Have the patient fill out an eating pattern questionnaire (e.g., Eating Pattern Questionnaire from the American Medical Association).[15]
  - Have the patient fill out a food diary for 3 to 7 days (e.g., Food and Activity Diary from the American Medical Association, a Web-based diary developed by the United States Department of Agriculture [USDA] is also available).[2]
- Evaluate for medical and psychiatric illnesses as well as surgical procedures that may affect energy or nutrient intake, absorption, or expenditure.
- Look for medications that may interact with nutrient absorption or stimulate appetite and cause weight gain.
- Screen for family history of conditions such as obesity, diabetes, and hyperlipidemia.
- Evaluate the patient's psychosocial environment and substance abuse (alcoholism) that may predispose to micronutrient deficiencies.
- Review of systems should include screening for changes in weight.

Physical Examination
- Vital signs: blood pressure, heart rate, temperature, height, weight, and a calculation of BMI.
- Physical examination in the malnourished patient should focus on general appearance, skin, hair, nails, mucous membranes, and the neurologic system.
- The evaluating physician should consider factors that affect nutrient intake, absorption, and metabolism (Table 22-9).

TABLE 22-9	Causes of Malnutrition	
Inadequate nutrient intake	**Malabsorption**	**Altered metabolism**
Limited finances	Pancreatic insufficiency	Fever
Ill-fitting dentures	Regional enteritis	Sepsis
Oral ulcers	Celiac disease	Cancer cachexia
Dysphagia	Whipple disease	AIDS wasting syndrome
Gastric ulcer	Gastrectomy	
Pulmonary disease with poor mechanics	Small bowel resection	
Depression	Bariatric surgery	
Anorexia nervosa	Protein-losing enteropathy	

Diagnostic Criteria

• Unintentional weight loss of 10% of body weight in the past 3 months
• BMI <18.5 kg/m^2

Diagnostic Testing

• Laboratory assessment in the malnourished patient may include individual micronutrient levels and evaluation of systemic disease if suspected (e.g., thyroid function, HIV status).
• **Serum albumin** level is not generally recommended, as a depressed level is not specific for malnutrition. It is often depressed in overhydration, acute illness, or chronic liver, renal, or cardiopulmonary disease.[16]

REFERENCES

1. Food and Nutrition Board. Institute of Medicine. Dietary Reference Intake Tables. Available at: http://fnic.nal.usda.gov/dietary-guidance/dietary-reference-intakes/dri-tables, last accessed 1/5/15.
2. ChooseMyPlate.gov. Volume 2013: United States Department of Agriculture, 2012.
3. Hausenloy DJ, Yellon DM. Targeting residual cardiovascular risk: raising high-density lipoprotein cholesterol levels. *Heart* 2008;94:706–714.
4. Padwal R, Li SK, Lau DC. Long-term pharmacotherapy for obesity and overweight. *Cochrane Database Syst Rev* 2003;(3):CD004094.
5. Fidler MC, Sanchez M, Raether B, et al. A one-year randomized trial of lorcaserin for weight loss in obese and overweight adults: the BLOSSOM trial. *J Clin Endocrinol Metab* 2011;96:3067–3077.
6. Martin CK, Redman LM, Zhang J, et al. Lorcaserin, a 5-HT(2C) receptor agonist, reduces body weight by decreasing energy intake without influencing energy expenditure. *J Clin Endocrinol Metab* 2011;96:837–845.
7. O'Neil PM, Smith SR, Weissman NJ, et al. Randomized placebo-controlled clinical trial of lorcaserin for weight loss in type 2 diabetes mellitus: the BLOOM-DM study. *Obesity (Silver Spring)* 2012;20:1426–1436.
8. Smith SR, Weissman NJ, Anderson CM, et al. Multicenter, placebo-controlled trial of lorcaserin for weight management. *N Engl J Med* 2010;363:245–256.
9. Allison DB, Gadde KM, Garvey WT, et al. Controlled-release phentermine/topiramate in severely obese adults: a randomized controlled trial (EQUIP). *Obesity (Silver Spring)* 2012;20:330–342.

10. Gadde KM, Allison DB, Ryan DH, et al. Effects of low-dose, controlled-release, phentermine plus topiramate combination on weight and associated comorbidities in overweight and obese adults (CONQUER): a randomised, placebo-controlled, phase 3 trial. *Lancet* 2011;377:1341–1352.

11. Garvey WT, Ryan DH, Look M, et al. Two-year sustained weight loss and metabolic benefits with controlled-release phentermine/topiramate in obese and overweight adults (SEQUEL): a randomized, placebo-controlled, phase 3 extension study. *Am J Clin Nutr* 2012;95:297–308.

12. Pavlou KN, Krey S, Steffee WP. Exercise as an adjunct to weight loss and maintenance in moderately obese subjects. *Am J Clin Nutr* 1989;49:1115–1123.

13. McWhirter JP, Pennington CR. Incidence and recognition of malnutrition in hospital. *BMJ* 1994;308:945–948.

14. Kotler D, Wang J, Pierson R. Studies of body composition in patients with acquired immunodeficiency syndrome. *The United Nations University Press: Food Nutr Bull* 1989;11:55–60.

15. Eating Pattern Questionnaire: American Medical Association, 2003.

16. Winter TA, O'Keefe SJ, Callanan M, et al. The effect of severe undernutrition and subsequent refeeding on whole-body metabolism and protein synthesis in human subjects. *J Parenter Enteral Nutr* 2005;29:221–228.

23

Laboratory Assessment of Kidney and Urinary Tract Disorders

Nima Naimi and Seth Goldberg

Urinalysis

Urinalysis is an integral part of the evaluation of kidney and urinary tract disease. It consists of two components:

- **Macroscopic examination**. This includes dipstick evaluation, which yields information regarding the physical and chemical properties of a urine sample, whereas microscopy provides for evaluation of formed elements in the urine.
- **Microscopic evaluation**. A microscopic evaluation of urine sediment should be performed in the presence of abnormal renal function, hematuria or proteinuria on macroscopy, or clinical concern for urinary tract infection. This analysis should be done personally instead of relying on the laboratory technologist report.

MACROSCOPIC EXAMINATION OF THE URINE

Specimen Collection and Testing Procedure

- Urine samples should be examined within 2 hours of collection, as urea breakdown into ammonia results in alkaline urine, which promotes cell lysis and cast degradation.
- Ideally, samples should be collected from midstream catch of an early-morning specimen. Alternatively, bladder catheterization, either transurethral or suprapubic, may be used, although it may cause hematuria. There is no proven benefit of cleaning the genitalia prior to the collection.
- First perform dipstick testing to interpret colorimetric reaction results. It is important to assess the color and clarity of urine as well.
- For microscopic evaluation, collect 10 to 15 mL of a freshly voided specimen and centrifuge at 1,500 to 3,000 rpm for 5 minutes. Most of the supernatant is then discarded and the sediment resuspended in the remaining fluid. Remove approximately 0.5 mL of supernatant using a pipette and apply one drop of this solution onto a clean glass slide and cover with a cover slip. View the sample with phase-contrast microscopy at 100× and 400× magnification to examine the formed elements in the urine.

Physical and Chemical Properties of Urine

Color

- Normal urine should appear pale yellow in color. Dilute specimens are lighter in color, and concentrated urine has an amber appearance.
- **Red urine** is seen with hematuria, hemoglobinuria, myoglobinuria, and porphyrinuria. The presence of blood on dipstick testing without red blood cells (RBCs) on microscopy is suggestive of myoglobinuria. Consumption of certain foods (beets, rhubarb, and blackberries) and drugs (phenytoin and rifampin) may also color the urine red.[1]
- **Brown urine** may be seen with fava beans, chloroquine, nitrofurantoin, levodopa, metronidazole or with jaundice.[1]

Clarity
- Normal urine is clear but turns turbid with any urine particles.
- Turbid urine is seen with organisms, cells, and casts in the urine. Urinary tract infections usually produce turbid urine.
- Other causes include hematuria, lipiduria, and metabolic disease (oxaluria, uricosuria).

Odor
- Normal urine does not have a strong odor.
- Foul-smelling urine may be encountered with urinary tract infections due to ammonia production.[1]
- Diabetic ketoacidosis is associated with fruity odor, and gastrointestinal-vesical fistulas may result in a fecal odor to urine.[1]

Specific Gravity
- Specific gravity refers to the relative density of urine with respect to water.
- Normal values range from 1.005 to 1.020.
- Specific gravity ≥ 1.020 is consistent with concentrated urine in the setting of volume depletion; higher values may suggest glycosuria or other osmotically active substances in the urine such as contrast material.[1]
- Values ≤ 1.005 suggest dilute urine, which may be seen in water intoxication and diabetes insipidus.
- A fixed specific gravity of 1.010 is often seen in intrinsic renal disease where the kidneys can neither concentrate nor dilute the urine. As a result, the urine is **isosthenuric** (i.e., it has the same osmolality as serum).
- Proteinuria (>7 g/dL) may cause falsely elevated specific gravity, and falsely decreased values may be seen with urine pH <6.5.

Urine pH
- The normal urine pH ranges from 4.5 to 8.0.
- Acidic urine is associated with metabolic acidosis (e.g., starvation ketosis, diabetic ketoacidosis), dehydration, and large protein loads. Respiratory acidosis can lead to compensatory metabolic alkalosis and decreased urine pH. Extrarenal bicarbonate losses (e.g., diarrhea) may promote urinary acidification.
- Alkaline urine is typically seen in distal renal tubular acidosis. Urea-splitting organisms (e.g., *Proteus* spp.) can raise urinary pH. Similarly, prolonged storage of urine results in conversion of urea to ammonia, and urinary pH increases.

Glucose
- In patients with preserved renal function and **serum glucose concentrations <180 mg/dL**, urine glucose is typically absent as it is almost completely reabsorbed in the proximal tubule.
- Dipstick analysis can provide qualitative information regarding the presence or absence of glycosuria.
- Urine glucose may be seen in diabetes mellitus, liver disease, pancreatic disease, Fanconi syndrome, and Cushing syndrome.

Protein
- Urine dipstick is the main screening test for proteinuria.
- The test is a pH-based assay, and **albumin is the primary protein identified**.
- False-positive results may be seen with highly concentrated specimens, alkaline urine, phenazopyridine, or quaternary ammonia compounds. False-negative tests are associated with dilute urine and nonalbumin proteins, including immunoglobulins and tubular proteins.
- A sulfosalicylic acid test may be used to identify nonalbumin proteins.

- If the dipstick test is positive, the protein should be measured using either a 24-hour protein excretion or a random protein-to-creatinine ratio (PCR) if the creatinine is at a stable baseline.

Hemoglobin
- The dipstick can detect **as few as four RBCs per high-power microscopic field** (HPF).
- **Free hemoglobin or myoglobin in urine**, as can be seen with hemolysis or rhabdomyolysis, catalyzes the same dipstick reaction. These conditions should be suspected when the urine dipstick is positive for occult blood in the absence of RBCs on microscopic examination of the urine sediment.
- False-negative tests result from the presence of substances such as ascorbic acid (ingestion of >200 mg/day vitamin C) that diminish the oxidizing potential of the reagent strip.
- Detection of hematuria by dipstick should always be confirmed by microscopic examination of the urine. The presence of dysmorphic RBCs or RBC casts (a so-called active urine sediment) or the coexistence of proteinuria suggests that the hematuria is of glomerular origin.

Leukocyte Esterase
- The detection of leukocyte esterase relies on the release of **esterases from lysed neutrophils**.
- False-positive results are seen when significant delay occurs between sampling and testing and when the sample is contaminated by vaginal cells.
- False-negative results occur with inhibition of granulocyte function, including glycosuria, proteinuria, high specific gravity, and high urinary concentrations of certain antibiotics (tetracycline, cephalexin, gentamicin).

Urine Nitrite
- Urine dipstick testing depends on **bacterial conversion of urinary nitrates into nitrite**.[1]
- While many gram-negative bacteria can reduce nitrates to nitrite, certain organisms, including *Enterococcus* spp., *Neisseria gonorrhoeae*, *Pseudomonas*, and mycobacteria, do not; this may result in negative results.
- False-negative results are also seen with insufficient bladder incubation time, low consumption of nitrates (found in vegetables), and reduction of nitrates to nitrogen by bacteria.
- The test has **low sensitivity but high specificity**.
- Both leukocyte esterase and nitrite testing must be combined with microscopic examination and clinical context to accurately diagnose urinary tract infections.

MICROSCOPIC EXAMINATION OF URINE

Red Blood Cells
- Presence of three or more RBCs/HPF on two of three urine specimens is diagnostic of microscopic hematuria.[1]
- **Dysmorphic RBCs** and RBC casts are suggestive of glomerular disease, whereas normal RBCs suggest nonglomerular bleeding in the urinary tract.
- Hematuria is discussed in further detail in Chapter 25.

White Blood Cells
- Urinary white blood cells (WBCs) are associated with either infection or inflammation.
- **Pyuria** is defined as more than five WBCs/HPF.
- Extraurinary inflammation, as seen in appendicitis, can also result in pyuria.
- Urine **eosinophils** may be seen in allergic interstitial nephritis, but this finding is neither sensitive nor specific. Urine eosinophils are also present with parasitic infection of the urinary tract (e.g., schistosomiasis), cholesterol emboli, chronic pyelonephritis, and prostatitis. Eosinophiluria is identified with Hansel staining of the urine.

Epithelial Cells

- Various types of epithelial cells are commonly encountered on urine microscopy.
- **Squamous epithelial cells** are large, flat cells with central nuclei; they are found in the distal urinary tract and are almost always contaminants.
- **Transitional epithelial cells** are small, pear-shaped cells lining the bladder and ureters. They may be seen after bladder catheterization but are also found in genitourinary malignancy.
- **Renal tubular epithelial cells** are notable for large nuclei; their presence suggests renal tubular injury.
- **Oval fat bodies** are lipid-laden renal epithelial cells. They are identified by the presence of a Maltese cross appearance on polarized light microscopy. Their presence is suggestive of nephrotic syndrome.

Casts

- Casts form when cells or other intraluminal debris (e.g., lipids, bacteria) are trapped within the **tubular protein matrix (Tamm-Horsfall protein)**. They often take the shape of the tubular lumen and represent a snapshot of the intraluminal environment.
- **Hyaline casts** are formed by Tamm-Horsfall proteins secreted by tubular epithelium into the tubular lumen. Tamm-Horsfall proteins accumulate into casts under states of volume depletion or acidic urine but may also occur in normal urine.
- **Granular casts** are formed by Tamm-Horsfall proteins and products of cellular break-down. Muddy brown granular casts may be seen in any renal disease, but in the right clinical context, they suggest a diagnosis of acute tubular necrosis (debris from tubular epithelial cell destruction).
- **RBC casts** are easily identified as tubular, orange-red structures on light microscopy. Their presence indicates glomerular hematuria.
- **WBC casts** consist of WBCs and tubular proteins trapped in the tubular lumen. These are seen with interstitial inflammation, including pyelonephritis, acute interstitial nephritis, and occasionally with glomerulonephritis.
- **Waxy casts** are formed from the degradation of other casts. They are smooth, well-defined structures visible without polarized light. Waxy casts are mainly seen in chronic kidney disease (CKD).
- **Fatty casts** are characterized by Maltese crosses visible under polarized light. Fatty casts are seen with ethylene glycol poisoning and nephrotic syndrome.

Organisms

- Bacteriuria is frequently encountered, as many urine specimens are not collected under sterile conditions. The clinical context of this finding aids in determining the presence of infection.
- Common bacterial causes of urinary tract infection include *E. coli*, *Staphylococcus saprophyticus* (especially in menstruating females), *Proteus mirabilis*, *Enterococcus* spp., group B *Streptococcus*, and other gram-negative bacillus infections (e.g., *Klebsiella* spp., *Citrobacter* spp., and *Pseudomonas* spp.).
- *Candida* spp. are frequently seen as contaminants from genital secretions or indwelling Foley catheter colonization.

Crystals

- A discussion of pathologic urinary crystals and nephrolithiasis may be found in Chapter 25.
- Acidic urine can result in precipitation of calcium oxalate or uric acid.
- Alkaline urine can result in precipitation of calcium phosphate or struvite (triple phosphate).
- Crystals may form from precipitation of drugs and drug metabolites (e.g., sulfadiazine, amoxicillin, ciprofloxacin, acyclovir, indinavir).

Assessment of Renal Function

ESTIMATION OF GFR

- Kidney function is best assessed by the glomerular filtration rate (GFR). The gold standard to measure GFR is infusion of an exogenous marker such as inulin; however, this technique is too cumbersome for clinical practice and thus only used for research purposes.
- Alternatively, the GFR can be estimated using creatinine-based equations or a 24-hour creatinine clearance. This estimation of GFR is accurate only if the serum creatinine (S_{Cr}) is stable and in steady state.

CREATININE AS A MARKER OF RENAL FUNCTION

- Creatinine is a metabolite of skeletal muscle and dietary meat that is freely filtered at the glomerulus and undergoes no significant tubular reabsorption. It is secreted to a small degree by the renal tubules into the urine. Its production is relative to an individual's muscle mass.
- Aging and weight loss contribute to reduced creatinine production rates.
- In patients with normal renal function, most of the creatinine elimination occurs by glomerular filtration. As renal function declines, creatinine elimination by tubular secretion may exceed filtration. Subsequently, **estimates of renal function based on creatinine overestimate actual GFR with worsening renal function**.
- Several medications are known to increase serum creatinine (S_{Cr}) by either inhibiting the secretion (trimethoprim, cimetidine) or increasing the production (fenofibrate).
- S_{Cr} varies inversely with GFR. Any elevation of S_{Cr} above the normal range (0.6 to 1.2 mg/dL) should alert the physician to the presence of reduced GFR and renal insufficiency.
- **Changes in plasma creatinine are not linearly related to renal function**. For example, an increase in creatinine from 1.0 to 1.5 signifies a greater decline in renal function than an increase from 2.0 to 2.5.
- Because S_{Cr} is a function of muscle mass and is dependent on age, gender, race, and size, it can often be difficult to assess the degree of renal impairment from S_{Cr} alone. Therefore, the following equations should be used to estimate the GFR.

THE COCKCROFT-GAULT CRCL FORMULA

- CrCl (mL/minute) = [(140 - age) × lean body weight (kg) × (0.85 if female)]/(72 × S_{Cr}).
- The Cockcroft-Gault formula was derived from studies on adult inpatient male patients. Problems with this formula include estimation of lean body weight and **overestimation of true GFR with worsening renal function**.[2]
- It takes age, ideal body weight, and gender into account to estimate GFR from a measurement of S_{Cr}.
- This formula estimates CrCl in mL/minute (normal, 100 to 125 mL/minute for males and 85 to 100 mL/minute for females).
- This rapid estimation of GFR is useful in adjustment of drug dosages for decreased renal function based on S_{Cr}.

THE MODIFICATION OF DIET IN RENAL DISEASE EQUATIONS

- GFR = $186 \times S_{Cr}^{-1.154} \times age^{-0.203} \times$ (1.210 if black) × (0.742 if female).
- The modification of diet in renal disease equation (MDRD) was developed in a mostly white outpatient CKD population. In patients with GFR <60 mL/minute/1.73 m^2, the equation accurately estimates renal function.[3] However, the MDRD is less reliable in patients with normal renal function as it underestimates the GFR.

- The MDRD cannot be generalized in patients with diabetes, patients >70 years of age, and nonwhite patients.
- The abbreviated equation uses age, serum creatinine, gender, and race.

CHRONIC KIDNEY DISEASE EPIDEMIOLOGY COLLABORATION EQUATION

- GFR $= 141 \times \min(S_{Cr}/\kappa,1)^{\alpha} \times \max(S_{Cr}/\kappa,1)^{-1.209} \times 0.993^{Age} \times (1.018 \text{ if female}) \times (1.159 \text{ if black})$, where κ is 0.7 for females and 0.9 for males, α is -0.329 for females and -0.411 for males, min indicates the minimum of S_{Cr}/κ or 1, and max indicates the maximum of S_{Cr}/κ or 1.[4]
- The Chronic Kidney Disease Epidemiology Collaboration Equation (CKD-EPI) was developed in an effort to create a more generalizable equation than the MDRD.
- It has been studied in a much larger and diverse population than the other two equations.
- In comparison studies with the MDRD, the CKD-EPI has been shown to be more generalizable, more accurate in estimating GFR, and more accurate in assessing prognosis.
- Current Kidney Disease Improving Global Outcomes (KDIGO) guidelines recommend the CKD-EPI equation for evaluation of CKD.

TWENTY-FOUR–HOUR URINE COLLECTION FOR CrCl

- A 24-hour urine CrCl is preferable to the above equations in extremes of age and weight, pregnancy, individuals with normal GFR, and malnutrition.
- Patients should be instructed to discard their first morning urine and then begin the 24-hour urine collection, ending the collection with inclusion of the following morning's first void.
- The amount of total creatinine in the collection can be used to assess the adequacy of the collection; an adequate 24-hour urine collection contains 15 to 20 mg/kg creatinine for females and 20 to 25 mg/kg for males.
- Accuracy may be altered by incorrect collection of the urinary specimen or hypersecretion of creatinine in advanced kidney disease.

CYSTATIN C

- Cystatin C is a low molecular weight protein that is part of the cysteine protease inhibitor family. It is produced at a constant rate by all nucleated cells and freely filtered by the glomerulus. Once in the proximal tubules, it is catabolized by the epithelial cells. Therefore, it cannot be used to measure clearance.
- Because it is **not secreted** in the tubules and is less affected by muscle mass and diet, cystatin C was thought to be a better marker to estimate GFR than creatinine. Many factors, however, have been found to affect its level, such as adiposity, diabetes, and inflammation.
- Equations that use cystatin C are not more accurate than creatinine-based estimates of GFR.
- **The most accurate estimation of GFR is obtained when using an equation that combines both cystatin C and creatinine**, especially around a GFR of 60 mL/minute/1.73 m².[5]

Proteinuria

GENERAL PRINCIPLES

- Patients with normal renal function excrete <150 mg of total protein or <30 mg of albumin in 24 hours.

- Proteinuria is defined as **protein excretion of >150 mg/day**, while nephrotic syndrome is defined as protein excretion >3.5 g/day associated with hypoalbuminemia, edema, lipiduria, and hyperlipidemia. Nephrotic-range proteinuria refers to urine protein excretion >3.5 g/day without the other findings.
- Albuminuria is now used to further classify the level of CKD as it is a marker of severity and is associated with progression of kidney disease.[6]
- **Treatment of proteinuria may slow progression of kidney disease and reduce the risk of cardiovascular disease**.
- If proteinuria is detected on a dipstick test, the test should be repeated after at least a week to rule out transient proteinuria. If the repeat test is negative, no further workup is needed.
- Transient proteinuria (usually <1 g/day) can occur with fever, emotional stress, heavy physical exercise, urinary tract infection, or acute medical illness.
- Orthostatic proteinuria should also be ruled out. It is defined by an elevated protein excretion in the upright position, which normalizes while the patient is supine. The diagnosis is usually made in patients younger than 30 and carries no increased risk of kidney disease. A normal first-void PCR may effectively rule out the diagnosis.
- Once proteinuria is confirmed, it should be quantified.
- Patients with persistent albuminuria (>300 mg/day) or proteinuria (>500 mg/day) should be referred to a nephrologist. In cases of unexplained proteinuria or hematuria, a biopsy is usually required to make a definitive diagnosis and to initiate disease-specific therapy.

DIAGNOSIS

Clinical Presentation

- Focus on signs and symptoms of conditions associated with proteinuria, such as hypertension, diabetes mellitus, or connective tissue diseases.
- All medications should be reviewed (prescription, illicit, over the counter, herbal). Nonsteroidal anti-inflammatory drugs (NSAIDs) are associated with a variety of renal diseases and should be discontinued in the presence of proteinuria pending further evaluation.
- Clinical features of malignancies, especially multiple myeloma and lymphoma, should be sought. Furthermore, solid organ malignancies are associated with glomerulonephritis.
- Findings consistent with infections, such as HIV, viral hepatitis, and bacterial endocarditis, should be evaluated, as all these can cause glomerular disease.
- A complete family history should be obtained.

Diagnostic Testing

Urine Reagent Strip

- The urine reagent dipstick is frequently used as the initial screening test for proteinuria as it is quick and inexpensive. It detects albumin at concentrations >10 to 20 mg/dL, which equates to approximately 300 to 500 mg of protein in 24 hours.
- The test is only semiquantitative, has low sensitivity for nonalbumin proteins (e.g., light chains of multiple myeloma), has variability among different manufacturers, and is dependent on hydration.[6]
- False positives can occur within 24 hours of iodinated radiocontrast infusion or with high urine pH.
- Any patient with persistent proteinuria should undergo a quantification study.

Twenty-Four–Hour Urine Collection for Protein

- The 24-hour urine collection, when obtained correctly, remains the reference point to accurately quantify the amount of daily protein excretion in the urine.
- Concurrent collection of urine creatinine should also be done to ensure the completeness of the collection.

- Although the gold standard, this test is cumbersome for patients and frequently leads to an inaccurate/incomplete urine collection.

Spot Urine Albumin-to-Creatinine or Protein-to-Creatinine Ratio
- The latest KDIGO guidelines recommend using the albumin to creatinine ratio (ACR) as the initial testing for proteinuria in CKD.[7] ACR is preferred over PCR as it is more sensitive for kidney disease in CKD. PCR should still be used in certain cases, such as inpatients with monoclonal gammopathies.
- These tests use a random spot urine sample for protein or albumin (mg/dL) and creatinine (mg/dL) concentrations to calculate a unitless ratio. The creatinine must be at a stable baseline. For best results, an early-morning urine sample should be used.
- ACR of 30 to 300 mg/g is referred to as **moderately increased** (formerly micro-albuminuria) and ACR >300 mg/g is referred to as **severely increased** (formerly macroalbuminuria).
- The results can be unreliable in patients at either extremes of muscle mass. Also, the amount of proteinuria varies throughout the day, being higher during the day than at night.

Other Laboratories
- Urine sediment should be carefully examined for other signs of glomerular disease, such as dysmorphic RBCs, RBC casts, and oval fat bodies.
- Obtain a complete blood count (CBC), basic metabolic profile (BMP) with GFR estimation, albumin, and quantification of the protein with either a spot urine or 24-hour collection.
- If multiple myeloma is considered, a urine and serum protein electrophoresis with immu-nofixation and serum free light chains should be ordered.
- If a connective tissue disease or vasculitis is suspected, a complete autoimmune workup is required (Chapter 24).

Imaging
A renal ultrasound should also be obtained to assess the renal and urinary tract architecture. The finding of symmetrically small kidneys (<10 cm) suggests CKD. Notable exceptions include the kidneys of diabetic nephropathy, HIV-associated nephropathy, polycystic kidney disease, and deposition disorders, in which the kidneys may be enlarged.

REFERENCES

1. Simerville JA, Maxted WC, Pahira JJ. Urinalysis: a comprehensive review. *Am Fam Physician* 2005;71:1153–1162.
2. Poggio ED, Wang X, Greene T, et al. Performance of the modification of diet in renal disease and Cockcroft-Gault equations in the estimation of GFR in health and in chronic kidney disease. *J Am Soc Nephrol* 2005;16:459–466.
3. Levey AS, Bosch JP, Lewis JB, et al. A more accurate method to estimate glomerular filtration rate from serum creatinine: a new prediction equation. Modification of Diet in Renal Disease Study Group. *Ann Intern Med* 1999;130:461–470.
4. Madero M, Sarnak MJ. Creatinine-based formulae for estimating glomerular filtration rate: is it time to change to chronic kidney disease epidemiology collaboration equation? *Curr Opin Nephrol Hypertens* 2011;20:622–630.
5. Inker LA, Schmid CH, Tighiouart H, et al. Estimating glomerular filtration rate from serum creatinine and cystatin C. *N Engl J Med* 2012;367:20–29.
6. Lamb EJ, MacKenzie F, Stevens PE. How should proteinuria be detected and measured? *Ann Clin Biochem* 2009;46:205–217.
7. Kidney Disease: Improving Global Outcomes (KDIGO) CKD Work Group. KDIGO 2012 clinical practice guideline for the evaluation and management of chronic kidney disease. *Kidney Int Suppl* 2013;3:1–150.

Acute Kidney Injury

GENERAL PRINCIPLES

- Acute kidney injury (AKI) is a clinical syndrome denoted by an abrupt decline (within 48 hours) in glomerular filtration rate (GFR) sufficient to decrease the elimination of nitrogenous waste products (urea and creatinine) and other uremic toxins.[1]
- Clinically, AKI is often further divided into oliguric or nonoliguric subtypes based on urine flow (500 mL/day or 0.5 mL/kg/hour for 6 hours).[2]
- AKI is generally a disease of the hospitalized patient with approximately 13% of all hospitalized patients meeting the diagnostic criteria for AKI.[3]
- AKI needs to be quickly recognized and the underlying etiology determined.

Etiology and Pathophysiology

Prerenal Azotemia

- Prerenal azotemia refers to conditions that lead to impaired renal perfusion with a resultant fall in glomerular capillary filtration pressure. The renal parenchymal function is generally preserved.
- The most common scenario of diminished renal perfusion is in the setting of **reduced effective circulating volume**, which results in concentrated urine (urine osmolality >500 mOsm/kg) with low urine sodium (<10 mmol/L). Causes include true hypovolemia, decreased cardiac output, and liver cirrhosis.
- However, **preferential renal vasoconstriction** may lead to a prerenal state in certain situations, even with normal or elevated systemic blood pressure (BP), including NSAIDs and calcineurin inhibitors (e.g., cyclosporine and tacrolimus).
- **Radiocontrast agents**, which typically occur in patients with underlying renal impairment. Other **risk factors** include diabetic nephropathy, advanced age (>75 years), heart failure, volume depletion, high or repetitive doses of radiocontrast agent, and high osmolar contrast agents.[4] **Prophylactic measures** include temporarily holding diuretics and administering saline-based fluids.
- **Endotoxin** associated with bacterial infection is also associated with prerenal AKI.

Intrinsic Renal Causes of Acute Renal Kidney Injury

- The most common cause of AKI due to intrinsic renal disease is acute tubular necrosis (ATN).
  - Common causes of ATN are listed in Table 24-1.
  - ATN is usually considered to be due to ischemic or nephrotoxic injury.[5,6]
  - The most important toxic materials that lead to ATN are drugs.[7]
- Other important disease processes such as glomerular disease, acute interstitial nephritis, and small vessel disease (e.g., vasculitis and renal atheroembolism) may also lead to AKI.

Postrenal Failure

- Ureteral obstruction (e.g., calculus, tumor, clot, sloughed papillae, and external compression)
- Bladder outlet obstruction (e.g., prostatic hypertrophy, neurogenic bladder, carcinoma, and urethral stricture)

TABLE 24-1	Some Causes of Toxic Acute Tubular Necrosis

Exogenous toxins	Endogenous toxins
Drugs (e.g., gentamicin, amphotericin B, acyclovir)	Hemoglobin and myoglobin
Recreational drugs (e.g., cocaine, phencyclidine [PCP], amphetamine)	Uric acid
Radiocontrast	Immunoglobulin light chains
Toxic chemicals (e.g., ethylene glycol, carbon tetrachloride)	
Biologic poisonous material (e.g., snake venom)	

DIAGNOSIS

Clinical Presentation

History
- **Urine history**
  - Establish urine volume and recent trends.
  - Elicit any history of hematuria, proteinuria, dysuria, or pyuria.
  - Urgency, frequency, dribbling, and incontinence, especially in elderly men, may direct to prostatic disease.
- **Drug history**
  - Look for nephrotoxins such as NSAIDs, angiotensin-converting enzyme (ACE) inhibitors, angiotensin receptor blockers (ARBs), aminoglycosides, or radiocontrast agents.
  - The history should include over-the-counter formulations and herbal remedies or recreational drugs.
- **Volume status**
  - History of thirst or orthostatic lightheadedness may suggest intravascular depletion.
  - Weight gain, ankle swelling, orthopnea, or paroxysmal nocturnal dyspnea may signify fluid retention.
  - Look for the possible causes of **fluid loss.**
    - Gastrointestinal: diarrhea, vomiting, and prolonged nasogastric drainage
    - Renal: diuretics and osmotic diuresis in hyperglycemia or hypercalcemia
    - Dermal: burns and extensive sweating
    - Third spacing: acute pancreatitis, ascites, and muscle trauma
- Other potential causes
  - Chronic liver disease may cause **hepatorenal syndrome**.
  - Hepatitis C with purpura may suggest cryoglobulinemia.
  - Arthralgias, skin rash, and oral ulcers may suggest a connective tissue disorder.
  - Sinusitis, cough, and hemoptysis may alert the physician to the possibility of granulomatosis with polyangiitis (formerly Wegener granulomatosis) or Goodpasture syndrome.
  - A history of recent sore throat or significant skin infection may suggest acute poststreptococcal glomerulonephritis.
  - Low back pain and anemia may suggest multiple myeloma.
  - Myalgias, dark-colored urine, and the appropriate clinical scenario (crush injury, exercise, immobilization) may suggest rhabdomyolysis.

Physical Examination
- Orthostatic vital signs, mucous membrane and skin turgor, and examination of jugular veins can assess the patient's fluid balance. Looking for sacral edema in a supinepositioned patient is also important.

- The presence of an S3, pulmonary crackles, and pitting edema suggests volume overload.
- The presence of an abdominal bruit suggests renovascular disease.
- Pelvic examination in females and rectal examination in both females and males may detect a cause of postrenal obstruction.
- The kidney can be palpable in cases of hydronephrosis or polycystic kidney disease.

Diagnostic Testing

Laboratories

- Routine **urinalysis and microscopic analysis** of urine should always be done and are often helpful in determining the cause of AKI. Usually, the urine is bland in prerenal and uncomplicated postrenal AKI, while an abnormal urinalysis and active sediment suggest an intrinsic renal cause.
  - Prerenal AKI: usually bland, with occasional hyaline casts
  - ATN: muddy brown granular casts, epithelial cells, and epithelial cell casts
  - Glomerulonephritis: dysmorphic red blood cells (RBCs) and RBC casts
  - Acute interstitial nephritis: eosinophils, other white blood cells (WBCs), and WBC casts
- In prerenal states, tubular function is intact, and the kidney avidly retains sodium, usually resulting in low urine sodium and a **fractional excretion of sodium (FE_{Na})** of <1%. FE_{Na} is particularly helpful in oliguric AKI (Table 24-2).

$$FE_{Na} = \left[\left(U_{Na} \times P_{Cr} \right) / \left(P_{Na} \times U_{Cr} \right) \right] \times 100$$

where U = urine, P = plasma, Na = sodium, and Cr = creatinine.

- Because loop diuretics force natriuresis, calculation of FE_{Na} is misleading in patients who are taking these agents. The **fractional excretion of urea (FE_{urea})** of <30% to 35% is suggestive of prerenal azotemia (Table 24-2).

$$FE_{urea} = \left[\left(U_{urea} \times P_{Cr} \right) / \left(BUN \times U_{Cr} \right) \right] \times 100$$

where U_{urea} = urine urea, P = plasma, BUN = blood urea nitrogen (mg/dL), and Cr = creatinine.

Imaging

- Ultrasonography exhibits high sensitivity (90% to 98%) but a lower specificity (65% to 84%) for the detection of urinary tract obstruction.[5] It can also measure the echotexture (increased echogenicity suggests more chronic damage) and kidney size (a marked difference may suggest renovascular disease).
- Compared with renal ultrasonography, **noncontrast CT** is superior in the evaluation of ureteral obstruction since it can define the level of obstruction and demarcate retroperitoneal fibrosis or a retroperitoneal mass.

TABLE 24-2	Laboratory Tests in the Differentiation of Oliguric Prerenal Azotemia from Oliguric Intrinsic Acute Tubular Necrosis				
Diagnosis	Plasma BUN/Cr	U_{Na}	FE_{Na} (%)	U_{osm}	U/P_{Cr}
Prerenal azotemia	>20	<20	<1	>500	>40
Oliguric ATN	<10–15	>40	>1	<350	<20

FE_{Na}, fractional excretion of sodium; Plasma BUN/Cr, plasma blood urea nitrogen to creatinine ratio; U_{Na}, urine sodium concentration; U_{osm}, urine osmolality; U/P_{Cr}, urine to plasma creatinine ratio.

Diagnostic Procedures

Renal biopsy is reserved for patients in whom the cause of intrinsic AKI is unclear or in cases of unexplained proteinuria or hematuria where immunosuppressive therapy is being considered.

TREATMENT

Nondialytic Therapy

- **Volume expansion**: Prompt and effective restoration of effective circulating volume is the key in prerenal azotemia due to true hypovolemia.
- **Avoidance of nephrotoxins**: Contrast media should be avoided when possible. ACE inhibitors, ARBs, diuretics, and NSAIDs should be held when there is a sudden decline in renal function.
- **Electrolyte management**: Hyperkalemia is a potentially lethal complication of AKI. Hyperphosphatemia and hypocalcemia are also common in AKI.
  - Rule out pseudohyperkalemia by repeating a whole-blood potassium. Consider drawing the sample without the use of a tourniquet or fist clenching.
  - If the patient has thrombocytosis or marked leukocytosis, the sample may be drawn in a heparinized tube.
  - Obtain a stat ECG and arterial blood gases (ABG) if acidosis is a concern.
  - Review the patient's medication list and stop all exogenous K^+ and potentially offending drugs.
  - **Acute treatment** is necessary for severe hyperkalemia.
  - **Calcium gluconate** 10%, 10 mL IV over 2 to 3 minutes, decreases cardiac membrane excitability but does not alter the potassium concentration. The effect occurs in minutes but lasts only 30 to 60 minutes. It can be repeated after 5 to 10 minutes if the ECG does not change. Use with extreme caution in patients receiving digoxin.
  - **Insulin**, 10 units of regular insulin IV, causes an intracellular shift of K^+ in 10 to 30 minutes. The effect lasts for several hours. **Glucose, 50 g IV (2 ampules D50), should be administered concurrently to prevent hypoglycemia.**
  - **β_2-Adrenergic agonists** can be used to cause an intracellular shift of K^+.
  - **Diuretics** (e.g., furosemide 40 to 120 mg IV) enhance K^+ excretion provided renal function is adequate.
  - **Cation exchange resins** (sodium polystyrene sulfonate, Kayexalate) enhance K^+ excretion from the gastrointestinal tract. Kayexalate may be given PO (15 to 30 g) or as a retention enema (30 to 50 g). The effect may not be evident for several hours and lasts 4 to 6 hours. Doses may be repeated every 4 to 6 hours as needed. The oral preparation is preferred given reports of intestinal necrosis in select patients after rectal administration.
  - **$NaHCO_3$**, 1 ampule (50 mEq) IV, can also be used to cause an intracellular shift of K^+, and the effect can last several hours. Its effect is minimal in organic acidoses. Patients with end-stage renal disease (ESRD) seldom respond and may not tolerate the Na^+ load.
  - **Dialysis** may be necessary for severe hyperkalemia when other measures are ineffective and for patients with renal failure.
- **Acid-base disorders**: Metabolic acidosis is a common complication of AKI. If severe, alkali therapy may be required.
  - Severe acidosis (pH < 7.20) may require treatment with parenteral $NaHCO_3$. Rapid infusion should be considered only for very severe acidosis.
  - The bicarbonate deficit may be estimated as follows:

$$\left[HCO_3^-\right] \text{ deficit } (mEq/L) = \left[0.5 \times \text{body weight } (kg)\right] \times \left(24 - \text{measured } \left[HCO_3^-\right]\right)$$

  - Overaggressive correction should be avoided to prevent overshoot alkalosis.
  - Hypernatremia and fluid overload can occur with $NaHCO_3$ administration.
  - Serum electrolytes, including calcium, should be followed closely.

- **Nutrition support** is an important facet of conservative care.
- Treatment for specific causes of AKI
  - Immunosuppressive agents for glomerulonephritis or vasculitis
  - Systemic anticoagulation for renal artery or vein thrombosis
  - Plasmapheresis for hemolytic-uremic syndrome (HUS)/thrombotic thrombocytopenic purpura

Dialytic Therapy for Acute Renal Failure

Indications for initiation of dialytic support in acute renal failure include the following:

- Severe hyperkalemia, metabolic acidosis, or volume overload refractory to medical therapy
- Uremic syndrome with uremic pericarditis, encephalopathy, or seizures
- Need to start total parental nutrition (volume/solute issues)
- Overdose/intoxications
- Refractory hypercalcemia
- Refractory hyperuricemia

Glomerulopathy

GENERAL PRINCIPLES

- Glomerular diseases are manifestations of primary kidney pathology or representations of kidney involvement of a multisystem disease.
- The etiology of many glomerular diseases remains unknown.
- Glomerular disease may be asymptomatic and found on routine patient evaluation for systemic diseases or in patients noted to have hypertension (HTN), edema, proteinuria, and/or hematuria (Fig. 24-1).[1]

DIAGNOSIS

Clinical Presentation

- The presentation of some glomerulopathies can be **asymptomatic**.
  - **Isolated proteinuria**: A daily protein excretion of >150 mg is abnormal. When proteinuria exceeds 3.5 g/day, it is termed nephrotic range and is highly likely to be caused by

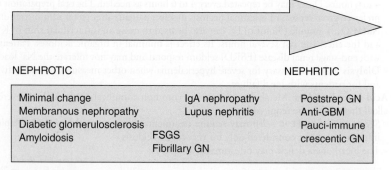

NEPHROTIC   **NEPHRITIC**

Minimal change	IgA nephropathy	Poststrep GN
Membranous nephropathy	Lupus nephritis	Anti-GBM
Diabetic glomerulosclerosis		Pauci-immune
Amyloidosis	FSGS	crescentic GN
	Fibrillary GN	

Figure 24-1 **Spectrum of glomerular diseases with nephrotic and nephritic features.** FSGS, focal segmental glomerulosclerosis; GBM, glomerular basement membrane; GN, glomerulonephritis; strep, streptococcal. (From Khalid SA. Overview and approach to the patient with glomerular disease. In: Cheng S, Vijayan A, eds. *The Washington Manual Nephrology Subspecialty Consult*, 3rd ed. Philadelphia, PA: Lippincott Williams & Wilkins; 2012:192.)

a glomerular lesion. **Microalbuminuria** is excretion of 30 to 300 mg albumin per day and is not typically detected on routine urine dipstick. This test is commonly used in diabetic subjects to help identify patients at risk of developing nephropathy.
- **Isolated hematuria** is classified as either microscopic, referring to more than two RBCs per high power field (HPF) in spun urine, or macroscopic, referring to visible **tea-colored** (brown/red) urine. In patients with glomerular disease, macroscopic hematuria is usually not associated with pain. The presence of dysmorphic RBCs and/or RBC casts in the urine sediment would be highly suggestive of a glomerular source of hematuria.
- The presence of **proteinuria with hematuria** is a stronger indicator of an underlying glomerular disease process.
- The **nephritic syndrome** presents with **proteinuria <3.5 g/day, edema, hematuria with dysmorphic RBC and/or casts**, renal failure with or without oliguria, and HTN.
- The **nephrotic syndrome** is characterized by presence of **proteinuria >3.5 g/day, hypo-albuminemia <3.5 g/dL, hyperlipidemia, lipiduria, and edema**. It is associated with an increased risk of:
  - **Atherosclerosis** and hyperlipidemia.
  - Thromboembolic events due to underlying **hypercoagulability** secondary to urinary loss of antithrombotic proteins, including proteins C and S, and antithrombin III. Venous thromboembolic disease is more common than arterial thrombosis.
  - **Infection** due to urinary loss of immunoglobulins.
- Rapidly progressive glomerulonephritis (RPGN) is an acute presentation of glomerular injury leading to renal failure, which develops **in days to weeks**. This is a severe manifestation of the nephritic syndrome. The key pathologic finding in RPGN is formation of **cellular crescents** within the Bowman space. When this involves more than 50% of the glomeruli, it is commonly referred to as **crescentic GN**.
- **Chronic glomerulonephritis** is a slowly progressive glomerular disease that leads to renal failure **over a period of months to years**. It is suggested by HTN, proteinuria >3 g/day, chronic renal insufficiency, and small atrophic kidneys.

History
- Ask about symptoms like joint pain, rash, peripheral and/or periorbital edema, foamy urine, and hematuria. Patients with RPGN may have in addition symptoms of fever, nose bleeds, hemoptysis or vague symptoms of hair loss, fatigue, and weight loss.
- Past history focuses on history of malignancies and infections. Timing of infection can be very helpful. IgA nephropathy will have hematuria within 1 to 3 days after onset of respiratory symptoms as opposed to postinfectious GN, which develops 1 to 3 weeks after a streptococcal upper respiratory tract infection and 5 to 6 weeks after a skin infection.
- Some GN have a familial nature like Alport syndrome (renal failure associated with hearing loss), thin basement membrane disease, IgA nephropathy, focal segmental glomerulosclerosis (FSGS), and atypical HUS.
- Medication use including prescription, over-the-counter medications, and herbal supplements should be evaluated. Many drugs and toxins may be associated with glomerular disease.
  - NSAIDs are associated with minimal change disease.
  - Penicillamine, gold, NSAIDs, and mercury are associated with membranous nephropathy.
  - Heroin has previously been associated with FSGS.
  - Cyclosporine, tacrolimus, and mitomycin C are associated with thrombotic microangiopathy.
  - Various malignancies are associated with glomerular disease.
- Review of systems should cover multisystem diseases associated with glomerular disease such as HTN, diabetes mellitus (DM), systemic lupus erythematosus (SLE), amyloid, and vasculitis.

Physical Examination

- **Periorbital edema** in the mornings is a highly suggestive feature of the nephrotic syndrome. Facial edema is most often absent in heart failure or in patients with liver cirrhosis due to the inability of these patients to lie flat.
- **Xanthelasmas** may be present due to hyperlipidemia associated with nephrotic syndrome.
- **Muehrcke bands** (white bands in fingernails parallel to the lunula) may also be present from hypoalbuminemia in patients with nephrotic syndrome.[8]
- Palpable purpura may be seen in cryoglobulinemia, vasculitis, or SLE.
- Malar rash can be seen in patients with SLE.
- Evaluation for piercing and skin tattoos may give a clue to underlying hepatitis or HIV, both of which can be associated with glomerular disease.

Differential Diagnosis

Minimal Change Disease

- Minimal change disease (MCD) is defined by the presence of nephrotic syndrome, the absence of histologic glomerular abnormality by light microscopy, and evidence of podocyte foot process effacement by electron microscopy.
- Most commonly presents in children between ages of 2 and 7 years, but the disease may occur at any age.
- Most cases are idiopathic. However, in a number of patients, the onset is preceded by allergic reaction, vaccination, or viral infection. Around 20% of the patients have a history of atopy.[9] Secondary causes include the following:
  - Drugs: NSAIDs, lithium, interferon-α
  - Infections: HIV, syphilis
  - Malignancies: Hodgkin lymphoma, rarely non-Hodgkin lymphoma, and solid tumors
- Onset of nephrotic syndrome is typically abrupt. Creatinine is generally normal at presentation but can be elevated in some adults.
- Urine sediment is usually bland. Complement levels are normal. Renal biopsy is required for diagnosis. Glomeruli appear normal on light microscopy, with no immunoglobulin or complement deposition on immunofluorescence. Presence of foot process effacement is seen on electron microscopy.
- Complications of MCD include infection, peritonitis, thromboembolism, and acute renal failure, especially in the setting of hypovolemia.

Focal and Segmental Glomerulosclerosis

- FSGS is defined by glomerular lesions characterized by segments of sclerosis in only a portion (segmental) of some glomeruli (focal). FSGS has become an important form of glomerular disease in the US due to its increasing cause of ESRD.[10] It can be classified as primary or secondary FSGS.
- **Primary idiopathic FSGS**
  - The most common cause of idiopathic nephrotic syndrome in adults. The disease is markedly more common in African Americans.
  - Pathogenesis remains unclear, but the presence of a circulating permeability factor called soluble urokinase plasminogen activator receptor (suPAR) has been seen in nearly 60% to 80% of adult patients with primary FSGS.[11] Circulating suPAR affects podocyte maturation and function thereby leading to damage at the glomerular filtration barrier.
  - FSGS presents most often as nephrotic syndrome but may also present in 20% to 30% as persistent nonnephrotic range proteinuria, HTN, microscopic hematuria, and renal insufficiency.
  - There is frequent progression to ESRD, up to 50% at 10 years.
  - Diagnosis requires renal biopsy. Multiple histologic variants of FSGS have been described. The so-called tip lesion variant has a better prognosis, while the collapsing variant is associated with worse outcomes.

- **Secondary FSGS** occurs as an adaptive response to glomerular hyperfiltration or podocyte injury. Podocyte injury can be caused by many factors like viral infection, drugs, or genetic mutation affecting the structural integrity of the podocytes.
  - ○ **HIV-associated nephropathy**: Up to 95% of cases occur in African Americans. Renal ultrasound shows enlarged kidneys with increased echogenicity. The collapsing form of FSGS is most notably associated with HIV.
  - ○ **Reduced renal mass** (unilateral renal agenesis, renal ablation, and renal allograft): This initially leads to an adaptive hyperfiltration, which over time causes glomerular HTN and FSGS.
  - ○ **Hypoxemia** in the setting of sickle cell anemia, congenital pulmonary disease, or cyanotic congenital heart disease leads to glomerular enlargement and subsequently causes FSGS.
  - ○ **Toxins** from impurities in heroin have been known to cause podocyte damage and an FSGS pattern.
  - ○ **Chronic vesicoureteral reflux.**
  - ○ **Morbid obesity.**
  - ○ **Genetic forms** of FSGS occur due to mutations in genes affecting podocyte and slit diaphragm structures. Variation in the APOL1 gene, (codes for apolipoprotein L-1), a protective mechanism against *Trypanosoma brucei brucei*, has been associated with FSGS in the presence of HTN among African Americans.[12]

Membranous Nephropathy
- Membranous nephropathy (MN) is a glomerular disease characterized by subepithelial immune deposits of IgG and complement along the glomerular basement membrane with characteristic spike pattern seen on methenamine silver staining.
- MN represents the most common cause of idiopathic nephrotic syndrome in adults >60 years of age and the second most common cause (after FSGS) of the nephrotic syndrome in all adults.
- The pathogenesis of MN remains unclear, but recent experiments have identified circulating antibodies to the M-type phospholipase A_2 receptor (anti-PLA$_2$R antibody) in 70% of patients with idiopathic MN.[13] Another antibody targeting neutral endopeptidase (NEP) has been attributed to the development of congenital MN. Secondary causes of MN include the following:
  - ○ Malignancies (colon, kidney, lung) account for the majority of secondary MN. Nephrotic syndrome may precede clinical manifestations of malignancy by up to 2 years.[1]
  - ○ Autoimmune diseases including SLE, type 1 DM, rheumatoid arthritis, and myasthenia gravis.
  - ○ Infections such as hepatitis B, hepatitis C, and syphilis.
  - ○ Drugs including NSAIDs, gold, and penicillamine.
- About 80% of patients with MN present with overt nephrotic syndrome. Microscopic hematuria may be seen in up to 50% of adults. Serum complement levels are normal in idiopathic MN.
- Deep vein thrombosis, especially renal vein thrombosis, is more common in MN than in other forms of nephrotic syndrome.

Membranoproliferative Glomerulonephritis
- Histopathologically, membranoproliferative glomerulonephritis (MPGN) is characterized by diffuse mesangial proliferation, thickening of the capillary loops due to reduplication of glomerular capillary basement membrane (double-contour or tram track), subendothelial immune deposits, and mesangial hypercellularity. Most cases are associated with circulating immune complexes and low serum complements.[9]
- Based on the histomorphologic pattern, there are three types of MPGN.[14]
  - ○ Type 1: discrete immune deposits in the mesangium and subendothelial space. This is frequently associated with hepatitis C infection, **cryoglobulinemia**, or endocarditis.

○ Type 2: continuous, intramembranous, ribbon-like deposits. It is often called **dense-deposit disease**. This can be associated with partial lipodystrophy, C3 nephritic factor, and factor H or I deficiency with complement consumption.[9]
○ Type 3: diffuse subepithelial and subendothelial deposits within the glomerular basement membrane.
• MPGN can manifest as microscopic hematuria and proteinuria, nephritic syndrome, nephrotic syndrome, or chronic progressive GN. The majority of patients have HTN.
• MPGN almost always is associated with low serum C3 and/or C4 levels.
• Primary MPGN is a diagnosis of exclusion after potential secondary causes like hepatitis infection, HIV/AIDS, infective endocarditis, collagen vascular disease, malignancy, or chronic liver disease have been excluded.

IgA Nephropathy and Henoch-Schönlein Purpura
• IgA nephropathy (also known as Berger disease) is a mesangial proliferative GN characterized by diffuse mesangial deposition of IgA.
• IgA nephropathy is **the most common primary GN globally**.
• There is a higher incidence in Asia and Europe, which may be due to difference in biopsy practices for isolated microscopic hematuria.
• Pathogenesis of IgA nephropathy remains unclear. Half of the patients have a preceding infection. There is reduced galactosylation of the *O*-linked hinge region sugar of circulating IgA1. This leads to production of IgG antibodies against the circulating abnormal IgA predisposing to formation of immune complexes and mesangial deposition.[15]
• IgA nephropathy can present as episodic hematuria, asymptomatic microscopic hematuria with variable degrees of proteinuria, or uncommonly as a rapidly progressive crescentic disease. Hematuria is seen within 1 to 3 days following upper respiratory infection. This distinguishes IgA nephropathy from poststreptococcal GN, in which the hematuria is delayed by 1 to 3 weeks.
• ESRD develops in 25% to 30% of patients within 20 years of diagnosis. Presence of uncontrolled HTN, persistent proteinuria >1 g/day, impaired renal function, and older age at diagnosis are risk factors for progression.[16]
• Approximately 30% to 50% of patients have increased serum IgA levels, but levels do not correlate with disease activity. Complement levels are usually normal.
• **Henoch-Schönlein purpura** is a syndrome with IgA nephropathy and systemic small vessel vasculitis caused by IgA deposits. It presents with arthralgia, purpuric skin rash, abdominal pain, or gastrointestinal bleeding. It predominantly affects children.

Glomerulonephritis in Multisystem Disorders
• **Systemic lupus erythematosus**
○ Lupus nephritis is an immune complex–mediated complication of SLE that presents with various histologic patterns described by the 2003 International Society of Nephrology and Renal Pathology Society, based on the degree of glomerular involvement (Table 24-3).
○ Renal biopsy plays a critical role in diagnosis and management of patients with lupus nephritis but remains a topic of controversy in predicting outcomes and prognosis.[17] Classically, the proliferative forms of SLE (Classes III and IV) are associated with an increased risk of renal failure.
○ About 50% to 60% of patients with lupus have renal involvement during their disease course. Lupus nephritis may manifest as benign asymptomatic hematuria, proteinuria, or even fulminant renal failure.[1]
○ Serum complement levels are usually low in the majority of patients because of classic complement pathway activation.[18]
• **Pauci-immune glomerulonephritis** is a group of small vessel vasculitides characterized by the presence of necrotizing crescents with minimal or no immune complex deposits.

TABLE 24-3 Abbreviated (ISN/RPS) Classification of Lupus Nephritis (2003)

Class	Definition
I	Minimal mesangial lupus nephritis
II	Mesangial proliferative lupus nephritis
III	Focal lupus nephritis[a]
IV	Diffuse segmental (IV-S) or global (IV-G) lupus nephritis[b]
V	Membranous lupus nephritis[c]
VI	Advanced sclerosing lupus nephritis

Indicate and grade (mild, moderate, severe) tubular atrophy, interstitial inflammation and fibrosis, severity of arteriosclerosis, or other vascular lesions.
[a]Indicate the proportion of glomeruli with active and with sclerotic lesions.
[b]Indicate the proportion of glomeruli with fibrinoid necrosis and cellular crescents.
[c]Class V may occur in combination with class III or IV in which case both will be diagnosed.
ISN/RPS, International Society of Nephrology/Renal Pathology Society.

- The majority (80%) of the patients have positive circulating antineutrophil cytoplasmic antibodies (ANCA) and hence are also called ANCA-associated vasculitis.
- Pauci-immune GN includes granulomatosis with polyangiitis (GPA, formerly called as Wegener granulomatosis), microscopic polyangiitis (MPA), eosinophilic granulomatosis with polyangiitis (EGPA, formerly called Churg-Strauss syndrome), and renal limited vasculitis.[19]
- Patients can present with nonspecific symptoms of malaise, weight loss, fever, and arthralgia.
- Renal manifestations include hematuria, varying degrees of proteinuria, and dysmorphic RBCs with RBC casts.
- Disease-specific manifestations:
  - GPA: sinusitis, nasopharyngeal mucosal ulceration, hemoptysis, purpura, and renal involvement. C-ANCA and proteinase 3 (PR3) are positive in 65% to 90% of patients with active disease. Serum complement levels are normal.
  - EGPA: asthma, peripheral eosinophilia, and renal involvement. P-ANCA and myeloperoxidase (MPO) are associated with EGPA.
  - MPA: generally associated with renal involvement and absence of granulomas.
- **Goodpasture disease** is suggested by the presence of antiglomerular basement membrane (anti-GBM) antibody along with a clinical presentation of pulmonary-renal syndrome consisting of hemoptysis, pulmonary infiltrates, and/or RPGN.
  - Anti-GBM antibodies are directed against the noncollagenous-1 domain of the α-3 chain of type IV collagen.
  - This disease is characterized by focal necrotizing crescentic GN in association with circulating anti-GBM antibodies in the blood and linear staining of IgG along the glomerular basement membrane.
  - Approximately 30% of patients with Goodpasture disease are P-ANCA positive.
- **Poststreptococcal glomerulonephritis** (PSGN) is an immune complex–mediated GN characterized by renal deposition of complement C3 and IgG as subepithelial humps on electron microscopy. It is associated with low serum C3 and CH50 and occurs following an infection with nephritogenic strains of group A or, sometimes, group C streptococci.
  - PSGN is principally a disease of children, but has been increasingly reported in older patients occurring 1 to 3 weeks after pharyngitis or 5 to 6 weeks after impetigo. Incidence of PSGN has progressively declined in the industrialized countries.

- ○ Clinical presentation consists of hematuria manifesting as **tea-colored urine**, edema, HTN, and oliguria. Prognosis is excellent in children and less favorable in adults.
- ○ Laboratory tests include antibodies to streptococcal antigens (antistreptolysin-O and anti-DNase B) and hypocomplementemia.
- ○ **Atypical postinfectious GN** is increasingly reported following staphylococcal and gram-negative infections. It is more commonly seen in patients with underlying diabetes. Clinical presentation is more severe than PSGN with a greater number of patients progressing to ESRD. Predominance of IgA deposition and C3 can be seen on renal biopsy with no subepithelial humps.[9]
- **Thrombotic microangiopathies** (TMA) is a syndrome characterized by microangiopathic hemolytic anemia (MAHA), thrombocytopenia, and varying degrees of organ dysfunction.
- ○ TMA can be seen in a variety of clinical conditions including thrombotic thrombocytopenic purpura (TTP), HUS, malignant HTN, scleroderma, antiphospholipid syndrome (APLA), HIV infection, and secondary to medications like calcineurin inhibitors and clopidogrel.
- ○ Diagnostic criteria for TTP include MAHA, thrombocytopenia, fever, neurologic signs, and renal failure. **Low circulating levels or antibodies against ADAMTS13** lead to increased circulating ultralarge vWF (ULvWF) consequently causing platelet activation and aggregation.
- ○ **HUS is classically associated with diarrheal infection** caused by exotoxins produced by *Escherichia coli* (O157:H7 serotype) or *Shigella dysenteriae* type 1.
- ○ **Atypical HUS (aHUS) is caused by dysregulation of the complement system.**[20] Absence of diarrhea and leukocytosis with clinical features of HUS and hypocomplementemia should raise the suspicion of aHUS.[9]
- **Amyloidosis** is characterized by the deposition of extracellular, insoluble, polymeric protein fibrils.
- ○ Classification is based on the type of protein precursor that forms the amyloid fibril. Renal involvement is most often seen in primary amyloidosis (AL) and systemic secondary (AA) amyloidosis.
- ○ Protein precursor for AL amyloid is light chain and hence can be seen in patients with multiple myeloma.
- ○ Clinical features include proteinuria with or without microscopic hematuria and renal insufficiency. Monoclonal light chains can be detected by measuring serum free light chains (SFLC) and serum or urine protein electrophoresis with immunofixation.[21]
- ○ **Congo red stain** will show an **apple-green birefringence** if AL amyloid is present on biopsy specimen.
- ○ Prognosis of AL amyloidosis is poor with a median survival of <2 years.

Diagnostic Testing

Laboratories

- Tests should include assessment of renal function (blood urea nitrogen [BUN], serum Cr), urinalysis, and microscopic examination of the urine sediment.
- The amount of urine protein should be quantified. A spot urine protein to creatinine ratio can give a rough estimation of 24-hour urine protein excretion when the creatinine is at a stable baseline. A 24-hour urine collection for protein provides a more accurate estimate especially in patients with acute renal failure.
- Presence or absence of RBC casts or dysmorphic RBCs aids in making the diagnosis of glomerular disease.
- Certain serologic tests should be considered (Table 24-4).
- Measurement of C3, C4, and CH50 is particularly helpful in limiting the differential diagnosis (Table 24-5).

TABLE 24-4	Serologic Tests for Glomerulonephritis
Glomerular disease	**Serologic tests**
Lupus nephritis	ANA, anti–double-stranded DNA antibody (dsDNA), C3, C4
Cryoglobulinemia	Cryoglobulins and rheumatoid factor, C3, C4
Goodpasture disease	Anti-GBM antibody, ANCA
Pauci-immune vasculitis	ANCA, MPO, PR3
Poststreptococcal GN	Antistreptolysin-O antibody (ASO), anti-DNaseB, C3, C4
Hepatitis-associated MPGN	Hepatitis B and C serologies, cryoglobulins, C3, C4
HIV-associated nephropathy	HIV antibodies
Amyloidosis and light chain deposition disease	Serum and urine protein electrophoresis, immunofixation, sFLC

ANA, antinuclear antibody; ANCA, antineutrophil cytoplasmic antibody; GBM, glomerular basement membrane; GN, glomerulonephritis; HIV, human immunodeficiency virus; MPGN, membranoproliferative glomerulonephritis; MPO, myeloperoxidase; PR3, proteinase 3; sFLC, serum free light chain.

Imaging
- **Renal ultrasound** has a role in the workup of glomerulopathy including confirming the presence of two kidneys, ruling out obstruction or anatomic abnormalities, and assessing kidney size.
- Atrophic small kidneys (<9 cm) suggest chronic kidney disease (CKD) and should limit the use of kidney biopsy or aggressive immunosuppressive therapies.
- Large kidneys (>14 cm) can be seen in nephrotic syndrome associated with diabetes, HIV infection, or deposition disorders such as amyloidosis.

Diagnostic Procedures
Renal biopsy is usually required to establish a definitive diagnosis. This can be done with the help of ultrasound, CT guidance, or rarely via a transjugular approach.

TABLE 24-5	Complement Measurements in Glomerulonephritis	
Pathway affected	**Complement changes**	**Glomerular disease**
Classical pathway activation	C3 ↓, C4 ↓, CH50 ↓	Lupus nephritis Mixed essential cryoglobulinemia MPGN type 1
Alternate pathway activation	C3 ↓, C4 normal, CH50 ↓	Poststreptococcal GN GN associated with other infections Atypical HUS MPGN type II

GN, glomerulonephritis; HUS, hemolytic-uremic syndrome; MPGN, membranoproliferative glomerulonephritis.
Data from Floege J, Johnson RJ, Feehally J. *Comprehensive Clinical Nephrology*, 4th ed. Philadelphia, PA: Mosby; 2010.

TREATMENT

- General treatment of glomerular disease addresses control of proteinuria, edema, HTN, and hyperlipidemia.
- Patients with proteinuria should be treated with **ACE inhibitors or ARBs** to a goal proteinuria of <1 g/day. Side effects with these agents include hyperkalemia and rising serum Cr (elevation ≤30% is acceptable).
- **Aggressive HTN control** is essential for patients with glomerular disease. BP goals are <135/80 mm Hg and can be achieved with a combination of diuretics and the above agents.
- Edema is controlled with dietary **sodium restriction** and **judicious use of diuretics**.
- Treatment of hyperlipidemia consists of the use of **statins**.
- Identification and treatment of the secondary cause of the glomerulopathy is very important.
- Specific treatments of the primary glomerulopathies are complex and require a nephrology consultation.
  - **MCD**: Corticosteroids are the first-line agents, with adults typically requiring a longer course (up to 16 weeks) to achieve remission.
  - **Primary FSGS**: High-dose daily or alternate day steroids for 8 to 16 weeks. Cyclosporine is used in patients with steroid-resistant cases. Secondary FSGS is not responsive to immunosuppressive therapy, and treatment is directed at the underlying condition. The use of antiviral HIV therapy has significantly reduced the incidence of HIV-associated nephropathy.
  - **MN**: Indolent cases may only require conservative antiproteinuric therapy with ACE inhibitors or ARBs. When immunosuppressive therapy is required, corticosteroids with daily cytotoxic therapy (e.g., cyclophosphamide) are used most commonly. Rituximab has also been used for treatment.
  - **MPGN**: Corticosteroids, with or without cytotoxic therapy, can be used in primary cases. MPGN associated with hepatitis C is responsive to antiviral therapy.
  - **IgA nephropathy**: Therapy is based on severity of hematuria and proteinuria, GFR, and histopathology. Fish oil and immune-modulating agents have been used with varying degrees of success in patients with refractory proteinuria.
  - **PSGN**: Therapy is generally supportive. Treatment of streptococcal infection with penicillin should be included even if no persistent infection is present in order to decrease antigenic load.
  - **Lupus nephritis**: Management is highly dependent on the type and severity. Classes I and II generally do not require specific therapy for renal manifestations. Treatment for classes III, IV, and V typically includes corticosteroids and cytotoxic immunosuppressive therapy.
  - **Pauci-immune GN**: Corticosteroids and cytotoxic agents are commonly used. Plasmapheresis is used if patients have associated pulmonary hemorrhage or are dialysis dependent.
  - **Goodpasture and anti-GBM disease**: Plasmapheresis along with corticosteroids and cytotoxic agents are generally indicated when renal function can be salvaged.
  - **TTP**: Plasmapheresis remains the first-line therapy. Corticosteroids are helpful in patients suspected to have antibodies against ADAMTS13.
  - **HUS**: Treatment is supportive in diarrheal cases of typical HUS. Antibiotics are not recommended.
  - **AL amyloid**: Treatment is directed at the underlying disease and may involve melphalan and corticosteroids.

Chronic Kidney Disease

GENERAL PRINCIPLES

- According to current estimates, approximately 26 million American adults have chronic kidney diseases (CKD). The most common causes of CKD and ESRD are DM and HTN.

- Risk factors for CKD include the following: advanced age, low income/education, US ethnic minority status (African American, Native American, Hispanic, Asian, or Pacific Islander), family history of CKD, DM, HTN, autoimmune diseases, systemic infections, urinary tract abnormalities, cancer, prior AKI, reduction in kidney mass, and exposure to certain drugs and toxins.[22]
- Identifying and treating CKD early is critical, as disease progression is associated with increased mortality, hospitalization, and cardiovascular events.
- Most patients with CKD have a fairly constant progressive decline in GFR over time. However, some patients may experience stabilization or remission.
- The rate of decline for an individual patient can be somewhat difficult to predict but is known to be dependent on the type of kidney disease. Other factors associated with a faster rate of decline include African American race, lower baseline kidney function, male gender, and older age.[17]
- Acute declines in GFR are not unusual in the course of CKD and may be caused by factors such as volume depletion, radiocontrast, NSAIDs, some antimicrobials (e.g., aminoglycosides, amphotericin B), cyclosporine, tacrolimus, and urinary tract obstruction.
- There is a strong association between CKD and cardiovascular disease. Modifiable risk factors (e.g., HTN, dyslipidemia, DM, and tobacco use) should be treated aggressively.

Definition

- According to the 2003 National Kidney Foundation guidelines on Chronic Kidney Disease, CKD is defined as either kidney damage or decreased GFR for at least 3 months' duration.[22]
- Markers of kidney damage include proteinuria, urinary tract abnormalities on imaging, and abnormal urinary sediment or urinary chemistries.

Classification

- The National Kidney Foundation staging for CKD is presented in Table 24-6.[22]

TABLE 24-6	Staging of Chronic Kidney Disease		
Stage	Description	GFR (mL/minute/1.73 m²)	Action
1	Kidney damage with normal GFR	>90	Diagnosis and treatment; slow progression
2	Kidney damage with mildly decreased GFR	60–89	Estimate progression
3	Moderately decreased GFR	30–59	Evaluate and treat complications
4	Severely decreased GFR	15–29	Prepare for renal replacement therapy
5	Kidney failure	<15	Assess needs for renal replacement therapy

GFR, glomerular filtration rate.
Modified from National Kidney Foundation. K/DOQI clinical practice guidelines for chronic kidney disease: evaluation, classification, and stratification. *Am J Kidney Dis* 2002;39(2 suppl 1): S1–S266.

- The goals of management of CKD evolve as the severity progresses.
  - Stages 1 and 2 CKD: preventing disease progression and treating underlying etiologies of kidney damage
  - Stage 3 CKD: managing complications that present at this level of dysfunction
  - Stage 4 CKD: treating complications of CKD and planning for initiation of renal replacement therapy
- As discussed in Chapter 23, various equations can be used to estimate the GFR when the creatinine is at a stable baseline.

DIAGNOSIS

- The basic diagnostic evaluation is discussed in detail in Chapter 23 and in the preceding sections of this chapter.
- The specific type of kidney disease dictates its treatment and prognosis.
- Renal function should be assessed to determine the stage of disease. The rate of decline of renal function can be assessed by ongoing measurements of serum Cr (e.g., plotting the inverse of serum Cr against time). The rate of decline can subsequently be used to estimate the interval to the onset of kidney failure.[22]
- Comorbidities that can accelerate the rate of decline of renal function should be identified and treated (e.g., DM, HTN).
- Patients with diabetes should be screened annually for albuminuric kidney disease.
- Screening should consist of spot urine albumin/Cr ratio, serum Cr, and estimation of GFR.
- **Microalbuminuria** is defined as an albumin/Cr ratio of 30 to 300 mg/g.[23]
- **Macroalbuminuria** is defined as an albumin/Cr ratio of >300 mg/g.
- Symptoms and signs of the complications of renal dysfunction must be identified.
  - **Uncontrolled HTN** can accelerate decline in renal function by increasing intraglomerular pressure. Furthermore, inappropriate sodium retention exacerbates preexisting HTN in patients with CKD.
  - **Anemia** of CKD is due to decreased erythropoietin production that usually occurs once GFR is <30 mL/minute/1.73 m^2. Anemia is associated with poorer outcomes in CKD.[24]
  - **Secondary hyperparathyroidism** occurs as an adaptation to (a) active vitamin D deficiency, (b) phosphorus retention due to decreased GFR, and (c) hypocalcemia due to reduced active vitamin D. Elevated parathyroid hormone (PTH) can result in increased bone turnover, placing patients at high risk for fractures. Serum levels of calcium, phosphorus, and intact plasma PTH should be measured in all patients with CKD and GFR <60 mL/minute/1.73 m^2.
  - **Metabolic acidosis** may develop with decreasing GFR as the kidney is less effective in excreting acid loads. Acidosis is present in most patients when the estimated GFR is below 30 mL/minute/1.73 m^2. Deleterious effects of metabolic acidosis include bone demineralization, insulin resistance, and increased protein catabolism. Serum bicarbonate is used as a surrogate marker of acidosis and should be measured every 3 to 6 months as CKD progresses.[25]
- Because of the strong association between CKD and cardiovascular disease, modifiable risk factors (e.g., HTN, dyslipidemia, DM, tobacco use) should be identified.
  - Dyslipidemia is common in CKD, and patients should be **screened with a fasting lipid profile annually**.[26]
  - Those with hyperlipidemia should be evaluated for potential causes such as nephrosis, hypothyroidism, excess alcohol consumption, chronic liver disease, and medications.

TREATMENT

Treatment of CKD is multifaceted and includes the following:

- Specific therapy directed at the etiology of the kidney disease (see above)
- Slowing the loss of kidney function
- Treatment of the complications of loss of kidney function
- Prevention and treatment of cardiovascular disease and its risk factors
- Preparation for renal replacement therapy
- Renal replacement therapy (hemodialysis, peritoneal dialysis, transplantation)

Hypertension

- Lifestyle modifications are usually insufficient to achieve BP goals in CKD, and multiple antihypertensives are often required.
- Control of HTN is particularly important in patients with diabetes.
- The Eighth Report of the Joint National Committee (JNC 8) BP goal for patients with CKD is the same as for the general population, <140/90.[27]
- The Kidney Disease: Improving Global Outcomes (KDIGO) Working Group, however, recommends a more strict goal of <130/80 for patients with CKD not on dialysis and with albuminuria ≥30 mg/day (or albumin/creatinine ratio ≥30 mg/g or proteinuria ≥150 mg/day). Data most strongly supports this goal for those with albuminuria ≥300 mg/day. The more lenient goal of <140/90 is recommended by KDIGO when albuminuria is <30 mg/day.[28]
- The National Kidney Foundation accepts these recommendations as reasonable but points out the lack of quality supporting data for the more stringent goals, particularly in those with moderate albuminuria (i.e., 30 to 300 mg/g).[29]
- KDIGO recommends that an ACE inhibitor or an ARB are first-line therapy in patients with albuminuria ≥30 mg/day (or albumin/creatinine ratio ≥30mg/g), particularly in those with concurrent DM.[28] The data most strongly supports this recommendation in those with albuminuria ≥300 mg/day.
  - They reduce intraglomerular pressures and hence slow the progression of renal dysfunction.
  - After starting ACE inhibitors or ARBs, serum K^+ and Cr levels should be checked within 1-2 weeks. **An increase in creatinine of up to 30% is acceptable** after starting these agents. Repeat measurements after dose adjustments.
- **Diuretics** are often effective adjuvant agents for BP control.
  - Thiazide diuretics are ineffective once GFR is <30 mL/minute/1.73 m^2, while higher doses of loop diuretics can reduce BP.
  - Reasonable starting doses include furosemide 40 mg PO bid or bumetanide 1 mg PO bid.

Diabetes Mellitus

- In patients with type 1 and type 2 diabetes mellitus (DM), lowering the A1C levels to approximately 7.0% will delay progression of the microvascular complications of diabetes, including diabetic kidney disease.[23]
- Reducing the A1C to approximately 7.0% may also reduce the rate of decline of GFR.
- Refer to the Chapter 20 for details regarding the treatment of DM.

Dyslipidemia

- Treatment of dyslipidemia in CKD should follow the 2013 guidelines of the American College of Cardiology (ACC) and the American Heart Association (AHA).[30]
- Currently, many consider ESRD to be a coronary artery disease equivalent.
- Lowering low-density lipoprotein cholesterol (LDL-C) with statin-based therapies reduces the risk of major atherosclerotic events, but not all-cause mortality, in patients with CKD including those with diabetes.[23]
- Refer to the Chapter 11 for details on the treatment of dyslipidemia.

Anemia

- **The goal hemoglobin (Hgb) range is 10 to 11 g/dL**. Recent studies have demonstrated that artificially increasing the Hgb above 13 g/dL in patients with CKD may result in increased risk of myocardial ischemia, stroke, blood clots, and death.[24,31]
- **Iron stores should be repleted** before initiating therapy with erythropoiesis-stimulating agents (ESAs) and should be monitored every 3 months during ESA therapy.
  - Transferrin saturation should be corrected to levels >25% to 30%.[24]
  - Iron can be given for ferritin levels <1,200 ng/dL if there is no evidence of iron overload.
  - Repletion can be in oral or IV form. Ferrous sulfate 325 mg PO bid to tid can be attempted. Oral formulations are best absorbed in an acid environment on an empty stomach; hence, patients on antireflux medications may require increased doses.
  - If response to oral iron is inadequate, or if patients cannot tolerate oral iron, then iron dextran may be given intravenously. This is usually prescribed in a nephrologist's office, with a 25-mg test dose given first to monitor for adverse events. If tolerated, 1,000 mg can be given IV. Other IV preparations such as iron sucrose or sodium ferric gluconate can also be used, but these require several smaller doses over several days to total 1 g of iron.
- Treatment with ESAs can be initiated if the Hgb level remains <10 g/dL after iron deficiency has been corrected.
  - Initial treatment options include epoetin alfa at 50 to 100 units/kg SC three times per week or darbepoetin alfa 0.45 µg/kg SC every 1 to 2 weeks. Subsequent dosing should be guided by Hgb levels.
  - Rates of Hgb increase are dose dependent, usually <1 g Hgb/week.
- Hgb should be measured at least monthly during ESA treatment to prevent fluctuation outside the goal range.

Secondary Hyperparathyroidism

- Treatment of secondary hyperparathyroidism is approached in a stepwise fashion by (a) reducing phosphorus intake, (b) supplementing nutritional vitamin D (25-OH), and (c) treating with vitamin D analogue ($1,25\text{-OH}_2$). Target levels for PTH can be found in Table 24-7.
- **Phosphorus intake** can be reduced by either dietary restriction or phosphate binders.[25]
  - Dietary intake should be limited to 800 to 1,000 mg/day.
  - Calcium-based binders (calcium carbonate and calcium acetate) may be used if dietary restriction of phosphate is insufficient.
  - The total dose of elemental calcium provided by the calcium-based phosphate binders should not exceed 1,500 mg/day.
- **Nutritional vitamin D (25-OH) deficiency should be** corrected.[25]
  - If the serum level is <30 ng/mL, supplementation with ergocalciferol should be initiated.

TABLE 24-7	Target PTH Goals in CKD	
CKD stage	Intact PTH goal	Frequency of PTH measurement in untreated patients
Stage 3	35–70 pg/mL	Yearly
Stage 4	70–110 pg/mL	Every 3 months
Stage 5	150–300 pg/mL	Every 3 months

CKD, chronic kidney disease; PTH, parathyroid hormone.
Modified from National Kidney Foundation. K/DOQI clinical practice guidelines for bone metabolism and disease in chronic kidney disease. *Am J Kidney Dis* 2003;42(4 suppl 3): S1–S201.

- ○ Vitamin D insufficiency (16 to 30 ng/mL) is treated with ergocalciferol 50,000 IU PO monthly for 3 months.
- ○ Mild deficiency (5 to 15 ng/mL) is treated with ergocalciferol 50,000 IU PO every other week for 3 months.
- ○ Severe deficiency (<5 ng/mL) is treated with ergocalciferol 50,000 IU PO weekly for 3 months.
- ○ Vitamin D levels should be reassessed at the conclusion of treatment.
- ○ Once the patient is replete, continue supplementation with either monthly ergocalciferol 50,000 IU or vitamin D 1,000 to 2,000 IU daily.
- ○ If the serum levels of corrected total calcium exceed the upper limit of the normal range, vitamin D therapy should be temporarily discontinued.
- If PTH levels remain above goal (Table 24-7) after vitamin D levels are replete, **active vitamin D treatment** can be used to further reduce PTH levels.[25]
  - ○ Therapy with an active oral vitamin D sterol (e.g., calcitriol) is indicated when serum levels of 25-OH vitamin D are >30 ng/mL and plasma levels of intact PTH are above the target range for the CKD stage. The typical starting dose of calcitriol is 0.25 μg PO daily.
  - ○ Vitamin D sterol should be given only to patients with serum levels of corrected total calcium <9.5 mg/dL and serum phosphorus <4.6 mg/dL.
  - ○ During treatment, serum levels of calcium and phosphorus should be monitored at least every month for the first 3 months and then every 3 months thereafter. Plasma PTH levels should be measured at least every 3 months. Active vitamin D therapy should be held if PTH falls below the target range, calcium is >9.5 mg/dL, or phosphorus is >4.6 mg/dL.
  - ○ Vitamin D sterol treatment is also indicated for dialysis patients with PTH >300 pg/mL. Overcorrection of the intact PTH should be avoided, as this may result in adynamic bone disease.

Metabolic Acidosis

In stage 3, 4, and 5 CKD, the goal serum bicarbonate is ≥22 mEq/L.[25] When the serum bicarbonate level is <20 mEq/L, alkali salts, such as sodium bicarbonate 650 to 1,300 mg PO bid to tid, may be started.

Nutrition

- Patients with stage 3 and stage 4 CKD may benefit from nutritional consultation.
- Nutritional goals are summarized in Table 24-8, but individualized patient therapy is most appropriate.
- While current recommendations suggest reducing dietary protein intake to minimize urea production, patients with CKD are at increased risk of malnutrition. Hypoalbuminemia is a marker of increased mortality in ESRD patients, and low serum albumin is a contraindication to peritoneal dialysis. Current guidelines recommend measuring albumin every 1 to 3 months.[32]

TABLE 24-8	Nutrition Goals for Patients with Stage 3 and 4 CKD
Nutritional item	**Goal**
Sodium	2 g/day
Protein	0.6–0.75 g/kg/day
Total calories	35 kcal/kg/day
Phosphorus	800–1,000 mg/day
Potassium	2–3 g/day

Data from K/DOQI, National Kidney Foundation. Clinical practice guidelines for nutrition in chronic renal failure. *Am J Kidney Dis* 2000;35(6 suppl 2):S1–S140.

REFERRAL

- Patient referral to a nephrologist should occur once the GFR is <30 mL/minute/1.73 m²; furthermore, referral may also be appropriate in patients with stage 3 CKD in whom further decline is anticipated.
- Late nephrology referral is associated with poorer outcomes and increased cost of care.
- Patients with stage 4 CKD should be referred for early vascular access for hemodialysis.
  - Arteriovenous fistulas are preferred for hemodialysis, as they have lower risks of infection, lower incidence of thrombosis, and higher flow rates than arteriovenous grafts (AVGs). Arteriovenous fistulas require an average of 3 to 4 months to mature after placement.
  - AVGs are preferred to indwelling catheters, as these have lower risks of infection and better flow rates compared with catheters. AVGs require approximately 3 to 6 weeks to mature before use.
- Nephrology consultation may aid in guiding the decision to initiate renal replacement therapy.
  - Patients with eGFR below 15 mL/minute/1.73 m² should be monitored regularly and dialysis started when symptoms of uremia develop. A higher threshold may be used in diabetics, as they tend to tolerate uremia poorly and are frequently troubled by sodium retention and fluid overload.
  - Signs and symptoms of uremia, HTN, refractory metabolic disturbances, and volume overload may contribute to a decision to initiate dialysis at higher GFR.
  - **Malnutrition** in the setting of a higher GFR may drive the decision to initiate dialysis even in the absence of severe electrolyte abnormalities.

REFERENCES

1. Feehally J, Floege J, Johnson RJ. *Comprehensive Clinical Nephrology*, 4th ed. Philadelphia, PA: Mosby; 2010.
2. Chertow GM, Burdick E, Honour M, et al. Acute kidney injury, mortality, length of stay, and costs in hospitalized patients. *J Am Soc Nephrol* 2005;16:3365–3370.
3. Lafrance JP, Miller DR. Defining acute kidney injury in database studies: the effects of varying the baseline kidney function assessment period and considering CKD status. *Am J Kidney Dis* 2010;56:651–660.
4. Lin J, Bonventre JV. Prevention of radiocontrast nephropathy. *Curr Opin Nephrol Hypertens* 2005;14:105–110.
5. Schrier RW, Wang W, Poole B, et al. Acute renal failure: definitions, diagnosis, pathogenesis, and therapy. *J Clin Invest* 2004;114:5–14.
6. Bonventre JV, Weinberg JM. Recent advances in the pathophysiology of ischemic acute renal failure. *J Am Soc Nephrol* 2003;14:2199–2210.
7. Agha IA. Acute renal failure. In: Agha IA, Green GB, eds. *Washington Manual Nephrology Subspecialty Consult*. Philadelphia, PA: Lippincott Williams & Wilkins; 2004:37–55.
8. Fawcett RS, Linford S, Stulberg DL. Nail abnormalities: clues to systemic disease. *Am Fam Physician* 2004;69:1417–1424.
9. Ponticelli C, Glassock RJ. *Treatment of Primary Glomerulonephritis*, 1st ed. New York, NY: Oxford University Press; 1997.
10. D'Agati VD, Kaskel FJ, Falk RJ. Focal segmental glomerulosclerosis. *N Engl J Med* 2011;365:2398–2411.
11. Wei C, Trachtman H, Li J, et al. Circulating suPAR in two cohorts of primary FSGS. *J Am Soc Nephrol* 2012;23:2051–2059.

12. Genovese G, Friedman DJ, Ross MD, et al. Association of trypanolytic ApoL1 variants with kidney disease in African Americans. *Science* 2010;329:841–845.

13. Beck LH Jr, Bonegio RG, Lambeau G, et al. M-type phospholipase A2 receptor as target antigen in idiopathic membranous nephropathy. *N Engl J Med* 2009;361:11–21.

14. Sethi S, Fervenza FC. Membranoproliferative glomerulonephritis—a new look at an old entity. *N Engl J Med* 2012;366:1119–1131.

15. Lai KN. Pathogenesis of IgA nephropathy. *Nat Rev Nephrol* 2012;8:275–283.

16. D'Amico G. Natural history of idiopathic IgA nephropathy: role of clinical and histological prognostic factors. *Am J Kidney Dis* 2000;36:227–237.

17. Giannico G, Fogo AB. Lupus nephritis: is the kidney biopsy currently necessary in the management of lupus nephritis? *Clin J Am Soc Nephrol* 2013;8:138–145.

18. Cameron JS. Lupus nephritis. *J Am Soc Nephrol* 1999;10:413–424.

19. Falk RJ, Gross WL, Guillevin L, et al. Granulomatosis with polyangiitis (Wegener's): an alternative name for Wegener's granulomatosis. *J Am Soc Nephrol* 2011;22:587–588.

20. Noris M, Remuzzi G. Atypical hemolytic-uremic syndrome. *N Engl J Med* 2009;361:1676–1687.

21. Mayo MM, Johns GS. Serum free light chains in the diagnosis and monitoring of patients with plasma cell dyscrasias. *Contrib Nephrol* 2007;153:44–65.

22. KDOQI, National Kidney Foundation. KDOQI clinical practice guidelines for chronic kidney disease: evaluation, classification, and stratification. *Am J Kidney Dis* 2002;39(2 suppl 1):S1–S266.

23. Chobanian AV, Bakris GL, Black HR, et al. The seventh report of the joint national committee on prevention, detection, evaluation, and treatment of high blood pressure: the JNC 7 Report. *JAMA* 2003;289:2560–2572.

24. KDOQI, National Kidney Foundation. KDOQI clinical practice guideline and clinical practice recommendations for anemia in chronic kidney disease: 2007 update of hemoglobin target. *Am J Kidney Dis* 2007;50:471–530.

25. KDOQI, National Kidney Foundation. KDOQI clinical practice guidelines for bone metabolism and disease in chronic kidney disease. *Am J Kidney Dis* 2003;42(4 suppl 3):S1–S201.

26. KDOQI, National Kidney Foundation. KDOQI clinical practice guidelines for management of dyslipidemias in patients with kidney disease. *Am J Kidney Dis* 2003;41(4 suppl 3):S1–S91.

27. James PA, Oparil S, Carter BL, et al. 2014 evidence-based guideline for the management of high blood pressure in adults: report from the panel members appointed to the Eighth Joint National Committee (JNC 8). *JAMA* 2014;311:507–520.

28. Kidney Disease: Improving Global Outcomes (KDIGO) Blood Pressure Work Group. KDIGO clinical practice guideline for the management of blood pressure in chronic kidney disease. *Kidny Int Suppl* 2012;2:337–414.

29. Taler SJ, Agrawal R, Bakris GL, et al. KDOQI US commentary on the 2012 KDIGO clinical practice guideline for management of blood pressure in CKD. *Am J Kidney Dis* 2013;62:201–213.

30. Stone NJ, Robinson JG, Lichtenstein AH, et al. 2013 ACC/AHA guideline on the treatment of blood cholesterol to reduce atherosclerotic cardiovascular risk in adults: a report of the American College of Cardiology/American Heart Association Task Force on Practice Guidelines. *Circulation* 2014;129:S1-45.

31. Singh AK, Szczech L, Tang KL, et al. Correction of anemia with epoetin alfa in chronic kidney disease. *N Engl J Med* 2006;355:2085–2098.

32. KDOQI, National Kidney Foundation. KDOQI clinical practice guidelines for nutrition in chronic renal failure. *Am J Kidney Dis* 2000;35(6 suppl 2):S1–S140.

Hematuria

GENERAL PRINCIPLES

- Hematuria, or blood in the urine, is common in the outpatient setting.
- Concomitant findings, such as pain, renal injury, and proteinuria, help to localize the site of injury along the genitourinary tract.
- Persistent hematuria may be a sign of serious disease and should not be ignored.

Definition

- Hematuria is the presence of red blood cells (RBCs) in urine.
- Gross hematuria is visible to the naked eye and often manifests as red, pink, or cola-colored urine.
- Microscopic hematuria is defined by the American Urological Association (AUA) as the presence of ≥3 RBCs/high-power field (HPF) on microscopic examination of one properly collected, noncontaminated urinalysis in the absence of obvious benign cause.[1]
- Microscopic hematuria should be confirmed on two out of three midstream clean-catch urine samples before proceeding with further workup.

Classification

- Hematuria is generally categorized based on the source of the blood.
- Blood that enters the urinary content at the glomerular filtration barrier is classified as **glomerular hematuria** and can be associated with any of the following findings:
  - ○ Dysmorphic RBCs
  - ○ Cellular casts
  - ○ Proteinuria (>0.5 g/24 hours)
- Blood that is introduced to the urinary content at any other site in the urinary tract is classified as nonglomerular.

Epidemiology

- Prevalence of microscopic hematuria ranges between 2.4% and 31.1% depending upon the demographics and the underlying risk factors of study population.[1]
- Risk of underlying malignancy varies between 2% and 11% with microscopic hematuria as compared to 15% and 22% with gross hematuria.[2]

Etiology
A brief summary of the causes of hematuria can be found in Table 25-1.[3,4]

Risk Factors
It is impossible to generalize risk factors for hematuria since there are so many different causes. However, common risk factors for hematuria associated with urinary tract malignancy are summarized in Table 25-2.[1]

TABLE 25-1   Causes of Hematuria

Source of hematuria		Causes
Nonglomerular origin	Upper urinary tract	Hypercalciuria
		Hyperuricosuria
		Interstitial nephritis
		Nephrolithiasis
		Papillary necrosis
		Polycystic kidney disease
		Pyelonephritis
		Renal cell carcinoma
		Renal infarction
		Renal vein thrombosis
		Sickle cell disease/trait
		Transitional cell carcinoma (renal pelvis/ureter)
		Trauma
	Lower urinary tract	Benign bladder and ureteral polyps
		Bladder cancer
		Cystitis, prostatitis, urethritis
		Prostate cancer/benign prostatic hypertrophy
		Schistosomiasis
		Trauma
		Urethral or meatal stricture
Glomerular origin		Hereditary nephritis (Alport syndrome)
		IgA nephropathy
		Loin pain-hematuria syndrome
		Primary or secondary glomerulonephritis
		Thin basement membrane nephropathy (benign familial hematuria)
Unknown		Menstrual contamination
		Factitious hematuria
		Exercise-induced hematuria
		Excessive anticoagulation
		Benign uncertain recurrent microscopic hematuria

Data from Cohen RA, Brown RS. Clinical practice. Microscopic hematuria. *N Engl J Med* 2003;348:2330–2338.

TABLE 25-2   Risk Factors for Urinary Tract Malignancy

Male gender
Age (>35 years)
History of smoking (past or current)
Exposure to chemicals or dyes
History of gross hematuria
History of urologic disease
Irritative voiding symptoms
History of pelvic irradiation
Chronic urinary tract infections
History of exposure to chemotherapy (e.g., cyclophosphamide)

DIAGNOSIS

The diagnosis of hematuria can be made by serial visual or microscopic assessments of the urine to confirm the persistent presence of blood. The purpose of the ensuing workup is to localize the cause of the hematuria and provide the appropriate treatment.

Clinical Presentation

History
- Although many causes of hematuria are asymptomatic, a detailed history can often identify symptoms that are suggestive of specific causes of hematuria.
- Pain:
  - Colicky pain at the costovertebral angle (CVA) or flank with radiation to the groin may indicate a ureteral stone but can be associated with blood clot or sloughed renal papilla.
  - A history of dysuria or urinary frequency suggests a urinary tract infection (UTI).
- Urine flow: urinary hesitancy, dribbling, or weak urinary stream accompanies bladder obstruction from an enlarged prostate, stone, or tumor.
- Timing:
  - Cyclical hematuria in women raises concern for genitourinary tract endometriosis.
  - A history of heavy physical activity may explain transient (<48 hours) microscopic hematuria but does not exclude other underlying pathologic conditions.
- Family history: A family history of hematuria can often be found in individuals with kidney stones, polycystic kidney disease, or congenital disease of the glomerular basement membrane, such as thin basement membrane disease and Alport syndrome.
- Associated illnesses:
  - Patients on anticoagulation may have hematuria from nonglomerular sites of bleeding.
  - Individuals with sickle cell disease or trait can develop renal diseases with hematuria.
  - Infections
    - A history of hematuria 1 to 2 weeks after pharyngitis or skin infection suggests post-streptococcal glomerulonephritis (PSGN).
    - IgA nephropathy can present with episodic gross hematuria in the setting of upper respiratory infections (URI).
    - Bacterial endocarditis, sepsis, abscesses, or infection of an indwelling foreign body can be associated with a proliferative glomerulonephritis. Other infections such as viral hepatitis (hepatitis B and C) and syphilis can also cause a variety of glomerulopathies.
  - Autoimmune diseases: immune complex–mediated glomerular diseases such as systemic lupus erythematosus or systemic vasculitis can present with arthritis, arthralgias, fever, or rashes.

Physical Examination
- Thorough physical examination including vital signs (especially blood pressure) and assessment of volume status is important. The presence of edema and hypertension favors a glomerular cause of hematuria.
- Fever, CVA tenderness, or suprapubic tenderness may suggest infection.
- Polycystic kidney or distended bladder may be palpable on abdominal examination.
- Skin rashes, arthritis, or heart murmurs can often be seen with systemic vasculitis, autoimmune glomerulonephritis, and infectious glomerulonephritis.
- Digital rectal examination helps with diagnosis of prostate enlargement, masses, or tenderness.
- Vaginal examination should be performed in women to exclude vaginal bleeding.

Diagnostic Testing

An overview of the workup for hematuria is summarized in Figure 25-1.

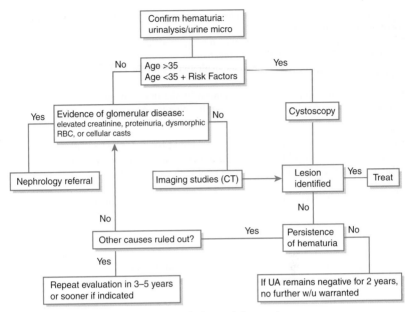

Figure 25-1 Algorithm for the evaluation of microscopic hematuria.

Laboratories

- The urinalysis (dipstick and micro) is the initial test for diagnosis and confirmation of hematuria. The urinalysis is able to distinguish true hematuria from urine that is discolored due to chemical pigments, food metabolites, or medications (e.g., bilirubin, porphyrins, beets, blackberries, blueberries, levodopa, metronidazole, nitrofurantoin, pyridium, phenytoin, rifampin).[5]
- The urine evaluation can also help differentiate glomerular from nonglomerular hematuria.
  - The dipstick is able to detect significant excretion of negatively charged proteins. While it may miss microalbuminuria seen in the earliest stages of nephropathy, a positive urine dipstick is suggestive of glomerular damage and should be further assessed by an estimate of renal function and quantification of proteinuria.
  - Urine microscopy can detect the presence of dysmorphic RBCs and cellular casts. When coupled with proteinuria (≥0.5 g/day) and/or renal insufficiency, it suggests renal parenchymal disease and warrants further nephrologic workup.
- Further laboratory testing can be guided based on history, physical examination, and initial lab testing.
  - Urine culture is indicated if pyuria or bacteriuria is present. Repeat urinalysis 6 weeks after appropriate antimicrobial therapy.
  - Hemoglobin electrophoresis evaluates for suspected sickle cell disease or trait.
  - Antinuclear antibody, antineutrophil cytoplasmic antibody, antiglomerular basement membrane antibodies, complement levels, cryoglobulins, HIV testing, and viral hepatitis serology are used for evaluation of glomerular hematuria.
  - Urine cytology is used for patients at risk for genitourinary malignancies but not for routine screening. If positive, cystoscopy is warranted.

Imaging

- Imaging should be performed in patients with no evidence of glomerular hematuria.
- CT scan with and without intravenous (IV) contrast is currently the preferred initial imaging modality. It has excellent sensitivity for stones and solid masses. In patients with

a contraindication to CT (contrast allergy, pregnancy, renal insufficiency), MRI with and without IV contrast can be considered.
- Ultrasonography is an effective and safe imaging modality in patients with contraindications to CT/MRI and is preferred in pregnancy.
- Retrograde pyelogram (RPG) provides an alternative for the evaluation of upper genitourinary tracts.
- Intravenous urography (IVU) was traditionally the initial imaging modality of upper urinary tracts but has been largely replaced by other methods.

Diagnostic Procedures
- Per the 2012 AUA guidelines, cystoscopy should be performed on all patients with hematuria ≥35 years old, with or without risk factors for urinary tract malignancy. Patients <35 years should have cystoscopy if underlying risk factors for malignancy are present.[1]
- Referral to nephrology with a possible kidney biopsy is indicated if glomerular pathology is suspected.

TREATMENT

- The treatment of hematuria is entirely dependent on the cause.
- See Chapter 24 for treatment of glomerulonephritis.

FOLLOW-UP

- A patient with a history of persistent microscopic hematuria and two consecutive negative annual urinalyses does not need any further urinalysis or other evaluation.[1]
- For persistent microscopic hematuria after negative workup, yearly urinalysis should be conducted.[1]
- Repeat evaluation in 3 to 5 years should be considered for persistent or recurrent microscopic hematuria after initial negative workup.[1]

Nephrolithiasis

GENERAL PRINCIPLES

Kidney stones are crystalline structures in the urinary tract that have achieved sufficient size to cause symptoms or be visible by radiographic imaging techniques.

Epidemiology
- Nephrolithiasis is a common condition that affects men twice as often as women (lifetime risk of 12% vs. 6%).[6]
- The peak age of onset is the third decade, with increasing incidence until age 70.
- Prevalence is influenced by age, sex, race, body size, and geographic distribution.

Classification
- **Calcium stones account for approximately 80% of all stones** and are composed of calcium oxalate, calcium phosphate, or both.[7] Calcium stones are usually idiopathic but can occur with primary hyperparathyroidism, medullary sponge kidney, or distal renal tubular acidosis.
- Uric acid and struvite stones comprise the majority of the remainder.
- **Uric acid stones** form in the setting of uric acid overproduction, low urinary volume, and persistently acidic urine pH.

- **Struvite stones (triple phosphate)** occur under conditions of high urinary pH and increased ammonia production, reflecting infection with urea-splitting organisms (e.g., *Proteus mirabilis, Klebsiella* spp.). *Escherichia coli* does not produce urease.[8,9] Struvite stones are usually composed of magnesium ammonium phosphate (struvite) or carbonate apatite and are often in the shape of a staghorn, as they grow rapidly and typically extend to involve more than one calyx. They often occur in paraplegic or quadriplegic patients because of increased predisposition to UTIs. Staghorn calculi are associated with increased rates of chronic kidney disease.
- Rarely poorly soluble drugs (e.g., triamterene, indinavir) can form stones.

Risk Factors

Risk factors for nephrolithiasis include family history, primary hyperparathyroidism, renal tubular acidosis, recurrent UTIs, inflammatory bowel disease, obesity, gout, diabetes, hot climates, high-protein and high-sodium diet, low fluid intake, and perhaps a high dietary fructose.[6,10]

DIAGNOSIS

Clinical Presentation

- The clinical spectrum of nephrolithiasis ranges from incidental radiologic diagnosis of otherwise asymptomatic disease to severe symptoms, such as flank pain (renal colic), hematuria, UTIs, or even renal failure.
- **Asymptomatic** disease: Patients with nephrolithiasis may be asymptomatic for years.
- **Renal colic:** Renal colic is typically abrupt in onset, colicky in nature, and localized to the flank area. The pain often radiates into the groin and the testicles or labia. Hematuria, urinary frequency, urgency, nausea, and vomiting are common associated symptoms. Staghorn calculi do not generally present in this fashion.[8]
- **Hematuria:** Passage of a stone through the urinary tract may lead to hematuria (gross or microscopic). It can occur even in otherwise asymptomatic patients.
- **Renal failure:** Acute renal failure may result if the obstruction is bilateral or if it obstructs a solitary functional kidney. Chronic obstruction or recurrent nephrolithiasis can lead to chronic kidney disease.
- Patients with staghorn calculi may be asymptomatic but can present with recurrent UTIs, gross hematuria, abdominal pain, fever, and urosepsis.[8]
- It is important to remember that renal colic can mimic other etiologies of acute abdomen (e.g., acute appendicitis, intestinal obstruction, ectopic pregnancy, cholecystitis). They should be ruled out in the appropriate clinical setting.

Diagnostic Testing

Laboratories
- In the acute setting, laboratory studies should include an assessment of renal function with serum creatinine and serum electrolytes.
- As calcium-based stones occur most frequently, the initial evaluation involves an assessment of calcium homeostasis, beginning with serum calcium and intact parathyroid hormone levels.
- Serum uric acid can be checked if uric acid stones are suspected.
- A microscopic assessment of the urine and/or passed stone fragment is mandatory to identify crystals in the urine.
  - Calcium oxalate: envelope-shaped crystals
  - Triple phosphate: coffin lid–shaped crystals
  - Calcium phosphate: small rosettes
  - Cystine: hexagons
  - Uric acid: polymorphic (rhomboid, rosettes, lemon shaped or four-sided whetstones)

- Metabolic evaluation:
  - Patients with recurrent calcium stones or a single noncalcium stone should undergo more extensive evaluation, including at least two 24-hour urine studies for measurement of urine volume, pH, calcium, citrate, creatinine, and sodium. This evaluation identifies metabolic characteristics that put the patient at risk for recurrent stone formation.
  - These urine studies should not be performed within 3 to 4 weeks of an acute stone episode or in the presence of a UTI.
  - A quantitative 24-hour urine for cysteine should be collected if the composition of the stone is unknown.

Imaging
- Helical CT scan (without contrast) is currently the gold standard for diagnosis of nephrolithiasis and has largely replaced other modalities.
- Plain radiography may visualize radiopaque stones, but it is clearly limited by its inability to detect radiolucent stones (e.g., uric acid stones) or provide additional data regarding the urinary tract.
- IVU is more sensitive but entails administration of nephrotoxic contrast.
- Ultrasound is an alternative imaging modality for the diagnosis of nephrolithiasis and hydronephrosis, especially in patients who cannot receive radiation. Presence of small stones may go undetected, and the exact level of obstruction may not be clearly delineated with ultrasound.

TREATMENT

Acute Management
- The treatment of acute renal colic consists of analgesia, relief of obstruction, and control of infection (if present).
- The urine should be strained to retrieve the stone for analysis.
- The rate of spontaneous stone passage is dependent on stone size and location.
  - If the stone is <5 mm, conservative management is adequate, as 80% to 90% of these stones pass spontaneously.[9,11]
  - Stones 5 to 7 mm pass spontaneously only 50% of the time, and stones >7 mm rarely pass spontaneously.
  - Stones <7 mm can be managed conservatively if there is no evidence of obstruction or infection, and the pain can be controlled with oral analgesic agents.
- Fluid administration should be titrated to achieve a urine output of roughly 2.5 L/day to assist with passage of stone.
- Nifedipine and peripheral β-blockers may improve the rate of stone passage (referred to as medical expulsive therapy).[12]
- If there is evidence of hydronephrosis or multiple stones, a follow-up imaging study, such as helical CT, is warranted.[12]
- Complete obstruction, UTI, urosepsis, and uncontrollable pain are indications for expedited stone removal.
  - A urology consultation should be obtained.
  - Treatment modalities include extracorporeal shockwave lithotripsy, percutaneous nephrolithotomy, ureteroscopic removal, surgery, and chemolysis.[12]

Lifestyle/Risk Modification
- **Dietary counseling should be provided to all patients with kidney stones to prevent further stone formation**.
- Fluid intake should be increased to maintain adequate urine flow rates and to lower the urine solute concentration. Suggested target urine volume for patients with nephrolithiasis is >2.5 L/day.

- Dietary calcium intake should be kept within the normal range (800 to 1,000 mg/day). **Calcium restriction may result in impaired bone mineralization and may actually increase the risk for nephrolithiasis** by increasing the absorption and urinary excretion of oxalate.[7,13]
- Low-sodium diet (100 mEq or 2.3 g/day) should be followed to decrease urinary calcium.[7]
- A low-oxalate diet may decrease urinary oxalate.[8] Oxalate is present in beets, rhubarb, spinach, greens, okra, tea, chocolate, cocoa, and nuts.
- A low-protein diet increases urine pH, decreases uric acid excretion, and may also decrease urinary calcium excretion.[7]

Chronic Management

Calcium Stones

- **Hypercalciuria** (>4 mg/kg/day) is most often due to increased gastrointestinal absorption of calcium but may also be caused by impaired renal tubular calcium reabsorption or excessive skeletal resorption as in primary hyperparathyroidism.
  - Patients should maintain a normal calcium intake (800 to 1,000 mg/day).
  - They should ensure adequate fluid intake and consume a salt-restricted diet.
  - Thiazide diuretics (e.g., hydrochlorothiazide 25 to 50 mg PO daily) increase calcium reabsorption and are frequently used in this setting.[7,14]
- **Hypocitraturia** (<250 mg/day) is a frequent finding.
  - Citrate is a potent inhibitor of calcium oxalate precipitation.
  - Citrate excretion can be enhanced by therapy with potassium citrate, starting at a dose of 10 mEq two to three times daily.
- **Hyperoxaluria** (>40 mg/day) often responds to dietary restriction.
  - Patients with small bowel malabsorption due to intrinsic disease (e.g., inflammatory bowel disease) or jejunoileal bypass may absorb excessive oxalate, resulting in enteric hyperoxaluria.
  - Dietary restriction of oxalate and oxalate binders such as oral calcium carbonate or cholestyramine may be useful. Follow-up 24-hour urine collection should be obtained within 2 to 4 weeks of initiating supplemental calcium therapy to monitor for hypercalciuria.
  - Primary hyperoxaluria is due to a genetic enzyme defect in amino acid metabolism in which excess oxalate is produced. These patients have nonenteric hyperoxaluria that does not respond to dietary manipulation.
  - **Hyperuricosuria** (>750 mg/day) may also result in calcium stone formation as uric acid crystals can serve as a nidus for calcium oxalate or calcium phosphate precipitation. Allopurinol has been shown to decrease calcium stone formation in the setting of hyperuricosuria.[7]

Uric Acid Stones

- Conservative therapy involves maintenance of urine volumes of >2.5 L/day through oral hydration, dietary protein/purine restriction (e.g., meat, fish, and poultry), and alkalinization of urine to pH 6.5 to 7.0 with an oral alkali preparation, such as potassium citrate.
- Allopurinol, 300 mg PO daily, can be used to achieve target excretion of uric acid <600 mg/day.
- Probenecid and other uricosuric drugs should be avoided, as they may increase the risk of uric acid or calcium stones.

Cystine Stones

- In general, a nephrologist should follow patients with cystine stones.
- High fluid intake (3 to 4 L/day) and consistent alkalinization (pH >7.5 using potassium citrate, sodium citrate, and sodium bicarbonate) are required to increase solubility and prevent stones.
- Cystine-binding drugs (e.g., penicillamine, tiopronin, and captopril) may be necessary.[15]

Struvite Stones

- For antimicrobial therapy to be effective, the infected stone must be removed surgically, percutaneously, or by extracorporeal shockwave lithotripsy.
- For poor surgical candidates, chemolysis is possible, but it is unlikely to be effective on its own.[9]

REFERENCES

1. Davis R, Jones JS, Barocas DA, et al. Diagnosis, evaluation and follow-up of asymptomatic microhematuria (AMH) in adults: AUA guideline 2012. *J Urol* 2012;188: 2473–2481.
2. Gkougkousis EG, Jain S, Mellon JK. Urologic issues for the nephrologist. In: Floege J, Johnson R, Feehally J., eds. *Comprehensive Clinical Nephrology*, 4th ed. Missouri, MO: Elsevier; 2010:720–723.
3. Cohen RA, Brown RS. Clinical practice. Microscopic hematuria. *N Engl J Med* 2003; 348:2330–2338.
4. Juran PJ. Approach to hematuria. In: Cheng S, Vijayan A., eds. *Nephrology Subspecialty Consult*, 3rd ed. Philadelphia, PA: Lippincott Williams & Wilkins; 2012:31–38.
5. Emmett M, Fenves AZ, Schwartz JC. Approach to the patient with kidney disease. In: Taal MW, Chertow GM, eds. *Brenner and Rector's the Kidney*, 9th ed. Philadelphia, PA: Elsevier; 2012:844–847.
6. Curhan GC. Epidemiology of stone disease. *Urol Clin North Am* 2007;34:287–293.
7. Delvecchio FC, Preminger GM. Medical management of stone disease. *Curr Opin Urol* 2003;13:2–33.
8. Healy KA, Ogan K. Pathophysiology and management of infectious staghorn calculi. *Urol Clin North Am* 2007;34:363–374.
9. Miller OF, Kane CJ. Time to stone passage for observed ureteral calculi: a guide for patient education. *J Urol* 1999;162:688–690.
10. Tracy CR, Pearle MS. Update on the medical management of stone disease. *Curr Opin Urol* 2009;19:200–204.
11. Coll DM, Varanelli MJ, Smith RC. Relationship of spontaneous passage of ureteral calculi to stone size and location as revealed by unenhanced helical CT. *AJR Am J Roentgenol* 2002;178:101–113.
12. Preminger GM, Tiselius HG, Assimos DG, EAU/AUA Nephrolithiasis Guideline Panel. 2007 guideline for the management of ureteral calculi. *J Urol* 2007;178:2418–2434.
13. Borghi L, Schianchi T, Meschi T, et al. Comparison of two diets for the prevention of recurrent stones in idiopathic hypercalciuria. *N Engl J Med* 2002;346:77–84.
14. Escribano J, Balaguer A, Pagone F. Pharmacological interventions for preventing complications in idiopathic hypercalciuria. *Cochrane Database Syst Rev* 2009;(1):CD004754.
15. Mattoo A, Goldfarb DS. Cystinuria. *Semin Nephrol* 2008;28:181–191.

General Infectious Diseases

Enrique Cornejo Cisneros and Susana M. Lazarte

RESPIRATORY TRACT INFECTIONS

Acute Rhinosinusitis

GENERAL PRINCIPLES

- Defined as inflammation of the mucosa of the nasal passage and paranasal sinuses lasting up to 4 weeks.
- **The most common etiology is a viral upper respiratory infection.** Bacteria can secondarily infect an inflamed sinus cavity, but this only accounts for 0.5% to 2% of cases.[1]
- **Since management of an acute viral rhinosinusitis (AVRS)** is supportive, the main focus for the clinician should be in **identifying** those cases with **acute bacterial rhinosinusitis (ABRS)**.
- The most common bacteria associated with ABRS are *Streptococcus pneumoniae*, *Haemophilus influenzae*, and *Moraxella catarrhalis*.
- Complications of ABRS are very uncommon and include orbital cellulitis, cavernous sinus thrombosis, osteomyelitis, meningitis, and brain abscess. These complications represent medical emergencies that require hospitalization.

DIAGNOSIS

Clinical Presentation

- The diagnosis is clinical. Acute rhinosinusitis of any etiology presents with three major symptoms: nasal congestion or blockage, purulent rhinorrhea, and facial pain or pressure.[2,3]
- AVRS symptoms typically peak within 2 to 3 days of onset, decline gradually thereafter, and disappear within 10 to 14 days. Any pattern that deviates from the "classical" viral disease progression could suggest bacterial infection.
- Three criteria help distinguish ABRS from AVRS[4]:
  - Persistent signs and symptoms lasting for ≥10 days.
  - Severe symptoms for 3 to 4 consecutive days **at the beginning** of illness: high fever (≥39°C) **and** purulent rhinorrhea or facial pain.
  - "Double sickening": new onset of fever or increased nasal discharge following a typical viral upper respiratory tract infection (URI) that lasted 5 to 6 days and was initially improving.

Diagnostic Testing

- Imaging studies such as plain radiographs and CT scans are of little diagnostic value in uncomplicated acute rhinosinusitis. **An abnormal radiographic finding cannot distinguish a viral from bacterial etiology.**[5]
- Cultures obtained by sinus aspiration are not indicated for uncomplicated ABRS. They could be performed if the patient has failed to respond to initial empiric antimicrobial therapy.

TREATMENT

- Intranasal saline irrigation with either physiologic or hypertonic saline can be beneficial in symptomatic control, although the evidence supporting it is still very weak.[4]
- Topical or systemic decongestants, antihistamines, and mucolytics are frequently used for symptom control. However, there are no significant data to support their use. Topical decongestants should not be used for more than 3 consecutive days to avoid rebound congestion.
- Intranasal corticosteroids have been shown to provide a modest relief in symptoms when compared to placebo and should be strongly considered in patients with allergic rhinitis.[6]
- Management of AVRS is **supportive**.
- If ABRS is diagnosed, antibiotic therapy may be started. It is important, however, to note that many patients will improve without antibiotic therapy. The recommended initial duration of empiric therapy is 5 to 7 days.[4]
- First-line antimicrobial agents:
  - Amoxicillin-clavulanate 500 mg/125 mg PO tid or 875 mg/125 mg PO bid
  - Doxycycline 100 mg PO bid or 200 mg PO once a day
- If symptoms worsen after 48 to 72 hours of initial empiric antimicrobial therapy or if they fail to improve after 3 to 5 days, second-line agents may be considered.[4]
- Second-line antimicrobial agents:
  - Amoxicillin-clavulanate 2,000 mg/125 mg PO bid
  - Levofloxacin 500 mg PO once a day
  - Moxifloxacin 400 mg PO once a day
- If second-line agents are used, duration of therapy can be extended to 7 to 10 days.

Pharyngitis

GENERAL PRINCIPLES

- Acute pharyngitis is one of the most common conditions encountered in primary care. **Most cases are of viral etiology**, benign, and self-limited.
- The major treatable causative agent is **group A streptococcus (GAS)**. Approximately 10% to 20% of sore throats yield positive cultures for GAS.[7]
- Other less common causes of acute bacterial pharyngitis include *Corynebacterium diphtheriae*, *Neisseria gonorrhoeae*, *Chlamydophila pneumoniae*, and *Mycoplasma pneumoniae*, among others.
- When evaluating patients with sore throat, it is also important to consider the possibility of infectious mononucleosis (Epstein-Barr Virus) or acute retroviral syndrome (HIV).

DIAGNOSIS

Clinical Presentation

Symptoms include sore throat, odynophagia, fever, and malaise. When caused by a virus, typical symptoms of a URI can also be present (nasal congestion, rhinorrhea, hoarseness, cough). Exam may reveal pharyngeal erythema, tonsillar exudates, or anterior cervical adenopathy.

Diagnostic Criteria

The **Centor clinical scoring system** can help to identify those patients who have a higher likelihood of GAS pharyngitis (Table 26-1).[7,8] However, **clinical features alone do not reliably discriminate between GAS and viral pharyngitis**. These criteria should be used in conjunction with other diagnostic tests for GAS.

TABLE 26-1	Modified Centor Criteria to Diagnose Group A Streptococcal Pharyngitis

Criteria	Point
Tonsillar exudates	1
Tender anterior cervical adenopathy	1
Temperature >38°C	1
Absence of cough	1
Age 3–14	1
Age 15–44	0
Age ≥ 45	−1

Score	Risk of GAS infection (%)	Action
0	1–2.5	No testing. No antibiotics
1	5–10	May choose to test
2	11–17	Perform testing,
3	28–35	antibiotics if positive
4–5	51–53	Empiric antibiotics

Data from McIsaac WJ, White D, Tannenbaum D, et al. A clinical score to reduce unnecessary antibiotic use in patients with sore throat. *CMAJ* 1998;158:75–83.

Diagnostic Testing

- Throat cultures are 90% to 95% sensitive but can take 18 to 24 hours or more to yield results.[9,10]
- **Rapid antigen detection tests (RADTs)** can be done at the office and are highly specific (approximately 95%). However, the sensitivity is variable (70% to 95%).[9,10]
- RADT should be performed in patients with a Centor score of 2 to 3. There is no need for further testing for a Centor score <2.[7,9]
- Routine use of throat culture for the diagnosis of GAS after a negative RADT is not recommended in adults.[9,10]
- Antistreptococcal antibody titers are not recommended for routine diagnosis of acute pharyngitis, as they reflect past but not current events.[10]

TREATMENT

- Treatment of **acute viral pharyngitis** is **supportive**.
- The goals of therapy for GAS pharyngitis are to reduce duration and severity of symptoms, to reduce the risk of complications such as rheumatic fever or peritonsillar abscess, and to reduce transmission to close contacts.
- Recommended duration of therapy is 10 days.
- Preferred treatment options include the following:
  - Benzathine penicillin G 1.2 million units IM for one dose
  - Penicillin V 500 mg PO bid or 250 mg PO four times daily
  - Amoxicillin 500 mg PO tid
- For patients with penicillin allergy, treatment options include cefadroxil or cephalexin (only if allergic reaction is not anaphylaxis), clarithromycin or azithromycin (for 5 days), or clindamycin.

Acute Bronchitis

GENERAL PRINCIPLES

- Acute bronchitis is a self-limited inflammation of the large airways of the lung that is characterized by cough without pneumonia.[11]

- **Viruses account for the majority of cases (>90%)** and include influenza, parainfluenza, respiratory syncytial virus, coronavirus, adenovirus, rhinovirus, and human metapneumovirus.
- The role of bacteria in acute bronchitis is unclear, but implicated species include *Bordetella pertussis*, *Mycoplasma pneumoniae*, and *Chlamydophila pneumoniae*. As a group, these agents account for 5% to 10% of uncomplicated acute bronchitis in adults.[12]
- Of all the etiologic agents that cause acute bronchitis, **influenza virus** and ***Bordetella pertussis*** require special attention because of their morbidity and treatment options.
- For pertussis (whooping cough), universal childhood vaccination is recommended. It has been proven that immunization during childhood wears off over time. Therefore, adults aged 19 to 64 years should receive a single booster administration with Tdap (acellular pertussis vaccine combined with tetanus toxoid and reduced diphtheria toxoid). In addition, adults aged 65 years and older who have not previously received Tdap should receive a single booster administration with Tdap.

DIAGNOSIS

Clinical Presentation

- Patients present with cough lasting more than 5 days, which may be associated with sputum production. **Cough may last up to 3 weeks for an episode of acute bronchitis**.
- **Purulent sputum** is common and results from sloughing off of the bronchial epithelium. It is **not necessarily an indication of a bacterial rather than a viral infection**.
- While evaluating a patient with acute cough, the clinician should be careful in ruling out more serious conditions, such as pneumonia. The presence of abnormal vital signs and abnormal findings on chest examination (e.g., rales, egophony, fremitus) raises concern for pneumonia.
- **Pertussis (whooping cough)** should be suspected after ≥2 weeks of cough that then becomes paroxysmal (succession of coughs without inspiration), is associated with an inspiratory "whoop" between paroxysms, and may be associated with posttussive emesis. **The disease can be mild, and the characteristic "whoop" may be absent in previously immunized patients.**

Diagnostic Testing

- Routine sputum cultures are not recommended since bacterial pathogens only play a minor role in acute bronchitis.
- Influenza testing should be considered based on seasonal patterns of influenza and patient presentation.
- Testing for pertussis includes nasopharyngeal culture and polymerase chain reaction (PCR).
- Chest radiography (CXR) is not indicated in the absence of abnormal vital signs or concerning physical exam findings. The exception is cough in the elderly patient, in which pneumonia could have a more subtle presentation.

TREATMENT

- **Treatment is largely supportive in patients with acute bronchitis.**
- Antivirals for influenza should be considered if influenza infection is confirmed within 24 to 48 hours of onset of symptoms.
- **Routine antibiotic treatment of uncomplicated acute bronchitis is not recommended, regardless of duration of cough.** Multiple randomized trials have failed to support a significant role for antibiotic therapy in acute bronchitis.[11–13]
- The one circumstance for which evidence supports antibiotic treatment of uncomplicated acute bronchitis is when there is suspicion of pertussis.[12]

- **Treatment of pertussis can decrease the duration and severity of cough if started within 2 weeks of symptom onset.** Treatment is also important to reduce the spread of the infection.
- Treatment regimens for pertussis in adults[14]:
  - Erythromycin 500 mg PO four times daily for 14 days
  - Clarithromycin 500 mg PO bid for 7 days
  - Azithromycin 500 mg PO once on day 1, followed by 250 mg PO once a day on days 2 to 5
- In case of allergy or intolerance to macrolides, trimethoprim-sulfamethoxazole (TMP-SMX) 160 to 800 mg PO bid for 14 days may be used.[14]
- Postexposure prophylaxis for pertussis is indicated for close contacts within 3 weeks of the onset of cough in the index case. The regimens are the same as for the treatment of pertussis.

Influenza

GENERAL PRINCIPLES

Definition

- Influenza is caused by infection with one of three subtypes of circulating RNA viruses: influenza A, B, or C.
- Influenza C virus causes a mild respiratory illness, and its diagnosis, treatment, and prevention are generally not pursued.
- Two important concepts in influenza pathogenesis are antigenic drift and antigenic shift:
  - Antigenic drift:
    - Results from point mutations in the envelope glycoproteins (**h**emagglutinin or **n**euraminidase) within a strain, which occur season to season
    - Can lead to outbreaks of variable extent and severity
    - Vaccine changed annually to account for antigenic drift
  - Antigenic shift:
    - Results from complete changes in the **h**emagglutinin or **n**euraminidase, creating a new strain (e.g., from H2N2 to H3N2)
    - Can lead to epidemics and pandemics
- Complications from influenza include primary influenza viral pneumonia, exacerbation of underlying medical conditions (e.g., pulmonary or cardiac disease), secondary bacterial pneumonia (*S. pneumoniae, S. aureus, H. influenzae*), sinusitis, and otitis media.

Epidemiology

- Influenza is predominantly seasonal with the Northern Hemisphere affected from November to April and the Southern Hemisphere affected May to September.
- Spread from person to person occurs primarily through large-particle respiratory droplet transmission, which requires close contact. Contact with respiratory droplet–contaminated surfaces is another possible source of transmission.
- Certain groups are at **increased risk of severe disease or death** secondary to influenza virus infection. These groups include elderly persons (age >65), persons with chronic medical conditions, immunocompromised persons, and pregnant women.

Prevention

- The current recommendation for influenza vaccination in the US is for annual administration to patients at least 6 months of age in the absence of contraindications to influenza vaccine.
- Contraindications include previous severe reaction to an influenza vaccination, severe allergy to chicken eggs, history of Guillain-Barré syndrome (GBS) within 6 weeks following receipt of influenza vaccine, and being moderately or severely ill (with or without fever).

- Following recommendations for influenza vaccination is especially important for high-risk individuals, their close contacts, and health care workers.
- The U.S. Centers for Disease Control and Prevention (CDC) offers annual guidelines for influenza vaccination (http://www.cdc.gov/flu, last accessed December 29, 2014).

DIAGNOSIS

Clinical Presentation

Most patients with influenza exhibit an acute, uncomplicated, self-limiting course, and some may even be asymptomatic. Symptoms may include abrupt onset of fever, headache, myalgia, and malaise, associated with manifestations of an URI.

Diagnostic Testing

- Respiratory specimens for diagnosis should be obtained preferably within 5 days of illness onset, as viral shedding in immunocompetent patients will be substantially decreased after that time.[15]
- Several diagnostic options are available:
  ○ Viral culture is the gold standard. Results take days to come back. Used for public health surveillance.
  ○ Immunofluorescence: slightly lower sensitivity and specificity than culture, but results available within hours. Performance depends on laboratory expertise.
  ○ RT-PCR: more sensitive than culture. Results available within 4 to 6 hours. Differentiates between types and subtypes.
  ○ Rapid antigen testing: convenient and fast, with results in 10 to 30 minutes. Significantly lower sensitivity than RT-PCR and culture.

TREATMENT

- Clinical trials have shown that early antiviral treatment can shorten the duration of symptoms, can shorten the duration of hospitalization, and may reduce the risk of complications from influenza.[15,16]
- **Clinical benefit is stronger if therapy is started within 48 hours of illness onset.**[15,16]
- However, treatment of any person with confirmed or suspected influenza who requires hospitalization is recommended, even if the patient presents >48 hours after illness onset.[16]
- **Adamantanes**: amantadine and rimantadine. These are only effective against influenza A. Due to high levels of resistance in the US, CDC no longer recommends its use.[16]
- **Neuraminidase inhibitors**: zanamivir and oseltamivir.
  ○ Effective against both influenza A and B
  ○ Oseltamivir: 75 mg PO bid for 5 days
  ○ Zanamivir: two 5-mg inhalations (10 mg total) bid for 5 days
- Postexposure chemoprophylaxis may be considered in close contacts of a confirmed or suspected case of influenza during that person's infectious period if those contacts are at high risk for complications of influenza. It should **only** be used when antivirals can be started **within 48 hours** of the most recent exposure. Options include
  ○ Oseltamivir: 75 mg PO once a day for 10 days
  ○ Zanamivir: two 5-mg inhalations (10 mg total) once a day for 10 days
- Influenza viruses and their susceptibility to antiviral medications evolve rapidly. Physicians should keep abreast of patterns of influenza circulation and susceptibility in their communities. Updated information in the US can be found on the CDC website: http://www.cdc.gov/flu (last accessed December 29, 2014).

Community-Acquired Pneumonia

GENERAL PRINCIPLES

Etiology

- **Community-acquired pneumonia (CAP)** is an infection of the lung parenchyma acquired outside of hospitals or extended-care facilities.
- Bacteria are the most common cause of CAP. The most common pathogens involved are *Streptococcus pneumoniae*, *Mycoplasma pneumoniae*, *Haemophilus influenza*, and *Chlamydophila pneumoniae*.
- Less common causes include *Legionella* spp., *Staphylococcus aureus*, Enterobacteriaceae, and *Pseudomonas aeruginosa*.
- The most common cause of viral CAP in adults is influenza.

Prevention

- Two types of pneumococcal vaccines are approved for use in the US for prevention of noninvasive and invasive pneumococcal infections: pneumococcal polysaccharide vaccine (PPSV23) and pneumococcal protein-conjugate vaccine (PCV13).
- PPSV23 is recommended for all adults ≥65 years of age and in persons 19 to 64 years of age who have a condition that increases the risk of pneumococcal disease (including cigarette smoking, chronic lung disease, chronic heart disease, diabetes, among others).
- PCV13 is recommended (in addition to PPSV23) for use in individuals aged 19 or older with functional or anatomic asplenia, immunocompromising conditions, cerebrospinal fluid leaks, cochlear implants, or advanced kidney disease. In late 2014 the Advisory Committee on Immunization Practices (ACIP) recommended PCV13 for all adults ≥65 years.

DIAGNOSIS

Clinical Presentation

- Common symptoms include fever, cough, sputum production, dyspnea, and pleuritic chest pain. Malaise, anorexia, chills, and abdominal complaints are also frequent.
- **Clinical features of pneumonia may be lacking or altered in elderly patients.** Confusion or delirium could be the initial presentation in the elderly.
- On exam, audible rales may be present. If a consolidation develops, bronchial breath sounds, dullness, egophony, and whispered pectoriloquy are associated findings.
- Tachypnea and hypotension are ominous findings and warrant more rapid evaluation.

Diagnostic Testing

- A CBC often reveals a leukocytosis with a leftward shift.
- A CXR should be obtained in all patients suspected of having pneumonia. The presence of an infiltrate on CXR is diagnostic of pneumonia when clinical features are supportive.
- The radiographic appearance of CAP may include lobar consolidation, interstitial infiltrates, or cavitation.
- **Routine testing for microbiologic diagnosis is usually not indicated in the outpatient setting**, since most patients do well with empiric antibiotic therapy.
- Exceptions may apply if clinical or epidemiologic clues raise suspicion for specific pathogens that would alter empiric therapy.
- Consider the following tests in selected patients in the appropriate clinical scenario: rapid antigen test for influenza, urinary antigen test for *Legionella*, urinary antigen test for pneumococcus, and sputum for acid-fast staining.
- Pretreatment sputum Gram stain and culture are useful only when quality specimens can be obtained.

TREATMENT

- The decision as to whether the patient can be safely treated as an outpatient or needs admission to the hospital can be assisted by the use of severity-of-illness scores such as the **Pneumonia Severity Index (PSI)**[17] (Table 26-2) or the **CURB-65 score**[18] (Table 26-3).
- Most patients will have a good response to empiric antibiotic therapy; however, treatment should always be tailored to provide narrow coverage if the etiologic agent is known.
- The following are risk factors associated with **drug-resistant *Streptococcus pneumoniae* (DRSP)**: age > 65 years; β-lactam, macrolide, or fluoroquinolone therapy within the last 3 months; alcoholism; medical comorbidities; immunosuppressive therapy or illness; and exposure to a child in a daycare center.

TABLE 26-2	Pneumonia Severity Index

Characteristic	Point			
Demographic factors				
Male	0			
Female	−10			
Age	1/year			
Nursing home resident	10			
Comorbidities				
Neoplasia	30			
Liver disease	20			
Heart failure	10			
Cerebrovascular disease	10			
Renal disease	10			
Physical exam				
Altered mental status	20			
Respiratory rate ≥30/minute	20			
Systolic blood pressure <90 mm Hg	20			
Temperature <35°C or ≥40°C	15			
Heart rate ≥125/minute	10			
Laboratory findings				
Arterial pH <7.35	30			
Urea ≥30 mg/dL	20			
Sodium <130 mmol/L	20			
Glucose ≥250 mg/dL	10			
Hematocrit <30%	10			
PaO_2 <60 mm Hg	10			
Radiographic findings				
Pleural effusion	10			
Total points		**Class**	**Mortality (%)**	**Management**
0		I	0.1	Outpatient
≤70		II	0.6	Outpatient
71–90		III	0.9	Brief inpatient
91–130		IV	9.3	Inpatient
>130		V	27.0	Inpatient

Data from Fine MJ, Auble TE, Yealy DM, et al. A prediction rule to identify low-risk patients with community-acquired pneumonia. *N Engl J Med* 1997;336:243–50.

TABLE 26-3 | **CURB-65 Score**

Criteria	Point	
Confusion	1	
Urea >20 mg/dL	1	
Respiratory rate >30/minute	1	
Blood pressure (systolic <90 mm Hg or diastolic ≤60 mm Hg)	1	
Age ≥**65**	1	

Score	Mortality (%)	Management
0	0.7	Outpatient
1	2.1	Outpatient
2	9.2	Inpatient
3	14.5	Consider intensive care unit
4	40	Consider intensive care unit
5	57	Consider intensive care unit

Data from Lim WS, van der Eerden MM, Laing R, et al. Defining community acquired pneumonia severity on presentation to hospital: an international derivation and validation study. *Thorax* 2003;58:377–82.

- Comorbidities including chronic heart, lung, liver, or renal disease, diabetes mellitus, malignancy, and asplenia should be taken into account when choosing empiric antibiotic therapy.
- Empiric regimen for previously healthy patients, with no use of antimicrobials within the previous 3 months and with no risk factors for DRSP: macrolide **or** doxycycline.[19]
- Empiric regimen for patients with comorbidities, use of antimicrobials within the previous 3 months, or risk factors for DRSP infection[19]:
  - A respiratory fluoroquinolone
  - A β-lactam **plus** a macrolide
  - A β-lactam **plus** doxycycline (less evidence than macrolide combination)
- The following are the suggested oral doses for the abovementioned antimicrobial agents:
  - Macrolides: azithromycin, 500 mg on day one followed by 4 days of 250 mg a day; clarithromycin, 500 mg bid; and erythromycin: 250 mg every 6 hours
  - Doxycycline: 100 mg bid
  - Respiratory fluoroquinolones: levofloxacin, 750 mg daily; moxifloxacin, 400 mg daily; gemifloxacin, 320 mg daily
  - β-Lactams: amoxicillin, 1,000 mg tid; amoxicillin-clavulanate, 2,000 mg/125 mg PO bid; cefpodoxime, 200 mg bid; cefuroxime, 500 mg bid
- **The minimum duration of therapy is 5 days.** Patients should be afebrile for 48 to 72 hours and clinically stable before stopping antibiotic therapy.
- Patients with CAP should be appropriately vaccinated for influenza and pneumococcal infection.
- Smoking cessation should be a goal for all patients with CAP who smoke.

COMPLICATIONS

Complications from CAP include bacteremia with extrapulmonary infection, parapneumonic effusion, empyema, necrotizing pneumonia, and lung abscess.

Tuberculosis

GENERAL PRINCIPLES

- **Tuberculosis (TB)** is a systemic disease caused by *Mycobacterium tuberculosis*. It is one of the most common infectious causes of death worldwide.
- TB most commonly affects the lungs; however, any organ or tissue can be involved. Extrapulmonary TB accounts for 14% to 25% of reported cases globally.[20]
- TB is transmitted by aerosolized droplets that deposit in the alveoli after inhalation. The bacilli proliferate in the alveolar macrophages and spread to lymph nodes. Subsequent hematogenous dissemination leads to seeding in extrapulmonary locations.
- TB infection can be immediately cleared, lead to primary disease, evolve to latent infection, or reappear as reactivation disease (most common presentation).
- Risk factors associated with TB include malnutrition, immunosuppression (HIV, transplant, tumor necrosis factor [TNF]-α inhibitors), systemic disease (diabetes, renal disease, malignancy), substance abuse, close household contact of a patient with TB, birth in a TB-endemic area, and exposure to crowded settings with poor ventilation.

DIAGNOSIS

Clinical Presentation

- **Pulmonary TB** most commonly presents with **productive cough**, which may be accompanied by other respiratory symptoms (shortness of breath, chest pain, hemoptysis) and/or **constitutional symptoms** (e.g., loss of appetite, weight loss, fever, night sweats, and fatigue).
- **Tuberculosis suspect**: patient with symptoms or signs suggestive of TB, most commonly an otherwise unexplained productive cough for more than 2 to 3 weeks.
- **Definite tuberculosis:** patient with *Mycobacterium tuberculosis* identified from a clinical specimen, either by culture or by a nucleic acid amplification test.

Diagnostic Testing

- Patients meeting clinical and/or epidemiologic criteria for TB should have a CXR. Reactivation TB typically involves focal infiltration of the apical-posterior segments of the upper lobes or the superior segment of the lower lobes.
- All patients with CXR findings suggestive of TB should have sputum specimens (coughed and induced or from bronchoscopy) submitted for microbiologic examination.
- **All patients suspected of having pulmonary TB should have at least two, and preferably three, sputum specimens obtained for microscopic examination.** When possible, at least one early-morning specimen should be obtained (sputum collected at this time has the highest yield).[21]
- **Acid-fast bacteria** observed on stained sputum specimens may represent *M. tuberculosis* or nontuberculous mycobacteria. Thus, acid-fast staining should be confirmed by culture or molecular testing.
- For all patients suspected of having extrapulmonary TB, appropriate specimens from the suspected sites of involvement should be obtained for microscopy, culture, and histopathologic examination.
- **All patients with suspected or confirmed TB should have testing for HIV.**

TREATMENT

- Treatment guidelines are available through the World Health Organization (www.who.int) and the Infectious Diseases Society of America (IDSA) (www.idsociety.org, last accessed December 29, 2014).

- The goals of therapy are eradication of *M. tuberculosis* infection, preventing TB relapse, preventing development of drug resistance, and preventing TB transmission.
- Treatment should be undertaken with the guidance of an expert and may include hospitalization to initiate therapy, patient education, and respiratory isolation.
- **Directly observed therapy (DOT)** is considered the standard of care. This allows confirmation of completion of therapy and prevents emergence of drug resistance.
- **The local public health authorities should be notified of all cases of TB so that contacts can be identified and arrangements for DOT can be made.**
- Initial therapy for tuberculosis should include four drugs: isoniazid (H), rifampin (R), pyrazinamide (Z), and ethambutol (E).
- All TB treatment regimens include an initial intensive phase and a continuation phase. Recommended doses for first-line drugs can be found in Table 26-4.[20]
- The WHO recommends a standard regimen for new TB patients (presumed, or known, to have drug-susceptible TB) that includes a 2-month initial phase with all four drugs followed by a 4-month continuation phase with isoniazid and rifampicin: 2HRZE/4HR.[20]
- The optimal dosing frequency for new TB patients is daily throughout the course of therapy. The WHO offers two alternatives to this regimen[20]:
  - Daily intensive phase followed by three times weekly continuation phase [2HRZE/4(HR)$_3$], provided that each dose is directly observed
  - Three times weekly dosing throughout therapy [2(HRZE)$_3$/4(HR)$_3$], provided that every dose is directly observed and the patient is **not** living with HIV or living in an HIV-prevalent setting
- To minimize neurotoxicity, supplemental pyridoxine should be provided (25 to 50 mg daily) in patients taking isoniazid.
- HIV-positive patients should be treated with the same regimens. Some experts recommend prolonged therapy (8 months or more) in certain circumstances. Treatment requires the supervision of an HIV specialist.
- Extrapulmonary TB should be treated with the same regimens as pulmonary TB. However, experts recommend 9 months of therapy for TB of bone and joints and 9 to 12 months of therapy for TB meningitis. In TB meningitis, ethambutol could be replaced by streptomycin.
- Unless drug resistance is suspected, adjuvant corticosteroid treatment is recommended for TB meningitis and pericarditis.

TABLE 26-4	Recommended Doses of First-Line Antituberculosis Drugs for Adults			
	Recommended dose			
	Daily		**Three times per week**	
Drug	Dose and range (mg/kg body weight)	Maximum (mg)	Dose and range (mg/kg body weight)	Maximum (mg)
Isoniazid	5 (4–6)	300	10 (8–12)	900
Rifampin	10 (8–12)	600	10 (8–12)	600
Pyrazinamide	25 (20–30)	—	35 (30–40)	—
Ethambutol	15 (15–20)	—	30 (25–35)	—

Data from WHO. *Treatment of Tuberculosis: Guidelines*, 4th ed. Geneva, Switzerland: World Health Organization; 2010.

SPECIAL CONSIDERATIONS

- **Multidrug-resistant tuberculosis (MDR-TB):** resistance to at least isoniazid and rifampin.
- **Extensively drug-resistant tuberculosis (XDR-TB):** resistance to isoniazid, rifampin, and fluoroquinolones, as well as aminoglycosides (amikacin, kanamycin) or capreomycin, or both.
- An assessment of the likelihood of drug resistance should be performed for all patients. **The most critical risk factor for MDR-TB is prior TB treatment.** Other risk factors include contact with a proven MDR case, patients who remain sputum smear positive at month 2 or 3 of therapy, and HIV infection.
- **Treatment of MDR-TB and XDR-TB requires a TB expert**.

MONITORING/FOLLOW-UP

- For smear-positive pulmonary TB patients treated with first-line drugs, sputum smear microscopy should be performed at completion of the intensive phase of treatment.
  - If the specimen obtained at the end of the intensive phase (month 2) is smear positive, sputum smear microscopy should be repeated at the end of month 3.
  - If the specimen obtained at the end of month 3 is smear positive, sputum culture and **drug susceptibility testing (DST)** should be performed.[21]
- All new pulmonary TB patients who were smear positive at the start of treatment should have sputum specimens for smear microscopy at the end of months 5 and 6.
- **Cure:** A patient whose sputum smear or culture was positive at the beginning of the treatment but who was smear or culture negative in the last month of treatment and on at least one other occasion.[20]
- **Treatment failure:** A patient whose sputum smear or culture is positive at 5 months or later during treatment, or a patient found to harbor a MDR strain at any point during treatment, whether they are smear negative or positive.[20] Patients who fail treatment should be managed by a TB expert.
- Follow-up radiographic examinations are usually unnecessary and might be misleading.

Latent Tuberculosis

GENERAL PRINCIPLES

Mycobacterium tuberculosis infection can be contained by host defenses and remain latent. **Latent TB infection (LTBI)** has the potential to progress to active disease at any time. The lifetime risk of progression is 10%.

DIAGNOSIS

- Latent TB patients are asymptomatic.
- **The goal of screening for LTBI is to identify patients at increased risk for developing active TB and who would, therefore, benefit from treatment.** These include the following:
  - Close contacts of patients with pulmonary TB
  - Health care workers and other occupations with exposure to patients with active TB
  - Recent immigrants (within 5 years) from high-prevalence countries
  - Patients with abnormal CXR with signs of healed TB
  - Patients with silicosis, intravenous drug use, diabetes mellitus, HIV, end-stage renal disease, lymphoma, leukemia, and head and neck malignancy

TABLE 26-5	Tuberculin Skin Test Interpretation

Reaction size (mm)	Risk group
≥5	HIV, recent contacts of a TB case, CXR consistent with prior TB, immunosuppressed patients
≥10	Recent (≤5 years) immigrants from endemic areas, IVDU, residents and employees of high-risk congregate settings (e.g., homeless shelters, prisons, nursing homes, hospitals), mycobacteria laboratory personnel, patients with chronic medical illnesses (e.g., silicosis, DM, ESRD, leukemia/lymphoma, malabsorption, low body weight), children <4 years of age, or infants, children, and adolescents exposed to adults at high risk
≥15	Persons with no risk factors for TB

CXR, chest radiograph; IVDU, intravenous drug users; DM, diabetes mellitus; ESRD, end-stage renal disease; TB, tuberculosis.

- ○ Patients with transplant, chemotherapy, or other major immunosuppressive conditions
- ○ Treatment with TNF-α inhibitors or systemic glucocorticoids
- ○ Conditions associated with rapid weight loss or chronic malnutrition
- Screening for LTBI is done by **tuberculin skin testing (TST)** or by **interferon-gamma release assays (IGRAs)**. A positive screening test without active disease is indicative of LTBI.
- The tuberculin material used for skin testing is **purified protein derivative (PPD)**, injected using the Mantoux technique. The test is interpreted by reading (at 48 to 72 hours) the transverse diameter of the area of induration (not erythema) at the site of injection.
- Interpretation of TST can be found in Table 26-5.[22]
- Close contacts of patients with active TB with a nonreactive TST should have a repeat test after 10 weeks.
- **Bacillus Calmette-Guérin (BCG)** vaccination in the 1st year of life has been reported to be a source of false-positive results on TST. Of note, BCG vaccination causes **no significant effect on TST after 10 years or more**. In contrast to TST, IGRAs are not affected by BCG vaccination status.

TREATMENT

- Two regimens are now jointly recommended for the treatment of LTBI by the CDC:[22,23]
  - ○ Isoniazid 5 mg/kg/day (maximum 300 mg) for 9 months
  - ○ Isoniazid 15 mg/kg (maximum 900 mg) plus rifapentine, both given once a week by **DOT** for 12 weeks
- The isoniazid-rifapentine regimen is only recommended for patients with LTBI aged ≥12 years and who have factors that are predictive of TB developing (e.g., recent exposure to contagious TB, conversion from negative to positive on TST or IGRA, and radiographic findings of healed pulmonary TB). The regimen is not recommended for HIV-positive patients who are receiving antiretroviral therapy.
- The weekly dose of rifapentine according to body weight is 300 mg (10 to 14 kg), 450 mg (14.1 to 25 kg), 600 (25.1 to 32 kg), 750 (32.1 to 49.9 kg), and 900 (≥50 kg).
- Patients taking isoniazid should receive supplemental pyridoxine (25 to 50 mg daily) to minimize neurotoxicity.
- Treatment of LTBI after MDR-TB and XDR-TB exposure is a complex issue and should be undertaken with the guidance of a TB expert.

URINARY TRACT INFECTIONS

Uncomplicated Urinary Tract Infections in Women

GENERAL PRINCIPLES

- Uncomplicated **urinary tract infection (UTI)** refers to cystitis and pyelonephritis in premenopausal, nonpregnant women with no known urologic abnormalities or comorbidities.
- UTI is the most common bacterial infection encountered in the ambulatory care setting in the US, accounting for 8.6 million visits (84% by women) in 2007. The self-reported annual incidence of UTI in women is 12%.[24]
- **The vast majority of episodes of uncomplicated UTI are caused by *Escherichia coli*** (75% to 95%). Other pathogens include *Klebsiella pneumoniae, Staphylococcus saprophyticus,* and *Proteus mirabilis.* Isolation of *Enterococcus faecalis,* and *Streptococcus agalactiae* could represent contamination of the urine specimen.
- The pathogenesis involves bacteria from the bowel or the vagina colonizing the periurethral mucosa and ascending through the urethra to the bladder. Pyelonephritis occurs when pathogens ascend to the kidneys through the ureters or, less commonly, when pathogens are seeded by hematogenous spread (e.g., *Staphylococcus aureus* or *M. tuberculosis*).
- Risk factors include previous history of UTI, sexual intercourse, use of spermicides, and a history of UTI in a first-degree female relative.

DIAGNOSIS

- **Cystitis:** symptoms include dysuria, frequency, urgency, suprapubic pain, or hematuria.
- **Pyelonephritis**: symptoms include fever (>38°C), chills, flank pain, costovertebral angle tenderness, nausea, or vomiting. Symptoms of cystitis may or may not be present.
- A urine dipstick test can detect leukocyte esterase (enzyme released by leukocytes) or nitrite (converted from urinary nitrate by Enterobacteriaceae). The presence of either of these predicts UTI with a sensitivity of 75% and a specificity of 82%.[24]
- Microscopic examination can be done in a voided midstream urine specimen to detect the presence of pyuria, defined as ≥10 leukocytes/mm^3 in uncentrifuged urine or >5 leukocytes/high-power field (HPF) in a centrifuged sediment. **Pyuria is present in almost all women with acute cystitis or pyelonephritis**.
- Urine cultures can be performed to confirm the presence of bacteriuria and to evaluate the antimicrobial susceptibility of the pathogen involved.
- **A urine culture is not necessary for the diagnosis of uncomplicated cystitis**, given the reliability of patient symptoms in establishing the diagnosis. The combination of dysuria and frequency without vaginal discharge or irritation raises the probability of cystitis in a woman to more than 90%.[25]
- **A urine culture must be obtained in all patients suspected of having pyelonephritis**, and treatment should be adjusted based on antimicrobial susceptibility results. A urine culture is also warranted if symptoms are atypical, if there is failure to respond to initial therapy, or if there is recurrence of symptoms within a month of prior treatment.
- The traditional definition of a positive urine culture is ≥10^5 colony-forming units (CFUs)/mL together with pyuria, obtained from voided midstream urine. It has been suggested that this criterion is appropriate for pyelonephritis but may lack sensitivity to diagnose cystitis. If culture is indicated for the diagnosis of cystitis, a lower threshold of ≥10^2 CFU/mL may increase the sensitivity for detection in symptomatic women, with a positive predictive value of 88%.[26]

TREATMENT

- Treatment guidelines from the IDSA emphasize the importance of considering the ecologic adverse effects of antimicrobial agents when selecting a treatment regimen. These effects include the selection and subsequent colonization or infection with multidrug-resistant organisms.
- Local antimicrobial susceptibility patterns of *E. coli* should be considered in empiric antimicrobial selection.
- For uncomplicated **cystitis**, studies suggest a **20% TMP-SMX resistance** prevalence as the threshold at which this agent is no longer recommended for empiric treatment.[27]
- For **pyelonephritis**, a **10% fluoroquinolone resistance** prevalence is the threshold for using an alternative agent in conjunction with or in place of a fluoroquinolone, based on expert opinion.[27]
- Empiric therapy of uncomplicated cystitis can be found in Table 26-6.[27]
- **Acute uncomplicated pyelonephritis can be treated in the outpatient setting.** However, admission is warranted in severe disease with high fever, pain, marked debility, hemodynamic instability, and poor PO tolerance or if there is concern about compliance with therapy.
- Empiric therapy of uncomplicated pyelonephritis in the outpatient setting can be found in Table 26-7.[27]

TABLE 26-6 Empiric Therapy of Uncomplicated Cystitis in Women

Antimicrobial regimen	Comments
First-line therapy **Nitrofurantoin** (monohydrate/macrocrystals): 100 mg bid for 5 days	Limited effects on microbiological ecology. Contraindicated if creatinine clearance <60 mL/minute. Avoid if pyelonephritis is suspected
TMP-SMX: 1 double-strength tablet (160/800 mg) bid for 3 days	Avoid if used within the prior 3 months
Fosfomycin trometamol: 3 g single dose (3 g sachet)	Inferior efficacy compared to other first-line agents
Pivmecillinam: 400 mg bid for 3 to 7 days	Not available in the US
Second-line therapy **Fluoroquinolones:** Ciprofloxacin (250 mg bid) or levofloxacin (250 mg daily) in 3-day regimens	Propensity for adverse effects on microbiological ecology. Reserve for uses other than acute cystitis
Oral β-lactams: Amoxicillin-clavulanate, cefpodoxime, cefdinir, or cefaclor, in 3- to 7-day regimens	Have less efficacy and more adverse effects

TMP-SMX, trimethoprim-sulfamethoxazole.

| TABLE 26-7 | Outpatient Empiric Therapy of Uncomplicated Pyelonephritis in Women |

Antimicrobial regimen	Comments
Fluoroquinolones: Ciprofloxacin (500 mg PO bid or 1,000 mg extended-release PO daily) for 7 days or levofloxacin (750 mg PO daily) for 5 days	An initial one-time dose of ciprofloxacin 400 mg IV is optional. Alternatives include ceftriaxone 1 g or a consolidated 24-hour dose of an aminoglycoside
TMP-SMX: 1 double-strength tablet (160/800 mg) bid for 14 days	If susceptibility is unknown, an initial IV dose of a long-acting parenteral antimicrobial, such as ceftriaxone 1 g or a consolidated 24-hour dose of an aminoglycoside, is recommended
Oral β-lactams: Specific agents not listed in IDSA guidelines. Treatment for 10 to 14 days	An initial IV dose of a long-acting parenteral antimicrobial, such as ceftriaxone 1 g or a consolidated 24-hour dose of an aminoglycoside, is recommended

TMP-SMX, trimethoprim-sulfamethoxazole.

- Empiric therapy of pyelonephritis requiring inpatient admission should include intravenous antibiotics such as a fluoroquinolone, an aminoglycoside (with or without ampicillin), an extended-spectrum cephalosporin or extended-spectrum penicillin (with or without an aminoglycoside), or a carbapenem. The choice between these agents should be based on local resistance data, and the regimen should be adjusted based on susceptibility results.[27]
- **Follow-up urine cultures are not needed in patients with acute cystitis or pyelonephritis whose symptoms resolve on antibiotics.**
- Symptomatic therapy of severe dysuria with phenazopyridine (100 to 200 mg tid) can be considered. Symptoms usually respond to antibiotics within 48 hours.

SPECIAL CONSIDERATIONS

- Antimicrobial prophylaxis has been shown to reduce the risk of UTI recurrence by approximately 95% in women who have had three or more UTIs in the past 12 months or two or more UTIs in the past 6 months.[24]
- Postcoital antimicrobial prophylaxis includes a single dose of nitrofurantoin 50 to 100 mg, TMP-SMX 40/200 mg, or cephalexin 250 mg.
- Continuous antimicrobial prophylaxis includes a daily bedtime dose of nitrofurantoin 50 to 100 mg, TMP-SMX 40/200 mg, or cephalexin 125 to 250 mg. Fosfomycin 3-g sachet every 10 days is also an option.

Uncomplicated Urinary Tract Infections in Men

GENERAL PRINCIPLES

- Uncomplicated UTI refers to cystitis and pyelonephritis in men with no known urologic abnormalities or comorbidities.

- **Uncomplicated UTI are much less common in men than in women**. This is thought to be due to the greater length and drier surrounding environment of the male urethra, as well as the antibacterial properties of prostatic fluid.[28]
- The etiologic agents causing uncomplicated UTI in men are similar to those in women. *Escherichia coli* is the most common causative organism.
- Risk factors include insertive anal intercourse, intercourse with a female partner colonized with uropathogens, and lack of circumcision.[28]
- In a patient without an obvious risk factor, further evaluation for predisposing conditions (e.g., anatomic abnormalities) should be considered.
- Prostatitis should be suspected in men with recurrent cystitis.

DIAGNOSIS

- Symptoms of uncomplicated cystitis or pyelonephritis in men are similar to those in women.
- The differential diagnosis includes urethritis in sexually active men with genital lesions or urethral discharge, as well as prostatitis in patients with fever, chills, pelvic pain, or obstructive urinary symptoms.
- A urine dipstick test can detect the presence of leukocyte esterase or nitrite. Microscopic examination can be done to detect the presence of pyuria.
- **A urine culture must be obtained in all male patients suspected of having an uncomplicated UTI.** A positive urine culture is defined as $\geq 10^4$ CFU/mL, obtained from voided midstream urine.[28] A posttreatment urine culture to document urinary tract sterility is recommended in men.

TREATMENT

- Duration of therapy for uncomplicated cystitis should be for a minimum of 7 days.[28] Treatment options include TMP-SMX, 1 double-strength tablet (160/800 mg) bid; ciprofloxacin, 500 mg bid; and levofloxacin, 500 mg PO daily.
- Duration of therapy for uncomplicated pyelonephritis should be 10 to 14 days.[28] Recommended antimicrobial agents and their doses are the same as the ones described for women. See Table 26-7.

Complicated Urinary Tract Infections

GENERAL PRINCIPLES

- A complicated UTI is the one associated with an underlying condition that increases the risk of infection or of failing therapy.
- Conditions that suggest a potential complicated UTI[29]:
  - Presence of an indwelling urethral catheter, stent, or nephrostomy tube
  - Intermittent bladder catheterization
  - An obstructive uropathy of any etiology
  - Vesicoureteric reflux or other functional abnormalities
  - Urinary tract modifications, such as an ileal loop or pouch
  - Renal insufficiency and transplantation, diabetes mellitus, and immunodeficiency
  - Peri- and postoperative UTI
  - Chemical or radiation injuries of the uroepithelium
- *Escherichia coli* is the most common causative organism. Other pathogens include *Proteus mirabilis*, *Klebsiella pneumoniae*, *Pseudomonas* spp., *Serratia* spp., *Enterococcus*, and staphylococci.

DIAGNOSIS

Pyuria and bacteriuria may be absent if the infection does not communicate with the collecting system (i.e., if there is an obstruction). Urine cultures and susceptibility testing should always be obtained prior to therapy.

TREATMENT

- Therapy involves selecting an appropriate antimicrobial regimen and managing the underlying urologic abnormality (when possible).
- Empiric therapy should be based on culture and susceptibility results.
- Complicated cystitis can be managed as an outpatient. However, hospitalization could be required depending on illness severity. Treatment is recommended for 7 to 14 days.
- Patients with complicated pyelonephritis should be initially managed as inpatients. Treatment is recommended for 14 days.
- Recommended initial empiric regimens[29]:
  - Fluoroquinolones: ciprofloxacin or levofloxacin
  - Aminopenicillin (amoxicillin or ampicillin) plus β-lactamase inhibitor
  - Cephalosporins: cefuroxime, ceftriaxone, and cefotaxime
  - Aminoglycoside: gentamicin and tobramycin
- Recommended empiric regimens for severe infection or in case of initial treatment failure (within 1 to 3 days) should include coverage for *Pseudomonas* spp.[29]:
  - Fluoroquinolones: ciprofloxacin or levofloxacin
  - Piperacillin plus β-lactamase inhibitor
  - Cephalosporins: ceftazidime, cefepime
  - Carbapenem: imipenem, meropenem
  - Aminoglycoside plus fluoroquinolone

Asymptomatic Bacteriuria

- Asymptomatic bacteriuria is defined as isolation of a specified quantitative count of bacteria in an appropriately collected urine specimen obtained from a patient without symptoms or signs of UTI.[30]
- In asymptomatic women:
  - Two consecutive voided urine specimens with isolation of the same bacterial strain in quantitative counts $\geq 10^5$ CFU/mL

  or
  - A single catheterized urine specimen with one bacterial species isolated in a quantitative count $\geq 10^2$ CFU/mL
- In asymptomatic men:
  - A single, clean-catch voided urine specimen with one bacterial species isolated in a quantitative count $\geq 10^5$ CFU/mL

  or
  - A single catheterized urine specimen with one bacterial species isolated in a quantitative count $\geq 10^2$ CFU/mL
- Screening for and treatment of asymptomatic bacteriuria is **only** recommended in the following situations[30]: pregnant women, before transurethral resection of the prostate, and before other urologic procedures for which mucosal bleeding is anticipated.

- Screening for or treatment of asymptomatic bacteriuria is **not** recommended for the following persons: premenopausal nonpregnant women, diabetic women, older persons living in the community, elderly institutionalized subjects, persons with spinal cord injury, and catheterized patients while the catheter remains in situ.
- Antimicrobial treatment of asymptomatic women with catheter-acquired bacteriuria that persists 48 hour after indwelling catheter removal may be considered.

SKIN AND SOFT TISSUE INFECTIONS

Cellulitis and Erysipelas

GENERAL PRINCIPLES

- Cellulitis and erysipelas are skin infections that are not secondary to an underlying suppurative focus, such as abscesses, septic arthritis, or osteomyelitis. However, cellulitis can be associated with purulent drainage or exudates in the absence of a drainable abscess.
- Erysipelas involves the upper dermis and superficial lymphatics, while cellulitis involves the deeper dermis and subcutaneous fat.
- Erysipelas is usually caused **by β-hemolytic streptococci**, more commonly group A (i.e., *S. pyogenes*). Groups C and G have also been implicated. Group B streptococci and *S. aureus* are less frequent.
- Cellulitis **without** purulent drainage or exudate is more commonly caused by β-hemolytic streptococci. Less frequently, *S. aureus* (both methicillin-sensitive and methicillin-resistant strains) is the causative agent.
- Cellulitis presenting **with** purulent drainage or exudate is more commonly caused by **community-acquired methicillin-resistant *Staphylococcus aureus* (CA-MRSA)**, representing up to 59% of cases presenting to emergency departments in the US.[31]
- These infections arise when there is disruption of the skin barrier. However, breaches in the skin are not always clinically apparent and may be unnoticed.
- Predisposing conditions include previous cutaneous damage, edema from venous insufficiency or lymphatic obstruction, obesity, or previous cutaneous infection (e.g., impetigo, tinea).[32] Diabetes, arterial insufficiency, eczema, and intravenous drug use also predispose to infection.
- Risk factors associated with CA-MRSA can be found on Table 26-8.[31,33]

DIAGNOSIS

- Both erysipelas and cellulitis present as rapidly spreading areas of erythema, warmth, and edema, sometimes associated with lymphangitis and inflammation of the regional lymph nodes.
- Vesicles, bullae, petechiae, and ecchymoses can be found occasionally.
- The most common site of infection is the lower extremities.
- Erysipelas has the distinctive feature of being a raised lesion with sharply demarcated borders. Cellulitis generally lacks sharp demarcated borders. It can present with or without purulent drainage or exudates, in the absence of a drainable abscess.
- The differential includes contact dermatitis, stasis dermatitis, deep venous thrombosis, acute gout, drug reactions, insect bites, early herpes zoster, and erythema migrans. Physicians must also maintain a high index of suspicion for severe processes such as

TABLE 26-8	Risk Factors Associated with Community-Acquired Methicillin-Resistant *Staphylococcus aureus* (CA-MRSA) Skin and Soft Tissue Infections

Use of antibiotics in the past month
Presence of an abscess
Presence of a lesion attributed to a spider bite
Previous history of MRSA infection
Household or day care contact with a patient with a similar skin infection
Men who have sex with men
Incarcerated persons
Military personnel
Athletes, particularly in contact sports
Intravenous drug users
Native Americans or Pacific Islanders

necrotizing fasciitis, as the initial presentation can be quite benign (see section on necrotizing fasciitis).
• Blood cultures are positive in ≤5% of cases.[34] Cultures from needle aspiration of intact
skin or from punch biopsies have variable results and are generally not helpful. In the case
of cellulitis associated with purulent drainage or exudates, cultures should be obtained
to guide therapy.

TREATMENT

• A large proportion of patients can be treated with oral medications. Parenteral therapy is
indicated for severely ill patients or for those unable to tolerate oral medications.
• For uncomplicated cellulitis, 5 to 10 days of antibiotic therapy is recommended in
the outpatient setting.[35] For severe disease, a longer course of antibiotics may be
warranted.
• Efforts should be made to treat any underlying predisposing condition.
• Elevation of the affected extremity aids in healing by promoting gravity drainage of the
edema and inflammatory substances.
• Erysipelas:
  ○ Therapy should cover β-hemolytic streptococci. Penicillin remains the treatment of
  choice. Therapeutic options for erysipelas are summarized in Table 26-9.
  ○ If there is high suspicion for **methicillin-sensitive *Staphylococcus aureus* (MSSA)**
  infection, a penicillinase-resistant semisynthetic penicillin or a first-generation cepha-
  losporin should be used.
• Nonpurulent cellulitis:
  ○ Empiric therapy should cover β-hemolytic streptococci and MSSA.
  ○ Empiric coverage for CA-MRSA is recommended in patients who do not respond
  to β-lactam therapy, in those with systemic toxicity, or in those with risk factors for
  CA-MRSA (see Table 26-8).
  ○ Therapeutic options for nonpurulent cellulitis are summarized in Table 26-10.
• Purulent cellulitis:
  ○ Empiric therapy should cover CA-MRSA, pending culture results.
  ○ Empiric therapy to cover β-hemolytic streptococci is likely unnecessary.
  ○ If parenteral therapy is needed, vancomycin is the treatment of choice.
  ○ Therapeutic options for purulent cellulitis are summarized in Table 26-11.

TABLE 26-9	Empiric Antimicrobial Therapy for Erysipelas	
	β-Hemolytic streptococci coverage	β-Hemolytic streptococci and MSSA coverage
Oral therapy	Penicillin V (500 mg q6h) Amoxicillin (500 mg q8h)	Dicloxacillin (500 mg q6h) Cephalexin (500 mg q6h)
Parenteral therapy	Penicillin G (1–2 million units q6h)	Nafcillin or oxacillin (1–2 g q4h) Cefazolin (1 g q8h)
Penicillin allergy	Clindamycin (300–450 mg PO q8h or 600 mg IV q8h)	

TABLE 26-10	Empiric Antimicrobial Therapy for Nonpurulent Cellulitis	
	β-Hemolytic streptococci and MSSA coverage	β-Hemolytic streptococci and CA-MRSA coverage
Oral therapy	Dicloxacillin (500 mg q6h)	Clindamycin (300–450 mg PO q8h)
	Cephalexin (500 mg q6h)	Amoxicillin (500 mg q8h) **plus** TMP-SMX (1–2 double-strength tablets bid)
	Clindamycin (300–450 mg PO q8h)	Amoxicillin (500 mg q8h) **plus** tetracycline (doxycycline or minocycline 100 mg q12h) Linezolid (600 mg bid)
Parenteral therapy	Nafcillin or oxacillin (1–2 g q4h) Cefazolin (1 g q8h) Clindamycin (600 mg q8h)	Clindamycin (600 mg q8h) Linezolid (600 mg bid)

TABLE 26-11	Empiric Antimicrobial Therapy for Purulent Cellulitis

Oral therapy
Clindamycin (300–450 mg PO q8h)
TMP-SMX (1–2 double-strength tablets PO bid)
Tetracycline (doxycycline or minocycline 100 mg PO q12h)
Linezolid (600 mg PO bid)

Parenteral therapy
Vancomycin (15–20 mg/kg q12h)
Clindamycin (600 mg q8h)
Daptomycin (4 mg/kg q24h)
Linezolid (600 mg bid)
Ceftaroline (600 mg bid)
Tigecycline (100 mg once, then 50 mg q12h)
Telavancin (10 mg/kg every 24 hour)

Abscesses, Furuncles, and Carbuncles

GENERAL PRINCIPLES

- Cutaneous abscesses are collections of pus within the dermis and deeper cutaneous tissues.
- Furuncles (boils) are collections of pus that form at the site of hair follicles, in which suppuration extends through the dermis into the subcutaneous tissue. Carbuncles are coalesced furuncles.
- Cutaneous abscesses are typically polymicrobial, containing bacteria that constitute the normal regional skin flora, often combined with organisms from adjacent mucous membranes.[34]
- *Staphylococcus aureus* is the predominant agent isolated from cutaneous abscesses, with CA-MRSA representing up to 61% of isolates in patients presenting to emergency departments in the US.[31]
- Furuncles and carbuncles are usually caused by MSSA or MRSA.[34] Furuncles and carbuncles can also be caused by other organisms, including *Pseudomonas aeruginosa* (hot tub or whirlpool exposure), atypical mycobacteria (nail salon footbaths), or *Candida* spp. (immunosuppressed, broad-spectrum antibiotic exposure).

DIAGNOSIS

- Cutaneous abscesses usually present as **painful, tender, and fluctuant red nodules**. These lesions can have an overlying pustule and are often associated with surrounding erythema and swelling.
- Furuncles have a similar appearance, with a hair emerging through the pustule. Carbuncles present as a coalescent inflammatory mass with pus draining from multiple follicular orifices.
- Fever, chills, and systemic toxicity are unusual with cutaneous abscesses. These manifestations are more common with carbuncles.
- Gram stain and culture are useful to tailor antibiotic therapy when indicated.

TREATMENT

- For cutaneous abscesses, **the primary treatment involves incision and drainage** of the pus, as well as probing the cavity to break up any loculation. **Antibiotic therapy is usually not necessary for simple abscesses.**
- For small furuncles, moist heat to promote drainage is usually sufficient. Larger furuncles and all carbuncles require incision and drainage.
- Antibiotics are recommended for cutaneous abscesses, carbuncles, and furuncles in the following circumstances[35]:
  - Severe or extensive disease involving multiple sites
  - Rapid progression with associated cellulitis
  - Signs and symptoms of systemic disease
  - Associated comorbidities or immunosuppression
  - Extremes of age
  - Abscess in areas difficult to drain completely (face, hand, genitalia)
  - Associated septic phlebitis
  - Lack of response to incision and drainage alone
- Empiric antibiotic therapy for cutaneous abscesses, carbuncles, and furuncles should include coverage for CA-MRSA. If antibiotics are started, therapy should be tailored according to culture and susceptibility results. Recommended duration of therapy is 5 to 10 days. Empiric therapeutic options can be found in Table 26-11.

Impetigo

GENERAL PRINCIPLES

- Impetigo is a contagious epidermal skin infection caused by β-hemolytic streptococci and/ or *S. aureus*. It can be classified into bullous and nonbullous forms.
- It most commonly occurs among children aged 2 to 5 years, although older children and adults may also be affected.
- The infection spreads easily among individuals in close contact and is usually facilitated by warm and humid conditions.
- *Staphylococcus aureus* (both MSSA and MRSA) is the most common cause of both forms of impetigo. β-Hemolytic streptococci (mainly *S. pyogenes*) can cause nonbullous impetigo, either alone or in combination with *S. aureus*.[34]
- Poststreptococcal glomerulonephritis may be a complication of impetigo caused by certain strains of *S. pyogenes*. However, it is unclear if treatment of impetigo prevents this sequela. Rheumatic fever has not been reported after streptococcal impetigo.

DIAGNOSIS

- Impetigo usually occurs on exposed areas of the body, most frequently the face and extremities. There are usually multiple well-localized, painful lesions.
- **Bullous impetigo:** superficial vesicles that enlarge to form flaccid bullae filled with clear yellow fluid that leaves a thin brown crust when ruptured.
- **Nonbullous impetigo:** the most common form. Papules that evolve into vesicles surrounded by erythema. The lesions later become pustules that break down to form the **characteristic thick golden crusts**. The process usually takes 4 to 6 days.
- **Ecthyma:** ulcerative form of impetigo with lesions extending into the dermis.

TREATMENT

- Antibiotic therapy should cover for both β-hemolytic streptococci and MSSA. If there is significant concern for CA-MRSA (see Table 26-8), empiric coverage should be modified accordingly. Duration of therapy is 7 to 10 days.
- Topical therapy is as effective as oral systemic antibiotics and may be used when lesions are limited in number. Topical agents include mupirocin 2%, tid for 7 days, and retapamulin 1%, bid for 5 days.[34,36]
- Empiric systemic therapy for both β-hemolytic streptococci and MSSA includes any one of the following:
  - Dicloxacillin 500 mg PO every 6 hour
  - Cephalexin 500 mg PO every 6 hour
  - Amoxicillin-clavulanate 875/125 mg PO bid
  - Clindamycin 300 to 450 mg PO every 8 hour (use in case of β-lactam allergy)
- Options for empiric systemic therapy of CA-MRSA can be found in Table 26-11.

Necrotizing Fasciitis

GENERAL PRINCIPLES

- Necrotizing fasciitis (NF) is a subcutaneous infection that tracks along superficial and deep fascial planes and is characterized by rapid progression and high mortality.
  - **Type I:** polymicrobial infection (average five organisms per lesion) caused by aerobic and anaerobic bacteria.

○ **Type II:** usually caused by GAS, either alone or in combination with other bacteria, most commonly *S. aureus.*
• The infection usually develops from an initial break in the skin related to trauma, surgery, or other predisposing lesions. The initial lesion is seen in 80% of cases, and many times, it is trivial. There is no visible skin lesion in up to 20% of patients.[34]
• **Risk factors:**
  ○ **Type I:** usually associated with surgical procedures involving the bowel or penetrating abdominal trauma, decubitus ulcers or perianal abscesses, IV drug use, and spread from a Bartholin abscess or a minor vulvovaginal infection.
  ○ **Type II:** often associated with a history of skin trauma. An underlying predisposing condition such as diabetes, arteriosclerotic vascular disease, or venous insufficiency with edema is frequently present.

DIAGNOSIS

• **NF is a surgical emergency, and early diagnosis is crucial.** The physician should keep a high index of suspicion in the proper clinical setting as the overlying superficial tissue can initially appear unaffected.
• In the initial phases, the affected area may be erythematous, swollen, and exquisitely tender.
• The following clinical features should suggest the presence of necrotizing fasciitis[34]:
  ○ Severe, constant pain, out of proportion from physical findings
  ○ Gas in the soft tissues, detected by palpation or imaging
  ○ Edema that extends beyond the margin of erythema
  ○ Cutaneous anesthesia
  ○ Skin necrosis
  ○ Systemic toxicity (fever, leukocytosis, delirium, renal failure)
  ○ Rapid spread of skin changes while on antibiotics
• Ultimately, the diagnosis of NF is established surgically, with direct examination of the involved tissues.
• Imaging studies have variable degrees of sensitivity and specificity and should not delay surgery.

TREATMENT

Any patient with clinical findings suspicious for an early necrotizing soft tissue infection should be admitted to the hospital. Surgical evaluation should be obtained immediately for drainage and debridement.

Animal and Human Bite Wounds

GENERAL PRINCIPLES

• Dog bites are the most common animal bites, accounting for 80% to 90% of cases.
• Human bite wounds often result from aggressive behavior and are frequently more serious than animal bites.
• These wounds are polymicrobial. The predominant pathogens are the oral flora of the biting animal, along with human skin flora.
• *Pasteurella* species are isolated from 50% of dog bite wounds and 75% of cat bite wounds. Staphylococci, streptococci, and anaerobic bacteria are also isolated after bites from both animals. *Capnocytophaga canimorsus* can cause bacteremia and fatal sepsis after animal bites, especially in patients with asplenia or underlying hepatic disease.[34]

- Human bite wounds reflect the normal oral flora of the biter, with streptococci (especially viridans streptococci) present in 80% of wounds. Other causative agents include staphylococci, *Haemophilus* species, *Eikenella corrodens*, and anaerobes. Human bites also have the potential to transmit various viral diseases, such as herpes, hepatitis B and C, and HIV infection.
- Infectious complications of bite wounds include septic arthritis, osteomyelitis, subcutaneous abscess formation, tendonitis, and, rarely, bacteremia.

DIAGNOSIS

- Dog bites can cause a wide variety of lesions, from minor abrasions to tissue avulsions and crush injuries.
- Cat bites often cause deep puncture wounds, frequently evolving into anaerobic abscesses. When these types of wounds occur in the hand, there is high risk for septic arthritis or osteomyelitis.
- Human bite wounds can be classified into **occlusive bite wounds**, occurring when teeth are closed forcibly and break the skin, or **clenched fist injuries**, which occur when the fist of one person strikes the teeth of another.
- Occlusive bite wounds can be seen as a semicircular or oval area of erythema or bruising. Clenched fist injuries usually imply wounds overlying the metacarpophalangeal joints.

TREATMENT

- Initial wound management with irrigation (sterile normal saline) and debridement is essential.
- **Primary closure is generally contraindicated.** Scarring and disfigurement related to facial wounds may, however, necessitate primary closure.
- Antibiotic therapy should be given empirically for 7 to 10 days. Therapeutic options include any one of the following:
  - Amoxicillin-clavulanate 875/125 mg PO bid
  - Doxycycline 100 mg PO bid
  - Penicillin V 500 mg PO q 6 h **plus** clindamycin 300 mg PO tid
  - Cefuroxime 500 mg PO bid **plus** clindamycin 300 mg PO tid
  - TMP-SMX 160/800 mg PO bid **plus** clindamycin 300 mg PO tid
- A tetanus (Td) booster should be given if indicated (i.e., more than 10 years since last booster).
- Rabies prophylaxis should be considered for all feral and wild animal bites and in geographic areas where there is a high prevalence of rabies. It is not routinely indicated for domestic dog and cat bites. The local department of health should be consulted about the risks and benefits of rabies prophylaxis.[34]

Spider Bites

GENERAL PRINCIPLES

- Very few species of spiders are medically important. The most important clinical syndromes resulting from spider bite are
  - **Latrodectism:** caused by widow spiders (***Latrodectus* spp.**)
  - **Loxoscelism:** caused by recluse spiders (***Loxosceles* spp.**)
- Widow spiders:
  - Have a worldwide distribution. In the US, the species more commonly implicated in latrodectism are *L. mactans* and *L. hesperus*.[37]
  - They are generally shiny black and could be identified by red or orange markings (hourglass or dot shaped) on their ventral abdomen.

- Recluse spiders:
  - Most commonly located in North America and South America. The majority of cases of loxoscelism in North America are attributed to *L. reclusa* and *L. deserta*. In South America, most cases are attributed to *L. laeta*, *L. intermedia*, and *L. gaucho*.[37]
  - They are usually brown and could be identified by violin-shaped markings on their dorsal surface.

DIAGNOSIS

- The diagnosis of spider bite is usually clinical, based on a **clear history** of a spider biting the patient and then being **identified**. Spider bites are usually **single lesions**.
- **Latrodectism**:
  - The bite lesion can present as blanched circular patch with surrounding erythema. A central punctum can be visualized.
  - Causes local, regional, or generalized pain associated with nonspecific symptoms and autonomic effects. Diaphoresis can be observed at the bite site or in an asymmetric regional distribution.
  - Severe envenomation can manifest as nausea, vomiting, headache, tachycardia, hypertension, muscle fasciculation or spasm, and patchy localized paralysis. Abdominal wall rigidity can be present. Rare complications include priapism, cardiomyopathy, shock, or pulmonary edema.
- **Loxoscelism**:
  - **Cutaneous form:** initial local pain and erythema. The lesion can develop central pallor. Severe forms have gradual increase in pain and can progress into a necrotic ulcer after 72 hours.
  - **Systemic form:** less common. Can present with fever, headache, nausea, vomiting, and myalgia. It is characterized by intravascular hemolysis and renal failure. Thrombocytopenia and rhabdomyolysis can also develop.

TREATMENT

- **Most cases will only require local wound care.**
- A tetanus (Td) booster should be given if indicated.
- Pain control with nonopioid and opioid analgesics is recommended.
- If bacterial superimposed infection is suspected, appropriate antibiotic coverage for cellulitis should be initiated.
- **Latrodectism**:
  - Benzodiazepines could be used for muscle spasms.
  - The use of antivenom is controversial and is usually reserved for severe cases. If use of antivenom is considered, consultation with a medical toxicologist is recommended.
- **Loxoscelism:**
  - Dapsone has been suggested to prevent the development of necrosis according to evidence from animal models. However, prospective trials in humans are lacking. Dapsone is contraindicated if the patient has glucose-6-phosphate dehydrogenase (G6PD) deficiency.
  - Antivenoms are only available in Brazil, Argentina, Peru, and Mexico. However, the benefit from antivenom use has not been well established through randomized clinical trials. If use of antivenom is considered, consultation with a medical toxicologist is recommended.

Herpes Zoster

GENERAL PRINCIPLES

- **Varicella-zoster virus (VZV)** causes two distinct syndromes: primary infection presents as **varicella** (chickenpox), and subsequent reactivation of latent VZV presents as **herpes zoster** (shingles).
- VZV is transmitted from person to person by direct contact or by aerosolization of virus from skin lesions.
- Primary varicella is a contagious and usually benign illness that occurs in epidemics mainly among susceptible children. After its resolution, latent infection develops within the sensory dorsal root ganglia.
- Reactivation of the virus leads to herpes zoster, which involves a localized cutaneous eruption with dermatomal distribution.
- The lifetime risk of herpes zoster is estimated to be 10% to 20%.[38]
- The main risk factors include **increasing age** (risk doubles after age 50), **altered cell-mediated immunity, and HIV infection**.
- Complications of herpes zoster in immunocompetent patients include postherpetic neuralgia, bacterial skin infection, encephalitis, myelitis, and cranial and peripheral nerve palsies. In immunosuppressed patients, complications include disseminated herpes zoster (more than two dermatomes) and zoster encephalitis. These cases should be treated with intravenous acyclovir and hospitalization.

DIAGNOSIS

- Abnormal skin sensations precede the rash by 1 to 5 days, ranging from tingling or itching to severe pain. Pain of variable severity occurs in virtually all patients with acute herpes zoster.[38]
- The **rash** is **unilateral** (does not cross the midline), has a **dermatomal distribution**, and is characterized by erythematous papules that evolve into vesicles and pustules. The lesions later crust after a period of 7 to 10 days.
- The thoracic and lumbar dermatomes are the most commonly involved sites. Lesions overlap adjacent dermatomes in 20% of cases.
- **Herpes zoster ophthalmicus:** VZV reactivation within the trigeminal ganglion. Potential sight-threatening condition.
- **Ramsay Hunt syndrome (herpes zoster oticus):** VZV reactivation within the geniculate ganglion. Triad of ipsilateral facial paralysis, ear pain, and vesicles in the auditory canal.
- Diagnosis is essentially clinical. If diagnostic uncertainty exists, culture, direct immunofluorescence assay, or PCR of vesicular fluid can assist in the diagnosis.

TREATMENT

- Goals of antiviral therapy include accelerating healing, limiting the severity and duration of pain, and reducing complications.
- Antiviral agents include acyclovir, 800 mg PO q4h (five times daily); famciclovir, 500 mg PO q8h (three times daily); and valacyclovir, 1,000 mg PO q8h (three times daily). These agents have demonstrated clinical benefit when started **within 72 hours** of the onset of rash. Recommended duration of therapy is 7 days.
- Herpes zoster ophthalmicus requires evaluation by an ophthalmologist and usually involves initial parenteral therapy.

TRAVEL MEDICINE

Pretravel Consultation

- Primary care physicians should be able to provide advice for low-risk travel destinations, but referral to an infectious disease specialist or travel clinic is preferred.[39]
- If these are not available, then the primary care provider should be able to identify high-risk travel by assessing:
  ○ Country or area of destination
  ○ Purpose of travel and activities planned, for example, extreme sports (risk of falls, weather, insect exposure) and medical/missionary work (risks of needle sticks, exposure to transmissible diseases)
  ○ Travel and lodging accommodations: access to running water, food safety, and exposure to insect bites (e.g., mosquito nets in malaria areas)
  ○ Patient's medical problems and medications that may contribute to increased risk for acquiring infections or other travel-related complications (e.g., immunosuppressed status, age, risk for dehydration/heat stroke in hot weather, photosensitivity due to medications and interactions with potential prophylactic drugs to be taken)
- Pretravel consultation does not only pertain to infections that the patient is at risk of acquiring but also includes advice regarding personal safety, prevention of sunburns or other extreme weather effect, and safe sex measures.
- Specific topics to discuss include management of traveler's diarrhea, malaria prophylaxis and insect avoidance, and personal safety among other more specific concerns depending on the patient's destination.
- For more specific and detailed information, follow CDC recommendations for US travelers, which can be found at www.cdc.gov/travel (last accessed April 14, 2014), and select the country of destination. This includes latest vaccination recommendations and information on any recent travel advisory or outbreak.
- Additional advisories related to travel destinations can be obtained through the U.S. Department of State's website (www.travel.state.gov, last accessed December 29, 2014).
- For a brief overview of recommendations regarding prevention and counseling of the most common infections to consider, depending on the travel destination, see Table 26-12.
- **Pretravel vaccination:**
  ○ Depends on the destination (including specific region within a country), the season, and activity the patient will be doing.
  ○ A detailed immunization history should be obtained, since not all recommended vaccines may be required.
  ○ Some patients may require **polio** vaccination or booster immunization.
  ○ Tetanus-diphtheria-acellular pertussis (Tdap) booster should also be administered.
- For the most common immunizations, see Table 26-12.
- Rabies vaccine may be considered only in patients who will be in close contact with at risk mammals in specific areas of the world.

The Returning Traveler

- In the case of the ill returning traveler, the provider must recognize that the infection may have been acquired during travel. If so, the provider can start the initial diagnostic workup and treatment while referring the patient to a travel medicine clinic as appropriate.

TABLE 26-12 Summary of Most Common Travel Associated Diseases

Disease	Organism	Characteristics	Prophylaxis	Notes
Dengue	Dengue virus	Fever, rash, severe cases: thrombocytopenia, anemia	Mosquito bite avoidance	Tropical areas, water containers
Malaria	*Plasmodium falciparum, P. vivax, P. malariae*	Fever, chills, rigors, headache, anemia, altered mental status	Mosquito bite avoidance, chemoprophylaxis (table)	*Plasmodium* susceptibilities vary geographically. Prophylactic regimens need to be tailored accordingly
Yellow fever	Yellow fever virus	Fever, jaundice, rash, myalgia	Yellow fever vaccine—available in travel clinics and local health departments	Contraindicated in immunosuppressed patients. Check destination country requirements
Typhoid fever	*Salmonella typhi*	Fever, headaches, hepatosplenomegaly	Typhoid fever vaccine: live (oral) and IM (inactivated) Bottled water, avoid fresh/raw vegetables, fruits	Live vaccine (oral) available in pharmacies with prescription US not for immunosuppressed
Hepatitis A	Hepatitis A virus (HAV)	Fever, jaundice, hepatomegaly, myalgia	Vaccination, at least first dose prior to travel. Bottled water, avoid fresh/raw vegetables, fruits	Fecal-oral transmission; can cause fulminant disease
Hepatitis B	Hepatitis B virus (HBV)	Rarely acute illness; chronic hepatitis, potential for hepatocellular carcinoma	Vaccination, at least partially, unless vaccinated previously	Main risk factor in travel: needlesticks, blood products, sexual
Meningitis	Meningococcus	Acute meningitis: fever, headache, confusion	Meningococcal vaccine, if not previously immunized	Sub-Saharan Africa (meningitis belt) In US, most young adults vaccinated

- Common diseases should be excluded, such as influenza, CAP, *S. aureus, or S. pyogenes* skin infections. HIV should always be explored as a possibility in a returning traveler with fever, lymphadenopathy, sore throat, and/or rash.
- Specific infectious diseases should be considered according to returning destination, for example, malaria or dengue in tropical countries, tick-borne diseases from Eastern Europe, and encephalitis in Southeast Asia.
- Therefore, visiting the CDC website (www.cdc.gov/travel, last accessed December 29, 2014) may be helpful for assessment of the returning traveler who presents with a suspicious disease.

Traveler's Diarrhea

GENERAL PRINCIPLES

- Traveler's diarrhea (TD) is usually a benign, self-limited illness of 3 to 5 days duration, but its sudden onset during travel can be quite disruptive. **It is by far the most common illness of travelers.**
- **The primary care provider should discuss prevention and treatment.**
- The most common pathogen is enterotoxigenic *E. coli,* which causes watery diarrhea that can lead to dehydration. Other common pathogens include *Salmonella* spp. (nontyphi), *Campylobacter* sp., and *Shigella* spp.
- Norovirus has to be considered in cruise trips, since it been associated with several travel-related outbreaks especially in this type of travel, due to the nature of sanitation and confinement.
- Other pathogens include parasites, of which *Giardia lamblia* is the most common.
- **Prevention centers on avoiding contaminated food and water.** Encouraging common sense practices such as eating thoroughly cooked or peeled foods and drinking only bottled or filtered water will minimize the incidence of disease.
  - **Antibiotic prophylaxis with systemic antibiotics such as ciprofloxacin is not routinely recommended in the prevention of traveler's diarrhea,** mainly due to systemic adverse effects and emergence of antimicrobial resistance.
  - Rifaximin is minimally absorbed systemically and has been associated with effective reduction of traveler's diarrhea in trips <3 weeks' duration.[40]
  - Antibiotic prophylaxis is recommended mainly in those at very high risk of developing TD or those patients whose underlying conditions put them at risk of severe complications and dehydration.

DIAGNOSIS

True disease is defined as **three or more loose stools in 24 hours along with fever, nausea, vomiting, or abdominal cramping.** Etiologic workup is usually not warranted during travel, unless the symptoms are severe in which case the patient should seek local medical care.

TREATMENT

- **Every traveler should be educated regarding the prevention, recognition, and treatment of diarrhea** that occurs during his or her trip.
- Hydration is the mainstay of treatment. Patients should be advised that if they are unable to drink fluids, they should seek prompt local medical attention. Likewise, if fever or blood in the stool is present, local medical care should be sought.

- Patients **without fever or blood in their stool** can manage their diarrhea symptomatically with **loperamide**. **Bismuth subsalicylate** can be used as a second-line agent, and patients should be advised to bring it with them.
- **Antimicrobial agents** can shorten the duration of disease by up to a day and may be provided to patients to bring with them.
  - First-line therapy is typically a **fluoroquinolone** (ciprofloxacin 500 mg PO bid for 1 to 3 days).
  - Azithromycin 1,000 mg for one dose is a second-line agent, especially in areas such as Asia and parts of Latin America where fluoroquinolone resistance is increasing among *Campylobacter* spp.[41]

Malaria

- Malaria is commonly caused by *Plasmodium falciparum* and *P. vivax*, with *P. falciparum* causing more severe disease and *P. vivax* causing relapsing disease.
- Prophylactic regimens vary from region to region according to the susceptibility of *Plasmodium* sp. to different antimicrobials. Therefore, the consulting provider should go to the CDC website to become acquainted with the most updated data prior to suggesting a regimen. When deciding on a regimen, it should be individualized to the traveler's comorbidities, preferences, and contraindications, if any.
- Malaria presents as a nonspecific illness with severe fevers, chills, headache, nausea, vomiting, and myalgia. Malaria by *P. falciparum* is an emergency given the risk for severe disease with central nervous system involvement; thus, prompt diagnosis and management are key.
- If suspected, a **thick and thin blood smear** should be ordered.
- A detailed history of adherence to malaria prophylaxis should be obtained.
- A summary of CDC recommendations for prophylactic regimens in the traveler from the US is presented in Table 26-13.

TABLE 26-13	Summary of CDC Recommendations for Malaria Prophylaxis for Travelers from the US	
Drug	**Dosing**	**Precautions**
Chloroquine (for chloroquine sensitive areas only)	500 mg (salt) PO weekly Start: 1–2 weeks prior to travel Finish: 4 weeks after travel	Itching, bitter taste, retinal or visual field deficits
Atovaquone/proguanil	250/100 mg PO daily Start: 1–2 days prior to travel Finish: 1 week after travel	Gastrointestinal upset
Mefloquine (mefloquine sensitive areas only)	250 mg PO weekly Start: 1 week prior to travel Finish: 4 weeks after travel	Night terrors Caution with seizures, psychosis, depression, or cardiac conduction disturbances
Doxycycline	100 mg PO daily Start: 1–2 days prior to travel Finish: 4 weeks after travel	Photosensitivity Contraindicated in children and pregnancy

DIARRHEAL ILLNESS

GENERAL PRINCIPLES

- Infectious diarrhea remains among the **top five causes of morbidity and mortality in the world**.
- In the US, it remains an important concern for public health, as evidenced by repeated nationwide recalls of contaminated foods determined to be the source of outbreaks. It can be caused by virus, bacteria, and parasites (protozoa).
- Diarrhea is defined as the passage of three or more stools in a day, which are of decreased consistency than usual for the individual.[42] In general, infectious diarrhea can be classified as follows:
  - **Acute watery diarrhea**: <14 days (e.g., Norovirus, Rotavirus, *Vibrio* spp.).
  - **Acute bloody diarrhea**, also known as **dysentery** (i.e., Shiga toxin–producing *E. coli, Campylobacter* spp., *Shigella* spp.).
  - **Persistent diarrhea**: between 14 and 30 days duration. Parasites should be ruled out in the appropriate context.
  - **Chronic diarrhea**: more than 30 days duration, less likely of infectious origin.
- Viral etiologies remain the most common cause of acute infectious diarrhea and are usually self-limited but pose a high risk for dehydration and spread.
- *Salmonella* spp., enterohemorrhagic *E. coli* (Shiga toxin producing), and *Clostridium perfringens* are among the most common bacterial pathogens associated with foodborne outbreaks.[43]
- *Clostridium difficile*–associated diarrhea has been increasing and is no longer considered exclusively a nosocomial infection. The wide use of broad-spectrum antibiotics in the community along with the presence of a more virulent strain have contributed to its emergence as a cause of acute infectious diarrhea in the ambulatory practice and in groups previously not considered at risk.[44]
- The most common causes of infectious diarrhea are presented in Table 26-14.

DIAGNOSIS

- As for many infectious diseases, the clinical presentation and exposure/epidemiologic history will guide the diagnostic workup. Travel history, food exposures, occupational exposures, and immune status should be reviewed.
- Stool culture should only be ordered if[42]
  - Severe disease: fever, mucous, >1-day duration
  - Bloody diarrhea
  - Immunosuppressed: >65 years, HIV, transplant patient, steroids, TNF inhibitors
  - Hospitalized <3 days
  - Positive lactoferrin test
- Currently, several pathogens can be detected by immunoassays in stool, such as rotavirus, *Giardia lamblia,* and *Cryptosporidium.*
- Stool examination for ova and parasites should be ordered if the patient is from a developing country or a returning traveler with consistent clinical picture, appropriate exposure, and persistent or chronic diarrhea and in patients with HIV/AIDS.

TREATMENT

Rehydration

- The initial assessment should include an evaluation of the patient's hydration status.
- **Rehydration should be prompt.** For the majority of adult patients with **mild-to-moderate dehydration,** soups and juices are generally sufficient.

TABLE 26-14 Summary of the Most Common Diarrheal Illnesses Worldwide

Etiology	Clinical presentation	Source/transmission	Treatment	Notes
Viral				
Norovirus	Vomiting and diarrhea of 24- to 48-hour duration	Fecal-oral, foodborne Frequent source of outbreaks Most common pathogen in foodborne outbreaks Mainly winter-spring	Self-limited, supportive, hydration	Associated with outbreaks in cruise ships, schools Hand and environmental hygiene for control
Rotavirus	Watery diarrhea 3–5 days, can be severe	Fecal-oral, mainly summer Children and day care centers usual source of outbreak	Aggressive hydration, supportive	Diagnostic assays available Rotavirus vaccination in children
Bacterial				
Escherichia coli	**Enterotoxigenic *E. coli*:** watery diarrhea **Shiga toxin–producing *E. coli*:** bloody diarrhea, fever, abdominal pain HUS	Fecal-oral, foodborne Associated with undercooked meat and foodborne outbreaks	Supportive, antibiotics in traveler May need admission, IV hydration Avoid antibiotics	See traveler's diarrhea Severe disease, consult ID specialist Antibiotics may worsen HUS
Non-typhi *Salmonella* spp.	Inflammatory and watery diarrhea, fever, abdominal pain	Foodborne: eggs, poultry, vine-stalk vegetables Reptiles can be carriers	Supportive, unless immunocompromised	Antibiotics may prolong the carrier state
Salmonella typhi/paratyphi	Typhoid fever: systemic febrile illness	Contaminated raw foods, fecal-oral, developing countries	Fluoroquinolones	Diarrhea not a prominent feature
Campylobacter jejuni	Abdominal pain, fever, bloody diarrhea in children	Poultry, waterborne outbreaks	Usually self-limited Severe cases: FQ macrolides	Associated with reactive arthritis, Guillain-Barre syndrome
Listeria monocytogenes	Severe diarrhea, fever, sepsis	Unpasteurized dairy products, undercooked deli meats, vegetables	Immunocompetent: no antibiotics, self-limited Immunosuppressed, pregnant women: admission, IV ampicillin	High mortality in high-risk groups: pregnant, >65 years old, immunosuppressed

(Continued)

TABLE 26-14 Summary of the Most Common Diarrheal Illnesses Worldwide *(Continued)*

Etiology	Clinical presentation	Source/transmission	Treatment	Notes
Vibrio spp.	Severe watery diarrhea	Contaminated water, fish products, fecal-oral shellfish (Gulf coast)	Supportive, aggressive hydration. May need IV resuscitation (*V. cholerae*)	*Vibrio cholerae*: developing countries, summer outbreaks
Shigella spp.	Bloody, mucoid diarrhea, fever, cramps, tenesmus	Fecal-oral, contaminated food	Ciprofloxacin 500 mg PO bid for 5 days	Very-low-infective dose
Protozoal *Giardia lamblia*	Foul smelling floating diarrhea, malabsorption, abdominal pain	Fecal-oral, contaminated water	Metronidazole 500 mg PO tid for 5 days	More common in developing countries, returning traveler; may cause persistent diarrhea; stool diagnostic immunoassay available
Cryptosporidium spp.	Watery diarrhea, severe in HIV (+) patients.	Contaminated water, farms, swimming pools	Self-limited in immunocompetent host HIV: antiretroviral therapy, nitazoxanide	Immune reconstitution essential Stool immunoassay for diagnosis, microscopy
Cyclospora cayetanensis	Abdominal pain, diarrhea, anorexia	Foodborne, waterborne Associated with food recalls: raspberries, vegetables	TMP-SMX 160/800 mg PO bid for 7 days	If suspected, order acid-fast stain of stool
Entamoeba histolytica	Abdominal pain, bloody diarrhea Majority asymptomatic but carriers	Fecal-oral, developing countries	Metronidazole 500 mg PO tid for 7–10 days followed by intraluminal agent (iodoquinol, paromomycin) Also tinidazole, nitazoxanide	Treat asymptomatics too Can cause persistent diarrhea, anemia Diagnosis: microscopy, serology
Other parasites not included: *Isospora belli*, *Microsporidium* spp.	Suspect in immunocompromised patients, HIV+ patients			

HUS, hemolytic-uremic syndrome; FQ, fluoroquinolones; TMP-SMX, trimethoprim-sulfamethoxazole.

- For more **moderate-to-severe dehydration,** patients should be encouraged to consume oral rehydration solutions with glucose-based electrolyte solutions.
  - The World Health Organization and United Nations Children's Fund oral rehydration solution consists of the following: 2.6 g NaCl, 13.5 g glucose, 1.5 g KCl, and 2.9 g trisodium citrate all in 1 L of water (total osmolality 245 mOsm/kg).
  - Similar commercial oral rehydration products are available (e.g., Pedialyte). These products contain sodium, potassium, and carbohydrate and have an appropriate osmolality (approximately 200 to 300 mOsm/kg).
  - **Intravenous therapy** should be administered to those who are obtunded or unable to tolerate oral therapy.

Empiric Treatment

- **The majority of disease lasts <1 day and is of viral etiology, making antimicrobial therapy of no benefit.**[42]
- **Unnecessary harm can occur from misuse of antimicrobials,** including prolonged carriage of *Salmonella* spp., worsening hemolytic-uremic syndrome from induction of Shiga toxin production, or development of *C. difficile* colitis.
- **Loperamide** is an antimotility agent that is not systemically absorbed. It can often limit the symptoms of acute diarrhea, but it **should not be used during disease caused by known or suspected invasive organisms (as evidenced by bloody diarrhea).** Complications of loperamide therapy include worsening of HUS and toxic megacolon.
- Nonpharmacologic therapies are of varying benefit.
  - **Strict handwashing for exposed and infected persons is imperative in limiting the spread of disease.**
  - The BRAT (bananas, rice, applesauce, toast) diet is of no proven benefit.
  - Dairy avoidance is important given the potential for transient lactase deficiency.
- Specific therapy is presented in Table 26-14.

Clostridium difficile Infection

General Principles

- *Clostridium difficile* infection (CDI) is caused by cytotoxin production, resulting in the formation of colonic pseudomembranes and inflammatory colitis.
- Disease is usually associated with **prior antibiotic use,** and more recently, a more virulent strain of *C. difficile* is increasing in frequency in the community.[44]
- Main risk factors include hospitalization, history of recent hospitalization, recent antibiotic use, and immunosuppression.
- Most patients have a history of antibiotic use in the prior 3 to 5 days, but it could be as remote as 90 days prior to symptoms.
- Disease is usually recognized by the onset of diarrhea in the appropriate clinical setting.
- Prevention of CDI is important.
  - **Proper hand hygiene, contact precautions, and isolation of the patient with active diarrhea are the most effective ways to prevent spread to others**.
  - Of note, commercially available alcohol-based hand sanitizers do not eliminate the spores and thus are not recommended as an adequate hand hygiene method for the prevention of *C. difficile* transmission.[45,46]
  - Patients should be instructed to disinfect surfaces at home with a 10% bleach solution, even if they are not visibly soiled, to kill the spores and prevent reinfection.[46,47]
  - Patients who require prolonged or repeated systemic antibiotic therapy for other reasons may require concomitant treatment with either metronidazole or oral vancomycin to prevent relapse.[45]

○ Ultimately, the best way to prevent emergence of *C. difficile* is **to avoid the indiscriminate use of broad-spectrum antibiotics in the community**.
- Recurrent CDI from either relapse or reinfection has been reported in up to 25% of the cases.[45]

DIAGNOSIS

- Common symptoms include liquid stools with abdominal pain, fever, mucus, and/or blood, almost always preceded by antimicrobial use or recent hospital discharge.
- Diarrhea can be severe and lead to volume depletion quickly, especially in the elderly and immunosuppressed.
- It may present solely as constipation, which can be an ominous sign since the patient may be developing **toxic megacolon**, which constitutes an emergency as perforation may be imminent.
- Leukocytosis is usually present, and hypoalbuminemia can be a sign of severe disease.[47]
- Diagnosis is made most often by detection of toxin A and/or B in the stool, for which several techniques are available, with variable sensitivity and specificity.[45] These include PCR for both toxins, enzyme immunoassay of toxins A/B, cell culture toxicity, and detection of hypervirulent 027 strain. For the treating provider, it is important to remember that the assay should test for both toxins, since disease can be present with either isolated toxin.
- Toxin assays should only be ordered on loose stools.
- There is no benefit in ordering the test more than once in a patient in whom CDI is suspected.[45]
- In severely ill patients who require hospitalization, endoscopic diagnosis may be required to prove the presence of pseudomembranes, which also confirms the diagnosis.

TREATMENT

- The first step in the management of CDI is to stop the antimicrobials the patient may be on during the onset of diarrhea.
- In the outpatient setting, either oral metronidazole or oral vancomycin can be used, since its equivalence has been shown in nonsevere disease.[44,45] Metronidazole is usually preferred over oral vancomycin due to cost reasons.
- **Metronidazole 500 mg orally every 8 hours and vancomycin 125 mg orally every 6 hours** are the recommended doses.
- Vancomycin should be the agent of choice in severe cases.[45,47]
- **Note that higher doses of oral vancomycin have not proven to be more effective, and thus, 125 mg is preferred**.
- **The duration of treatment in mild-to-moderate disease is 10 to 14 days**.
- Newer antibiotics approved for the management of CDI (rifaximin, fidaxomicin) are not recommended as first-line therapy for the first episode or first recurrence.
- Studies on the use of probiotics have had mixed results regarding their role in prevention of CDI.[45]
- **The first recurrence should be treated the same way as the initial episode,** unless a more severe presentation warrants hospitalization or changing from metronidazole to vancomycin.[45] For further recurrences, oral vancomycin is the drug of choice, and a prolonged taper is recommended. A consultation with an infectious diseases specialist is advised in these cases.

SUPERFICIAL FUNGAL INFECTIONS

Tinea Versicolor

- The most common skin fungal infection **not caused** by dermatophytes is **tinea versicolor**, which is caused by *Malassezia* spp.
- It typically presents as hypopigmented or erythematous macules in trunk, which in most cases are nonpruritic or tender. In darker-skinned patients, macules may be hyperpigmented.
- See Chapter 41 for information on diagnosis and treatment.

INFECTIONS BY DERMATOPHYTES

- Dermatophytes (*Trichophyton* spp.) are the most common fungi causing infection of the skin, hair, and nails. In isolation, they rarely cause severe disease, but they can play a role in the development of more severe bacterial infections.
- Tinea infections are named by their location and include tinea pedis (athlete's foot), tinea cruris (jock itch), tinea capitis (scalp ringworm), tinea corporis (ringworm), tinea faciei, tinea barbae, and tinea unguium (i.e., onychomycosis).
  - Usually present as areas of mild inflammation with pain and itching.
  - The margin of the infection is usually the area of most intense inflammation, and central clearing is frequently seen.
  - Tinea pedis usually starts in the interdigital spaces and may spread to the dorsum or lateral aspect of the foot. The skin may crack and become macerated.
  - **Onychomycosis** is a common dermatophyte infection of the nails. The nails become thickened and discolored (white, yellow, or brown).
- **Visualization of fungi on microscopic examination of skin scrapings** can generally provide the diagnosis. Ultraviolet light can help identify infected hairs for further evaluation. Fungal culture can also be useful.
- Treatment of tinea and onychomycosis is discussed in detail in Chapter 41.

SPOROTRICHOSIS

- Sporotrichosis is a subcutaneous infection caused by *Sporothrix schenckii* and presents as a nodular, pustular skin lesion.
- It is found in decaying plant matter, and infections are frequently linked to gardening.
- Ulcers may or may not be painful. It usually spreads via the lymphatic vessels, which accounts for streaking, regional lymph node swelling, and secondary ulcerations.
- Pulmonary disease is a rare manifestation.
- Diagnosis is made by visualization on skin biopsy and culture.
- Although the lesions are rarely life threatening, treatment is usually indicated.
- **Oral itraconazole** (200 mg solution daily for 3 to 6 months) has largely replaced potassium iodide (1 to 2 drops three times daily for 3 to 6 months) as the treatment of choice in the developed world.
- Pulmonary disease should be treated more aggressively because of its progressive nature.

CANDIDAL INFECTIONS

- *Candida* spp. are normally present in the gastrointestinal tract. They are frequently recovered from bladder catheters, sputum, skin, and the female genital tract.
- **Isolation of these organisms does not necessarily represent true infection**.

- Pathologic infections caused by *Candida* spp. can range from cutaneous to severe systemic disease.
- This discussion will focus only on frequently encountered outpatient infections.

Candiduria

- Candiduria is frequently observed but **rarely clinically significant.**
- Prior antibiotic use and genitourinary (GU) tract manipulation are risk factors for candiduria.
- **Treatment is not necessary in every patient with candiduria**.
- Without treatment, healthy patients generally clear the yeast in their urine.
- **Only symptomatic patients** (e.g., dysuria), **neutropenic or posttransplant patients, and those undergoing GU tract manipulations should be treated**.
- **Fluconazole** 200 mg daily for 7 to 14 days will reduce the duration of candiduria.

Oral Candidiasis

- Thrush is frequently seen in **immunosuppressed patients,** patients with diabetes, patients treated with antibiotics and inhaled corticosteroids, and children.
- Presents as curd-like patches on the tongue and buccal mucosa. Lesions can be scraped off leaving an erythematous lesion that may bleed.
- Esophageal disease may occur independently of oral disease and presents as severe odynophagia.
- Clinical exam is generally sufficient for diagnosis.
- Treatment with topical therapy such as **clotrimazole** troches (10 mg five times daily) and **nystatin** (4 to 6 mL of 100,000 units/mL qid) is generally effective.
- Oral **fluconazole** (100 mg daily for 7 to 14 days) may be needed for **recurrent disease** and is usually indicated at higher doses (200 to 400 mg daily) for esophageal disease.

Candidal Vaginitis

- Candidal vaginitis is a common infection occurring in patients with diabetes , with recent antibiotic use, and in pregnancy. This injection is discussed in more detail in Chapter 3.
- Oral contraceptives may also increase the risk of colonization, and cessation of oral contraceptives may be needed to cure recurrent cases.
- Patients present with dysuria, vaginal discharge, and erythema of the external genitalia.
- Visualization of yeast on a wet preparation of vaginal fluid aids in diagnosis, though empiric treatment is often recommended.
- **Topical therapy** (e.g., nystatin, miconazole, clotrimazole, terconazole) is sufficient for uncomplicated disease.
- **Fluconazole** 150 mg for one dose is also an approved therapy but can be more expensive. Many patients will find it to be much more convenient.

DEEP FUNGAL INFECTIONS

Histoplasmosis

GENERAL PRINCIPLES

- Histoplasmosis, caused by *Histoplasma capsulatum*, occurs worldwide.
- In the US, infection is mostly seen in the Ohio and Mississippi River valleys.[48]
- Risk factors include visits to caves with bat droppings and exposure to construction zones, bird droppings, or contaminated soil in endemic areas.
- Transmission is airborne, and depending on the patient's immune status, the patient may develop disease or present with lower respiratory symptoms, which usually resolve within 1 month.

- In this case, the only sequelae may be calcified nodules seen in the lungs on radiography or asymptomatic mediastinal lymphadenopathy.
- Acute infection can disseminate, and complications may arise such as fibrosing mediastinitis, arthritis and arthralgias, hepatic involvement, and erythema nodosum.
- Clinical resolution appears to depend on cell-mediated immunity.

DIAGNOSIS

- Diagnosis can be made by histopathologic visualization, growth in culture, or high titers on **complement fixation assays (serologic testing)**.[48]
- Detection of *Histoplasma* antigen in the urine is useful primarily in disseminated disease and in patients with HIV/AIDS.

TREATMENT

- Treatment is usually not needed for mild-to-moderate disease.[48]
- Persistent symptoms may require treatment, which can be accomplished with **itraconazole** 200 mg solution tid for 3 days and then once daily for 6 to 12 weeks.[48]
- Severe disease requires hospitalization and initial treatment with IV **amphotericin B.**
- Chronic cavitary disease requires prolonged treatment with itraconazole and monitoring of drug levels.

Blastomycosis

GENERAL PRINCIPLES

- Blastomycosis is caused by the dimorphic fungus *Blastomyces dermatitidis.*
- It is commonly found in the southeast and south central US as well as the Great Lakes region and territories around the St. Lawrence River.
- Patients acquire infection via inhalation of conidia.
- Acute infection can mimic influenza or pneumonia.
- It can also present in an indolent fashion, being confused with TB or malignancy due to its ability to form mass-like lesions.
- Extrapulmonary sites of infection include bone, skin, and the GU tract.
- Cutaneous involvement may be the only sign of infection, which consists of violaceous verrucous raised lesions on the upper extremities or face.

DIAGNOSIS

- Diagnosis is based on isolation of the fungus in culture from a biopsy specimen.[49]
- The diagnosis should be sought in patients with history of weight loss, night sweats, and lower respiratory symptoms, with or without skin lesions in the appropriate epidemiologic area.
- A presumptive diagnosis can be made on histopathologic findings, revealing the classic **broad-based budding yeast.**
- Serologic testing is unreliable and plays only a supportive role.[49]

TREATMENT

- Treatment has reduced the mortality associated with blastomycosis from >90% to <10%.
- Mild-to-moderate disease can be treated with **itraconazole** (200 to 400 mg PO daily for a minimum of 2 months). Most patients require at least 6 months of therapy.[49]

- Severe disease requires hospitalization and prolonged treatment with **amphotericin B,** which can be changed to itraconazole after the patient has improved.
- Given difficulties with absorption of itraconazole, one should consider **monitoring drug levels.**
- The **oral solution has better absorption than tablets,** which need to be taken with food or after drinking an acidic beverage.

Coccidioidomycosis

GENERAL PRINCIPLES

- Coccidioidomycosis, otherwise known as valley fever, is caused by *Coccidioides immitis* or *C. posadasii.*
- In the US, infection is endemic to the southwestern region.
- Patients present 1 to 3 weeks after exposure with an acute illness indistinguishable from bacterial pneumonia that resolves spontaneously; however, some patients may experience prolonged fatigue.
- Patients with acute self-limited disease may have symptoms similar to an upper respiratory infection.
- Complications include dissemination to the central nervous system (CNS), skin, and bone. In a minority of patients, chronic disease or lung nodules may develop. Patients may also have a rash similar to erythema multiforme or erythema nodosum.
- Latent infections and reactivation can occur in immunosuppressed patients.
- Transmission is airborne, and even a short stay in an endemic area may be sufficient to cause infection and disease.

DIAGNOSIS

- Detailed residence and travel history should be obtained in any patient presenting outside of an endemic area.
- CXRs can reveal multiple nodules with hilar adenopathy.
- **Serologic testing** (complement fixation antigen) is more reliable than in other endemic mycoses.[50]
- Definitive diagnosis is made by **culture** of the organism from a pulmonary sample.[50]
- The microbiology laboratory should be notified if one is attempting to recover coccidioidomycosis through culture as this pathogen is a select agent per the CDC.

TREATMENT

- Acute infection in otherwise healthy individuals does not necessarily require treatment.
- Patients with immunosuppression, diabetes, or underlying cardiopulmonary disease should receive treatment.
- **Itraconazole or fluconazole** at doses of 200 to 400 mg daily for three to six is recommended.[50]
- For severe disease or disease in pregnancy, **amphotericin B** is the treatment of choice.

Cryptococcosis

GENERAL PRINCIPLES

- Cryptococcosis is caused by *Cryptococcus neoformans,* a yeast distributed throughout the world in soil. Various other species exist but rarely cause disease in humans.
- Infection begins with inhalation of spores; exposure to bird droppings is a common risk factor.

- Pulmonary infection presents as cough, fever, dyspnea, and multiple nodular lung densities.
- Disease is more common in immunosuppressed patients, such as HIV-infected patients, those on chronic steroids, chronic TNF-α inhibitors, and pregnant women.
- Meningitis commonly occurs, and all patients with pulmonary disease should have a lumbar puncture performed to evaluate for CNS disease.
- Patients with CNS disease can present with various symptoms, but generally all patients complain of severe headache.

DIAGNOSIS

- Diagnosis is made by **culture** or positive **cryptococcal antigen** titer on the serum or cerebrospinal fluid.[51]
- When none of these tests are available, then India ink preparations should be used to identify encapsulated yeast on direct microscopic examination.
- Patients who undergo lumbar puncture should have an opening pressure documented.

TREATMENT

- Treatment for pulmonary disease is **fluconazole** 200 to 400 mg daily for 6 to 12 months. Itraconazole is a second-line agent.[51]
- Treatment of disseminated cryptococcal disease should be conducted with the aid of a specialist and usually requires hospitalization.

TICK-BORNE DISEASE

- Common tick-borne diseases in the US include **ehrlichiosis, anaplasmosis, Lyme disease, Rocky Mountain spotted fever (RMSF), and babesiosis.** Each is endemic in various geographical regions based on tick distribution.
- Other diseases transmitted by ticks within the US include the following:
  - **Tularemia:** acquisition of *Francisella tularensis* via ticks is thought to be the most common way Americans contract the disease.
  - **Colorado tick fever:** a Coltivirus infection transmitted by the wood tick *Dermacentor andersoni,* in the Western coast states and Colorado area.
  - **Tick-borne relapsing fever:** *Borrelia* spp. infection transmitted by *Ornithodoros* spp. ticks.
  - **Tick paralysis:** caused by tick salivary neurotoxins rather than by transmission of a microbial infection. Many tick species have been implicated.
  - **Southern tick-associated rash illness** (STARI) is an entity that can strongly resemble Lyme disease but typically occurs in areas where Lyme disease is uncommon. In spite of the name, it also occurs in the Mid-Atlantic states and the Midwest. There is currently no diagnostic test.
- Tick-borne diseases peak in the spring through fall but can occur any time during the year.
- **Knowledge of disease distribution and patient travel history to endemic areas is important to diagnosis.**
- In the primary care setting, the role of the provider should be to identify a probable tick or arthropod-borne disease in order to consult an infectious diseases specialist and/or admit if needed.
- In this section, only the most common tick-borne diseases in the US will be discussed, since they may present with frequency in the primary care setting.

Lyme Disease

GENERAL PRINCIPLES

- Lyme disease is the most common tick-borne disease in North America and Europe.
- In the US, Lyme disease is caused by *Borrelia burgdorferi*; other *Borrelia* species are the pathogens in the rest of the world.
- Lyme disease occurs with more frequency **throughout the northeastern US as well as north central states**.
- It is transmitted by the tick *Ixodes scapularis* (deer tick), which is also the vector for babesiosis and anaplasmosis.
- The most common acute presentation is a **single cutaneous lesion** (erythema migrans) with systemic symptoms such as **fever, myalgia, and arthralgia**.
- If untreated, complicated Lyme can include **neurologic disease** (neuroborreliosis) and/ or **cardiac disease**, most typically presenting with second- or third-degree heart block.
- **Post–Lyme disease syndrome** (PTLDS) consists of chronic/recurrent subjective constitutional or neurologic symptoms (e.g., fatigue, malaise, headache, arthritis, myalgia, and poor concentration, third nerve palsy) **after appropriately treated Lyme disease**.[52] It is not felt to be a manifestation of persistent infection.
- The best way to prevent Lyme disease is by avoiding tick bites, wearing appropriate clothing and using tick repellent when tick exposure is possible, and performing daily tick checks.
- Widespread chemoprophylaxis with antibiotics is not recommended, given the low incidence of Lyme disease among the population of patients with known tick bites.
- Per the guidelines of the IDSA, a **single dose of doxycycline 200 mg** should be given to patients in whom an *Ixodes* sp. tick is removed after 36 hours (by witnessed time or degree of tick engorgement) in areas where the prevalence of *B. burgdorferi* infection of ticks is at least 20%.[52]
- These recommendations require that health care providers in endemic areas are able to identify *Ixodes* ticks and their different stages.

DIAGNOSIS

- In the setting of a tick bite or **appropriate epidemiologic background,** the diagnosis is clinical but can be confirmed with serologic testing.[52]
- Many patients do not recall a specific tick bite; therefore, known tick bites are not necessary for making the diagnosis.

Clinical Presentation

- Acutely, the patient presents with a rash (**erythema migrans,** EM) occurring 7 to 10 days after tick exposure. Classically, this lesion is at least 5 cm in biggest diameter, which starts as a red papule and clears in the center as it enlarges. The lesion is unique, though other secondary similar lesions may appear.
- In addition to the EM rash, patients may develop fevers, constitutional symptoms, and adenopathy.
- Chronic forms (i.e., not previously treated) of disease may present as **second- or third-degree heart block, chronic oligoarthritis, subacute encephalopathy, or axonal polyneuropathy**.
- PTLDS **should not** be considered in patients who do not have a convincing history of previously treated Lyme disease.[52]

Diagnostic Testing

- The CDC recommends a two-tier process. Initially, an enzyme immunodiffusion analysis (EIA, ELISA) or immunofluorescence (IFA) is done, and if positive or equivocal, it is confirmed by Western blot.

- **Positive ELISA must be confirmed by Western blot analysis.**[52]
- **Serology alone should not be the sole means of diagnosis and should not be used as a screening test in unselected populations.**

TREATMENT

- **First-line treatment of acute disease is doxycycline** (100 mg PO bid) for 14 days to decrease duration and prevent development of late manifestations of disease.
- Doxycycline has the added advantage of effectively treating *Anaplasma phagocytophilum*, which is transmitted by the same deer tick.
- Alternative agents include cefuroxime or ceftriaxone.
- Those with meningitis and/or carditis require more aggressive, often inpatient, treatment.
- Cardiac disease due to Lyme disease is treated with 28 days of IV ceftriaxone.

Rocky Mountain Spotted Fever

GENERAL PRINCIPLES

- RMSF fever is caused by *Rickettsia rickettsii* transmitted by the dog tick *Dermacentor variabilis*.
- It was originally isolated from the northern regions of the Rocky Mountains in the US; however, the **disease is most prevalent in the Atlantic coastal states and south central US.**
- Disease begins 5 to 7 days after tick exposure.
- It can be a lethal disease; the diagnosis should be recognized early so that treatment can be initiated promptly.

DIAGNOSIS

- Diagnosis rests largely on the clinical syndrome:
  - Patients initially present with marked constitutional symptoms (e.g., fever, malaise, fatigue, arthralgia, myalgia, headache, anorexia, nausea, and emesis).
  - **Rash begins on the 3rd to 5th day of symptoms.**
  - Typically, it starts as a **maculopapular eruption** (later becoming petechial) on the extremities, specifically the wrists and ankles and often involving the palms and soles, and progresses toward the trunk.[53]
  - A minority of patients never develop the characteristic rash (i.e., "spotless").
- A history of tick exposure in a patient with these symptoms in the right epidemiologic area is sufficient to initiate treatment.
- Failure to initiate prompt treatment can lead to severe disease with meningeal involvement, respiratory failure, renal dysfunction, and death.
- **Acute and convalescent serologies** can confirm the diagnosis.[53]
- Direct immunofluorescence of skin lesions can aid in diagnosis.
- Additional laboratory abnormalities may include elevated transaminases, leukopenia, and thrombocytopenia. All may be seen in ehrlichiosis and anaplasmosis, adding further difficulty in differentiation. PCR techniques are under development.

TREATMENT

- Early treatment (often before the rash develops) reduces overall mortality.[53]
- **Doxycycline** (100 mg bid) should be initiated promptly when disease is suspected.
- Patients severely ill with RMSF require hospital admission.

Ehrlichiosis and Anaplasmosis

GENERAL PRINCIPLES

- **Human granulocytic anaplasmosis (HGA)** is caused by *A. phagocytophilum* and is transmitted by *Ixodes* spp. It is commonly found in the northeastern parts of the US. It is more common than ehrlichiosis.
- **Human monocytic ehrlichiosis (HME)** is caused by *Ehrlichia chaffeensis* and is transmitted by the Lone Star tick, *Amblyomma americanum*. In the US, it mainly occurs in the South Central, Southeastern, and Mid-Atlantic states.
- More severe infection appears to occur in the immunocompromised patients.
- Since they have the same vector, coinfection with anaplasmosis and Lyme disease can occur in the appropriate geographic area.

DIAGNOSIS

- As in other tick-borne diseases, **clinical suspicion is the most important step in the diagnosis**.
- Patients may present with a nonspecific febrile illness (e.g., malaise, fatigue, myalgias, and headache) after tick exposure, though they may not remember exposure or contact to a tick. Neurologic symptoms and signs are also possible.
- **Rash is much less common than with RMSF,** particularly so with HGA.[52]
- **Common laboratory findings include thrombocytopenia, leukopenia, and elevated transaminases.**
- Any of these findings in a febrile patient in the summer months in endemic areas should raise suspicion of these entities and prompt empiric treatment.
- Severe complications include seizure, coma, renal failure, cardiopulmonary failure, and clinical picture similar to the systemic inflammatory response syndrome.
- Diagnosis can be made by **acute and convalescent serologies.**[52]
- **PCR** testing is available with good sensitivity and specificity when obtained prior to administration of antimicrobial therapy.[52] When available, this should be the test of choice.
- As these organisms are typically found within macrophages, a peripheral smear showing **intracellular morulae** may be seen, aiding in the diagnosis.

TREATMENT

- The mainstay of treatment is **doxycycline** 100 mg bid for 10 days, which is also effective for the frequent alternative diagnosis of RMSF and possible coexistent Lyme disease.[52]
- Patients should rapidly respond to therapy.
- Rifampin therapy (300 mg PO bid) can be used as an alternative in less severe anaplasmosis.

Babesiosis

GENERAL PRINCIPLES

- Babesiosis, a malaria-like illness, is caused by the intraerythrocytic parasite, *Babesia microti,* and is found mainly in the northeastern US. It is transmitted by *I. scapularis.*
- Blood transfusion is also a possible means of infection.

- Asplenia is a major risk factor for severe disease.
- The majority of infections in immunocompetent hosts are probably asymptomatic.
- Possible coinfection with Lyme disease and ehrlichiosis should be considered.

DIAGNOSIS

- In symptomatic patients, fever, malaise, and headache usually begin 1 week after tick exposure.
- Severe hemolytic anemia, renal failure, and hypotension can develop in some patients.
- Hepatosplenomegaly may occur.
- Laboratory findings include those compatible with hemolysis (e.g., anemia, abnormal red cell morphology, elevated lactic dehydrogenase, and decreased haptoglobin), thrombocytopenia, elevated transaminases, and hyperbilirubinemia.
- Diagnosis can be made by identification of ring forms on blood smear.
- Serologic assays can be of benefit.

TREATMENT

- First-line therapy is with **atovaquone** (750 mg PO every 12 hours) **plus azithromycin** (500 to 1,000 mg on day 1 and then 250 mg PO daily) **or clindamycin** (300 to 600 mg every 8 hours) for 4 to 10 days.[52]
- Severe disease should be treated with quinine plus clindamycin.

FEVER OF UNKNOWN ORIGIN

- Temperature must be >38.3°C on several occasions over a period >3 weeks with a diagnosis remaining uncertain after 1 week of hospitalization.
- Given the changes in delivery of medical care, the requirement for hospitalization in the developed world has become less stringent.
- Finding the correct diagnosis in these situations can be challenging, and it is of utmost importance to **avoid excessive and unnecessary testing as well as empiric antimicrobial therapy.** Both of these errors can be misleading and cause increased morbidity for the patient.
- **So long as the patient is not acutely ill, there is no need to rush to empiric therapy.** Reassurance should be provided.
- Case series suggest >200 potential causes. A systematic approach to evaluate for more common causes of FUO is important and an algorithm has been proposed by Mourad et al.[54]
- Commonly, disease has been classified into three categories: malignancy, connective tissue disease/vasculitis, and infectious.
- **Malignancy:**
  - Of the many potential malignant causes of fever, lymphoma is probably the most common.
  - Clinical clues include night sweats, weight loss, and lymphadenopathy.
  - CT scanning of the chest, abdomen, and pelvis may be of benefit.
  - In addition, bone marrow biopsy can be considered.
- **Connective tissue diseases/vasculitis:**
  - Multiple autoimmune diseases have been implicated in causing FUO.
  - Rheumatoid arthritis and systemic lupus erythematosus are common causes as well as granulomatosis with polyangiitis (Wegener) so laboratory testing for antinuclear antibody (ANA), rheumatoid factor (RF), or antinuclear cytoplasmic antibody (ANCA) should be done in these cases.
  - Results of CT scanning may provide clues to accessible lesions for biopsy as well.

- **Infectious:**
  - The most common infections to consider include tuberculosis and subacute endocarditis in the developed world.
  - Workup for infectious causes includes CXR, CBC, blood cultures, sedimentation rate, C-reactive protein, and blood cultures.
  - Echocardiogram can be useful in evaluating for cardiac vegetations. A panorex radiograph should also be considered since dental abscess can be a cause of fever.
- **Other causes:**
  - Frequently, a medication that the patient is already taking may be the cause of fever. Any nonessential medications should be discontinued.
  - Blood clots are another frequent cause of fever, and Doppler ultrasounds of the lower extremities may be helpful.

IMMUNOSUPPRESSION

- The topic of infections in a non–HIV-infected patient who is immunocompromised is quite complex and cannot be covered in its entirety in the scope of this chapter. See Chapter 27.
- This section aims to give a very brief overview of common infections in this population as well as when to suspect immunodeficiencies in adult patients.
- Many patients who have undergone transplantation (solid organ or bone marrow) remain under close supervision of the transplant team. This is especially true in the highly vulnerable and complex posttransplantation period, which can last up to 1 year after transplant.
- Much disease is managed by or with the help of specialists. Severe disease can develop quickly, and care frequently requires an inpatient setting.

Antitumor Necrosis Factor Agents

- Immune-modulating therapy has become commonplace in the management of various autoimmune processes.
- TNF is a major cytokine in the control of disease, but its misdirection is thought to be involved in the pathophysiology of inflammatory disorders.
- TNF seems to exert its effect by activating natural killer cells and CD8⁺ lymphocytes.
- The most concerning infection in patients receiving anti-TNF agents is reactivated TB.
  - Patients should have PPD testing performed before initiating therapy with anti-TNF agents.
  - Should they have a PPD ≥5 mm, therapy for latent infection (after active infection has been ruled out) should be initiated before starting anti-TNF therapy.
  - There is no need to delay anti-TNF therapy until treatment of latent infection has been completed.

Primary Immunodeficiencies

One of the more challenging diagnoses for clinicians is that of primary immunodeficiencies. These relatively common processes tend to have obscure presentations and are frequently overlooked as potential underlying disease states. In addition, their complexity and various forms are difficult to fully comprehend. Often times, simple treatments such as monthly intravenous immune globulin can reduce the number of infections that patients endure.

DEFICIENCIES IN B-CELL FUNCTION AND ANTIBODY PRODUCTION

- These relatively common conditions typically present as recurrent sinopulmonary disease, but could present with bronchiectasia or urinary problems.
- Recurrent infections with encapsulated organisms (e.g., streptococci) are another clue.

- Primary B-cell dysfunction may be a cause of failure to respond to vaccines.
- **Common variable immunodeficiency** is perhaps the most important primary immune deficiency of adults, and its etiology is based on various defects in B-cell differentiation and varying degrees of T-cell dysfunction.
- Other diseases in this class of deficiency include **IgA deficiency** (also quite common), hyper-IgM syndrome, Good syndrome, and individual IgG subclass deficiencies. The latter conditions tend to be relatively asymptomatic.
- When suspected, a simple screen of immunoglobulin levels can be helpful in identifying underlying processes. Additional testing of immune globulin subsets or specific vaccine responses can further delineate the diagnosis.
- Treatment by monthly intravenous immune globulin injections can reduce the number of recurrent infections.

OTHER IMMUNODEFICIENCIES

- Adults can present with primary deficiencies commonly uncovered in childhood such as adenosine deaminase deficiency, Job syndrome (hyper-IgE syndrome), chronic granulomatous disease, and leukocyte adhesion defects. Age should not be an absolute factor in ruling out such diseases.
- The presentation of these processes is quite diverse; however, recurrent pyogenic abscesses can be one clue.
- Opportunistic infections in HIV-negative patients may also prompt evaluation.
- Recurrent mycobacterial infections or *Salmonella* infections may lead one to suspect a deficiency in interferon-γ. This group of genetic disorders is quite rare.
- Testing of lymphocyte and neutrophil function may be necessary as defects in cytokine production or oxidative bursts can be easily identified and can uncover the deficiency.

REFERENCES

1. Gwaltney JM Jr. Acute community-acquired sinusitis. *Clin Infect Dis* 1996;23: 1209–1225.
2. Rosenfeld RM, Andes D, Bhattacharyya N, et al. Clinical practice guideline: adult sinusitis. *Otolaryngol Head Neck Surg* 2007;137:S1–S31.
3. Meltzer EO, Hamilos DL. Rhinosinusitis diagnosis and management for the clinician: a synopsis of recent consensus guidelines. *Mayo Clin Proc* 2011;86:427–443.
4. Chow AW, Benninger MS, Brook I, et al. IDSA clinical practice guideline for acute bacterial rhinosinusitis in children and adults. *Clin Infect Dis* 2012;54:e72–e112.
5. Gwaltney JM Jr, Phillips D, Miller D, et al. Computed tomographic study of the common cold. *N Engl J Med* 1994;330:25–30.
6. Zalmanovici Trestioreanu A, Yaphe J. Intranasal steroids for acute sinusitis. *Cochrane Database Syst Rev* 2013;12:CD005149.
7. McIsaac WJ, White D, Tannenbaum D, et al. A clinical score to reduce unnecessary antibiotic use in patients with sore throat. *CMAJ* 1998;158:75–83.
8. McIsaac WJ, Kellner JD, Aufricht P, et al. Empirical validation of guidelines for the management of pharyngitis in children and adults. *JAMA* 2005;291:1587–1595.
9. Pelucchi C, Grigoryan L, Galeone C, et al. Guideline for the management of acute sore throat. *Clin Microbiol Infect* 2012;18(suppl 1):1–27.
10. Shulman ST, Bisno AL, Clegg HW, et al. Clinical practice guideline for the diagnosis and management of group A streptococcal pharyngitis: 2012 update by the Infectious Diseases Society of America. *Clin Infect Dis* 2012;55:e86–e102.
11. Wenzel RP, Fowler AA III. Acute bronchitis. *N Engl J Med* 2006;355:2125–2130.
12. Gonzales R, Bartlett JG, Besser RE, et al. Principles of appropriate antibiotic use for treatment of uncomplicated acute bronchitis: background. *Ann Intern Med* 2001;134:521–529.

13. Smith SM, Fahey T, Smucny J, et al. Antibiotics for acute bronchitis. *Cochrane Database Syst Rev* 2014;(3):CD000245.

14. Tiwari T, Murphy TV, Moran J. Recommended antimicrobial agents for the treatment and postexposure prophylaxis of pertussis: 2005 CDC Guidelines. *MMWR Recomm Rep* 2005;54(RR-14):1–16.

15. Harper SA, Bradley JS, Englund JA, et al. Seasonal influenza in adults and children-diagnosis, treatment, chemoprophylaxis, and institutional outbreak management: clinical practice guidelines of the Infectious Diseases Society of America. *Clin Infect Dis* 2009;48:1003–1032.

16. Fiore AE, Fry A, Shay D, et al. Antiviral agents for the treatment and chemoprophylaxis of influenza—recommendations of the Advisory Committee on Immunization Practices (ACIP). *MMWR Recomm Rep* 2011;60(1):1–24.

17. Fine MJ, Auble TE, Yealy DM, et al. A prediction rule to identify low-risk patients with community-acquired pneumonia. *N Engl J Med* 1997;336:243–250.

18. Lim WS, van der Eerden MM, Laing R, et al. Defining community acquired pneumonia severity on presentation to hospital: an international derivation and validation study. *Thorax* 2003;58:377–382.

19. Mandell LA, Wunderink RG, Anzueto A, et al. Infectious Diseases Society of America/American Thoracic Society consensus guidelines on the management of community-acquired pneumonia in adults. *Clin Infect Dis* 2007;44:S27–S72.

20. WHO. *Treatment of Tuberculosis: Guidelines*, 4th ed. Geneva, Switzerland: World Health Organization; 2010.

21. Hopewell PC, Pai M, Maher D, et al. International standards for tuberculosis care. *Lancet Infect Dis* 2006;6:710–725.

22. American Thoracic Society. Targeted tuberculin testing and treatment of latent tuberculosis infection. *Am J Respir Crit Care Med* 2000;161:S221–S247.

23. Centers for Disease Control and Prevention. Recommendations for use of an isoniazid-rifapentine regimen with direct observation to treat latent *Mycobacterium tuberculosis* infection. *MMWR Morb Mortal Wkly Rep* 2011;60:1650–1653.

24. Hooton TM. Uncomplicated urinary tract infection. *N Engl J Med* 2012;366:1028–1037.

25. Bent S, Nallamothu BK, Simel DL, et al. Does this woman have an acute uncomplicated urinary tract infection? *JAMA* 2002;287:2701–2710.

26. Stamm WE, Counts GW, Running KR, et al. Diagnosis of coliform infection in acutely dysuric women. *N Engl J Med* 1982;307:463–468.

27. Gupta K, Hooton TM, Naber KG, et al. International clinical practice guidelines for the treatment of acute uncomplicated cystitis and pyelonephritis in women: a 2010 update by the Infectious Diseases Society of America and the European Society for Microbiology and Infectious Diseases. *Clin Infect Dis* 2011;52:e103–e120.

28. Hooton TM, Stamm WE. Diagnosis and treatment of uncomplicated urinary tract infection. *Infect Dis Clin North Am* 1997;11:551–581.

29. Grabe M, Bjerklund-Johansen TE, Botto H, et al. Guidelines on urological infections. European Association of Urology 2013. http://www.uroweb.org/guidelines/online-guidelines/. Last accessed December 29, 2014.

30. Nicolle LE, Bradley S, Colgan R, et al. Infectious Diseases Society of America guidelines for the diagnosis and treatment of asymptomatic bacteriuria in adults. *Clin Infect Dis* 2005;40:643–654.

31. Moran GJ, Krishnadasan A, Gorwitz RJ, et al. Methicillin-resistant *S. aureus* infections among patients in the emergency department. *N Engl J Med* 2006;355:666–674.

32. Dupuy A, Benchikhi H, Roujeau JC, et al. Risk factors for erysipelas of the leg (cellulitis): case–control study. *BMJ* 1999;318:1591–1594.

33. Daum RS. Skin and soft-tissue infections caused by methicillin-resistant *Staphylococcus aureus*. *N Engl J Med* 2007;357:380–390.

34. Stevens DL, Bisno AL, Chambers HF, et al. Practice guidelines for the diagnosis and management of skin and soft-tissue infections. *Clin Infect Dis* 2005;41:1373–1406.

35. Liu C, Bayer A, Cosgrove SE, et al. Clinical practice guidelines by the Infectious Diseases Society of America for the treatment of methicillin-resistant *Staphylococcus aureus* infections in adults and children. *Clin Infect Dis* 2011;52:e18–e55.

36. Koning S, van der Wouden JC, Chosidow O, et al. Efficacy and safety of retapamulin ointment as treatment of impetigo: randomized double-blind multicentre placebo-controlled trial. *Br J Dermatol* 2008;158:1077–1082.

37. Gnann JW Jr, Whitley RJ. Herpes zoster. *N Engl J Med* 2002;347:340–346.

38. Isbister GK, Fan HW. Spider bite. *Lancet* 2011;378:2039–2047.

39. Hill DR, Ericsson CD, Pearson RD, et al. The practice of travel medicine: guidelines by the Infectious Diseases Society of America. *Clin Infect Dis* 2006;43:1499–1539.

40. DuPont HL. Therapy for and Prevention of Traveler's Diarrhea. *Clin Infect Dis* 2007;45:S78–S84.

41. DuPont HL. Azithromycin for self-treatment of traveler's diarrhea. *Clin Infect Dis* 2007;44:347–349.

42. Guerrant RL, Van Gilder T, Steiner TS, et al. Practice guidelines for the management of infectious diarrhea. *Clin Infect Dis* 2001;32:331–351.

43. Gould LH, Walsh KA, Vieria AR, et al. Surveillance for Foodborne Disease Outbreaks—U.S., 1998–2008. *MMWR Surveill Summ* 2013;62:S1–S34.

44. Kelly CP, LaMont JT. Clostridium difficile—more difficult than ever. *N Engl J Med* 2008;359:1932–1940.

45. Zar FA, Bakkanagari SR, Moorthi KM, et al. A comparison of vancomycin and metronidazole for the treatment of *Clostridium difficile*-associated diarrhea, stratified by disease severity. *Clin Infect Dis* 2007;45:302–307.

46. Cohen SH, Gerding DN, Johnson S, et al. Clinical practice guidelines for *Clostridium difficile* infection in adults: 2010 update by the Society for Healthcare Epidemiology of America (SHEA) and the Infectious Diseases Society of America (IDSA). *Infect Control Hosp Epidemiol* 2010;31:431–445.

47. Gerding DN, Muto CA, Owens RC. Measures to control and prevent *Clostridium difficile* infection. *Clin Infect Dis* 2008;46:S43–S49.

48. Wheat LJ, Freifeld AG, Kleiman MB, et al. Clinical practice guidelines for the management of patients with histoplasmosis: 2007 update by the Infectious Diseases Society of America. *Clin Infect Dis* 2007;45:807–825.

49. Chapman SW, Brasher RW Jr, Campbell GD Jr, et al. Practice guidelines for the management of patients with blastomycosis. *Clin Infect Dis* 2000;30:679–683.

50. Galgiani JN, Ampel NM, Blair JE, et al. Coccidioidomycosis. *Clin Infect Dis* 2005;41:1217–1223.

51. Saag MS, Graybill RJ, Larsen RA, et al. Practice guidelines for the management of cryptococcal disease. *Clin Infect Dis* 2000;30:710–718.

52. Wormser GP, Dattwyler RJ, Shapiro ED, et al. The clinical assessment, treatment, and prevention of Lyme disease, human granulocytic anaplasmosis, and babesiosis: clinical practice guidelines by the Infectious Diseases Society of America. *Clin Infect Dis* 2006;43:1089–1134.

53. Dantas-Torres F. Rocky Mountain spotted fever. *Lancet Infect Dis* 2007;7:724–732.

54. Mourad O, Palda V, Detsky AS. A comprehensive evidence-based approach to fever of unknown origin. *Arch Intern Med* 2003;163:545–551.

27 HIV Infection and Sexually Transmitted Diseases

Youngjee Choi, Courtney Chrisler, and Hilary E. L. Reno

HIV INFECTION AND AIDS

GENERAL PRINCIPLES

- Human immunodeficiency virus (HIV) type 1 is a human retrovirus that infects T lymphocytes and other cells that bear the CD4 surface marker. Infection leads to lymphopenia, CD4 lymphocyte deficiency and dysfunction, impaired cell-mediated immune response, and polyclonal B-cell activation with impaired B-cell responses to new antigens.
- This immune derangement gives rise to the acquired immunodeficiency syndrome (AIDS), which is characterized by opportunistic infections and unusual malignancies.
- Transmission is primarily by sexual and parenteral routes.
- Major risk groups include sexual contacts of infected individuals, intravenous (IV) drug users, and children born to HIV-infected mothers.
- Because management of HIV-infected patients is a complex and rapidly evolving field, this viral infection is best managed in close coordination with an expert. The information presented here is not intended as a substitute for expert care. Excellent sources of information for physicians who wish to familiarize themselves with HIV care include http://www.aidsinfo.nih.gov and hivinsite.ucsf.edu (last accessed 1/5/15).

DIAGNOSIS

Clinical Presentation

- Patients may be symptomatic at the time of diagnosis if they have been chronically infected. Recommendations are to screen all sexually active people for HIV. It is estimated that over 20% of people with HIV are not aware that they are infected.
- Patients with HIV infection may also present acutely near the time of seroconversion.
- Symptoms that should lead to a suspicion for HIV include recurrent oral candidiasis, lymphadenopathy, weight loss, fevers, night sweats, and chronic diarrhea.
- Abnormal laboratory findings may include anemia, thrombocytopenia, leukopenia, hypertriglyceridemia, low high-density lipoprotein (HDL) cholesterol levels, and elevated immunoglobulin levels.
- **Diagnosis is established with an HIV antibody assay and/or HIV RNA viral load.** HIV antibody assays are often nonreactive in acute HIV infection, while circulating HIV RNA viral load is very elevated. If suspicion is high for acute infection, HIV RNA viral load should be checked.
- **Primary HIV infection** (acute retroviral syndrome) often presents as a mononucleosis-like syndrome, with fever being the most common presenting symptom (>75% of patients). Other common symptoms include headache, rash, fatigue, and lymphadenopathy. As many as 90% of acutely infected patients experience at least some symptoms of the acute retroviral syndrome and may be identified as candidates for early therapy.

- Initial infection with HIV type 1 less commonly presents with neurologic manifestations such as aseptic meningitis, Guillain-Barré syndrome, spinal vacuolar myelopathy, peripheral neuropathy, and subacute encephalitis.
- Acute HIV infection is often not recognized in the primary care setting because of the nonspecific symptoms. Maintaining a high index of suspicion and knowing the appropriate testing modality (i.e., HIV viral load) are critical for diagnosis during this time period.

Diagnostic Testing

- Initial assessment of patients should determine the degree of immunodeficiency by measuring the absolute CD4 T-lymphocyte count (normal range for adults is 600 to 1,500 cells/μL^3). Along with comorbidities and AIDS-defining illnesses, **CD4 count is used to stratify those needing antiretroviral therapy (ART) and prophylactic therapy against opportunistic infections**.
- **The most important initial laboratory tests are the CD4 count and HIV RNA viral load**.
- Given that HIV drug resistance is transmitted as much as 6% to 16% of the time, an HIV genotype should also be performed at baseline to evaluate for critical mutations.
- As HIV is a sexually transmitted disease (STD), it is important to evaluate for other STDs including gonorrhea, chlamydia, syphilis, and the viral hepatitides.
- It is also important to have baseline **blood counts, basic chemistry values, liver function testing, urinalysis, fasting lipid profile, and glucose** testing to monitor for HIV complications and possible medication toxicities. Many of these laboratory tests should be repeated every 3 to 6 months as part of routine monitoring prior to initiating ART and once ART is initiated or modified. Unless abnormal, urinalysis, fasting lipid profile, and glucose testing can be repeated annually. In addition, baseline testing for antibodies to opportunistic infections such as cytomegalovirus (CMV) and toxoplasmosis may be helpful.
- Finally, all HIV-infected individuals should have baseline and annual testing for TB with a **tuberculin skin test** (TST) or interferon-gamma release assay (IGRA).

TREATMENT

- **ART should be offered to all HIV-infected individuals**, with the strongest evidence for those with CD4 count <500 cells/μL^3 and expert opinion suggesting treatment for CD4 count >500 cells/μL^3.[1,2]
  - Regardless of CD4 count, ART should be started in the following conditions: pregnancy, history of an AIDS-defining illness, HIV-associated nephropathy, and hepatitis B coinfection.
  - **Typical ART regimens** for initial therapy consist of a triple-drug combination: a pair of nucleoside or nucleotide reverse transcriptase inhibitors (NRTI) plus a drug from a second class (see Table 27-1).
  - Selecting a drug regimen should be individualized based on resistance testing, toxicity (e.g., hyperbilirubinemia and nephrolithiasis with atazanavir), comorbidities (e.g., pregnancy or hepatitis B coinfection), pill burden, dosing frequency, and potential drug-drug interactions. See aidsinfo.nih.gov and the 2012 International Antiviral Society-USA Panel guidelines for additional risks and benefits to various agents.[1,2]
  - Additional information on drug regimens based on resistance testing can be found at hivdb.stanford.edu (last accessed 1/6/15). Consultation with an HIV expert is recommended.
- **Prophylactic treatment against various organisms** is recommended for HIV-infected patients and is largely based on the CD4 count.[3]

TABLE 27-1	Preferred ART Regimens

Tenofovir and emtricitabine (dual NRTIs) plus one of the following agents:
Efavirenz (NNRTI)
Atazanavir (PI) plus ritonavir (PI)[a]
Darunavir (PI) plus ritonavir (PI)[a]
Raltegravir (InSTI)

[a]The addition of ritonavir is used to boost the level of the PI it is given with.
ART, antiretroviral therapy; NRTI, nucleos(t)ide reverse transcriptase inhibitor; NNRTI, nonnucleoside reverse transcriptase inhibitor; PI, protease inhibitor; InSTI, integrase strand transfer inhibitor.
Data from Panel on Antiretroviral Guidelines for Adults and Adolescents. Guidelines for the use of antiretroviral agents in HIV-1-infected adults and adolescents. 2012;1-240. Available at: http://aidsinfo.nih.gov/contentfiles/adultandadolescentgl.pdf, last accessed 12/6/15.

- Prophylaxis against **pneumocystis pneumonia** (PCP) is indicated when the CD4 count is <200 cells/μL^3, when the percent of CD4 lymphocytes is <20% of the total lymphocyte count, or if the patient has thrush regardless of CD4 count. Appropriate regimens are trimethoprim-sulfamethoxazole (TMP-SMX) one double-strength tablet daily or dapsone 100 mg daily.
- Prophylaxis against **toxoplasmosis** is indicated when the CD4 count is <100 cells/μL^3 (TMP-SMX for PCP prophylaxis is adequate).
- For patients with CD4 counts of <50 cells/μL^3, weekly azithromycin (1,200 mg) should be given as prophylaxis against *Mycobacterium avium* **complex** (MAC).
- For patients with CD4 counts <50 cells/μL^3, eye examinations should be conducted to evaluate for **CMV retinitis.**
- If immune reconstitution with ART occurs with sustained CD4 counts of >200 cells/μL^3 for 3 months, PCP and MAC prophylaxis can be discontinued.
- **Immunizations** such as annual influenza vaccine, pneumococcal vaccine, and hepatitis B vaccine (if seronegative) should also be offered, although immunologic response with CD4 counts <200 cells/μL^3 may be poor.[4] Patients who are men who have sex with men (MSM) or have chronic liver disease should also be considered for hepatitis A vaccination.[3] Vaccination for human papillomavirus (HPV) has not yet been established.[5]
- HIV is an STD, and therefore, the Centers for Disease Control and Prevention (CDC) recommends **annual screening for other STDs** including gonorrhea, chlamydia, and syphilis. More frequent screening is indicated in patients with high-risk behavior.
- Female patients with HIV should receive **screening for cervical cancer** with Pap smears at least annually.
- Because **TB** is an important complication of HIV infection, screening is warranted at the time of initial assessment and annually via TST or IGRA. Patients often become anergic as their immune deficiency progresses. Chest radiography should be performed as an alternative diagnostic procedure.

COMPLICATIONS

Viral Infections

Cytomegalovirus Reactivation
- CMV reactivation is common in patients with advanced AIDS (CD4 count <100 cells/μL^3).
- Manifestations include viremia with fever and constitutional symptoms, chorioretinitis, esophagitis, gastritis, enterocolitis, pancreatitis, acalculous cholecystitis, bone marrow suppression, necrotizing adrenalitis, and upper and lower respiratory tract infections.

- End-organ disease is seen most often when CD4 counts are <50 cells/μL[3].
- **Ganciclovir** 5 mg/kg IV or **valganciclovir** 900 mg PO every 12 hours is an effective induction therapy for chorioretinitis and gastrointestinal (GI) disease but is associated with significant hematologic toxicity.[3] Blood cell counts should be monitored for neutropenia. Concomitant granulocyte colony–stimulating factor can be used as a possible means of ameliorating ganciclovir myelotoxicity.
- Relapse after drug discontinuation is common, usually necessitating maintenance therapy until CD4 counts are >100 cells/μL[3] for 6 months.
- Patients with retinitis who are intolerant of systemic ganciclovir may benefit from intravitreal administration of the drug by an experienced ophthalmologist.
- Foscarnet is indicated for ganciclovir-resistant CMV or those failing ganciclovir therapy.

Other Herpesviridae
- **Herpes simplex virus-2** (HSV-2), but not HSV-1, has been identified more commonly in HIV-infected individuals than in HIV-negative individuals.
  - HSV-2 likely facilitates the transmission of HIV by providing a portal of entry (e.g., the genital ulcer) and by increasing HIV viral shedding in the genital tract.
  - HSV-2 coinfection has also been found to speed the progression of HIV to AIDS.
  - HSV infection has been associated with esophagitis, proctitis, pulmonary disease, and large, atypical, persistent cutaneous ulcerations.
  - **IV acyclovir** is usually effective for these problems, but relapses are frequent and individuals may require chronic HSV suppression.[3]
- **Varicella-zoster virus** may cause typical dermatomal lesions or disseminate. Recurrent disease, meningoencephalitis, and cranial neuritis have been reported. **Acyclovir** 800 mg PO five times per day or **famciclovir** 500 mg PO tid is the treatment of choice.
- Evidence of **Epstein-Barr virus** (EBV) infection is common in patients with AIDS, particularly oral hairy leukoplakia, a benign condition on the lateral aspect of the tongue.
  - Oral **acyclovir** may be effective but should be reserved for symptomatic cases.
  - EBV is also associated with central nervous system (CNS) lymphomas in individuals with advanced AIDS (generally CD4 count <50 cells/μL[3]).
  - Effective therapy for EBV-related malignancies includes ART.

JC Virus
- JC virus is a polyomavirus that is associated with **progressive multifocal leukoencephalopathy** (PML).
- Diagnosis is made by characteristic clinical features, MRI, and polymerase chain reaction (PCR) testing of cerebrospinal fluid (CSF) for JC virus. Detection of JC virus via PCR is needed for definite diagnosis, but has low sensitivity due to low viremia in the setting of ART.[6]
  - PML is characterized by subacute (weeks to months) progressive neurologic deficits including altered mental status, visual loss, weakness, and gait abnormalities.
  - MRI is the imaging modality of choice and reveals multifocal white matter hyperintensities on T2-weighted and fluid-attenuated inversion recovery (FLAIR) images.
  - No effective therapy has been identified; however, the course may be significantly altered by immune reconstitution via ART.[2]

Human Papillomavirus
- HPV causes a wide spectrum of disease in HIV-infected patients, from transient infection to **anogenital warts (HPV types 6 and 11) and squamous cell cancers (HPV types 16 and 18)**.
- HIV-infected women have a 5% to 10% increase in **cervical intraepithelial neoplasia** over HIV-negative women. Risk of more advanced cervical cancer increases with lower CD4 counts.

- Likewise, **anal intraepithelial neoplasia** is more common in HIV-infected men.
- Although usually asymptomatic, cervical, vaginal, or anal lesions may cause pain or spotting.
- **Annual pelvic examinations and cervical Pap smears** are recommended in HIV-infected women with referral and additional testing as indicated by abnormal results.
- The role of anal pap smears in HIV-infected patients, especially MSM, is under investigation.
- There are now two vaccines available for HPV (bivalent for types 16 and 18 and quadrivalent for types 6, 11, 16, and 18).
- **The efficacy of the HPV vaccine in HIV infection is unknown**, but the vaccine appears to be safe and produces a robust immune response.[5] It may be reasonable to vaccinate individuals aged 9 to 26 years old, as is recommended for HIV-negative individuals.

Bacterial Infections
Bacterial Pneumonia
- Bacterial pneumonias occur with increased frequency and are a common cause of morbidity.
- Pneumonias are usually due to ***Streptococcus pneumoniae, Staphylococcus aureus,*** or ***Haemophilus influenzae.***
- Pneumonia due to gram-negative enteric organisms occurs in advanced HIV disease.
- Chest radiographs may reveal typical lobar pneumonia, but diffuse interstitial infiltrates similar to PCP have been reported.

Syphilis
- The natural history of syphilis may be altered by HIV infection.
- Reactivation of previously treated disease, active disease with negative serology, asymptomatic neurosyphilis, and relapse after standard therapy have been reported. The optimal management of syphilis in this setting remains unclear.
- Current guidelines suggest **at least annual screening for syphilis in HIV-infected individuals** and more frequently in patients with high-risk behavior. Additional information on diagnosis is provided later in this chapter.
- Lumbar puncture is reserved for seropositive patients with neurologic symptoms. There are also data to support performing lumbar puncture in HIV-infected individuals with a serum rapid plasma reagin (RPR) titer >1:32 or CD4 count <350 cells/μL[3].
- Up to 20% of HIV-infected individuals will remain serofast after successful treatment of syphilis; serum RPR or Venereal Disease Research Laboratory (VDRL) remains reactive at a low titer, generally <1:8. The clinical relevance of this is unclear, but a fourfold rise in titer above this serofast baseline is indicative of reinfection or reactivation and may warrant a lumbar puncture to investigate for neurosyphilis.

Bacterial Diarrhea
- Bacterial diarrhea due to ***Salmonella*** spp., ***Campylobacter*** spp., and ***Shigella*** spp. is more common in HIV patients, particularly MSM.
- Nontyphoidal salmonellae (especially *Salmonella typhimurium*) are associated with invasive disease that often recurs or persists despite appropriate antibiotics.
  - Preferred treatment is **ciprofloxacin** for 7 to 14 days for diarrhea or 4 to 6 weeks for bacteremia.
  - Initial IV therapy should be followed by long-term oral suppressive therapy based on susceptibility testing; relapse may occur as soon as therapy is discontinued.
- Campylobacter diarrhea is treated with ciprofloxacin, but resistance is increasing.
- Shigellosis treatment is with ciprofloxacin or TMP-SMX.

Mycobacterial Infections

Tuberculosis

- TB can occur at any CD4 count, but extrapulmonary manifestations occur with increased frequency in patients with lower CD4 counts.
- In the developing world, TB is the most prominent AIDS-defining illness, and in the developed world, TB is most commonly diagnosed in substance abusers, immigrants from high-prevalence countries, and the urban poor.
- Atypical radiographic patterns and extrapulmonary disease are quite common; apical cavitary disease is uncommon in advanced HIV disease.
- See Chapter 26 for the treatment of TB.
- After ruling out active disease, **isoniazid** for 9 months should be considered in any HIV-infected patient with a reactive (>5-mm induration) TST or positive IGRA. Pyrazinamide plus rifampin for 2 months is an alternative, although there are significant drug interactions with ART and rifampin.

Mycobacterium Avium Complex

- MAC is one of the most frequent opportunistic pathogens in patients with advanced AIDS (usually CD4 count <50 cells/μL[3]).
- Generalized infection and GI disease are the most common manifestations.
- The organism can be cultured from sputum, blood, bone marrow, and tissue from the GI tract.
- Treatment with **clarithromycin, ethambutol, and rifabutin** is often effective.[3]
- For patients with CD4 counts <50 cells/μL[3], MAC prophylaxis therapy should be initiated with either azithromycin 1,200 mg PO weekly or clarithromycin 500 mg PO bid.

Fungal Infections

Candidiasis

- Persistent oral, esophageal, and vaginal infections are common; dissemination is rare in the absence of other risk factors such as IV catheters.
- The severity and frequency of mucocutaneous candidiasis increase with declining immune function.
- **Oral thrush** is effectively treated with topical therapy: **clotrimazole** troches PO five times per day for 14 days.[3]
- Frequently recurring thrush can be prevented with fluconazole 100 mg PO daily.
- **Esophagitis** should be treated with **fluconazole** (200 mg one time followed by 100 mg daily for 14 days; higher doses up to 400 mg daily may be required in some patients).
- **Vaginal candidiasis** can be treated with antifungal vaginal suppositories as discussed later in this chapter.

Cryptococcosis

- *Cryptococcus neoformans* is the most common cause of fungal CNS disease in patients with AIDS.
- Symptoms may be mild; therefore, **the threshold for performing a lumbar puncture should be low.**
- Lumbar puncture results include elevated opening pressure (often >200 mm H_2O), lymphocyte predominant pleocytosis, and low glucose. However, normal CSF parameters occur in as many as 25% of AIDS patients with cryptococcal meningitis, so a **cryptococcal antigen should be sent for all AIDS patients in whom a lumbar puncture is performed.**
- Repeat lumbar puncture is indicated for clinical deterioration as well as relief of elevated opening pressures, which are associated with poor outcomes.
- Initial treatment is with IV **amphotericin B and flucytosine** for 2 weeks, followed by **fluconazole** 400 mg daily for 8 to 10 weeks.[3]

- Following acute treatment, **maintenance therapy** is required with fluconazole 200 mg daily until CD4 count is >200 cells/µL[3].
- Response is usually monitored clinically and is generally slow.

Histoplasmosis

- *Histoplasma capsulatum* is an important pathogen in patients with AIDS from endemic areas and may cause disseminated disease and septicemia. The organism's endemic areas include the Ohio and Mississippi river valleys in the US, Central and South America, parts of southern Europe, Africa, eastern Asia, and Australia.
- Diagnosis is made by sending a **urine *H. capsulatum* antigen**; the organism can also be cultured from blood and bone marrow.
- Pancytopenia may result from bone marrow involvement.
- Treatment includes a 12-week induction phase with a subsequent long-term maintenance phase to complete 1 year of therapy.
- A cumulative dose of **amphotericin B** 1.5 to 2.0 g is given initially for severely ill patients. For patients who are intolerant of amphotericin B, liposomal amphotericin B can be considered. **Itraconazole** is effective for induction in milder disease. Itraconazole is also used for the maintenance phase.[3]

Coccidioidomycosis

- *Coccidioides* spp. infections occur in patients with AIDS from endemic areas (southwestern US and northern Mexico).
- In immunocompetent hosts, primary infection is a self-limited acute pneumonia known as **valley fever**.
- Extensive pulmonary disease with extrapulmonary spread, including meningitis and lymphadenopathy, is common in AIDS patients.
- **Fluconazole** 400 mg daily is usual treatment, with amphotericin B as an alternative therapy.[3]
- Lifelong maintenance treatment is required for coccidioidal meningitis.

Pneumocystis Pneumonia

- *Pneumocystis jiroveci* pneumonia remains the most common opportunistic infection in patients with AIDS and a leading cause of morbidity and mortality.
- Presenting symptoms include progressive dyspnea, fever, and cough; early disease may have a subtle presentation and a normal chest radiograph.
- **The treatment of choice for PCP is TMP-SMX** 5 mg/25 mg/kg PO or IV every 6 to 8 hours for 21 days.[3]
  - Anemia or rashes can occur in AIDS patients who are treated with TMP-SMX but may not require a change in therapy.[8]
  - For patients who do not tolerate TMP-SMX, **dapsone-trimethoprim, clindamycin-primaquine, and pentamidine** are other options.
- In patients with well-documented PCP and moderate-to-severe disease (arterial oxygen pressure <75 torr on room air), **adjunctive use of steroids** prevents adult respiratory distress syndrome and leads to a survival benefit.[9] **Prednisone** (or equivalent methylprednisolone) 40 mg PO bid for 5 days, followed by 40 mg PO daily for 5 days, followed by 20 mg PO daily for the duration of antipneumocystis therapy is recommended.

Protozoal Infections

Toxoplasma Reactivation

- *Toxoplasma gondii* typically presents in HIV-infected patients with CD4 counts <100 cells/µL[3].
- It is characterized by multiple CNS lesions presenting as encephalitis with headache, confusion, fever, and focal neurologic findings. Extracerebral toxoplasmosis has also been reported.

- Treatment with **sulfadiazine** 25 mg/kg PO every 6 hours (or TMP-SMX 5 mg/25 mg/kg PO or IV every 6 to 8 hours) plus **pyrimethamine** 100 to 150 mg PO on day 1 and then 50 to 75 mg PO daily often results in improvement, but **indefinite therapy is needed to prevent relapse.**[3] **Folinic acid** 5 to 10 mg PO daily can be added to minimize hematologic toxicity.
- For patients with sulfonamide allergy, clindamycin 600 mg PO four times per day can be substituted.

Diarrheal Diseases

- ***Cryptosporidium*** spp., ***Isospora belli***, and ***Cyclospora cayetanensis*** may all cause severe and prolonged diarrheal illness in patients with AIDS. *Isospora belli* is most frequently seen in MSM.
- Diagnosis of cryptosporidiosis is by microscopy, immunoassay, or PCR. Diagnosis of isosporiasis and cyclosporiasis requires acid-fast staining and other specific staining techniques.
- **No therapy has proved to be effective for cryptosporidiosis** besides immune reconstitution through ART (CD4 count >100 cells/μL[3]). **TMP-SMX treats isosporiasis and cyclosporiasis.**[3]

Neoplasms

- Neoplasms associated with AIDS include **non-Hodgkin lymphoma** and **Kaposi sarcoma. Primary CNS lymphomas** are common and may be multicentric. The treatment of these conditions is beyond the scope of this manual.
- As noted above, women should receive annual screening for **cervical cancer.** In addition, there is growing literature on the need for anal screening in both men and women.

Metabolic Complications

- There are a myriad of metabolic consequences from HIV as well as ART.[10]
- Dyslipidemia is characterized by hypertriglyceridemia and low HDL cholesterol levels.
  - Among ART, ritonavir causes the most lipid derangements. Atazanavir appears to provide improvement in the lipid profile.
  - Treatment of choice is **atorvastatin** or **pravastatin**, due to relatively lower drug interactions with ART. Of note, efavirenz reduces inhibition of HMG-CoA reductase activity; therefore, higher doses of statins may be needed for efficacy.
- Peripheral lipoatrophy (thin extremities), central obesity, and buffalo humps are some prominent features of **lipodystrophy**. Avoiding certain older-generation ARTs (NRTIs such as stavudine and zidovudine) as well as dietary changes and exercise are strategies to improve lipodystrophy.
- Mechanisms leading to **insulin resistance** include lipodystrophy, hepatic steatosis, chronic inflammation from HIV, and ART (particularly protease inhibitors). **Metformin** and **rosiglitazone** have been shown to improve insulin sensitivity.

SEXUALLY TRANSMITTED DISEASES

- A standardized, thorough evaluation including a complete history and physical is important in the diagnosis of STDs.
- History should include the presence or absence of genital drainage or discharge; dysuria; sores or other lesions (including warts, growths, or bumps) on or near the genitalia; any rash; testicular pain or discomfort; abdominal, rectal, or pelvic pain; the presence of any oral or pharyngeal symptoms; and any known drug allergies.
- A detailed sexual history should also be taken and include whether the patient has sex with men, women, or both; number of sexual partners in the past year; sites of sexual contact (vaginal, penile, oral, rectal); condom use; known exposure to STDs; and, for women, menstrual history and history of pregnancy.

- Physical examination must be complete and include the lower abdomen, palpation of inguinal area for lymphadenopathy, thorough external genitalia examination, and appropriate pelvic examination for women and visual examination of the urethra in men.
- Patients diagnosed with an STD should be screened for others, particularly for HIV.
- Counseling for the prevention of STDs is also recommended for all sexually active adults, and barrier methods should be encouraged.
- Partner notification, evaluation, and treatment, if indicated, are also essential.
- Treatment recommendations discussed in this section were adapted from the CDC STDs guidelines.[11]

URETHRITIS AND CERVICITIS SYNDROMES

- A variety of infections, most notably gonorrhea and chlamydia, cause urethritis in men and cervicitis in women.
- Symptoms in men generally include purulent urethral discharge and dysuria. In women, vaginal discharge may occur, but many patients are asymptomatic.
- Diagnosis is supported by physical exam and appropriate microbiologic testing. Additionally, a diagnosis of urethritis or cervicitis is supported by Gram stain of urethral or vaginal secretions showing >5 WBCs per high-power field in men or >10 WBCs per high-power field in women.

Gonorrhea

- Gonorrhea is caused by infection with *Neisseria gonorrhoeae* and is a common cause of urethritis in men and cervicitis in women. It can also cause oropharyngeal or rectal infection in patients with sexual contact in those areas. Less commonly, it causes disseminated infection resulting in bacteremia, pustular skin lesions, tenosynovitis, septic arthritis, and/or perihepatitis.
- Gram stain of urethral, endocervical, or anal samples showing gram-negative diplococci is diagnostic. *Neisseria gonorrhoeae* can also be cultured from urethral, endocervical, anal, or oropharyngeal samples. Nucleic acid hybridization tests of swab specimens and nucleic acid amplification testing of urine or swab specimens have better sensitivity than Gram stain or culture techniques.
- Recommended treatment for uncomplicated gonococcal infection is **single-dose ceftriaxone (250 mg IM)** in addition to **azithromycin (1 g PO) or doxycycline (100 mg PO bid for 7 days)** given the high rate of emerging resistance and chlamydial coinfection.
- **Cefixime and quinolones are no longer recommended for the treatment of gonorrhea** secondary to increased antimicrobial resistance.[12]
- Therapy may be initiated before results of diagnostic testing are available.
- Patients with disseminated gonococcal infection should be referred for hospital admission for IV antibiotics. The diagnostic evaluation often includes cultures of blood, mucosal sites, skin lesions, and joint aspirates.

Chlamydia

- *Chlamydia trachomatis* is a major cause of urethritis and cervicitis, but asymptomatic infection is also common. It can also cause oropharyngeal or rectal infection in patients with sexual contact in those areas.
- Nucleic acid amplification tests are the most sensitive assays, but a variety of testing methods are available including cell culture, direct immunofluorescence, enzyme immunoassay (EIA), and nucleic acid hybridization assays. Urethral, cervical, oropharyngeal, or rectal swabs or urine specimen may be tested depending on suspected sites of exposure and infection.

- Treatment is **single-dose azithromycin (1 g PO) or doxycycline (100 mg PO bid for 7 days).**
- Treatment may be initiated before confirmatory testing results are available.

Nongonococcal Urethritis and Mucopurulent Cervicitis

- Nongonococcal urethritis (NGU) and mucopurulent cervicitis (MPC) are clinical syndromes that mimic infection with *N. gonorrhoeae* but are caused by other pathogens.
- Organisms that cause NGU or MPC include *C. trachomatis, Mycoplasma genitalium, Mycoplasma hominis, Ureaplasma urealyticum, Trichomonas vaginalis,* and occasionally HSV.
- The recommended therapeutic approach is to provide adequate coverage for possible *C. trachomatis* infection with either **single-dose azithromycin (1 g PO) or doxycycline (100 mg PO bid for 7 days)** and then treatment for *T. vaginalis* with **single-dose metronidazole (2 g PO)** if patients fail to respond.

VAGINITIS AND VAGINOSIS SYNDROMES

- **Bacterial vaginosis** is a clinical syndrome of bacterial overgrowth that produces malodorous vaginal discharge and pruritus. Diagnosis and treatment are discussed in Chapter 3.
- **Trichomoniasis** is an STD caused by the parasite *T. vaginalis* and may be more common than *C. trachomatis* and *N. gonorrhea.* It may be a cause of NGU in men and a profuse, purulent vaginal discharge in women. Further diagnosis and treatment is discussed in Chapter 3.
- **Vulvovaginal candidiasis** ("yeast infection") is suggested by the presence of vulvovaginal soreness, dyspareunia, vulvar pruritus, external dysuria, and thick or "cheesy" vaginal secretions. See Chapter 3 for diagnosis and treatment.

GENITAL ULCER SYNDROMES

Syphilis

GENERAL PRINCIPLES

- Syphilis is a systemic infection caused by *Treponema pallidum.*
- **Primary syphilis** is characterized by one or more **painless, superficial ulcerations** (chancres). These lesions are seen in genital, anorectal, or pharyngeal sites.
  - A chancre typically has raised, sharply demarcated borders; a red, smooth, nontender base; and scant serous secretions.
  - Regional lymphadenopathy may be present.
  - The average time between exposure and chancre development is 3 weeks.
  - Spontaneous resolution of lesions generally occurs in 3 to 6 weeks, even without treatment.
- **Secondary syphilis** typically occurs 6 weeks after exposure and is characterized by a **macular, maculopapular, or papular rash** that can involve the palms, soles, and flexor areas of the extremities. Any body site, including mucous membranes, may be involved.
- **Tertiary syphilis** is rare and refers to development of mucocutaneous/osseous lesions (gummas) or cardiovascular lesions (aortitis).
- **Neurosyphilis** may present with variable neurologic manifestations including syphilitic meningitis, cranial nerve dysfunction, stroke, altered mental status, loss of vibration sense, auditory abnormalities, or uveitis. CNS involvement can occur during any stage of syphilis.

- **Latent syphilis** is infection that is diagnosed serologically in the absence of primary or secondary symptoms.
  - Early disease (<1 year) is differentiated from late disease (>1 year) for treatment purposes.
  - If a negative serology within the past year cannot be documented, the patient should be treated for late latent disease.

DIAGNOSIS

- Dark-field microscopy of lesion exudate or tissue is the definitive method for diagnosis, but this is seldom available and is insensitive.
- Two types of serologic tests are used for diagnostic purposes: nontreponemal tests (RPR and VDRL) and treponemal tests (e.g., fluorescent treponemal antibody absorbed [FTA-ABS] tests and the *T. pallidum* passive particle agglutination [TP-PA] assay). Both types of tests have limitations, and so they are used in a complementary manner to support the diagnosis.
- RPR and VDRL are often reactive within 1 to 2 weeks of onset of the chancre, but up to 30% may have negative RPR at the time of initial examination (chancre present). Titers decline after treatment, and the tests may become nonreactive with time.
- False-positive nontreponemal tests occur in a variety of conditions (e.g., autoimmune disease, pregnancy, older age, and intravenous drug use).
- When a patient has a reactive RPR or VDRL, confirmatory testing by FTA-ABS or TP-PA is recommended.
- CSF analysis is indicated if there is concern for neurosyphilis. In cases of neurosyphilis, CSF abnormalities may or may not be present. The VDRL in the CSF is the standard serologic test for CSF and is highly specific but insensitive. CSF FTA-ABS is less specific for neurosyphilis but is highly sensitive.
- All patients with syphilis should be tested for HIV.

TREATMENT

- **Penicillin is the treatment of choice** for all stages of syphilis.
- For pregnant patients with a history of penicillin allergy, penicillin skin testing and desensitization are recommended, because alternative regimens do not treat the fetus.
- **For primary, secondary, and early latent infection (<1 year duration):**
  - **Single-dose benzathine penicillin G (2.4 million units IM)** is recommended.
  - Effective alternatives include doxycycline (100 mg PO bid for 14 days) or tetracycline (500 mg PO qid for 14 days). Azithromycin (2 g PO once) can be used with caution in non-MSM and nonpregnant women if treatment with penicillin or doxycycline is not feasible. Ceftriaxone (1 g daily either IM or IV for 10 to 14 days) has been effective in trials, but the optimal dose and duration of therapy have not been defined.
  - Follow-up and repeat serology should be done at 6 and 12 months.
  - The RPR should show a fourfold decrease in titer within 6 months of treatment.
  - One must consider treatment failure or reinfection if symptoms persist or recur or if nontreponemal titer increases fourfold.
- **For late syphilis (>1-year duration—except neurosyphilis):**
  - **Benzathine penicillin G (2.4 million units IM weekly for 3 weeks)** is recommended.
  - Alternatives are tetracycline (500 mg PO qid for 28 days) or doxycycline (100 mg PO bid for 28 days).
  - Repeat serologies should be conducted at 6, 12, and 24 months.
  - Evaluate for neurosyphilis if the nontreponemal titer increases fourfold, if initially high titer ≥1:32 fails to fall fourfold in 12 to 24 months, or if signs or symptoms of neurosyphilis develop.

- **For neurosyphilis:**
  - **Aqueous penicillin G (18 to 24 million units daily IV, 3 to 4 million units every 4 hours for 14 days)** is recommended.
  - Limited data suggest that ceftriaxone 2 g daily either IM or IV for 10 to 14 days may be an effective alternative treatment.
  - Repeat serologies at 3, 6, 12, and 24 months and follow-up lumbar puncture at 6-month intervals are indicated until the CSF cell count is normal.
  - Retreatment should be considered if cell count has not decreased at 6 months or CSF is not entirely normal at 2 years.
- HIV-positive patients with syphilis require closer clinical follow-up with clinical examination at 1 week and repeat serology in 3, 6, 9, 12, and 24 months and then yearly, even if RPR becomes negative.

Herpes

GENERAL PRINCIPLES

- Herpes simplex virus (HSV) causes a chronic, lifelong latent infection and can cause episodic symptoms during periods of viral reactivation.
- HSV types 1 and 2 can be sexually transmitted, but most genital infections are caused by HSV-2.
- HSV typically produces **painful grouped vesicles** on or near the genitalia. Over several days, the lesions evolve into shallow ulcers, which generally heal within 1 to 2 weeks.
- Most patients with genital HSV are asymptomatic or have mild or nonspecific symptoms.
- Extragenital lesions of HSV may develop in the buttock, groin, or thigh areas.
- HSV can also cause neurologic syndromes including encephalitis, aseptic meningitis, transverse myelitis, and sacral radiculopathy. Disseminated disease, hepatitis, and pneumonitis may also occur, particularly in immunocompromised hosts.
- HSV recurrences usually cause fewer lesions and less frequent occurrence of systemic symptoms than are seen during primary genital HSV infection.
- Reactivation of HSV-1 is less frequent, and almost all patients with HSV-2 experience recurrence, though the rates decrease over time.

DIAGNOSIS

- Clinical diagnosis relies on detection of grouped, tender vesicular or pustular lesions on an erythematous base. Lymphadenopathy, fever, headache, myalgias, urethritis, or cervicitis is variably present.
- Cell culture and PCR are the preferred testing methods for HSV.
- HSV PCR is a more sensitive method for diagnosis and is available for samples from oral or genital lesions, CSF, and ocular fluid.

TREATMENT

- Recommended treatments for genital HSV outbreaks:
  - Acyclovir, 400 mg PO tid or 200 mg PO five times a day for 7 to 10 days
  - Famciclovir, 250 mg PO tid for 7 to 10 days
  - Valacyclovir, 1 g PO bid for 7 to 10 days
- Early treatment usually reduces the symptomatic interval and may result in accelerated healing.
- Suppressive therapy may be recommended for patients with recurrent symptomatic infection.
  - Acyclovir, 400 mg PO bid
  - Famciclovir, 250 mg PO bid
  - Valacyclovir, 500 mg PO bid or 1 g PO daily

- Continuation of suppressive therapy should be reevaluated on a yearly basis.
- Patients should be counseled that **therapy decreases but does not eliminate the risk of transmitting HSV to their sexual partners and that they may be infectious even when they have no visible ulcers.**
- Patients with severe HSV disease, including those with CNS disease and those that require hospitalization, should receive IV therapy.

Chancroid

GENERAL PRINCIPLES

- Chancroid is caused by infection with *Haemophilus ducreyi*.
- Chancroid is distributed worldwide, with concentrations in Africa and the Caribbean, but the incidence has declined in the United States. Clusters occur in New York City and the Gulf Coast states, where most cases are in non-Caucasian uncircumcised men or are associated with prostitute contact.
- The typical lesions are **painful, nonindurated, excavated genital ulcers with undermined borders.** Tender, enlarged inguinal lymph nodes are often present. Fever and other systemic symptoms are generally absent.
- The incubation period is usually 5 to 7 days.

DIAGNOSIS

- Laboratory diagnosis relies on culture or Gram stain from a lymph node aspirate, but culture techniques are <80% sensitive and require special media. Identification of small, gram-negative bacilli on Gram stain provides a presumptive diagnosis.
- Clinical diagnosis may be made in patients with typical clinical features and for whom syphilis and HSV have been excluded.

TREATMENT

- Treatment is **single-dose azithromycin** (1 g PO), **single-dose ceftriaxone** (250 mg IM), **ciprofloxacin** (500 mg PO bid for 3 days), **or erythromycin** base (500 mg PO qid for 7 days).
- The patient should be reexamined in 3 to 7 days to assess for clinical improvement. Large ulcers may take more than 2 weeks to heal, and scarring may result despite successful therapy.

Lymphogranuloma Venereum

GENERAL PRINCIPLES

- Lymphogranuloma venereum is caused by *C. trachomatis* serovars L1, L2, or L3, which predominantly infect the lymphatic tissue.
- Historically, this infection has occurred in underdeveloped tropical and subtropical areas, but outbreaks in Europe and the United States have been reported, mostly in MSM.
- The **primary stage is often unnoticed** and consists of a self-limited ulcer at the inoculation site, after which, a secondary invasive stage occurs with varied complications based on the original location of inoculation.
- The **inguinal syndrome** occurs after inoculation at the genital mucosa and produces tender inguinal lymphadenopathy and even buboes, which may spontaneously rupture.

- The **anorectal syndrome** occurs via infection of the rectal mucosa and results in proctitis and inflammation of the surrounding lymphatic tissue. Chronic, colorectal fistulas and strictures may occur.
- Infection may also occur via the pharyngeal mucosa and result in the **pharyngeal syndrome**.

DIAGNOSIS

- Diagnosis is largely clinical.
- Genital and lymph node specimens can be tested for *C. trachomatis* by culture, direct immunofluorescence, or nucleic acid detection.
- PCR-based testing of lesion swab or bubo aspirate can differentiate LGV from non-LGV *C. trachomatis*, but this testing is not widely available.
- Chlamydial serology, though not type specific, may be supportive if the titer is high, although acute and convalescent sera are preferred.

TREATMENT

- Recommended **treatment is doxycycline (100 mg PO bid for 3 weeks).** Alternatively, erythromycin base (500 mg PO qid for 3 weeks) may be used.
- Azithromycin 1 g PO once weekly for 3 weeks and fluoroquinolone-based treatments may also be effective, but clinical data are lacking.

Granuloma Inguinale

GENERAL PRINCIPLES

- Granuloma inguinale (also known as donovanosis, with reference to characteristic intracellular inclusions called Donovan bodies) is a progressive ulcerative condition caused by the intracellular gram-negative bacterium *Klebsiella granulomatis* (formerly known as *Calymmatobacterium granulomatis* or *Donovania granulomatis*).
- It is endemic to India, Papua New Guinea, southern Africa, and central Australia. Rare cases are reported in the United States via foreign travel.
- Presents as **painless, slowly progressive, beefy-red ulcers** without associated lymphadenopathy. The typical ulcers are often highly vascular and bleed easily on contact.
- Hypertrophic, necrotic, and sclerotic variants have been described.
- Extragenital infection can occur with extension of infection into the pelvis and dissemination to the intra-abdominal organs, to bones, or in the mouth.

DIAGNOSIS

Clinical diagnosis may be supported by tissue crush preparation or biopsy showing classic bipolar-staining **Donovan bodies**. The organism cannot be grown in standard culture media.

TREATMENT

- First-line recommended treatment is **doxycycline** (100 mg PO bid). Alternatives include TMP-SMX (160 mg/800 mg PO bid), ciprofloxacin (750 mg PO bid), azithromycin (1,000 mg once per week), or erythromycin base (500 mg PO qid).
- Duration of therapy for any agent is at least 3 weeks and until all lesions have completely healed.
- Addition of an aminoglycoside (e.g., gentamicin, 5 mg/kg IV daily) may be considered if lesions do not respond after the first few days of oral therapy.

EXOPHYTIC PROCESSES

Human Papillomavirus

GENERAL PRINCIPLES

- HPV can result in a wide variety of epithelial manifestations including common, plantar, flat/juvenile warts.
- 90% of **anogenital warts** (condylomata acuminata) are also caused by HPV subtypes 6 and 11.
- Serotypes 16 and 18 are associated with approximately 70% of all **cervical cancers**. HPV is also linked to the development of anal intraepithelial neoplasia and invasive squamous cell carcinoma.
- Most HPV infections are asymptomatic and most clear spontaneously.

DIAGNOSIS

- The diagnosis of anogenital warts is usually made by inspection, which reveals typical flesh-colored "cauliflower" or wart-like masses, usually involving the external genitalia, perineum, or perianal area. The lesions are typically asymptomatic, but minor complaints such as pruritus may be present.
- The differential diagnosis includes molluscum contagiosum or condyloma lata (secondary syphilis).
- A weak acetic acid solution (3% to 5%) can be used to highlight exophytic warts on the skin surface. The lesions turn white as the solution dries (do not apply to mucous membranes).
- A dermatologic consultation may be desirable for evaluation and biopsy of a lesion.
- Cervical cytology should be performed for women with diagnosed HPV infection and for female partners of infected men.

TREATMENT

- The treatment of warts is typically with application of liquid nitrogen, podophyllin, or trichloroacetic acid.
- **Liquid nitrogen** (cryotherapy) is applied by a 10- to 15-second spray followed by a thaw and a single repeat application.
- **Trichloroacetic acid,** 80% to 90%, is very caustic and physically destroys the lesions after repeated applications. It may be used during pregnancy.
- **Podophyllin,** 10% to 25% in tincture of benzoin, is applied once or twice a week and washed off 1 hour after each application. Podophyllotoxin is an antimitotic agent.
- Home therapy with podofilox, imiquimod, or sinecatechins can also be tried.
- **Surgical removal** of warts may be necessary for extensive disease.
- There are now two approved HPV vaccines, one for serotypes 16 and 18 and a quadrivalent vaccine for serotypes 16 and 18 as well as serotypes 6 and 11. The divalent vaccine is currently indicated for women aged 13 to 26 years, and the quadrivalent vaccine can also be used in males 9 to 26 years of age.

Molluscum Contagiosum

GENERAL PRINCIPLES

- Molluscum contagiosum is a benign papular lesion caused by the molluscum contagiosum virus (a poxvirus), of which there are four types, MCV-1 to MCV-4.

- It can be transmitted sexually or nonsexually through close physical contact and is more common in children.
- In healthy patients, it is a self-limited infection and lesions usually resolve spontaneously.
- HIV positivity is a significant risk factor, and HIV-positive patients may have more widespread, larger lesions.

DIAGNOSIS

- Typical lesions are firm, small (1- to 5-mm diameter), **fleshy papules that are often umbilicated.** A firm white "pearl" is sometimes expressed on compression, followed by bleeding from the lesion.
- Very similar skin lesions may occur with disseminated *C. neoformans* or less commonly by *H. capsulatum.*
- Standard histology (molluscum bodies) or electron microscopy (visualization of poxvirus particles) can be used for a specific diagnosis.

TREATMENT

- Successful treatment of lesions may be with liquid nitrogen or trichloroacetic acid in the same fashion as described for warts.
- For those with concomitant HIV infection, more aggressive treatment and referral to a dermatologist may be appropriate. However, resolution usually occurs with treatment of the underlying HIV disease and immune reconstitution.

ECTOPARASITIC INFECTIONS

Pediculosis Pubis

- Pediculosis pubis, also known as pubic lice and crabs, is caused by the crab louse, *Phthirus pubis.*
- The parasite infests the pubic hair and causes intense itching in the pubic area.
- Nits or live lice may be visible to the human eye.
- Recommended first-line treatment entails topical **permethrin 1% cream rinse** or pyrethrins with piperonyl butoxide applied to the affected areas and washed off after 10 minutes.
- Alternatives for suspected treatment failures include topical malathion or systemic ivermectin.
- Bedding and clothing should be decontaminated, and sexual partners should also be evaluated and treated.

Scabies

- Scabies is caused by infestation with the mite *Sarcoptes scabiei* and is typically transmitted by skin-to-skin contact. The mite burrows into the skin, typically on the hands, feet, wrists, elbows, back, buttocks, and external genitals, causing intense allergic itching and sometimes small pimple-like bumps along the burrowing trails.
- Recommended treatments include topical **permethrin** cream (5%) or systemic ivermectin 200 µg/kg orally once and then repeated in 2 weeks time.
- Treatment with 1% lindane may be used as an alternative treatment but should not be used as first line, given concerns for drug toxicity.
- Bedding and clothing should be decontaminated, and sexual partners and household contacts should be evaluated and treated.

SYSTEMIC SEXUALLY TRANSMITTED DISEASE SYNDROMES

Pelvic Inflammatory Disease

GENERAL PRINCIPLES

- Pelvic inflammatory disease (PID) is a spectrum of upper genital tract infection. It may include any combination of **endometritis, salpingitis, tubo-ovarian abscess, and pelvic peritonitis.**
- *Neisseria gonorrhoeae* and *C. trachomatis* are the most common sexually transmitted causes, although infections are often polymicrobial involving normal flora of the female GU tract.
- Most cases occur proximate to the menses.
- Risk factors include multiple sexual partners, age 15 to 25 years, recent intrauterine device (IUD) placement, and prior PID.

DIAGNOSIS

- PID is characterized by lower abdominal or pelvic pain; adnexal, uterine, or cervical motion tenderness; and systemic signs and symptoms of infection. Other signs and symptoms may include dyspareunia, vaginal discharge, and menorrhagia or metrorrhagia.
- The differential diagnosis is extensive and includes several causes of acute abdomen such as appendicitis, ectopic pregnancy, septic abortion, and ovarian torsion.
- All patients with PID should be tested for pregnancy and HIV.
- Radiography, including ultrasound and CT, may assist with making a diagnosis of PID, but sensitivity is variable depending on the extent of the disease.

TREATMENT

- Treatment regimens should include **broad-spectrum antimicrobial coverage, including coverage for *N. gonorrhoeae* and *C. trachomatis***, vaginal flora and anaerobes, such as *Bacteroides* spp.
- Patients with mild-moderately severe PID may be treated as outpatients, but others require admission for IV antibiotics and occasionally surgical intervention.
- CDC **guidelines for hospital admission** should be reviewed prior to consideration of outpatient treatment. They are as follows:
  - Other surgical emergencies (e.g., appendicitis) cannot be excluded.
  - The patient is pregnant.
  - Outpatient therapy has failed.
  - The patient is unable to follow or tolerate outpatient treatment.
  - The illness is severe, with nausea, vomiting, and high fever.
  - Tubo-ovarian abscess is strongly suspected.
- Duration of therapy is typically at least 2 weeks but may be longer in severe cases.
- Recommended **parenteral regimens** include **cefotetan 2 g IV q12 hours or cefoxitin 2 g IV q6 hours plus doxycycline 100 mg orally or IV every 12 hours or clindamycin 900 mg IV q8 hours plus gentamicin** dosed based on body weight and renal function.
- **Outpatient treatment** should include single-dose **ceftriaxone** (250 mg IM) or cefoxitin 2 g IM with probenecid 1 g orally **plus doxycycline** (100 mg PO bid for 14 days) **with or without metronidazole** (500 mg PO bid for 14 days). **A follow-up examination within 72 hours is essential** to ensure that an adequate response to therapy has occurred.
- Intrauterine devices should be removed if present.

Hepatitis B Virus

- Refer to Chapter 30 for a detailed discussion of hepatitis B.
- Hepatitis B can be transmitted sexually, parenterally, or from mother to child during pregnancy. Epidemiologic studies suggest that in the United States, 40% to 60% of cases of HBV infection are sexually transmitted.
- Symptoms of infection may include malaise, fever, loss of appetite, abdominal pain, nausea, vomiting, jaundice, dark urine, arthralgias, or polyarthritis, but up to 50% of people may be asymptomatic.
- The physical examination may detect right upper quadrant abdominal tenderness, hepatic enlargement, or scleral or cutaneous jaundice.
- Laboratory diagnostic studies should include serologic testing for HBV, including hepatitis B surface antigen. Other useful diagnostic tests may include hepatitis A IgM, hepatitis C virus enzyme–linked immunosorbent assay test, complete blood count, and liver function tests.
- Treatment for acute HBV is supportive.
- Hepatitis B **vaccination is recommended** for all unvaccinated adolescents and for all unvaccinated adults at risk for infection.

REFERENCES

1. Panel on Antiretroviral Guidelines for Adults and Adolescents. Guidelines for the use of antiretroviral agents in HIV-1-infected adults and adolescents. http://www.aidsinfo.nih.gov. 2012;1–240. http://www.aidsinfo.nih.gov/guidelines/. Last accessed 1/6/15.
2. Thompson MA, Aberg JA, Hoy JF, et al. Antiretroviral treatment of adult HIV infection: 2012 recommendations of the International Antiviral Society-USA Panel. *JAMA* 2012;308:387–402.
3. Kaplan JE, Benson C, Holmes KH, et al. Guidelines for prevention and treatment of opportunistic infections in HIV-infected adults and adolescents: recommendations from CDC, the National Institutes of Health, and the HIV Medicine Association of the Infectious Diseases Society of America. *MMWR Recomm Rep* 2009;58:1–207.
4. Overton ET. An overview of vaccinations in HIV. *Curr HIV/AIDS Rep* 2007;4:105–113.
5. Hecht FM, Luetkemeyer A. Immunizations and HIV. hivinsite.ucsf.edu. 2011. hivinsite.ucsf.edu/InSite?page=kb-03-01-08. Last accessed 1/6/15.
6. Brew BJ, Davies NW, Cinque P, et al. Progressive multifocal leukoencephalopathy and other forms of JC virus disease. *Nat Rev Neurol* 2010;6:667–679.
7. Muñoz N, Bosch FX, de Sanjosé S, et al. Epidemiologic classification of human papillomavirus types associated with cervical cancer. *N Engl J Med* 2003;348:518–527.
8. Sattler FR, Cowan R, Nielsen DM, et al. Trimethoprim-sulfamethoxazole compared with pentamidine for treatment of Pneumocystis carinii pneumonia in the acquired immunodeficiency syndrome. A prospective, noncrossover study. *Ann Intern Med* 1998;109:280–287.
9. Bozzette SA, Sattler FR, Chiu J, et al. A controlled trial of early adjunctive treatment with corticosteroids for Pneumocystis carinii pneumonia in the acquired immunodeficiency syndrome. *N Engl J Med* 1990;323:1451–1457.
10. Chow DC, Day LJ, Souza SA, et al. Metabolic complications of HIV therapy. hivinsite.ucsf.edu. 2006. http://hivinsite.ucsf.edu/InSite?page=kb-03-02-10. Last accessed 1/6/15.
11. Workowski KA, Berman SM. Centers for Disease Control and Prevention Sexually transmitted diseases treatment guidelines, 2010. *MMWR Recomm Rep* 2010;59:1–116.
12. Centers for Disease Control and Prevention (CDC). Update to CDC's sexually transmitted diseases treatment guidelines, 2010: oral cephalosporins no longer a recommended treatment for gonococcal infections. *MMWR Recomm Rep* 2012;61:590–594.

Dysphagia and Odynophagia

GENERAL PRINCIPLES

- The swallowing mechanism consists of the pharynx, cricopharyngeus (upper esophageal sphincter), body of the esophagus, and lower esophageal sphincter.
- **Dysphagia** is a sense of difficulty with the passage of food or liquid from the pharynx to the stomach. Dysphagia can be divided into oropharyngeal or esophageal dysphagia. These groups can be further subdivided into mechanical causes or neuromuscular causes. Dysphagia is distinct from **globus**, which is a subjective feeling of fullness in the throat not related to eating.
- **Odynophagia** is the presence of pain on swallowing that may or may not accompany dysphagia.

DIAGNOSIS

Clinical Presentation

History
- Progressive difficulty in swallowing solid foods but not liquids indicates mechanical obstruction such as malignancy or benign stricture. Dysphagia is distinct from **globus**, which is a subjective feeling of fullness in the throat not related to eating. Intermittent dysphagia for solids, usually meat or bread, can result from a lower esophageal ring, known as Schatzki ring.[1]
- When hoarseness follows the onset of dysphagia, involvement of the recurrent laryngeal nerve by oropharyngeal or esophageal cancer should be considered.
- Symptoms located in the lower part of the sternum are most likely due to abnormality in the distal esophagus. Otherwise, subjective localization of dysphagia is nonspecific.
- Unintended weight loss associated with dysphagia suggests carcinoma. Risk factors for esophageal cancer include heavy tobacco and alcohol use and long-standing gastroesophageal reflux.
- Tracheobronchial aspiration may occur in those with tracheoesophageal fistula, brainstem neuromuscular diseases, achalasia, or severe gastroesophageal reflux.
- A history of chronic heartburn associated with dysphagia is usually present in peptic strictures. These individuals may describe chronic antacid use.
- Chest pain may occur in those with severe reflux, accounting for half of noncardiac chest pain.[2]
- Odynophagia is frequently related to esophageal infections or pill ulcers.
- Hiccups can be associated with a lesion in the distal esophagus causing diaphragmatic irritation or gastric or esophageal distention from aerophagia.

Physical Examination
- Oral pharyngeal examination should focus on finding evidence of thrush or lesions of pemphigus or epidermolysis bullosa.
- Examination of the neck may reveal structural defects such as thyromegaly, spinal deformity, and neck masses.

- Skin examination is important for features of collagen vascular disease including scleroderma or CREST syndrome (**C**alcinosis, **R**aynaud phenomenon, **E**sophageal dysmotility, **S**clerodactyly, and **T**elangiectasias), which is associated with dysphagia and impaired peristalsis.

Differential Diagnosis

- Infections including candidal, herpetic, or other viral esophagitis must be considered in patients who describe odynophagia. Acute **odynophagia** can be secondary to esophagitis or ulcers from pills such as tetracycline, potassium tablets, bisphosphonates, ferrous sulfate, quinidine, and nonsteroidal anti-inflammatory agents (NSAIDs).
- The differential diagnosis/causes of dysphagia are presented in Table 28-1.[3]

Diagnostic Testing

- When esophageal dysphagia is suspected, **endoscopy** is the initial test to visualize the mucosa directly with biopsy of suspicious lesions and/or biopsy of the midesophagus for eosinophilic esophagitis.

TABLE 28-1 Causes of Dysphagia

Location	Mechanism	Causes
Esophageal	Mechanical	Peptic stricture
		Previous radiation therapy resulting in stricture
		Schatzki ring
		Webs
		Cancer
		Erosive esophagitis
		Extrinsic compression (e.g., mediastinal tumor, thoracic aortic aneurysm, left atrial enlargement)
		Foreign body
		Eosinophilic esophagitis
Esophageal	Neuromuscular	Achalasia
		Diffuse esophageal spasm
		Nutcracker esophagus
		Scleroderma
Oropharyngeal	Mechanical	Oropharyngeal tumors
		Zenker diverticulum
		Postsurgical or postradiation change
		External compression (e.g., goiter, cervical osteophytes, cervical esophageal rings/webs)
		Decreased saliva/dry mouth
Oropharyngeal	Neuromuscular	Cerebrovascular accident
		Cricopharyngeal achalasia
		Parkinson disease
		Multiple sclerosis
		Myasthenia gravis
		Amyotrophic lateral sclerosis
		Polymyositis/dermatomyositis
		Other neuromuscular disorders

- **Barium swallow** can be used to identify structural defects in patients at high risk for sedation and those taking anticoagulants.
- **Modified barium swallow** is used to evaluate oropharyngeal dysmotility and aspiration.
- **Laryngoscopy** can identify oropharyngeal lesions.
- **Esophageal manometry** is the test of choice when esophageal motor disease is suspected.

TREATMENT

- Gastroesophageal reflux disease (GERD) should be treated with **proton pump inhibitors**.[4]
- Esophageal strictures or rings can be treated with endoscopy by **bougienage** (the passage of dilators with or without guidewire assistance) or balloon dilators.
- Achalasia can be treated with the following:
  - ○ **Pneumatic dilatation** via fluoroscopic and endoscopic visualization.
  - ○ Heller **myotomy** (surgical procedure that dissects the smooth muscle of the hypertensive lower esophageal sphincter).
  - ○ **Botulinum toxin** injection can be used for those at high risk for other interventions. The effects of botulinum toxin injection are temporary, usually lasting 3 to 6 months.
- **Eosinophilic esophagitis** can be treated with aggressive acid suppression, elimination diets, and/or swallowed fluticasone.
- Odynophagia may be treated symptomatically with opioid analgesic agents or topical viscous lidocaine.
  - ○ Pill ulcers are generally self-limited.
  - ○ Infectious causes of odynophagia should be treated with appropriate antimicrobials.

Nausea and Vomiting

DIAGNOSIS

Clinical Presentation

History
- The initial evaluation should determine the duration and severity of symptoms.
- Association with certain triggers including smells, tastes, emotional or physical stress, headaches, and abdominal pain should be noted.
- If abdominal pain is the main symptom, refer to the Abdominal Pain section of this chapter for the differential diagnosis.
- Nausea and/or vomiting associated with right upper quadrant (RUQ) or epigastric pain could be secondary to biliary colic, pancreatitis, cholecystitis, peptic ulcer disease, or acute viral hepatitis.
- Initial periumbilical pain that relocates to the right lower quadrant accompanied by nausea and vomiting is suggestive of appendicitis.
- Left lower quadrant pain in the presence of vomiting may be secondary to diverticulitis.
- Flank pain along with fever and vomiting may indicate pyelonephritis.
- Occurrence soon after meals can be a result of gastric outlet obstruction.
- Vomiting that is delayed after meals and consists of partially digested food or food consumed several hours earlier may indicate gastroparesis (particularly in diabetics) or intestinal obstruction.
- Vomiting undigested food (regurgitation) is seen with a Zenker diverticulum (pharyngoesophageal diverticulum) and achalasia, which are also associated with severe halitosis.
- Presence of diarrhea may indicate an infectious gastroenteritis.

Physical Examination
- Evaluate for orthostatic hypotension defined by fall of systolic blood pressure of 20 mm Hg or 10 mm Hg diastolic with positional change, which may be present in persistent vomiting due to volume depletion.
- Decreased skin turgor or dry mucous membranes are signs of significant fluid losses.
- Severe halitosis may be associated with intestinal obstruction, gastroparesis, gastrocolic fistula, bacterial overgrowth, achalasia, and Zenker diverticulum.
- Oral examination may reveal poor dentition and enamel erosion in those with eating disorders such as bulimia.
- High-pitched bowel sounds may suggest small bowel obstruction, while succussion splash (the movement of gastric fluid within the stomach heard on auscultation) may be seen in gastric outlet obstruction or gastroparesis.
- Palpation to find areas of tenderness, abdominal masses, or Murphy sign.

Differential Diagnosis
The differential diagnosis of nausea and vomiting is presented in Table 28-2.

Diagnostic Testing
Laboratories
- Serum chemistries evaluating electrolytes, bilirubin, amylase, lipase, alkaline phosphatase, and transaminases. Hyponatremia and azotemia may cause nausea and vomiting. Hyponatremia and hyperkalemia can be seen in adrenal insufficiency. Check AM cortisol if adrenal insufficiency is suspected.
- Complete blood cell count (CBC) evaluating for leukocytosis indicating acute inflammation or infection as well as anemia indicating possible blood loss within the gastrointestinal (GI) tract.
- Pregnancy test should be obtained in women of childbearing age.

Imaging
- If nausea and vomiting are associated with pain, an **obstructive series** is important to identify intestinal obstruction, air-fluid levels, bowel gas pattern, and free air.
- Upper GI **endoscopy** can detect mechanical sources of nausea and vomiting. If negative, a small bowel exam should be considered, such as small bowel follow-through, capsule endoscopy, or CT enterography.
- Radionuclide **gastric-emptying scan** and manometry can evaluate for motility disorders of the stomach.
- **CT** may be obtained to evaluate for intra-abdominal processes, such as pancreatitis or appendicitis.
- CT scan or MRI of the brain may be pertinent if an intracranial process is suspected.

TREATMENT

- Identify and treat underlying process, using antiemetic agents to temporarily alleviate symptoms.
  - Prochlorperazine starting at 5 to 10 mg PO tid/qid or 25-mg suppositories every 12 hours.
  - Promethazine starting at 12.5 to 25 mg PO every 4 to 6 hours or 25-mg suppositories every 4 to 6 hours.
  - Also, refer to Chapter 36 for a more detailed discussion of antiemetic therapy.
- Prokinetic medication such as metoclopramide may be used for delayed gastric emptying; the starting dose is 10 mg PO/IM/IV 1 hour before meals and at bedtime.
  - Mechanical obstruction must be **excluded before** using prokinetics.
  - **Metoclopramide should not be used for prolonged periods and/or in high doses**, particularly in the elderly, because of the risk of drug-induced tardive dyskinesia.

TABLE 28-2 Causes of Nausea and Vomiting

Gastrointestinal
Gastroenteritis
Toxin mediated (e.g., *Staphylococcus aureus*, *Bacillus cereus*)
Viral (e.g., rotaviruses, enteric adenovirus, Norwalk agent)
GI tract obstruction (any cause, any level)
Esophageal webs/rings/achalasia/cancer
Gastric cancer/gastroparesis/pyloric stenosis/outlet obstruction
Intestinal cancer
Adhesions
Intussusception
Hernia
Volvulus
Zenker diverticulum (regurgitation)
Gastroesophageal reflux disease (regurgitation)
Peptic ulcer disease
Appendicitis
Ileus
Colonic pseudoobstruction
Inflammatory bowel disease
Toxic megacolon
Eosinophilic gastroenteritis
Constipation
Hepatitis
Passive hepatic congestion
Cholecystitis/choledocholithiasis
Pancreatitis
Pancreatic cancer
Peritonitis
Mesenteric ischemia

Central nervous system
Increased intracranial pressure
Tumor
Hemorrhage/infarct/associated edema (e.g., cerebellar, brainstem)
Cerebral vein and dural sinus thrombosis
Pseudotumor cerebri
Meningitis/encephalitis
Hydrocephalus (congenital, acquired, and many causes)
Migraine headache
Seizure disorders

Labyrinthine disorders
Motion sickness
Vestibular neuronitis
Acute labyrinthitis

Endocrine disorders
Diabetic ketoacidosis
Adrenal insufficiency
Hypercalcemia/hyperparathyroidism

Functional
Nonulcer dyspepsia
Irritable bowel syndrome
Cyclic vomiting syndrome

Psychiatric disorders
Eating disorders
Somatization disorder
Depressive disorders
Anxiety disorders
Rumination syndrome

Medications/toxins
Chemotherapeutic agents
Nonsteroidal anti-inflammatory agents (NSAIDs)
Opiate analgesics
Colchicine
Antibiotics (e.g., erythromycin, metronidazole, sulfa drugs, and tetracycline)
Cardiovascular drugs (e.g., β-blockers, calcium channel blockers, diuretics, digoxin)
Central nervous system agents (e.g., antidepressants, benzodiazepines, medications for Parkinson disease, anticonvulsants)
Estrogen replacement or hormone therapy
General anesthetics
Other drugs (e.g., theophylline, iron)
Ethanol
Many poisons
Narcotic withdrawal

Other
Pregnancy
Hyperemesis gravidarum
Pyelonephritis
Nephrolithiasis
Myocardial infarction
Uremia
Acute glaucoma
Radiation therapy
Acute intermittent porphyria

Data from Quigley EM, Hasler WL, Parkman HP. AGA technical review on nausea and vomiting. *Gastroenterology* 2001;120:263–286.

- A number of serotonin receptor inhibitors, such as ondansetron, or antagonists of substance P/neurokinin-1 receptors, such as aprepitant, are frequently used in nausea and emesis related to chemotherapy.
- Indications for hospitalization:
  ○ Clinical evidence of severe volume depletion
  ○ Electrolyte derangements that require correction under monitored conditions
  ○ Patients at extremes of age and those with diabetes and/or accompanying debilitating illnesses

Dyspepsia

GENERAL PRINCIPLES

- Persistent or recurrent discomfort or pain located in the upper abdomen. Pain can be accompanied by bloating, heartburn, nausea, and food intolerance.
- Divided into two categories: **peptic ulcer disease and nonulcer dyspepsia.**

DIAGNOSIS

Clinical Presentation

History
- Pain in the preprandial state or nocturnal pain that results in awakening several hours after ingestion of food is suspicious for peptic ulcer disease. Similar pain that is relieved by food is suggestive of a duodenal ulcer.
- Pain from nonulcer dyspepsia is difficult to distinguish from ulcer-related dyspepsia.
- Pain radiating to the back and somewhat improved on leaning forward suggests pancreatitis, perforated peptic ulcer, or leaking abdominal aneurysm.
- Pain referred to the right scapula may originate in the gallbladder or from any process causing diaphragmatic irritation.
- Constipation, diarrhea, tenesmus, or nonspecific lower abdominal discomfort in association with upper abdominal complaints may be due to irritable bowel syndrome.
- Early satiety can result from ulcers at the gastric outlet or infiltrating tumors creating reduced gastric wall compliance.
- Fear of eating because of subsequent abdominal pain is suggestive of mesenteric ischemia or intestinal angina.
- History of peptic ulcer disease, gastric surgery, cigarette smoking, or alcohol use are risk factors for the development of dyspepsia.
- Early satiety, recurrent vomiting, or bloating that is not accompanied by visible distention or pain may indicate dysmotility.
- Aerophagia is excess swallowing of air that results in fullness, belching, or reflux-like symptoms relieved by repetitive belching. Aerophagia is usually psychiatric in origin.
- **Red flags**: weight loss, GI bleeding, recurrent vomiting, dysphagia, and NSAID use.

Physical Examination
- Abdominal tenderness to palpation is nonspecific and may be seen in most disorders that cause dyspepsia. RUQ tenderness increased by palpation with inspiration (Murphy sign) indicates cholecystitis.
- Evaluate for peritoneal signs such as guarding and rebound tenderness (i.e., discomfort induced by movement of an irritated peritoneum during the release of pressure from palpation).
- Jaundice suggests a hepatic or biliary process.
- Evaluate for blood in stool.

Diagnostic Testing

Laboratories

CBC looking for anemia, if GI bleeding is suspected, and leukocytosis indicating possible intra-abdominal infection.

Diagnostic Procedures

- **Endoscopy** of the upper GI tract is indicated for those with alarm symptoms, for new-onset dyspepsia in a patient over 50, and for whom trials of acid-suppressing medications are inadequate.[5]
- *Helicobacter pylori* **testing** is appropriate if mucosal abnormalities, such as peptic ulcers, erosive gastropathy, or duodenitis, are detected, or in the case of documented prior peptic ulcer disease and mucosa-associated lymphoid tissue (MALT) lymphoma.
- **Upper GI** barium radiographs are reserved for patients who cannot undergo endoscopy.
- Gastroparesis can be demonstrated by **gastric-emptying scintigraphy** but must be interpreted in conjunction with the clinical setting.
- Transabdominal **ultrasound** can be used to evaluate for liver and biliary tract abnormalities.

TREATMENT

- Peptic ulcer disease should be managed with acid suppression. **Documentation of healing is recommended for gastric ulcer.**[6] *Helicobacter pylori* **should be tested for and eradicated if found.**
- Nonulcer dyspepsia may not respond to specific treatment but may improve with acid suppression or neuromodulators such as tricyclic antidepressants. In those with alarm symptoms or new-onset dyspepsia after age 50, upper endoscopy is warranted.[7]
- **Reflux should be treated symptomatically** with regularly scheduled proton pump inhibitors as well as weight reduction, dietary changes, and elevation of the head of bed.[4]
- Dysmotility-like dyspepsia may benefit from prokinetic agents such as metoclopramide. Metoclopramide should not be used for prolonged periods and/or in high doses, particularly in the elderly, because of the risk of drug-induced tardive dyskinesia.

Abdominal Pain

GENERAL PRINCIPLES

One of the most valuable diagnostic tools in evaluating the patient with abdominal pain is the history. The location and features of pain are useful in narrowing the differential diagnosis to an organ (e.g., hepatobiliary, gastric, and intestinal) as well as to a cause (e.g., inflammation, infection, obstruction, ischemia, and neurogenic).

DIAGNOSIS

Clinical Presentation

History

- The initial evaluation should focus on the chronology of events and determine the duration of symptoms (e.g., acute [Table 28-3] or chronic [Table 28-4]).
- The first consideration for a patient with acute abdominal pain is whether they can be evaluated in an outpatient setting or whether an emergency room is more appropriate.
- Some causes of abdominal pain can be well localized, particularly if they result from inflammation in the parietal peritoneum (Table 28-3).
- Substernal chest pressure or pain can be indicative of esophageal disorders. This can result in pain that radiates to the neck, jaw, arms, and back and may mimic cardiac angina.

TABLE 28-3 Common Causes of Acute Abdominal Pain by Location

Right upper quadrant
Budd-Chiari syndrome
Cholecystitis, cholangitis, choledocholithiasis
Congestive heart failure with hepatic
   congestion
Fitz-Hugh-Curtis syndrome
Hepatic abscess
Hepatic cancer
Hepatitis
Sickle hepatic crisis
Subdiaphragmatic abscess
Referred: myocardial infarction, pericarditis,
   pneumonia, pleural effusion/empyema,
   pulmonary embolism

Left upper quadrant
Gastritis, gastric ulcer
Pancreatitis
Splenic flexure ischemia
Splenic infarct/rupture/abscess
Referred: myocardial infarction,
   pericarditis, pleural effusion/
   empyema, pneumonia, pulmonary
   embolism

Right lower quadrant
Appendicitis
Bladder distension
Cecal volvulus
Ectopic pregnancy
Endometriosis
Infectious colitis
Infectious terminal ileitis
Inflammatory bowel disease
Inguinal hernia
Mesenteric adenitis
Neutrophilic colitis (typhlitis)
Pancreatitis
Pelvic inflammatory disease
Psoas abscess
Pyelonephritis
Renal pathology
Right ureteric calculus
Ruptured ovarian cyst
Salpingitis
Septic sacroiliitis
Testicular torsion

Left lower quadrant
Bladder distention
Diverticulitis
Ectopic pregnancy
Endometriosis
Infectious colitis
Inflammatory bowel disease
Inguinal hernia
Left ureteric calculus
Pancreatitis
Pelvic inflammatory disease
Psoas abscess
Pyelonephritis
Renal pathology
Rupture ovarian cyst
Salpingitis
Septic sacroiliitis
Sigmoid volvulus
Testicular torsion

Central abdominal pain
Aortic dissection/ruptured aortic aneurysm
Gastroenteritis, gastritis
Gastroesophageal reflux disease
Mesenteric ischemia
Pancreatitis
Peptic ulcer disease
Small bowel obstruction
Referred: myocardial infarction, pericarditis,
   pleural effusion/empyema, pneumonia,
   pulmonary embolism

Diffuse abdominal pain
Acute infectious peritonitis
Acute noninfectious peritonitis
Appendicitis
Diverticulitis
Familial Mediterranean fever
Hemorrhagic pancreatitis
Inflammatory bowel disease
Mesenteric ischemia
Perforated ulcer (gastric or duodenal)
Sickle cell crisis
Small bowel obstruction
Spontaneous bacterial peritonitis
Toxic megacolon
Metabolic: acute adrenal insufficiency,
   diabetic ketoacidosis, porphyria

Data from Yamada T, Alpers DH, Laine L, et al. *Textbook of Gastroenterology*, 4th ed.
Philadelphia, PA: Lippincott Williams & Wilkins; 2003.

TABLE 28-4	Causes of Chronic Abdominal Pain

Pancreaticobiliary disease
Chronic pancreatitis (particularly with chronic alcohol use)
Sphincter of Oddi dysfunction/biliary dyskinesia

Inflammatory disease
Celiac disease (often with diarrhea)
Eosinophilic gastrointestinal disorders
Familial Mediterranean fever
Hereditary angioedema/C1 inhibitor deficiency/dysfunction
Inflammatory bowel disease

Infectious disease
Chronic Giardiasis
Liver abscess
Schistosomiasis
Whipple disease (often with diarrhea)

Motility disorders
Constipation
Gastroparesis

Intermittent obstructive disease
Adhesions
Crohn disease
Internal or abdominal wall hernia
Intussusception

Other gastrointestinal
Drug-induced dyspepsia
Gastroesophageal reflux disease (GERD)
Peptic ulcer disease

Vascular disease
Celiac artery compression syndrome (postprandial)
Intestinal ischemia (postprandial)
Polyarteritis nodosa and other forms of vasculitis
Superior mesenteric artery syndrome

Neoplastic
Colon cancer
Gastric cancer
Hepatic cancer
Pancreaticobiliary neoplasm

Metabolic
Acute intermittent porphyria
Adrenal insufficiency
Heavy metal (lead) poisoning
Lactose intolerance

Neurologic disease
Abdominal cutaneous nerve entrapment syndrome
Abdominal epilepsy
Abdominal migraine
Postherpetic neuralgia
Radiculopathy (diabetes, spinal cord compression/fractures)

Musculoskeletal
Myofascial abdominal wall pain (trigger points)
Painful rib syndrome

Functional bowel disease
Irritable bowel syndrome
Nonulcer dyspepsia

Gynecologic disease
Dysmenorrhea (related to menstrual cycle)
Endometriosis (often related to menstrual cycle)
Mittelschmerz (related to menstrual cycle)
Ovarian cancer
Ovarian cysts
Somatization disorder
Uterine fibroids

- Epigastric discomfort may be secondary to a process affecting the stomach, duodenum, and pancreas, while stretching of the liver capsule or gallbladder distention or inflammation can result in RUQ pain. Small bowel obstruction and appendicitis may localize to the periumbilical area. Colonic pain may be localized to the lower abdomen but can be generalized. Abdominal disease causing inflammation under the diaphragm can produce referred pain in the shoulder.
- Non-GI abdominal pain can result from the following:
  - Urinary tract disease (e.g., cystitis, pyelonephritis, obstructive uropathy, and nephrolithiasis) is often associated with dysuria or hematuria and can cause pain in the flanks or suprapubic area as well as abdominal discomfort.

- ○ Pleural, pulmonary, or pericardial etiologies may cause upper abdominal pain.
  - ○ Gynecologic etiologies must be considered in women with lower abdominal symptoms (Tables 28-3 and 28-4).
- Description of pain that is sharp, tearing, and cutting may indicate an acute process, whereas descriptors such as gnawing, burning, dull, or boring point toward a chronic process.
- Colic describes pain with a waxing and waning intensity.
- Certain movements can generate abdominal pain due to musculoskeletal disorders or nerve root compression.
- Pain that is worse while supine may indicate pancreatic disease.
- Postprandial pain may indicate a process such as cholecystitis, pancreatitis, bowel obstruction, or gastric ulcer. In contrast, pain from duodenal ulcers generally improves with food ingestion. Intestinal angina may be associated with a fear of eating due to pain and result in weight loss.
- Nausea and emesis are nonspecific symptoms and can occur in association with abdominal pain due to a number of causes. Diarrhea associated with nausea and emesis suggests an infectious source.Hiccups can result from distention of the esophagus or stomach or irritation of the diaphragm.
- Patients should be questioned about changes in bowel movements, stool caliber, and stool volume. Constipation can result in diffuse abdominal discomfort, while diarrhea can be accompanied by cramping. Patients with alternating complaints of diarrhea and constipation may have irritable bowel syndrome.
- GI bleeding raises concern for ulcers, infections, inflammation, or ischemia. Melena (dark, tarry stool) usually signals an upper GI source, although it can occur during right-sided colonic bleeding or small bowel bleeding. Hematochezia (bright red blood from the rectum) usually reflects a colonic source but sometimes presents during massive upper bleeding.
- Menstrual cycles, irregularity, or abnormalities in bleeding may cause abdominal pain or worsening of underlying GI disorders. Symptoms of inflammatory bowel disease or irritable bowel syndrome can clearly worsen during and around the time of menses. Pain that follows a close pattern of menstrual cycles may be due to underlying endometriosis.
- Psychiatric causes should be considered in patients with underlying depression and anxiety, after organic causes are eliminated.
- **Red flags**: pain that awakens the patient from sleep, fever, prolonged severe pain of more than several hours duration, persistent vomiting, changes in patterns or location, significant alterations in appetite or mental status, unintentional weight loss, and GI bleeding.

Physical Examination
- Inspection and assessment for signs of systemic illness such as cachexia, pallor, severity of distress, presence of ascites, masses, prior surgical procedures, or other abnormalities, and presence of cutaneous findings of underlying cirrhosis.
- Auscultation for presence or absence of bowel sounds. High-pitched sounds may indicate bowel obstruction, whereas absence of sounds may be a feature of ileus or peritonitis.
- Tympanic percussion can indicate gas-filled or dilated loops of bowel. Dullness may indicate a mass or ascites, particularly if percussed in the flanks. Dullness below the left costal margin may indicate splenomegaly, and dullness below the right costal margin may indicate hepatomegaly.
- Palpation for the detection of hepatomegaly or splenomegaly. Palpation for masses, localized tenderness, or ascites. **Murphy sign** is tenderness to palpation in the RUQ, which induces a midinspiratory pause in breathing, and is suggestive of cholecystitis.
- Mesenteric ischemia classically presents with pain that is out of proportion to findings on physical examination.
- Signs worrisome for surgical abdomen include guarding and peritoneal signs (rebound tenderness or a rigid abdomen), fever, Murphy sign, iliopsoas sign (hyperextension of right hip causing abdominal pain associated with appendicitis or terminal ileal disease, absent or high-pitched bowel sounds.)

Diagnostic Testing

Laboratories
- CBC, looking for the following: leukocytosis suggesting acute inflammatory response; anemia, which can indicate GI bleeding; and thrombocytopenia suggesting liver disease.
- Serum chemistries evaluating electrolytes, bilirubin, amylase, lipase, alkaline phosphatase, and transaminases
- Urinalysis to assess hydration, proteinuria, infection, and renal disease

Imaging
- **Plain films** (obstructive series) are easy, inexpensive, and low risk. They can detect obstruction or perforation (free air under the diaphragm). However, when there is no real concern for obstruction or perforation, plain films are rarely diagnostic.
- **Ultrasound** to evaluate for organomegaly, masses, ascites, or biliary tract disease.
- **CT scan** may be more sensitive in detecting intra-abdominal processes.

Diarrhea

GENERAL PRINCIPLES

- A subjective increase in the frequency of stools as well as liquid consistency may be described as diarrhea by patients.
- Diarrhea is defined as stool quantity that exceeds 200 g/24-hour period.
- Diarrhea that has been present for <2 to 4 weeks is classified as acute, while chronic diarrhea describes symptoms of >4 weeks.

DIAGNOSIS

Clinical Presentation

History
- Relation to eating can be important in determining if the diarrhea is due to an osmotic or secretory cause, as the latter does not improve with fasting (Table 28-5).
- Nighttime diarrhea could indicate organic causes including infectious, secretory, inflammatory, or diabetic diarrhea. Functional diarrhea such as irritable bowel syndrome tends not to disturb the patient during sleep.
- Ascertain if the patient has had recent travel or contact with others at work, home, or otherwise who have similar symptoms.
- Blood, mucus, or pus in the stool and/or fever may indicate an invasive bacterial pathogen.
- Localized abdominal pain to the lower quadrants or rectum in the presence of bleeding, tenesmus, and weight loss are features of inflammatory bowel disease. Tenesmus is the sense of incomplete rectal evacuation accompanied by pain, cramping, and involuntary straining and strongly suggests proctitis. Pain is more commonly associated with Crohn disease than ulcerative colitis. Nonspecific diffuse pain or discomfort may be reported with irritable bowel syndrome.
- Patients with steatorrhea (fat malabsorption) often describe light-colored loose stools that are difficult to flush and stick to the toilet bowl. Fatty food intolerance may be observed in disorders of pancreatic exocrine insufficiency.
- Nighttime visual impairment and bone pain may be associated with fat-soluble vitamin malabsorption of vitamins A and D, respectively.
- Frequent small volumes of stool output with urgency suggest distal colorectal pathology, whereas larger volumes with less frequency suggest small bowel or proximal colonic disorders.

Physical Examination
- Dehydration should be assessed: orthostatic hypotension and pulse changes, poor skin turgor, and dry mucous membranes.

TABLE 28-5   Causes of Chronic Diarrhea

Osmotic/malabsorptive diarrhea	Secretory diarrhea	Inflammatory diarrhea
Causes		
Ingestion of unabsorbed solutes	Hormonal	Crohn disease
Lactose intolerance	VIPoma	Ulcerative colitis (multifactorial)
Medications (e.g., sorbitol, antacids, magnesium laxatives)	Watery diarrhea-hypokalemia-achlorhydria (WDHA) syndrome	Eosinophilic gastroenteritis
Maldigestion	Zollinger-Ellison (gastrinoma)	Intestinal ischemia
Chronic intestinal ischemia	Carcinoid	
Short bowel syndrome/ bacterial overgrowth	Bile salt malabsorption	
Gastrocolic fistula	Pancreatic cholera	
Mucosal transport defects/ mucosal disease	Collagen vascular disease	
Celiac sprue	Intestinal lymphoma	
Whipple disease		
Acrodermatitis enteropathica		
Lymphatic obstruction		
Chronic pancreatitis		
Signs and symptoms		
Moderate volume of stool	Voluminous stool	Moderate amount of stool (possibly with blood and mucus)
Improved with fasting	Little change with fasting	Little change with fasting
Weight loss	Nighttime symptoms	Weight loss
Signs of nutrient deficiency		Extraintestinal manifestations (arthritis, erythema nodosum, ocular signs)
Diagnosis		
Increased osmolar gap (measured osmolality is 100 mOsm greater than twice the sum of stool cations [K and Na])	Stool osmolality approximates serum osmolality 24-hour stool quantity >1 L	Colonoscopy with mucosal biopsy
Sometimes acidic stool pH	Usually neutral stool pH	Upper endoscopy
Fecal fat >7–10 g/ 24 hours (in steatorrhea)	VIP, vasoactive intestinal polypeptide	Angiography

Differential Diagnosis

- Sugar substitutes and sugar-free candy or chewing gum containing sorbitol, mannitol, or olestra are a common cause of diarrhea.
- Antibiotic use within the preceding 8 weeks is a predisposing factor for *Clostridium difficile*–associated pseudomembranous colitis,[8] although infection can occur in the absence of predisposing factors.
- Acute diarrhea is usually infectious (also see Chapter 26).
  - Viruses such as Norovirus in adults and older children and rotavirus in young children.
  - Enterotoxigenic bacteria such as *Escherichia coli* (traveler's diarrhea), *Bacillus cereus*, *Clostridium perfringens*, and *Staphylococcus aureus*.
  - Enteropathic agents, which can be invasive, include *Campylobacter*, *Salmonella*, *Shigella*, and certain species of *Yersinia*.
  - Protozoa including *Giardia* species, which can be acquired from spring or well water consumption, as well as amebiasis being common in travelers and homosexual men.
- Bloody diarrhea may be secondary to the following:
  - Invasive infections particularly *Campylobacter* and *Shigella*.
  - Acute onset of watery diarrhea that becomes bloody within 24 to 48 hours and is accompanied by fever suggests hemorrhagic colitis caused by *E. coli* O157:H7.
  - Inflammatory bowel disease.
  - Drug-induced colitis.
  - Mesenteric ischemia.
  - Ischemic colitis.
- Diverticular diarrhea can have features of left lower quadrant discomfort, rectal urgency, pain with defecation, tenesmus, and fever.
- Fecal impaction may paradoxically cause diarrhea in the elderly or in those who consume opioid pain medications with small liquid stool leakage around an impacted hard stool.
- Several categories of chronic diarrhea exist including osmotic, secretory, malabsorptive, and inflammatory (Table 28-5).
- Dumping syndrome is voluminous diarrhea occurring shortly after eating, commonly seen in postgastrectomy states. Within a few hours, some may experience the latent phase characterized by weakness, light-headedness, flushing, and hypoglycemia due to reactive insulin release.
- Irritable bowel syndrome can be characterized by alternating features of diarrhea and constipation with abdominal pain and frequently coexists with depression or anxiety.
- Diabetic diarrhea occurs in those with poorly controlled and/or long-standing diabetes and usually coexists with other signs of peripheral neuropathy.
- Factitious diarrhea is the surreptitious use of laxatives resulting in severe watery diarrhea, nausea, vomiting, and weight loss. The majority of these individuals are women <30 years of age who have eating disorders or middle-aged women with extensive medical histories who derive secondary gain from being chronically ill.[9]
- Significant intestinal resection, particularly segments of the ileum that exceed 100 cm, can result in malabsorption and a bile acid–induced diarrhea.[10]
- Microscopic colitis manifests as chronic diarrhea with few associated symptoms and is divided into lymphocytic colitis or collagenous colitis.

Diagnostic Testing

Laboratories

- Electrolytes, blood urea nitrogen (BUN), and creatinine can assist in identifying severity of dehydration or metabolic acidosis.
- CBC to assess for anemia or leukocytosis.
- Thyroid-stimulating hormone (TSH) level in those with chronic diarrhea.

- Presence of elevated IgA anti–tissue transglutaminase antibody is highly sensitive and specific for celiac sprue.[11,12] About 10% of celiac sprue patients have selective IgA deficiency, so total IgA levels should be checked as well.
- Stool should be examined for the following: ova, parasites, and culture; *C. difficile* toxin; fecal leukocytes, which are nonspecific but indicate inflammatory cause; stool electrolytes and osmolality to calculate osmotic gap; and Sudan staining of stool for fat (if abnormal, obtain 24-hour stool specimen for fat and volume).

Diagnostic Procedures
- **Sigmoidoscopy** with biopsies for infectious and inflammatory colitis can be a useful tool for those who have had diarrhea for >1 week. If initially negative or if colitis is present, a full colonoscopy may be necessary to determine the extent of involvement.
- **Colonoscopy** with terminal ileum exam is frequently performed to evaluate chronic diarrhea. It is highly sensitive for inflammatory bowel disease, microscopic colitis, and diverticular disease.
- **Upper endoscopy with small bowel biopsies** can be performed in chronic diarrhea to identify celiac sprue histologically. Alternatively, serologic testing can be performed, and upper endoscopy is performed only if serology is abnormal.

TREATMENT

- **Oral rehydration** with noncaffeinated and nonalcoholic products is preferred, but intravenous fluid administration may be necessary.
- **Antidiarrheal medications**
  - Kaolin and pectin-containing agents may add bulk to stool.
  - Bismuth subsalicylate has antisecretory, antimicrobial, and anti-inflammatory properties.
  - Loperamide is initially given as 4 mg dose followed by 2-mg capsules with a maximum of 8 mg/day.
  - Diphenoxylate plus atropine can be given as 5 mg initially and then 2.5 mg after each loose stool to a maximum of 20 mg/day.
  - Systemically absorbed opiates are sometimes given including tincture of opium (0.6 mL every 4 hours), belladonna/opium (1 suppository every 12 hours), and codeine (30 - 60 mg PO every 4 hours).
  - **All of these agents impair intestinal motility and should be avoided in bacterial infectious states, as they may delay clearance of the organism.**
- **Anticholinergic agents** such as atropine and hyoscyamine products are useful to some, particularly with cramping that accompanies diarrhea.
- **Bulk-forming substances** such as psyllium and methylcellulose may ameliorate functional diarrhea but are otherwise rarely effective in controlling symptoms.
- **Cholestyramine** can improve refractory diarrhea of malabsorption or bile acid–induced diarrhea, which can occur as a result of distal small bowel resections.
- **Antibiotics are not required for most acute infectious diarrhea**, as it is usually self-limited. Severe **traveler's diarrhea** that presents as dysentery with bloody stools with/without fever may require antibiotics (discussed in Chapter 26).

Constipation

GENERAL PRINCIPLES

- Constipation is the subjective feeling of infrequent stools or difficulty in passing stools. Absolute inability to pass stools can be referred to as obstipation.

- By ROME III criteria for functional constipation ≥2 of the following must be present: straining during ≥25% of defecations, lumpy or hard stools in ≥25% of defecations, sensation of incomplete evacuation for ≥25% of defecations, sensation of anorectal obstruction/blockage for ≥25% of defecations, manual maneuvers to facilitate ≥25% of defecations (e.g., digital evacuation, support of the pelvic floor), and <3 defecations per week.[13]
- The frequency of bowel movements may decrease with age.

DIAGNOSIS

Clinical Presentation
History
- Significant alterations in bowel habits without previous problems should alert the clinician to search for organic causes. Intermittent constipation may be due to medications, dietary habits, or functional bowel disease. Unrelenting symptoms should be investigated for serious illness such as obstruction from a mass.
- Patients with a rectal mass may sometimes describe a gradual reduction of stool caliber and often have accompanying hematochezia.
- Constipation in association with pain could indicate either inflammatory or obstructive causes such as: diverticulitis (left lower quadrant pain), anal fissures (anorectal pain), inflammatory colitis (diffuse pain), thrombosed external hemorrhoids (anal pain), and cancer. Cramping abdominal pain associated with bloating relieved by defecation may indicate irritable bowel syndrome if organic pathology has been excluded.
- Digital manipulation through either the vagina or the rectum may be described by the patient as a routine practice to induce bowel movements.

Physical Examination
Abdominal examination evaluating for distention, tenderness, and masses. Tympanic distention may indicate ileus or obstruction. Perineal and rectal examination to identify external deformities, such as rectal prolapse and hemorrhoids. Digital examination of the rectum assessing for fissures, distal fixed stenosis, masses, or fecal impaction as well as to test perineal sensation, rectal sphincter tone, and reflexes.

Differential Diagnosis
- Medications including narcotic analgesics, calcium channel blockers, anticholinergic agents, iron supplements, and many others.
- Constipation that accompanies urinary incontinence, particularly in postmenopausal women, could indicate the following: abnormal pelvic floor relaxation, rectocele, and cystoceles.
- Inadequate intake of fiber or fluid (6 to 8 glasses daily).
- Colonic inertia.
- Constipation—predominant irritable bowel syndrome.
- Colorectal neoplasia.
- Stricture (postoperative, diverticular, and radiation).
- Hypothyroidism.
- Neurologic/autonomic dysfunction (e.g., diabetes, Parkinson disease, Hirschsprung disease).

Diagnostic Testing
Laboratories
Serum electrolytes, particularly low potassium and magnesium, and abnormally low or high calcium levels, may become clinically significant. Thyroid studies to evaluate for hypothyroidism. Hyperglycemia may identify diabetics who have delayed transit time.

Diagnostic Procedures
- In the setting of new-onset or progressive constipation (especially in those >50 years of age), **colonoscopy** is essential to evaluate for colon cancer or strictures. **Melanosis coli**, a dark pigmentation that is most often seen in the distal colon, may be seen during colonoscopy in patients who use excess laxatives.
- **Barium enema** may be helpful when combined with flexible sigmoidoscopy to exclude obstructive colonic process in patients who are unable to undergo colonoscopy.
- **Obstructive series and abdominal CT** may evaluate for obstruction and megacolon (grossly dilated colon with significant abdominal distention).
- **Proctoscopy** may be useful to identify rectal pathology such as hemorrhoids, fissures, and masses.
- **Anorectal manometry** is used to identify anorectal dyssynergia and pelvic floor dysfunction.
- **Defecography** is a radiologic procedure that is helpful in identifying rectocele and pelvic floor dysfunction.

TREATMENT

- Treatment of constipation symptoms presumes that serious etiologies have been excluded.
- For **mild** symptoms
  - Increased fiber and fluid intake increases stool bulk and intestinal motility, which is generally only effective for mild constipation or constipation alternating with diarrhea. Most individuals with mild constipation are able to achieve a positive response with 20 to 30 g of daily fiber supplementation.[14]
  - Bulk-forming fiber supplements can be used.
    - Psyllium (e.g., Metamucil, 1 tsp in liquid or packet with liquid PO bid-qid)
    - Methylcellulose (e.g., Citrucel, 1 tbsp in 8 oz water qd-tid)
    - Polysaccharide derivatives (e.g., FiberCon, 1 g qid prn; 500-, 625-, and 1,000-mg tablets accompanied by 4 to 6 glasses of water)
  - Stool softeners including docusate (100 mg PO bid) can be used along with bulk-forming therapy for maintenance.[15]
- For **moderate** symptoms
  - Hyperosmolar agents
    - Polyethylene glycol (17 g PO qid) is well tolerated and available over the counter.
    - Lactulose (15 to 30 g PO every 2 to 3 hours prn) can cause bloating, which may be limiting.
  - Emollient laxatives may be used; however, mineral oil (15 to 45 mL PO every 6 to 8 hours) should be used with caution because of the risk of aspiration and lipid pneumonia.
  - Saline laxatives
    - Magnesium citrate (200 mL PO qid); **should not be used with impaired renal function**.
    - Fleet phospho soda if no contraindications; **should not be used with impaired renal function**.
- For **severe** symptoms
  - Stimulant laxatives
    - Castor oil (15 to 60 mL qid)
    - Cascara (1 tsp [5 mL] PO bid)
    - Senna (2 tsp [10 mL] PO bid)
    - Bisacodyl (10 to 15 mg PO qid-bid)
    - Lubiprostone (24 mcg PO bid)
    - Colchicine (0.6 mg PO bid). It is important to remember, however, that the margin between therapeutic and toxic is rather narrow with this drug and it **should not be used in patients with impaired renal function**.[16–18]

○ Enemas
  ▪ Saline enemas (120 to 240 mL)
  ▪ Tap water enemas (500 to 1,000 mL)
  ▪ Oil-retention enemas such as cottonseed with docusate
- **Routine long-term use of stimulant laxatives should be avoided.**
- Surgical treatment for rectal deformities, intestinal obstruction and masses, resuspension of rectal intussusception or prolapsed, and pelvic floor disorders.

Anorectal Disorders

DIAGNOSIS

Clinical Presentation

- Evaluation for anal pruritus, pain with defecation, bleeding, and fever
- Association with underlying constipation, inflammatory bowel disease, or other medical illness
- Evaluation of bowel habits, incontinence, and rectal pain changing with position
- Simple visual inspection after spreading the buttocks can often identify a tear, lesion, or fluctuant mass with purulence.
- Digital examination of the rectum for impacted stool, anal sphincter tone, blood, fissure, or mass.
- A lateral or anterior fissure found on examination may suggest Crohn disease, proctitis, leukemia, syphilis, tuberculosis, or carcinoma, but can be benign as well. Posterior fissures are often benign and self-limited.

Differential Diagnosis

- **External hemorrhoids** (below dentate line) manifesting as anal pruritus and sometimes pain. Severe pain may occur with thrombosis of an external hemorrhoid. **Internal hemorrhoids** (above dentate line) may produce mild discomfort, but significant pain is seen primarily in prolapse and strangulation. Bleeding from internal hemorrhoids is usually minimal but may be alarming to patients. It tends to be bright red in color and is found on the outside of stool, on toilet paper, or in the toilet bowl.
- **Anal fissure** is a linear tear of the anal canal tissue and is often associated with pain and rectal bleeding.
- **Perirectal fistula** characterized as a chronic purulent, foul-smelling discharge from the rectum, or a small opening in the perineum is found with Crohn disease. Perirectal abscess should raise suspicion for Crohn disease or immunosuppression.
- **Rectal prolapse** manifests as extrusion of the rectum during defecation and may need manual reduction by the patient. This is often seen in women and may be associated with urinary symptoms.
- **Rectosigmoid intussusception** presents with hematochezia and pain.
- **Proctalgia fugax** is characterized by sudden brief episodes of severe rectal pain occurring along the midline. Symptoms are typically mild and are a result of levator ani musculature spasm.
- **Fecal incontinence** with episodes of rectal urgency and fecal soiling of garments.
- **Pruritus ani** is the itching sensation of the anus or perianal skin. It is a manifestation of residual fecal material, hemorrhoids, rectal fistula, anal fissures, malignancy, psoriasis, or ingestion of certain foods. It can also be caused by infection with pinworms, scabies, pubic lice, and certain sexually transmitted diseases.

Diagnostic Testing

- **Anoscopy** is used to evaluate for anal fissures with 90% of lesions found at the posterior midline.
- Direct visualization via **sigmoidoscopy or colonoscopy** may be necessary to evaluate for hemorrhoids, perirectal fistula, intussusception, malignancy, or inflammatory bowel disease.

- Perineal sensory disturbances, identifiable by nerve conduction studies, can be a sign of low back injury or degenerative disk disease with nerve damage.
- Endoscopic ultrasound can assess the sphincter for mechanical disruption.

TREATMENT

- Increased **dietary fiber**, resulting in softer bulky stools and less straining, as well as **stool softeners, analgesic suppositories, and warm sitz baths** given two to three times a day can alleviate most anorectal pain.[19]
- Topical nitroglycerin or injection with botulinum toxin has achieved temporary relaxation of sphincter tone to permit healing of anal fissures.[20]
- Antibiotics such as ciprofloxacin and metronidazole may aid in healing of perirectal fistulas, but additional medical therapy may be needed when due to Crohn disease.
- Pelvic floor muscle strengthening with biofeedback can be used in appropriate patients.
- Patients with proctalgia fugax benefit from reassurance and symptomatic relief with local heat and massage.
- Pruritus ani benefits from the following treatment:
  ○ Antimicrobial therapy for the specific organism, if indicated
  ○ Oral antihistamines for nocturnal symptoms
  ○ Short-term topical treatment with hydrocortisone cream 1% (not to exceed 2 weeks' duration) or zinc oxide ointment
- Surgical intervention
  ○ Persistent, symptomatic hemorrhoids may require endoscopic band ligation or hemorrhoidectomy.
  ○ Chronic anal fissures require anal sphincterotomy.
  ○ Excision and drainage of perirectal fistulas.
  ○ Incision and drainage of perirectal abscesses.
  ○ Reduction of rectal prolapse or frequent partial prolapse.
  ○ Refractory fecal incontinence.

Approach to Abnormal Liver Chemistries

GENERAL PRINCIPLES

- Laboratory evaluation should be interpreted in conjunction with the clinical history and physical examination. A full discussion of liver diseases is presented in Chapter 30.
- Liver test abnormalities can be grouped into the following categories:
  ○ **Hepatocellular disease**: aspartate aminotransferase (AST) and alanine aminotransferase (ALT) elevated more than bilirubin and alkaline phosphatase
  ○ **Cholestatic disease**: bilirubin and alkaline phosphatase elevated more than AST and ALT

DIAGNOSIS

Clinical Presentation
History
- Screen for exposure to hepatitis A, B, or C, and obtain history of blood transfusions, intravenous drug use, and sexual contacts.
- The constellation of RUQ pain, fever, and jaundice is known as **Charcot triad** and suggests acute cholecystitis. The addition of altered mental status and hypotension to this triad is known as **Reynolds pentad** and can indicate ascending cholangitis.
- Pain in the midabdomen that radiates to the back suggests acute pancreatitis, which is most commonly caused by choledocholithiasis and may be accompanied by abnormal liver tests.

- Rapid intense RUQ pain may also imply choledocholithiasis, particularly in those with prior cholelithiasis or cholecystectomy.
- Evaluate for nonspecific symptoms including nausea, vomiting, chills, fevers, anorexia, and weight loss. Fatigue alone is frequently reported as the primary presenting symptom in patients with liver disease.
- Dark urine is often noted earlier than jaundice and is an indication of increased urobilinogen due to biliary obstruction or hepatocellular dysfunction.
- Pruritus is usually generalized and present in almost all cases of jaundice that exceed 3 to 4 weeks' duration.
- Painless jaundice should raise suspicion for pancreaticobiliary disorders, as neoplasms of the pancreatic head may result in extrahepatic biliary obstruction.
- Acute onset of abnormal liver tests may indicate hemolysis or biliary tract obstruction.
- Abdominal pain may reflect stretching of the liver capsule from a space-occupying lesion.
- Congestive heart failure and passive hepatic congestion can account for up to 10% of all jaundice in those >60 years of age.[21]

Physical Examination
- Evaluate for **stigmata of chronic liver disease** such as parotid gland enlargement, spider angiomas (most commonly found on the trunk), palmar erythema, Dupuytren contractures (fibrous contractures of the palmar fascia), gynecomastia, hepatomegaly or small liver size, splenomegaly, caput medusa, testicular atrophy, and ascites.
- **Fever** can be found in acute and chronic illness and may be suggestive of infection.
- **Hepatomegaly** >15 cm in span can be found in passive congestion, malignant or fatty infiltration, or other infiltrative disorders.
- **Splenomegaly** is found in patients with portal hypertension and cirrhosis and may also be found in those with hemolysis and a vast array of hematologic disorders and malignancies.
- **Murphy sign** (RUQ tenderness palpated during inspiration) may indicate cholecystitis. **Palpable distended gallbladder** without tenderness (Courvoisier sign) is commonly found in pancreaticobiliary malignancy with obstruction.
- **Ascites** may be present in cirrhosis of various causes and intra-abdominal malignancy as well as congestive heart failure and pancreatitis.
- Cutaneous findings include xanthomas, which may be seen in chronic cholestasis of primary biliary cirrhosis. Gray-bronze discoloration of the skin may suggest hemochromatosis with hepatic involvement. Urticaria may be a sign of acute hepatitis B infection.

Differential Diagnosis
The differential diagnosis for abnormal liver tests is presented in Table 28-6.[22]

Diagnostic Testing
Laboratories
Evaluate for hemolysis with a CBC, peripheral blood smear, reticulocyte count, lactate dehydrogenase, haptoglobin, and indirect bilirubin.
- **Bilirubin:**
  ○ Impaired excretion of bilirubin results in an increase in the conjugated form, and clinical icterus presents if the total bilirubin level exceeds 2.5 mg/dL.
  ○ Bilirubin elevation can be prolonged despite convalescence of the acute illness.
  ○ An isolated indirect hyperbilirubinemia that does not exceed 5 mg/dL with normal transaminases and no indication of hemolysis may be the result of a benign familial disorder known as Gilbert syndrome, in which hyperbilirubinemia occurs in response to fasting and physiologic stress.

TABLE 28-6 Causes of Abnormal Liver Tests

Hepatocellular disease

Drugs/toxins
Acetaminophen, with the use of as
little as 4 g/day in an individual with
prior liver disease, can result in
hepatocyte damage
Herbal agents
Vitamin A
NSAIDs
Propylthiouracil
Antidepressants (e.g., duloxetine,
sertraline, phenelzine)
General anesthetics
Antimicrobials (e.g., sulfonamides,
erythromycin, isoniazid,
antifungals)
Anticonvulsants (e.g., phenytoin,
carbamazepine)
Many others (particularly with
idiosyncratic drug reactions)
Certain occupational exposures
can result in hepatotoxicity with
exposure to chemicals such as
arsenic in many industrial settings
and in organic gardening as well
as insecticides for agricultural
workers

Alcohol use
Daily consumption that exceeds
80 g (72 oz beer, 9 oz liquor, or
30 oz wine) for 10–15 years can
lead to cirrhosis in men, while lower
levels possibly 20–40 g/day for
women

Hepatitis
Viral (A, B, C, D, E, Epstein-Barr virus,
cytomegalovirus)
Autoimmune hepatitis

Others
Hemochromatosis
Wilson disease
α-1-Antitrypsin deficiency
Shock liver

Cholestatic disease

Intrahepatic causes
Viral hepatitis
Alcoholic liver disease
Drugs
Antimicrobials (nitrofurantoin, floxins,
macrolides, amoxicillin-clavulanic
acid, and other penicillin-based
antibiotics)
Anabolic steroids
Oral contraceptives
Sulfonylureas
Phenothiazines (e.g., chlorpromazine,
prochlorperazine)
Malignancy such as hepatocellular
carcinoma, lymphoma, or other
masses
Sepsis
Abscesses
Pregnancy
Primary biliary cirrhosis
Primary sclerosing cholangitis
Sarcoidosis
Amyloidosis
Pregnancy
Total parenteral nutrition

Extrahepatic causes
Choledocholithiasis
Cholangiocarcinoma
Pancreatitis
Pancreatic cancer or pseudocyst
Papillary stenosis
Primary sclerosing cholangitis

NSAIDs, nonsteroidal anti-inflammatory agents.

- **Prothrombin Time:**
  - Impaired liver synthesis of vitamin K–dependent coagulation factors in the extrinsic pathway results in an abnormal PT.
  - Cirrhosis, hepatitis, and cholestatic syndromes may produce prolonged PT, which, as a result, can serve as a useful prognostic indicator in patients with cirrhosis.
- **Albumin:**
  - Another measure of the liver's synthetic function.
  - Half-life of 20 days, which makes it better indicator of chronic liver disease.
  - Low levels may be present in some patients with poor nutrition, but the finding is nonspecific and should not be used independently to assess a patient's nutritional status or liver function.
  - Loss of this protein can occur through the GI tract or kidneys.
  - Dilutional effect should also be considered in volume overload states, in normal pregnancy, and in acute or chronic inflammatory states.
- **Aminotransferases:**
  - AST can be released into the blood from numerous tissues, including liver, cardiac and skeletal muscle, kidney, and brain.
  - ALT is more specific to the liver, and serum levels rise with hepatocyte death.
  - Elevations in the thousands can be seen in viral hepatitis and toxin- or ischemia-induced hepatic injury.
  - Elevation of AST and ALT in a ≥2:1 ratio, high serum γ-glutamyl transpeptidase (GGT), and an elevated mean corpuscular volume of red cells are highly suspicious for alcoholic liver disease.
  - Injury from alcohol almost never results in elevations that exceed 10 times the normal values.
- **Alkaline phosphatase:**
  - Elevated serum levels can arise from processes that affect the liver, skeletal system, intestines, placenta, kidneys, and leukocytes.
  - GGT levels can differentiate between biliary and other sources of alkaline phosphatase.
  - The largest increases are seen in cholestatic syndromes and intrahepatic and extrahepatic biliary ductal obstruction.
  - Markedly increased levels without associated liver disease are sometimes seen in congestive heart failure, bone diseases, and Hodgkin lymphoma.
- Elevated antimitochondrial antibody (AMA) indicates primary biliary cirrhosis.
- Elevated anti–smooth muscle antibody (ASMA) and antinuclear antibody and immunoglobulins indicate autoimmune hepatitis.
- Elevated iron studies suggest hemochromatosis.
- Viral hepatitis panel can diagnose viral etiologies.
- α-Fetoprotein (AFP) is used as a screening test for hepatocellular malignancy in patients with cirrhosis.[23]

Diagnostic Procedures
- **Ultrasound** should be used initially for rapid evaluation of the biliary system. Sensitivity is 95% for detection of cholelithiasis and acute cholecystitis and identifying ductal dilation.
- **CT scan** should be obtained for liver parenchyma examination as well as for distinction between stones, tumors, and stricture.
- **Endoscopic retrograde cholangiopancreatography (ERCP)** is most useful in diagnosing and treating obstructive jaundice in the setting of choledocholithiasis, cholangitis, intra- and extrahepatic strictures, and pancreatic ductal disease. **Magnetic resonance cholangiopancreatography (MRCP)** is also useful diagnostically but has no therapeutic use.
- **Liver biopsy** is helpful in diagnosing the etiology of liver disease in those with abnormal enzymes for >6 months, assuming obstruction is excluded.

- If ascites is present, consider **paracentesis** to check the following:
  - Cell count to rule out infection.
  - Serum ascites-albumin gradient (SAAG, the difference between serum and ascites albumin measurements); values of >1.1 indicate portal hypertension.
  - Cytology to evaluate for malignancy.

TREATMENT

Treatment depends on the underlying illness. See Chapter 30 for specific management.

REFERENCES

1. Jalil S, Castell DO. Schatzki's ring: a benign cause of dysphagia in adults. *J Clin Gastroenterol* 2002;35:295–298.
2. Hewson EG, Sinclair JW, Dalton CB, et al. Twenty-four-hour esophageal pH monitoring: the most useful test for evaluating noncardiac chest pain. *Am J Med* 1991;90:576–583.
3. Domenech E, Kelly J. Swallowing disorders. *Med Clin North Am* 1999;83:97–113.
4. DeVault KR, Castell DO. Updated guidelines for diagnosis and treatment of gastroesophageal reflux disease. *Am J Gastroenterol* 2005;100:190–200.
5. Talley NJ, Vakil NB, Moayyedi P. American Gastroenterological Association technical review on the evaluation of dyspepsia. *Gastroenterology* 2005;129:1756–1780.
6. Cohen J, Safdi MA, Deal SE, et al.; ASGE/ACG Taskforce on Quality in Endoscopy. Quality indicators for esophagogastroduodenoscopy. *Am J Gastroenterol* 2006;101:886–891.
7. Fisher RS, Parkman HP. Management of nonulcer dyspepsia. *N Engl J Med* 1998;339:1376–1381.
8. Hurley BW, Nguyen CC. The spectrum of pseudomembranous enterocolitis and antibiotic-associated diarrhea. *Arch Intern Med* 2002;162:2177–2184.
9. Ewe K, Karbach U. Factitious diarrhoea. *Clin Gastroenterol* 1986;15:723–740.
10. Potter GD. Bile acid diarrhea. *Dig Dis* 1998;16:118–124.
11. Carroccio A, Vitale G, Di Prima L, et al. Comparison of anti-transglutaminase ELISAs and an anti-endomysial antibody assay in the diagnosis of celiac disease: a prospective study. *Clin Chem* 2002;48:1546–1550.
12. Rostom A, Dubé C, Cranney A, et al. The diagnostic accuracy of serologic tests for celiac disease: a systematic review. *Gastroenterology* 2005;128:S38–S46.
13. Longstreth GF, Thompson WG, Chey WD, et al. Functional bowel disorders. *Gastroenterology* 2006;130:1480–91.
14. Soffer EE. Constipation: an approach to diagnosis, treatment, referral. *Cleve Clin J Med* 1999;66(1):41–46.
15. Schiller LR. Clinical pharmacology and use of laxatives and lavage solutions. *J Clin Gastroenterol* 1999;28(1):11–18.
16. Frame PS, Dolan P, Kohli R, Eberly SW. Use of colchicine to treat severe constipation in developmentally disabled patients. *J Am Board Fam Pract* 1998;11:341–6.
17. Verne GN, Davis RH, Robinson ME, et al. Treatment of chronic constipation with colchicine: dandomized, double-blind, placebo-controlled, crossover trial. *Am J Gastroenterol* 2003;98:1112–6.
18. Raghavi SA, Shabani S, Mehramiri A, et al. Colchicine is effective for short-term treatment of slow transit constipation: a double-blind placebo-controlled clinical trial. *Int J Colorectal Dis* 2010;25:389–94.
19. Herzig DO, Lu KC. Anal fissure. *Surg Clin North Am* 2010;90:33–44.

20. Dhawan S, Chopra S. Nonsurgical approaches for the treatment of anal fissures. *Am J Gastroenterol* 2007;102:1312–1321.
21. Qureshi WA. Intrahepatic cholestatic syndromes: pathogenesis, clinical features and management. *Dig Dis* 1999;17:49–59.
22. Zimmerman HJ. Update of hepatotoxicity due to classes of drugs in common clinical use: non-steroidal drugs, anti-inflammatory drugs, antibiotics, antihypertensives, and cardiac and psychotropic agents. *Semin Liver Dis* 1990;10(4):322–338.
23. Frank BB. Clinical evaluation of jaundice. A guideline of the Patient Care Committee of the American Gastroenterological Association. *JAMA* 1989;262:3031–3034.

29 Gastroesophageal Reflux Disease

C. Prakash Gyawali and Amit Patel

GENERAL PRINCIPLES

- Gastroesophageal reflux disease (GERD) is a condition characterized by symptoms or tissue damage from reflux of gastric contents into the esophagus or beyond.
- Population surveys indicate that GERD is very common, with 10% to 20% of the general population reporting at least weekly symptoms.[1,2]
- There are several barriers to reflux of gastric contents into the esophagus.[3,4]
  - Resting tone in the lower esophageal sphincter (LES) keeps the gastroesophageal junction closed in between swallows.
  - The diaphragmatic crura, normally aligned with the LES, pinch the gastroesophageal junction during inspiration to prevent reflux when intrathoracic pressure is negative relative to the atmosphere.
  - Any refluxed material is promptly returned back into the stomach by secondary peristaltic waves initiated by local esophageal neural reflexes.
  - Residual acidic material in the mucosa is neutralized by saliva, which is alkaline.
- Despite these measures, physiologic reflux occurs in most individuals, typically after meals.
- Inappropriate transient LES relaxation (TLESR) is the most frequent mechanism of reflux, in healthy people as well as patients with GERD.[3,4]
  - The LES is designed to relax immediately at the initiation of a swallow.
  - A TLESR is said to occur inappropriately when the LES relaxes in between swallows.
  - Several triggers, including a full stomach and the presence of a hiatus hernia, may precipitate frequent TLESRs, which in turn can lead to reflux of gastric contents into the esophagus.
- Low tone in the LES is seen in approximately a quarter of reflux patients, wherein the barrier to gastroesophageal reflux is weak.[3,4]
  - A prototype condition associated with extremely low LES tone is scleroderma, where fibrosis of the esophageal smooth muscle leads to near-absent tone in the LES and hypomotility or aperistalsis in the esophageal body.
  - Certain medications and food items that lower LES tone include the following anticholinergics, smooth muscle relaxants, caffeine, theophylline, alcohol, and fatty or greasy foods.
- A **hiatus hernia** results when the diaphragmatic crura are not snug against the gastroesophageal junction, allowing a pouch of stomach to prolapse proximal to the crura.[3,4]
  - The typical axial hiatus hernia slides up and down through the diaphragmatic hiatus. The presence of a hiatus hernia disrupts the physiologic barrier to gastroesophageal reflux by several mechanisms. First, the anatomic integrity of the barrier formed by close alignment of the diaphragmatic crura and the closed LES is lost. A pouch of gastric mucosa is now above the level of the diaphragmatic pinch, which can serve as a reservoir for gastric (acidic) secretions that can easily reflux when the patient lays supine. Finally, local neural reflexes may be affected by the presence of the hiatus hernia, allowing for a higher frequency of inappropriate LES relaxations.
  - The larger the hiatus hernia, the higher the likelihood for reflux.
  - However, **not every patient with a hiatus hernia has GERD, and not every patient with GERD has a hiatus hernia.**

DIAGNOSIS

Clinical Presentation

- Heartburn is the most frequent reflux symptom, described by patients as a retrosternal or epigastric burning sensation.[4] The discomfort may radiate upward to the neck, to the shoulders, or even to the back.
- Acid reflux often occurs in the postprandial state but can sometimes occur at night and awaken the patient from sleep.
- Eating or taking an antacid promptly relieves the symptom by neutralizing refluxed acid.
- Heartburn may be associated with regurgitation of a sour, bitter liquid with an acidic taste.
- Bending over, laying supine, and wearing tight garments over the abdomen may provoke both heartburn and regurgitation in some instances.
- Mucosal inflammation in the esophagus from acid reflux can also prompt the sensation of dysphagia in some patients, which may improve with acid-suppressive therapy.
- Atypical presentations can occur.
  - Over the past few decades, several atypical reflux symptoms have been identified. It is important to recognize atypical symptoms, as they may occur even when typical symptoms are absent.[5]
  - The most significant atypical symptom is **chest pain**, which is important because chest pain may indicate concomitant cardiac disease. Conversely, cardiac disease needs careful exclusion before chest pain is attributed to GERD in appropriate age groups. In older patients, both GERD and coronary artery disease can coexist. Despite documenting correlation of reflux with chest pain, many patients continue to worry about cardiac disease, making noncardiac chest pain an important cause for health care expenditure.
  - **Wheezing and asthma** have also been linked to reflux, especially adult-onset symptoms in the absence of an allergic component. There are two mechanisms by which reflux can result in asthma. Regurgitation of gastric contents to the pharynx and tracheal microaspiration. Triggering of a reflex bronchospasm in susceptible individuals by smaller amounts of acid in the distal esophagus. When correlation between bronchospastic symptoms and reflux exists, adequate management of GERD can lead to better treatment outcomes. Other pulmonary symptoms and disorders linked to reflux include cough, interstitial fibrosis, and aspiration pneumonia.
  - Other supraesophageal manifestations of reflux disease include hoarseness, throat clearing, dental erosions, and posterior laryngitis. Dyspeptic symptoms, nausea, and back pain may also have etiologic links to GERD in certain situations.

Differential Diagnosis

Eosinophilic Esophagitis

- Eosinophilic esophagitis (EoE) is a chronic condition characterized by eosinophil infiltration of the esophageal mucosa and submucosa, leading to mucosal inflammation, fibrosis, and luminal narrowing.[6,7]
- Annual incidence rates vary between 0.1 and 1.2 per 10,000. It is seen most often in young men.[8]
- Presenting manifestations can be obstructive (dysphagia, recurrent food bolus impactions) or perceptive (heartburn, chest pain). Solid food dysphagia is the most common presenting symptom.[9]
- On endoscopy, the esophageal lumen may be narrowed with a corrugated trachea-like appearance.[10] However, similar endoscopic features have been described in other esophageal disorders and are not pathognomonic for EoE.
- Esophageal biopsies should therefore be obtained whenever EoE is suspected, regardless of esophageal endoscopic appearance.[10] With few exceptions, biopsies should demonstrate >15 eosinophils/high-power field to establish a diagnosis of EoE.[9]

- Topical steroids should be considered for both initial and maintenance therapy in EoE patients. Topical treatment is available in both inhaled and viscous forms. Recommended initial dose of inhaled treatment is 440 to 880 µg of fluticasone puffed and swallowed through metered dose inhaler twice daily. Viscous treatment consists of mixing 1 g of budesonide with ten 1-g packets of sucralose. The mixture is then swallowed, and patients should not eat or drink for 30 minutes after drug ingestion.[9,11–13]
- Proton pump inhibitors (PPIs) are effective adjunctive treatment options for EoE.[9]
- Esophageal dilation is a treatment option in healthy adult patients with anatomic esophageal narrowing, followed by a course of topical steroids to reduce inflammation and decrease remodeling. Patients with EoE are not at greater risk for perforation when compared to patients with other causes of esophageal stricture undergoing dilatation.[14,15]
- Patients with EoE have high rates of concurrent asthma, allergic rhinitis, eczema, and food allergy. A thorough evaluation by an allergist or immunologist is recommended for diagnosis and treatment of concurrent atopic diseases.[9]

Infectious Esophagitis
- **Candida esophagitis** is the most frequent infectious esophagitis seen in immunocompromised individuals.[16]
  - Other risk factors include esophageal stasis (strictures, achalasia, and neoplasia), antibiotic use, steroid use, diabetes, and malnutrition.
  - Endoscopic evaluation reveals whitish exudates and plaques in the esophagus; fungal hyphae can be seen on cytology.
  - If an immunocompromised patient has esophageal symptoms (dysphagia and odynophagia) and oropharyngeal thrush is encountered, empiric therapy with **fluconazole** (100 mg daily for 14 days) or **nystatin** (100,000 units/mL, 5 mL tid for 14 to 21 days) can be empirically initiated, reserving endoscopy for refractory symptoms.
- **Herpes esophagitis** can occur in both immunocompetent and immunocompromised hosts.[16]
  - A history of cold sores is frequently elicited.
  - Patients present with severe odynophagia, resulting in food aversion.
  - Endoscopic evaluation may reveal grouped vesicles or ulcers, biopsies from which may reveal intracytoplasmic inclusions.
  - Therapy consists of **acyclovir** for 10 to 14 days.
- **Cytomegalovirus esophagitis** is only seen in immunocompromised hosts, typically after solid organ transplants and in advanced AIDS with low CD4 counts.[16] Endoscopy typically reveals deep ulcers, and biopsies demonstrate typical intranuclear inclusions.

Pill Esophagitis
- Pill esophagitis is usually seen in conjunction with esophageal stasis, strictures, and hypomotility disorders.[17]
- Presentation may include heartburn, chest pain, and odynophagia.
- Frequent locations for pill esophagitis are the aortic arch and the LES.
- Usual culprits include quinidine, tetracycline, doxycycline, nonsteroidal anti-inflammatory drugs, and alendronate.

Functional Heartburn and Chest Pain
Perceptive esophageal symptoms similar to that seen with GERD can be encountered in patients with visceral hyperalgesia.[18] Symptoms may overlap with nonerosive reflux disease, functional heartburn, and functional chest pain.

Diagnostic Testing
Proton Pump Inhibitor Trial
- **The most convenient and cost-effective approach for diagnosis of GERD is by initiating a therapeutic trial of PPI therapy.**[19]

- This approach has been studied using omeprazole (40 mg before breakfast and 20 mg before supper) for 1 week in patients with typical symptoms.
- Symptom resolution predicts good diagnostic accuracy with a sensitivity of 78% and specificity of 54% in meta-analyses.[20]
- Patients with atypical symptoms require double doses of PPIs and longer therapeutic trials, as long as 1 month for atypical chest pain and 3 to 6 months for supraesophageal symptoms.[5]

Endoscopy
- Esophagitis is visualized in only 50% to 60% of GERD patients with typical symptoms if endoscopy is performed prior to initiation of antireflux therapy; the number goes down to <10% if adequate antireflux therapy has already been initiated.[21,22]
- The frequency of finding visible esophagitis is lower in patients with atypical symptoms (30% for asthma, 15% to 20% for atypical chest pain, and ≤15% for laryngeal symptoms) even under ideal circumstances.
- Therefore, the best use of endoscopy is to evaluate for complications and to **screen for Barrett esophagus.**[19,21]
- Patients with **alarm symptoms** (dysphagia, weight loss, anemia, or family history of esophageal cancer) or with a long history of reflux symptoms (>5 years), older patients (>45 years), or those failing to respond adequately to antisecretory therapy are offered endoscopy, typically performed after the patient has been taking a PPI for 8 to 12 weeks. The purpose of the procedure is, therefore, to evaluate for ongoing erosive esophagitis, alternate causes of esophagitis (e.g., EoE and infectious esophagitis), strictures, Barrett esophagus, and esophageal neoplasia.

Ambulatory pH Monitoring
- Ambulatory pH monitoring is considered the **gold standard for quantifying esophageal acid exposure.**[19,23] The test is not used to diagnose GERD but rather to quantify the degree of acid exposure in patients referred for antireflux surgery, patients with atypical symptoms, and patients not responding to seemingly adequate antireflux measures. Ambulatory pH monitoring allows not just measurement of acid exposure time, but also correlation of symptoms to reflux events.
- There are two techniques of pH monitoring, **catheter-based monitoring** with one or two pH sensors and **wireless monitoring**, where a pH sensor capsule attached to the esophageal mucosa communicates recorded pH to a receiver worn by the patient.
- The test is performed off antireflux therapy (off PPIs for a week, H_2 receptor blockers for 3 days, and antacids for 24 hours) to quantify acid exposure time, to correlate symptoms to reflux events, for preoperative evaluation prior to antireflux procedures, and in patients with persistent GERD despite antireflux surgery.[24]
- Testing on twice a day PPI therapy allows assessment of adequacy of treatment in patients with persistent symptoms despite therapy. This indication is now served best by esophageal impedance-pH testing as described below.
- The wireless pH system allows for longer duration of pH monitoring and better patient tolerability, without loss of accuracy.[25] Longer monitoring improves sensitivity of symptom-reflux association tests and addresses day-to-day variation in acid exposure.[26] The capsule is placed 6 cm above the squamocolumnar junction following upper endoscopy. Contraindications include stricture, severe esophagitis, varices, history of bowel obstruction, and pacemakers or defibrillators.
- Ambulatory pH monitoring only measures acidic elements in the refluxate, but impedance monitoring assesses reflux irrespective of the pH of the refluxate.[23,27] Impedance is measured by passing minute electrical currents through pairs of electrodes implanted on a catheter. Changes in the resistance to flow of current indicate presence of liquid refluxate or air (e.g., belch), and direction of movement of the change distinguishes swallows

from reflux events. Impedance catheters typically have a pH sensor for distal esophageal pH measurement. Impedance-pH monitoring is an attractive option for patients with ongoing symptoms despite antireflux therapy, especially if symptoms are regurgitation predominant.

Esophageal Manometry
- Esophageal manometry contributes little to the diagnosis of GERD but may define patho-physiologic mechanisms in patients with impaired esophageal peristalsis or low LES resting tone.[19,23,28]
- Manometry is often performed **prior to antireflux surgery** to assess adequacy of esophageal peristaltic performance and to exclude potentially confounding diagnoses such as achalasia.
- Esophageal manometry is used to locate the LES for placement of catheter-based pH and impedance-pH probes (placed 5 cm proximal to the LES).

Barium Esophagogram
Barium contrast esophagograms provide accurate anatomic information and delineate even subtle strictures or narrowings. Barium studies are **not accurate for the diagnosis of GERD** and should not be used for this indication.[21,29]

Other Diagnostic Procedures
Other specialized esophageal investigative studies used in the research setting include the Bernstein test, balloon distension studies, esophageal planimetry, high-definition ultrasound, and transit time measurements.

TREATMENT

Medications
Acidic gastric contents are corrosive to the esophageal mucosa. The basis of pharmacologic treatment is to reduce gastric acidity and render the refluxate less corrosive.

Proton Pump Inhibitors
- **The standard of acid-suppressive therapy is the PPI.**[19,30]
- PPIs are administered 30 to 60 minutes before a meal to allow the agent to circulate in the blood stream when the proton pumps are activated by a meal. PPIs then bind to the proton pump and render them inactive, thereby lowering gastric acidity for 12 to 18 hours. For continued efficacy, these agents have to be administered daily, prior to breakfast if used once a day and additionally prior to supper if used twice a day.
- PPIs are remarkably safe; minor side effects include abdominal pain and diarrhea. Fundic gland polyps may develop in some patients on long-term acid suppression.[31] Concern for rare side effects arises from prolonged continued use, but reports are limited, and long-term studies continue to establish overall safety of these agents.[32]
- These rare side effects include small intestinal bacterial overgrowth, *Clostridium difficile* colitis, vitamin B_{12} malabsorption, and calcium malabsorption leading to osteopenia and hip fractures in susceptible individuals.[33–35]
- Commonly available PPIs are listed in Table 29-1.

Histamine-2 Receptor Antagonists
- H_2 receptor antagonists also lower gastric acid secretion and may be effective in patients with intermittent or mild symptoms.
- H_2 receptor antagonists have been used in addition to PPI therapy in patients with nocturnal breakthrough symptoms.
- These agents may be **subject to tachyphylaxis**, which may affect continued efficacy.
- Side effects include drug interactions and rarely thrombocytopenia and confusion.

TABLE 29-1	Typical Doses of Antisecretory Medications for GERD
Drug	**Dosage**
Proton pump inhibitors	
Esomeprazole (Nexium)	20–40 mg daily/bid
Lansoprazole (Prevacid)	15–30 mg daily/bid
Dexlansoprazole (Dexilant)	60 mg daily
Omeprazole (Prilosec, generic)	20–40 mg daily/bid
Omeprazole with NaHCO$_3$ (Zegerid)	20–40 mg daily/bid
Pantoprazole (Protonix)	40 mg daily/bid
Rabeprazole (Aciphex)	20 mg daily/bid
Histamine-2 receptor antagonists	
Cimetidine (Tagamet, generic)	200–400 mg bid
Famotidine (Pepcid, generic)	20–40 mg bid
Ranitidine (Zantac, generic)	150–300 mg bid

GABA Agonists
- GABA agonists such as baclofen reduce TLESRs, the most common mechanism of reflux in both healthy individuals and GERD patients.
- Baclofen has been associated with decreased upright acid exposure times as well as significant improvement in belching, regurgitation, and overall reflux symptoms.
- Baclofen has also been shown to be a useful adjunct therapy in patients with nighttime heartburn and/or sleep complaints despite PPI therapy.[36,37]

Promotility Agents
- **There are no effective promotility agents appropriate for management of GERD symptoms currently on the market.**[19]
- Metoclopramide is sometimes prescribed to improve LES tone and enhance gastric emptying but is associated with frequent side effects, including irritability and extrapyramidal dysfunction. Benefit for reflux has not been systematically demonstrated.

Surgical Management
- Antireflux surgery performed by an experienced surgeon is an alternate option to pharmacologic management in patients with well-documented GERD.[19]
- Patients with large hiatus hernias, low LES resting tone, and regurgitation-predominant symptoms appear to benefit most from this approach.
- Good to excellent results can be expected in patients who respond to PPI therapy, especially when there is good symptom-reflux correlation on ambulatory pH monitoring. Antireflux surgery can also be considered in patients intolerant of PPIs.
- Antireflux surgery has similar efficacy to PPI therapy when considering remission rates at 5 years. Breakthrough reflux symptoms may develop in some, especially after 5 to 10 years, and supplemental antisecretory therapy may be required.[38] It is estimated that the cost of antireflux surgery compares with that of pharmacologic therapy in approximately 10 years.
- Benefits of surgery must also be weighed against the possible adverse effects. New symptomatic postoperative dysphagia occurs in approximately 6% of patients undergoing antireflux surgery. However, early postoperative dysphagia is not associated with poorer long-term reflux control after surgery.[39,40]

Lifestyle Modification
- Lifestyle modification measures make physiologic sense but are **not considered adequate by themselves for management of symptomatic reflux disease**. Rather, these measures are recommended in conjunction with pharmacologic therapy.[19]

- These measures include the following:
  - Avoid large meals.
  - Avoid eating 2 to 3 hours before lying down.
  - Avoid foods and beverages that can decrease the lower esophageal sphincter pressure (e.g., chocolate, peppermint, caffeine, and alcohol).
  - Individual patients should avoid foods that worsen their symptoms—common examples include acidic foods, spicy foods, and fatty foods, but this is not necessarily consistent from patient to patient.
  - Avoid tight-fitting garments.
  - Lose weight.
  - Elevate the head of the bed (placement of four to six in blocks underneath the front legs of the bed is preferred to propping the head up with pillows).
  - Quit smoking and decrease alcohol use.

COMPLICATIONS

Mucosal Erosion/Strictures

- Mucosal erosions are seen in the esophagus in approximately 60% of patients with typical reflux symptoms prior to initiation of antireflux therapy. These erosions can be circumferential and associated with ulcerations in 10% to 15%. Healing of ulcerated areas can lead to luminal narrowing and **stricture formation**.
- When dysphagia results, esophageal dilation is of value.[41] Continued acid suppression with a PPI may delay recurrence of peptic esophageal strictures.
- Dilation can be performed with through-the-scope endoscopic balloons or bougies, either passed blindly (Maloney dilators) or over a guide wire (Savary dilators).
- Refractory strictures that recur within short intervals may benefit from steroid injection into the rents created by dilation, which may prolong intervals between dilations.

Barrett Esophagus

- In genetically susceptible individuals, acid reflux can trigger a change in the distal esophageal mucosal lining from the normal squamous cell lining to incomplete intestinal metaplasia, termed Barrett esophagus.[19,42,43]
- This is characterized visually as a change in color from normal pearly white to salmon pink, either in a circumferential fashion or as slivers of changed mucosa (also called "tongues") extending proximally from the gastroesophageal junction.
- Barrett esophagus is seen most frequently in middle-aged Caucasian males who are obese, smoke, and consume alcohol.[44]
- The overall prevalence of Barrett esophagus is thought to be about 5% to 15% in the GERD population and about 1% to 2% in the general population.[44,45]
- The significance of Barrett esophagus is the **small but real risk of progression to high-grade dysplasia and esophageal adenocarcinoma.** The risk of progression from high-grade dysplasia to esophageal adenocarcinoma is approximately 10% per year.[46]
- The incidence of esophageal adenocarcinoma has been rising over the past few decades and has overtaken squamous cell cancer as the most frequent esophageal cancer in Caucasian males.
- Although Barrett esophagus is asymptomatic, erosive disease and adenocarcinoma both can lead to symptoms of dysphagia, anemia, and rarely weight loss, making these **alarm symptoms** necessitating endoscopic evaluation of the esophagus.
- Most authorities agree that patients with established Barrett esophagus should undergo surveillance high-resolution endoscopy with biopsies every 1 to 3 years to assess for dysplastic changes that are suggestive of degeneration toward malignancy.[42]
- At least two experienced gastrointestinal pathologists should evaluate all biopsies when diagnosis of dysplasia is considered. Extent of dysplasia can correlate with progression to cancer.[46]

- If **high-grade dysplasia** is encountered, intervention is needed:
  - Esophagectomy remains an option but is not the only therapy available.
  - Endoscopic options include photodynamic therapy, radiofrequency ablation, endoscopic mucosal resection, endoscopic thermal, and cryotherapy.
  - Endoscopic mucosal resection should treat all suspected areas of high-grade dysplasia and early esophageal adenocarcinoma.
  - Any mucosal irregularity, including nodularity or ulceration, requires intense biopsy and endoscopic mucosal resection if possible, to exclude adenocarcinoma. Endoscopic ultrasound may help further characterize mucosal nodules.
  - Radiofrequency ablation is the best ablative technique for treating flat high-grade dysplasia and residual Barrett esophagus mucosa after focal endoscopic mucosal resection.[46,47] Follow-up screening endoscopies are required at suggested intervals of 2, 5, and 10 years.[46]
  - When high-grade dysplasia is unifocal, repeat surveillance after 3 months of aggressive PPI therapy can be an option, as mucosal inflammation can rarely lead to histopathologic findings mimicking dysplasia. The risk of development of adenocarcinoma is 30% with high-grade dysplasia.
- **Low-grade dysplasia** is monitored with more frequent endoscopic biopsy surveillance, typically every 6 months initially, which can subsequently be extended to every 12 months in the absence of progression.
- All patients with Barrett esophagus are maintained on PPI therapy, mainly to heal esophagitis proximal to the Barrett segment, but also because Barrett esophagus is an accurate indicator of abnormal acid exposure times.

Extraesophageal Complications

Extraesophageal complications of GERD include laryngitis, tracheal stenosis, interstitial pneumonitis, aspiration pneumonia, dental erosions, worsening of asthma, and chronic cough. It is not completely clear if reflux of gastric contents can contribute to laryngeal cancer.

REFERENCES

1. Dent J, El-Serag HB, Wallander MA, et al. Epidemiology of gastroesophageal reflux disease: a systematic review. *Gut* 2005;54:710–717.
2. Locke GR III, Talley NJ, Fett SL, et al. Prevalence and clinical spectrum of gastroesophageal reflux: a population based study in Olmstead County, Minnesota. *Gastroenterology* 1997;112:1448–1456.
3. Galmiche JP, Janssens J. The pathophysiology of gastro-oesophageal reflux disease: an overview. *Scand J Gastroenterol Suppl* 1995;211:7–18.
4. Richter JE. Gastroesophageal reflux disease. In: Yamada T, Alpers DH, Kaplowitz N, Laine L, et al., eds. *Textbook of Gastroenterology*, 4th ed. Philadelphia, PA: Lippincott Williams & Wilkins; 2003:1196–1224.
5. Richter JE. Extraesophageal presentations of gastroesophageal reflux disease: an overview. *Am J Gastroenterol* 2000;95:S1–S3.
6. Katzka DA. Eosinophilic esophagitis. *Curr Opin Gastroenterol* 2006;22:429–432.
7. Dellon E, Aderogu A, Woosley JT, et al. Variability in diagnostic criteria for eosinophilic esophagitis: a systematic review. *Am J Gastroenterol* 2007;102:2300–2313.
8. Abonia PJ, Rothenberg ME. Eosinophilic esophagitis: rapidly advancing insights. *Annu Rev Med* 2012;63:421–434.
9. Liacouras CA, Furuta GT, Hirano I, et al. Eosinophilic esophagitis: updated consensus recommendations for children and adults. *J Allergy Clin Immunol* 2011;128:3–20.
10. Kim HP, Vance RB, Shaheen NJ, et al. The prevalence and diagnostic utility of endoscopic features of eosinophilic esophagitis: a meta-analysis. *Clin Gastroenterol Hepatol* 2012;10:988–996.

11. Peterson KA, Thomas KL, Hilden K, et al. Comparison of esomeprazole to aerosolized, swallowed fluticasone for eosinophilic esophagitis. *Dig Dis Sci* 2010;55:1313–1319.
12. Dellon ES, Sheikh A, Speck O, et al. Viscous topical is more effective than nebulized steroid therapy for patients with eosinophilic esophagitis. *Gastroenterology* 2012;143:321–324.
13. Dohil R, Newbury R, Fox L, et al. Oral viscous budesonide is effective in children with eosinophilic esophagitis in a randomized, placebo-controlled trial. *Gastroenterology* 2010;139:418–429.
14. Bohm ME, Richter JE. Review article: esophageal dilation in adults with eosinophilic esophagitis. *Aliment Pharmacol Ther* 2011;33:748–757.
15. Jacobs JW, Spechler SJ. A systematic review of the risk of perforation during esophageal dilation for patients with eosinophilic esophagitis. *Dig Dis Sci* 2010;55:1512–1515.
16. Wilcox CM. Esophageal infections and disorders associated with acquired immunodeficiency syndrome. In: Yamada T, Alpers DH, Kaplowitz N, et al., eds. *Textbook of Gastroenterology*, 4th ed. Philadelphia, PA: Lippincott Williams & Wilkins; 2003: 1225–1237.
17. Winstead NS, Bulat R. Pill esophagitis. *Curr Treat Options Gastroenterol* 2004;7:71–76.
18. Gyawali CP, Clouse RE. Approach to dysphagia, odynophagia and noncardiac chest pain. In: Yamada T, Alpers DH, Kalloo AN, et al., eds. *Principles of Clinical Gastroenterology*. Hoboken, NJ: Wiley-Blackwell; 2008:62–83.
19. DeVault KR, Castell DO. Updated guidelines for the diagnosis and treatment of gastroesophageal reflux disease. *Am J Gastroenterol* 2005;100:190–200.
20. Numans ME, Lau J, de Wit NJ, et al. Short-term treatment with proton-pump inhibitors as a test for gastroesophageal reflux disease: a meta-analysis of diagnostic test characteristics. *Ann Intern Med* 2004;140:518–527.
21. Lichtenstein DR, Cash BD, Davila R, et al. Role of endoscopy in the management of gastroesophageal reflux disease. *Gastrointest Endosc* 2007;66:219–224.
22. Pilotto A, Franceschi M, Leandro G, et al. Long-term clinical outcome of elderly patients with reflux esophagitis: a six-month to three-year follow-up study. *Am J Ther* 2002;9:295–300.
23. Hirano I, Richter JE. ACG practice guidelines: esophageal reflux testing. *Am J Gastroenterol* 2007;102:668–685.
24. Richter JE, Pandolfino JE, Vela MF, et al. Utilization of wireless pH monitoring technologies: a summary of the proceedings from the Esophageal Diagnostic Working Group. *Dis Esophagus* 2013;26:755–765.
25. Roman S, Mion F, Zerbib F, et al. Wireless pH capsule-yield in clinical practice. *Endoscopy* 2012;44:270–276.
26. Pandolfino JE, Kwiatek MA. Use and utility of the Bravo pH capsule. *J Clin Gastroenterol* 2008;42:571–578.
27. Sifrim D, Holloway R, Silny J, et al. Acid, nonacid, and gas reflux in patients with gastroesophageal reflux disease during ambulatory 24-hour pH-impedance recordings. *Gastroenterology* 2001;120:1588–1598.
28. Kahrilas PJ, Quigley EM. Clinical esophageal pH recording: a technical review for practice guideline development. *Gastroenterology* 1996;110:1982–1996.
29. Johnston BT, Troshinsky MB, Castell JA, et al. Comparison of barium radiology with esophageal pH monitoring in the diagnosis of gastroesophageal reflux disease. *Am J Gastroenterol* 1996;91:1181–1185.
30. Miner P, Katz PO, Chen Y, et al. Gastric acid control with esomeprazole, lansoprazole, omeprazole, pantoprazole, and rabeprazole: a five way crossover study. *Am J Gastroenterol* 2003;98:2616–2620.
31. Jalving M, Koornstra JJ, Wesseling J, et al. Increased risk for fundic gland polyps during long term proton pump inhibitor therapy. *Aliment Pharmacol Ther* 2006;24:1341–1349.

32. Klinkenberg-Knol E, Nelis F, Dent J, et al. Long-term omeprazole treatment in resistant gastroesophageal reflux disease. *Gastroenterology* 2000;118:661–669.

33. Howden CW. Vitamin B12 levels during prolonged treatment with proton pump inhibitors. *J Clin Gastroenterol* 2000;30:29–33.

34. Dial S, Delanye JAC, Barkun AN, et al. Use of gastric acid-suppressive agents and the risk of community acquired *Clostridium difficile*-associated disease. *JAMA* 2005;294:2989–2995.

35. Yang Y-X, Lewis JD, Epstein S, et al. Long-term proton pump inhibitor therapy and risk of hip fracture. *JAMA* 2006;296:2947–2953.

36. Cossentino MG, Mann K, Armbruster SP. Randomised clinical trial: the effect of baclofen in patients with gastroesophageal reflux—a randomised prospective study. *Aliment Pharmacol Ther* 2012;35:1036–1044.

37. Orr WC, Goodrich D, Wright S, et al. The effect of baclofen on nocturnal gastro-esophageal reflux and measures of sleep quality: a randomized, cross-over trial. *Neurogastroenterol Motil* 2012;24:553–559.

38. Galmiche JP, Hatlebakk J, Attwood S, et al. Laparoscopic antireflux surgery vs esome-prazole treatment for chronic GERD: the LOTUS randomized clinical trial. *JAMA* 2011;305:1969–1977.

39. Kahrilas PJ, Shaheen NJ, Vaezi MF. American Gastroenterological Association medical position statement on the management of gastroesophageal reflux disease. *Gastroenterology* 2008;135:1383–1391.

40. Makris KI, Cassera MA, Kastenmeier AS, et al. Postoperative dysphagia is not predictive of long-term failure after laparoscopic antireflux surgery. *Surg Endosc* 2012;26:451–457.

41. Spechler SJ. AGA technical review on treatment of patients with dysphagia caused by benign disorders of the distal esophagus. *Gastroenterology* 1999;117:233–254.

42. Wang KK, Sampliner RE. Updated guidelines 2008 for the diagnosis, surveillance and therapy of Barrett's esophagus. *Am J Gastroenterol* 2008;103:788–797.

43. Nelsen EM, Hawes RH, Iyer PG. Diagnosis and management of Barrett's esophagus. *Surg Clin North Am* 2012;92:1135–1154.

44. Westhoff B, Brotze S, Weston A, et al. The frequency of Barrett's esophagus in high-risk patients with chronic GERD. *Gastrointest Endosc* 2005;61:226–231.

45. Ronkainen J, Aro P, Storskrubb T, et al. Prevalence of Barrett's esophagus in the general population: an endoscopic study. *Gastroenterology* 2005;129:1825–1831.

46. Bennett C, Vakil N, Bergman J, et al. Consensus statements for management of Barrett's dysplasia and early-stage esophageal adenocarcinoma, based on Delphi process. *Gastroenterology* 2012;143:336–346.

47. Garman KS, Shaheen NJ. Ablative therapies for Barrett's esophagus. *Curr Gastroenterol Rep* 2011;13:226–239.

30

Hepatobiliary Diseases

Claire Meyer, Amit Patel, and Mauricio Lisker-Melman

VIRAL HEPATITIS

Hepatitis A

GENERAL PRINCIPLES

- Hepatitis A is caused by an **RNA virus (picornavirus)** and is acquired and spread via **the fecal-oral route**.
- The hepatitis A virus (HAV) causes acute hepatitis, defined as the sudden onset of significant aminotransferase elevation as a consequence of diffuse necroinflammatory liver injury, which can vary from mild illness to acute liver failure. **There is no chronic form of hepatitis A.**
- Although the annual reported incidence of hepatitis A is around 1.5 million, the actual incidence may be as much as 10-fold higher.[1] The morbidity and mortality of this infection increase with increased age of onset.
- Most cases of hepatitis A resolve in 4 to 8 weeks. Prolonged cholestatic disease, characterized by persistent jaundice and waxing and waning liver enzymes, is more frequently seen in adults.
- Prophylaxis
  - **Preexposure prophylaxis:** Vaccination is recommended for high-risk populations, including men who have sex with men, residents and staff of institutions that serve the mentally disabled, restaurant workers, and residents of and travelers to endemic areas.
  - **Postexposure prophylaxis:** For nonimmune patients who are exposed to hepatitis A, immunoprophylaxis is available in the form of hepatitis A immune globulin (0.2 mL/kg). The hepatitis A vaccine has also been shown to be effective as postexposure prophylaxis. The immune globulin or the vaccine should be given within 2 weeks of exposure.[2]

DIAGNOSIS

- Hepatitis A can be asymptomatic, particularly in children and young adults.
- Common but nonspecific clinical manifestations of hepatitis A include malaise, fatigue, pruritus, headache, abdominal pain, myalgias, arthralgias, nausea, vomiting, anorexia, and fever.
- The diagnosis of acute hepatitis A is based on identification of IgM antibodies to HAV. Presence of IgG antibodies to HAV, in the absence of an acute hepatitis, suggests the recovery phase after acute hepatitis A or immunity to HAV.

TREATMENT

Patients can usually be treated supportively on an outpatient basis, but hospitalization may be required for those who are unable to maintain hydration. Emergent liver transplant evaluation should be considered for patients in whom acute liver failure develops.

Hepatitis B

GENERAL PRINCIPLES

- The hepatitis B virus (HBV) is a **DNA virus of the hepadnavirus family**. Eight genotypes (A through H) have been identified.
- **In the US, the virus is most commonly transmitted through horizontal transmission** via injection drug use and sexual contact. In Asia, vertical transmission (mother to child) continues to be a major public health problem.[3]
- **HBV can cause both acute and chronic hepatitis**.
- Two billion people worldwide have serologic evidence of past or present infection, with approximately 400 million being chronic carriers.
- Progression from acute to chronic disease occurs in about 90% of children infected before age 6 but in only 5% to 10% of those who acquire the virus as adults.
- Patients with acute hepatitis B have an excellent prognosis if they do not progress to chronic state.
- Prognosis in chronic hepatitis B is related to the level of activity (biochemical and histologic) and persistence of viral replication. For chronic hepatitis B patients, the cumulative 5-year incidence of progression to cirrhosis ranges from 8% to 20%. Hepatocellular carcinoma (HCC) is detected in 5% to 10% of patients with chronic hepatitis B with or without cirrhosis.
- Prophylaxis
  - **Preexposure prophylaxis:** HBV vaccination should be considered for everyone, but particularly individuals who belong to high-risk groups, including patients on hemodialysis, injection drug users, individuals with multiple sexual partners, men having sex with men, household and heterosexual contacts of HBV carriers, residents and employees of residential care facilities, travelers to endemic regions, and individuals born in areas of high or intermediate prevalence (e.g., Alaska, Southern Asia, Africa, South Pacific Islands, and the Amazon).
  - **Postexposure prophylaxis:** Infants born to hepatitis B surface antigen–positive mothers should receive the hepatitis B vaccine and hepatitis B immunoglobulin (HBIG) within 12 hours of birth. Susceptible sexual partners of individuals with HBV and those with needlestick injuries should receive HBIG and the first dose of the hepatitis B vaccine within 48 hours of exposure. A second dose of HBIG should be administered 30 days after exposure and the vaccination schedule completed.

DIAGNOSIS

- Acute hepatitis B can be asymptomatic, particularly in children and young adults. Common but nonspecific clinical manifestations include malaise, fatigue, pruritus, headache, abdominal pain, myalgias, arthralgias, nausea, vomiting, anorexia, and fever.
- Extrahepatic, unusual presentations include polyarteritis nodosa, glomerulonephritis, cryoglobulinemia, serum sickness-like illness, papular acrodermatitis (predominantly in children), and aplastic anemia.
- Chronic hepatitis B is defined as persistent viral activity (serologic or molecular studies) for at least six months from diagnosis. As in acute hepatitis, symptoms may vary. Chronic hepatitis B can progress to cirrhosis and HCC.
- Based on biochemical, serologic, molecular, and histologic criteria, chronic hepatitis B infection is a dynamic process that occurs in different phases (see Table 30-1).

TABLE 30-1	Use of HBV Markers in Clinical Practice					
Test	Acute hepatitis B	Resolved acute hepatitis B	High replication chronic HBV	Low replication chronic HBV	HBV precore mutant	Vaccination
HBsAg	+	–	+	+	+	–
HBeAg	+	–	+	+	–	–
Anti-HBs	–	+	–	–	–	+
Anti-HBe	–	+	–	+	+	–
IgM anti-HBc	+	–	+	–	–	–
IgG anti-HBc	–	+	+	+	+	–
HBV DNA	>10^5 copies/mL	Negative	>10^5 copies/mL	10^2–10^4 copies/mL	>10^4 copies/mL	Negative
ALT/AST	+++	Normal	+++	Normal	+/++	Normal

ALT, alanine transaminase; AST, aspartate transaminase; HBc, hepatitis B core antigen; HBeAg, hepatitis B e antigen; HBsAg, hepatitis B surface antigen; HBV, hepatitis B virus.

TREATMENT

- **Acute hepatitis B**: Patients can usually be treated supportively on an outpatient basis.
- **Chronic hepatitis B**
  - Current indications for treatment include patients with chronic hepatitis B (e antigen positive and negative) with HBV DNA >2,000 IU/mL and/or elevated ALT with necroinflammation and fibrosis on liver biopsy. Patients with cirrhosis, both compensated and decompensated, should be treated even with normal ALT levels or HBV DNA <2,000 IU/mL.[4]
  - Entecavir, tenofovir, and pIFN-α are first-line treatment agents.[5] The goal of treatment is viral suppression or eradication to prevent progression to cirrhosis and HCC. Treatment end points include clearance of HBV DNA, hepatitis B e antigen and hepatitis B surface antigen seroconversion (loss of antigen and production of antibody), and normalization of liver enzymes and histology.

Hepatitis C

GENERAL PRINCIPLES

- The hepatitis C virus (HCV) is an **RNA virus of the Flavivirus family**. There are six genotypes (1 to 6) and multiple subtypes (a, b, c, etc.). Genotype 1 is the most common in the United States (75%).
- **HCV is a common blood-borne infection** that is often transmitted by intravenous and intranasal drug use.
- **HCV can cause both acute and chronic hepatitis**.
- There are approximately 180 million HCV carriers worldwide. In the United States, about 4 million people are infected with HCV and 50% to 75% are unaware of their infection.[6]
- In industrialized countries, HCV accounts for 20% of cases of acute hepatitis, 70% of chronic hepatitis, 40% of cirrhosis, 60% of HCC, and 40% to 50% of liver transplantations.
- Male gender, older age at the time of infection, duration of infection, hepatic steatosis, heavy alcohol consumption, daily marijuana use, and coinfection with HIV have been identified as risk factors for fibrosis progression.
- Patients with cirrhosis due to hepatitis C develop HCC at a rate of approximately 1% to 4% per year.[7]

DIAGNOSIS

- Acute hepatitis can be asymptomatic, especially in children and young adults. Symptoms vary from mild illness to acute liver failure. Malaise, fatigue, pruritus, headache, abdominal pain, myalgias, arthralgias, nausea, vomiting, anorexia, and fever are common but nonspecific presentations.
- Chronic hepatitis C runs an indolent course, sometimes for decades, and its diagnosis requires a high index of suspicion. Fatigue is a common symptom. The disease may only become clinically apparent late in the natural course, when advanced liver disease develops. Patients with risk factors for HCV infection should be tested. In addition, the CDC recommends one-time screening for hepatitis C for all those born in the decades from 1945 through 1965.[8]
- Extrahepatic, unusual presentations include mixed cryoglobulinemia (10% to 25% of patients with HCV), glomerulonephritis, porphyria cutanea tarda, vasculitis, lymphoma, diabetes mellitus, and lichen planus.[9]
- The diagnosis of hepatitis C is based on a combination of liver chemistries, serologies, molecular studies, and histology.
- Antibodies against HCV (anti-HCV) may be undetectable for the first 8 weeks after infection. Antibodies do not confer immunity. The test has a sensitivity of 95% to 99%

and a lower specificity. A false-positive test (anti-HCV positive with HCV RNA negative) may occur in the setting of autoimmune hepatitis (AIH) or hypergammaglobulinemia. A false-negative test (anti-HCV negative with HCV RNA positive) may be seen in immunosuppressed individuals and in patients on hemodialysis.

- HCV RNA can be detected by PCR in serum as early as 1 to 2 weeks after infection (qualitative and quantitative assays). HCV RNA determination is useful for both diagnosis and treatment purposes.
- HCV genotype influences the duration, dosage, and response to treatment.
- Liver biopsy is useful to score the degree of inflammation (grade) and fibrosis (stage) in the liver of chronically infected patients. It also allows for assessment of the amount of liver steatosis and guides treatment decisions.

TREATMENT

- **Acute hepatitis C:** IFN-α (standard or pegylated) for 6 months has been associated with a high rate (98%) of sustained HCV RNA clearance.[10]
- **Chronic hepatitis C:** Treatment varies according to genotype. In patients with genotype 1, the standard of care is to use triple therapy including pegylated interferon (pIFN-α), ribavirin, and a protease inhibitor (PI). Boceprevir and telaprevir are the only two currently approved PIs (only for genotype 1 patients). In patients with genotype 2 or 3, a combination of pIFN-α and ribavirin is administered for 6 to 12 months.
- Multiple side effects are associated with these regimens. pIFN-α is associated with flu-like symptoms, neuropsychiatric disorders, and bone marrow suppression. Ribavirin is associated with hemolytic anemia and pulmonary symptoms. PIs are associated with anemia, rash, dysgeusia, diarrhea, and anal discomfort.
- pIFN-α should not be used in patients with decompensated cirrhosis or in patients with autoimmune conditions. Ribavirin is teratogenic and should not be used in pregnancy, in women of childbearing age who are not using birth control, in patients with chronic renal insufficiency, or in those who cannot tolerate anemia. PIs inhibit the hepatic cytochrome P450 enzymes and have extensive drug-drug interactions.

IMMUNE-MEDIATED LIVER DISEASE

Autoimmune Hepatitis

GENERAL PRINCIPLES

- AIH is **a chronic disorder characterized by inflammation of the liver associated with circulating autoantibodies and hypergammaglobulinemia**.
- There are two types of AIH. **Type 1** is the most common form (80%). It is associated with **ANA (antinuclear antibodies) and/or ASMA (anti–smooth muscle antibodies)**. **Type 2**, predominately seen in children and young adults, is associated with antibodies to liver/kidney/microsome type 1 (ALKM-1) and/or antibodies to cytosol type 1 (ALC-1).
- AIH affects all ethnic groups and occurs worldwide. In Norway and Sweden, for example, its prevalence is 11 to 17 per 100,000.[11]
- **Women are affected more than men** (gender ratio 3.6:1).

DIAGNOSIS

- An acute presentation, clinically similar to acute viral hepatitis, is observed in 30% to 40% of patients.

- Extrahepatic manifestations may be found in 30% to 50% and include synovitis, celiac disease, Coombs-positive hemolytic anemia, autoimmune thyroiditis, Graves disease, rheumatoid arthritis, ulcerative colitis, uveitis, and other autoimmune-mediated processes.
- The most common symptoms at presentation include fatigue, jaundice, myalgia, anorexia, diarrhea, acne, and right upper quadrant abdominal tenderness.
- Diagnostic criteria are based on autoantibodies, IgG levels, histologic changes, and the exclusion of viral hepatitis and other liver conditions.[12]
- Liver biopsy is essential for the diagnosis.

TREATMENT

- Goals of treatment include biochemical normalization and histologic remission.
- Treatment should be started in patients with elevated serum aminotransferase levels and hypergammaglobulinemia (aminotransferases >10 times upper limit of normal [ULN] or aminotransferases >5 times ULN and immunoglobulins ≥2 times ULN) or those with biopsy findings of interface hepatitis, bridging necrosis, or multiacinar necrosis.
- **Therapy is initiated with either prednisone monotherapy (40 to 60 mg/day) or a combination of prednisone and azathioprine (30 mg/day and 1 to 2 mg/kg/day, respectively).**[11]
- Prednisone is tapered with biochemical and clinical improvement. Some patients require lifelong low-dose therapy.
- Liver transplantation should be considered in patients with decompensated cirrhosis and those with AIH-mediated acute liver failure.
- Most adults (90%) have clinical and biochemical improvement within 2 weeks of beginning treatment. Remission is achieved in 80% of patients at 3 years.
- Relapses occur in at least 20% to 50% of patients after treatment discontinuation. Those patients require retreatment.

Primary Biliary Cirrhosis

GENERAL PRINCIPLES

- Primary biliary cirrhosis (PBC) is **a cholestatic disorder with autoimmune features and unknown etiology.**
- It is more commonly seen in women (90% to 95%) and in Caucasians.
- PBC is an indolent disease that progresses from laboratory abnormalities to increasing histologic damage, leading to fibrosis, cirrhosis, and liver failure.

DIAGNOSIS

- The clinical course is highly variable, with up to 50% to 60% of patients asymptomatic at the time of diagnosis. Fatigue, jaundice, and pruritus are often the most troublesome symptoms. While there are no exam findings that are specific for PBC, xanthomata and xanthelasma can be manifestations of underlying cholestasis.
- Extrahepatic manifestations include keratoconjunctivitis sicca (Sjögren syndrome), renal tubular acidosis, gallstones, thyroid disease, scleroderma, Raynaud phenomenon, CREST syndrome, and celiac disease.
- **Antimitochondrial antibodies are present in >90% of patients with PBC.** Typical biochemical features include elevated levels of alkaline phosphatase, total bilirubin, and cholesterol as well as elevations of IgM.
- Liver biopsy is helpful for both diagnosis and staging.

TREATMENT

- No curative therapy is available, but ursodeoxycholic acid (13 to 15 mg/kg/day) has been shown to improve laboratory abnormalities as well as survival.[13]
- Symptom-specific therapy for pruritus, steatorrhea, and malabsorption may be needed.
- Liver transplantation is an alternative in advanced liver disease.

Primary Sclerosing Cholangitis

GENERAL PRINCIPLES

- Primary sclerosing cholangitis (PSC) is **a cholestatic liver disease characterized by inflammation, fibrosis, and progressive obliteration of the extrahepatic and intrahepatic biliary tree**.
- PSC can be subdivided into those with small duct and large duct involvement. **Small duct disease** has typical histologic features of PSC with a normal cholangiogram. **Large duct, or classic, PSC** has characteristic strictures of the biliary ducts that can be detected by cholangiography.
- Most patients have involvement of both intrahepatic and extrahepatic ducts, with <25% having only intrahepatic involvement and <5% only extrahepatic disease.[14]
- Male to female ratio is 2:1, and peak incidence is approximately age 40.
- The clinical progression of PSC is unpredictable, but most patients have insidious progression to cirrhosis.
- Cholangiocarcinoma has a poor prognosis; however, perihilar cholangiocarcinoma may be an indication for liver transplantation in selected patients.

DIAGNOSIS

- Clinical manifestations include intermittent episodes of jaundice, hepatomegaly, pruritus, weight loss, and fatigue. Acute cholangitis is a frequent complication in patients with severe biliary strictures.
- Patients are at increased risk for cholangiocarcinoma, which develops in 10% to 30%.[15]
- **In 70% of patients with PSC, ulcerative colitis is an associated condition**. Crohn disease is less commonly associated with PSC.
- pANCA (perinuclear antineutrophil cytoplasmic antibody) is positive in 80% of cases. In contrast, ANA is only seen in 50% of patients.
- Imaging studies useful in the diagnosis of PSC include liver ultrasound, MRCP (magnetic resonance cholangiopancreatography), and ERCP (endoscopic retrograde cholangiopancreatography). Those studies typically show ductal dilation, strictures, or irregularities of the intrahepatic or extrahepatic bile ducts. ERCP is also useful to obtain brushings to evaluate for associated malignancy.
- While liver biopsy is not the gold standard for the diagnosis of PSC, it is helpful to exclude other diseases and for staging.

TREATMENT

- **No specific drug treatments have been shown to alter disease progression.** Ursodeoxycholic acid is not currently recommended for therapy.[14]
- Acute cholangitis should be managed with antibiotics and endoscopic therapy (dilation and stenting of dominant strictures).
- Symptom-specific therapy for pruritus, steatorrhea, and malabsorption may be needed.
- Liver transplantation is an alternative in advanced liver disease.

METABOLIC LIVER DISEASE

Nonalcoholic Fatty Liver Disease

- Nonalcoholic fatty liver disease (NAFLD) is an increasingly common metabolic disorder of the liver strongly **associated with diabetes mellitus type 2, the metabolic syndrome, obesity, and dyslipidemia.**[16]
- The disorder can range from the benign accumulation of triglyceride in hepatocytes (simple steatosis) to the nonalcoholic steatohepatitis (NASH) characterized by steatosis with hepatocellular ballooning plus lobular inflammation. The proportion of patients with NAFLD who will progress to NASH is unknown. For patients with NASH, progression to cirrhosis occurs in approximately 11% over a 15-year period.[17]
- NAFLD has an estimated prevalence of 6% to 14% in the general population in the US.[18]
- **NAFLD should be considered in the differential diagnosis of patients with elevated liver enzymes, particularly those with the metabolic syndrome.**
- Imaging studies, including ultrasound, CT, and MRI, may show steatosis, but the presence of inflammation can only be determined by liver biopsy.
- Weight loss improves liver histology, and bariatric surgery can be considered in morbidly obese patients.[16] Discontinuation of medications associated with NAFLD (e.g., amiodarone, corticosteroids, and total parenteral nutrition) should also be considered.

Alpha-1 Antitrypsin Deficiency

- Alpha-1 antitrypsin (α1AT) is a PI. α1AT deficiency is an **autosomal recessive** disorder that damages the liver through the accumulation of misfolded α1AT in hepatocytes and damages the lungs through uninhibited proteolysis, resulting in cirrhosis and emphysema.
- Patients with low serum α1AT levels (<10% to 15% of normal) should undergo α1AT genotype testing. The M allele gives rise to the normal PI, while S and Z are the most common deficiency alleles. The genotypes associated with liver disease are SZ, ZZ, and possibly MZ.[19] Patients who are homozygous for the Z allele may develop chronic hepatitis, cirrhosis, or HCC at a rate of 10% to 15% in the first 20 years of life.
- Diagnosis requires liver biopsy showing periportal hepatocytes with intracellular globules.
- No specific drug therapy exists for α1AT-associated liver disease.
- Liver transplantation in patients with decompensated cirrhosis normalizes α1AT production.

Hereditary Hemochromatosis

GENERAL PRINCIPLES

- Hereditary hemochromatosis is characterized by increased iron absorption and toxic deposition of iron into parenchymal cells of various tissues. It can be caused by mutations that affect any of the proteins that limit the entry of iron into the blood.
- **Ninety percent of individuals with hereditary hemochromatosis are homozygous for the mutation C282Y in the HFE gene on chromosome 6.** However, not all patients with the mutation develop iron overload.[20] There are other conditions, not linked to the C282Y mutation, associated with iron overload or high ferritin, suggesting that other proteins in the iron metabolism process are defective.
- Patients with a family history of hemochromatosis in a first-degree relative due to an HFE gene mutation should be screened for hemochromatosis.[21]

- Noncirrhotic patients appropriately treated for hereditary hemochromatosis have an excellent prognosis. **The survival rate in appropriately treated noncirrhotic patients is identical to that of the general population.**
- Patients with cirrhosis or advanced fibrosis are at increased risk for the development of HCC despite therapy and should be routinely screened for HCC.

DIAGNOSIS

- Patients with hereditary hemochromatosis may be asymptomatic or may develop hepatic dysfunction (including cirrhosis), bronzing of the skin, diabetes, cardiomyopathy, arthritis, and hypogonadism.
- **Transferrin saturation (serum iron divided by the total iron-binding capacity) $\geq$45% and/or elevated ferritin are suggestive of hemochromatosis and should be further investigated with HFE mutation analysis.**[21]
- Indications for liver biopsy in patients with an HFE gene mutation include ferritin >1,000 μg/L and elevated transaminases.
- MRI is the modality of choice for noninvasive quantification of iron storage in the liver.

TREATMENT

- Treatment consists of phlebotomy (500 mL blood) every 1 to 2 weeks until the ferritin is 50 to100 μg/L. The need for maintenance phlebotomy varies.[21]
- For patients who cannot tolerate phlebotomy, iron chelation with deferoxamine may be an alternative. Side effects include gastrointestinal distress, visual and auditory impairments, and muscle cramps. Deferoxamine is only given IV, IM, or SC. Deferasirox is another alternative in the treatment of iron overload and is given orally.[22]

Wilson Disease

GENERAL PRINCIPLES

- **Wilson disease is an autosomal recessive disorder (ATP7B gene on chromosome 13) leading to progressive copper overload.** Incidence is 1 in 30,000 with a female to male ratio of 2:1 and an age at presentation ranging from 6 to 20 years.
- The gene mutation in Wilson disease results in accumulation of copper in the liver and ultimately liver injury. In addition, copper is also deposited in other organs, notably the brain, kidneys, and cornea.
- First-degree relatives of patients diagnosed with Wilson disease should be screened for this condition.

DIAGNOSIS

- Presentation of liver disease in Wilson disease ranges from asymptomatic to acute liver failure.
- Extrahepatic manifestations include neuropsychiatric symptoms, gold-brown rings at the periphery of the cornea on slit-lamp examination (Kayser-Fleischer rings), Coombs-negative hemolytic anemia, renal tubular acidosis, arthritis, and osteopenia.
- **Low serum ceruloplasmin of <20 mg/dL (seen in 85% of patients) and elevated 24-hour urine copper level of >100 mcg/24 hours suggest the diagnosis.**[23]
- Liver biopsy with a copper level >250 mcg/g (dry weight) is consistent with Wilson disease.

TREATMENT

- **Copper-chelating agents (including D-penicillamine, trientine, and zinc salts) block the intestinal absorption of copper and are used to treat Wilson disease.**[23] While zinc and trientine are well tolerated, D-penicillamine is associated with several side effects including hypersensitivity, bone marrow suppression, proteinuria, systemic lupus erythematosus, and Goodpasture syndrome.
- Patients presenting with fulminant liver failure should be considered for liver transplant.
- Liver transplant in patients with Wilson disease without neurologic symptoms carries an excellent prognosis.

ALCOHOLIC AND DRUG-INDUCED LIVER DISEASE

Alcohol-Induced Liver Disease

GENERAL PRINCIPLES

- Alcohol is, when used in excess, a hepatotoxin capable of inducing a spectrum of diseases including fatty liver, alcoholic hepatitis, and alcoholic cirrhosis. **In the US, excessive alcohol consumption is the third leading preventable cause of death and 50% of all cases of cirrhosis are due to alcohol abuse**.
- Patients with fatty liver are generally asymptomatic and may have hepatomegaly and mild transaminase elevations (typically with an AST:ALT ratio >2:1).
- Alcoholic hepatitis ranges from asymptomatic to quite severe, with fever, abdominal pain, jaundice, complications of portal hypertension and, in some cases, liver failure and death.
- Alcoholic cirrhosis is typically micronodular and results from chronic alcohol consumption. The sensitivity of the liver to damage from alcohol varies widely. Among patients with heavy alcohol consumption, only 6% to 41% progress to cirrhosis.[24]

DIAGNOSIS

- A thorough history is essential; **self-reports of alcohol consumption may be underestimates.**
- Patients with suspected alcoholic liver disease should be evaluated for coexisting causes of liver injury. Liver biopsy may be helpful if alternative diagnoses are being considered.
- Severity of alcoholic hepatitis can be estimated by using a discriminant function.[25]

$$(DF) = (4.6 \times [\text{measured PT} - \text{control PT}]) + \text{bilirubin (mg / dL)}$$

- **A DF of >32 defines a severe alcoholic hepatitis and is associated with a high 30-day mortality**.
- **In-hospital mortality of severe alcoholic hepatitis is approximately 50%.**

TREATMENT

- **The cornerstone of treatment is abstinence from alcohol**. Abstinence from alcohol may reverse fatty liver and lead to biochemical improvement in patients with alcoholic cirrhosis.
- In alcoholic hepatitis, medical therapies include **corticosteroids and pentoxifylline**. Corticosteroids (prednisolone 40 mg daily for 4 weeks) should be considered in subjects with alcoholic hepatitis and a DF of ≥32 or encephalopathy. Potential contraindications

to steroids include infection, gastrointestinal bleeding, and pancreatitis.[26] Pentoxifylline (400 mg tid for 4 weeks) decreases cytokine production and is an alternative for patients in whom steroids are contraindicated.[27] In addition, good nutrition is an essential component of treatment.

• Patients with decompensated alcoholic cirrhosis may be considered for transplant when they have demonstrated sustained abstinence from alcohol (>6 months) and enrollment in a rehabilitation program.

DRUG-INDUCED LIVER INJURY

GENERAL PRINCIPLES

• **Drug-induced liver injury (DILI) may be intrinsic or idiosyncratic.** Intrinsic hepatotoxicity is a direct, dose-dependent drug effect. Idiosyncratic hepatotoxicity includes hypersensitivity reactions and altered drug metabolism, which are variable and not predictable.
• Incidence of DILI is estimated to be between 1 in 10,000 and 1 in 100,000. A searchable database of medications and supplements associated with liver injury is available online (http://livertox.nih.gov, last accessed April 18, 2014). DILI accounts for up to 10% of all adverse drug reactions and represents 10% of hepatology consultations.
• DILI is a frequent cause of acute jaundice, and it is the **most common cause of acute liver failure in the US. Jaundice in DILI is a poor prognostic indicator**, with a case fatality rate of 10% to 50%.[28]
• Use of herbal and dietary supplements is common in the US. Like other pharmaceuticals, these supplements may exhibit hepatotoxicity, manifested as transient abnormalities of liver enzymes or acute or chronic hepatitis.

DIAGNOSIS

• **Clinical presentation of DILI ranges from asymptomatic elevation of liver enzymes to fulminant hepatic failure.**
• A high index of suspicion is essential to suspect DILI. A thorough interview with the patient and his/her relatives and a review of pharmacy records are essential to define the drugs, herbs, or dietary supplements involved in the liver injury.
• Diagnostic criteria include clinical suspicion, temporal relationship between drug exposure and liver injury, and resolution of injury after discontinuing the offending agent.
• Patterns of liver biochemistry abnormalities in DILI include hepatocellular (AST and ALT >2× ULN), cholestatic (alkaline phosphatase and conjugated bilirubin >2× ULN), and mixed (hepatocellular and cholestatic).

TREATMENT

Treatment involves stopping the offending agent, instituting supportive measures and, when applicable (e.g., acetaminophen), use of drug-specific therapy.[28]

Acetaminophen Hepatotoxicity

GENERAL PRINCIPLES

• Acetaminophen is a safe and effective analgesic and antipyretic if consumed at the recommended dose of <4 g/day. However, it is the most common cause of acute liver failure in the US (suicide attempts or therapeutic misadventures).[29]

- **The toxicity of acetaminophen is dose dependent.** Overdose is defined as >150 mg/kg in children and >10 to 15 g in adults. Toxicity can actually occur at doses <10 g.
- Toxicity is due to the metabolism of acetaminophen to toxic N-acetyl-p-benzoquinone imine (NAPQI). At usual doses, NAPQI is quickly detoxified by conjugation with glutathione.
- Hepatotoxicity is not increased in the setting of nonalcoholic chronic liver disease. In chronic ethanol abusers, the repetitive use of supratherapeutic doses of acetaminophen is linked to liver toxicity.
- Drugs that induce CYP2E1 enzymes (carbamazepine, phenytoin, phenobarbital, isoniazid, and rifampin) can produce liver injury in the absence of acetaminophen overdose.

DIAGNOSIS

- Patients may present asymptomatically; symptoms of toxicity may not develop until 1 to 2 days after ingestion. Initial symptoms are nonspecific and include anorexia, malaise, nausea, and vomiting, followed by right upper quadrant pain.
- Subsequently, hepatic failure develops, including jaundice, encephalopathy (cerebral edema), and coagulopathy. Renal failure can also develop at this point, due to drug-induced acute tubular necrosis and dehydration.
- Differential diagnosis includes gastroenteritis, acute cholecystitis, pancreatitis, alcoholic hepatitis, viral hepatitis, Reye syndrome, shock liver, and other forms of drug/herb hepatotoxicity.
- The Rumack-Matthew nomogram is used to predict the likelihood of hepatotoxicity given the serum acetaminophen level obtained and the time since consumption.[29]
- Serum aminotransferases begin to rise sharply about 12 hours after ingestion. Peak levels occur at about 72 hours and are frequently >3,000 IU/L.
- Hepatic synthetic function declines as hepatotoxicity progresses (e.g., prolonged PT, hyperbilirubinemia, hypoalbuminemia, and hypoglycemia). Acidosis, azotemia, and electrolyte disturbances may occur.

TREATMENT

- Treatment involves the prompt administration of N-acetylcysteine (NAC) (a glutathione precursor) to protect the liver against the toxic metabolites of acetaminophen.[29] If the patient presents with acute liver failure, treatment should be administered in intensive care units of hospitals with liver transplant programs.
- **Treatment should begin ideally within 8 to 10 hours postingestion, but may be beneficial up to 24 hours**.
- NAC is given orally or intravenously.
  - Oral: Loading dose of 140 mg/kg followed by a maintenance dose of 70 mg/kg every 4 hours for a total of 17 doses over 72 hours.
  - Intravenous: Loading dose of 150 mg/kg IV over 15 minutes followed by a maintenance dose of 50 mg/kg over 4 hours followed by 100 mg/kg over 16 hours. Other IV dosage regimens have also been suggested.
- Patients who present late (>10 hours after ingestion) may benefit from longer treatment durations than those described above.
- Prompt administration of N-acetylcysteine is associated with a good outcome. Unfortunately, many patients present for medical care late, once the toxic effects are established and the acute liver failure is too advanced to be reversed by simple administration of NAC.
- Careful attention should be paid to detecting cerebral edema and correcting fluid, electrolyte, and acid-base abnormalities.
- **Liver transplantation should be considered in patients with liver failure that continues to progress despite adequate treatment.**[29]

TUMORS OF THE LIVER

Adenoma

- Hepatic adenomas are rare, benign epithelial liver tumors commonly associated with a history of **oral contraceptive (OC) use** and **androgen steroid therapy**. Usually located in the right hepatic lobe, roughly three-fourths of adenomas are **solitary**.[30]
- The incidence of liver adenomas is estimated to be 0.1 per year per 100,000 and has **grown to be 3 to 4 per 100,000 in long-term OC users**.[31]
- Hepatic adenomas, especially those that are larger, may present with **upper abdominal pain**. Adenomas >5 cm in diameter have an increased risk of **spontaneous bleeding**. Hepatic adenomas have a risk of **malignant transformation** that has been calculated at 4% to 10%.[32]
- Diagnosis is usually based on the clinical setting with the assistance of imaging studies. In particular, contrast CT scans may show early-phase peripheral enhancement followed by centripetal flow during the portal venous phase.[33]
- **OC cessation** may lead to regression and even complete resolution of hepatic adenomas.[34]
- Because of the risk of hemorrhage, rupture, and malignant transformation, **surgical resection** is typically recommended for adenomas >5 cm in diameter.[35]

Hemangioma

- Hepatic hemangiomas, the **most common benign liver tumors**, are nonepithelial lesions usually discovered incidentally.[36]
- Approximately three-fourths are found in females. Female sex hormones (endogenous or exogenous) may exert influence over the growth of hemangiomas, but significant enlargement still only occurs in a minority of patients.[37]
- Although typically of minimal clinical concern, hemangiomas measuring >10 cm in diameter may be symptomatic (right upper quadrant abdominal pain, nausea, or early satiety).
- Giant hepatic hemangiomas may be associated with the Kasabach-Merritt syndrome, which is characterized by fibrinolysis, thrombocytopenia, coagulopathy, and a fatal outcome in up to 30% of patients and often represents an indication for liver transplantation.
- Diagnosis of liver hemangiomas is made on imaging.
- As most hemangiomas remain stable in size, **surgical indications are typically limited** to symptomatic patients with giant hemangiomas.[38]

Focal Nodular Hyperplasia

- Focal nodular hyperplasia (FNH) is a benign liver tumor that is usually **solitary** (but may be multiple in 20% of cases) and <5 cm in diameter. FNH is the second most common benign liver tumor after hemangiomas and is found predominantly in females in a roughly 10:1 ratio.[39]
- It is thought that FNH arises in response to arterial malformations as hyperplastic lesions. While controversial, current OC (low-dose estrogen) use is not associated with FNH lesions. Moreover, pregnancy does not affect the clinical behavior of FNH.[40]
- Diagnosis is made with imaging modalities; CT and MRI are particularly specific for FNH with typical features. However, imaging similarities have been described with liver adenomas and even HCCs. Therefore, when findings are atypical, invasive diagnostic measures (liver biopsy) should be considered.[41]
- FNH has **no known malignant potential** and only very rarely ruptures or bleeds. Most FNH lesions remain stable in size, and a minority may regress. Given the absence of

malignant potential, stability of most lesions, possibility of lesion regression, and especially low risk of rupture, FNH is almost always **managed conservatively**.[42]
- Resection should be considered for patients with symptomatic FNH (large and subcapsular lesions), lesions with atypical radiologic characteristics, and lesions that increase in size.

Hepatocellular Carcinoma

GENERAL PRINCIPLES

- HCC represents an increasingly common complication of liver disease.
- **Cirrhosis is present in 80% to 90% of patients with HCC**.
- Over 500,000 individuals worldwide are diagnosed each year with HCC (fifth most common cancer in men and the seventh most common cancer in women). Roughly half occur in the setting of chronic HBV infection.[43] Nearly 85% of cases of HCC occur in **developing countries**.[44]
- **In the US, up to half of all cases of HCC occur in the setting of HCV infection**. Other associated conditions include alcoholic cirrhosis, α_1AT deficiency, and hemochromatosis.[45]
- Early diagnosis is essential, as surgical resection and liver transplantation can improve long-term survival with 5-year disease-free survival exceeding 50%. Advanced HCC has a dismal prognosis with a 5-year survival of 0% to 10%.

DIAGNOSIS

- Clinical presentation is proportional to the stage of disease. HCC may present with right upper quadrant abdominal pain, weight loss, and hepatomegaly. HCC should be suspected in a cirrhotic patient who develops manifestations of liver decompensation.
- The diagnosis of HCC can often be made with **imaging**. In patients with suspicious imaging findings, an **elevated serum α-fetoprotein** >400 is highly predictive of HCC. Liver biopsy can be considered for patients at risk for HCC with suspicious liver lesions >1 cm with noncharacteristic imaging features.
- Since patients with cirrhosis are at the highest risk for developing HCC, **surveillance ultrasonography or cross-sectional imaging is recommended for cirrhotics every 6 months** to allow diagnosis at early stages. Serum α-fetoprotein should not be used as the only screening modality.[46]

TREATMENT

- Oral systemic chemotherapy with sorafenib may be used as palliative therapy for advanced-stage HCC. In patients with advanced HCC, median survival and radiologic progression were 3 months longer for patients treated with sorafenib compared to placebo.[47]
- **Transarterial chemoembolization (TACE) or transarterial radioembolization (TARE)** may be used for palliation in intermediate-stage or multifocal HCC or to downstage HCC to meet the Milan criteria.[46]
- Local radiofrequency or alcohol ablation therapy is best for very early-stage HCC or early-stage HCC not amenable to surgical resection or transplantation.[48]
- The best candidates for surgical resection are those with small solitary tumors in the absence of cirrhosis or in those with cirrhosis with well-preserved liver function.
- **Liver transplantation** represents a curative treatment, but patients must meet the Milan criteria to be eligible for transplantation (solitary nodule ≤5 cm or three nodules each ≤3 cm).

Cholangiocarcinoma

- Cholangiocarcinoma is a malignancy affecting the intrahepatic and extrahepatic bile ducts. It represents the second most common primary hepatic cancer behind HCC.
- Men are more frequently affected, and it typically presents in the seventh decade of life. Risk factors include **PSC**, bile duct cysts, hepatolithiasis, toxins (e.g., thorotrast), and parasitic infections (e.g., hepatobiliary flukes).[49]
- Since tumors are often locally advanced at presentation, **prognosis is poor** with 5-year survival rates of 5% to 10%.
- When symptomatic (often late in the natural history), cholangiocarcinomas may present with symptoms of **bile duct obstruction** and right upper quadrant abdominal pain.[50]
- **Serum CA 19-9** is often elevated, but has **limited specificity** for cholangiocarcinoma.[51]
- Imaging can identify ductal dilation or a dominant stricture, but may not always identify the primary tumor. Ideal imaging modalities include MRCP and ERCP, which afford the opportunity for visualization of the biliary tree as well as diagnosis (via brush cytology, biopsy, and/or fluorescence in situ hybridization [FISH]).
- **Surgical resection** represents a chance for cure, though postsurgical cancer recurrence remains a concern. Radiation and chemotherapy have not been shown to enhance survival for inoperable tumors. Liver transplantation in combination with neoadjuvant chemoradiotherapy can represent an option for selected perihilar cholangiocarcinomas. Palliation may involve biliary drainage via stents or photodynamic therapy.[52]

CIRRHOSIS

GENERAL PRINCIPLES

- Cirrhosis is characterized by the diffuse replacement of liver cells by **fibrotic tissue**, leading to nodular-appearing distortion of the normal liver architecture.
- Although **chronic viral infection, alcoholic liver disease, and NASH** account for the majority of cases of cirrhosis, other causes may include AIH, drug-induced hepatotoxicity, venoocclusive disease, Wilson disease, hemochromatosis, and α1AT deficiency. In some instances, no etiology for cirrhosis is identified; in which case, it is categorized as cryptogenic.

DIAGNOSIS

The diagnosis of cirrhosis typically lies in the **recognition of its complications**. The main complications of cirrhosis include portal hypertension (esophageal and gastric varices, portal hypertensive gastropathy and colopathy, gastric antral vascular ectasia, ascites and spontaneous bacterial peritonitis [SBP], hepatorenal syndrome [HRS]), hepatic encephalopathy, and HCC.

COMPLICATIONS

Portal Hypertension

- Portal hypertension represents the **primary complication** of cirrhosis and is characterized by increased resistance to portal flow and increased portal venous inflow. Portal hypertension is established by measuring the pressure gradient between the hepatic vein and the portal vein (normal approximately 3 mm Hg). Clinical consequences of portal hypertension typically appear when the portosystemic pressure gradient exceeds 10 mm Hg.[53]

- Ultrasonography, CT, and MRI showing cirrhosis, splenomegaly, collateral venous circulation, and ascites may indicate portal hypertension.
- Upper endoscopy can reveal varices (esophageal or gastric), portal hypertensive gastropathy, or gastric antrum vascular ectasia (GAVE).

Esophageal and Gastric Varices

- Esophageal and gastric varices are asymptomatic sequelae of portal hypertension until they rupture. **Upper gastrointestinal bleeding** secondary to variceal rupture is the most common lethal complication of cirrhosis.
- In 50% of patients with cirrhosis, varices are present. Predictors of bleeding risk include **variceal size, red wale marks on varices, and severity of liver dysfunction.** Variceal hemorrhage happens at a yearly rate of 5% to 15% and is associated with a mortality rate of 20% at 6 weeks.[54]
- **Screening esophagogastroduodenoscopy (EGD) should be performed at the time of diagnosis of cirrhosis**.
  - In patients with compensated cirrhosis without varices, EGD should be repeated in 3 years. In patients with low-risk small varices that have not bled, EGD should be repeated in 2 years.[55]
  - However, if small varices are present in the setting of increased risk for hemorrhage (decompensated cirrhosis or red wale marks) or medium or larger varices are present, indefinite treatment with **nonselective β-blockers,** such as propranolol or nadolol, decreases the risk of variceal bleeding. **Endoscopic variceal ligation (EVL)** may be equivalent to β-blockade for preventing the first variceal hemorrhage in high-risk varices and should be especially considered in patients with contraindications to or noncompliance with β-blockade.[56]
- After variceal hemorrhage, secondary prophylaxis with **both** nonselective β-blockade and EVL should be used.
- **Transjugular intrahepatic portosystemic shunt (TIPS)** can be considered for recurrent episodes of variceal hemorrhage. Surgical shunts are now rarely performed.

Ascites and Spontaneous Bacterial Peritonitis

- Ascites is the accumulation of fluid (>25 mL) within the peritoneal cavity. While commonly due to portal hypertension, other causes of ascites may include peritoneal carcinomatosis, heart failure, tuberculosis, myxedema, pancreatic disease, nephrotic syndrome, trauma to the lymphatic system or ureters, and serositis.
- Clinical presentation may range from ascites detected only by imaging to a distended, bulging, and sometimes tender abdomen. Physical exam can reveal shifting dullness, dullness to flank percussion, palpable fluid wave, and umbilical hernia.
- The initial laboratory investigation of ascitic fluid should include an ascitic fluid cell count and differential, ascitic fluid total protein, and serum-ascites albumin gradient (SAAG). An **SAAG value of >1.1 g/dL** is consistent with ascites secondary to portal hypertension.[57]
- First-line treatment of cirrhotic ascites includes **sodium restriction (2 g/day)** and **combination diuretics** (typically oral spironolactone starting at 100 mg PO qd and oral furosemide starting at 40 mg PO qd).[58]
- Patients should be observed closely for signs of dehydration, electrolyte disturbances, encephalopathy, muscle cramps, and renal insufficiency. NSAIDs may blunt the effects of diuretics and increase the risk of renal dysfunction. Care must also be taken to avoid salt substitutes rich in potassium.
- Ascites is considered **refractory** when unresponsive to maximal doses of diuretics (spironolactone 400 mg/day and furosemide 160 mg/day) or if the patient is unable to tolerate diuretic therapy. Refractory ascites may require treatment with serial large-volume paracentesis or TIPS. Moreover, referral for liver transplantation should be expedited.[59]

- **Spontaneous bacterial peritonitis** (SBP) is an infectious complication of portal hypertension–related ascites defined as ascitic fluid containing **>250 neutrophils/mm³**. SBP may be asymptomatic. Cirrhotic patients with ascites and evidence of any clinical deterioration should undergo diagnostic paracentesis and be treated with empiric antibiotics. These patients typically require hospitalization. Regarding SBP prophylaxis, norfloxacin 400 mg PO qd is the treatment of choice and should be given indefinitely to any patient who has been diagnosed with SBP.[60]

Portosystemic Encephalopathy

- Portosystemic encephalopathy (PSE) is characterized by altered consciousness and disordered neuromuscular activity in patients with acute or chronic hepatic failure or portosystemic shunting. While its pathogenesis is controversial, PSE probably results from disordered clearance of neurotransmitters and gut-derived toxins. Excess ammonia, in particular, may lead to astrocyte swelling and cerebral edema.[61]
- Common precipitants of PSE may include noncompliance with medications, specifically lactulose; azotemia; opioids or sedative-hypnotic medications; acute liver failure; acute gastrointestinal bleeding; alkalosis (diuretics or diarrhea); constipation; infection; high-protein diet; progressive hepatocellular dysfunction; and portosystemic shunts (surgical or TIPS).
- PSE may be graded by the clinical West Haven criteria. The following grades may overlap and quickly change:
  - Grade I: shortened attention span, trivial lack of awareness, mild confusion, tremor
  - Grade II: lethargy, disorientation, inappropriate behavior, subtle personality change
  - Grade III: somnolence to semistupor (responsive to verbal stimuli), severe confusion
  - Grade IV: coma (unresponsive to stimuli)
- Physical examination findings may include altered mental status, asterixis (flapping tremor not specific to PSE), or hyperactive reflexes.[62]
- Management of PSE includes supportive care, identification of precipitating factors, elimination of sedative or hypnotic medications, and the reduction of gut-derived nitrogenous products.[63] Medications include nonabsorbable disaccharides or antibiotics. Lactulose may be titrated to produce three to five soft bowel movements daily. Moreover, nonabsorbed oral antibiotics, such as rifaximin 550 mg PO bid, may also be used. Neomycin and metronidazole are used less often than rifaximin due to their attendant toxicities.[64]

Hepatopulmonary Syndrome

- Hepatopulmonary syndrome presents as dyspnea and hypoxemia due to pulmonary vasodilation as a result of liver disease.
- Physical exam findings may include **platypnea** (shortness of breath when upright) or **orthodeoxia** (decrease in arterial oxygenation when upright).
- Agitated saline contrast echocardiography (bubble study) may show the early appearance of intravenous microbubbles in the left atrium (within 2 to 3 heartbeats).
- Management of hepatopulmonary syndrome includes supplemental oxygen; resolution is typically seen with liver transplantation.[65]

Hepatorenal Syndrome

- HRS represents functional renal impairment in the setting of acute or chronic liver disease. Precipitants may include systemic infection, SBP, and therapeutic paracentesis (especially without volume expansion).[66]
- **Type I HRS** involves rapidly progressive oliguric renal failure with serum creatinine doubling to ≥2.5 mg/dL in less than 2 weeks, whereas **type II HRS** is a steady and relentless deterioration in renal function associated with refractory ascites and a median survival of 6 months.[67]

- HRS is characterized by **major criteria**: renal failure in the absence of other causes (shock, infection, nephrotoxins, renal outflow obstruction), failure to improve after intravenous volume expansion, and absence of proteinuria >500 mg/day. **Additional criteria** include low urine volume <500 mL/day, low urine sodium concentration <10 mEq/L, urine osmolality greater than plasma osmolality, urine red blood cells <50/hpf, and serum sodium concentration <130 mEq/L.[68]
- Upon the suspicion for or diagnosis of HRS, patients should be admitted for inpatient workup and treatment. Treatments for HRS may include systemic vasoconstrictors (terlipressin, octreotide, midodrine) with plasma expansion. TIPS placement and hemodialysis may represent treatment alternatives to be used in selected patients. Ultimately, liver transplantation is curative.

LIVER TRANSPLANTATION

GENERAL PRINCIPLES

- Liver transplantation represents an effective option for irreversible acute or chronic liver failure, especially when available therapies have failed. The explosive growth in the number of liver transplants in the US over the past several decades has had a favorable impact on chronic liver disease mortality. Survival rates in the US after liver transplantation at 1, 3, and 5 years are 88%, 80%, and 75%, respectively.[69]
- Allocation for liver transplantation is based on the **Model for End-Stage Liver Disease (MELD) score**, which aims to provide donor organs for listed patients with the greatest short-term (3-month) mortality. The MELD score calculation variables are serum bilirubin, international normalized ratio (INR), and serum creatinine. MELD score calculators are readily available online.[70]

INDICATIONS

- Patients should be evaluated for transplant when they reach a **MELD score of ≥15**.
- Liver transplantation evaluation includes multidisciplinary comprehensive physical, physiologic, and psychosocial assessments to address the following 3 concerns: (a) Will liver transplant offer the best chance for long-term survival? (b) Are there any comorbid medical or psychosocial conditions that may outweigh the benefits of transplantation? (c) What is the urgency of transplant (informed by the MELD score)?
- Contraindications to liver transplantation include extrahepatic malignancy, hepatic malignancy with macrovascular or diffuse tumor invasion, active extrahepatic infection, active substance abuse, severe comorbid conditions (especially cardiopulmonary), psychosocial factors likely to preclude recovery, technical and/or anatomical barriers, and brain death.[71]

IMMUNOSUPPRESSION

- Posttransplant immunosuppression aims to prevent the immune system from rejecting the allograft while preserving physiologic defenses against infection and neoplasia.[72]
- Classes of immunosuppressants with attendant concerns include the following:
  - **Corticosteroids** are typically weaned off within 3 to 6 months posttransplant, though they are used as first-line therapy for acute cellular rejection. Side effects of steroids can include hypertension, glucose intolerance, dyslipidemia, central obesity, osteoporosis, avascular necrosis, adrenal suppression, and poor wound healing.

- **Calcineurin inhibitors (CNI),** such as cyclosporine and tacrolimus, represent the foundation of maintenance immunosuppression and are used in >95% of transplant centers on discharge. Classic adverse effects include nephrotoxicity, neurotoxicity (especially with tacrolimus), hypertension, and hyperlipidemia.
- **Mycophenolate mofetil** is notable for its lack of renal toxicity and can be used with low-dose CNI in renal-sparing protocols. Adverse effects can include diarrhea and bone marrow suppression.
- **mTOR inhibitors**, such as sirolimus (SRL) and everolimus (EVL), are rarely used as first-line therapy but may be used in patients with CNI-induced nephrotoxicity. Side effects can include proteinuria, increases in cholesterol and triglycerides, interstitial pneumonitis, and early posttransplant hepatic artery thrombosis.

POSTTRANSPLANT COMPLICATIONS

- Early posttransplant complications typically stem from issues of allograft function, surgical anatomy, or infection. Early complications include **acute cellular rejection** (often managed with steroids), **biliary disease** (such as anastomotic stricture), **hepatic artery thrombosis** (may require retransplantation), or **infection**.
- Posttransplant immunosuppression increases the risk for malignancy (skin and nonskin cancers), cardiometabolic conditions (such as the metabolic syndrome and its components), and infection.[73] Clinicians should, therefore, screen regularly for malignancy, hypertension, diabetes, dyslipidemia, cardiovascular disease, renal disease, and bone mineral density.[74]
- **Chronic rejection** is a late complication.

OUTPATIENT BILIARY AND PANCREATIC DISEASES

Cholelithiasis

GENERAL PRINCIPLES

- Cholelithiasis is a common phenomenon, with an estimated prevalence of 10%.
- Gallstones are typically cholesterol stones, brown stones, or black stones.
  - **Cholesterol stones**, which account for over three-fourths of biliary stones in Westernized societies, are associated with risk factors of female gender, obesity, Native American ethnicity, rapid weight loss, and estrogen therapy.
  - **Brown pigment stones** form when bacteria in the biliary tree deconjugate bilirubin, forming insoluble calcium bilirubinate.
  - **Black pigment stones** typically develop in cirrhosis or chronic hemolytic states, such as sickle cell disease, thalassemias, or hereditary spherocytosis.[75]
- Biliary sludge appears to be capable of producing biliary symptoms and should be managed in same fashion as gallstones.[76]

DIAGNOSIS

- **Approximately 80% of gallstones are asymptomatic** (with many found incidentally); however, complications from obstruction of the biliary tree may develop in a minority of patients.[77]
- **Uncomplicated biliary colic** is the most common manifestation and is characterized by several hours of right hypochondrium or epigastric pain often radiating to the right shoulder as well as intolerance to fried or fatty foods.[78]

- Complications include acute cholecystitis, choledocholithiasis, ascending cholangitis, gallstone pancreatitis, and gallstone ileus.
- **Ultrasound** is the most frequently used test for cholelithiasis, with greater sensitivity than CT.

TREATMENT

- Given that most gallstones are asymptomatic, laparoscopic **cholecystectomy** is only indicated to prevent recurrent symptoms and complications from symptomatic gallstones. Patients at high risk for gallbladder carcinoma, such as those with calcified or "porcelain" gallbladders and those of Native American descent, should be considered for cholecystectomy even in the absence of symptoms.
- Dissolution therapy with **ursodeoxycholic acid** may be an option for patients with symptomatic cholesterol gallstones who are not surgical candidates. Extracorporeal biliary shock wave lithotripsy is now rarely utilized.

Chronic Pancreatitis

GENERAL PRINCIPLES

- Chronic pancreatitis represents **irreversible** morphologic and functional damage to the pancreas from **progressive inflammatory changes**.
- Causes of chronic pancreatitis include the following:
  - **Alcohol** is the most common cause in Westernized societies, though only 5% to 10% of alcoholics develop chronic pancreatitis.
  - **Genetic syndromes,** such as **cystic fibrosis** or **hereditary pancreatitis** (autosomal dominant).
  - **Ductal obstruction** from stones, trauma, neoplasia, or sphincter of Oddi dysfunction.
  - **Autoimmune conditions** such as systemic lupus erythematosus, Sjögren syndrome, inflammatory bowel disease, and autoimmune pancreatitis.
  - **"Tropical" pancreatitis** typically occurs in young people in impoverished areas of Africa and Asia, though its cause is unknown.
  - **Idiopathic** pancreatitis accounts for 30% to 40% of chronic pancreatitis.[79]

DIAGNOSIS

- Clinical presentation is classically **recurrent attacks of dull upper abdominal pain** that may radiate to the midback or scapula and be associated with nausea and vomiting.
- The diagnosis of chronic pancreatitis is typically made clinically. **Amylase and lipase may be normal or only mildly elevated,** and laboratory testing for pancreatic exocrine function can be complex.
- **Pancreatic calcifications** may be seen on abdominal plain films in up to 30% of patients with pancreatitis. Their presence does not correlate with disease severity. While imaging with ultrasound or CT is relatively sensitive for chronic pancreatitis, MRCP, endoscopic ultrasound (EUS), and ERCP are the best imaging studies for diagnosis and management.

TREATMENT

- **Alcohol cessation** is paramount.
- **Pain** is the symptom that most frequently requires treatment.
  - **Analgesia** with nonopioids and opioids is often needed.
  - **Pancreatic enzyme supplementation** reduces pancreatic stimulation and may decrease pain but should be used with acid suppression to minimize acid degradation.
  - **Octreotide**, a somatostatin analog, may aid with pain relief.
  - **Celiac plexus nerve block** is a treatment alternative in refractory cases.

- ○ Surgical drainage (pancreaticojejunostomy), surgical resection, lithotripsy, or endoscopic stent placement can be considered.[80]
- Pancreatic insufficiency occurs when >80% to 90% of pancreatic function is compromised, resulting in **steatorrhea (fat malabsorption)** and/or **glucose intolerance** (exocrine and endocrine pancreatic insufficiency, respectively). Malabsorption is typically managed with a low-fat diet and pancreatic enzyme replacement therapy (along with acid suppression).
- Pancreatic **pseudocysts** may be asymptomatic. They develop in 10% of chronic pancreatitis, may rupture or become infected, and require endoscopic, radiologic, or surgical drainage.
- **Pancreatic ascites** is notable for a high ascitic fluid amylase concentration, and treatment may be nonoperative (aspiration or diuretics) or operative.
- **Bile duct or duodenal obstruction** typically presents with pain and often requires endoscopic or surgical intervention.
- **Splenic vein thrombosis** may occur due to adjacent inflammation and should be suspected in patients with gastric varices. Splenectomy may be necessary in those with bleeding varices.

Pancreatic Cancer

GENERAL PRINCIPLES

- **Pancreatic ductal adenocarcinoma** ranks fourth among cancer-related deaths in the US. The overall **5-year survival rate for pancreatic cancer is <5%**. Less than 10% of pancreatic cancers are localized at diagnosis. More than 80% of pancreatic cancers are diagnosed after the age of 60 years.[81]
- The causes of pancreatic cancer are not well known, but the risk of pancreatic cancer in smokers is approximately three times that in nonsmokers. Other risk factors may include male sex, age >45 years, African American ethnicity, chronic pancreatitis, heavy alcohol consumption, family history of pancreatic cancer, BRCA2 mutations, history of partial gastrectomy, obesity, and diabetes.[82]
- Universal screening is controversial and not currently recommended.
- About two-thirds of pancreatic cancers occur in the **head of the pancreas** (where they can cause obstructive cholestasis), with the remainder in the body or tail.

DIAGNOSIS

- The classic symptoms of pancreatic cancer are **painless jaundice**, **pain** (dull, deep epigastric or right upper quadrant) and **weight loss** (anorexia from pain, cachexia from proinflammatory cytokines, and malabsorption from pancreatic insufficiency). Other presentations may include dysglycemia, pancreatitis, gastrointestinal bleeding, emesis, or thrombophlebitis (Trousseau sign).
- Upon suspicion, **imaging** frequently establishes the diagnosis. CT predicts surgical resectability with 80% to 90% accuracy. **ERCP** allows for tissue diagnosis and/or stent placement for biliary obstruction. EUS may be used, especially if no mass is seen on CT or for fine needle aspiration (FNA).[83] Diagnostic testing may include the **CA 19-9** level (tumor marker with limited sensitivity and specificity for pancreatic cancer).

TREATMENT

- When surgical resection is possible, a **Whipple procedure** (cephalic pancreaticoduodenectomy) may be performed for tumors of the pancreatic head, whereas a distal pancreatectomy and splenectomy may be performed for tumors of the pancreatic body or tail.
- For nonresectable pancreatic cancer, palliative options include endoscopically placed **stents to relieve biliary obstruction**, chemoradiation (typically with 5-fluorouracil or gemcitabine), and derivative surgical procedures.

REFERENCES

1. Franco E, Meleleo C, Serino L, et al. Hepatitis A: epidemiology and prevention in developing countries. *World J Hepatol* 2012;4:68–73.
2. Victor JC, Monto AS, Surdina TY, et al. Hepatitis A vaccine versus immune globulin for postexposure prophylaxis. *N Engl J Med* 2007;357:1685–1694.
3. Margolis HS, Alter MJ, Hadler SC. Hepatitis B: evolving epidemiology and implications for control. *Semin Liver Dis* 1991;11:84–92.
4. European Association for the Study of the Liver. EASL clinical practice guidelines: management of chronic hepatitis B. *J Hepatol* 2009;50:227–242.
5. Lok AS, McMahon BJ. Chronic hepatitis B: update 2009. *Hepatology* 2009;50:661–662.
6. Rein DB, Smith BD, Wittenborn JS, et al. The cost-effectiveness of birth-cohort screening for hepatitis C antibody in U.S. primary care settings. *Ann Intern Med* 2012;156:263–70.
7. El-Serag HB. Epidemiology of viral hepatitis and hepatocellular carcinoma. *Gastroenterology* 2012;142:1264–1273.
8. Smith BD, Morgan RL, Beckett GA, et al. Hepatitis C virus testing of persons born during 1945–1965: recommendations from the Centers for Disease Control and Prevention. *Ann Intern Med* 2012;157:817–822.
9. Koff RS, Dienstag JL. Extrahepatic manifestations of hepatitis C and the association with alcoholic liver disease. *Semin Liver Dis* 1995;15:101–109.
10. Jaeckel E, Cornberg M, Wedemeyer H, et al. Treatment of acute hepatitis C with interferon alfa-2b. *N Engl J Med* 2001;345:1452–1457.
11. Manns MP, Czaja AJ, Gorham JD, et al. Diagnosis and management of autoimmune hepatitis. *Hepatology* 2010;51:2193–2213.
12. Hennes EM, Zeniya M, Czaja AJ, et al. Simplified criteria for the diagnosis of autoimmune hepatitis. *Hepatology* 2008;48:169–176.
13. Lindor KD, Gershwin ME, Poupon R, et al. Primary biliary cirrhosis. *Hepatology* 2009;50:291–308.
14. Chapman R, Fevery J, Kalloo A, et al. Diagnosis and management of primary sclerosing cholangitis. *Hepatology* 2010;51:660–678.
15. Maggs JR, Chapman RW. An update on primary sclerosing cholangitis. *Curr Opin Gastroenterol* 2008;24:377–383.
16. Chalasani N, Younossi Z, Lavine JE, et al. The diagnosis and management of nonalcoholic fatty liver disease: practice guideline by the American Association for the Study of Liver Diseases, American College of Gastroenterology, and the American Gastroenterological Association. *Hepatology* 2012;55:2005–2023.
17. Angulo P. Long-term mortality in nonalcoholic fatty liver disease: is liver histology of any prognostic significance? *Hepatology* 2010;51:373–375.
18. Clark JM. The epidemiology of nonalcoholic fatty liver disease in adults. *J Clin Gastroenterol* 2006;40:S5–S10.
19. Fairbanks KD, Tavill AS. Liver disease in alpha 1-antitrypsin deficiency: a review. *Am J Gastroenterol* 2008;103:2136–2141.
20. Olynyk JK, Cullen DJ, Aquilia S, et al. A population-based study of the clinical expression of the hemochromatosis gene. *N Engl J Med* 1999;341:718–724.
21. Bacon BR, Adams PC, Kowdley KV, et al. Diagnosis and management of hemochromatosis: 2011 practice guideline by the American Association for the Study of Liver Diseases. *Hepatology* 2011;54:328–343.
22. Maxwell KL, Kowdley KV. Metals and the liver. *Curr Opin Gastroenterol* 2012;28:217–22.
23. Roberts EA, Schilsky ML. Diagnosis and treatment of Wilson disease: an update. *Hepatology* 2008;47:2089–111.

24. Mandayam S, Jamal MM, Morgan TR. Epidemiology of alcoholic liver disease. *Semin Liver Dis* 2004;24:217–232.

25. Maddrey WC, Boitnott JK, Bedine MS, et al. Corticosteroid therapy of alcoholic hepatitis. *Gastroenterology* 1978;75:193–199.

26. O'Shea RS, Dasarathy S, McCullough AJ. Alcoholic liver disease. *Am J Gastroenterol* 2010;105:14–32.

27. Akriviadis E, Botla R, Briggs W, et al. Pentoxifylline improves short-term survival in severe acute alcoholic hepatitis: a double-blind, placebo-controlled trial. *Gastroenterology* 2000;119:1637–1648.

28. Navarro VJ, Senior JR. Drug-related hepatotoxicity. *N Engl J Med* 2006;354:731–739.

29. Larson AM. Acetaminophen hepatotoxicity. *Clin Liver Dis* 2007;11:525–548.

30. Bonder A, Afdhal N. Evaluation of liver lesions. *Clin Liver Dis* 2012;16:271–283.

31. Paradis V. Benign liver tumors: an update. *Clin Liver Dis* 2010;14:719–729.

32. Reddy K, Schiff E. Approach to a liver mass. *Semin Liver Dis* 1993;13:423–435.

33. Grazioli L, Federle M, Brancatelli G, et al. Hepatic adenomas: imaging and pathologic findings. *Radiographics* 2001;21:877–892.

34. Aseni P, Sansalone C, Sammartino C, et al. Rapid disappearance of hepatic adenoma after contraceptive withdrawal. *J Clin Gastroenterol* 2001;33:234–236.

35. Barthelmes L, Tait I. Liver cell adenoma and liver cell adenomatosis. *HPB (Oxford)* 2005;7:186–196.

36. Gandolfi L, Leo P, Solmi L, et al. Natural history of hepatic haemangiomas: clinical and ultrasound study. *Gut* 1991;32:677–680.

37. Glinkova V, Shevah O, Boaz M, et al. Hepatic haemangiomas: possible association with female sex hormones. *Gut* 2004;53:1352–1355.

38. Giulante F, Ardito F, Vellone M, et al. Reappraisal of surgical indications and approach for liver hemangioma: single-center experience on 74 patients. *Am J Surg* 2011;201:741–748.

39. Nahm C, Ng K, Lockie P, et al. Focal nodular hyperplasia—a review of myths and truths. *J Gastrointest Surg* 2011;15:2275–2283.

40. Mathieu D, Kobeiter H, Maison P, et al. Oral contraceptive use and focal nodular hyperplasia of the liver. *Gastroenterology* 2000;118:560–564.

41. Choi J, Lee H, Yim J, et al. Focal nodular hyperplasia or focal nodular hyperplasia-like lesions of the liver: a special emphasis on diagnosis. *J Gastroenterol Hepatol* 2011;26:1004–1009.

42. Kuo Y, Wang J, Lu S, et al. Natural course of focal nodular hyperplasia: a long-term follow-up study with sonography. *J Clin Ultrasound* 2009;37:132–137.

43. El-Serag H. Hepatocellular carcinoma. *N Engl J Med* 2011;365:1118–1127.

44. El-Serag H. Epidemiology of viral hepatitis and hepatocellular carcinoma. *Gastroenterology* 2012;142:1264–1273.

45. Davis G, Alter M, El-Serag H, et al. Aging of hepatitis C virus (HCV)-infected persons in the United States: a multiple cohort model of HCV prevalence and disease progression. *Gastroenterology* 2010;138:513–521.

46. Bruix J, Sherman M. Management of hepatocellular carcinoma: An update. American Association for the Study of Liver Diseases Practice Guideline. *Hepatology* 2011;53:1020–1022.

47. Llovet J, Ricci S, Mazzaferro V, et al. *N Engl J Med* 2008;359:378–390.

48. Forner A, Llovet J, Bruix J. Hepatocellular carcinoma. *Lancet* 2012;379:1245–1255.

49. Tyson G, El-Serag H. Risk factors for cholangiocarcinoma. *Hepatology* 2011;54:173–184.

50. De Groen P, Gores G, LaRusso N, et al. Biliary tract cancers. *N Engl J Med* 1999;341:1368–1378.

51. Sinakos E, Saenger A, Keach J, et al. Many patients with primary sclerosing cholangitis and increased serum levels of carbohydrate antigen 19-9 do not have cholangiocarcinoma. *Clin Gastroenterol Hepatol* 2011;9:434–439.

52. Khan S, Thomas H, Davidson B, et al. Cholangiocarcinoma. *Lancet* 2005;366: 1303–1314.

53. Merkel C, Montagnese S. Hepatic venous pressure gradient measurement in clinical hepatology. *Dig Liver Dis* 2011;43:762–767.

54. Garcia-Tsao G, Sanyal A, Grace N, et al. Prevention and management of gastroesophageal varices and variceal hemorrhage in cirrhosis. *Hepatology* 2007;46:922–938.

55. Bosch J, Abraldes J, Groszmann R. Current management of portal hypertension. *J Hepatol* 2003;38:S54–S68.

56. Lay C, Tsai Y, Lee F, et al. Endoscopic variceal ligation versus propranolol in prophylaxis of first variceal bleeding in patients with cirrhosis. *J Gastroenterol Hepatol* 2006;21:413–419.

57. Runyon B, Montano A, Akriviadis E, et al. The serum-ascites albumin gradient is superior to the exudate-transudate concept in the differential diagnosis of ascites. *Ann Intern Med* 1992;117:215–220.

58. Runyon B. Management of adult patients with ascites due to cirrhosis: an update. *Hepatology* 2009;49:2087–2107.

59. Saab S, Nieto J, Lewis S, et al. TIPS versus paracentesis for cirrhotic patients with refractory ascites. *Cochrane Database Syst Rev* 2006;(4):CD004889.

60. Gines P, Angeli P, Lenz K, et al. EASL clinical practice guidelines on the management of ascites, spontaneous bacterial peritonitis, and hepatorenal syndrome in cirrhosis. *J Hepatol* 2010;53:397–417.

61. Prakash R, Mullen K. Mechanisms, diagnosis and management of hepatic encephalopathy. *Nat Rev Gastroenterol Hepatol* 2010;7:515–525.

62. Cash W, McConville P, McDermott E, et al. Current concepts in the assessment and treatment of hepatic encephalopathy. *QJM* 2010;103:9–16.

63. Riordan S, Williams R. Treatment of hepatic encephalopathy. *N Engl J Med* 1997;337: 473–479.

64. Bass N, Mullen K, Sanyal A, et al. Rifaximin treatment in hepatic encephalopathy. *N Engl J Med* 2010;362:1071–1081.

65. Rodriguez-Roisin R, Krowka M. Hepatopulmonary syndrome—a liver-induced lung vascular disorder. *N Engl J Med* 2008;358:2378–2387.

66. Cardenas A. Hepatorenal syndrome: a dreaded complication of end-stage liver disease. *Am J Gastroenterol* 2005;100:460–467.

67. Arroyo V, Guevara M, Gines P. Hepatorenal syndrome in cirrhosis: pathogenesis and treatment. *Gastroenterology* 2002;122:1658–1676.

68. Arroyo V, Gines P, Gerbes A, et al. Definition and diagnostic criteria of refractory ascites and hepatorenal syndrome in cirrhosis. *Hepatology* 1996;23:164–176.

69. Murray K, Carithers R. AASLD practice guidelines: evaluation of the patient for liver transplantation. *Hepatology* 2005;41:1407–1432.

70. Wiesner R, Edwards E, Freeman R, et al. Model for end-stage liver disease (MELD) and allocation of donor livers. *Gastroenterology* 2003;124:91–96.

71. O'Leary J, Lepe R, Davis G. Indications for liver transplantation. *Gastroenterology* 2008;134:1764–1776.

72. Pillai A, Levitsky J. Overview of immunosuppression in liver transplantation. *World J Gastroenterol* 2009;15:4225–4233.

73. Watt K, Pedersen R, Kremers W, et al. Long-term probability of and mortality from de novo malignancy after liver transplantation. *Gastroenterology* 2009;137:2010–2017.

74. Laish I, Braun M, Mor E, et al. Metabolic syndrome in liver transplant recipients: prevalence, risk factors, and association with cardiovascular events. *Liver Transpl* 2011;17:15–22.

75. Johnston D, Kaplan M. Pathogenesis and treatment of gallstones. *N Engl J Med* 1993; 11:412–421.
76. Jungst C, Kullak-Ublick G, Jungst D. Gallstone disease: microlithiasis and sludge. *Best Pract Res Clin Gastroenterol* 2006;20:1053–1062.
77. Thistle J, Cleary P, Lachin J, et al. The natural history of cholelithiasis: the National Cooperative Gallstone Study. *Ann Intern Med* 1984;101:171–175.
78. Festi D, Sottili S, Colecchia A, et al. Clinical manifestations of gallstone disease: evidence from the multicenter Italian study on cholelithiasis (MICOL). *Hepatology* 1999;30: 839–846.
79. Steer M, Waxman I, Freedman S. Chronic pancreatitis. *N Engl J Med* 1995;332: 1482–1490.
80. Warshaw A, Banks P, Fernandez-del Castillo C. AGA technical review: treatment of pain in chronic pancreatitis. *Gastroenterology* 1998;115:765–776.
81. Shaib Y, Davila J, El-Serag H. The epidemiology of pancreatic cancer in the United States: changes below the surface. *Aliment Pharmacol Ther* 2006;24:87–94.
82. Hassan M, Bondy M, Wolff R, et al. Risk factors for pancreatic cancer. *Am J Gastroenterol* 2007;102:2696–2707.
83. Hidalgo M. Pancreatic cancer. *N Engl J Med* 2010;362:1605–1617.

GENERAL PRINCIPLES

- Ulcerative colitis (UC) and Crohn disease (CD) are chronic inflammatory disorders of the gastrointestinal (GI) tract categorized under the spectrum of inflammatory bowel disease (IBD). Though the underlying etiology of IBD is not precisely known, genetic, environmental, and immune factors all play a role.
- Clinical history and physical examination in combination with objective findings from laboratory studies, radiology, endoscopy, and pathology are used to diagnose IBD.[1–3]
- IBD occurs at a high enough prevalence that most primary care physicians care for one or more IBD patients in their own practice. Therefore, understanding the nomenclature, clinical features, and basic management strategies of IBD is important.
- Key principles for the primary care clinician include 1) recognizing the clinical disease presentation, the cyclical nature of disease activity, and common extraintestinal disease manifestations; 2) understanding general treatment strategies including limiting the frequency and duration of corticosteroid use and smoking cessation for CD; 3) assisting in managing disease comorbidities including osteoporosis and anxiety/depression.
- **UC is defined by mucosal inflammation limited to the colon**. Inflammation most typically involves the distal rectum and extends proximally in a **circumferential and contiguous** distribution. The nomenclature for UC describes the extent of inflammation and is important in determining medical therapy (Table 31-1).
  - **Bloody diarrhea with associated rectal urgency and tenesmus** (sense of incomplete defecation) **is the hallmark presentation of active UC.**
  - Disease severity is characterized by patient symptoms.
    - **Mild disease:** <4 stools per day and no signs of systemic toxicity.
    - **Moderate disease:** 4–6 stools per day and minimal signs of systemic toxicity.
    - **Severe disease:** >6 stools per day with signs of systemic toxicity (fever, tachycardia, anemia, and increased erythrocyte sedimentation rate).
    - **Fulminant disease:** >10 stools per day, continuous bleeding, abdominal tenderness or distention, and dilation on radiographic imaging.
    - Clinical manifestations of UC are compared with those of CD in Table 31-2.
  - Patients with UC can develop **toxic megacolon** (which can also be caused by infectious or toxin-mediated colitis). Precipitating factors include electrolyte abnormalities, opiates, and other antimotility agents. Life-threatening complications of toxic megacolon include perforation, hemorrhage, and sepsis.
- **CD is characterized by transmural intestinal inflammation** that can involve any part of the GI tract from the oropharynx to the anus.
  - Inflammatory changes are usually **asymmetric and discontinuous** with **skip areas** (normal tissue separating diseased intestinal segments).
  - CD is described by **location** (ileal, colonic, and ileocolonic) and **behavior** (penetrating [fistulae, abscesses], stricturing, inflammatory, or perianal disease).
  - The manifestations of CD vary with the degree and segment of intestinal involvement.
    - Upper GI tract involvement may present as oral ulcers, gum pain, odynophagia, dysphagia, or gastric outlet obstruction.

TABLE 31-1	Classifying Disease Extent in Ulcerative Colitis
Proctitis	Inflammation limited to the **rectum**
Distal colitis or proctosigmoiditis	Inflammation extending to the **midsigmoid colon**
Left-sided colitis	Inflammation extending to the **splenic flexure**
Extensive colitis	Inflammation extending **beyond the splenic flexure but sparing the cecum**
Pancolitis	Continuous inflammation from **rectum to cecum**
Backwash ileitis	**Ileal inflammation** in association with pancolitis

- Small bowel and colonic symptoms include diarrhea, abdominal pain, weight loss, obstructive symptoms, and fever.
- Gross rectal bleeding occurs less commonly than in UC. Many CD patients do not have diarrhea and, in fact, may trend toward constipation early in an obstructive process.
  - Disease severity assessment is more difficult than with UC and is sometimes complicated by concurrent irritable bowel syndrome. With that caveat noted, classification system for CD includes the following.
    - **Mild-moderate disease:** Outpatients able to tolerate oral intake without signs of dehydration, abdominal pain, systemic toxicity, or weight loss of >10%.
    - **Moderate-severe disease:** Patients who have failed therapy for mild-moderate disease or have abdominal pain, nausea/vomiting, and signs of systemic toxicity such as fevers, dehydration, anemia, or weight loss of >10%.

TABLE 31-2	Comparison of Crohn Disease and Ulcerative Colitis	
	Crohn disease	**Ulcerative colitis**
Scope of disease	Entire GI tract; ileum most common	Rectum and proximally
Clinically	Abdominal pain or mass, diarrhea, weight loss, vomiting, perianal disease	Rectal bleeding, diarrhea, passage of mucus, crampy pain, tenesmus, urgency
Endoscopy	Rectal sparing, skip lesions, aphthous ulcers, cobblestoning, linear ulceration	Rectal involvement, continuous, friability, loss of vascularity
Radiology	Small bowel and terminal ileal disease, segmental, strictures, fistulae	Colon disease, loss of haustra, continuous ulceration, no fistulae
Histology	Transmural disease, aphthous ulcers, noncaseating granulomas	Abnormal crypt architecture, superficial inflammation
Cigarette smoking	Increases risk of disease, recurrence rate, decreases time to surgery, and lessens therapeutic efficacy	Current smoking decreases risk

Modified from Iskandar H, Ciorba MA. Inflammatory bowel disease. In: Gyawali CP, ed. *The Washington Manual Gastroenterology Subspecialty Consult*, 3rd ed. Philadelphia, PA: Lippincott Williams & Wilkins; 2012:169–179.

- **Severe-fulminant disease:** Persistent symptoms despite corticosteroid use or patients with high fevers, cachexia, persistent vomiting, intestinal obstruction, surgical abdomen, or abscess formation.
- **Remission:** Asymptomatic patients or those who have responded to medical or surgical intervention without evidence of residual/recurrent disease (not on steroids).
  - Patients with CD can also develop **toxic megacolon**.

Epidemiology

- IBD can develop at any age; peak incidence rates occur between 15 and 30 years of age.
- Though all races are affected, the incidence rates are higher in white Northern Europeans and North Americans.
- The prevalence of IBD in the United States is[4]
  - CD: 58 to 241/100,000
  - UC: 34 to 263/100,000

Risk Factors

- Patients with a first-degree relative with IBD have an increased risk of having IBD themselves.
- Current smokers have a lower risk of developing UC. Former smokers, however, have a 1.7-fold increased risk for UC over lifetime nonsmokers.
- Smoking is associated with an increased risk of CD, increased chance of disease recurrence, and reduced therapeutic efficacy.
- Though no single microbe causes IBD, concomitant infections (intestinal and extraintestinal) as well as antibiotic use can exacerbate IBD.

Associated Conditions

- IBD can be associated with **extraintestinal manifestations** (EIMs), which often correlate to colonic IBD activity.[5] EIMs occur more frequently in UC than CD.
- **Musculoskeletal**
  - **Central arthropathies** (**ankylosing spondylitis** and **sacroiliitis**) associated with IBD are progressive conditions and tend to correlate poorly with IBD activity.
  - **Pauciarticular peripheral arthritis** correlates well with colonic inflammation. Asymmetric large joint (knees, hips, ankles, wrists, and elbows) involvement is typical.
  - **Polyarticular peripheral arthritis** is symmetric, involves smaller joints (fingers and toes), and may occur independent of IBD activity.
  - **Osteoporosis** risk is increased in IBD patients presumably due to cumulative steroid use, malabsorption, low body weight, and relative hypogonadism related to disease activity. Guidelines suggest using dual-energy x-ray absorptiometry (DEXA) testing to screen for osteoporosis in all postmenopausal women with IBD and those individuals who have received prolonged or frequent courses of corticosteroids. All patients with disease severe enough to require steroids at least once should take supplemental vitamin D (800 IU) daily along with 1,000 to 1,500 mg calcium supplementation.
- **Dermatologic**
  - **Erythema nodosum** (EN) is a painful, poorly demarcated, nodular lesion that tends to be bilateral but asymmetric. It is closely related to IBD activity, and treatment of the underlying disease resolves EN lesions.
  - **Pyoderma gangrenosum** (PG) is a debilitating skin disease characterized by irregular, blue-red ulcers with purulent necrotic bases. Lesions are usually found on the lower extremities, buttocks, abdomen, and face. PG can develop independent of IBD activity. A high index of suspicion for PG should exist for patients with poorly healing skin lesions.
  - **Aphthous ulcers** in the oropharynx occur in 10% to 30% of patients with IBD.

- **Ocular**
  - ○ **Episcleritis** is a painless inflammation of the eye's surface. Visual acuity is not affected, and episodes tend to coincide with IBD flares.
  - ○ **Uveitis** is an inflammation of the eye that can be painful and associated with decreased visual acuity. It does not always coincide with disease activity. Uncontrolled uveitis can cause permanent ocular damage.
  - ○ Prompt referral to an eye specialist is necessary for all new changes in vision or eye complaints in the setting of IBD.
- **Hepatobiliary**
  - ○ **Gallstones** may develop in patients with CD due to malabsorption of bile salts in the ileum.
  - ○ **Primary sclerosing cholangitis** (PSC) is more commonly associated with UC than CD and is a chronic inflammatory disease of the bile ducts (refer to Chapter 30). Endoscopic retrograde cholangiopancreatography (ERCP) or magnetic resonance cholangiopancreatography (MRCP) reveals strictures of intrahepatic and extrahepatic ducts. Patients with PSC have an increased risk of developing cholangiocarcinoma and colitis-associated cancer.
- **Vascular**: The risk of venous and arterial thrombosis is increased in patients with IBD and can be a major source of mortality.
- **Renal**: Nephrolithiasis (calcium oxalate stones) can occur with CD. Hyperoxaluria is common and related to fat malabsorption, which increases the amount of dietary oxalate available for absorption in the colon.

DIAGNOSIS

Clinical Presentation

History
- A thorough history is the first step in diagnosing IBD and defining disease severity.
- Questions should be aimed at abdominal symptoms, systemic signs of toxicity, family history of IBD, medication history, smoking history, and the presence of EIMs.
- UC primarily presents with bloody diarrhea, urgency, tenesmus, and abdominal pain.
- CD patients primarily present with abdominal pain, weight loss, fatigue, and sometimes fever. Diarrhea and rectal bleeding are less common than in UC, but can be significant.

Physical Examination
- Fever, hypotension, and tachycardia are signs of systemic toxicity.
- High-pitched or absent bowel sounds may suggest obstruction.
- Peritoneal signs (rebound, guarding, and rigidity) suggest intestinal perforation.
- A right lower quadrant mass is often palpable in patients with active ileal CD.
- A careful rectal and perianal examination is important. Skin tags, fistulae, and anal fissures suggest perianal CD.
- With toxic megacolon, the colon rapidly dilates to >5 to 6 cm and the abdomen is distended and painful. As the name implies, patients appear quite toxic (e.g., fever, hypotension, and tachycardia). Steroids may mask some of these signs.
- Ocular, skin, and musculoskeletal exams identify EIMs of IBD.

Differential Diagnosis

The differential diagnosis of IBD is extensive, including infection, neoplasia, ischemia, and other inflammatory conditions (Table 31-3).

Diagnostic Testing

Laboratories
- No specific laboratory test confirms IBD; however, several autoantibodies have been detected in IBD patients, including perinuclear antineutrophil cytoplasmic antibody (P-ANCA) and anti–*Saccharomyces cerevisiae* antibodies (ASCA).

TABLE 31-3	Differential Diagnosis for Irritable Bowel Disease

Infectious etiologies

Bacterial	Mycobacterial	Viral
Salmonella spp.	Tuberculosis	Cytomegalovirus
Shigella spp.	Mycobacterium avium	Herpes simplex
Toxigenic Escherichia coli		HIV

	Parasitic	Fungal
Campylobacter spp.	Amebiasis	Histoplasmosis
Yersinia spp.	Isospora belli	Candidiasis
Clostridium difficile	Trichuris trichiura	Aspergillosis
Gonorrhea	Hookworm	
Chlamydia trachomatis	Strongyloidiasis	

Noninfectious etiologies

Inflammatory	Medications	Neoplasias
Appendicitis	NSAIDs	Lymphomas
Diverticulitis	Chemotherapy	Carcinomas (colon, small bowel)
Microscopic colitis		
Ischemic colitis		
Radiation enteritis		
Behçet disease		

HIV, human immunodeficiency virus; IBD, inflammatory bowel disease; NSAID, nonsteroidal anti-inflammatory drug.
Modified from Iskandar H, Ciorba MA. Inflammatory bowel disease. In: Gyawali CP, ed. *The Washington Manual Gastroenterology Subspecialty Consult*, 3rd ed. Philadelphia, PA: Lippincott Williams & Wilkins; 2012:169–179.

- Initial evaluation should include complete blood cell count (evaluate for anemia and leukocytosis); comprehensive metabolic panel (evaluate for metabolic derangements); erythrocyte sedimentation rate; and C-reactive protein (measure of active inflammation), calcium, vitamin D, vitamin B_{12}, iron studies.
- Antibody panels (ASCA/pANCA) sometimes aid in clinical decision making.
- Stool studies (*Clostridium difficile* toxin, culture, ova, and parasites) are important to look for infectious etiologies that may mimic IBD.

Imaging
- Urgent CT scans are used for patients presenting with systemic toxicity and significant abdominal complaints to examine for signs of obstruction, perforation, or megacolon.
- Elective small bowel follow-through computerized tomography enterography (CTE) or magnetic resonance enterography (MRE) are frequently ordered to look for strictures, abscesses, and fistulae and to assess disease activity.

Diagnostic Procedures
- Endoscopy is used to differentiate between CD and UC, while also allowing for determination of disease location, extent, and severity.

- Histology in UC shows inflammation confined to the mucosa and superficial submucosa. The crypt architecture is distorted (branching), and basal lymphoid aggregations and plasma cells are often present.
- Inflammation in CD is transmural with crypt abscesses and noncaseating granulomas. Microscopic skip areas also occur.

TREATMENT

Medications
- The goals of medical management of CD and UC are to induce and maintain remission.[4,5]
- Disease location and the nature of extraintestinal complaints influence choice of therapy. The goal is to maximize benefit while minimizing the chances of drug toxicity.
- Prior to initiating immunosuppressive/immunomodulator therapy, concurrent infection (hepatitis B, *C. difficile*, and TB) should be ruled out. Also, ensure influenza, hepatitis B, and pneumococcal immunizations are up to date. Tobacco screening/cessation counseling should be a part of this discussion as well.
- Treatment of toxic megacolon consists of complete bowel rest, correction of dehydration and electrolyte abnormalities, discontinuation of all drugs that can reduce motility, and high-dose steroids. Surgery may be necessary for those unresponsive to medical management or for those with perforation or severe hemorrhage.

Antibiotics
- **Ciprofloxacin** and **metronidazole** are often used to treat perianal, fistulizing, and mildly active CD of the colon.
- Peripheral neuropathy is an important toxicity of prolonged metronidazole use. Tendon rupture has been reported with ciprofloxacin use.

Aminosalicylates
- 5-Aminosalicylates (5-ASA) drugs are often the first-line therapies to treat patients with **mild-to-moderate UC.**
- Various formulations of 5-ASA compounds are available and are generally well tolerated. **Mesalamine** and **balsalazide** are the formulations available in the United States.
- Mesalamine as a suppository or enema is effective treatment for proctitis and left-sided colitis.
- A small percentage of patients are intolerant of 5-ASA, which results in a paradoxical increase in diarrhea.
- Sulfasalazine (a 5-ASA prodrug) is a less expensive alternative medication and has demonstrated efficacy for colonic disease and IBD-associated peripheral arthropathy. Its use is dose limited by the **sulfa moiety.**

Corticosteroids
- While undesirable in both side effect profile and the inability to maintain remission, **steroids are commonly used to induce remission in moderate-to-severe IBD**.
- The need to initiate steroids portends a poor prognosis. An increase in frequency of usage or prolonged usage generally signals the need for an immunomodulatory drug to be initiated (see below).
- Steroid dependency (i.e., symptoms flare with decreased doses) or steroid resistance (i.e., symptoms persist despite increasing doses of steroids) occurs in 50% of patients.
- Locally delivered/released steroids reduce systemic side effects. Enteric-coated budesonide is used in ileal/ileocolonic CD due to terminal ileum and right colon delivery. Suppositories and enemas are useful in proctitis and left colon disease.
- **Steroids are ineffective as maintenance therapy** and lead to significant side effects including metabolic, psychiatric, ocular, GI, and osseous side effects.

- Steroids are usually started at a dose of 1 mg/kg and continued until remission of symptoms. A slow taper (over 2 to 3 months) is then initiated; more rapid taper typically leads to recurrence of symptoms.

Immunomodulators
- Immunomodulators such as **6-mercaptopurine (6-MP)** and its prodrug **azathioprine (AZA)** are widely used in the management of IBD to maintain steroid-free disease remission. Therapeutic effect may take 3 to 5 months of continued use.
- Immunomodulators are typically initiated in patients unable to wean from steroids and in those requiring >1 course of steroids per year.
- **Bone marrow suppression** can occur; thus the need for routine CBCs.
- **Checking a thiopurine methyltransferase (TPMT) activity level is standard of care** prior to immunomodulator initiation to identify patients at risk for severe bone marrow suppression.
- Thiopurine metabolite (6-TGN/6-MMP) levels provide information on medication adherence, adequacy of therapeutic levels (6-TGN), and risk for hepatotoxicity (6-MMP).
- **Idiosyncratic pancreatitis** occurs in approximately 1% to 3% of patients. If pancreatitis develops, the drug should be immediately discontinued. Repeat challenge with either 6-MP or AZA is contraindicated.
- Other immunosuppressant drugs, including **methotrexate** (for CD) and **cyclosporine** (in UC), have been used successfully to manage moderate-to-severe IBD.
- Use of these drugs during **pregnancy** remains controversial. It is generally considered that the risk-to-benefit ratio favors continuation of AZA/6-MP over possible recurrence of disease activity during pregnancy. Methotrexate and cyclosporine are contraindicated during pregnancy.

Tumor Necrosis Factor Alpha Antagonists
- Tumor necrosis factor alpha antagonists (anti–TNF-α) are indicated **for moderate-to-severe or steroid-dependent disease**.
- Infliximab, adalimumab, and certolizumab pegol are FDA-approved anti–TNF-α therapies for CD. Infliximab and adalimumab are approved for the therapy of UC.
- If a patient responds to induction dosing regimen by 8 to 12 weeks, long-term maintenance dosing is recommended.
- Prior to starting treatment, latent tuberculosis and occult hepatitis B must be ruled out.
- Adverse effects include acute and delayed infusion reactions, injection site reactions, infection, an increased risk of lymphoma, and perhaps nonmelanoma skin cancer.

Surgical Management
- Indications for surgery include severe GI hemorrhage, toxic megacolon, perforation, medically refractory disease, recurrent/persistent obstructions, significant fistulizing disease, and abscess.
- **Total colectomy is curative for UC.** Surgery for CD involves resection limited to diseased segments.
- UC patients with colonic carcinoma, high-grade dysplasia, or multifocal low-grade dysplasia found during surveillance colonoscopy should also be referred for total colectomy.
- Postcolectomy, many patients opt to have an ileal pouch created in lieu of a permanent ileostomy. **Pouchitis** occurs in up to 50% of patients—typical symptoms include increased stool frequency, abdominal cramping, rectal urgency, rectal bleeding, incontinence, and fever.
  - Antibiotics (ciprofloxacin or metronidazole) are effective therapy for pouchitis.
  - Recurrent or refractory pouchitis may represent misdiagnosed CD. Pouch excision is required in approximately 5% of patients.
  - Cuffitis is inflammation due to a short "cuff" of retained rectal mucosa and is treated with topical steroid or 5-ASA suppositories.
- **Postoperative recurrence of CD is common.** Smoking has been associated with an accelerated time to disease recurrence postoperatively in CD patients.

SPECIAL CONSIDERATIONS

Treatment of Extraintestinal Manifestations of IBD

- Treatments for ankylosing spondylitis and sacroiliitis include analgesics, exercise, sulfasalazine, methotrexate, or anti-TNF therapy (Chapter 33).
- Treatment of the underlying colitis tends to improve pauciarticular peripheral arthritis. The course of polyarticular peripheral arthritis is more protracted, often requiring immunosuppressants for treatment.
- Low bone density and vitamin D deficiency are common in patients with IBD, particularly CD. Steroid therapy intensifies these complications. Adequate vitamin D and calcium supplementation is suggested for all IBD patients.
- Treatment of the underlying disease results in improvement of EN lesions. PG calls for aggressive local wound care, and systemic steroids are often required. Aphthous ulcers tend to resolve with disease remission.
- Treatment of episcleritis consists of controlling the underlying disease flare as well as topical steroids. Topical steroids are the primary treatment for uveitis.
- Treatment of PSC includes endoscopic dilation of symptomatic strictures. Patients with severe disease may ultimately require liver transplantation (refer to Chapter 30).
- Inpatients should be given thromboembolism prophylaxis with heparin products (unless severe bleeding is present) and avoid immobilization and prolonged indwelling catheters.

Cancer Surveillance

- Patients with IBD have an **increased risk of developing colorectal cancer**.
- A family history of colon cancer and concurrent PSC elevates the risk even further.
- Cancer risk is related to IBD disease duration (after 8 to 10 years), extent, and severity.
- The current recommendation is to begin colorectal cancer screening after 8 to 10 years of disease. **Surveillance colonoscopies should be performed every 1 to 2 years**.
- Patients with PSC should begin surveillance colonoscopies at the time of diagnosis.
- Patients with high-grade dysplasia or multifocal low-grade dysplasia seen on colon biopsies should be referred to a colorectal surgeon.

REFERENCES

1. Baumgart DC, Sandborn WJ. Crohn's disease. *Lancet* 2012;380:1590–1605.
2. Danese S, Fiocchi C. Ulcerative colitis. *N Engl J Med* 2011;365:1713–1725.
3. Kornbluth A, Sachar DB. Ulcerative colitis practice guidelines in adults: American College of Gastroenterology, Practice Parameters Committee. *Am J Gastroenterol* 2010;105:501–523.
4. Kappelman MD, Rifas-Shiman SL, Kleinman K, et al. The prevalence and geographic distribution of Crohn's disease and ulcerative colitis in the United States. *Clin Gastroenterol Hepatol* 2007;5:1424–1429.
5. Rothfuss KS, Stange EF, Herrlinger KR. Extraintestinal manifestations and complications in inflammatory bowel diseases. *World J Gastroenterol* 2006;12:4819–4831.

32 Irritable Bowel Syndrome

Sagar R. Shroff and Gregory Sayuk

GENERAL PRINCIPLES

- Irritable bowel syndrome (IBS) is a functional gastrointestinal disorder characterized by abdominal pain or discomfort associated with defecation or a change in bowel habit and features of disordered defecation (constipation and/or diarrhea).
- IBS is one of several functional GI syndromes defined by symptom-based criteria, listed in Table 32-1.[1,2]

Classification

- Several historical diagnostic criteria for IBS exist, with the Rome III criteria (Table 32-2) representing the most recent and encompassing criteria.[1] It should be noted that these criteria were devised primarily as a tool for devising clinical studies in the area. However, when applied to clinical practice, they have a high positive predictive value (>95%).
- Although they are not necessary for IBS diagnosis, several supporting symptoms (Table 32-3) help to solidify the diagnosis and further characterize the disorder into IBS with constipation (IBS-C), IBS with diarrhea (IBS-D), mixed IBS (IBS-M), or unsubtyped IBS (IBS-U).

Epidemiology

- IBS is frequently seen in both primary care and specialty care settings and is one of the most common diagnoses seen by gastroenterologists.[3]
  - Estimates place the prevalence of IBS anywhere from 1% to 20% worldwide.
  - Systematic reviews suggest that 10% to 15% of the adult US population are affected with IBS.[4]
  - Population surveys of adults have shown IBS to be more prevalent in women than in men with a ratio of 3 to 4:1.
  - Symptom onset tends to occur between the ages of 20 and 40 but can occur at any age. When considering a new diagnosis of IBS in older individuals, exclusion of other mimicking conditions is requisite (e.g., celiac disease, inflammatory bowel disease, and small intestinal bacterial overgrowth [SIBO]).
- Surveys from both the United States and United Kingdom report an average disease duration of 11 years, although about one-third of patients have symptoms for even longer periods.
- As few as one in three individuals affected with IBS in the United States actually seek medical attention, and the vast majority of these are managed by their primary care physician. Still, the cost to society is considerable, accounting for approximately 3.6 million physician visits and $1.6 billion in direct medical costs each year.
- The burden on the patient is also considerable with health-related quality-of-life (HRQOL) scores similar to patients with diabetes and worse than patients with chronic kidney disease and gastroesophageal reflux disease.[5]

Pathophysiology

- No single pathophysiologic abnormality has been found that adequately explains the manifestations of IBS. Given the symptomatic basis on which the diagnosis is made, more than one pathophysiologic mechanism likely plays a role. Multiple factors, including

---

TABLE 32-1 The Functional Gastrointestinal Disorders (From Rome III)

Functional esophageal disorders
Heartburn
Chest pain of presumed esophageal origin
Dysphagia
Globus

Functional gastroduodenal disorders
Functional dyspepsia
Belching disorders
Nausea and vomiting disorders
Rumination syndrome

Functional bowel disorders
Irritable bowel syndrome
Functional bloating
Functional constipation
Functional diarrhea
Unspecified functional bowel disorder

Functional abdominal pain syndrome

Functional gallbladder and sphincter of Oddi (SO) disorders
Functional gallbladder disorder
Functional biliary SO disorder
Functional pancreatic SO disorder

Functional anorectal disorders
Functional fecal incontinence
Functional anorectal pain
Functional defecation disorders

TABLE 32-2 The Rome III Irritable Bowel Syndrome Criteria

Recurrent abdominal pain or discomfort at least 3 days per month in the last 3 months associated with two or more of the following:

1. Improvement with defecation
2. Onset associated with a change in frequency of stools
3. Onset associated with a change in form (appearance) of stool

---

TABLE 32-3 Supportive Symptoms of Irritable Bowel Syndrome

Abnormal stool frequency (*abnormal* defined more than three bowel movements per day or fewer than four bowel movements per week)
Abnormal stool form (lumpy/hard or loose/watery stool)
Abnormal stool passage (straining, urgency, or feeling of incomplete evacuation)
Passage of mucus
Bloating or feeling of abdominal distention

abnormalities of intestinal motility, visceral hypersensitivity, GI tract inflammatory processes, disturbances along the brain-gut axis, and psychological factors, have been examined as potentially causative in IBS.[6]

- A portion of patients with IBS will exhibit exaggerated motility and sensory responses to stressors, meals, and balloon inflation in the GI tract; however, these are neither uniformly identifiable in IBS patients nor consistently reproducible in the same individual.

- IBS may result from sensitization of afferent neural pathways from the gut such that normal intestinal stimuli induce pain.

- Intestinal inflammation also has been hypothesized as playing a role in the development of IBS, particularly as it relates to persistent neuroimmune interactions following infectious gastroenteritis (so-called postinfectious IBS); approximately one-third of patients with IBS report symptom onset after an episode of acute gastroenteritis.

- The role of SIBO or lower levels of bacterial colonization (intestinal dysbiosis) in the development of IBS has been a focus of recent investigations, but its role remains to be fully understood.[7]

- The central nervous system (and its interpretation of peripheral enteric nerve signals) is receiving increasing attention in investigational settings because of the potential mechanistic significance in IBS.

DIAGNOSIS

Clinical Presentation

- IBS is a symptom-based diagnosis. Patients should report abdominal discomfort and a temporal association with alterations in stool pattern, improvement with bowel movement, or both.

- IBS diagnosis requires an element of chronicity (per Rome criteria, ≥3 days per month over the preceding 3 months), with symptom onset at least 6 months prior to diagnosis.

- **The diagnosis of IBS should be made after organic or structural causes have been considered**, necessitating a careful search for **alarm symptoms** before establishing a diagnosis of IBS.
  - Important alarm symptoms include unintentional weight loss of ≥10 pounds, recurrent fever, persistent diarrhea, hematochezia, age >50 years at onset of symptoms, male sex, and family history of GI malignancy, inflammatory bowel disease, or celiac sprue.
  - A brief history of rapidly progressive symptoms suggests organic disease. The presence of any alarm features warrants a more detailed investigation before diagnosing as IBS.

- Likewise, the physical examination should be focused to exclude organic disease.
  - Diffuse abdominal tenderness is commonly present because of the heightened visceral sensitivity noted in this population.
  - Physical examination alarm signs include the presence of thyroid abnormalities, organomegaly, abdominal masses, lymphadenopathy, perianal disease, or heme-positive stool.

Diagnostic Testing

- **Laboratory and invasive testing should be kept to a minimum in the absence of alarm symptoms**, because extensive or repetitive investigations may be costly and serve only to reinforce illness behavior.

- Initial laboratory testing should include a complete blood count (CBC), erythrocyte sedimentation rate (ESR), thyroid-stimulating hormone (TSH), and fecal occult blood test (FOBT).

- **Testing for celiac sprue should be considered in all IBS patients** (particularly in IBS-D and IBS-M) with IgA anti–tissue transglutaminase test (anti-tTG IgA).

- Complete metabolic profile and stool for culture and *Clostridium difficile* toxin or PCR testing can be ordered if the pretest probability is high enough, but are likely low yield for the majority of IBS patients.
- **Colonoscopy and EGD typically are unnecessary in young patients presenting with classic features of IBS without any alarm symptoms**.
  - Colonoscopy should be performed in all patients >50 or those with positive FOBT.
  - In cases of IBS-D or IBS-M, random colonoscopic biopsies should be performed to exclude microscopic colitis.

TREATMENT

- The approach to therapy in IBS is multifaceted and should be tailored to the patient given the individual's constellation and severity of symptoms.
- **Two key factors** determine therapy: dominant symptoms (diarrhea, constipation, pain, others) and symptom severity (intensity, effects on quality of life).
- Current management approaches include behavioral modification, dietary changes, peripherally acting agents, centrally acting agents, and psychological-behavioral therapy.

Medications

- Cases with mild or intermittent symptoms can be managed with symptomatic treatment using peripherally acting agents administered on an as-needed basis.
- Patients with moderate symptoms (as designated by intermittent interference with daily activities) may benefit from regular use of peripheral agents as an initial approach, with the option of introducing centrally acting agents if this approach fails.
- Patients with severe symptoms (regular interference with daily activities, and concurrent affective, personality, and psychosomatic disorders) benefit from combinations of peripheral and central agents but may also need contemporary pharmaceutical agents and psychological approaches to manage their overlapping affective, personality, and psychosomatic disorders.
- Although medical therapy is available and new drugs are currently in development, IBS is a long-term condition with exacerbations and remissions, and medications should be minimized to the extent possible.
- **Opioids have no role in the management of IBS**. The use of opioids actually may worsen IBS symptoms and provoke so-called narcotic bowel syndrome.[8]
- Given the lack of identifiable biomarkers, trials of medications are frequently part of the IBS diagnostic process. These trials should be pursued for at least 4 weeks (and ideally 12 weeks) before moving on to different therapy.
- If failure to respond to a single agent in a drug class is experienced, response to a different drug in the same class may still be observed.
- It is important to recognize the substantial (up to 50%) placebo response rates present in this patient population.
- **Patient education and reassurance** while establishing a therapeutic relationship are cornerstones in the management of this condition. The strength of the physician-patient relationship translates into higher rates of patient satisfaction and fewer return visits.
- Table 32-4 summarizes general management principles for patients with IBS or other functional bowel disorders.

Peripherally Acting Agents

Therapies for Constipation-Predominant IBS

- Increasing the amount of **dietary fiber** is a simple, inexpensive option in mild IBS-C and can be instituted as an early approach.
  - Limited randomized controlled studies seem to show some benefit in global symptom relief with this approach.[9]
  - Whole grains, fruits, nuts, and vegetables are natural sources of fiber.

TABLE 32-4	General Approach to Irritable Bowel Syndrome and the Functional Bowel Disorders

Minimize invasive testing targeted to exclude other disorders as appropriate
Avoid repetitive testing unless necessary
Determine patient expectations and goals
Provide education and reassurance with emphasis on benign nature of condition
Dietary modifications (minimize lactose/FODMAPS) and fiber supplementation
    are first-line therapies
Medications should be used in more persistent or difficult cases
Oral or psychological interventions for refractory and motivated patients
    with IBS

FODMAPS, fermentable, oligo-, di-, and monosaccharides and polyols.

- ○ Supplements include psyllium, methylcellulose, and guar gum.
- ○ Our preference is the use of soluble fiber products.
- ○ In patients who complain of bloating or gas, fiber supplementation can be associated with an increase in those symptoms and slow titration along with the exclusion of flatulogenic foods should be encouraged.
- **Osmotic laxatives** such as milk of magnesia, sorbitol, lactulose, or polyethylene glycol also may be considered in patients with IBS-C.
  - ○ Currently randomized controlled trial data supporting their use are lacking.
  - ○ Nonabsorbable carbohydrates such as lactulose and sorbitol can induce abdominal pain and bloating symptoms when used chronically and are probably best reserved as second-line agents.
  - ○ Polyethylene glycol can be safely used for chronic constipation on a maintenance basis.
- **Lubiprostone** is a chloride channel activator indicated in the treatment of IBS-C in women at a dose of 8 mcg twice daily.
  - ○ Lubiprostone has shown benefit in reducing global IBS symptom scores and increasing spontaneous bowel movements.[9,10]
  - ○ Side effects include nausea, diarrhea, and headache, which can be improved by taking the medication with food.
  - ○ Women of childbearing age should have a negative pregnancy test before starting lubiprostone therapy and should be capable of complying with effective contraception while on this medication.
- **Linaclotide** is a guanylate cyclase-C agonist, which functions as a secretogogue, and is approved for use in IBS-C at a dose of 290 mcg per day. Phase III clinical trials suggest a potential pain benefit to this medication in addition to its effect on bowel transit. Primary side effect is diarrhea.[11]
- **Tegaserod** is a partial 5-HT-4 receptor agonist that exerts GI stimulatory effects and had been indicated for short-term treatment of women with constipation-predominant symptoms. Use is limited to prescription by gastroenterologists for women <55 years of age with IBS-C or chronic constipation due to a small, but significant increase in cardiovascular events found through clinical trial data.[12]

Therapies for Diarrhea-Predominant IBS (IBS-D)

- The antidiarrheal **loperamide** taken 2 to 4 mg up to qid, no more than 12 mg/day, is the only agent with randomized, controlled data supporting its use in IBS-D. Based on its mechanism of action, diphenoxylate-atropine 2.5 mg/0.025 mg up to qid may also be used.[9] No effect on bloating or abdominal pain.
- **Cholestyramine** taken 4 g with meals and **colesevelam** 625 mg up to two times daily with meals can be considered as adjuncts or for early use in diarrheal symptoms exacerbated by cholecystectomy.

- **Alosetron**, a selective $5\text{-}HT_3$ receptor antagonist that slows colonic transit, is approved for treatment of women with IBS-D. Alosetron requires a patient use agreement and prescriber registration with the manufacturer because of rare cases of ischemic colitis and severe constipation with its use. Reserved only for those who have failed to respond to conventional therapy, but can be quite effective.[13]
- **Anticholinergic or antispasmodic agents** often are used in all classes of IBS, though are most useful in the setting of IBS-D.
  - Anticholinergic medications function as antidiarrheal agents by decreasing intestinal transit and modulating bowel secretory function, but also reduce pain by relaxing the smooth muscle of the gut.
  - **Hyoscyamine**, 0.125 to 0.25 mg PO q4h PRN, no more than 1.5 mg/day or **dicyclomine** 10 to 20 mg PO q6h.
  - The synthetic anticholinergics **glycopyrrolate** 1 to 2 mg two to three times a day and **methscopolamine** 2.5 to 5 mg twice a day also are available and have less CNS side effect potential than other antispasmodics.
  - These agents are most useful in patients with postprandial symptoms of abdominal pain, bloating, diarrhea, or fecal urgency. They should be prescribed in a way that circumvents symptoms, such as before meals.
  - These agents often become less effective with chronic use.
  - Limited data also exist supporting the use of several herbal preparations, including peppermint oil as an antispasmodic agent.[9,14]
- The use of antibiotic regimens in IBS recently has generated considerable interest.
  - Gut-selective antibiotics such as rifaximin (550 mg three times daily) or neomycin (500 mg twice daily) have been proposed for use in patients with IBS for whom bacterial overgrowth is suspected, particularly in those with significant gas-bloat symptoms.[15]
  - Studies do demonstrate significant improvement in overall symptoms and bloating, but at high cost, and therefore best used for those refractory to other therapies.
  - Given the modest sensitivity and specificity of hydrogen and methane breath testing, empiric use of antibiotics in the proper clinical setting is advocated, rather than a test-and-treat approach.
- Dietary interventions have demonstrated considerable benefit and are safe, easy options to consider. Higher rates of lactose intolerance are encountered in IBS patients, and a trial of lactose withdrawal should be considered. Moderation of consumption of foods containing fermentable oligo-, di-, and monosaccharides and polyols (FODMAPS) also has proven beneficial in clinical trials.[16]

Centrally Acting Agents

- **Antidepressant medications** are most useful in patients with chronic and refractory abdominal pain symptoms.
- They are particularly helpful with those who have concomitant psychiatric and somatic complaints, although their efficacy appears to be independent of any direct influence on these comorbid conditions.
- Patient perceptions and expectations should be adequately addressed in using antidepressants in the management of IBS in order to optimize compliance.
- **Tricyclic antidepressants** (TCAs), such as nortriptyline or amitriptyline, are the best-studied agents.[17]
  - TCAs are used in doses much lower than those traditionally used in depression management (starting dose, 10 to 25 mg qhs, titrate up by 25 mg every week to symptom relief as tolerated).
  - The anticholinergic properties of TCAs may be beneficial in IBS-D but should not dissuade use in patients with constipation or mixed pattern presentations.

○ Side effects can include weight gain, sedation, dry mouth, urinary difficulties, sexual dysfunction, and dizziness.

○ Individuals experiencing such side effects may tolerate use of agents with fewer anticholinergic effects, such as desipramine.

• **Selective serotonin reuptake inhibitors** (SSRIs) and serotonin norepinephrine reuptake inhibitors (SNRIs) increasingly also are being used in IBS and appear to be nearly as effective as TCAs.[17]

○ Start at the lower range of usual psychiatric doses and titrate up to symptom relief as tolerated.

○ The SNRIs venlafaxine and duloxetine are good first-line options in patients with pain-predominant symptom patterns.

○ Citalopram may be a good option because of its side effect profile and its beneficial effect on colonic tone and sensitivity.

○ Paroxetine may be useful in patients with IBS-D because of its greater anticholinergic effect.

○ Fluoxetine may be useful in patients with IBS-C because it decreases abdominal discomfort, bloating, and increases bowel movements.

Other Nonpharmacologic Therapies

• Psychological and behavioral therapies, such as **cognitive-behavioral therapy** (CBT), are particularly useful in IBS management, especially in patients who correlate an increase in severity of symptoms with life stressors.[18,19]

• CBT and hypnotherapy both have been demonstrated to be beneficial in IBS in randomized controlled trials, particularly with respect to its positive influence on global well-being.

• Although response is sporadic, factors favoring a good response include high patient motivation, overt psychiatric symptoms, and intermittent pain exacerbated by stress and/or anxiety.

REFERENCES

1. Drossman DA, Corazziari E, Tally NJ, et al., eds. *Rome III: The Functional Gastrointestinal Disorders. Diagnosis, Pathophysiology and Treatment: A Multinational Consensus*, 3rd ed. McLean, VA: Degnon Associates; 2006.

2. Whitehead WE, Palsson O, Jones KR. Systematic review of the comorbidity of irritable bowel syndrome with other disorders: what are the causes and implications? *Gastroenterology* 2002;122:1140–1156.

3. Russo MW, Gaynes BN, Drossman DA. A national survey of practice patterns of gastroenterologists with comparison to the past two decades. *J Clin Gastroenterol* 1999;29:339–343.

4. Grundmann O, Yoon SL. Irritable bowel syndrome: epidemiology, diagnosis and treatment: an update for health-care practitioners. *J Gastroenterol Hepatol* 2010;25:691–699.

5. Gralnek I, Hays RD, Kilbourne A, et al. The impact of irritable bowel syndrome on health-related quality of life. *Gastroenterology* 2000;119:654–660.

6. Gunnarson J, Simren M. Peripheral factors in the pathophysiology of irritable bowel syndrome. *Dig Liver Dis* 2009;41:788–793.

7. Posserud I, Stotzer PO, Bjornsson ES, et al. Small intestinal bacterial overgrowth in patients with irritable bowel syndrome. *Gut* 2007;56:802–808.

8. Grunkemeier DMS, Cassara JE, Dalton CB, et al. The narcotic bowel syndrome: clinical features, pathophysiology, and management. *Clin Gastroenterol Hepatol* 2007;5:1126–1139.

9. Brandt LJ, Chey WD, Fox-Orenstein AE, et al. An evidence-based position statement on the management of irritable bowel syndrome. *Am J Gastroenterol* 2009;104 (suppl 1):S1–S35.

10. Johanson JF, Ueno R. Lubiprostone, a locally acting chloride channel activator, in adult patients with chronic constipation: a double-blind, placebo-controlled, dose-ranging study to evaluate efficacy and safety. *Aliment Pharmacol Ther* 2007;25:1351–1361.

11. Chey WD, Lembo AJ, Lavins BJ, et al. Linaclotide for irritable bowel syndrome with constipation: a 26-week, randomized, double-blind, placebo-controlled trial to evaluate efficacy and safety. *Am J Gastroenterol* 2012;107:1702–1712.

12. Tack J, Müller-Lissner S, Bytzer P, et al. A randomised controlled trial assessing the efficacy and safety of repeated tegaserod therapy in women with irritable bowel syndrome with constipation. *Gut* 2005;54:1707–1713.

13. Andresen V, Montori VM, Keller J, et al. Effects of 5-hydroxytryptamine (serotonin) type 3 antagonists on symptom relief and constipation in nonconstipated irritable bowel syndrome: a systematic review and meta-analysis of randomized controlled trials. *Clin Gastroenterol Hepatol* 2008;6:545–555.

14. Spanier JA, Howden CW, Jones MP. A systematic review of alternative therapies in the irritable bowel syndrome. *Arch Intern Med* 2003;163:265–274.

15. Pimentel M, Lembo A, Chey WD, et al. Rifaximin therapy for patients with irritable bowel without constipation. *N Engl J Med* 2011;364:22–32.

16. Gibson PR, Shepherd SJ. Food choice as a key management strategy for functional gastrointestinal symptoms. *Am J Gastroenterol* 2012;107:657–666.

17. Ford AC, Talley NJ, Schoenfeld PS, et al. Efficacy of antidepressants and psychological therapies in irritable bowel syndrome: systematic review and meta-analysis. *Gut* 2009;58:367–378.

18. Drossman DA, Toner BB, Whitehead WE, et al. Cognitive-behavioral therapy versus education and desipramine versus placebo for moderate to severe functional bowel disorders. *Gastroenterology* 2003;125:19–31.

19. Lackner JM, Brasel AM, Quigley BM, et al. Rapid response to cognitive behavioral therapy predicts outcome in patients with irritable bowel syndrome. *Clin Gastroenterol Hepatol* 2010;8:426–432.

Rheumatologic Diseases

Jonathan J. Miner and Richard D. Brasington

Approach to the Patient with Painful Joints

GENERAL PRINCIPLES

- The initial evaluation of a patient with painful joints is focused on ruling out emergent versus nonemergent causes of arthritis.
- While early diagnosis and treatment of most causes of arthritis are important to ensure the best possible outcome, infectious causes of arthritis such as septic arthritis and endocarditis require emergent evaluation and treatment.
- A logical approach to the evaluation of painful joints includes categorizing as either **monoarticular** arthritis or **polyarticular** arthritis based on the number of joints involved.

DIAGNOSIS

An algorithmic approach to the diagnosis of monoarticular and polyarticular arthritis is presented in Figures 33-1 and 33-2, respectively.[1]

Clinical Presentation

History

- Characteristic **inflammatory symptoms** include swelling, heat, redness, morning stiffness, stiffness after inactivity (the so-called gelling phenomenon), and sometimes fever.
- **Mechanical symptoms** include pain with activity that is relieved with rest, minimal morning stiffness, joint locking or giving out, and lack of swelling or heat.
- **Location** of pain can help provide clues as to the etiology.
  - History of **precedent traumatic** injury might suggest degenerative arthritis of the joint, whereas the classic presentation of podagra with inflammation of the first metatarsophalangeal (MTP) joint suggests gout.
  - Osteoarthritis (OA) tends to affect knees, hips, and the first carpometacarpal joint in the hand.
  - Multiple pain complaints and diffuse tender points suggest a chronic pain syndrome such as fibromyalgia or depression.

Physical Examination

- **Gait**: Observing the patient walking away, turning, and walking back can help localize the source of pain.
- **Hand**: Have the patient make a fist and inspect the dorsum of the hand; observe supination; and inspect the palm of the hands. Look carefully at each of the joints, and palpate the metacarpophalangeal joints for swelling or tenderness.
- **Shoulder**: Ask the patient to put both hands together above the head and observe any abnormal movement of the scapula; put both hands behind the head; and put both hands behind the back (normally, the thumb tip can reach the tip of the scapula).
- **Cervical spine**: Have the patient touch the tip of the chin to chest, look up, and look over each shoulder.
- **Lower spine**: Ask the patient to bend forward to touch the toes without bending the knees, and observe movement of the lumbar spine (normally, there should be reversal of lordosis with flexion of the lumbar spine).

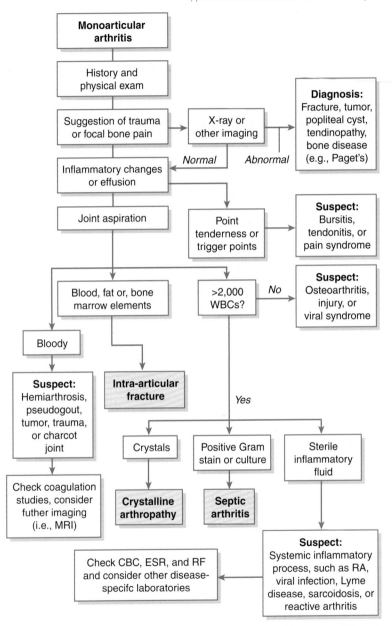

Figure 33-1 Evaluation of monoarticular arthritis. CBC, complete blood count; ESR, erythrocyte sedimentation rate; RA, rheumatoid arthritis; RF, rheumatoid factor; WBC, white blood cells. Modified from Guidelines for the initial evaluation of the adult patient with acute musculoskeletal symptoms. American College of Rheumatology Ad Hoc Committee on Clinical Guidelines. *Arthritis Rheum* 1996;39:1–8.

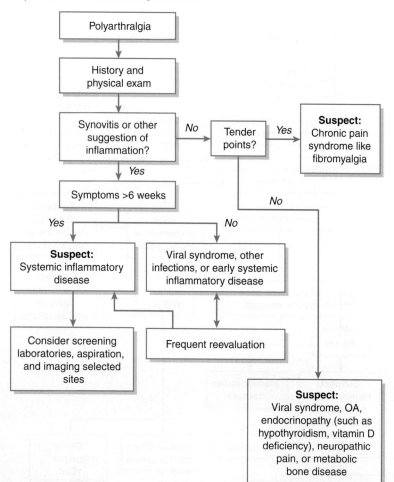

Figure 33-2 Evaluation of polyarthralgia. Modified from Guidelines for the initial evaluation of the adult patient with acute musculoskeletal symptoms. American College of Rheumatology Ad Hoc Committee on Clinical Guidelines. *Arthritis Rheum* 1996;39:1–8.

- **Hip**: The FABER maneuver (flexion-abduction-external rotation) is performed by first having the patient put his or her heel on the contralateral knee; the examiner then presses down on the medial knee, putting the hip into external rotation. The important finding is where pain is elicited. Pain in the groin is indicative of hip joint pathology, but pain may also be elicited from the SI joint and the lateral aspect of the hip from the trochanteric bursa.
- **Knee**: The patient should be able to straighten the knee fully and flex it so the heel almost touches the buttocks. Look for symmetry and effusions. The patella can be held in place with one hand and normally should have little give. In the presence of an effusion, one can elicit a bulge sign.
- **Ankle**: One should look for limitations in flexion and extension and inversion and eversion.

Diagnostic Testing

Laboratories

- Few rheumatology tests are designed to serve as independent diagnostic tools, and test results must always be interpreted in a clinical context.
- **Erythrocyte sedimentation rate** (ESR) is a **very nonspecific** indicator of inflammation and is often elevated due to increased fibrinogen during inflammation. Anemia, kidney disease (especially proteinuria), and aging can all elevate the ESR in the absence of inflammation.
- **C-reactive protein** (CRP) is an acute-phase reactant and a component of the innate immune system; levels rise rapidly with inflammation and infection and fall quickly as inflammation resolves.
  ○ Unlike the ESR, the CRP is not influenced by anemia and abnormal erythrocytes.
  ○ Today, most laboratories perform a high-sensitivity assay for the presence of CRP that can identify minute increases.
- **Rheumatoid factor** (RF) is an immune complex of immunoglobulin (Ig) M that binds to the Fc portion of IgG and is elevated in approximately 80% of patients with rheumatoid arthritis (RA). However, RF can also be elevated in Sjögren syndrome, sarcoidosis, chronic infections, and other conditions where immune complexes are formed.
- **Anticitrullinated protein antibodies (ACPA or anti-CCP)** recognize a posttranslational modification of proteins that is thought to occur in the synovium of patients with RA. The assay is now routinely performed, has a higher specificity for the diagnosis of RA, and may be predictive of progressive joint disease.[2]
- **Antineutrophil cytoplasmic antibody** (ANCA): ANCA detects antibodies against neutrophils and is reported as either a cytoplasmic pattern (c-ANCA) or a perinuclear pattern (p-ANCA).
  ○ A positive ANCA test is only significant when confirmatory ELISA demonstrates that the c-ANCA represents anti–proteinase-3 (PR3) or the p-ANCA represents antimyeloperoxidase (MPO).
  ○ Antibodies against PR3 are specific for granulomatosis with polyangiitis (GPA, formerly known as Wegener granulomatosis).
  ○ Antibodies against MPO are less specific and are seen in conditions such as microscopic polyangiitis and Goodpasture syndrome (in up to 30% of patients).
- The **antinuclear antibody** (ANA) test detects antibodies that bind to nuclear antigens. ANA is a **very sensitive test** for patients with systemic lupus erythematosus (SLE, sensitivity >95%) and may be abnormal in many other autoimmune diseases such as scleroderma, Sjögren syndrome, and polymyositis. However, **because the specificity of the ANA is low, a positive ANA alone is seldom useful.** Furthermore, this highly sensitive test produces many confusing false positives and should only be obtained in patients whose clinical presentation suggests lupus or a related disease.
- **Antibodies to extractable nuclear antigens (ENA)**: This test encompasses a panel of saline-soluble nuclear antigens. This panel detects four autoantibodies: anti-SM (Smith, SLE), anti-RNP (ribonucleoprotein, SLE, and mixed connective tissue disease), and SSA and SSB (Sjögren syndrome, SLE, and neonatal lupus). SSA and SSB are also known as anti-Ro and anti-La, respectively.
- **Anti–Scl-70 antibodies**: Directed against topoisomerase I and associated with diffuse scleroderma.
- **Anticentromere antibodies**: Directed against 70/13-kDa proteins that make up the centromere complex and associated with limited scleroderma. This is the discretely speckled pattern on the ANA test.
- **Anti–Jo-1 antibodies**: Directed against histidyl tRNA synthetase and associated with myositis with interstitial lung disease, arthritis, and mechanic's hands (known as the antisynthetase syndrome).
- Table 33-1 presents an overview of the various autoantibodies and their disease associations.[3]

TABLE 33-1 Autoantibodies and Disease Associations

Disease	ANA	Pattern	RF	dsDNA	Sm	SS-A/Ro	SS-B/La	Scl-70	Centromere	Jo-1	RNP
Systemic lupus erythematosus	>95%	P,H,S,N	20	50–70	30	35	15	0	0	0	30–50
Rheumatoid arthritis	15%–35%	H	80–85	<5	0	10	5	0	0	0	10
Sjögren syndrome	>90%	H,S	75	<5	0	55	40	0	0	0	15
Diffuse scleroderma	>90%	S,N,H	25–33	0	0	5	1	40	<5	0	30
Limited scleroderma	>90%	S,N,H,C	25–33	0	0	5	1	<15	60–80	0	30
Polymyositis and dermatomyositis	75%–95%	S,N,H	33	0	0	0	0	0	0	20–30	0
Mixed connective tissue disease	>95%	S,H	0	0	0	<5	<5	0	0	0	100

C, centromere; H, homogenous or diffuse; P, peripheral or rim; N, nucleolar; S, speckled.
Data from Klippel JH, ed. *Primer on the Rheumatic Diseases*, 12th ed. Atlanta, GA: Arthritis Foundation; 2001.

TABLE 33-2	Classification of Synovial Fluid		
Type of fluid	Special features	Leukocytes/mm³	Example conditions
Normal	Clear, colorless, viscous	<200	Healthy adult
Noninflammatory	Clear, yellow, viscous	200–2,000	Osteoarthritis, trauma
Inflammatory	Cloudy, yellow, decreased viscosity	2,000–100,000	Rheumatoid arthritis, crystalline arthropathy, seronegative arthritis, etc.
Septic	Purulent, markedly decreased viscosity	Usually >50,000 (>95% PMNs)	Septic arthritis

Synovial Fluid Evaluation
- Obtaining synovial fluid from a patient with undiagnosed arthritis, particularly monoarticular arthritis, can be very beneficial.
- The synovial fluid is often characterized by number of cells (especially polymorphonuclear leukocytes [PMNs]), viscosity, and color.
- A Gram stain plus culture and the presence or absence of crystals can confirm the diagnosis (Table 33-2).

Imaging
- Radiographic changes are common, even in early forms of arthritis.
- The distribution, appearance, severity, and other features of the radiography can help limit the differential diagnosis (Table 33-3).

Osteoarthritis

GENERAL PRINCIPLES

- The typical joints involved in primary OA are lower cervical spine, lower lumbar spine, first carpometacarpal joint of the thumb, proximal interphalangeal joints (Bouchard nodes), distal interphalangeal (DIP) joints (Heberden nodes), hip, knee, and first MTP joint.
- Primary OA is rarely seen in the following locations and, if present here, should raise the suspicion for secondary causes (trauma, inflammatory arthritis, etc.): metacarpophalangeal joints, shoulders, elbows, wrists, and ankles.

DIAGNOSIS

- **History** consists of mechanical pain (i.e., pain that is worse with activity and relieved with rest). Morning stiffness may be present, but usually lasts for <30 to 60 minutes.
- **Examination** reveals reduced range of motion, mild swelling, and bony hypertrophy. Small-to-moderate effusions may be present in the knee. Crepitus may be observed with range-of-motion examination.
- **Laboratory tests** are noncontributory except to rule out other causes of arthritis. Synovial fluid if drawn tends to have <2,000 cells/mm³.
- **Radiographic** findings are indicated in Table 33-3.

TABLE 33-3 Radiographic Changes by Disease

	Osteoarthritis	Rheumatoid arthritis	Seronegative spondyloarthropathy	Gout	Septic arthritis
Alignment	Affected late	Affected late	Affected late	Typically not affected	Can be altered early
Distribution	Hips, knees, ankles, and the PIP, DIP, CMC of hands	Symmetric MCP, MTP, wrists	SI joint involvement and lower spine	1st MTP classic, but all joints possible	Knees, ankles, but all joints possible
Erosions	None (except in erosive OA)	Symmetric, marginal, and 50% of patients have them at 2 years.	Can occur and are marginal and at sites of tendon insert	"Mouse bite" erosions with "overhanging edges" and a "punched out" appearance	Loss of cortical line; a destructive process
Periarticular osteoporosis	Absent	Present	Absent	Absent	Often present
Joint space	Narrowed	Narrowed in affected joints	Narrowed in affected joints	Preserved	May be narrowed
Special features	Extra bone formation with osteophytes is common; subchondral sclerosis	Feet may be affected prior to hands	Ankylosis of the spine with enthesitis and syndesmophytes	Erosions tend to occur late and in patients with tophaceous gout	May have no changes at all in mild disease

CMC, carpometacarpal; DIP, distal interphalangeal; MCP, metacarpophalangeal; MTP, metatarsophalangeal; OA, osteoarthritis; PIP, proximal interphalangeal; SI, sacroiliac.

TREATMENT

Guidelines for the treatment of OA have been published by the American College of Rheumatology (ACR).[4]

Medications

- **Acetaminophen** at doses of 1,000 mg tid is often helpful and may be as beneficial as nonsteroidal anti-inflammatory drugs (NSAIDs) for some patients. **Maximum total daily dose should not exceed 2,000 mg in those with significant liver disease.**
- **NSAIDs** including those that are selective inhibitors of cyclooxygenase-2 (COX-2) are commonly prescribed and have been specifically demonstrated to relieve the signs and symptoms of OA. Patients may require a trial of several of these agents to find the most efficacious. Major toxicities include but are not limited to the following:
  - **Gastrointestinal (GI) toxicity** particularly if certain risk factors are present (e.g., age ≥65, oral steroids/anticoagulant use, and history of ulcer disease/GI bleeding).[3] The use of celecoxib or a proton pump inhibitor (PPI) along with a nonselective NSAID may dramatically reduce this risk.[5]
  - **Nephrotoxicity** and nephrogenic sodium retention.
  - **Cardiovascular risks.** Recent placebo-controlled trials have demonstrated an increased risk of thrombotic cardiovascular events such as myocardial infarction (MI) and strokes with COX-2 selective NSAIDs.[6] It is likely that this cardiovascular risk extends to all NSAIDs.
- **Topical capsaicin, diclofenac, and lidocaine** can improve symptoms particularly if few joints are involved.
- Analgesics such as tramadol and opiates are sometimes indicated. With chronic opiate use, tolerance typically develops, requiring progressively higher doses.

Joint Injections

Intra-Articular Steroids

- Intra-articular steroids have been used for the treatment of OA since the 1950s and are routinely performed by general practitioners. Their use should be limited to those with training in the procedure.
- Available steroid preparations include triamcinolone hexacetonide (fluorinated), triamcinolone acetonide (fluorinated), methylprednisolone acetate (nonfluorinated), and dexamethasone.
- **Dose varies based on location,** and no controlled studies exist to guide therapy. General guidelines are as follows:
  - Large joint (knee and shoulder), 40 to 80 mg (1 to 2 mL)
  - Medium joint (wrist, ankle, elbow), 30 mg
  - Small spaces (metacarpophalangeal and proximal interphalangeal joints, tendon sheaths), 10 mg
- **Precautions:**
  - Do not inject through cellulitis or psoriatic skin lesion.
  - **Do not inject the same joint more than three to four times a year.**
  - Infections can occur but are rare, occurring in only 6 of >100,000 procedures in one classic series.[7]
  - Steroid-induced crystalline arthritis can occur because the steroid preparations involve crystalline glucocorticoid. The reactions usually occur within 24 hours after injection and last 2 to 3 days similar to gout, while septic arthritis from an injection tends to occur >48 hours after the injection.

Hyaluronic Acid Analog Injections

- The most commonly used preparation is hylan G-F 20, which can be given as a single injection that is administered once every 6 months.

- Early studies have shown efficacy equal to naproxen in the treatment of OA, but a large meta-analysis of several studies showed little benefit.[8] It is possible that a subset of patients may benefit, and this therapy can be considered in patients with early disease.
- Iatrogenic joint infection, postinjection inflammation (pseudoseptic reaction), and aspiration-proven pseudogout can complicate hyaluronate injections.

Nonpharmacologic Measures

- Nonpharmacologic measures include weight loss, use of a cane or walker, braces and other orthotics, and acupuncture.
- Exercise with and without formal physical therapy. Muscle strength surrounding an affected joint can help stabilize the joint, relieve pain, and possibly reduce progression of joint space narrowing.

Surgery

- Orthopedic consultation for joint replacement of hip, knee, or shoulder should be considered for patients who have exhausted conservative options.
- The timing of surgery is a complicated decision but is primarily based on the severity of the patient's symptoms.

Rheumatoid Arthritis

GENERAL PRINCIPLES

- RA, the prototypical inflammatory arthritis, affects approximately 1% of the population and accounts for a significant degree of morbidity in affected patients.
- RA is a chronic, polyarticular inflammatory arthritis with a symmetric distribution that affects the hands and feet.
- The etiology is still not well understood, but identification and characterization of biologic mediators of the inflammatory response associated with RA has led to the development of new treatments.[9]

DIAGNOSIS

The ACR has specified criteria associated with RA (Table 33-4).[10] These criteria help outline the symptoms at presentation, but all may not be present in the early course of the disease.

Extra-Articular Manifestations

- **Pulmonary**: RA can cause several types of pulmonary disease such as isolated rheumatoid lung nodules, pleural effusions, or interstitial lung disease, which can progress to fibrosis.
- **Felty syndrome** is a syndrome of seropositive RA, neutropenia, and splenomegaly. It usually occurs in patients with long-standing severe disease and can result in increased risk of infection.
- **Ocular**: Severe ocular dryness (keratoconjunctivitis sicca) is the most common ocular problem. Scleritis with a painful red eye that may lead to a thinning of the sclera indicates severe refractory disease and often requires aggressive treatment both systemically and topically.
- **Vasculitis**: Rheumatoid vasculitis can affect any blood vessel, but the most common manifestation is distal arteritis ranging from nail fold infarcts to gangrene of the fingertips.
- **Cardiovascular risk**: Chronic inflammation may play a role in the pathophysiology of atherosclerosis. Patients with chronic inflammatory conditions have been shown to be at increased risk of macrovascular complications such as stroke and MI. Indeed, the same is true for RA, and aggressive therapy to reduce cardiovascular risks is an important aspect of RA management.[11]

TABLE 33-4	ACR 2010 Criteria for the Classification of Acute Rheumatoid Arthritis

Classification criteria for RA (score-based algorithm: Add scores of categories A–D. A score of greater than or equal to 6/10 is needed for classification of a patient as having definite RA).

A. Joint involvement:

1 large joint = 0 points

2–10 large joints = 1 point

1–3 small joints (with or without involvement of large joints) = 2 points

4–10 small joints (with or without involvement of large joints) = 3 points

>10 joints (at least 1 small joint) = 5 points

B. Serology (at least 1 test result is needed for classification)

Negative RF and negative ACPA = 0 points

Low-positive RF or low-positive ACPA = 2 points

High-positive RF or high-positive ACPA = 3 points

C. Acute-phase reactants (at least 1 test result is needed for classification)

Normal CRP and normal ESR = 0 points

Abnormal CRP or abnormal ESR = 1 point

D. Duration of symptoms:

<6 weeks = 0 points

6 weeks or longer = 1 point

Modified from Aletaha D, Negoit T, Silman AJ, et al. *Ann Rheum Dis* 2010;69:1580–1588.

Diagnostic Testing

Laboratories

• Refer to Approach to the Patient with Painful Joints above regarding RF, ACPA, ESR, and CRP.

• Complete blood count (CBC), CMP, and hepatitis panel (to rule out hepatitis C as a cause of a positive RF and arthralgias as well as to avoid using hepatotoxic medications in patients with chronic viral hepatitis) should also be performed.

Imaging

• Classical findings on plain radiography include soft tissue swelling, joint space loss, peri-articular osteoporosis, and erosions (which eventually develop in the large majority of patients). Musculoskeletal ultrasound can be useful in demonstrating synovial proliferation and inflammation prior to radiographic abnormalities.

• Baseline chest radiography is warranted given the possibility of pulmonary involvement.

TREATMENT

Many aspects of RA diagnosis and treatment can be managed in the primary care setting including establishing the diagnosis early, documenting baseline activity, educating patients, initiating NSAID therapy, referral for physical/occupational therapy, and prescribing disease-modifying therapy within 3 months of diagnosis (e.g., corticosteroids, hydroxychloroquine, sulfasalazine, or methotrexate [MTX]). Patients should be reassessed frequently and referred to a rheumatologist if the response is inadequate.[12] **Early treatment with disease-modifying antirheumatic drugs (DMARDs) has the potential to retard the progression of disease**.

Medications

Most patients with RA benefit symptomatically from the use of NSAIDs, but they **do not prevent the progression** of bone and cartilage damage.

Glucocorticoids

- Glucocorticoids (especially prednisone) in low doses are extremely effective for promptly reducing the symptoms of RA and can be considered to help patients recover their previous functional status.
- Unfortunately, short courses of oral corticosteroids produce only interim benefit and chronic therapy is often required to manage symptoms and prevent progression of disease.
- Corticosteroids are particularly helpful in treating patients with severe functional impairment or while awaiting clinical response from a slow-acting DMARD.
- Side effects of corticosteroids are many and include hyperglycemia, adrenal insufficiency, osteopenia, and avascular necrosis. If a dose equivalent to 5 mg or greater of prednisone is to be used for longer than 3 months, then a bisphosphonate should be used to prevent bone loss in the absence of contraindications.[13]
- **Intra-articular steroids** are particularly useful in patients with a flare of RA in a monoarticular or oligoarticular pattern.

Hydroxychloroquine

- Hydroxychloroquine is indicated for mild-to-moderate RA.
- It is effective at doses of 400 mg PO daily not to exceed 6 mg/kg but is contraindicated in patients with renal or hepatic insufficiency.
- The side effect of macular toxicity is extremely unusual at these doses and rarely occurs before 5 years of treatment. Nonetheless, an ophthalmologist should perform a baseline examination and monitor the patient at least annually.

Sulfasalazine

- Sulfasalazine is also indicated for mild-to-moderate RA and in those who are poor candidates for methotrexate therapy.
- It should be initiated at 500 mg PO bid and gradually increased to 1,000 to 1,500 mg PO bid.
- GI intolerance is common and may be reduced with an enteric-coated preparation.
- It is contraindicated in those allergic to sulfa antibiotics and those with glucose-6-phosphate dehydrogenase deficiency. Severe/fatal skin reactions have occurred.
- Monitoring of liver tests and blood counts is required.

Methotrexate

- MTX is **generally considered to be the DMARD of choice** for most RA patients. The usual maintenance dose is 7.5 to 20 mg/week orally.
- If MTX is at least partially effective, it should be continued as other agents are added.
- Common side effects include stomatitis, nausea, diarrhea, and thinning of the hair. It is teratogenic.
- Supplementation with folic acid at doses of 1 to 3 mg PO daily can reduce side effects, although efficacy may be somewhat attenuated.
- Serious adverse reactions include hepatotoxicity, lung toxicity, and bone marrow suppression.
- **MTX should only be prescribed by those experienced in its use,** and careful monitoring of liver tests, serum creatinine, and blood counts is required. It should be used with great caution in the elderly and those with reduced renal function.

Leflunomide

- Leflunomide is a pyrimidine synthesis inhibitor that has been shown to have efficacy comparable to that of MTX in the treatment of RA and may be used in combination with MTX.

- Common side effects include diarrhea, rash, and alopecia. It is teratogenic.
- Monitoring of liver tests and blood counts is required due to the risk of hepatotoxicity and bone marrow suppression. **Leflunomide should only be prescribed by those experienced in its use.**

Tofacitinib

- Tofacitinib is a small molecule inhibitor of JAK2, a kinase that operates downstream of multiple cytokines and growth factors. Tofacitinib has shown similar efficacy to methotrexate and adalimumab and has been effective in patients who have failed other therapies.
- Side effects include headache, nausea, vomiting, and diarrhea. Elevated cholesterol and transaminase levels as well as neutropenia can occur.
- Tofacitinib requires regular monitoring of blood counts, liver enzymes, and cholesterol. **Tofacitinib should only be prescribed by those experienced in its use.**

Biologic DMARDs

- **Etanercept** (Enbrel) is a human fusion protein consisting of both the soluble tumor necrosis factor receptor and the Fc component of IgG.
- **Infliximab** (Remicade), **adalimumab** (Humira), **golimumab** (Simponi), and **certolizumab** (Cimzia) are monoclonal antibodies against TNF-α.
- **Anakinra** (Kineret) is a recombinant interleukin-1 (IL-1) receptor antagonist.
- **Abatacept** (Orencia) is a selective costimulation modulator (inhibitor) and a fusion protein consisting of an IgG Fc fused to the CTLA4 extracellular domain. Studies have shown it to be efficacious in patients who have failed prior treatment with anti-TNF therapy.[14]
- **Rituximab** (Rituxan) is a chimeric monoclonal antibody against CD20 and results in the destruction of B cells. This agent has been shown to be efficacious in patients with inadequate responses to TNF inhibitors.[15]
- **Tocilizumab** (Actemra) is a monoclonal antibody against the interleukin-6 (IL-6) receptor.
- Consideration of biologic DMARDs is appropriate for patients unresponsive to oral DMARDs.
- Toxicities of the biologic DMARDs include opportunistic infections, disseminated TB, drug-induced lupus, worsened heart failure, demyelinating syndromes, colon perforation, and possibly increased risk of lymphoma.

Combination Therapy

- Combination regimens of multiple DMARDs or DMARDs plus biologic agents may be particularly effective in RA.[9] **Such combined therapy should only be done in conjunction with a rheumatologist.**
- Data show that virtually all DMARDs and biologic DMARDs are more effective when combined with MTX

Other Nonpharmacologic Therapies

- **Occupational therapy** usually focuses on the hand and wrist and can help patients with splinting, work simplification, activities of daily living, and assistive devices.
- **Physical therapy** assists in stretching and strengthening exercises for large joints such as the shoulder and knee, gait evaluation, and fitting with crutches and canes.
- Moderate exercise is appropriate for all patients and can help to reduce stiffness and maintain joint range of motion.
- In general, an exercise program should not produce pain for >2 hours after its completion.

Surgical Management

Orthopedic surgery to correct hand deformities and replace large joints such as the hip, knee, and shoulder should also be considered when pain cannot be controlled adequately with medications.

Infectious Arthritis and Septic Bursitis

GENERAL PRINCIPLES

- Infectious arthritis is generally categorized into gonococcal and nongonococcal infection.
- The usual presentation is with fever and acute monoarticular arthritis, although multiple joints may be affected by hematogenous spread of pathogens.
- **Nongonococcal** infectious arthritis in adults tends to occur in patients with previous joint damage or compromised host defenses.
  - Nongonococcal septic arthritis is caused most often by *Staphylococcus aureus* (60%) and *Streptococcus* spp.
  - Gram-negative organisms are less common, except with IV drug abuse, neutropenia, concomitant urinary tract infection, and prosthetic joints.
- **Gonococcal arthritis** is more common than nongonococcal septic arthritis and is the most common cause of monoarticular arthritis in patients between the ages of 20 and 30.[16] The clinical spectrum of disease often includes migratory or additive polyarthralgias, followed by tenosynovitis or arthritis of the wrist, ankle, or knee, and asymptomatic dermatitis on the extremities or trunk.
- **Nonbacterial infectious arthritis** is common with many viral infections, especially hepatitis B, rubella, mumps, infectious mononucleosis, parvovirus, enterovirus, adenovirus, and HIV. Hepatitis C infection is associated with the formation of cryoglobulinemia, which can present as a polyarticular inflammatory arthritis with glomerulonephritis, cutaneous vasculitis, and mononeuritis multiplex.
- Septic bursitis, usually involving the olecranon or prepatellar bursa, can be differentiated from septic arthritis by localized, fluctuant superficial swelling with relatively painless joint motion (particularly extension). Most patients have a history of previous trauma to the area or an occupational predisposition (e.g., so-called housemaid's knee and writer's elbow). *Staphylococcus aureus* is the most common pathogen.

DIAGNOSIS

- **Joint fluid examination, including Gram stain of a centrifuged pellet, and culture are mandatory to make a diagnosis and to guide management.**
- A joint fluid leukocyte count is useful diagnostically and as a baseline for serial studies to evaluate response to treatment.
- Cultures of blood and other possible extra-articular sites of infection **also** should be obtained.
- In contrast to nongonococcal septic arthritis, Gram staining of synovial fluid and cultures of blood or synovial fluid are often negative in gonococcal arthritis.

TREATMENT

- Hospitalization is indicated to ensure drug compliance and careful monitoring of the clinical response.
- IV antimicrobials provide good serum and synovial fluid drug concentrations. **Oral antimicrobials are not appropriate as initial therapy,** and there is no role for intra-articular antibiotic therapy.
- Arthrocenteses should be performed daily or as often as necessary to prevent reaccumulation of fluid and monitor response to therapy.
- General supportive measures include splinting of the joint, which may help to relieve pain. However, prolonged immobilization can result in joint stiffness.

Medications

- An NSAID or selective COX-2 inhibitor is often useful to reduce pain and to increase joint mobility but should not be used until response to antimicrobial therapy has been demonstrated by symptomatic and laboratory improvement.
- **Initial therapy is based on the clinical situation and a carefully performed Gram stain**, which reveals the organism in approximately 50% of patients.[17]
  - With a positive Gram stain, antibiotic coverage can be adjusted accordingly.
  - With a nondiagnostic Gram stain, antibiotics should be selected to cover *S. aureus*, *Streptococcus* spp., and *Neisseria gonorrhoeae* in otherwise healthy patients, whereas broad-spectrum antibiotics are appropriate in immunosuppressed patients.
  - IV antimicrobials are usually given for at least 2 weeks, followed by 1 to 2 weeks of oral antimicrobials, with the course of therapy tailored to the patient's response. Infectious disease consultation can be helpful for treatment.
- Treatment for gonococcal arthritis begins with an intravenous antibiotic for the first 1 to 3 days, generally ceftriaxone, 1 g daily or ceftizoxime, 1 g every 8 hours.
  - Response to IV antibiotics is usually noted within the first 24 to 36 hours of treatment.
  - After initial clinical improvement, therapy is continued with an oral antibiotic to complete 7 to 10 days of treatment.
  - Ciprofloxacin, 500 mg bid, or amoxicillin/clavulanate, 500/875 mg bid, can be used, although resistance to fluoroquinolones is increasing and decisions regarding treatment should be based on regional guidelines.[18]
- Viral arthritides are generally self-limited, lasting for <6 weeks, and respond well to a conservative regimen of rest and NSAIDs.
- Septic bursitis should be treated with aspiration, which should be repeated if fluid reaccumulates. Oral antibiotics and outpatient management are usually appropriate, and surgical drainage is rarely indicated.

Surgical Management

Surgical drainage or arthroscopic lavage and drainage are indicated in the following circumstances:

- A septic hip that cannot easily be accessed by arthrocentesis
- Joints in which the anatomy, large amounts of tissue debris, or loculation of pus prevent adequate needle drainage
- Septic arthritis with coexistent osteomyelitis
- Joints that do not respond in 4 to 6 days to appropriate therapy and repeated arthrocenteses
- Prosthetic joint infection

Gout

GENERAL PRINCIPLES

- Deposition of microcrystals in joints and periarticular tissues results in gout, pseudogout, and basic calcium phosphate (BCP) disease.[19]
- Gout is caused by the accumulation of excess amounts of uric acid in the body, leading to deposition of monosodium urate crystals when levels exceed solubility.
- Gout can produce four distinct clinical syndromes: acute gouty arthritis, chronic tophaceous gout, urate nephropathy, and urate nephrolithiasis.
- All complications of gout result from hyperuricemia. **In 90% of cases, this occurs as a result of underexcretion of urate**.
- Risk factors include male sex, hypertension, hyperlipidemia, obesity, renal dysfunction, alcohol, dehydration, and drugs (e.g., low-dose salicylates, diuretics, ethambutol, pyrazinamide, levodopa, cyclosporine, and tacrolimus).[20]

DIAGNOSIS

Clinical Presentation

- Acute gouty arthritis presents with acute pain and swelling, usually of a single joint.
- Commonly affected joints include the great toe MTP joint (i.e., podagra), ankle, knee, and wrist.
- Episodes often occur at night and frequently accompany acute medical illnesses, postsurgical periods, dehydration, fasting, or heavy alcohol consumption.
- Pain is severe, and immediate medical attention to provide pain relief is essential.
- Periarticular involvement is rare at presentation but may occur in long-standing cases.
- Intense periarticular inflammation with desquamation of skin may give the appearance of cellulitis.

Diagnostic Testing

- Gout is diagnosed by polarized microscopy of synovial fluid demonstrating bright, negatively birefringent, needle-shaped crystals (often found within a PMN).
- Cell counts of synovial aspirates are usually consistent with an inflammatory arthritis (white cells in the tens of thousands, mostly PMNs).
- Aspiration of superficial tophi with a 25-gauge needle can also provide diagnostic material.

TREATMENT

NSAIDs

- **NSAIDs are particularly effective and are the treatment of choice for acute gout**.
- They should be started in maximal doses and tapered over several days once the gouty flare has subsided.
- A common high-dose NSAID regimen is indomethacin 50 mg PO qid given for several days until relief is obtained, followed by 50 mg tid for 2 to 3 days, 50 mg bid for 2 to 3 days, 50 mg/day for a few days, and then discontinue.
- Naproxen, ibuprofen, sulindac, and other NSAIDs are also effective and are generally better tolerated than high-dose indomethacin.

Colchicine

- The current approved dose of colchicine for acute gout is 1.2 mg PO then 0.6 mg 1 hour later as needed. Avoid this treatment in patients on colchicine prophylaxis and taking a CYP3A4 inhibitor. Dose adjustment is not needed for renal impairment but should not be repeated for 2 weeks. For patients on hemodialysis, only 0.6 mg should be given and not repeated.
- **The traditional dose of colchicine every hour is obsolete and should not be used**.
- IV colchicine is no longer available.

Glucocorticoids

- Oral steroids can be used when other therapies are contraindicated. Prednisone initiated at 60 mg/day and tapered rapidly can provide adequate symptomatic relief while avoiding toxicities of long-term steroid use.
- Intra-articular aspiration and corticosteroid injection is appropriate for large joints and is an excellent choice for patients who are not good candidates for NSAIDs. Because the knee joint often has a tense effusion, aspiration of as much fluid as possible can bring immediate relief, followed by injection of 1 to 2 mL corticosteroid with an equal volume of 1% lidocaine. A volume of 1 mL is appropriate for the ankle.

Biologic Therapy

Pegloticase (Krystexxa) is a pegylated, recombinant uricase that can be administered to patients with chronic tophaceous gout who have had persistent disease and elevated uric acid despite maximum therapy with other uric acid–lowering medications. Patients must be tested for glucose-6-phosphate dehydrogenase deficiency prior to administration. Pegloticase should only be prescribed by those experienced in its use.

Prophylactic Treatment

- Prophylactic treatment is advisable when patients have recurrent attacks several times per year.
- **Colchicine**, 0.6 mg once or twice daily, may be used (dose must be reduced for renal insufficiency or concomitant CYP3A4 inhibitors). Low-dose NSAIDs such as indomethacin, 25 mg bid, or naproxen, 250 mg bid, are another option. In patients with multiple recurrent attacks, uric acid–lowering therapy may be beneficial.
- **Xanthine oxidase inhibitors (allopurinol and febuxostat)** reduce uric acid production and are much easier to administer than probenecid.
  - Xanthine oxidase inhibitors are indicated for recurrent attacks that are not controlled with colchicine or NSAIDs.
  - Other indications for xanthine oxidase inhibitors include the presence of tophi, renal stones, and severe hyperuricemia (>13 mg/dL).
  - **Asymptomatic hyperuricemia should not be treated with these medications**.
  - A starting dose of allopurinol 100 mg/day can be increased after 2 to 4 weeks to 300 mg/day. Sometimes, higher doses (400 to 600 mg/day) are required. In the setting of renal impairment, starting dose should be 50 mg. The correct dose is that which reduces the serum uric acid to <6 mg/dL.
  - Febuxostat should be started at 40 mg daily and may be increased to 80 mg daily if necessary. There are no data for higher doses or for use in patients with creatinine clearance <30.
  - Xanthine oxidase inhibitors should not be started during an acute attack as they may cause a severe flare of the disease. Administration of prophylactic colchicine or low-dose NSAIDs before initiation of uric acid–lowering therapy may prevent the gouty attacks that sometimes accompany the initiation of allopurinol treatment. It is not necessary to discontinue use of a urate-lowering medication if a gout attack occurs after it is started.
  - These medications are usually well tolerated, although a **severe hypersensitivity syndrome** can occur, especially with renal insufficiency and diuretic use.
- **Probenecid** prevents tubular reabsorption of uric acid and can be used to enhance urinary excretion of uric acid provided that the baseline 24-hour urinary uric acid is 600 mg or less.
  - If the 24-hour uric acid is >600 mg, increasing the urinary excretion of uric acid may precipitate uric acid kidney stones.
  - Probenecid can be initiated at 500 mg PO daily and increased as needed, not exceeding 3,000 mg in three divided doses.
  - Normal renal function is necessary for probenecid to be effective.
  - Salicylates at any dose antagonize the effect of probenecid.
- A 12-year study of 730 patients with gout suggested that high levels of meat and seafood in the **diet** are associated with an increased risk of gout, whereas dairy products may be protective. The level of purine-rich vegetables and total protein intake was not associated with an increased risk of gout.[21]

Pseudogout

- Pseudogout is caused by deposition of **calcium pyrophosphate crystals** and tends to occur more often in elderly individuals.
- It may be precipitated by surgery and has been associated with hypothyroidism, hyperparathyroidism, diabetes, and hemochromatosis.

- Like gout, pseudogout tends to cause monoarticular attacks, **especially in large joints**.
- Symmetric involvement of the hands may mimic RA.
- Periarticular inflammation can be severe, mimicking cellulitis.
- Polarized microscopy of synovial fluid reveals **rhomboid-shaped crystals that are positively birefringent**.
- Radiographic studies may demonstrate **chondrocalcinosis** (especially knee, wrist, and symphysis pubis) but alone are not diagnostic of pseudogout.
- Treatment is the same as for gout, except that there is no role for uric acid–lowering therapy. Joint aspiration, alone or with steroid injection, often provides immediate relief of pain.

Apatite Deposition Disease

- Apatite deposition disease may present with periarthritis or tendonitis, particularly in the elderly and in patients with chronic renal failure.
- An episodic oligoarthritis may also occur, and apatite disease should be suspected when no crystals are present in the synovial fluid.
- Erosive arthritis may be seen, particularly in the shoulder (e.g., Milwaukee shoulder, a syndrome of large shoulder effusion, rotator cuff pathology, and the presence of basic calcium phosphate [BCP] crystals in synovial fluid).
- Hydroxyapatite complexes and BCP complexes can be identified only by electron microscopy, mass spectroscopy, or alizarin red staining, none of which are readily available to the clinician.
- The treatment of apatite disease is similar to that for pseudogout, except that recent studies suggest that early intervention and washing out the joint may help prevent progression of the disease.[22]
- Referral to orthopedic surgery may be required.

Systemic Lupus Erythematosus

GENERAL PRINCIPLES

- SLE is a multisystem autoimmune disease of unknown etiology that commonly occurs in women of childbearing age. There is clearly a genetic predisposition.
- Manifestations of SLE are protean, and organ systems involved may include skin, heart, lungs, nervous system, kidneys, hematopoietic system, and joints.
- African-Americans and Hispanics have a worse prognosis.
- SLE can occur in the elderly, but when it does, it is usually milder.

DIAGNOSIS

Clinical Presentation

- The ACR has proposed 11 criteria for the diagnosis of SLE (Table 33-5).[23]
- For inclusion in clinical studies, a diagnosis requires that at least four of them be present at some point through the course of the disease. These criteria may be used to aid in the clinical diagnosis of lupus, recognizing that having four criteria in isolation is neither necessary nor sufficient for the diagnosis.[23]

Diagnostic Testing

- The **ANA is highly sensitive** and is positive in virtually all patients with SLE. Therefore, **a negative ANA is useful to exclude SLE**; however, a positive ANA test alone is of little significance in the absence of clinical evidence of disease, regardless of how high the titer.
- **Antibodies to double-stranded DNA are very specific** for SLE, especially when present at high titers.

TABLE 33-5	Systemic Lupus Erythematosus Classification Criteria Definitions

Criteria	Description
Malar rash	Fixed erythema, flat or raised, sparing the nasolabial folds
Discoid rash	Raised patches, adherent keratotic scaling, follicular plugging; older lesions may cause scarring
Photosensitivity	Skin rash from sunlight
Oral or nasopharyngeal ulcers	Usually painless
Arthritis	Nonerosive, inflammatory in two or more peripheral joints
Serositis	Pleuritis or pericarditis
Renal disorder	Persistent proteinuria or cellular casts
Neurologic disorder	Seizures or psychosis
Hematologic	Hemolytic anemia, leukopenia (<4,000/mm^3), lymphopenia (<1,500/mm^3), or thrombocytopenia (<100,00/mm^3)
Immunologic disorder	Antibodies to dsDNA or
	Antibodies to Sm or
	Antiphospholipid antibodies: IgG/IgM antibodies or positive lupus anticoagulant test results or false-positive serologic test results for syphilis
Antinuclear antibody	Present

dsDNA, double-stranded (native) deoxyribonucleic acid; Sm, Smith nuclear antigen.
Modified from Tan EM, Cohen AS, Fries JF, et al. *Arthritis Rheum* 1982;25:1271–1277.

- High levels of anti-DNA antibody can correlate with disease activity, especially with lupus nephritis. Therefore, quantitative anti-DNA titers are sometimes useful in monitoring disease flares and response to treatment. However, lupus often occurs in the absence of anti-DNA antibodies.
- **Anti-Sm** is **very specific** for SLE although it is positive in a minority of patients.
- **Serum complement measures, C3 and C4,** are sometimes abnormal in active SLE, especially in the setting of nephritis, and may rise and fall with disease activity.
- **Antiphospholipid antibodies** are important in diagnosing the **antiphospholipid syndrome (APS)**, characterized by fetal loss, venous and arterial thromboses, CNS events, and thrombocytopenia.[24]
  - Diagnosis of APS is relevant, as the treatment may necessitate lifelong anticoagulation.
  - Anticardiolipin and beta2-glycoprotein-I antibodies are measured by ELISA. IgG antibodies in significant titer are more predictive of clinical events than are IgM or IgA.
  - **False-positive Venereal Disease Research Laboratory test (VDRL) or rapid plasma reagin (RPR) can be caused by the presence of APA reacting with the cardiolipin substrate.** The fluorescent treponemal antibody absorption test should be negative, although a low-titer beaded pattern is sometimes observed.
  - **The lupus "anticoagulant"** (LAC) is not specific for lupus and despite its name promotes coagulation. The activated thromboplastin time (PTT) assay does not correct with the addition of normal plasma, but does correct when phospholipid is added in excess to neutralize the APA. The dilute Russell Viper venom time (dRVVT) is another test for LAC that does not require a prolonged PTT.
  - A positive LAC or high-titer IgG anticardiolipin antibody is more predictive of clinical events than the other tests.

TREATMENT

- Treatment for SLE is dependent on the clinical scenario.
- For patients without life- or organ-threatening disease, initiation of conservative therapy is appropriate: sunscreen and sun avoidance, topical steroids for isolated skin lesions, and hydroxychloroquine for arthralgias and fatigue.
- More severe cases of SLE may require more aggressive therapy. In general, prednisone in moderate (15 to 30 mg/day) or higher (40 to 60 mg/day) doses is usually the first-line therapy for a moderate-to-severe lupus flare. Steroid-sparing therapies are frequently needed when flares are recurrent. Such therapies include:
  - Mycophenolate mofetil.
  - Azathioprine.
  - Methotrexate or leflunomide.
  - Cyclophosphamide for life-threatening disease.
  - Belimumab, a monoclonal antibody that inhibits B-cell–activating factor.
  - B-cell depletion with rituximab is widely thought to benefit a subset of patients with SLE although randomized clinical trials have yet to confirm this.
  - Immunoablation with or without stem cell transplantation for refractory disease is still considered to be an investigational approach.

Symptom-Specific Treatments

- **Arthritis** often responds to NSAIDs, although they must be used with caution in patients with decreased renal function. The addition of prednisone in low doses (5 to 10 mg/day) may be necessary. Long-term treatment with hydroxychloroquine or MTX helps control arthritis (see the "Rheumatoid Arthritis" section).
- **Rashes** may respond to topical corticosteroids (fluorinated topical steroids on the face should be avoided because of the risk of subcutaneous atrophy). If topical agents are not effective, systemic corticosteroids may be needed. Hydroxychloroquine is often beneficial in the long-term management of rash and may help to reduce the need for corticosteroids.
- **Oral ulcers** can be treated with dental paste that contains benzocaine (Orabase B) or triamcinolone (Kenalog in Orabase) or an over-the-counter anesthetic oral rinse (e.g., Ulcer Ease).
- Mild cases of **pleuritis and pericarditis** sometimes respond to NSAIDs, whereas more severe cases require corticosteroids.
- The treatment of **renal disease** is complicated.[25]
  - For most serious renal lesions, periodic monthly cyclophosphamide has traditionally been administered, although MMF is being used more frequently as first-line therapy.
  - High doses of corticosteroids, administered either orally or intravenously, are also commonly used in the acute setting as cyclophosphamide, and mycophenolate mofetil may take weeks to reach peak efficacy.
- For **hematologic manifestations**, such as hemolytic anemia, severe leukopenia, or thrombocytopenia, corticosteroids in moderate-to-high doses are required.
- **Neuropsychiatric disease** is difficult to assess because there is no laboratory test or physical finding that can unequivocally support the diagnosis of lupus affecting the central nervous system. The diagnosis is based on clinical factors and is a diagnosis of exclusion. Aggressive treatment with high-dose steroids may be necessary to help control symptoms.

Seronegative Spondyloarthropathies

GENERAL PRINCIPLES

- The spondyloarthropathies are a group of articular disorders characterized by involvement of the axial skeleton with a negative RF.[26]

- These disorders include ankylosing spondylitis, reactive arthritis, psoriatic arthritis, and arthritis associated with inflammatory bowel disease.
- **Ankylosing spondylitis**, the prototype of the spondyloarthropathies, is diagnosed in men much more commonly than in women, partly because the spine symptoms in women tend to be more subtle. Associated acute iritis produces severe eye pain and blurred vision and requires urgent referral to an ophthalmologist.
- **Reactive arthritis** occurs after infectious syndromes such as nongonococcal urethritis or infectious diarrhea with *Shigella* spp., *Salmonella* spp., or *Yersinia enterocolitica*. A reactive arthritis syndrome of urethritis, arthritis, and conjunctivitis was previously referred to as Reiter syndrome.
- **Psoriatic arthritis** has five basic presentations: spinal predominance, polyarticular small joint involvement, oligoarticular asymmetric large joint involvement, DIP joint predominance, and the rare arthritis mutilans with telescoping digits. In general, the severity of joint disease does not parallel that of the skin disease, except for the DIP pattern, which correlates with nail abnormalities.
- **Ulcerative colitis and Crohn disease** may be accompanied by inflammatory arthritis of two types. The peripheral joint variety tends to parallel the activity of the bowel disease, whereas the spondylotic pattern typically has an independent course of the bowel disease.
- **Axial spondyloarthropathy** is a relatively new term that includes patients with axial-predominant spondyloarthropathy with and without radiographic evidence of sacroiliitis.

DIAGNOSIS

Clinical Presentation

History
- The characteristic history is that of **inflammatory back pain**. Five distinguishing symptoms include gradual onset, onset before the age of 40 years, morning stiffness, improvement with mild exercise, and duration >3 months.
- When **peripheral joint involvement** is present, it is typically asymmetric and oligoarticular, generally in the lower extremities.
- Inflammation generally occurs where tendons insert on bone (**enthesopathy**) and produces so-called sausage digits of individual fingers and toes (dactylitis), plantar fasciitis, and Achilles tendonitis.
- Nonarticular symptoms may include aphthous stomatitis, ocular inflammation such as conjunctivitis and iritis, and aortic dilatation.

Physical Examination
- **Spine motion** may be simply assessed by having the patient bend forward with the knees extended and measuring the distance between the fingertips and floor (recognizing that hamstring tightness reduces the range of motion). To perform the modified Schober test, mark two points 10 cm cephalad to and 5 cm caudal to the sacral dimples of Venus. With forward flexion, the line between these points should increase by at least 5 cm.
- **Peripheral joints** should be checked for diffuse fusiform swelling of fingers and toes (sausage digits or dactylitis) and asymmetric swelling of large joints, especially the knees and ankles.
- **Ocular findings** in ankylosing spondylitis and reactive arthritis include redness and a pupil that reacts asymmetrically, indicating previous episodes of ocular inflammation resulting in synechiae.
- **Skin findings** in psoriasis are usually obvious, but the following areas should be specifically examined to look for subtle changes: the scalp, external auditory canal, umbilicus, and intergluteal cleft. It may be difficult to distinguish the skin findings of reactive arthritis from those of psoriasis.

Diagnostic Testing

- The **RF** is by definition negative, and the **ESR** is inconsistently elevated.
- Although the **human leukocyte antigen B27** is present in >90% of Caucasians with ankylosing spondylitis, its frequency is lower in other ethnic groups and in other spondyloarthropathies. It is present in approximately 8% to 10% of unaffected Caucasians.
- **Radiographs** to look for sacroiliitis include an anteroposterior view of the pelvis, sometimes supplemented by modified Ferguson views of the sacroiliac joints (taken with a 30-degree cephalad angle). Definite radiographic changes take years to develop. MRI of the SI joints enables diagnosis of early disease. Radiographs of peripheral joints may show periostitis.

TREATMENT

- **Physical therapy** to improve and maintain spinal motion is extremely important.
- **NSAIDs** are the mainstay of symptomatic treatment. High doses are generally required (e.g., indomethacin, 50 mg qid; naproxen, 500 mg tid).
- **Sulfasalazine** is efficacious in some patients for whom NSAIDs do not provide adequate relief (see the "Rheumatoid Arthritis" section).
- **MTX** has a well-established role in treating psoriatic arthritis and is sometimes effective for peripheral joint problems in the other spondylotic disorders. Patients with psoriasis have an increased risk of fibrosis and cirrhosis from methotrexate and should undergo liver biopsy at cumulative dose intervals of 2.5 to 3 g.
- The **TNF blockers** have been shown to be effective in providing symptomatic relief in ankylosing spondylitis and psoriatic arthritis.

Scleroderma

GENERAL PRINCIPLES

- Scleroderma is a poorly understood process that leads to pathologic changes of small-vessel vasculopathy (distinct from vasculitis), fibrosis, and proliferation of myofibroblasts in affected organs. The disease is characterized by fibrosis of the skin and internal organs, especially the lungs, heart, kidneys, and GI tract.
- The two major forms of this disease are (1) diffuse scleroderma and (2) limited scleroderma (known as the **CREST syndrome** which stands for **C**alcinosis, **R**aynaud phenomenon, **E**sophageal dysmotility, **S**clerodactyly, and **T**elangiectasias).

DIAGNOSIS

Clinical Presentation

- The diagnosis of scleroderma rests on the history and physical examination.
- Skin findings on physical examination are key to the diagnosis. Patients with diffuse as well as limited disease may have tight skin on the fingers as well as involvement of facial skin, most often around the mouth. In diffuse disease, the skin proximal to the elbows and knees is involved as well as loss of facial wrinkles and perioral fibrosis.
- **Raynaud phenomenon:**
  - Raynaud phenomenon is present in almost all patients with scleroderma.
  - The classic history is one of triphasic skin color change: pallor (vasospasm) followed by cyanosis (desaturation of tissue hemoglobin) followed by rubor (reactive hyperemia). Many patients note only two of these changes.
  - Cold temperatures, tobacco smoke, stress, and certain medications may provoke symptoms.

○ The nail fold capillaries can be visualized by coating the cuticle with a thin layer of clear surgical lubricant and looking through an ophthalmoscope set at +40. Dilatation or dropout of nail fold capillaries increases the likelihood that Raynaud phenomenon will evolve into a systemic rheumatic disease.[27]

Diagnostic Testing

• ANA is positive in most patients.
• **Anticentromere antibody** is a special subset of ANA, with a finely speckled pattern, and is seen in the majority of patients with limited disease.
• **Anti–Scl 70** is an antibody to topoisomerase that is quite specific for diffuse disease but is found in a minority of patients. This antibody is associated with interstitial lung disease and scleroderma renal crisis.

TREATMENT

• Treatment is largely supportive and organ system specific because there is no treatment that clearly alters the long-term course of this disease.
• The most important aspect of treatment of **Raynaud phenomenon** is protecting the hands from cold temperatures. Covering the head during cold weather is essential, because much of core body heat can be lost through the head, leading to lower body temperature in the extremities.
  ○ A variety of vasodilating calcium channel blockers (especially dihydropyridines such as nifedipine or amlodipine) help reduce recurrence and severity of symptoms.
  ○ Sildenafil and bosentan are not FDA approved for this indication, but may be effective in refractory cases.[28]
• Azotemia, proteinuria, and a microangiopathic hemolytic anemia can develop in patients with **scleroderma renal crisis**. Hypertension must be managed aggressively, and the angiotensin-converting enzyme (ACE) inhibitors are the drugs of choice for scleroderma renal crisis. Data presented at the American College of Rheumatology call into question the use of ACE inhibitors prior to development of scleroderma renal crisis. The use of ACE inhibitors has decreased the mortality due to renal crisis such that pulmonary disease is now the leading cause of death in these patients.
• **GI complications**:
  ○ **Gastroesophageal reflux** can be treated with proton pump inhibitors or high-dose histamine-2 receptor blockers. Surgery to correct reflux should be avoided in these patients because of coexisting motility disorders.
  ○ **Esophageal strictures** sometimes require mechanical dilatation.
  ○ **Malabsorption** due to bacterial overgrowth can be treated with broad-spectrum antibiotics.
• Limited data indicate that cyclophosphamide therapy can reduce the progression of **interstitial lung disease,** and studies are underway to evaluate MMF.[29]
• Many patients with systemic sclerosis may develop complications of **pulmonary hypertension**. Recent advances have been made in the treatment of pulmonary hypertension associated with scleroderma. Treatment options include sildenafil, bosentan, and other prostacyclin analogues.[30,31]
• **Coronary artery vasospasm** can cause angina that may be responsive to calcium channel blockers.

Sjögren Syndrome

GENERAL PRINCIPLES

Sjögren syndrome is a multisystem autoimmune disease characterized by dysfunction of exocrine glands. It may occur as a primary disorder or secondary to other rheumatic diseases such as RA, SLE, scleroderma, or inflammatory myopathy.

DIAGNOSIS

Clinical Presentation

History
- History is notable for the sicca symptoms of dry eyes and dry mouth.
- Parotid gland swelling may occur, and occasionally, patients have symptoms of pancreatic insufficiency with diarrhea and malabsorption.
- Symptoms of vaginal dryness may be present in women.

Physical Examination
- Eye exam may show a diminished corneal light reflex and reduced tear meniscus.
- Oral examination reveals a diminished or absent sublingual salivary pool, and the tongue and buccal mucosa may appear dry.
- The parotid and submandibular glands are sometimes enlarged.
- Inflammatory arthritis and cutaneous vasculitis may also be associated with Sjögren syndrome.
- Additionally, patients with Sjögren syndrome often have symptoms of Raynaud phenomenon.
- Enlargement of lymph nodes, liver, or spleen raises the suspicion of lymphoma, the incidence of which is increased 40-fold.

Diagnostic Testing
- Laboratory tests associated with Sjögren syndrome include ANA, RF, and SSA (anti-Ro) or SSB (anti-La) antibodies.
- Lymphocytic infiltration on biopsy of minor salivary glands from the inner surface of the lower lip helps support the diagnosis of Sjögren syndrome.

TREATMENT

- Artificial tears are helpful for **dry eye symptoms** and can be self-administered as needed. Optic cyclosporine has been shown to decrease symptoms of ocular dryness. For more severe cases, an ophthalmologist can accomplish temporary or permanent occlusion of the lacrimal puncta.
- Treatment of **dry mouth symptoms** is more challenging but important to reduce discomfort and the incidence of dental caries.
  - Conservative measures, such as increased oral water intake and chewing sugarless gum, can provide symptomatic relief.
  - Oral pilocarpine, 5 mg qid, or cevimeline, 30 mg tid, has been shown to increase saliva production and improve symptoms of oral dryness.
  - Various saliva substitutes are available over the counter but may be poorly tolerated.
- Hydroxychloroquine (see the "Rheumatoid Arthritis" section) is sometimes prescribed for various manifestations of Sjögren syndrome.
- Immunosuppressive agents may be required for involvement of major organs including vasculitis.

Vasculitis

GENERAL PRINCIPLES

- The clinical manifestations of vasculitis are protean. Fever, weight loss, mononeuropathy, rash, arthritis, abdominal pain, sinusitis, pulmonary hemorrhage, and glomerulonephritis are among the many presenting symptoms.

- Physical manifestations tend to be nonspecific, but skin lesions such as palpable purpura, livedo reticularis, and digital gangrene raise suspicion for vasculitis.
- Wrist-drop or foot drop is suggestive of mononeuropathy, another important clue to the presence of systemic vasculitis.

DIAGNOSIS

Specific Vasculitic Syndromes

- **Polyarteritis nodosa** includes many of the above symptoms but typically presents with hypertension, glomerulonephritis, abdominal pain, and mononeuropathy (commonly wrist-drop or foot drop). Onset may be gradual or sudden, and patients are systemically ill.
- **Giant cell arteritis** (GCA) presents with headache, visual disturbance, tongue and jaw claudication, and scalp tenderness. GCA is often associated with polymyalgia rheumatica (PMR).
- **Takayasu arteritis** affects the aorta and its branches. It occurs most commonly in young Asian women and is often detected by asymmetric pulses or blood pressure measurements. Other symptoms include headache, arm claudication, visual changes, and arthralgias.
- **Granulomatosis with polyangiitis** (formerly known as Wegener granulomatosis) presents with the classic triad of upper airway disease (sinusitis), lower airway disease (pulmonary hemorrhage), and glomerulonephritis. Limited granulomatosis with polyangiitis occurs without renal involvement.
- **Churg-Strauss vasculitis** is classically associated with severe asthma and systemic eosinophilia. Peripheral neuropathy, mononeuritis, and pulmonary and cutaneous involvement are common.
- **Cutaneous vasculitis** may be common to all subtypes of vasculitis and commonly presents with palpable purpura, usually in dependent areas of the lower extremities. Although often associated with systemic diseases, vasculitis may be limited to the skin.
- **Cryoglobulinemia**, frequently associated with hepatitis C, can present with purpura, arthritis, and glomerulonephritis.
- **Secondary vasculitis**: vasculitis may also occur secondary to other rheumatic diseases, such as RA and SLE, and should be suspected when symptoms include cutaneous vasculitis, peripheral neuropathies, or mesenteric ischemia.

Diagnostic Testing

- Laboratory findings are nonspecific, but anemia, elevated ESR, and urinalysis abnormalities (proteinuria, hematuria, and cellular casts) are often seen.
- c-ANCA that represents antibody to proteinase-3 is specific for granulomatosis with polyangiitis.
- Biopsy of affected tissues, such as skin, muscle, artery, and nerve, can be valuable in establishing the diagnosis. The gastrocnemius muscle and sural nerve are common sources of diagnostic material. Renal biopsy findings tend to be nonspecific (crescentic glomerulonephritis with negative immunofluorescence) and rarely include vasculitis.

TREATMENT

- Treatment depends on the specific diagnosis.
- **High-dose corticosteroids** (prednisone at 1 mg/kg/day) are usually effective, especially in the short term.
- **Cyclophosphamide** can also be used, in either a daily oral dose of 1 to 2 mg/kg/day or a monthly IV dose of 0.5 to 1 g/m^2.
- **Rituximab** has been shown to be as effective as cyclophosphamide for initial treatment of granulomatosis with polyangiitis.

- Vasculitis that is limited to the skin does not require potent immunosuppressive treatment, and therapies such as methotrexate, azathioprine, or even colchicine may be effective.

Polymyalgia Rheumatica and Giant Cell Arteritis

GENERAL PRINCIPLES

PMR and GCA represent a continuum of disease. A patient may have one or both diagnoses, and they can develop in either order. PMR and GCA occur after the age of 50 years, and the incidence increases with age.

DIAGNOSIS

Clinical Presentation

- The classic history for PMR is morning stiffness, worse in the neck, shoulder, and pelvic girdle region. The patient may complain of the inability to roll over in bed at night.
- GCA presents with headache, tongue or jaw claudication, scalp tenderness, and vision loss (typically amaurosis fugax).
- Systemic symptoms such as fever and weight loss may also occur in GCA.
- Physical examination of patients with PMR is most notable for a profound inability to abduct and elevate the shoulders in most cases. Synovitis, if present, should be minimal. Although an uncommon finding, in GCA, a tender, nodular superficial temporal artery with reduced or absent pulse strongly suggests the diagnosis.

Diagnostic Testing

- **Virtually all patients with PMR or GCA have an elevated ESR**. The high sensitivity of this test makes PMR/GCA unlikely with a normal ESR. CRP may also be elevated.
- A temporal artery **biopsy** should be performed in all patients in whom GCA is suspected. The pathologic findings of granulomatous inflammation with giant cells and fragmentation of the internal elastic lamina confirm the diagnosis. Because the temporal artery biopsy does not have 100% sensitivity, when the clinical presentation is convincing, a diagnosis of GCA may be made despite a negative biopsy.

TREATMENT

- Treatment for PMR is focused on relieving discomfort and improving quality of life.
- Although NSAIDs occasionally are effective for PMR, most patients require prednisone in doses of 10 to 15 mg/day for relief.
- Failure of the patient to improve dramatically and rapidly with low-dose corticosteroids should lead to reconsideration of the diagnosis of PMR.
- Treatment can be tapered over approximately 1 year, although some patients require longer treatment.
- **GCA must be treated aggressively as a systemic vasculitis**.
  - For suspicion of GCA, **high-dose prednisone must be initiated immediately** at approximately 60 mg daily to prevent the complication of irreversible vision loss.
  - Treatment **should not be delayed until a temporal artery biopsy** can be performed, because the diagnostic findings on biopsy can still be demonstrated several days after corticosteroid therapy has been started. Furthermore, patients may develop blindness during the first few days of therapy.
  - The dose of prednisone can be tapered slowly over several months, provided that the patient remains asymptomatic.
  - Methotrexate may be an effective steroid-sparing agent in some patients, although the evidence is conflicting.

Polymyositis and Dermatomyositis

GENERAL PRINCIPLES

- Polymyositis (PM) and dermatomyositis (DM) are both idiopathic inflammatory myopathies but have many distinctions.
- DM is associated with skin manifestations, but PM is not. Proximal myopathy is characteristic of both, but DM may sometimes occur without myositis.
- There does appear to be an association with malignancy in a minority of patients, more pronounced with DM.

DIAGNOSIS

Clinical Presentation

History
- The cardinal feature of myositis is **proximal muscle weakness** without pain. Typically, patients notice difficulty in getting out of a car, chair, or bathtub; climbing stairs; or using their arms above the head. Distal muscle strength should be normal except in inclusion body myositis, which tends to occur in older individuals.
- **Dysphagia** with nasal regurgitation may occur if there is weakness of the striated muscle of the upper esophagus.
- **Dyspnea** due to interstitial lung disease and joint pain from inflammatory arthritis may occur, especially in the antisynthetase syndrome (PM with anti–Jo-1 antibody).

Physical Examination
- The exam should focus on evidence of proximal muscle weakness, a sensitive test of which is the ability to raise the head from the supine position. Standing up from a chair with the arms folded across the chest and rising from a deep squat are other good tests for proximal weakness.
- Patients with dermatomyositis have typical skin findings such as a heliotrope rash on the eyelids, Gottron papules on the knuckles, and nail fold capillary abnormalities.
- Mechanic's hands are classically associated with the antisynthetase syndrome.

Diagnostic Testing

- Laboratory studies should include serum **muscle enzymes**, especially creatine phosphokinase (CK), which is elevated in virtually all cases of inflammatory myopathy. Elevations of aspartate aminotransferase (AST) and aldolase may occur but are less specific for muscle injury.
- Myositis-associated antibodies (such as anti–Jo-1, anti–MI-2, and anti-SRP) are primarily important for classifying diseases in research but sometimes can be helpful in atypical cases.
- Most patients should undergo **electromyography** (EMG) to look for the classic myopathic findings of fibrillations, positive sharp waves, and low-amplitude polyphasic motor unit potentials.
- **Muscle biopsy** can be done on the contralateral side, corresponding to the most abnormal area on the EMG. The biceps, deltoid, and vastus medialis are the muscles that are easily biopsied. MRI has recently been shown to help with identifying affected muscles for biopsy.

TREATMENT

- Treatment involves **high doses of corticosteroids**, either 1 mg/kg/day prednisone orally or pulse doses of methylprednisolone.
  - Sustained high doses for several months are usually required to control disease activity.

- ○ Normalization of CK levels precedes improvement in muscle strength by several weeks.
- ○ After several months of treatment, it is usually possible to taper the dose of prednisone, often to an every-other-day regimen.
- Patients whose disease cannot be controlled with corticosteroids can be treated with MTX or azathioprine as steroid-sparing agents.
- IV Igs can be beneficial, particularly in the short term.
- Other approaches to therapy include using immunomodulators such as mycophenolate, tacrolimus, cyclosporine, and rituximab as steroid-sparing agents.

Fibromyalgia

GENERAL PRINCIPLES

- Fibromyalgia is a common cause of musculoskeletal pain. It can be described as a soft tissue amplification syndrome, in which patients experience diffuse musculoskeletal pain.
- Data obtained by functional MRI indicate that pain input is processed differently in the brain in fibromyalgia patients, compared to controls.[32]

DIAGNOSIS

- **History suggestive** of fibromyalgia includes diffuse nonarticular pain, sleep disturbance resulting in nonrestorative sleep and fatigue, and accompanying symptoms such as headache, irritable bowel syndrome, paresthesias, depression, and vasomotor symptoms in the hands and feet.
- **Physical examination** is notable for tenderness to palpation in at least 11 of 18 predetermined tender points. Although the tender points were included in the initial ACR Classification Criteria for Fibromyalgia, opinion is divided as to whether tender points must be present to make the diagnosis.
- **Laboratory** studies are normal.

TREATMENT

- Treatment has three primary goals: improve sleep, relieve pain, and enhance physical conditioning.
- Non–habit-forming medications that aid in sleep include tricyclic antidepressants (e.g., amitriptyline, 10 to 50 mg qHS), trazodone (25 to 100 mg qHS), and cyclobenzaprine (10 to 20 mg qHS).
- Antidepressant medications (such as venlafaxine, duloxetine, and milnacipran) may also be beneficial. Duloxetine and milnacipran have been shown to be effective in reducing pain in fibromyalgia, regardless of whether depression is present.
- Gabapentin and pregabalin also reduce pain in fibromyalgia. Pregabalin is FDA approved for the treatment of fibromyalgia.
- NSAIDs and other analgesics may bring some relief of pain, but **opiates typically require escalating doses to control symptoms and are problematic in the chronic treatment of fibromyalgia**.
- An aerobic exercise program is essential and can be supplemented by stretching exercises.
- Cognitive-behavioral therapy programs are also effective.

REFERENCES

1. Guidelines for the initial evaluation of the adult patient with acute musculoskeletal symptoms. American College of Rheumatology Ad Hoc Committee on Clinical Guidelines. *Arthritis Rheum* 1996;39:1–8.

2. Nishimura K, Sugiyama D, Kogata Y, et al. Meta-analysis: diagnostic accuracy of anti-cyclic citrullinated peptide antibody and rheumatoid factor for rheumatoid arthritis. *Ann Intern Med* 2007;146:797–808.
3. Klippel JH, ed. *Primer on the Rheumatic Diseases*, 12th ed. Atlanta, GA: Arthritis Foundation; 2001.
4. Recommendations for the medical management of osteoarthritis of the hip and knee: 2000 update. American College of Rheumatology Subcommittee on Osteoarthritis Guidelines. *Arthritis Rheum* 2000;43:1905–1915.
5. Goldstein JL, Howard KB, Walton SM, et al. Impact of adherence to concomitant gastroprotective therapy on NSAID-related gastroduodenal ulcer complications. *Clin Gastroenterol Hepatol* 2006;4:1337–1345.
6. Stacy ZA, Dobesh PP, Trujillo TC. Cardiovascular risks of cyclooxygenase inhibition. *Pharmacotherapy* 2006;26:919–938.
7. Holander JL. 9 years of experience with steroid therapy, using intra-articular administration. *Hospital (Rio J)* 1963;64:491–495.
8. Lo GH, LaValley M, McAlindon T, Felson DT. Intra-articular hyaluronic acid in treatment of knee osteoarthritis: a meta-analysis. *JAMA* 2003;290:3115–3121.
9. O'Dell JR. Therapeutic strategies for rheumatoid arthritis. *N Engl J Med* 2004;350:2591–2602.
10. Aletaha D, Negoi T, Silman AJ, et al. 2010 rheumatoid arthritis classification criteria: an ACR/EULAR collaborative initiative. *Ann Rheum Dis* 2010;69:1580–1588.
11. Wolfe F, Freundlich B, Straus WL. Increase in cardiovascular and cerebrovascular disease prevalence in rheumatoid arthritis. *J Rheumatol* 2003;30:36–40.
12. Guidelines for the management of rheumatoid arthritis: 2002 update. American College of Rheumatology Subcommittee on Rheumatoid Arthritis Guidelines. *Arthritis Rheum* 2002;46:328–346.
13. Recommendations for the prevention and treatment of glucocorticoid-induced osteoporosis: 2001 update. American College of Rheumatology Ad Hoc Committee on Glucocorticoid-Induced Osteoporosis. *Arthritis Rheum* 2001;44:1496–1503.
14. Genovese MC, Becker JC, Schiff M, et al. Abatacept for rheumatoid arthritis refractory to tumor necrosis factor alpha inhibition. *N Engl J Med* 2005;353:1114–1123.
15. Edwards JC, Szczepanski L, Szechinski J, et al. Efficacy of B-cell-targeted therapy with rituximab in patients with rheumatoid arthritis. *N Engl J Med* 2004;350:2572–2581.
16. O'Brien JP, Goldenberg DL, Rice PA. Disseminated gonococcal infection: a prospective analysis of 49 patients and a review of pathophysiology and immune mechanisms. *Medicine (Baltimore)* 1983;62:395–406.
17. Pinals RS. Polyarthritis and fever. *N Engl J Med* 1994;330:769–774.
18. Update to CDC's sexually transmitted diseases treatment guidelines, 2006: fluoroquinolones no longer recommended for treatment of gonococcal infections. *MMWR Morb Mortal Wkly Rep* 2007;56:332–336.
19. Wise CM. Crystal-associated arthritis in the elderly. *Rheum Dis Clin North Am* 2007;33:33–55.
20. Kashyap AS, Kashyap S. Hormone replacement therapy and serum uric acid. *Lancet* 1999;354:1643–1644.
21. Choi HK, Atkinson K, Karlson EW, et al. Purine-rich foods, dairy and protein intake, and the risk of gout in men. *N Engl J Med* 2004;350:1093–1103.
22. Epis O, Caporali R, Scirè CA, et al. Efficacy of tidal irrigation in Milwaukee shoulder syndrome. *J Rheumatol* 2007;34:1545–1550.
23. Tan EM, Cohen AS, Fries JF, et al. The 1982 revised criteria for the classification of systemic lupus erythematosus. *Arthritis Rheum* 1982;25:1271–1277.
24. Wilson WA, Gharavi AE, Koike T, et al. International consensus statement on preliminary classification criteria for definite antiphospholipid syndrome: report of an international workshop. *Arthritis Rheum* 1999;42:1309–1311.

25. Weening JJ, D'Agati VD, Schwartz MM, et al. The classification of glomerulonephritis in systemic lupus erythematosus revisited. *Kidney Int* 2004;65:521–530.
26. Dougados M, van der Linden S, Juhlin R, et al. The European Spondyloarthropathy Study Group preliminary criteria for the classification of spondyloarthropathy. *Arthritis Rheum* 1991;34:1218–1227.
27. Spencer-Green G. Outcomes in primary Raynaud phenomenon: a meta-analysis of the frequency, rates, and predictors of transition to secondary diseases. *Arch Intern Med* 1998;158:595–600.
28. Heymann WR. Sildenafil for the treatment of Raynaud's phenomenon. *J Am Acad Dermatol* 2006;55:501–502.
29. Tashkin DP, Elashoff R, Clements PJ, et al. Cyclophosphamide versus placebo in scleroderma lung disease. *N Engl J Med* 2006;354:2655–2666.
30. Highland KB, Garin MC, Brown KK. The spectrum of scleroderma lung disease. *Semin Respir Crit Care Med* 2007;28:418–429.
31. Badesch DB, Tapson VF, McGoon MD, et al. Continuous intravenous epoprostenol for pulmonary hypertension due to the scleroderma spectrum of disease: a randomized, controlled trial. *Ann Intern Med* 2000;132:425–434.
32. Nebel MB, Gracely RH. Neuroimaging of fibromyalgia. *Rheum Dis Clin North Am* 2009;35:313–327.

34 Musculoskeletal Complaints

Ananth Arjunan and Ernie-Paul Barrette

Neck Pain

GENERAL PRINCIPLES

- Neck pain is an extremely common symptom, but most episodes are short lived and seldom require medical care.
- Those patients who come to medical attention generally need only conservative treatment. With conservative therapy, more than half of the patients have improvement in neck pain within 2 to 4 weeks, and the majority are asymptomatic by 2 to 3 months.
- By far, **most neck pain is not serious** and is musculoskeletal-biomechanical in origin, caused by minor trauma or age-related changes in the cervical spine. A much smaller number of patients have serious systemic diseases that affect the neck or have referred pain.
- **Strain/sprain/spasm** of the paracervical musculature is an especially common cause of acute nonspecific neck pain, particularly in younger patients. It may develop after a prolonged period in an awkward position, sudden jarring neck movement related to minor trauma, or activities that require new, unusual, or repetitive neck movements.
- **Acute flexion-hyperextension neck injury (whiplash)** occurs most commonly after a rear-end car collision.
  - For unclear reasons, whiplash tends to respond less well to therapy than do typical cervical sprains. After 12 months, 15% to 20% of patients remain symptomatic, with 5% severely affected.[1]
  - Facet (zygapophyseal) joint pain has been suggested to be the most common cause for chronic neck pain after whiplash. Imaging tests are unrevealing. Fluoroscopically guided, controlled diagnostic blocks of the painful joint may establish the diagnosis.
- **Osteoarthritis/spondylosis**: Degenerative cervical spine changes generally begin in the fourth decade of life.
  - Disc degeneration can result in posterior and lateral bulging.
  - Osteoarthritis develops in the zygapophyseal synovial joints. Osteophyte formation may occur, originating from the vertebral body, facet joints, and neural foramina margins. Occasionally, there is segmental instability or subluxation. This entire process is referred to as **cervical spondylosis**, and it is thought to be a common cause of chronic mechanical neck pain in older individuals.
  - Encroachment on the neural foramina and spinal canal may result in radiculopathy or cervical myelopathy.
- **Degenerative cervical disc disease** increases with age and may result in neck pain with or without radiculopathy. Acute cervical disc herniations may also cause neck pain or radiculopathy, or both.
- **Cervical radiculopathy** may be caused by multiple processes, most commonly acute disc herniation, chronic disc degeneration, and cervical spondylosis.
  - Radiculopathy is occasionally caused by a more serious condition such as malignancy or infection.
  - Thoracic outlet syndrome, brachial plexus disorders, and upper extremity peripheral nerve compression syndromes may mimic radicular symptoms.

- **Serious or systemic causes** of neck pain and/or radiculopathy are much less common and include vertebral osteomyelitis, epidural abscess, discitis, meningitis, rheumatoid arthritis (RA), spondyloarthropathies, polymyalgia rheumatica, fibromyalgia, and primary or metastatic tumors. Cervical fractures are generally the result of significant trauma and may or may not present with neurologic symptoms. Osteoporotic fractures of the cervical spine are unusual.
- **Other structures in the neck** may produce pain, such as thyroiditis, pharyngitis, retropharyngeal or peritonsillar abscess, and carotodynia.
- **Referred pain** to the neck may be the result of headaches, shoulder disorders, angina, esophageal disorders, and vascular dissection.

DIAGNOSIS

In most patients, a thorough but focused history and physical examination is the primary diagnostic tool. An important goal is to detect symptoms and signs that suggest a potentially serious condition or a neurologic urgency. In the absence of such findings, special diagnostic tests are generally not indicated.

Clinical Presentation
History
- The history should focus on the mode of onset, nature, and location of the pain.
- A history of trauma is important. Patients should also be asked about activities that may have preceded the pain (e.g., prolonged neck extension or flexion, twisting, new physical activity, sport, or job). Neck pain often does not develop until 12 to 24 hours after such activity.
- Acute neck pain that is unrelated to trauma suggests cervical strain or disc herniation (that may or may not be associated with radicular symptoms). Chronic neck pain with intermittent acute exacerbations (sometimes with radiculopathy) is often due to cervical spondylosis.
- Mechanical neck pain is typically exacerbated by movement and relieved by rest. Morning stiffness may be present in patients with an inflammatory arthropathy.
- Neurologic symptoms are a vital component of the history.
  - **Radiculopathy** may involve single, multiple, or bilateral roots. Sensory changes are usually more pronounced than motor symptoms. Patients may also complain of paresthesias that radiate from the neck into the arm. Weakness is the primary symptom of motor involvement. Extensive paralysis only occurs with multiple root involvement.
  - Symptoms of cervical **myelopathy** (due to severe cervical spondylosis) generally develop slowly and intermittently over weeks to months. Patients complain of upper and lower extremity weakness and sensory changes. Spastic paraparesis of the legs and loss of sphincter control may eventually develop.
  - In patients with RA, neck pain may indicate impending neurologic compromise. Subluxation of the C1–C2, atlantoaxial joint, can compress the spinal cord, resulting in sudden motor and sensory deficits at multiple levels.
- Symptoms or history suggestive of a serious etiology, such as malignancy or infection, should be carefully sought (e.g., fever, weight loss, very severe pain, pain unrelieved by rest, a history of cancer, long-term corticosteroid use, and IV drug use).

Physical Examination
- The physical examination should include the entire cervical spine and surrounding areas (e.g., shoulders and head) and an appropriate neurologic examination.
- The range of motion (ROM) of the neck normally decreases with age.
  - Lateral flexion of the neck may worsen radiculopathy symptoms, as may vertical pressure on the head (**Spurling maneuver**).

- ○ **Lhermitte sign**, an electric shock sensation down the spine into the arms and legs with bending forward on the cervical spine, may be seen in cervical myelopathy/cord compression.
- • Localized tenderness of the cervical spine and spasm of the paraspinal musculature may be present. The sensitivity and specificity of severe bony tenderness for fracture are unknown.
- • When the patient has neurologic complaints, a thorough neurologic examination is necessary.
  - ○ Not all patients with radiculopathy have demonstrable findings on examination.
  - ○ Cervical radiculopathy has characteristic sensory changes and motor weakness (Table 34-1).
  - ○ Motor weakness in the upper and lower extremities, spasticity, hyperreflexia, clonus, Babinski sign, and reduced sphincter tone are consistent with cervical myelopathy.

Diagnostic Testing

Imaging

- • **Plain radiography** of the cervical spine should be used judiciously in patients with non-specific mechanical neck pain.
  - ○ Use of plain radiographs in evaluating neck pain has two important limitations:
    - ▪ First, **cervical spondylosis is extremely common in asymptomatic individuals** and increases with age.
    - ▪ Second, plain radiographs are of **very limited value in assessing nerve root or spinal cord compression**.
    - ▪ Nonetheless, plain films should generally be done in patients with radiculopathy to evaluate for serious bony abnormalities.
  - ○ Plain cervical spine films are warranted when a serious disorder is suspected or in cases that are related to significant trauma.
  - ○ If plain films are unrevealing but strong suspicion still exists, other imaging studies, such as computed tomography (CT) or magnetic resonance imaging (MRI), should be done.
- • **CT or MRI** is recommended when tumor, infection, fracture, or other space-occupying lesion is strongly suggested by the clinical findings or in the setting of serious neurologic signs and symptoms.
  - ○ In the absence of severe or progressive neurologic symptoms, it is generally not necessary to do a CT or MRI for patients with typical radiculopathy.
  - ○ Many patients with cervical radiculopathy have substantial improvement in a few weeks.
  - ○ If symptoms have not improved with several months of conservative management and the patient is an appropriate potential candidate for surgery, CT or MRI may be useful.

TABLE 34-1	Features of Cervical Radiculopathy		
Nerve root	Area of sensory change	Motor weakness	Reflex
C5	Upper lateral arm	Shoulder abduction	Biceps
C6	Lower lateral forearm into thumb and index finger	Forearm supinators and pronators	Brachioradialis
C7	Dorsal and palmar surface of forearm into middle finger	Triceps and wrist extension flexion	Triceps
C8	Medial forearm into ring and little fingers	Intrinsic hand muscles	None

Electrodiagnostic Testing

Electrodiagnostic tests are usually not indicated in individuals with obvious radiculopathy. They are probably most useful when the cause of upper extremity pain is unclear, for example, differentiating C6 radiculopathy from median nerve entrapment, or if surgery is being considered.

TREATMENT

- Simple conservative therapy is appropriate for the majority of patients with nonspecific mechanical neck pain. In most cases, the pain improves in several weeks.
- **Modest activity restriction** is generally believed to be appropriate.
  - ○ Patients should avoid activities that worsen their neck pain.
  - ○ Bed rest is not indicated, and patients should be encouraged to continue most daily activities.
  - ○ Soft cervical collars are also frequently recommended and may reduce symptoms in some patients. These collars are not particularly effective at reducing neck motion but may serve as a reminder to the patient to limit movements that can increase pain. Rigid cervical collars should not be prescribed by the untrained.
- Pharmacotherapy with **acetaminophen or nonsteroidal anti-inflammatory drugs (NSAIDs)** may provide relief for nonspecific mechanical neck pain. **Opiate analgesics** may be an effective time-limited option for patients with acute severe neck pain. Some patients may find **muscle relaxants** effective, but sedation is a common side effect. Supportive data are limited for all of these medications.[2]
- **Neck mobilization and manipulation** appear to be effective for short-term and intermediate relief.[3]
- **Stretching and strengthening exercises** of the cervical and shoulder/thoracic area may be effective for chronic mechanical neck disorders.[4]
- There are very limited data regarding **electrotherapy and electromagnetic therapy**; a definitive statement of their effectiveness is not possible.[5]
- Simple application of **local heat or ice** is an option for symptomatic relief.
- Limited evidence suggests that **myofascial trigger point injections** with lidocaine may be effective.[2]
- **Acupuncture** appears to be moderately effective for chronic neck pain.[6]
- **Traction** has unclear efficacy for neck pain with or without radiculopathy due to the lack of high-quality data.[7]
- The medical benefit of **massage** is unknown.[8]
- **Surgery** has no role in the relief of neck pain secondary to cervical spondylosis in the absence of significant persistent neurologic involvement.
- **Whiplash** does not seem to respond as well to conservative treatments, but they are frequently used, and their effectiveness is unclear.[9]
  - ○ For patients with chronic cervical zygapophyseal joint pain after whiplash confirmed with double-blind placebo-controlled local anesthesia, percutaneous radiofrequency neurotomy may provide lasting relief.[10,11]
  - ○ A small study suggests that the acute treatment with high-dose methylprednisolone may be beneficial in preventing extensive sick leave after whiplash.[2,12]
- **Neck pain with radiculopathy** is generally treated in a manner similar to that of nonspecific mechanical neck pain.
  - ○ Patients with prolonged severe radicular symptoms may benefit from surgical decompression. Those who are agreeable to surgery and are medically appropriate surgical candidates can be referred to a neurosurgeon.
  - ○ Patients with persistent radicular pain secondary to cervical spondylosis may respond to fluoroscopically guided therapeutic selective nerve root block.[13]
- **Myelopathy** often requires surgical treatment and is best managed in conjunction with a neurosurgeon, neurologist, or both.

Low Back Pain

GENERAL PRINCIPLES

Epidemiology

- Low back pain (LBP) is an exceedingly common complaint, with a lifetime incidence of >70%.
- Patients present along a wide spectrum of pain and disability, which unfortunately often does not correlate well with the seriousness of the underlying etiology.
- The medical and societal costs are enormous (up to $50 billion a year), with the majority due to a small percentage of patients with temporary or permanent disability.
- There is an epidemiologic association between LBP and **obesity**. Whether or not losing weight reduces LBP is a largely unanswered question.
- There is also an association with **smoking,** but true cause and effect are unknown.[14–16]

Etiology

- Many of the etiologies of LBP are presented in Table 34-2.[17] The distribution of diagnoses varies somewhat among populations and degree of chronicity.
  - Regardless, the large majority of cases are due to mechanical causes with lumbar sprain/strain accounting for the biggest proportion (about 70%).
  - The pathologic corollary to sprain/strain is unknown, and the concept of skeletal muscle "spasm" is not universally accepted.
- Ultimately, in approximately 85% of cases, a specific diagnosis cannot be made, so-called **nonspecific musculoskeletal (or idiopathic) LBP**. Medical LBP specialists and surgeons will see a higher percentage of specific pathologies.[17]
- **Spondylosis** is a generalized degenerative change of the spine, including disc degeneration, with disc space narrowing and osteoarthritic changes of the facet joints. **Spondylosis is just as common in asymptomatic as in symptomatic individuals.** In general, LBP patients with spondylosis have the same prognosis as those without spondylosis.
- **Spondylolisthesis** is the forward movement of the body of one vertebra on the vertebra below it or on the sacrum. Minor degrees of spondylolisthesis are fairly common and usually asymptomatic. Individuals with LBP that is presumed to be secondary to spondylolisthesis usually follow a similar course as those with nonspecific LBP. When the slippage is severe, it may cause back pain and radiculopathy.
- **Lumbar disc herniation** is common and increases with age.
  - Of disc herniations, 95% occur at the L4–L5 or L5–S1 levels.
  - Disc herniation may result in LBP, sciatica, or both. However, disc herniations may also be totally asymptomatic.
  - Large midline disc herniations occasionally cause cauda equina syndrome.
- **Sciatica** refers to a symptom of sharp, burning pain radiating from the low back or buttock and into the posterolateral aspect of lower extremity and extends below the knee. It is most commonly caused by L5 or S1 radiculopathy.
- **Spinal stenosis** is usually caused by hypertrophy of the ligamentum flavum and facet joints, resulting in narrowing of the spinal canal, often at multiple levels.
  - This narrowing may result in entrapment of nerve roots, with resultant symptoms in the legs.
  - **Pseudoclaudication** or neurogenic claudication is characterized by back pain and numbness of the lower extremities that worsen with walking and extension of the spine. It is relieved with spinal flexion (bending forward).
- Several reputed conditions are not universally accepted as valid diagnoses, including discogenic LBP, facet joint syndrome, piriformis syndrome, and sacroiliac joint dysfunction (without sacroiliitis or spondyloarthropathy).[18–21] None has sufficiently distinct historical

TABLE 34-2	Etiologies of Low Back Pain

Mechanical or activity related

Lumbosacral myofascial strain, strain, spasm

Degenerative changes of the vertebrae, discs, facet joints (spondylosis)

Herniated intervertebral disc[a]

Lumbar spinal stenosis[a]

Discogenic low back pain[b]

Facet joint syndrome[b]

Sacroiliac joint dysfunction without sacroiliitis/spondyloarthropathy[b]

Osteoporotic compression fracture

Traumatic fractures

Other anatomical/congenital abnormalities

Spondylolisthesis

Kyphosis

Scoliosis

Medical conditions of the spine

Rheumatologic

Spondyloarthropathies (e.g., ankylosing spondylitis, psoriatic arthritis, reactive arthritis, inflammatory bowel disease related)

Rheumatoid arthritis

Neoplastic

Primary tumors

Metastatic disease (e.g., multiple myeloma, lymphoma, carcinoma)

Infectious

Discitis

Epidural abscess

Vertebral osteomyelitis

Metabolic

Paget disease

Referred pain

Vascular

Abdominal aortic aneurysm

Aortic dissection

Genitourinary

Nephrolithiasis

Pyelonephritis

Pelvic inflammatory disease

Endometriosis

Prostatitis

Gastrointestinal

Cholecystitis

Pancreatitis

Peptic ulcer disease

---

[a]Often associated with neurogenic leg pain.
[b]Validity of the diagnosis, method of precise diagnosis, and optimal unique management not universally accepted.
Data from Deyo RA, Weinstein JN. Low back pain. *N Engl J Med* 2001;26:153–159.

or physical findings allowing for certain diagnosis. All are reportedly substantiated by injection into the potentially pathogenic area. Gold standard tests are lacking. These diagnoses are made frequently by some clinicians and rarely or never by others. Their exact incidence and prevalence are unknown. Potentially effective and unique therapies are being investigated, but none has been clearly shown to be effective in randomized controlled trials.

• A very small number of patients have serious systemic diseases that affect the spine or have referred pain.

DIAGNOSIS

- In the vast majority of patients, the primary diagnostic tool is a careful but focused history and physical examination searching for **red flags** that suggest a potentially serious underlying condition or a neurologic urgency (Table 34-3).[22]
- In primary care, individual red flags may have a very high false-positive rate.[23,24]
- The red flags listed in Table 34-3 were initially described in reference to acute LBP; however, they have some validity with regard to chronic LBP as well.
- **In the absence of red flags, special diagnostic tests are rarely indicated during the 1st month of pain.**

Clinical Presentation

History
- Symptoms and historical features potentially suggestive of **malignancy** include current or prior malignancies, breast or prostate masses, smoking, family history of cancer, and systemic symptoms (e.g., weight loss, night sweats, fever, and decreased appetite).
- Symptoms and historical features potentially suggestive of **infection** include HIV, chronic use of steroids or other immunosuppressants, history of IV drug abuse, hemodialysis, osteomyelitis/abscess, endocarditis, fever, chills, and sweats.
- Those that suggest **fracture** include female sex, trauma relative to age, age >70 years, and prolonged steroid use.[23]
- Symptoms compatible with **cauda equina syndrome** include bowel and/or bladder dysfunction, saddle anesthesia, bilateral lower extremity sciatica, sensory changes, and/or weakness.
- Pain worst with standing is typical of lumbar **spinal stenosis**, while pain worst with sitting or flexing the spine suggests **disc herniation**.
- Associated leg pain with standing and ambulation may represent spinal stenosis–related **pseudoclaudication**. True claudication generally does not occur just with standing. Some patients with spinal stenosis will have leg pain only. Flexion of the spine may improve the symptoms. The discomfort typically lasts longer after walking than it does in true vascular claudication.
- **Sciatica** is most specifically defined as pain radiating down the posterolateral leg below the knee. The sensitivity of the symptom of sciatica, defined as pain radiating into the

TABLE 34-3	Red Flags of Low Back Pain

Age >50 years
History of cancer
Unexplained weight loss
Chronic steroid use
Pain duration >1 month
Pain unresponsive to treatment for 1 month
Pain unrelieved or worsened by rest
IV drug use
Urinary tract or other infection
Fever
Bladder dysfunction
Saddle anesthesia
Unilateral or bilateral major motor weakness
Significant trauma relative to age
Rapidly progressive severe radiculopathy

buttocks and down the leg below the knee, is sufficiently high (0.95) that its absence makes a clinically significant disc herniation unlikely.[25] Coughing, sneezing, and Valsalva maneuver can worsen sciatica secondary to disc herniation.

• Questions about personal or family history of spondyloarthropathies and RA may suggest these as potential causes. Morning stiffness may also provide a clue to these diagnoses.

• All patients should be asked about their occupational history, including current employment and exactly what kinds of physical activities are involved.

• There does not appear to be a relationship between leisure time sport or exercises, sitting, and prolonged standing/walking and LBP. Evidence is conflicting regarding home repair, gardening, whole-body vibration, nursing tasks, heavy physical work, and working with the trunk in a bent/twisted position.[26]

• Low job satisfaction and insufficient social support in the workplace are associated with the development of new-onset LBP.[27]

• The presence of nonorganic signs, high levels of maladaptive pain coping behaviors, high baseline functional impairment, psychiatric comorbidities, and low general health status have been shown to predict which patients with acute LBP will develop chronic LBP.[28] Interventions that break the cycle of fear and avoidance might be of benefit.[29]

Physical Examination

• Look for fever and tachycardia as potential clues to infection or inflammatory arthropathy.

• ROM, kyphosis, scoliosis, costovertebral angle tenderness, surgical scars, and spinal/paravertebral tenderness/spasm. Unfortunately, assessments of ROM and tenderness/spasm are not particularly reproducible nor are they sensitive or specific.[25]

• A thorough joint exam may reveal evidence of synovitis.

• Evaluate **peripheral pulses** to distinguish true claudication from pseudoclaudication.

• A rectal exam may reveal prostatitis or a prostate mass.

• Decreased perianal sensation or rectal tone is worrisome for spinal neurologic involvement.

• **Straight leg raise** (SLR) testing may be performed with the patient supine or sitting up; it is considered positive if reproduction or worsening of sciatic pain occurs at <60 degrees. The ipsilateral SLR has a high sensitivity (0.85) and low specificity (0.52), while the contralateral (crossed) SLR has a high specificity (0.84) and low sensitivity (0.30).[30]

• An abbreviated **neurologic examination** can be done in most patients without neurologic symptoms (Table 34-4).

• When neurologic symptoms other than sciatica are present, a complete neurologic examination is warranted. Patients with the **cauda equina syndrome** typically have saddle anesthesia, bilateral radicular findings, and decreased anal sphincter tone.

• Often referred to as "**Waddell signs**" or "nonorganic signs," the presence of three or more behavioral responses to being examined suggests that the patient does not have simply a straightforward physical problem.[31] These signs, however, do not exclude organic causes or do they specifically detect secondary gain and/or malingering.[32] True malingering is, in general, quite unusual.

  ○ Superficial tenderness
  ○ Nonanatomic tenderness
  ○ Pain on axial loading of the skull

TABLE 34-4	Neurologic Examination for Sciatica		
Nerve root	**Area of sensory change**	**Motor weakness**	**Reflex**
L4	Medial foot	Ankle dorsiflexion	Knee
L5	Dorsal foot	Great toe dorsiflexion	None
S1	Lateral foot	Plantar flexion, eversion	Ankle

○ Pain on passive rotation of the shoulders and pelvis
○ Sitting and supine straight leg raising discrepancy
○ Regional weakness
○ Regional sensory change
○ Inconsistent "overreaction" to examination (e.g., tremor, sweating, collapse, exaggerated verbalizing, inappropriate sighing, guarding, bracing, rubbing, insistence on standing or changing position, and questionable use of walking aids or equipment)

Diagnostic Testing

Assuming there are no red flags present, it is reasonable to hold off any imaging or laboratory tests for the 1st month because the majority of patients will be significantly improved during that period of time with or without intervention.

Laboratories

• The use of laboratory tests should be judicious and guided by the history and physical examination. The large majority of patients will not need any laboratory tests specifically for the purpose of elucidating the cause of LBP.
• If the history and physical examination suggest the possibility of serious diagnoses (e.g., malignancy, infection, rheumatologic, and conditions that can cause referred LBP), appropriate laboratory tests should be done.
• Some have advocated the erythrocyte sedimentation rate (ESR) as a nonspecific screening test for potentially serious and related conditions.[33]

Imaging

• A clinical guideline by the American College of Physicians advises against imaging in most patients with acute LBP. They stress that routine imaging has not been shown to improve clinical outcomes.
  ○ Early imaging may be linked to worse health outcomes and increased risk of surgery.
  ○ The radiation exposure from plain lumbar films is not inconsequential. For women, the gonadal irradiation from plain lumbar films is estimated to be equal to a plain chest film every day for several years.
  ○ They recommend imaging in patients with severe progressive neurologic deficits or signs or symptoms of a serious disorder, for example, malignancy, infection, cauda equina syndrome, fracture, or spinal cord compression.
  ○ For those with persistent pain and symptoms of radiculopathy or spinal stenosis, MRI (preferred) or CT should be considered only in patients who would be candidates for surgery or epidural steroid injections.[34]
• **Plain radiographs** of the lumbosacral spine correlate poorly with the presence of LBP. Many patients without back pain have degenerative changes, and many patients with back pain will have no or nondiagnostic radiographic abnormalities.
  ○ **Degenerative changes increase with age and are extremely common** in the elderly. Therefore, when degenerative changes are present, it is very difficult to know if they are causative.
  ○ Plain films cannot detect disc herniation, spinal stenosis, or nerve root impingement and may not clearly show evidence of infection or malignancy.
  ○ In the final analysis, **plain films will often be nondiagnostic** and generally do not detect abnormalities not already suggested by the history and physical examination. Nonetheless, when red flags are present, plain films are reasonable.[34]
  ○ In patients with very chronic LBP, the red flag of duration of >1 month should not be interpreted as a mandate for plain films.
  ○ Of course, clinical judgment may override these general guidelines at any time.
  ○ One study suggests that while patients may be more "satisfied" when plain films are done, short-term pain and other clinical outcomes are not improved.[35]

- The obvious advantages of **CT and MRI** over plain films are much clearer delineation of bony and soft tissue abnormalities.
  - Both are capable of disclosing disc herniation, spinal stenosis, nerve root and spinal cord compression, malignancy, fractures, and infection.
  - On the other hand, they also detect more nondiagnostic degenerative changes.[36–38]
  - Degenerative findings on MRI are poorly predictive of the subsequent development of LBP.[39,40]
  - This does not mean that such findings cannot be the cause of LBP in some patients.[41,42]

Diagnostic Procedures

- **Myelography and CT-myelography** are generally only indicated in special situations for preoperative planning in consultation with a surgeon.
- **Bone scintigraphy** is rarely needed in the diagnostic evaluation of patients with LBP. Bone scans may have a high yield for spinal metastases in patients with a known history of cancer. However, when they are positive, other diagnostic tests are usually required (i.e., CT or MRI).
- **Electrophysiologic tests** are usually not indicated in individuals with obvious radiculopathy or in those with only LBP. These tests appear to be most useful in the diagnostic evaluation of patients with leg pain when the diagnosis is unclear.

TREATMENT

In the absence of red flags, treatment for most patients with acute nonspecific LBP can be simple and conservative. Most patients improve in approximately 1 month with or without treatment. Pain that has persisted without improvement for more than a month should be reevaluated. The goals of treatment are to reduce pain, increase mobility, return to functioning at home, return to work, and prevent the development of chronic pain and disability.

Medications

- **Acetaminophen** is a reasonable first-line choice for the treatment of acute and chronic LBP.[43]
- **NSAIDs** are more effective than placebo in patients with acute nonspecific LBP.[43,44]
- **Tramadol** (50 to 100 mg qid) is a reasonable alternative for patients who fail to respond to or who cannot take nonselective or selective NSAIDs, but side effects are common (e.g., nausea, constipation, and drowsiness).
- **Muscle relaxants** have been shown to be superior to placebo for acute LBP.[43,45,46] The concept of muscle spasm is ill defined, and these drugs do not directly relax skeletal muscles. Their exact mechanism of action is unknown. There is insufficient evidence to suggest that one muscle relaxant is better than the others. Many patients will experience significant sedation.
- **Opiates** may be considered as a time-limited option for severe acute LBP. The use of opiates in chronic LBP continues to be controversial. Due to their substantial risk, experts recommend opiates for LBP only when their administration results in improved function rather than merely pain relief.[47,48]
  - Notwithstanding, chronic LBP is a very common nonmalignant reason for prescribing chronic opioids.
  - Long-term opioid use for LBP is associated with increased rates of substance abuse disorders and aberrant medication-taking behaviors.[48]
  - Patients should be carefully screened for opioid misuse and fully informed of the risks and benefits. A written plan (pain agreement/contract) may be helpful. All patients on chronic opioid therapy should be monitored with urine drug screens. For high-risk patients, urine drug screen testing is essential to rule out use of illicit drugs and confirm

adherence to the plan. Interpretation of urine drug screen testing is complex, and expert assistance is often required.

- **Antidepressants** may be useful in patients with chronic LBP with or without depression, though reviews have come to contradictory conclusions.[43,49]
  - Antidepressants that inhibit the uptake of norepinephrine (tricyclics) seem to produce moderate symptomatic benefit.
  - Based on limited evidence, pure selective serotonin reuptake inhibitors (SSRIs) do not appear to be effective.
  - Venlafaxine and duloxetine are SSRIs that also inhibit the uptake of norepinephrine—there is limited evidence to suggest that both may be effective for other chronic pain conditions.
  - Antidepressants are not indicated for the treatment of acute LBP.
  - Potential risks of therapy should be carefully considered especially in the elderly.
- **Anticonvulsants** are increasingly being used to modulate chronic LBP. Some supportive evidence is beginning to emerge, particularly regarding topiramate and gabapentin (for sciatica).[43,50,51]

Other Nonpharmacologic Therapies

- **Education**: The overall good prognosis of acute LBP should be stressed but not oversold. Although acute LBP may rapidly and completely resolve, it certainly does not always do so, and recurrences are common. Patients should be encouraged to notify the physician if symptoms change significantly. Intensive education may reduce pain.[42]
- In the occupational setting, **back school** appears to be effective for reducing pain and improving function.[53]
- **Bed rest** may actually delay recovery and potentially contribute to the development of chronic back pain. Patients with acute nonspecific LBP should be **advised to continue ordinary activities as much as possible.** Patients with sciatica also should be encouraged to go about daily activities as much as tolerated.[54]
- **Activity restriction**: It is reasonable to advise the patient to limit temporarily activities that are known to increase mechanical stress on the spine, including prolonged unsupported standing, heavy lifting, and bending or twisting the back while lifting.
- **Physical therapy (PT, trunk-strengthening exercises)** has not been clearly shown to be beneficial in acute LBP. However, exercise therapy is somewhat effective.[55,56]
- **Local heat or cold** may be efficacious and is relatively low cost with minimal risk of side effects, particularly low-level heat wraps.[57] Patients should be warned against sleeping with heating pads and placing ice in direct contact with the skin due to the potential for burns and frostbite.
- **Massage** might be beneficial for subacute or chronic LBP, but it can be relatively expensive.[58]
- **Spinal manipulation** (chiropractic) continues to engender controversy. Multiple reviews and meta-analyses have been published with somewhat differing conclusions. However, recent systematic reviews suggest that there is no benefit in acute LBP but may benefit chronic LBP when compared with other interventions.[56,59,60] The occurrence of adverse outcomes appears to be very rare.
- **Injection therapies** have been tried in multiple different areas of the spine, including the facet joints, the epidural space, and soft tissue (trigger points, acupuncture points, or ligaments). Corticosteroids, local anesthetics, and saline have all been used.
  - **Trigger point injections** are done fairly frequently. The theory of trigger points as a cause or perpetuator of LBP is controversial at best. Evidence is insufficient to recommend for or against their use in either acute or chronic LBP.[61]
  - **Facet joint injections** have been advocated for the treatment of the so-called facet joint syndrome. The syndrome is diagnosed clinically in patients with lumbar pain

that improves with the injection of corticosteroid or local anesthetic into or near the facet joints. The efficacy of such treatment is unclear but can be considered in selected patients with chronic LBP in whom more conservative treatment has failed.[61]

○ **Epidural steroid injections** have been recommended for subacute or chronic LBP with and without sciatica. Results from multiple studies have been conflicting. Epidural steroids can be considered for patients in whom conservative therapy has failed.[61]

○ **Prolotherapy** (proliferative injection therapy), the injection of an irritant solution intended to strengthen weakened lumbosacral ligaments), does not appear to be an effective sole treatment for chronic LBP.[62]

○ The efficacy of **sacroiliac joint injections** is unknown.

• Data regarding the utility of **acupuncture** are contradictory, but it may be effective for those with chronic LBP.[56,63,64]

• Data support the use of **cognitive-behavioral therapies** for subacute and chronic LBP.[56,65]

• **Multidisciplinary biopsychosocial therapy** attempts to address all aspects of LBP, involving physicians, psychologists, physical/occupational therapists, and social workers. It requires the patient to take part in a substantial amount of active therapies (>100 hours) that incorporate the concept of functional restoration. Though expensive and not widely available, it has been shown to be effective for chronic LBP.[66]

• **Lumbar supports** do not appear to be useful for preventing LBP, and their role in treatment is unclear.[67]

• **Traction** as a single therapy is ineffective for LBP with or without sciatica.[68]

• Data do not support the use of **transcutaneous electrical nerve stimulation (TENS)** for LBP.[69]

• Data regarding **therapeutic insoles** are severely limited. They do not appear to prevent back pain in relatively young, highly active populations. Efficacy in treating LBP is unknown.[70]

• **Nonsurgical spinal decompressive therapy** (e.g., Vax-D) is of unproven benefit.[71]

• Data regarding **low-level laser therapy** are insufficient to draw conclusions.[72]

• Radiofrequency denervation may be effective for facet joint syndrome.[11] Likewise, intradiscal radiofrequency thermocoagulation might be useful for discogenic LBP, but data are very limited.[73]

Surgical Management

• There is good evidence that **surgical discectomy** provides effective relief of sciatica for properly selected patients.[74–76]

○ The primary benefit of discectomy appears to be the more rapid relief of symptoms in those individuals in whom conservative therapy has failed.

○ Whether there is a significant difference in long-term outcomes is less clear.[77]

• Similarly, surgery for appropriately selected patients with lumbar **spinal stenosis** is effective, but the effect diminishes over time.[75,78,79] Surgical intervention for **spinal stenosis with spondylolisthesis** may also be effective.[80]

• Surgical treatment for **degenerative lumbar spondylosis** is especially controversial. Surgical treatments may include decompression, spinal fusion, or both. The data available are limited, sometimes of poor quality, and conflicting and often focus on technical rather than patient-centered outcomes. A 2009 review concluded that for nonradicular back pain associated with degenerative changes, spinal fusion is no more effective than intensive rehabilitation but more beneficial compared with standard nonsurgical therapies.[75] A 2013 review was more optimistic about the effects of fusion surgery for patients with disc degeneration.[81] Regardless, for the large majority, surgical intervention for nonspecific mechanical back should only be considered for those with prolonged pain who have failed all more conservative interventions and who are appropriate medical candidates.

Shoulder Pain

GENERAL PRINCIPLES

- The **glenohumeral (GH) joint** is very shallow and is the most commonly dislocated joint.
- The **rotator cuff** supports the GH joint and consists of the tendons of four muscles: supraspinatus, infraspinatus, teres minor, and subscapularis.
  - The tendons of these muscles blend with the shoulder joint capsule and insert on the greater and lesser tuberosities of the humeral head.
  - The rotator cuff muscles assist in internal and external rotation and depress the humeral head during shoulder elevation.
  - This action holds the humeral head down, minimizing impingement on the acromion process and the intervening tissues.
- The **subacromial bursa** lies deep to the deltoid muscle and superficial to the insertion point of the supraspinatus tendon. This bursa protects the rotator cuff from the acromion.
- The long head of the biceps originates from the **glenoid labrum**. The **biceps tendon** emerges from the GH joint through the bicipital groove.
- Patients with acute shoulder problems have a better prognosis than those with chronic shoulder pain.[82]
- **The shoulder impingement syndrome causes the majority of painful nontraumatic shoulder problems.** It is due to mechanical impingement of the rotator cuff structures by the humeral head against the subacromial structures. This is related to a continuum of inflammation, degeneration, and attrition of the rotator cuff structures, especially the supraspinatus tendon. As a result, the rotator cuff fails to prevent upward migration of the humeral head during shoulder elevation. Several interrelated conditions are involved in the impingement syndrome; all may occur simultaneously.
  - **Rotator cuff tendonitis** refers to a spectrum of changes that affect the tendons of the rotator cuff, particularly the supraspinatus. Acute inflammation with hemorrhage and edema can occur secondary to trauma or overuse, particularly in younger patients. Acute rotator cuff tendonitis is sometimes associated with calcification of the supraspinatus and biceps tendons (so-called **calcific tendonitis**). The pain of calcific tendonitis can be severe and may lead to a **frozen shoulder**. With aging, the tendons undergo degenerative changes and attenuation related to chronic inflammation and repeated mechanical insults.[83]
  - **Rotator cuff tears** can occur suddenly secondary to falling on an outstretched arm or with lifting a heavy object. Tears can also occur more indolently in older patients with attrition of the rotator cuff or with a chronic inflammatory condition such as RA or the Milwaukee shoulder (progressive, destructive shoulder arthropathy associated with bloody shoulder effusions and the deposition of hydroxyapatite crystals).
  - **Subacromial bursitis and bicipital tendonitis** may accompany rotator cuff tendonitis. In fact, it is often difficult to distinguish these entities, as they frequently occur simultaneously. Occasionally, the proximal biceps tendon **ruptures**.
- **Adhesive capsulitis (frozen shoulder)** may complicate any painful shoulder condition and has been associated with myocardial infarction, diabetes mellitus, apical lung cancer, cervical disc disease, metastatic lesions, and thyroid disease. However, such clinical associations are often lacking. The precise pathophysiology of adhesive capsulitis is not entirely clear but appears to involve initial hypervascular synovitis and subsequent fibrosis. What triggers this process is unknown.[84] It is not unusual for frozen shoulder to develop subsequently in the contralateral shoulder.
- **Osteoarthritis** does not commonly occur as a primary process in the GH joint, with two exceptions: (a) rapidly progressive osteoarthritis of the shoulder in elderly women and

(b) the Milwaukee shoulder. Secondary osteoarthritis may occur as a result of RA, trauma, repetitive manual labor, calcium pyrophosphate deposition disease, and long-standing rotator cuff tears (cuff tear/rotator arthropathy).

- **Shoulder instability and dislocation**: The shoulder joint is inherently unstable and the most commonly dislocated joint. Acute GH dislocation occurs most frequently in young active adults after a fall on an outstretched arm and results in anterior displacement of the humeral head. Recurrent dislocation is not unusual, with subsequent episodes requiring less force. Some patients have a chronic syndrome of GH instability with subluxation. This is often seen in athletes such as baseball pitchers.
- **Inflammatory arthropathies** such as RA and lupus can affect the GH joint.
- **Crystalline arthropathies** occasionally occur in the shoulder, such as the above-mentioned Milwaukee shoulder (hydroxyapatite crystals) and pseudogout/pyrophosphate arthropathy (calcium pyrophosphate dihydrate crystals). Gout is relatively rare.
- The **acromioclavicular joint** can also be painful due to sprain/separation and arthritic changes.
- **Referred pain** from the chest, abdomen, and cervical spine or from myocardial ischemia should be considered. With referred pain, intrinsic shoulder movement is not painful. Aching pain over the superior shoulder that involves the lateral upper arm or the medial border of the scapula is likely from **C5 cervical radiculopath**y.

DIAGNOSIS

Clinical Presentation

History
- Intrinsic shoulder pain is typically worse at night and aggravated by lying on the affected shoulder.
- Motion of the shoulder generally increases the discomfort, particularly full forward-flexed elevation and abduction to 90 degrees.
- A history of recent trauma, new physical activity, and prior dislocation are important.
- Patients with shoulder instability may complain that the shoulder has a disconcerting "going out" sensation.
- Referred pain tends to be poorly localized.
- **Impingement syndrome** patients may have a history of repetitive overhead arm motion. Pain tends to be focal and anterior, occurring at night or when the patient is lying on the shoulder. Activities such as throwing, working with arms overhead, and swimming aggravate the pain.
- **Adhesive capsulitis** is most common in women in the fifth and sixth decades of life. The key historical feature is a painful and significant reduction in ROM. The onset can be fairly acute or chronic. As the condition progresses, pain subsides, but the limitation of ROM may become quite severe. After months of symptoms, some patients have a slow progressive improvement in ROM.
- Individuals with **GH instability** complain of a chronic feeling of the shoulder "going out" with certain activities and sometimes pain. A history of significant trauma (usually related to sports) and pain is elicited from patients with acute **GH dislocation** and **acromioclavicular separation**.

Physical Examination
- Physical examination of the shoulder should include observation, palpation of the bony and soft tissues, assessment of passive and active ROM, strength testing, and certain provocative tests.
- Normal **abduction** of the internally rotated (palm down) shoulder is approximately 120 degrees and externally rotated (palm up) shoulder is 180 degrees.

- Normal **elevation** (forward flexion) of the shoulder is 180 degrees, **extension** 40 degrees, and **internal and external rotation** 90 degrees.
- If active ROM is limited, passive ROM should be carefully tested.
- Marked loss of both active and passive ROM is consistent with adhesive capsulitis.
- **Crepitus** during ROM may be appreciated with osteoarthritis.
- There are many named physical exam tests for the shoulder. The evidence that any one test is pathognomonic for a condition is poor.[85]
- **Cross-chest abduction** (touch the opposite shoulder) tests internal rotation and adduction.
- The **Apley scratch test** evaluates external rotation and abduction from above (scratch between the scapulae from above) or internal rotation and adduction from below.
- Patients with acute **anterior dislocation** have a loss of the shoulder's normally rounded appearance. The acromion process becomes the most lateral structure. A prominence of the humeral head is present anterior and inferior to the glenoid. ROM is painfully restricted. Patients with acute dislocation should have a detailed neurovascular examination, specifically the motor and sensory innervation of the axillary nerve.
- The **impingement sign** is elicited by passive forward flexion of the arm by the physician. Passive abduction to 90 degrees with internal rotation also causes pain. **Painful arc sign** is present when pain is elicited with between 80 and 120 degrees during abduction. Both suggest subacromial bursitis or rotator cuff tendonitis.
- The **apprehension sign** is elicited by having the patient place their arm in the throwing position. The examiner places one hand over the posterior shoulder and exerts pressure onto the wrist. The patient's apprehension is evident when shoulder instability is present.
- **Neer impingement sign**: With the patient in the seated position, elbow extended, and forearm pronated (humerus internally rotated), passively elevate (forward flex) the GH joint with the examiner's hand distal to the elbow while the other stabilizes the posterior aspect of the shoulder. Pain indicates a positive sign, especially near the end of the ROM. Sensitivity and specificity are estimated to be 0.72 and 0.60, respectively.[85]
- **Hawkins impingement sign**: With patient sitting or standing, grasp the arm at the elbow and wrist, flex the elbow and shoulder to 90 degrees, then passively internally rotate the shoulder. Pain, particularly at the end of the ROM, is a positive test—sensitivity 0.80 and specificity 0.56.[83]
- **Yocum test** consists of having the patient place the palm on the affected side on the opposite shoulder and then to raise the elbow without elevating the shoulder. Pain is indicative of impingement—sensitivity 0.79 and specificity 0.40.[86]
- The **drop arm sign** to demonstrate a rotator cuff tear is performed by assisting the patient in abducting and elevating the shoulder. When the examiner withdraws support of the upper arm, the patient is unable to hold the arm up if there is a complete tear of the rotator cuff.
- The **lift-off test** tests specifically for weakness of the subscapularis. The patient places the hand of the affected side on the small of the back, with the palm oriented posteriorly, and pushes against resistance. Normally, the patient should be able to push the examiner's hand away from the back.
- **Anterior instability** is most common and is suggested by pain with the **anterior apprehension test**.
  - With the patient supine, the shoulder is initially at 90 degrees of abduction and neutral rotation, and the arm is externally rotated (as in a throwing position). The examiner places one hand under the shoulder and applies pressure backward against the wrist.
  - The patient's discomfort is apparent through verbal and nonverbal cues.
  - The relocation test is performed immediately after the apprehension test. The examiner moves his or her hand from behind the shoulder to the front and applies pressure. Improvement in pain or impending dislocation is a positive test.
  - Impingement produces an apprehension sign, but it is not significantly altered by relocation.

- **The posterior apprehension test** is performed by having the patient flex the elbow and elevate the internally rotated shoulder to 90 degrees (hand on opposite shoulder). The examiner pushes backward onto the elbow, and apprehension is apparent.
- **Yergason sign** produces pain and tenderness over the bicipital groove with resisted supination of the forearm while the elbow is flexed and held at the side. Passive extension of the shoulder may also reproduce the pain of bicipital tendonitis.
- **Speed test** is thought to identify tendonitis/inflammation of the biceps tendon-superior labral complex. The patient flexes the shoulder at 30 degrees against resistance with the elbow extended and the forearm supinated. Pain is noted along the long head of the biceps brachii tendon. Estimated sensitivity and specificity for superior labral tears are 0.20 and 0.78, respectively.[85]
- Rupture of the biceps tendon is evident as the **Popeye sign**, a mass of contracted muscle midway between the shoulder and the elbow.

Diagnostic Testing

- In many cases, using a combination of history and specific examination tests will allow reasonable diagnostic accuracy. For example, for patients with a painful shoulder, the following three criteria help diagnose supraspinatus tendinopathy: age >39, painful arc sign, and self-report of popping or clicking. When 2 of 3 are present, the sensitivity and specificity are 0.75 and 0.81. When all three are present, the sensitivity and specificity are 0.38 and 0.99.[85]
- **Plain radiographs are not necessary or appropriate in the initial evaluation of every patient with shoulder pain**, especially if the history and physical examination suggest impingement.
  - In patients with no history of a fall or a shoulder deformity, plain radiographs are very unlikely to provide any useful information.
  - Anteroposterior (AP) views of the GH joint in internal and external rotation and an axillary view are typically done.
  - Arthritis of the GH and acromioclavicular joints and calcification of the rotator cuff tendons can be visualized. Osteoarthritis is indicated by joint space narrowing and, in more advanced cases, flattening of the humeral head, subchondral cysts, and marginal osteophytes.
  - Detection of shoulder dislocation may require special views.
  - Plain films should be obtained in patients who do not appear to be responding to conservative treatment for impingement syndrome. The primary value of a radiograph in this situation is to assess the degree of impingement, based on the vertical distance between the inferior aspect of the acromion and the superior aspect of the humeral head. Normally, the width of a ballpoint pen should fit in between the acromion and the humeral head. Narrowing of this space suggests that the patient has chronic rotator cuff disease, in which case conservative treatment may be inadequate.
  - Diffuse osteopenia is sometimes seen with adhesive capsulitis.
- **MRI**, or, in some centers, a diagnostic **ultrasound**, can assess the degree of supraspinatus tendon pathology. If the tendon is significantly narrowed or partially or completely torn, the patient should be referred to an orthopedist who is experienced in shoulder surgery.

TREATMENT

Impingement Syndrome

- Treatment goals are to reduce pain and improve shoulder function and ROM.
- The optimal management of impingement syndrome is unclear. However, in older patients with chronic shoulder pain, no history of an injury, and findings consistent with impingement syndrome, a trial of PT is reasonable. Imaging prior to PT for chronic shoulder pain is not necessary.

- Methodologically strong trials are limited and, therefore, it is difficult to provide evidence-based recommendations.
- The individual entities can be difficult to distinguish clinically, often coexist, and can overlap with other shoulder disorders. They are usually self-limited, and conservative treatments are generally sufficient. Some cases, however, are resistant to treatment, and recurrences can occur.
- **Relative rest of the shoulder** is reasonable. Patients should avoid activities and movements that aggravate the pain but must not stop moving the shoulder all together.
- **Gentle ROM exercises** are usually recommended to maintain ROM and avoid adhesive capsulitis. Pendulum exercises are easy for patients to do at home and consist of flexing at the waist 90 degrees, supporting the upper body on a low table, and loosely swinging the arm like a pendulum against gravity. The arc of movement is slowly increased over time.
- Referral to **PT** for careful strengthening of the shoulder muscles may be beneficial.[87]
- Evidence is insufficient to clearly support the use of **physiotherapy modalities** (e.g., ultrasound, laser, heat, cold, manipulation, and electrotherapy).[87]
- Application of **heat or ice** may be comforting.
- **NSAIDs** are probably effective for the pain of impingement syndrome.
- **Local corticosteroid injections** (subacromial bursa and rotator cuff region) may have a temporary benefit for adhesive capsulitis, rotator cuff disease, and subacromial bursitis, but evidence is limited.[88-91] Triamcinolone acetonide 40 mg is a typical dose for a larger joint. Repeated injections should be avoided. Potential complications of steroid injections include infections, skin atrophy, and tendon weakening and rupture. Steroid injections may be inadvisable for patients with more than small rotator cuff tears.
- **Referral to an orthopedist** who is experienced in shoulder surgery is appropriate for patients who would consider surgery and who have prolonged pain and limitation of function. Early referral should be considered for all patients with moderate-to-large rotator cuff tears.

Other Conditions

- Treatment for **adhesive capsulitis** is generally noninvasive including PT and NSAIDs.
  - Many patients will have resolution over 1 to 2 years.
  - **Corticosteroid injections** directly into the GH joint (usually done under fluoroscopy) may be of some benefit, particularly early in the course. Oral steroids may also provide short-term relief (<6 weeks).[92]
  - Arthroscopic capsular release is sometimes recommended for recalcitrant cases.
- **Osteoarthritis** treatment is also generally conservative, including NSAIDs and PT. Patients with advanced cases may require a total shoulder arthroplasty for pain relief.
- Treatment of **acute shoulder dislocation** is best handled by immediate orthopedic consultation.
- Patients with **chronic GH instability** are treated conservatively with a program of PT and avoiding activities that provoke subluxation. Surgery may be indicated for some young patients and for those with continued intolerable symptoms.

Elbow Pain

GENERAL PRINCIPLES

- Elbow pain is a fairly common complaint in the ambulatory setting. In general, only one of a few conditions is causative.
- **Lateral epicondylitis or tendinosis (tennis elbow)** is the most common cause of elbow pain. The condition is caused by chronic overuse of the wrist extensors and supinators that originate from the lateral epicondyle. This results in repetitive microtears and

angiofibroblastic degeneration or tendinosis of the origins of these muscles. No significant degree of inflammatory reaction appears to occur.[93]

- **Medial epicondylitis or tendinosis (golfer's elbow)** is very similar to but less common than lateral epicondylitis. It involves overuse and degenerative changes of the tendinous origins of the wrist flexor/pronator muscles at the medial epicondyle.

- **Ulnar nerve entrapment (cubital tunnel syndrome)** results from compression of the ulnar nerve as it passes behind the medial epicondyle through the cubital tunnel, where it is very superficial. Direct pressure, repetitive elbow bending, prolonged elbow flexion, elbow arthritis, diabetes, and certain occupations and activities have all been associated with the condition. A firm direct blow to this area produces the familiar "funny bone" sensation.

- **Olecranon bursitis (student's elbow)** is a common condition that results from acute inflammation of the olecranon bursa. This bursa does not connect with the synovial cavity of the elbow. The cause may be infectious or noninfectious. The most common infectious agent is *Staphylococcus aureus*. Common noninfectious causes include repetitive trauma, gout, pseudogout, and RA. It can be difficult to differentiate an infectious from a noninfectious inflammatory bursitis.

DIAGNOSIS

Clinical Presentation

History
- Patients usually complain of pain but may also report stiffness or swelling, or both.
- A history of acute trauma is important and may suggest fracture, dislocation, or tendon rupture.
- Repetitive overuse is a major cause of elbow pain, and patients should be asked about recreational and occupational activities.
- The specific location of the pain may be the key to proper diagnosis.
- Patients with **lateral epicondylitis** complain of lateral elbow pain that worsens with certain activities, usually related to sports (e.g., racquet sports) or other repetitive uses that involve wrist extension and power gripping (e.g., carpentry or lifting with the palm facing down). Tenderness may extend to the proximal lateral forearm. Symptoms may develop acutely or more slowly. A direct blow to the outside of the elbow can also trigger lateral epicondylitis.
- Patients with **medical epicondylitis** also complain of pain and tenderness but over the medial epicondyle that is worsened by certain activities. It too is often related to sports (golf and throwing activities) and work.
- A history of weakness and sensory changes should also be sought.
- With **ulnar nerve entrapment**, patients complain of medial elbow pain and sensory changes (numbness and paresthesias) in the ulnar nerve distribution, particularly the fourth and fifth digits. The symptoms may be worse at night. Weakness is sometimes reported.
- **Olecranon bursitis** typically presents with tender painful swelling of the posterior elbow that may develop acutely or more slowly. A history of trauma should be sought.

Physical Examination
- The elbow examination should include inspection, palpation, ROM, and neurologic assessment.
- The point of maximal tenderness should be determined if possible.
- The normal range of extension and flexion is 0 to 140 degrees. Normal supination and pronation are 80 degrees each way.
- The neck, shoulder, and wrist should be examined to evaluate for referred pain.

- With **lateral epicondylitis**, the diagnostic maneuver involves shaking hands on the affected side, cupping the patients elbow with your other hand, and moving your thumb over and just anterior to the lateral epicondyle. Reproducible pain at this site while the patient resists the shaking hand from supinating confirms the diagnosis.
- With **medial epicondylitis**, the tenderness expectedly increases over the medial epicondyle. The pain may be reproduced by resisted wrist flexion.
- **Ulnar entrapment** findings include sensory changes and weakness in the ulnar nerve distribution. Light touch and pinprick sensation are decreased in the ring and little fingers. Tapping the ulnar nerve where it passes behind the medial epicondyle causes pain along the inner elbow and paresthesias in the fourth and fifth digits (**Tinel sign**). Full elbow flexion can produce a similar result (**elbow flexion test**). Weakness in the abductor digiti minimi, which is innervated only by the ulnar nerve, may be seen. Testing is performed by having the patient place the palm on a desktop and moving the fifth digit across the desktop while the examiner applies resistance to this digit. Reduced grip strength and intrinsic hand muscle weakness may be present. With prolonged nerve compression, atrophy of the intrinsic muscles may be seen.
- With **bursitis**, the exam is most notable for an obvious swelling (goose egg) of the olecranon bursa, which may be quite large. **Infectious and noninfectious causes may be indistinguishable on examination.** Both can present with erythema, tenderness, and warmth. Marked findings are more likely to be traumatic or infectious in origin. Chronic or recurrent bursitis may be nontender.

Diagnostic Testing

- **Plain radiographs** of the elbow typically include the AP and lateral views.
  - In many cases, plain films are nondiagnostic (e.g., lateral and medial epicondylitis).
  - They should probably be done in all patients with significant acute trauma to evaluate for dislocation and fracture.
  - With ulnar nerve entrapment, they are generally unnecessary unless a bony abnormality causing nerve compression is suspected.
  - Special views are sometimes taken to evaluate the olecranon fossa and radial head.
- **CT and MRI** are occasionally indicated for better delineation of the bony and soft tissues.
- **Nerve conduction studies and electromyography** may be useful when the diagnosis of ulnar nerve entrapment is uncertain or surgery is being considered.
- When the olecranon bursa is acutely swollen, **aspiration** of the bursal fluid should be done to evaluate for infection. The fluid should be sent for Gram stain, culture, cell count, and crystal examination. Synovial fluid cell counts in infectious bursitis are generally lower (several thousand cells/mL) than in septic arthritis. The bursal fluid may be obviously bloody in cases of trauma.

TREATMENT

- Treatment of **lateral epicondylitis** is usually conservative.
  - **Relative rest** (i.e., initially avoiding the activities that cause pain) is appropriate.
  - Topical NSAIDs provide relief in the short term, while there is insufficient evidence to make recommendations for or against oral NSAIDs.[94]
  - A **compressive strap** worn just below the elbow (tennis elbow splint) might be useful, but data are contradictory.[95]
  - Some patients find local application of ice comforting.
  - Proper racquet size and backhand technique may also be of value.
  - **Local corticosteroid injection** (e.g., 40 mg triamcinolone) is an often-recommended alternative for patients who fail to respond to simple measures. It is generally believed to be effective, at least in the short term.[91]

- ○ Multiple other treatments are available, but their effectiveness is uncertain.[95]
- ○ Surgery is rarely necessary.
- Treatment of **medial epicondylitis** is similar to that of lateral epicondylitis. Local corticosteroid injection may be effective in the short term for those who do not respond to more conservative therapy, but due to the proximity of the nerve and artery, this is usually performed by an orthopedic surgeon.
- Treatment of **ulnar nerve entrapment** is also usually conservative.
  - ○ The elbow should be kept straight as much as possible. A **splint** can be worn at night to prevent flexion of the elbow during sleep.
  - ○ If possible, the patient's work environment should be altered to prevent further compression. A cushioning **elbow pad** can be worn to protect the nerve during work.
  - ○ A trial of **NSAIDs** is reasonable for pain.
  - ○ Surgery may be necessary for patients with recalcitrant symptoms.
- Aspiration of the olecranon bursa is not only diagnostic but also therapeutic for **olecranon bursitis**.
  - ○ Fluid reaccumulation is not unusual in noninfectious cases, and repeat aspiration may be necessary. A **compression dressing** can be applied to help prevent recurrence, and an elbow pad can be used to prevent trauma.
  - ○ **NSAIDs** are frequently given.
  - ○ **Injection of 20 mg methylprednisolone** into the bursa may also reduce recurrence in patients with nonseptic olecranon bursitis.[96] Corticosteroid injection is contraindicated in infectious bursitis.
  - ○ Empiric **antibiotic treatment** (e.g., dicloxacillin or a cephalosporin) should be given when infection is suspected with pending culture results. Daily aspiration is usually necessary for septic bursitis.

Wrist and Hand Pain

GENERAL PRINCIPLES

- Wrist and hand complaints are common in primary care. Because of their obvious functional importance, careful diagnosis and treatment are particularly important.
- **Stenosing tenosynovitis** is an inflammation and thickening of tendons, sheaths, and synovium in the hand, sometimes with nodular enlargement of the tendon. It is frequently related to repetitive overuse, particularly those activities that involve gripping.
- **Trigger finger or thumb** is caused by stenosing tenosynovitis of the flexor tendons of the fingers and thumb.
  - ○ **de Quervain tenosynovitis** is a very similar condition that affects the tendons and sheaths of the abductor pollicis longus and the extensor pollicis brevis.
  - ○ **Dupuytren contracture** is a fibroproliferative disorder that results in painless thickening and nodularity of the palmar aponeurosis. The flexor tendons of the hand are not primarily involved. The fibrosis of the palmar fascia draws the fingers (most commonly the ring and little finger) into flexion at the metacarpophalangeal (MCP) joint. The condition generally affects men >40 years and appears to have a strong genetic component. It is also associated with diabetes, alcoholism, repetitive trauma, and seizure disorders.
- **Carpal tunnel syndrome** (CTS) is the most frequently occurring entrapment neuropathy.
  - ○ It results from compression of the median nerve as it passes through the carpal tunnel.
  - ○ It is most common in middle-aged women and usually affects the dominant hand.
  - ○ CTS is known to occur with increased frequency in patients with diabetes, amyloidosis, renal failure on hemodialysis, RA and other arthropathies of the wrist, acromegaly, pregnancy, hypothyroidism, and previous wrist trauma. It is often related to repetitive overuse of the hands and wrists.

- **Ulnar nerve entrapment** can occasionally occur at the wrist as the nerve passes through the canal of Guyon. It may be caused by repetitive trauma (e.g., operating a jackhammer, using the hand as a hammer, and resting the ulnar side of the wrist and hand on the edge of a desk or keyboard) or a space-occupying lesion (e.g., ganglion or lipoma).
- **Arthritic conditions** of the wrist and hand are common. **RA** characteristically involves the wrist, MCP, and proximal interphalangeal joints. The erosive synovitis causes pain, stiffness, deformity, and loss of functionality. **Osteoarthritis** typically involves the distal interphalangeal and carpometacarpal joints (especially of the thumb). See Chapter 33 for a full discussion of the management of these conditions.
- **Infectious causes** of hand/finger pain include **paronychia and felons**. The latter are a more serious infection of the entire distal pulp of the fingertip. The most common organism is *S. aureus*. They are generally caused by a puncture wound to the thumb or index finger.
- **Subungual hematoma** is a very common traumatic cause of finger pain.

DIAGNOSIS

Clinical Presentation

History
- With **trigger finger/thumb**, digit extension is limited when the affected tendon catches on the pulley at the base of the digit. This results in pain with use, and the affected digit can become painfully stuck in flexion. The finger may need to be forcibly extended with the other hand, often with a painful and audible pop.
- Patients with **de Quervain tenosynovitis** complain of pain, tenderness, and swelling on the radial side of the wrist just proximal to the wrist crease in the region of the anatomic snuffbox. Ulnar deviation of the wrist and movement of the thumb exacerbate the pain, and a squeaking or creaking sensation may be described. Onset is often after overuse of the wrist and thumb (e.g., prolonged writing or carrying an infant car seat).
- Affected patients with **Dupuytren contracture** complain of painless nodules in the palm, an inability to extend the fingers fully, and difficulty in picking up large objects.
- Patients with **CTS** usually complain of an aching pain in the wrist and hand, which may radiate up the forearm. Intermittent paresthesias and numbness in the median nerve distribution (palmar surface of the thumb, index, long, and radial side of the ring fingers) are typical.
  - Less-than-classic descriptions of the location of discomfort are not unusual.
  - Symptoms are frequently worse at night and with overuse of the hands.
  - The patient may describe shaking out the hand to improve the symptoms (the flick sign). The sensitivity and specificity are low, however.[97]
  - Weakness, clumsiness, and a tendency to drop objects may also be reported.
  - Patients should be questioned about trauma, work-related duties, hobbies, and activities.

Physical Examination
- Palpation at the distal palmar crease in **trigger finger** may reveal a thickened tendon sheath or a tender nodule, or both, usually overlying the MCP joint of the affected finger.
- **Finkelstein sign** is diagnostic for **de Quervain tenosynovitis**. The patient makes a fist enclosing the thumb; if this does not produce pain, the examiner forces the wrist into ulnar deviation as an additional stress. Focal tenderness is usually present over the radial styloid.
- With **Dupuytren contracture**, examination reveals painless thickening and nodularity of the palmar fascia with flexion deformity of one or more fingers.

- In **CTS**, the examination classically reveals decreased sensation (hypalgesia) in the median nerve distribution, weakness of thumb abduction, and **Tinel and Phalen signs**.
  - In the Phalen maneuver, the wrists are held in unforced flexion for 30 to 60 seconds. Reproduction or worsening of the symptoms constitutes a positive sign.
  - Tinel sign is the development of paresthesias in the median nerve distribution when the median nerve is tapped at the distal wrist crease.
  - When compared with electrodiagnostic testing, however, Tinel and Phalen signs may have limited diagnostic value.[98]
  - Thenar atrophy can occur with long-standing CTS.

Diagnostic Testing

- **Radiographs** of the hands and wrists may provide diagnostic information, particularly if arthritis is suspected.
  - However, definitive changes may not be apparent until the disease has been present for an extended period of time.
  - In cases of significant trauma, plain films are usually mandatory.
- **Electrodiagnostic testing** (median nerve conduction) is generally thought to be the gold standard for CTS, but false positives and false negatives do occur. Such testing should be considered only when the diagnosis is uncertain or surgical treatment is being considered or in cases of work-related injury compensation.

TREATMENT

- Treatment of **trigger finger** initially consists of splitting the MCP joint in extension and a short course of NSAIDs. Corticosteroid injection (methylprednisolone, 15 to 20 mg) with lidocaine into the flexor digital tendon sheath can also be effective.[99] Recurrence is common, and surgical release may be required.
- **de Quervain tenosynovitis** is treated with a short opponens splint, supplemented by NSAIDs. Refractory cases may respond to corticosteroid injection (methylprednisolone, 20 to 30 mg) with lidocaine.[100] Surgical release is sometimes required.
- Apart from gently stretching the fingers, there is no known effective conservative treatment for **Dupuytren contracture**. Surgical treatment can be considered for the severely affected, but recurrences are common.
- Treatment for **CTS** is likewise initially conservative.
  - There is very limited evidence to support benefits of **wrist splint** (worn primarily at night), exercise and mobilization, and ultrasound therapy.[101–103]
  - Work-related **ergonomic modifications** should be undertaken if necessary.
  - If these simple measures fail, the patient can be referred for a single **corticosteroid injection** (40 mg triamcinolone) with lidocaine (10 mg) into the area close to the carpal tunnel, which may be effective for up to 4 weeks.[104]
  - Definitive treatment entails **surgical release**, a simple outpatient procedure in which the flexor retinaculum is incised, relieving the pressure on the median nerve. Surgery is very effective in treating CTS, provided that the diagnosis has been confirmed electro-diagnostically and is more effective than splinting.[105]

Hip Pain

GENERAL PRINCIPLES

- Hip pain has many potential causes, but only a few are common.
- Pain may emanate from the hip joint, periarticular soft tissues, pelvic bones, and sacroiliac joint or be referred from another location (usually the lumbosacral spine).

- **Osteoarthritis** of the hip joint is very common and increases with age. It is characterized by loss of the articular cartilage of the joint. Predisposing factors include childhood hip disorders, leg-length anomalies, and work that involves heavy lifting and carrying. The diagnosis and treatment of osteoarthritis are discussed in Chapter 33.
- **Trochanteric bursitis** is another common cause of hip pain. It can occur in association with iliotibial band syndrome, hip joint pathology, previous hip surgery, leg-length discrepancy, and mechanical back pain.
- **Avascular necrosis (osteonecrosis, AVN)** is the death of a variable amount of trabecular bone in the femoral head.
  - The precise pathophysiology is not known, but it is unusual in the absence of known risk factors, which include corticosteroid treatment (especially in those with lupus), alcoholism, trauma or prior fracture, RA, HIV infection, sickle cell disease, myeloproliferative disorders, and radiation.
  - A high index of suspicion should be maintained in patients with these risk factors. The condition may be bilateral.
  - Severe AVN can cause collapse of the femoral head.
- **Meralgia paresthetica** is an entrapment neuropathy caused by compression of the lateral femoral cutaneous nerve. It may be related to one or more factors, including obesity, pregnancy, diabetes, wearing tight garments around the waist (e.g., pantyhose, tool belts), local surgery, trauma, repetitive hip extension (joggers, cheerleaders who do splits frequently) and, rarely, intrapelvic masses.
- **Hip fractures** are particularly common in elderly women and usually occur at the femoral neck or the intertrochanteric area. They are associated with a high morbidity and mortality. Age, Caucasian race, female sex, osteoporosis, and falls are common predisposing factors.

DIAGNOSIS

Clinical Presentation

History
- Patients typically complain of painful limited ROM and difficulty ambulating.
- The location of the pain can be the key to proper diagnosis.
  - True hip joint pain usually affects the groin and radiates to the buttock. Bearing weight worsens the pain.
  - Buttock pain alone without groin pain is likely to originate in the low back, sacroiliac joint, or ischial tuberosity.
  - Lateral proximal thigh pain suggests trochanteric bursitis.
  - Anterolateral thigh pain suggests either lateral femoral cutaneous nerve entrapment or sciatica.
  - Pain that radiates down the posterior thigh is frequently due to lumbosacral radiculopathy.
- Patients with chronic progressive disease have increasing difficulty in ambulating and performing the activities of daily living.
- Patients with **trochanteric bursitis** complain of lateral hip pain that may radiate down the leg. The pain is worse with exercise and at night, especially when the patient lies on the affected side. Some patients complain of a limp.
- **AVN** pain tends to come on suddenly and can be severe, but the onset can be more gradual. A few patients may be asymptomatic. The pain is typically in the groin radiating to the buttocks and is increased with weight bearing.
- **Meralgia paresthetica** is remarkable for pain, burning, and dysesthesia in the groin and anterolateral thigh. The discomfort may extend to the lateral knee. No motor symptoms occur.
- Most patients with **hip fracture** report a fall and subsequent inability to walk. They have pain in the groin that radiates to the buttocks. A few patients may be able to walk with assistance, but pain increases with weight bearing.

Physical Examination
- The patient should be observed **standing and walking**. A limp or expression of pain may be demonstrative of the patient's complaint.
- The **abductor lurch (Trendelenburg gait)** suggests intra-articular hip pathology. The patient shifts weight over the affected leg to unload weakened abductors.
- The **Trendelenburg test** should be done. Ask the standing patient to raise the knee on the unaffected side so that weight is borne on the affected side. Normally, the pelvis elevates on the raised-knee side. A drop in the pelvis on the raised-knee side suggests weakness of the hip abductors on the straight-knee (affected) side.
- **Patrick test or the FABERE sign** (flexion-abduction-external rotation-extension) is performed by placing the supine patient's heel on the contralateral knee. The examiner then pushes the knee and thigh downward to put the hip into external rotation, producing pain in intrinsic hip disease. Pain in the groin on the side with the flexed knee suggests hip pathology, while pain in the contralateral buttock to the flexed knee suggests sacroiliac joint pathology.
- **Palpation** of the hip joint and surrounding area is done to elicit tenderness.
- **ROM** should be tested. Normal hip flexion is approximately 120 degrees; normal internal rotation is 30 degrees and external rotation 60 degrees. Hip joint pathology tends to affect internal rotation most.
- **Strength** of the adductors, abductors, and flexors should be tested. The lumbar spine and the sacroiliac joints should be examined.
- The groin is examined, looking for evidence of an inguinal or femoral hernia.
- Local tenderness over the trochanteric prominence can be demonstrated with **trochanteric bursitis,** and hip ROM should be unrestricted.
- With **AVN**, internal and external rotation of the hip is painful and sometimes reduced. The patient often has a limp.
- Examination in **meralgia paresthetica** usually reveals hypoesthesia or dysesthesia, or both, in the lateral femoral cutaneous nerve distribution. Examination of the hip is normal unless coexistent hip pathology is present.
- **Hip fracture** classically reveals an externally rotated, abducted, and foreshortened leg. Ecchymosis or hematoma formation may be present at the hip.
- Pulses should be evaluated to rule out vascular claudication or Leriche syndrome (aortoiliac occlusive disease).

Diagnostic Testing
- **Plain radiographs**, when indicated, should include AP and lateral views of the hip and an AP view of the pelvis.
- **CT or MRI** is occasionally needed to evaluate the hip further (e.g., occult hip fractures and osteonecrosis).
- Films in **AVN** may show sclerosis of the femoral head. Collapse of the femoral head is seen in advanced cases. If initial radiographs are normal, an MRI should be considered because of its high sensitivity for this diagnosis.
- **Hip fractures** are usually obvious, but plain films are occasionally negative. A bone scan, CT scan, or MRI may be necessary for diagnosis.

TREATMENT

- **Trochanteric bursitis** is slow to respond to therapy but almost never becomes chronic.
  ○ **NSAIDs** often provide symptomatic relief, and **PT** for modalities and iliotibial band stretching can be helpful. Patients should be encouraged to continue with stretching exercises at home.
  ○ A **corticosteroid injection** (30 to 40 mg methylprednisolone) with local anesthetic (3 mL/1% lidocaine) into the greater trochanteric bursa usually brings at least temporary relief.[106,107]

- Limited weight bearing with a cane or walker may be sufficient for some patients with **AVN**, but orthopedic consultation should always be obtained to evaluate the need for surgical core decompression or total hip arthroplasty. If corticosteroid therapy remains necessary, efforts should be made to reduce the dose as much as possible.
- For **meralgia paresthetica**, treatment consists of eliminating the source of nerve compression or repetitive trauma. Weight loss in obese patients can be effective.
- Treatment of **hip fractures** is almost always surgical, and an orthopedic consultation is mandatory. A patient with an osteoporotic fracture should have bone density measured by dual x-ray absorptiometry as a baseline and should be started on medications to increase bone density and decrease the risk of subsequent fracture (Chapter 3).

Knee Pain

GENERAL PRINCIPLES

- With normal use, the knee is subject to considerable wear and tear and is vulnerable to injury (often sports related). As such, knee pain is a common complaint. Degenerative disease, trauma, and inflammatory processes are the most frequent causes.
- **Osteoarthritis** of the knee is an extremely common condition and an important source of disability.
  - Important associations include age, wear and tear, obesity, genetic factors, prior trauma (e.g., fractures, ligamentous injuries that cause instability, and meniscal damage), and prior knee surgery. Osteoarthritis may affect any or all of the three compartments of the knee (medial and lateral tibiofemoral and patellofemoral).
  - The medial compartment is the most commonly involved.
  - The diagnosis and treatment of osteoarthritis are discussed in Chapter 33.
- The **inflammatory conditions** can be divided into **noninfectious and infectious** causes.
  - Noninfectious causes include **RA, lupus, psoriatic arthritis, reactive arthritis, gout, and pseudogout**.
  - The most common infectious causes are **gonococcal arthritis** (especially in sexually active young adults) and **S. aureus**. Extra-articular infections, previous damage to the joint, prosthetic joints, serious underlying chronic illness, immunosuppression, corticosteroid therapy, and IV drug use are predisposing factors for septic arthritis.
  - The treatment of inflammatory arthropathies is discussed in Chapter 33.
- **Patellofemoral pain syndrome** (PFPS) is characterized by retropatellar or peripatellar pain and crepitation with certain activities.
  - The condition is ill defined and poorly understood, but nonetheless **anterior knee pain** of this type is very common and may become chronic and limit activity.
  - Multiple associations and predisposing factors have been proposed, including overuse/overloading, maltracking of the patella, patellar subluxation, obesity, malalignment of the knee extensor mechanism, quadriceps weakness, and trauma. Many patients, however, have no such associations.
  - The relationship of PFPS to chondromalacia of the patella is controversial. PFPS can occur without chondromalacia, and patients with chondromalacia may have no symptoms.[108]
- **Ligamentous injuries** are generally seen after trauma in athletic young adults. These injuries comprise a spectrum from torn and stretched ligamentous fibers to complete tear or rupture. Collateral and cruciate ligament injuries can occur alone or together, with or without meniscal damage.
- **Meniscal tears** typically occur after a **twisting injury**, and the medial meniscus is much more commonly affected. This type of injury can occur in isolation or with a medial collateral or anterior cruciate ligament (ACL) tear, or both. Older individuals may experience a degenerative meniscal tear after minimal trauma.

- **Bursitis** can occur at several locations in the knee. Bursae are lined with synovium and produce a small amount of fluid that decreases friction between adjacent structures. Chronic overuse, trauma, and friction can result in inflammation.
  - **Prepatellar bursitis** is usually caused by repeated trauma involving a lot of kneeling (e.g., housemaid's knee and clergyman's knee).
  - The **pes anserine bursa** lies under the insertion of the hamstrings on the proximal medial tibia. It can become inflamed with overuse (e.g., walking or running) and in those with osteoarthritis of the knee.
- **Baker cyst** (popliteal cyst or semimembranosus-gastrocnemius bursitis) is a fluid-filled sac located in the popliteal fossa, usually on the medial side. It frequently connects with the joint cavity. It is often associated with knee effusions, posterior meniscal tears, and degenerative arthropathy.[109] It is also very common in RA.[110]
- **Iliotibial band friction syndrome** is a common overuse injury in runners and cyclists. Repetitive movement of a tight iliotibial over the lateral femoral condyle causes friction and pain, particularly with climbing stairs and running down hills.
- **Tibial tubercle apophysitis (Osgood-Schlatter disease)** generally presents in adolescents, with pain localized to the insertion of the patellar tendon at the tibial tubercle. It is often related to an ossicle of bone within the tibial tendon anterior to the tubercle. Pain usually resolves with time when the ossicle fuses with the underlying bone. Until that time, pain should limit athletic activity.

DIAGNOSIS

Clinical Presentation

History

- Knee disorders usually present with one or more of the following: pain, stiffness, swelling, redness, warmth, tenderness, giving way, locking, and cracking.
- Patients should be carefully asked about exacerbating activities, sports, and prior episodes of trauma. A history of pain in the contralateral knee or other joints, or both, can be important.
- With mechanical causes, pain is typically worsened with activity and improved with rest.
- Acute knee pain is often traumatic, and the mechanism of injury should be detailed. An audible pop is sometimes heard. Subacute and chronic knee discomfort is also common.
- The possibility of septic arthritis (discussed in detail in Chapter 33) should always be considered with acute monoarticular arthritis of the knee.
- Synovitis presents with pain, stiffness, and an effusion. Infection, gout, and pseudogout are the usual causes.
- **PFPS** patients complain of anterior knee pain with activities such as going down steps or hills, squatting, running, jumping, and prolonged sitting (the theater sign).
- **ACL tears** are usually caused by a significant **twisting injury**. A popping sensation may be described. Pain is immediate, quickly followed by the development of a large effusion, giving way, and great difficulty in walking.
- **Collateral ligament tears** usually follow an **abduction or adduction force** (medial or lateral collateral ligaments, respectively). These patients complain of pain, stiffness, and localized swelling. Most are able to ambulate after the injury.
- With **meniscal injuries**, patients usually report pain, swelling, and stiffness after a significant twisting injury. Pain may be referred to the popliteal area. Clicking, locking, or giving way may also be described. Most patients are able to walk after the injury.
- Many **Baker cysts** are asymptomatic, but swelling, tenderness, and fullness behind the knee may be reported. Very large cysts can cause significant pain and even neurovascular compromise because of the pressure on surrounding structures. Some cysts become symptomatic only when they rupture, producing redness, swelling, warmth, pain, and tenderness of the calf, which can be confused with a deep venous thrombosis.

Physical Examination

- Physical examination of the knee includes inspection, palpation, ROM, strength, and gait. Acute knee inflammation may make adequate examination difficult or impossible. Normal flexion of the knee is 135 degrees, and extension is 0 degrees.
- Inspection should compare the affected knee to the unaffected side. Subtle warmth is best appreciated by comparing side to side with the examiner's anterior wrist, which is more sensitive than the digits.
- The **bulge sign** can be used to detect **small knee effusions**.
  - The patient's knee is extended flat on the examination table.
  - Joint fluid is milked up into the suprapatellar pouch by moving the hand proximally along the medial side of the patella.
  - The fluid is then milked down into the medial knee by moving the hand from above the lateral side of the patella along the lateral knee and down to the tibia.
  - Excessive fluid creates a bulge medial to the patella.
- The **anterior drawer test** and **Lachman test** are used to test for **cruciate ligament instability**. Both knees should be tested for comparison.
  - The anterior drawer test is performed with the patient supine and the knee flexed to 90 degrees. The tibia is grasped with both hands and pulled anteriorly.
  - Lachman test is performed with the supine patient's knee in 20 degrees of flexion. The distal femur is stabilized with one hand, while the other hand pulls the tibia forward.
  - Excessive anterior displacement of the tibia and a less than sharp end point suggest ACL damage.
  - Lachman test is generally believed to be the more sensitive test, but the combination of both tests may be better still.[111,112]
- **Stability of the collateral ligaments** should be tested in 20 to 30 degrees of flexion and full extension. One hand stabilizes the lateral side of the knee, while the other hand applies abduction force to the distal leg, or one hand stabilizes the medial side of the knee, while the other hand applies adduction force to the distal leg. Excessive motion, usually with pain, signifies medial or collateral ligament damage.
- **McMurray test** can be used to detect meniscal tears. With the supine patient's knee in full flexion, the knee is slowly extended as the tibia is rotated internally and externally. A palpable or audible pop, often with pain, suggests a meniscal tear. This test is insensitive but fairly specific.[112] Combining McMurray test with **joint line tenderness** may improve diagnostic ability.[111,113]
- The examination with **osteoarthritis** often reveals tenderness along the joint line, a small effusion, crepitus during knee motion, and sometimes palpable osteophytes. Patients with significant medial compartment disease often have a varus (bowleg) deformity when standing. Less commonly, a valgus (knock-knee) deformity may occur with lateral compartment disease.
- With **PFPS**, crepitus and malalignment of the patella with flexion and extension (patella tracks too far laterally) can sometimes be appreciated. Some quadriceps atrophy may also be present. A knee effusion is infrequently seen. The **patellar compression test** supports the diagnosis. The examiner immobilizes the patella while the patient contracts the quadriceps muscle, pulling the patella proximally against the femoral condyles, reproducing the pain.
- The **prepatellar bursa** lies between the skin and the patella. It produces swelling directly above the patella. There may also be redness and warmth, suggesting an infectious process.
- With **pes anserine bursitis**, pain occurs on the anteromedial aspect of the knee, and the area is exquisitely tender.
- A **Baker cyst** may be appreciated as a prominence in the medial aspect of the popliteal fossa. In the situation of a ruptured cyst, inflammation of the calf occurs, potentially simulating thrombophlebitis.

Diagnostic Testing

- All new **knee effusions** that are warm and painful should be tapped. Removal of the synovial fluid is necessary to rule out a septic joint, gout, or pseudogout.
- **Plain radiographs** of the knee are frequently done as a part of the evaluation of knee pain, but they are not always necessary.
- If the history and physical examination suggest a periarticular problem, plain films are unlikely to be diagnostic and are generally unnecessary. When a significant mechanical articular problem is suggested by the history and physical examination, plain films may be helpful. The **Ottawa knee rules** can be used to determine, which patients with acute knee injuries require knee films (Table 34-5).[112,114]
- Standard films include AP and lateral views, and standing films should be obtained if possible.
- Detection of some fractures by plain radiography may require special views.
- With **PFPS**, radiographs of the patella (Merchant view) may show malalignment of the patella but are usually normal.
- Plain films cannot diagnose **ligamentous or meniscal damage** but can detect avulsion fractures.
- **MRI** detects meniscal tears but false positives can occur.
- Ultrasound can be used to visualize a **Baker cyst** and evaluate for thrombophlebitis of the leg. MRI can also be used to visualize a Baker cyst.

TREATMENT

- For a detailed discussion of the treatment of osteoarthritis, see Chapter 33.
- **Septic arthritis** demands swift and aggressive treatment to minimize joint destruction.
  - Unless there is an established noninfectious diagnosis, strong consideration should be given to admission for empiric antibiotics until the synovial fluid cultures are negative.
  - Definitive treatment of septic arthritis (Chapter 33) includes IV antibiotics (agent and duration determined by culture results), serial joint aspiration, and occasionally surgical drainage.
- For **PFPS**, relative rest, PT, acetaminophen, NSAIDs, and ice are reasonable treatment options for most patients. Quadriceps training is generally believed to be of potential value. Knee taping and knee braces are advocated by some. Surgery may be appropriate for a few patients (e.g., those with serious chondromalacia or marked patellar maltracking or subluxation).
- If **ligamentous injury** is suspected, referral to an orthopedist or sports medicine specialist should be obtained. Initial conservative treatment includes rest, ice, compression, elevation, NSAIDs, crutches, and a knee brace. More specific treatment and possible surgical intervention should be directed by the orthopedic consultant.
- Orthopedic consultation is reasonable for most patients with a **meniscal tear**. Many patients heal with conservative treatment, which includes rest, ice, compression, elevation,

TABLE 34-5	Ottawa Knee Rules

Obtain radiographs when any of the following factors are present:
Age >55
Tenderness at head of fibula
Isolated tenderness of patella
Inability to flex knee to 90 degrees

Data from Stiell IG, Wells GA, Hoag RH, et al. Implementation of the Ottawa Knee Rule for the use of radiography in acute knee injuries. *JAMA* 1997;278:2075–2079.

NSAIDs, and gradual return to activity. Surgery should be reserved for patients who continue to have pain or locking, or both. In the presence of osteoarthritis of the knee, surgical treatment for a torn meniscus may actually lead to an intensification of knee pain, necessitating a total knee arthroplasty.
- Patients with noninfectious **prepatellar bursitis** can be managed conservatively with avoidance of the inciting trauma, ice, and NSAIDs. When infection is likely or confirmed, antibiotic administration should be combined with daily aspiration of the bursa to confirm that the cell count falls and the Gram stain and culture become negative with treatment. Patients who are systemically ill should be admitted to the hospital for IV antibiotics. Surgical incision and drainage are rarely necessary.
- For **pes anserine bursitis**, conservative treatment with relative rest, ice, and NSAIDs is frequently helpful. Local corticosteroid injection may also be effective.
- Mild-to-moderately symptomatic unruptured **Baker cysts** can be treated with as-needed acetaminophen or NSAIDs. Some advocate knee joint aspiration (sometimes with corticosteroid injection) as effective treatment for more symptomatic individuals. Surgical treatment may be useful for a small number of patients. Ruptured cysts can be treated with relative rest, elevation, heat, and NSAIDs.

Ankle Pain

GENERAL PRINCIPLES

- **Ankle sprains** are one of the most common injuries encountered.
  - They are typically caused by inversion injuries and, therefore, usually involve the lateral ligaments.
  - The severity of sprains can range from minimal to quite severe.
  - Chronic ankle instability and recurrent injury after an ankle sprain is not uncommon.
- **Primary osteoarthritis of the tibiotalar (ankle) joint is rare**, but secondary osteoarthritis may develop after trauma or an inflammatory arthropathy such as RA.
- An ankle effusion suggests inflammatory arthritis, sarcoidosis, gout, or infection and should be aspirated to establish a diagnosis.

DIAGNOSIS

- Ankle sprain patients usually report a trip or fall that results in forced inversion of the ankle. Eversion injuries do occur but are much less common.
- Swelling, tenderness, and painful ambulation are common. Some patients have severe pain and possibly an inability to walk.
- **Examination** is notable for swelling, tenderness, and sometimes ecchymosis over the lateral collateral ligaments (deltoid ligament for an eversion injury). Swelling may extend to involve the entire ankle. The medial and lateral malleoli should be palpated for tenderness. Discomfort with attempted manual inversion is obvious. Weight bearing may or may not be possible.
- **Plain radiographs** of the ankle are not always necessary and are often overused. The **Ottawa ankle rules** (Table 34-6) can be successfully used to determine when ankle films are necessary to evaluate for fracture.[115]

TREATMENT

- Treatment for most ankle sprains is conservative consisting of rest, ice, compression, elevation, and NSAIDs. An air stirrup-type ankle brace can be used for added support. As tolerated, weight bearing is permissible, but some patients require crutches.

TABLE 34-6	Ottawa Ankle Rules

Obtain radiographs in patients with any pain in the malleolar zone and if any of the following are present:
Bony tenderness at the posterior edge or tip of the lateral malleolus
Bony tenderness at the posterior edge or tip of the medial malleolus
Inability to bear weight immediately after injury and take four steps in the emergency department

Data from Stiell IG, McKnight RD, Greenberg GH, et al. Implementation of the Ottawa ankle rules. *JAMA* 1994;271:827–832.

- When the patient can bear weight without pain, increased activity can begin. Continued use of an air stirrup brace should be encouraged.
- Organized PT for ankle strengthening after a sprain may be beneficial.
- Severe sprains require more intensive treatment, and an orthopedic consultation should be obtained for these patients.
- Use of an ankle support (semirigid orthosis or air stirrup) during sporting activities can reduce the risk of a recurrent sprain.[116]

Heel Pain

GENERAL PRINCIPLES

- **Plantar fasciitis** is the most common cause of plantar heel pain.
  ○ It is a painful inflammation of the insertion of the plantar fascia into the calcaneus.
  ○ Plantar fasciitis is more common with a pronated foot and a flattened longitudinal arch, obesity, and excessive walking.
  ○ Although it is usually an isolated problem, its presence may be a clue to a spondyloarthropathy such as reactive arthritis.
- **Achilles tendonitis** is a painful inflammatory condition of the Achilles tendon at or just proximal to its insertion onto the calcaneus.
  ○ It usually affects young athletic individuals (e.g., runners and dancers).
  ○ In older patients, degenerative changes in the tendon may be causative.
  ○ Inflammation in this enthesis may also indicate a spondyloarthropathy, such as ankylosing spondylitis or reactive arthritis.
  ○ Complete Achilles tendon rupture occasionally occurs.

DIAGNOSIS

- With **plantar fasciitis**, patients complain of pain under the heel, particularly when first rising in the morning or after a period of non–weight bearing. Physical examination discloses point tenderness over the plantar fascia insertion and for a short distance along the fascia.
- **Achilles tendonitis** is notable for the insidious onset of pain in the Achilles tendon that is typically worsened by activity. Patients sometimes report a squeaking or creaking during plantar flexion. Physical examination may reveal thickening and tenderness of the Achilles tendon. A protuberant posterolateral bony process of the calcaneus may also be present. Pump bumps (localized soft tissue swelling) may occur where the shoe contacts the posterior heel.
- Radiographs are generally unnecessary for either condition. **The actual clinical significance of heel spurs is uncertain.** Those with them may not have plantar fasciitis, and those with plantar fasciitis may not have them.

TREATMENT

- Treatment of **plantar fasciitis** is almost always conservative and initially consists of padding the foot, therapeutic insoles (can be purchased over the counter), NSAIDs, Achilles- and plantar-stretching exercises, and possible steroid injections.[117]
  - Conservative treatment may require several weeks to months to be significantly effective.
  - Dorsiflexion night splints may be effective for some patients.[117]
  - Local corticosteroid injections are sometimes used; however, there is only very limited quality evidence to support the use of this therapy.[117]
  - Data regarding the efficacy of extracorporeal shock wave therapy are conflicting.
  - A very few patients require more aggressive treatment and can be referred to a **podiatrist** or **orthopedic surgeon** if symptoms persist after prolonged conservative management.
- Treatment for **Achilles tendonitis** is likewise usually conservative and includes relative rest, heel lifts, ice, stretching exercises, and NSAIDs.
  - Corticosteroid injections are contraindicated because of the increased risk of tendon rupture.
  - Patients who are unresponsive to conservative management may benefit from an orthopedic or sports medicine consultation.

Mid- and Forefoot Pain

GENERAL PRINCIPLES

- **Hallux valgus** is the most common great toe malady and is characterized by the lateral movement of the first metatarsophalangeal (MTP) joint.
  - The medial head of the first metatarsal enlarges with bony hypertrophy, and the bursa over it becomes inflamed as a **bunion**.
  - A marked female predominance is seen, probably because of constricting footwear; there may also be a hereditary predisposition.
  - A similar condition may affect the lateral foot and fifth MTP joint and lead to bunionette formation.
- **Hallux rigidus** entails pain and stiffness of the osteoarthritic first MTP, which must extend with each step. It usually affects older individuals.
- **Metatarsalgia** is a general term for pain under one or more of the metatarsal heads.
  - It typically occurs when the pronated forefoot spreads out and the second, third, and fourth metatarsal heads begin to bear weight with resultant callus formation.
  - It may also be secondary to claw toe deformities (with distal migration of the plantar fat pad and subsequent exposure of the metatarsal heads) and cavus foot.
- **Morton neuroma** is characterized by pain in the web space between the third and fourth toes and is caused by compression on the interdigital nerve at this location.
- **Gout**, and less commonly **pseudogout**, can present as acute inflammation of the first MTP joint (**podagra**). Management of crystalline arthropathies is discussed in Chapter 33.
- **Stress fractures** (fatigue fractures) of the metatarsals occur as a result of repetitive overuse. They are common in runners and dancers, and a history of recent increase in the level of activity is common. The second and third metatarsals are most commonly affected.
- **Pes planus (flat feet)** per se is not always symptomatic, but chronically pronated feet often lead to pain and further deformity.
  - Flat feet may be related to multiple different foot problems, particularly **posterior tibial tendon dysfunction,** which is a common, but underdiagnosed, cause of ankle pain and foot deformity.
  - This is characterized by sudden or progressive loss of strength of the posterior tibialis tendon with secondary progressive **flatfoot deformity.**

○ The deformity is initially reversible but can become permanent.
○ Multiple etiologies are possible, including **avulsion/rupture** of the tendon (usually traumatic), **partial tendon tear** and elongation, and **tendonitis**.

DIAGNOSIS

- With **hallux valgus**, patients complain of pain, swelling, and deformity that are aggravated by shoes. Numbness over the medial aspect of the great toe may also be reported. Examination reveals medial deviation of the first metatarsal head and lateral deviation of the great toe phalanges. Impingement of the other toes is often present, and the second toe may override the great toe. Bunion formation is frequent, and there may be ulceration of the overlying skin.
- Restricted dorsiflexion of the first MTP is characteristic of **hallux rigidus** on examination.
- **Metatarsalgia** pain is often concentrated at the second metatarsal head.
- Plantar pain and dysesthesia of the affected toes are typical of **Morton neuroma**. Walking and high-heeled, constrictive shoes worsen the symptoms. Squeezing the metatarsal heads may reproduce the discomfort.
- A **stress fracture** presents as sudden or gradual onset of pain in the forefoot near the metatarsals, which can be tender.
- Plain radiographs can show the characteristic bony displacement of hallux valgus and typical osteoarthritic changes of hallux rigidus.
- Stress fractures are not detectable with plain radiographs during the first 2 weeks, but after that, callus may be seen. A bone scan is positive within the first week. MRI can detect very early stress fractures but is not usually required.

TREATMENT

- A shoe with a wide toe box is critical for symptom relief of **hallux valgus**, sometimes supplemented by an insole. Surgical treatment may be appropriate in patients who are unresponsive to conservative measures.
- A sole stiffener, such as a steel shank, reduces motion of the MTP joint and therefore reduces pain of **hallux rigidus**. A rocker-bottom sole can be used; however, it produces a gait that is difficult to get used to. Surgical arthrodesis, without a prosthetic implant, may be effective if conservative measures fail.
- Relief from **metatarsalgia** can often be provided with a metatarsal pad, inserted into the shoe such that weight bearing occurs proximal to the metatarsal heads. In the presence of coexisting foot problems, such as pronation or osteoarthritis, it may be better to order a full-contact, custom-molded insole into which a metatarsal pad can be incorporated.
- Properly fitting footwear with low heels can reduce pain from a **Morton neuroma**. A metatarsal pad may also be effective. Some advocate local corticosteroid injection. Surgery may be effective for patients who are unresponsive to conservative treatment.
- **Stress fractures** call for conservative treatment: rest, ice, and NSAIDs. Stiff-soled shoes should be worn. Patients who do not respond may need immobilization.

REFERENCES

1. Bogduk N, Teasell R. Whiplash: the evidence for an organic etiology. *Arch Neurol* 2000;57:590–591.
2. Peloso P, Gross A, Haines T, et al.; Cervical Overview Group. Medicinal and injection therapies for mechanical neck disorders. *Cochrane Database Syst Rev* 2007;(3):CD000319.

3. Gross A, Miller J, D'Sylva J, et al. Manipulation or mobilization for neck pain. *Cochrane Database Syst Rev* 2010;(1):CD004249.

4. Kay TM, Gross A, Goldsmith CH, et al. Exercises for mechanical neck disorders. *Cochrane Database Syst Rev* 2012;(8):CD004250.

5. Kroeling P, Gross A, Goldsmith CH, et al. Electrotherapy for neck pain. *Cochrane Database Syst Rev* 2009;(4):CD004251.

6. Trinh KV, Graham N, Gross AR, et al. Acupuncture for neck disorders. *Cochrane Database Syst Rev* 2006;(3):CD004870.

7. Graham N, Gross A, Goldsmith CH, et al. Mechanical traction for neck pain with or without radiculopathy. *Cochrane Database Syst Rev* 2008;(3):CD006408.

8. Patel KC, Gross A, Graham N, et al. Massage for mechanical neck disorders. *Cochrane Database Syst Rev* 2012;(9):CD004871.

9. Verhagen AP, Scholten-Peeters GG, van Wijngaarden S, et al. Conservative treatments for whiplash. *Cochrane Database Syst Rev* 2007;(2):CD003338.

10. Lord SM, Barnsley L, Wallis BJ, et al. Percutaneous radio-frequency neurotomy for chronic cervical zygapophyseal-joint pain. *N Engl J Med* 1996;335:1721–1726.

11. Niemisto L, Kalso E, Malmivaara A, et al. Radiofrequency denervation for neck and back pain. A systematic review of randomized controlled trials. *Cochrane Database Syst Rev* 2003;(1):CD004058.

12. Pettersson K, Toolanen G. High-dose methylprednisolone prevents extensive sick leave after whiplash injury. A prospective, randomized, double-blind study. *Spine (Phila Pa 1976)* 1998;23:984–989.

13. Slipman CW, Lipetz JS, Jackson HB, et al. Therapeutic selective nerve root block in the nonsurgical treatment of atraumatic cervical spondylotic radicular pain: a retrospective analysis with independent clinical review. *Arch Phys Med Rehabil* 2000;81:741–746.

14. Leboeuf-Yde C. Smoking and low back pain. A systematic literature review of 41 journal articles reporting 47 epidemiologic studies. *Spine* 1999;24:1463–1470.

15. Goldberg MS, Scott SC, Mayo NE. A review of the association between cigarette smoking and the development of nonspecific back pain and related outcomes. *Spine* 2000;25:995–1014.

16. Mikkonen P, Leino-Arjas P, Remes J, et al. Is smoking a risk factor for low back pain in adolescents? A prospective cohort study. *Spine* 2008;33:527–532.

17. Deyo RA, Weinstein JN. Low back pain. *N Engl J Med* 2001;344:363–370.

18. Zhou Y, Abdi S. Diagnosis and minimally invasive treatment of lumbar discogenic pain—a review of the literature. *Clin J Pain* 2006;22:468–481.

19. Cohen SP, Raja SN. Pathogenesis, diagnosis, and treatment of lumbar zygapophysial (facet) joint pain. *Anesthesiology* 2007;106:591–614.

20. Cohen SP. Sacroiliac joint pain: a comprehensive review of anatomy, diagnosis, and treatment. *Anesth Analg* 2005;101:1440–1453.

21. Foley BS, Buschbacher RM. Sacroiliac joint pain: anatomy, biomechanics, diagnosis, and treatment. *Am J Phys Med Rehabil* 2006;85:997–1006.

22. Chou R, Qaseem A, Snow V, et al. Diagnosis and treatment of low back pain: a joint clinic practice guideline from the American College of Physicians and the American Pain Society. *Ann Intern Med* 2007;147:478–491.

23. Henschke N, Maher CG, Refshauge KM, et al. Prevalence of and screening for serious spinal pathology in patients presenting to primary care settings with acute low back pain. *Arthritis Rheum* 2009;60:3072–3080.

24. Henschke N, Maher CG, Ostelo RW, et al. Red flags to screen for malignancy in patients with low-back pain. *Cochrane Database Syst Rev* 2013;(2):CD008686.

25. Deyo RA, Rainville J, Kent DL. What can the history and physical examination tell us about low back pain. *JAMA* 1992;268:760–765.

26. Bakker EW, Verhagen AP, van Trijffel E, et al. Spinal mechanical load as a risk factor for low back pain: a systematic review of prospective cohort studies. *Spine* 2009;34:E281–E293.

27. Hoogendoorn WE, van Poppel MN, Bongers PM, et al. Systematic review of psychosocial factors at work and private life as risk factors for back pain. *Spine* 2000;25:2114–2125.

28. Chou R, Shekelle P. Will this patient develop persistent disabling low back pain? *JAMA* 2010;303:1295–1302.

29. Pincus T, Vlaeyen JW, Kendall NA, et al. Cognitive-behavioral therapy and psychosocial factors in low back pain: directions for the future. *Spine* 2002;27:E133–E138.

30. Vroomen PC, de Krom MC, Knottnerus JA. Diagnostic value of history and physical examination in patients suspected of sciatica due to disc herniation: a systematic review. *J Neurol* 1999;246:899–906.

31. Waddell G, McCulloch JA, Kummel E, et al. Nonorganic physical signs in low-back pain. *Spine* 1980;5:117–125.

32. Fishbain DA, Cutler RB, Rosomoff HL, et al. Is there a relationship between nonorganic physical findings (Waddell signs) and secondary gain/malingering? *Clin J Pain* 2004;20:399–408.

33. van den Hoogen HM, Koes BW, van Eijk JT, et al. On the accuracy of history, physical examination, and erythrocyte sedimentation rate in diagnosing low back pain in general practice. A criteria-based review of the literature. *Spine* 1995;20:318–327.

34. Chou R, Qaseem A, Owens DK, et al. Diagnostic imaging for low back pain: advice for high-value health care from the American College of Physicians. *Ann Intern Med* 2011;154:181–189.

35. Kendrick D, Fielding K, Bentley E, et al. Radiography of the lumbar spine in primary care patients with low back pain: randomised controlled trial. *BMJ* 2001;322:400–405.

36. Wiesel SW, Tsourmas N, Feffer HL, et al. A study of computer-assisted tomography. I. The incidence of positive CAT scans in an asymptomatic group of patients. *Spine* 1984;9:549–551.

37. Jensen MC, Brant-Zawadzki MN, Obuchowski N, et al. Magnetic resonance imaging of the lumbar spine in people without back pain. *N Engl J Med* 1994;331:69–73.

38. Jarvik JJ, Hollingworth W, Heagerty P, et al. The Longitudinal Assessment of Imaging and Disability of the Back (LAIDBack) Study: baseline data. *Spine* 2001;26:1158–1166.

39. Borenstein DG, O'Mara JW Jr, Boden SD, et al. The value of magnetic resonance imaging of the lumbar spine to predict low-back pain in asymptomatic subjects: a seven-year follow-up study. *J Bone Joint Surg Am* 2001;83-A:1306–1311.

40. Jarvik JG, Hollingworth W, Heagerty PJ, et al. Three-year incidence of low back pain in an initially asymptomatic cohort: clinical and imaging risk factors. *Spine* 2005;30:1541–1548.

41. Cheung KM, Karppinen J, Chan D, et al. Prevalence and pattern of lumbar magnetic resonance imaging changes in a population study of one thousand forty-three individuals. *Spine* 2009;34:934–940.

42. Kjaer P, Leboeuf-Yde C, Korsholm L, et al. Magnetic resonance imaging and low back pain in adults: a diagnostic imaging study of 40-year-old men and women. *Spine* 2005;30:1173–1180.

43. Chou R, Huffman LH; American Pain Society; American College of Physicians. Medications for acute and chronic low back pain: a review of the evidence for an American Pain Society/American College of Physicians clinical practice guideline. *Ann Intern Med* 2007;147:505–514.

44. Roelofs PD, Deyo RA, Koes BW, et al. Non-steroidal anti-inflammatory drugs for low back pain. *Cochrane Database Syst Rev* 2008;(1):CD000396.

45. Browning R, Jackson JL, O'Malley PG. Cyclobenzaprine and back pain: a meta-analysis. *Arch Intern Med* 2001;161:1613–1620.

46. van Tulder MW, Touray T, Furlan AD, et al. Muscle relaxants for non-specific low back pain. *Cochrane Database Syst Rev* 2003;(2):CD004252.

47. Chou R, Fanciullo GJ, Fine PG, et al. Clinical guidelines for the use of chronic opioid therapy in chronic noncancer pain. *J Pain* 2009;10:113–130.

48. Martell BA, O'Connor PG, Kerns RD, et al. Systematic review: opioid treatment for chronic back pain: prevalence, efficacy, and association with addiction. *Ann Intern Med* 2007;146:116–127.

49. Urquhart DM, Hoving JL, Assendelft WW, et al. Antidepressants for non-specific low back pain. *Cochrane Database Syst Rev* 2008;(1):CD001703.

50. Muehlbacher M, Nickel MK, Kettler C, et al. Topiramate in treatment of patients with chronic low back pain: a randomized, double-blind, placebo-controlled study. *Clin J Pain* 2006;22:526–531.

51. Yaksi A, Ozgönenel L, Ozgönenel B. The efficiency of gabapentin therapy in patients with lumbar spinal stenosis. *Spine* 2007;32:939–942.

52. Engers A, Jellema P, Wensing M, et al. Individual patient education for low back pain. *Cochrane Database Syst Rev* 2008;(1):CD004057.

53. Heymans MW, van Tulder MW, Esmail R, et al. Back schools for non-specific low-back pain. *Cochrane Database Syst Rev* 2004;(4):CD000261.

54. Dahm KT, Brurberg KG, Jamtvedt G, et al. Advice to rest in bad versus advice to stay active for acute low-back pain and sciatica. *Cochrane Database Syst Rev* 2010;(6):CD007612.

55. Hayden JA, van Tulder MW, Malmivaara A, et al. Exercise therapy for treatment of non-specific low back pain. *Cochrane Database Syst Rev* 2005;(3):CD000335.

56. Chou R, Huffman LH. Nonpharmacologic therapies for acute and chronic low back pain: a review of the evidence for an American Pain Society/American College of Physicians clinical practice guideline. *Ann Intern Med* 2007;147:492–504.

57. French SD, Cameron M, Walker BF, et al. Superficial heat or cold for low back pain. *Cochrane Database Syst Rev* 2006;(1):CD004750.

58. Furlan AD, Imamura M, Dryden T, et al. Massage for low-back pain. *Cochrane Database Syst Rev* 2008;(4):CD001929.

59. Rubinstein SM, van Middelkoop M, Assendelft WJJ, et al. Spinal manipulative therapy for chronic low-back pain. *Cochrane Database Syst Rev* 2011;(2):CD008112.

60. Rubinstein SM, Terwee CB, Assendelft WJJ, et al. Spinal manipulative therapy for acute low-back pain. *Cochrane Database Syst Rev* 2012;(9):CD008880.

61. Staal JB, de Bie R, de Vet HC, et al. Injection therapy for subacute and chronic low-back pain. *Cochrane Database Syst Rev* 2008;(3):CD001824.

62. Dagenais S, Yelland MJ, Del Mar C, et al. Prolotherapy injections for chronic low-back pain. *Cochrane Database Syst Rev* 2007;(2):CD004059.

63. Furlan AD, van Tulder MW, Cherkin DC, et al. Acupuncture and dry-needling for low back pain. *Cochrane Database Syst Rev* 2005;(1):CD001351.

64. Cherkin DC, Sherman KJ, Avins AL, et al. A randomized trial comparing acupuncture, simulated acupuncture, and usual care for chronic low back pain. *Arch Intern Med* 2009;169:858–866.

65. Henschke N, Ostelo RWJG, van Tulder MW, et al. Behavioural treatment for chronic low-back pain. *Cochrane Database Syst Rev* 2010;(7):CD002014.

66. Karjalainen KA, Malmivaara A, van Tulder MW, et al. Multidisciplinary biopsychosocial rehabilitation for subacute low-back pain among working age adults. *Cochrane Database Syst Rev* 2003;(2):CD002193.

67. van Duijvenbode IC, Jellema P, van Poppel MN, et al. Lumbar supports for prevention and treatment of low back pain. *Cochrane Database Syst Rev* 2008;(2):CD001823.

68. Clarke JA, van Tulder MW, Blomberg SE, et al. Traction for low-back pain with or without sciatica. *Cochrane Database Syst Rev* 2007;(2):CD003010.
69. Khadilkar A, Odebiyi DO, Brosseau L, et al. Transcutaneous electrical nerve stimulation (TENS) versus placebo for chronic low-back pain. *Cochrane Database Syst Rev* 2008;(4):CD003008.
70. Sahar T, Cohen MJ, Ne'eman V, et al. Insoles for prevention and treatment of back pain. *Cochrane Database Syst Rev* 2007;(4):CD005275.
71. Macario A, Pergolizzi JV. Systematic literature review of spinal decompression via motorized traction for chronic discogenic low back pain. *Pain Pract* 2006;6:171–178.
72. Yousefi-Nooraie R, Schonstein E, Heidari K, et al. Low level laser therapy for nonspecific low-back pain. *Cochrane Database Syst Rev* 2008;(2):CD005107.
73. Helm S, Hayek SM, Benyamin RM, et al. Systematic review of the effectiveness of thermal annular procedures in treating discogenic low back pain. *Pain Physician* 2009;12:207–232.
74. Gibson JN, Waddell G. Surgical interventions for lumbar disc prolapse. *Cochrane Database Syst Rev* 2007;(2):CD001350.
75. Chou R, Baisden J, Carragee EJ, et al. Surgery for low back pain: a review of the evidence for an American Pain Society Clinical Practice Guideline. *Spine* 2009;34:1094–1109.
76. Weinstein JN, Lurie JD, Tosteson TD, et al. Surgical vs nonoperative treatment for lumbar disk herniation: the Spine Patient Outcomes Research Trial (SPORT) observational cohort. *JAMA* 2006;296:2451–2459.
77. Atlas SJ, Keller RB, Wu YA, et al. Long-term outcomes of surgical and nonsurgical management of sciatica secondary to a lumbar disc herniation: 10 year results from the Maine lumbar spine study. *Spine (Phila Pa 1976)* 2005;30:927–935.
78. Atlas SJ, Keller RB, Wu YA, et al. Long-term outcomes of surgical and nonsurgical management of lumbar spinal stenosis: 8 to 10 year results from the Maine lumbar spine study. *Spine* 2005;30:936–943.
79. Weinstein JN, Tosteson TD, Lurie JD, et al.; SPORT Investigators. Surgical versus nonsurgical therapy for lumbar spinal stenosis. *N Engl J Med* 2008;358:794–810.
80. Weinstein JN, Lurie JD, Tosteson TD, et al. Surgical versus nonsurgical treatment for lumbar degenerative spondylolisthesis. *N Engl J Med* 2007;356:2257–2270.
81. Phillips FM, Slosar PJ, Youssef JA, et al. Lumbar spine fusion for chronic low back pain due to degenerative disc disease: a systematic review. *Spine* 2013;38:E409–E422.
82. Reilingh ML, Kuijpers T, Tanja-Harfterkamp AM, et al. Course and prognosis of shoulder symptoms in general practice. *Rheumatology* 2008;47:724–730.
83. Hurt G, Baker CL Jr. Calcific tendinitis of the shoulder. *Orthop Clin North Am* 2003;34:567–575.
84. Hannafin JA, Chiaia TA. Adhesive capsulitis. A treatment approach. *Clin Orthop Relat Res* 2000;(372):95–109.
85. Hegedus EJ. Which physical examination tests provides clinicians with the most value when examining the shoulder? Update of a systematic review with meta-analysis of individual tests. *Br J Sports Med* 2012;46:964–978.
86. Silva L, Andréu JL, Muñoz P, et al. Accuracy of physical examination in subacromial impingement syndrome. *Rheumatology* 2008;47:679–683.
87. Green S, Buchbinder R, Hetrick S. Physiotherapy interventions for shoulder pain. *Cochrane Database Syst Rev* 2003;(2):CD004258.
88. Buchbinder R, Green S, Youd JM. Corticosteroid injections for shoulder pain. *Cochrane Database Syst Rev* 2003;(1):CD004016.
89. Arroll B, Goodyear-Smith F. Corticosteroid injections for painful shoulder: a meta-analysis. *Br J Gen Pract* 2005;55:224–228.
90. Koester MC, Dunn WR, Kuhn JE, et al. The efficacy of subacromial corticosteroid injection in the treatment of rotator cuff disease: a systematic review. *J Am Acad Orthop Surg* 2007;15:3–11.

91. Coombes BK, Bisset L, Vicenzino B. Efficacy and safety of corticosteroid injections and other injections for management of tendinopathy: a systematic review of randomised controlled trials. *Lancet* 2010;376:1751–1767.

92. Buchbinder R, Green S, Youd JM, et al. Oral steroids for adhesive capsulitis. *Cochrane Database Syst Rev* 2006;(4):CD006189.

93. Kraushaar BS, Nirschl RP. Tendinosis of the elbow (tennis elbow). Clinical features and findings of histological, immunohistochemical, and electron microscopy studies. *J Bone Joint Surg Am* 1999;81:259–278.

94. Green S, Buchbinder R, Barnsley L, et al. Non-steroidal anti-inflammatory drugs (NSAIDs) for treating lateral elbow pain in adults. *Cochrane Database Syst Rev* 2002;(2):CD003686.

95. Bisset L, Paungmali A, Vicenzino B, et al. A systematic review and meta-analysis of clinical trials on physical interventions for lateral epicondylalgia. *Br J Sports Med* 2005;39:411–422.

96. Smith DL, McAfee JH, Lucas LM, et al. Treatment of nonseptic olecranon bursitis. A controlled, blinded prospective trial. *Arch Intern Med* 1989;149:2527–2530.

97. Hansen PA, Micklesen P, Robinson LR. Clinical utility of the flick maneuver in diagnosing carpal tunnel syndrome. *Am J Phys Med Rehabil* 2004;83:363–367.

98. D'Arcy CA, McGee S. The rational clinical examination. Does this patient have carpal tunnel syndrome? *JAMA* 2000;283:3110–3117.

99. Peters-Veluthamaningal C, van der Windt DA, Winters JC, et al. Corticosteroid injection for trigger finger in adults. *Cochrane Database Syst Rev* 2009;(1):CD005617.

100. Peters-Veluthamaningal C, van der Windt DA, Winters JC, et al. Corticosteroid injection for de Quervain's tenosynovitis. *Cochrane Database Syst Rev* 2009;(3): CD005616.

101. Page MJ, Massy-Westropp N, O'Connor D, et al. Splinting for carpal tunnel syndrome. *Cochrane Database Syst Rev* 2012;(7):CD010003.

102. Page MJ, O'Connor D, Pitt V, et al. Exercise and mobilisation interventions for carpal tunnel syndrome. *Cochrane Database Syst Rev* 2012;(6):CD009899.

103. Page MJ, O'Connor D, Pitt V, et al. Therapeutic ultrasound for carpal tunnel syndrome. *Cochrane Database Syst Rev* 2012;(1):CD009601.

104. Marshall S, Tardif G, Ashworth N. Local corticosteroid injection for carpal tunnel syndrome. *Cochrane Database Syst Rev* 2007;(2):CD001554.

105. Verdugo RJ, Salinas RA, Castillo JL, et al. Surgical versus non-surgical treatment for carpal tunnel syndrome. *Cochrane Database Syst Rev* 2008;(4):CD001552.

106. Shbeeb MI, O'Duffy JD, Michet CJ Jr, et al. Evaluation of glucocorticosteroid injection for the treatment of trochanteric bursitis. *J Rheumatol* 1996;23:2104–2106.

107. Williams BS, Cohen SP. Greater trochanteric pain syndrome: a review of anatomy, diagnosis and treatment. *Anesth Analg* 2009;108:1662–1670.

108. Kannus P, Natri A, Paakkala T, et al. An outcome study of chronic patellofemoral pain syndrome. Seven-year follow-up of patients in a randomized, controlled trial. *J Bone Joint Surg Am* 1999;81:355–363.

109. Miller TT, Staron RB, Koenigsberg T, et al. MR imaging of Baker cysts: association with internal derangement, effusion, and degenerative arthropathy. *Radiology* 1996;201:247–250.

110. Andonopoulos AP, Yarmenitis S, Sfountouris H, et al. Baker's cyst in rheumatoid arthritis: an ultrasonographic study with a high resolution technique. *Clin Exp Rheumatol* 1995;13:633–636.

111. Solomon DH, Simel DL, Bates DW, et al. The rational clinical examination. Does this patient have a torn meniscus or ligament of the knee? Value of the physical examination. *JAMA* 2001;286:1610–1620.

112. Jackson JL, O'Malley PG, Kroenke K. Evaluation of acute knee pain in primary care. *Ann Intern Med* 2003;139:575–588.

113. Eren OT. The accuracy of joint line tenderness by physical examination in the diagnosis of meniscal tears. *Arthroscopy* 2003;19:850–854.
114. Stiell IG, Wells GA, Hoag RH, et al. Implementation of the Ottawa Knee Rule for the use of radiography in acute knee injuries. *JAMA* 1997;278:2075–2079.
115. Stiell IG, McKnight RD, Greenberg GH, et al. Implementation of the Ottawa ankle rules. *JAMA* 1994;271:827–832.
116. Handoll HH, Rowe BH, Quinn KM, et al. Interventions for preventing ankle ligament injuries. *Cochrane Database Syst Rev* 2001;(3):CD000018.
117. Thomas JL, Christensen JC, Kravitz SR, et al. The diagnosis and treatment of heel pain: a clinical practice guideline—revision 2010. *J Foot Ankle Surg* 2010;49:S1–S19.

35 Care of the Cancer Patient

Maria Q. Baggstrom

GENERAL PRINCIPLES

- Before treatment of a cancer patient is initiated, all patients should have a diagnosis of cancer based on tissue pathology and, if possible, a clinical, biochemical, or radiographic marker of disease should be identified to assess the results of therapy.
- **Stage** is a clinical or pathologic assessment of tumor spread. The major role of staging is to define the optimal therapy and prognosis in subsets of patients. Treatment plans are generally determined by the stage of the tumor. The role of local therapies, surgery, and radiation is determined by regional spread of disease. The role of systemic therapy, or chemotherapy, is also dependent on the stage of the tumor. In general, the probability of survival correlates well with tumor stage.
- The **grade** of a tumor defines its retention of characteristics compared to the cell of origin. It is designated as low, moderate, or high as the tissue loses its normal appearance. Although grade is important in determining prognosis for many tumors, it is not used as commonly as stage in defining treatment plans.
- **Performance status** is a gauge of a patient's overall functional status. Two scales are commonly used: the Karnofsky performance status scale and the Eastern Cooperative Oncology Group performance status scale (Table 35-1). Performance status is an essential component of the evaluation of cancer patients, as it helps predict response to treatment, duration of response, and survival. For most solid tumors, patients with poor performance status are unlikely to derive significant benefit from systemic chemotherapy. However, patients with tumors that respond dramatically to chemotherapy may benefit from this treatment, even if they have poor performance status.
- Cancers are broadly characterized as so-called liquid or solid malignancies.
  - **Leukemias and lymphomas comprise the liquid group.** The treatment of liquid tumors is usually chemotherapy or radiation therapy, or both.
  - **The solid tumors include tumors that arise from any solid organ or tissue.** Solid tumors are treated with surgery, radiation therapy, chemotherapy, or some combination of these modalities.
- **Chemotherapy** is administered in several different settings.
  - **Induction** chemotherapy is used to achieve a complete remission.
  - **Consolidation** chemotherapy is administered to patients who initially respond to treatment.
  - **Maintenance** therapy refers to low-dose, outpatient treatment used to prolong remissions; its use has proved effective in a few malignancies.
  - **Adjuvant** chemotherapy is given after complete surgical or radiologic eradication of a primary malignancy to eliminate any unmeasurable metastatic disease.
  - **Neoadjuvant** chemotherapy is given in the presence of local disease, before planned local therapy.
- Survival data are often reported in terms of median survival and 5-year survival and cause confusion among patients with newly diagnosed malignancies; these data must be conveyed to the patient with caution by the treating oncologist who can help interpret.

TABLE 35-1	Performance Status		

Karnofsky performance status scale		ECOG performance status scale	
%	Definition	Grade	Definition
100	Normal; no complaints; no symptoms of disease	0	Fully active, able to carry on all predisease activity without restriction
90	Able to carry on normal activity; minor signs or symptoms of disease	1	Restricted in physically strenuous activity but ambulatory and able to carry out work of a light or sedentary nature
80	Normal activity with effort; some signs or symptoms of disease		
70	Able to care for self; unable to carry on normal activity or to do active work	2	Ambulatory and capable of all self-care but unable to carry out any work activities; up and about >50% of waking hours
60	Requires occasional care for most needs	3	Capable of only limited self-care; confined to bed or chair; >50% of waking hours
50	Requires considerable assistance and frequent medical care		
40	Disabled; requires special care and assistance	4	Completely disabled; cannot carry out any self-care; totally confined to bed or chair
30	Severely disabled; hospitalization is indicated, although death is not imminent		
20	Very sick; hospitalization necessary; active supportive treatment necessary		
10	Moribund; fatal process progressing rapidly		
0	Dead	5	Dead

ECOG, Eastern Cooperative Oncology Group.
Data from Karnofsky DA, Burchenal JH. The clinical evaluation of chemotherapeutic agents in cancer. In: Macleod CM, ed. *Evaluation of Chemotherapeutic Agents*. New York: Columbia University Press; 1949:199–205; Oken MM, Creech RH, Tormey DC, et al. Toxicity and response criteria of the Eastern Cooperative Oncology Group. *Am J Clin Oncol* 1982;5:649–655.

- ○ **Median survival** equates to the period of time during which 50% of studied subjects are alive and 50% are dead.
- ○ **Five-year survival** means the percentage of patients studied who are alive at 5 years.

DIAGNOSIS

Breast Cancer

- Breast cancer develops in approximately 12% of women during their lifetime in the United States.
- A breast lump in a premenopausal woman is less likely to be cancerous than a breast lump in a postmenopausal woman.

- In a younger woman, a mass should be observed for 1 month to identify any cyclic changes that suggest benign disease.
- If the mass is still present, bilateral mammography should be performed. The accuracy of mammography to diagnose cancer in pre- and postmenopausal women is approximately 90%. **Nevertheless, a woman with a clinically suspicious lump and negative mammograms should undergo biopsy.**

Cancer of Unknown Primary Site

- Approximately 5% of cancer patients present with symptoms of metastatic disease, but no primary tumor site is identifiable on physical examination, routine laboratory studies, or chest radiography.
- The histopathologic cell type and the site of the metastasis should direct a search for the primary lesion.
- Immunohistochemical stains may identify specific tissue antigens that help define the origin of the tumor and guide subsequent therapy.
- If **cervical adenopathy** is also present:
  - This suggests cancer of the lung, breast, or head and neck, or lymphoma.
  - Initial evaluation usually includes panendoscopy (nasendoscopy, laryngopharyngoscopy, bronchoscopy, and esophagoscopy) and biopsy of any suspicious lesion before excision of the lymph node.
  - If squamous cell carcinoma is identified, the patient is presumed to have primary head and neck cancer and radiation therapy may be curative.
- If a **midline mass** in the mediastinum or retroperitoneum is identified:
  - In both sexes, this may represent an extragonadal germ cell cancer.
  - Elevations in AFP (alpha-fetoprotein) or β-HCG (human chorionic gonadotropin) further suggest this diagnosis.
  - This neoplasm is potentially curable.

Lymphoma

- Lymphoma is usually diagnosed by biopsy of an enlarged lymph node.
- Staging of Hodgkin disease and non-Hodgkin lymphoma is organized into four categories.
  - **Stage I** is localized to a single lymph node or group.
  - **Stage II** involves more than one lymph node group but confined to one side of the diaphragm.
  - **Stage III** is in the lymph nodes or the spleen and occurs on both sides of the diaphragm.
  - **Stage IV** involves the liver, lung, skin, or bone marrow.
- **B symptoms** include fever above 38°C, drenching night sweats, or a 10% weight loss within 6 months prior to diagnosis. These symptoms suggest bulky disease and a worse prognosis.
- **Hodgkin disease** usually presents with cervical adenopathy and spreads in a predictable manner along lymph node groups.
- **Non-Hodgkin lymphoma** is classified as low, intermediate, or high grade based on the histologic type.
  - Staging evaluation is the same as for Hodgkin disease, but non-Hodgkin lymphoma has a less predictable pattern of spread.
  - Advanced-stage disease (stage III or IV) is very common and can usually be diagnosed by computed tomography (CT) scan or bone marrow biopsy; exploratory laparotomy and lymphangiography are rarely necessary.

Leukemia

Acute Leukemias

- Patients may present with manifestations of cytopenias, including fatigue and dyspnea (anemia), cutaneous or mucosal hemorrhage (thrombocytopenia), and fever/infection (neutropenia).

- Patients may also present with leukemic infiltration of organs, manifested as lymphade-nopathy, splenomegaly (more common in acute lymphocytic leukemia), gingival hyper-plasia, and skin nodules (more common in acute myeloid leukemia).
- Leukemic **blasts** are usually present in the blood.
- **Bone marrow aspiration/biopsy** is performed to establish the diagnosis and often shows nearly complete replacement by blasts.
- **Flow cytometry and cytogenetics** must be performed on the bone marrow aspirate for classification and to provide prognostic information.

Chronic Leukemias
- **Chronic lymphocytic leukemia** (CLL) usually presents with lymphocytosis, lymphade-nopathy, and splenomegaly. Malignant cells resemble mature lymphocytes.
- **Chronic myelogenous leukemia** (CML) presents with leukocytosis and a left shift, as well as splenomegaly.
  - Thrombocytosis, basophilia, and eosinophilia are also common.
  - The diagnosis of CML is confirmed by demonstration of the **Philadelphia chromo-some (t9:22)**, which results in production of a hybrid protein (bcr-abl).
- **Hairy cell leukemia** represents only 2% to 3% of all adult leukemias.
  - Clinical presentation includes splenomegaly, pancytopenia, and infection.
  - Patients are at increased risk for bacterial, viral, and fungal infections, and have a unique susceptibility to atypical mycobacterial infections.
  - Bone marrow biopsy reveals infiltration by cells that have prominent cytoplasmic projec-tions (thus the name).

Multiple Myeloma
- Multiple myeloma (MM) is a malignant plasma cell disorder that is usually accompanied by a **serum or urine paraprotein**, or both.
- Presenting manifestations may include hypercalcemia, anemia, lytic bone lesions with bone pain, and acute renal failure.
- The initial evaluation should include a radiographic bone survey, bone marrow aspiration and biopsy, serum and urine protein electrophoresis, β_2-microglobulin, and quantitative immunoglobulins.

TREATMENT

General Principles of Chemotherapy
- **The advice of an oncologist and precise adherence to a treatment plan are mandatory because of the low therapeutic index of chemotherapeutic agents.** Specific agents are included in Table 35-2.
- The dosage of chemotherapy is usually based on body surface area. This is determined by body weight and height and should be adjusted when changes in weight occur.
- An assessment of a patient's disease status, determination of side effects from the pre-vious treatment, and a complete blood count should be obtained before each cycle of chemotherapy.
- Drug dosages often require adjustment for the following conditions: neutropenia, throm-bocytopenia, stomatitis, diarrhea, and limited metabolic capacity for the drug.
- **Oral drug administration**
  - May be accompanied by nausea and vomiting and may require antiemetic therapy.
  - For some agents, oral absorption is variable and may require special instructions regard-ing diet and other medications.
- **IV drug administration**
  - Should be performed by experienced personnel.

TABLE 35-2 | Chemotherapeutic Medications

Drugs	Toxicities
Antimetabolites	
Ara-C (cytarabine)	Myelosuppression, GI toxicity, conjunctivitis, cerebellar ataxia, pancreatitis, hepatitis
5-FU	Myelosuppression, stomatitis, diarrhea, cerebellar ataxia, chest pain, hand-foot syndrome
Capecitabine	Diarrhea, hand-foot syndrome
Methotrexate	Mucositis, prolonged reabsorption in patients with effusions, interstitial pneumonitis, hepatitis, renal failure
Pemetrexed	Prolonged reabsorption in patients with effusions, hand-foot syndrome, myelosuppression, fatigue
6-Mercaptopurine	Decreased metabolism in patients taking allopurinol, hepatic cholestasis, immunosuppression
Fludarabine	Myelosuppression, immunosuppression, tumor lysis syndrome
Cladribine (2-chlorode-oxyadenosine)	Myelosuppression
Gemcitabine	Fever, edema, flu-like symptoms, rash, pneumonitis, rare hemolytic uremic syndrome
Alkylating agents	
Busulfan	Interstitial pneumonitis, gynecomastia, reversible Addison-like syndrome
Chlorambucil	Myelosuppression
Cyclophosphamide	Hemorrhagic cystitis, hemorrhagic myocarditis, SIADH, secondary malignancies
Dacarbazine	Flu-like syndrome, fever, myalgias, facial flushing, malaise, elevations of hepatic enzymes
Ifosfamide	Hemorrhagic cystitis, neurologic toxicity, including seizures
Mechlorethamine (nitrogen mustard)	Skin irritant, drug rash
Melphalan	Idiosyncratic interstitial pneumonitis
Nitrosoureas (carmustine [BCNU] and lomustine [CCNU])	Myelosuppression, giddiness, flushing, phlebitis
Temozolomide	Nausea, vomiting, teratogenicity
Thiotepa	Myelosuppression
Antitumor antibiotics	
Anthracyclines (dauno-rubicin, doxorubicin, mitoxantrone, idarubicin)	Cardiomyopathy, bone marrow suppression, mucositis
Bleomycin	Severe allergic reactions with hypotension, interstitial pneumonitis, dermatologic toxicity
Mitomycin-C	Delayed myelosuppression, hemolytic-uremic syndrome
2-Deoxycoformycin (pentostatin)	Myelosuppression

(Continued)

TABLE 35-2 Chemotherapeutic Medications (*Continued*)

Drugs	Toxicities
Plant alkaloids	
Vincristine	Dose-limiting neuropathy, SIADH, Raynaud phenomenon
Vinblastine	Myelosuppression, myalgias, obstipation, transient hepatitis, SIADH
Vinorelbine	Myelosuppression, SIADH
Etoposide (VP-16)	Myelosuppression, hypersensitivity reactions, secondary malignancies
Teniposide (VM-26)	Myelosuppression, hypersensitivity reactions, alopecia, hypotension
Paclitaxel	Anaphylactoid reactions, myelosuppression, arthralgias, neuropathy, arrhythmias
Docetaxel	Third-space fluid collections, dermatologic toxicity, myelosuppression
Navelbine	Pain at IV injection site
Platinum-containing agents	
Cisplatin	Severe nausea and vomiting, neurotoxicity, renal toxicity, hypomagnesemia, ototoxicity
Carboplatin	Myelosuppression, neurotoxicity, ototoxicity, nephrotoxicity
Oxaliplatin	Sensory neuropathy, cold sensitivity
Other agents	
Hydroxyurea	Myelosuppression
L-Asparaginase	Allergic or anaphylactoid reactions, hemorrhagic pancreatitis, hepatic failure, encephalopathy
Procarbazine	Monoamine oxidase inhibitor, disulfiram-like effect
Topotecan	Myelosuppression, flu-like syndrome
Irinotecan	Severe diarrhea
Hormonal agents	
Tamoxifen and raloxifene	Hormone flare (bone pain, erythema, hypercalcemia), endometrial cancer, deep vein thrombosis
Aromatase inhibitors (anastrozole, letrozole, exemestane)	Hot flashes, night sweats
Progestational agents (megestrol acetate and medroxyprogesterone)	Weight gain, fluid retention, hot flashes, vaginal bleeding with discontinuation of therapy
Antiandrogens (flutamide and bicalutamide)	Nausea, vomiting, gynecomastia, breast tenderness
Targeted therapies	
Trastuzumab	Cardiomyopathy, embryo-fetal toxicity
Rituximab	Infusion-related reaction, tumor lysis syndrome, mucocutaneous reaction, PML
Ofatumumab	Infusion-related reaction, PML, hepatitis B reactivation, immunosuppression
Alemtuzumab	Immunodeficiency and opportunistic infections
Bevacizumab	Hypertension, proteinuria, serious bleeding or clotting events, GI perforations, RPLS

TABLE 35-2 Chemotherapeutic Medications (*Continued*)

Drugs	Toxicities
Cetuximab	Infusion reactions, rash, diarrhea, interstitial lung disease, hypomagnesemia, sudden death
Panitumumab	Infusion reactions, rash, diarrhea
Gemtuzumab	Nausea, fever, myelosuppression, tumor lysis, hypersensitivity reaction
Ibritumomab and iodine 131 tositumomab	Myelosuppression
Imatinib	Edema, nausea, rash, musculoskeletal pain, congestive heart failure
Erlotinib	Rash, diarrhea, interstitial lung disease
Sunitinib	Hypertension, fatigue, asthenia, diarrhea, hand-foot syndrome, hypothyroidism, congestive heart failure, adrenal insufficiency
Sorafenib	Hypertension, skin rash, diarrhea, hand-foot syndrome, hypophosphatemia
Lapatinib	Diarrhea, cardiac toxicity
Nonspecific immunotherapy	
Interferon-α	Nausea, vomiting, flu-like symptoms, headache
Aldesleukin (interleukin-2)	Fluid overload, hypotension, prerenal azotemia, elevation of liver enzymes
Chemopreventive agents	
Retinoids	Dry skin, cheilitis, hyperlipidemia, elevation of transaminases

BCNU, bis-chloronitrosourea or carmustine; CCNU, lomustine; GI, gastrointestinal; SIADH, syndrome of inappropriate antidiuretic hormone; PML, progressive multifocal leukoencephalopathy; RPLS, reversible posterior leukoencephalopathy syndrome.

- Care should be taken to ensure free flow of fluid to the vein and adequate blood return should be verified before instillation of chemotherapy.
- Infusions should be through a large-caliber, upper extremity vein. When possible, veins of the antecubital fossa, wrist, dorsum of the hand, and arm ipsilateral to an axillary lymph node dissection should be avoided.
- In patients with poor peripheral venous access or those who require many doses of chemotherapy, indwelling venous catheter devices should be considered.
- **Intrathecal chemotherapy**
  - Intrathecal (IT) chemotherapy is administered for the treatment of meningeal carcinomatosis or central nervous system (CNS) prophylaxis.
  - Side effects include acute arachnoiditis, subacute motor dysfunction, and progressive neurologic deterioration (leukoencephalopathy).
  - Impaired cognitive function and leukoencephalopathy occur more often when IT chemotherapy is combined with whole-brain radiation.
- **Intracavitary instillation**
  - Some chemotherapeutic agents can be instilled directly into the pleural or peritoneal spaces when indicated.
  - Systemic toxicities can be observed if the agent is systemically absorbed.
- **Intra-arterial chemotherapy**
  - Is advocated as a method of achieving high drug concentrations at specific tumor sites.
  - Although it is of theoretical advantage, there are no absolute indications for chemotherapy administered by this route.

Breast Cancer

Overview

- **Surgical options:** treatment is focused on local control and reducing the risk of systemic spread.
  - Local control with **tylectomy** (lumpectomy and axillary lymph node dissection) is as effective as a modified radical mastectomy. An axillary lymph node dissection should be included because it provides prognostic information and is of therapeutic value.
  - **Sentinel lymph node mapping** and dissection allow many women to be spared full axillary dissection. In this procedure, blue dye, a radiotracer, or both are injected around the tumor bed. The lymph node(s) that pick up the dye/tracer are excised. If no cancer cells are seen in these lymph nodes, further axillary dissection can be avoided.
- **Radiation therapy** is indicated for patients treated with tylectomy and for some individuals with axillary lymph node involvement. It can also be used for palliation of painful or obstructing metastatic lesions.
- **Systemic therapy** is given for two reasons in the treatment of breast cancer:
  - **Adjuvant therapy** is given to reduce recurrence risk following surgery (see below).
  - **Palliative therapy** is given to women with metastatic breast cancer to slow the progression of disease and to extend their lives (see below).
- **Hormone therapy** is used for women with estrogen receptor (ER)-positive and/or progesterone receptor–positive disease.
- **Trastuzumab** (Herceptin) is appropriate for women with **HER2/neu-positive** breast cancer.
- **Anthracycline-based chemotherapy** is potentially useful in all subtypes.

Adjuvant Therapy

- **The presence or absence of axillary lymph node metastases is the most important prognostic factor in breast cancer. All women with axillary nodal involvement should receive adjuvant therapy.**
- Women with node-negative breast cancer should also be considered for adjuvant therapy if the tumor is >1 cm, is ER negative or has overexpression of HER2.
- Chemotherapy should be considered in patients who are premenopausal, have cancers that are ER negative, or overexpress HER2.
- **Tamoxifen,** 20 mg PO daily for 5 years, is recommended for all ER-positive breast cancers in premenopausal women.[1]
- In postmenopausal women, the **aromatase inhibitors** (anastrozole, letrozole, and exemestane) have generally replaced tamoxifen for adjuvant hormone therapy.
- **Trastuzumab** has been found to be effective in the adjuvant treatment of women with HER2/neu-positive disease.[2]

Metastatic Disease

- Menopausal status, hormone receptor status, HER2-neu expression, and sites of metastatic disease dictate initial treatment.
- ER-negative breast cancer, lymphangitic lung disease, and liver metastasis seldom respond to hormonal manipulation and should be treated with chemotherapy.
- ER-positive disease is treated with hormonal manipulation.
  - Premenopausal women are initially treated with tamoxifen and a luteinizing hormone–releasing hormone (LHRH) agonist; postmenopausal women should receive a hormonal agent, such as tamoxifen or an aromatase inhibitor. If the disease responds to hormonal therapy, subsequent disease progression may respond to other hormonal agents.
  - Chemotherapy should be considered if there is no response to initial hormonal therapy or if progression occurs during subsequent hormonal manipulations.
- In HER2-overexpressing cancers, the addition of **trastuzumab** to first-line chemotherapy produced an improvement in survival compared to chemotherapy alone.[3]

- In women with more than one osteolytic metastasis, the monthly administration of zoledronic acid, 4 mg IV, produces an improvement in quality of life, greater response to therapy, fewer extravertebral fractures, and possibly a prolongation in survival.[4] Other bone modifying agents such as denosumab have also been recently approved.

Inflammatory and Unresectable Cancers
- Inflammatory breast cancer manifests as peau d'orange changes or erythema involving more than one-third of the chest wall.
- Because of the high likelihood of metastases at diagnosis, these patients and those with inoperable primary breast cancers are initially treated with chemotherapy.
- Subsequently, surgery and radiation therapies are used for maximal local control.

Lung Cancer
- Lung cancer is the most common cause of cancer death in the United States and is the most preventable given its relationship to cigarette smoking.
- Treatment is based on the histology and stage of the disease.

Small Cell Lung Cancer
- Small cell lung cancer (SCLC) is often responsible for a variety of **paraneoplastic syndromes** in addition to local symptoms.
- It is treated according to whether disease is **limited** (confined to one hemithorax and ipsilateral regional lymph nodes) **or extensive** stage.
  - For **limited disease**, combination chemotherapy and radiation therapy result in a 70% to 90% response rate, a median survival of 14 to 20 months, and a cure in 5% to 15% of patients.
  - With **extensive disease**, the median survival is 9 to 11 months, and **cures are rare**.
- For patients who achieve a complete remission with chemotherapy, **prophylactic whole-brain radiation therapy** has been shown to decrease the risk of central CNS metastases.[5]
- Radiation therapy to the chest as consolidation therapy may improve survival in limited disease but is not recommended in extensive disease except for palliation of local symptoms.

Non–Small Cell Lung Cancer
- **Whenever possible, surgical resection should be attempted for non–small cell lung cancer (NSCLC) because it affords the best chance of cure.**
- Survival rates after resection of NSCLC are improved using adjuvant chemotherapy with or without radiation therapy.
- For unresectable disease confined to the lung and regional lymph nodes, radiation therapy in combination with chemotherapy is the conventional treatment.
- In patients with metastatic disease, cisplatin-based combination chemotherapy may modestly improve survival.
- With nonsquamous histology, epidermal growth factor receptor (EGFR) mutation testing and anaplastic lymphoma kinase (ALK) testing should be performed since treatment with erlotinib or crizotinib, respectively, would be recommended in the first-line metastatic setting.

Gastrointestinal Malignancies
Esophageal Cancers
- Esophageal cancers are either squamous cell (associated with cigarette smoking and alcohol use) or adenocarcinoma (arising in Barrett esophagus).
- Surgical resection of the esophagus is recommended in small primary tumors and in selected patients after chemoradiation.
- Local control of unresectable cancers can be achieved with combined chemotherapy and radiation therapy.[6]

- In metastatic disease, trastuzumab should be added to chemotherapy for HER2-overexpressing esophageal adenocarcinoma in the first- and second-line settings.
- Palliation of obstructive symptoms can be accomplished by radiation therapy, dilation, prosthetic tube placement, or laser therapy.

Gastric Cancer
- Gastric cancer is usually adenocarcinoma and can be cured with surgery in the rare patient with localized disease.
- Adjuvant chemotherapy and concurrent radiation have been shown to improve outcomes in surgically resected gastric cancer.[7]
- Locally advanced but unresectable cancers may benefit from concomitant chemotherapy and radiation therapy.
- Chemotherapy may offer increased survival and quality of life in patients with metastatic disease. Trastuzumab should be added to chemotherapy in patients with HER2-overexpression.

Colon and Rectal Adenocarcinomas
- These cancers are primarily treated by surgical resection.
- In all patients who are undergoing surgical resection of colon or rectal cancer, a preoperative **carcinoembryonic antigen** level should be measured and followed. A persistently elevated or increasing level may indicate residual or recurrent tumor.
- A number of chemotherapy agents are available for the treatment of colorectal cancer. These include 5-FU, irinotecan, capecitabine, and oxaliplatin. Adjuvant chemotherapy is offered in stage III patients and in selected high-risk stage II patients.
- Rectal cancer that arises below the peritoneal reflection commonly recurs locally after surgery alone; postoperative radiation therapy and 5-FU are recommended.
- Three **monoclonal antibodies** have been approved for the treatment of metastatic colon cancer. Bevacizumab targets vascular endothelial growth factor (VEGF). Both cetuximab and panitumumab target EGFR. Also the multikinase inhibitor regorafenib is indicated in metastatic colon cancer.
- Selected patients with metastases confined to the liver may be candidates for liver resection.[8]

Anal Cancer
- **Chemotherapy with concurrent radiation therapy** appears to result in a higher cure rate than surgical resection and usually preserves the anal sphincter and fecal continence.[9]
- Surgical resection should be used only as salvage therapy.

Genitourinary Malignancies
Bladder Cancer
- In the United States, bladder cancer usually presents as **transitional cell carcinoma**. A variety of chemical carcinogens, including those in cigarette smoke, have been implicated.
- **Unifocal** tumors confined to the mucosa should be managed with cystoscopy and transurethral resection or fulguration, repeated at approximately 3-month intervals.
- **Multifocal** mucosal disease is treated with intravesicular bacillus Calmette-Guérin, thiotepa, or mitomycin-C.
- **Locally invasive** cancers should be resected.
- Adjuvant chemotherapy improves survival when regional lymph node involvement is confirmed in the cystectomy specimen.
- In metastatic or recurrent disease, the highest response rates are seen with cisplatin-containing regimens.

Prostate Cancer
- Prostate cancer is the most common cancer in men behind nonmelanoma skin cancer.
- Prostate-specific antigen is useful as a marker for recurrence, bulk of disease, and response to therapy and may detect asymptomatic early-stage disease.

- **Local control** of the primary lesion can be achieved with either prostatectomy or radiation therapy.
- In patients with **metastatic disease**, bilateral orchiectomy and LHRH analogs with or without an antiandrogen produce tumor regression in approximately 85% of patients for a median of 18 to 24 months.
  - Disease that has relapsed after hormonal therapy may respond to withdrawal of that antiandrogen.[10]
  - Anthracyclines, taxanes, vinblastine, estramustine, sipuleucel-T, and abitaterone are options in hormone-refractory disease.
- Anemia and bone pain dominate the advanced phases of this disease and are best relieved with transfusions, growth factors, and palliative radiation therapy.

Renal Cell Cancer
- Renal cell cancer is treated by **surgical resection**, which may be curative if disease is localized; no effective adjuvant therapy is available. Cytoreductive nephrectomy is offered in select stage IV patients.
- Multitargeted tyrosine kinase inhibitors (TKIs) (sunitinib, sorafenib, and pazopanib) have been approved for the treatment of metastatic renal cell cancer. These agents appear more active and better tolerated than previously available agents. Other options include temsirolimus, bevacizumab plus interferon, and high-dose interleukin-2.

Testicular Cancer
- Considered one of the most curable malignancies and should be treated aggressively.
- A patient suspected of having cancer of the testis should have tissue obtained only through an inguinal orchiectomy.
- The initial evaluation should include serum **α-fetoprotein** and **β-human chorionic gonadotropin** levels and a CT scan of the abdomen and pelvis.
- Most patients with **seminoma** should be treated with radiation therapy after primary treatment with orchiectomy.
- In **nonseminomatous germ cell cancer**, a retroperitoneal lymph node dissection should be performed for staging, except in the instance of bulky abdominal disease or pulmonary metastasis.
  - If **microscopic disease** is identified at surgery, two alternatives are acceptable: two cycles of postoperative chemotherapy or observation until relapse occurs followed by institution of chemotherapy.
  - With **gross metastatic disease**, cisplatin-based chemotherapy is curative for most germ cell cancers. If tumor markers normalize after chemotherapy but a radiographic mass persists, exploratory surgery should be performed. The lesion proves to be residual cancer in approximately one-third of the patients. Patients with residual cancer should receive additional chemotherapy.[11]
- Sperm banking should be discussed with patients of reproductive age prior to treatment.

Gynecologic Malignancies
Cervical Cancer
- The recognized risk factors are multiparity, multiple sexual partners, and infection with **human papillomavirus (HPV)**.
- **Carcinoma in situ** and superficial disease can be treated by endocervical cone biopsy.
- **Microinvasive disease** is treated with an abdominal hysterectomy.
- **Advanced local disease** (invasion of the cervix or local extension) is initially treated with surgery or radiation therapy, or both. The addition of chemotherapy to radiation therapy postoperatively is associated with improved survival.[12]
- Inoperable cancer can be controlled with radiation therapy; metastatic disease is treated with cisplatin-based chemotherapy.

- The **HPV vaccine** (covering types 6, 11, 16, & 18) is recommended for young women ages 9 to 26 in hopes of reducing the rates of cervical and vaginal carcinoma (see Chapter 5).

Ovarian Cancer
- Ovarian cancer is primarily a disease of postmenopausal women.
- Because symptoms are uncommon with localized disease, most patients present with advanced local disease, malignant ascites, or peritoneal metastases.
- **Surgical staging** and treatment include a total abdominal hysterectomy (TAH), bilateral oophorectomy, lymph node sampling, omentectomy, peritoneal cytology, and removal of all gross tumor. If the tumor is localized to the ovary, the surgery may be curative and further treatment is not routinely recommended. However, if microscopic foci of cancer are identified, chemotherapy is administered postoperatively.
- The serum marker **CA-125**, although not specific, is elevated in >80% of women with epithelial ovarian cancer and is a sensitive indicator of response and recurrence.

Endometrial Cancer
- The risks include obesity, nulliparity, early age at menarche, late age at menopause, polycystic ovaries, older age, Lynch syndrome, and the use of unopposed estrogens (including tamoxifen).
- Patients generally present with vaginal bleeding.
- Surgery TAH and bilateral salpingo-oophorectomy (BSO) and radiation therapy (tumor-directed external beam radiation and brachytherapy) are often curative.

Head and Neck Cancer

- Head and neck cancer is usually squamous cell.
- It may arise in a variety of sites, each of which has a different natural history.
- Early lesions can be cured with surgery, radiation therapy, or both.
- Despite aggressive surgical and radiation therapy, approximately 65% of patients with head and neck cancer have uncontrolled local disease.
- The addition of chemotherapy to radiation therapy improves the survival in patients with nasopharyngeal cancers and selected patients with other primary disease sites.[13]

Malignant Melanoma

- This should be considered when evaluating any changing or enlarging nevus. Suspicious lesions should be removed by **excisional biopsy**. Subsequently, a wide local excision is performed to remove possible vertical and radial spread of tumor.
- Deeper invasion is associated with a worse prognosis.
- Adjuvant interferon is an option for melanoma patients with nodal involvement.
- Systemic disease may respond to ipilimumab (monoclonal antibody targeting CTLA-4) or vemurafenib (targeting BRAF V600 mutation). Other options include dacarbazine, interferon-α, or high-dose interleukin-2.

Sarcomas

- Sarcomas are tumors arising from mesenchymal tissue and occur most commonly in soft tissue or bone.
- Initial evaluation should include a CT scan of the chest, as hematogenous spread to the lungs is common.

Soft Tissue Sarcoma
- Prognosis is primarily determined by tumor grade and not by the cell of origin.
- **Surgical resection** should be performed when feasible and may be curative.
- In low-grade tumors, local and regional recurrence is most common, and **adjuvant radiation therapy** may be of benefit.

- High-grade tumors often recur systemically but no advantage to the routine use of adjuvant chemotherapy has been demonstrated.
- In **metastatic disease**, doxorubicin, ifosfamide, and dacarbazine produce responses in 40% to 55% of patients. Targeted agents such as pazopanib, imatinib, and sunitinib have also shown therapeutic efficacy.

Osteogenic Sarcoma
- Osteogenic sarcoma is usually treated with neoadjuvant chemotherapy followed by surgical resection. If this results in a good response, further adjuvant chemotherapy is recommended. In patients who are not resectable after neoadjuvant chemotherapy, further chemotherapy or radiation are options.
- Treatment of isolated pulmonary metastasis by surgical resection is associated with long-term survival.

Kaposi Sarcoma
- In an immunocompetent patient, Kaposi sarcoma is generally a low-grade lesion of the lower extremities that is readily treated with **local radiation therapy or vinblastine**.
- When Kaposi sarcoma complicates organ transplantation or AIDS, it is more aggressive and may arise in visceral sites.
- **Liposomal doxorubicin** alone is as effective as combination chemotherapy for palliation.[14] Paclitaxel is another systemic option.

Lymphoma
Hodgkin Disease
- **Treatment is based on the presenting stage of the disease;** the cell type is relatively unimportant in the natural history and prognosis.
- Initial staging evaluation includes a CT scan of the chest, abdomen, and pelvis, PET/CT, and bilateral bone marrow biopsies to determine the clinical stage of the disease.
- **Stages IA and IIA (favorable disease)** are treated with a combination of chemotherapy and radiation or chemotherapy alone as an alternative treatment option.
- **Stage IA and IIA (unfavorable disease) and IIIA** disease are treated with chemotherapy followed by consolidative radiation therapy.
- All **Stage IV** patients should receive combination chemotherapy followed by consolidative radiation, if the patient presented with bulky mediastinal disease.
- When **B symptoms** are present, chemotherapy is recommended regardless of the stage.

Non-Hodgkin Lymphoma
- **Low-grade lymphoma**
  ○ It often involves the bone marrow at diagnosis but the disease has an **indolent course.**
  ○ Because this tumor is **not curable with standard chemotherapy,** treatment can be delayed until the patient is symptomatic (i.e., watch and wait).
  ○ **Radiation therapy** or an alkylating agent (e.g., cyclophosphamide) can be used to ameliorate symptoms.
  ○ Radiation therapy may produce long-term complete remission in stage I or II disease.
  ○ **Rituximab** produces an objective response in approximately 50% of patients with follicular lymphoma without the usual toxicities of chemotherapy in the elderly or infirm.
- **Intermediate-grade lymphoma**
  ○ This has a more aggressive course, usually does not involve the bone marrow at diagnosis, and **can be cured with chemotherapy.**
  ○ Complete response rates exceed 80%.
  ○ Features associated with a lower likelihood of cure include an elevated lactate dehydrogenase level, stage III/IV disease, age >60 years, more than one extranodal site, and poor performance status.

- **High-grade lymphoma**
  - This subtype includes Burkitt and lymphoblastic lymphoma, the **most aggressive subtypes** that have a high frequency of CNS and bone marrow involvement.
  - Cerebrospinal fluid (CSF) cytology should be included as part of the initial evaluation.
  - Combination chemotherapy is the mainstay of treatment and should include CNS prophylaxis, if the CSF is cytologically free of tumor.
  - If tumor cells are seen in the CSF, additional therapy may be indicated.
  - Prophylaxis to prevent **tumor lysis syndrome** should be initiated before induction chemotherapy.

Leukemia
Acute Leukemias
- **Acute myeloid leukemia (AML)**
  - Acute myeloid leukemia constitutes approximately 80% of adult acute leukemia.
  - Approximately 50% to 80% of patients achieve complete remission with **induction chemotherapy** that includes cytarabine (cytosine arabinoside [ara-C]) and daunorubicin.
  - **Consolidation therapy** is given with at least one additional cycle of chemotherapy, which is typically ara-C at a dose of 10 to 30 times that used for induction (high-dose ara-C). High-dose ara-C consolidation results in cure in approximately 30% to 40% of patients <60 years of age.
  - Pretreatment factors associated with a low (<10%) chance for cure includes the following: preceding myelodysplastic syndrome, prior exposure to radiation, benzene, or chemotherapy, and adverse cytogenetic abnormalities.
  - For these high-risk patients, allogeneic stem cell transplant in first remission increases the likelihood of cure.
- **Acute promyelocytic leukemia**
  - Acute promyelocytic leukemia is characterized by a chromosomal translocation (t[15;17]) that results in a hybrid protein (PML-RAR).
  - Induction treatment with oral **tretinoin** (all-trans retinoic acid) plus chemotherapy results in complete remission in >90% of patients.
  - After consolidation chemotherapy, approximately 75% of patients are cured.
- **Acute lymphocytic leukemia**
  - Typically a disease of childhood with a median age at diagnosis of 13 years. It represents only 20% of all leukemias in adults.
  - For adults, **induction and consolidation** involve treatment with multiple chemotherapeutic agents over a period of approximately 6 months followed by at least 18 months of lower-dose **maintenance** chemotherapy.
  - To prevent CNS relapse, patients receive **IT chemotherapy** and either cranial radiation or CNS-penetrating chemotherapy.
  - Approximately 60% to 80% of adults achieve complete remission, with about 30% to 40% cured. Increasing age, higher white blood cell count, and longer time to remission are associated with reduced survival. **Cytogenetics** is crucial in determining prognosis and **allogeneic stem cell transplantation** during the first remission should be considered in patients with a poor prognosis.

Chronic Leukemias
- **Chronic lymphocytic leukemia**
  - Treatment of CLL is similar to that for low-grade lymphoma except that **fludarabine** appears to be more active than alkylating agents.
  - Median survival is approximately 6 to 8 years.
  - Anemia and thrombocytopenia are associated with shortened survival.
  - As in low-grade lymphoma, patients are treated for control of symptoms or cytopenias.

- Because CLL is accompanied by immunodeficiency, life-threatening infections may occur. Therefore, febrile patients must be evaluated carefully.
- **Autoimmune hemolytic anemia or immune thrombocytopenia** may develop as complications of CLL and are treated with **glucocorticoids** (e.g., prednisone, 1 mg/kg PO daily) or chemotherapy, or both.
- CLL may transform to an intermediate or high-grade lymphoma (**Richter transformation**).
- **Chronic myelogenous leukemia**
  - During the stable phase of the CML, the disease can be controlled, and most patients are asymptomatic.
  - **Imatinib** is an orally administered medication designed specifically to inhibit the BCR-ABL tyrosine kinase. Because imatinib is highly active and has few toxicities, it is currently the **first-line therapy** for this disease. Even blast-phase CML or Philadelphia chromosome–positive acute leukemia may respond to imatinib. Responses in this setting are generally of relatively short duration.
  - Next generation TKIs **nilotinib and dasatinib** are also first-line therapy options.
  - Allogeneic transplant is appropriate in patients with blast phase, patients with BCR-ABL mutations resistant to all TKIs, and those intolerant of all TKIs.
- **Hairy cell leukemia**
  - For hairy cell leukemia, a single 7-day course of **chlorodeoxyadenosine** (cladribine) produces remission in >90% of patients.
  - Although this drug is not curative, 5-year progression-free survival exceeds 50%.

Multiple Myeloma
- Treatment of MM depends on whether the patient is a candidate for stem cell transplant. Steroids such as dexamethasone or prednisone are included in all treatment regimens. Alkylating agents such as melphalan are not recommended for transplant candidates.
- Local radiation therapy can be used to relieve painful bone lesions, and zoledronic acid, 4 mg IV every month decreases skeletal complications.
- **Thalidomide and lenalidomide** are immunomodulatory agents that have been shown to be effective in MM.
  - Because thalidomide can cause severe fetal malformations, prescribing this medication requires participation in a prescriber program.
  - Prophylaxis with anticoagulation agents is also recommended.
- **Bortezomib** (Velcade) is a proteasome inhibitor that degrades ubiquitinated proteins which has shown activity in MM.
- Treatment options include various combinations of the above-mentioned agents with adjustment based on whether a patient is a transplant candidate.
- After induction chemotherapy, consolidation with high-dose therapy and **autologous stem cell transplant** improves survival.

COMPLICATIONS

Complications Related to Tumor
Brain Metastasis
- Patients with parenchymal brain metastasis may present with headache, mental status changes, weakness, or focal neurologic deficits. Papilledema is observed in only 25% of patients.
- In individuals with malignancy, a CT scan of the head showing one or more round, contrast-enhancing lesions surrounded by edema is usually sufficient for the diagnosis. If cancer has not been diagnosed previously, tissue should be obtained from the brain lesion or a more accessible site before radiation therapy is initiated.

- Therapy with **dexamethasone,** 10 mg IV or PO, should be initiated to decrease cerebral edema and should be continued at a dosage of 4 to 6 mg PO every 6 hours throughout the course of **radiation therapy,** or longer if symptoms related to edema persist.
- Subsequent therapy depends on the number and location of the brain lesions as well as the prognosis of the underlying cancer.
- Patients with a chemotherapy-responsive neoplasm and a solitary accessible lesion should be considered for surgical resection.
- **All patients who have not received prior radiation therapy should be given whole-brain radiation therapy.**
- **Meningeal carcinomatosis** should be suspected in a cancer patient with headache or cranial neuropathies.
  - ○ This pattern of spread is most often seen with lung cancer, breast cancer, melanoma, or lymphoma.
  - ○ The diagnosis is confirmed by cytology of the CSF.
  - ○ A CT scan of the head should be performed to rule out parenchymal metastases or hydrocephalus before a lumbar puncture is performed.
  - ○ Local radiation therapy or IT chemotherapy may provide temporary relief of symptoms.

Spinal Cord Compression
- Spinal cord compression is most commonly caused by hematogenous spread of cancer to the vertebral bodies followed by expansion into the spinal canal or ischemia of the spinal cord.
- The most common malignancies causing spinal cord compression are breast, lung, and prostate cancer, but the diagnosis should be considered in any patient with cancer who complains of back pain.
- **Magnetic resonance imaging** is the imaging modality of choice to assess for acute cord compression.
- **Treatment involves urgent neurosurgical and radiation oncology consultation in addition to high-dose corticosteroid therapy.**

Superior Vena Cava Obstruction
- Most commonly caused by cancers that arise in or spread to the mediastinum, such as lymphoma or lung cancer.
- The compressed superior vena cava leads to swelling of the face or trunk, chest pain, cough, and shortness of breath. A mediastinal mass may compromise the airway.
- Dilated superficial veins of the chest, neck, or sublingual area suggest an engorged collateral circulation.
- The presence of a mass on chest radiograph or CT scans usually confirms the diagnosis.
- If the histologic origin of the obstruction is unknown, tissue can be obtained for diagnosis via bronchoscopy or mediastinoscopy.
- Therapy is directed at the underlying disease.
- Neoplasms that are not responsive to chemotherapy are treated with **radiation therapy.**[15]

Malignant Pericardial Effusions
- Most malignant pericardial effusions result from cancer of the breast or lung.
- Initial presentations range from dyspnea to acute cardiovascular collapse due to cardiac tamponade requiring emergency pericardiocentesis.
- After cardiovascular stabilization, some patients may improve with treatment if the tumor is chemotherapy sensitive.
- When the pericardial effusion is a complication of uncontrolled disease, palliation can be achieved by **pericardiocentesis** with sclerosis.
- Subxiphoid **pericardiotomy** can be performed in patients whose effusions do not respond to other treatment.

Malignant Pleural Effusions
• Malignant pleural effusions develop as a result of pleural invasion by tumor or obstruction of lymphatic drainage.
• When systemic control is impossible and reaccumulation of fluid occurs rapidly after drainage, removal of the fluid followed by instillation of a **sclerosing agent** into the pleural space is recommended.
• Resistant effusions can be controlled with **pleurectomy** or placement of an **indwelling pleural catheter**, which can be used to drain pleural fluid as needed.

Malignant Ascites
• Most commonly caused by peritoneal carcinomatosis and best controlled by systemic chemotherapy.
• Therapeutic paracenteses can provide symptomatic relief.
• Intraperitoneal instillation of chemotherapy has been used but is not routinely recommended.

Bone Metastases
• Bone metastases can result in spontaneous (pathologic) fractures.
• Prophylactic surgical pinning and radiation therapy may be indicated.
• Bone modifying agents (e.g., zoledronic acid, pamidronate, and denosumab) can also protect against skeletal-related events.

Paraneoplastic Syndromes
• Are complications of malignancy not directly caused by a tumor mass effect and are presumed to be mediated by either secreted tumor products or the development of autoantibodies.
• Paraneoplastic syndromes can affect virtually every organ system, and, in most cases, successful treatment of the underlying malignancy eliminates these effects.
• **Metabolic complications**
  ○ **Hypercalcemia** is the most common metabolic complication in malignancy and can cause mental status changes, gastrointestinal (GI) discomfort, arrhythmias, and constipation.
  ○ The **syndrome of inappropriate antidiuretic hormone** (SIADH) should be considered in a euvolemic cancer patient with unexplained hyponatremia. Although a variety of neoplasms have been described in association with SIADH, SCLC is most often responsible.
  ○ **Cancer-related anorexia and cachexia** (CRCA):
    ▪ A clinical syndrome of anorexia, distortion of taste perception, and loss of muscle mass.
    ▪ The asthenic appearance of patients is more often related to tumor type than to tumor burden.
    ▪ Mirtazapine 15 to 30 mg PO daily has been used as an appetite stimulant and is a promising agent in CRCA treatments.[16] Other appetite stimulants include corticosteroids, cannabinoids, and promotility agents such as metoclopramide.
• **Neuromuscular complications**
  ○ **Dermatomyositis**, more often than polymyositis, has been associated with a variety of malignancies, including NSCLC and colon, ovarian, and prostate cancers.
    ▪ Successful treatment of the underlying malignancy may result in resolution of the symptoms.
    ▪ In a patient with no known malignancy, an exhaustive search for a malignancy is not recommended because a primary malignancy is found in <20% of patients.[17]
  ○ **Lambert-Eaton myasthenic syndrome** is characterized by proximal muscle weakness, decreased or absent deep tendon reflexes, and autonomic dysfunction.

- Electromyography using high-frequency nerve stimulation may show posttetanic potentiation.
- **SCLC** is most often associated with this syndrome, and effective chemotherapy may result in improvement.
- Worsening symptoms have been reported with the use of calcium channel antagonists; these agents are contraindicated in this syndrome.[18]

- **Hematologic complications**
  - Although cytopenias occur more often as a complication of treatment or marrow involvement with cancer, elevated blood counts may be explained by paraneoplastic syndromes.
  - **Erythrocytosis** is a rare complication of hepatoma, renal cell cancer, and benign tumors of the kidney, uterus, and cerebellum. Debulking the tumor with surgery or radiation therapy generally results in resolution of the erythrocytosis. Occasionally, therapeutic phlebotomy is indicated.
  - **Granulocytosis** (leukemoid reaction) in the absence of infection is seen with cancers of the stomach, lung, pancreas, and brain, as well as lymphoma. Because the neutrophils are mature and seldom exceed $100,000/mm^3$, complications are rare and intervention is generally unnecessary.
  - **Thrombocytosis** in patients with cancer may be caused by splenectomy, iron deficiency, acute hemorrhage, or inflammation; treatment is usually not necessary.

- **Thromboembolic complications**
  - Mucin-secreting adenocarcinomas of the GI tract and lung cancer have been associated with a **hypercoagulable state**, resulting in recurrent venous and arterial thromboembolism.
  - Nonbacterial **thrombotic (marantic) endocarditis**, usually involving the mitral valve, may also occur.
  - Heparin anticoagulation or low molecular weight heparin should be instituted, as well as treatment of the underlying cancer.[19]

- **Glomerular injury**
  - Glomerular injury has been observed as a paraneoplastic syndrome.
  - **Minimal change disease** is often associated with lymphoma, especially Hodgkin disease.
  - **Membranous glomerulonephritis** is more often seen with solid tumors.
  - The process can be reversed with treatment of the underlying cancer.

- **Clubbing and hypertrophic osteoarthropathy**
  - This includes polyarthritis and periostitis of long bones.
  - Most often observed in NSCLC but also seen with lesions that are metastatic to the mediastinum.
  - Some improvement in the osteoarthropathy can be achieved with nonsteroidal anti-inflammatory drugs (NSAIDs), but definitive therapy requires treatment of the underlying malignancy.

- **Fever**
  - Fever may accompany lymphoma, renal cell cancer, and hepatic metastasis.
  - Once an infectious etiology for the fever has been excluded, NSAIDs (e.g., ibuprofen, 400 mg PO every 6 hours, or indomethacin, 25 to 50 mg PO tid) may provide symptomatic relief.

Complications Related to Treatment

Cancer treatments can cause serious or life-threatening toxicity. The most common and predictable toxicities are to the rapidly proliferating cells of hematopoietic and mucosal tissue. Because repair of these tissues cannot be accelerated, palliation during the healing process is the primary goal.

Complications of Radiation Therapy
- Toxicity is related to the location of the therapy, total dose delivered, and rates of delivery. Large-dose fractions of radiation are associated with greater toxicity to the normal tissues encompassed in the radiation field.
- **Acute toxicity**
  - Develops within the first 3 months of therapy and is characterized by an inflammatory reaction in the tissue receiving radiation.
  - Such toxicity may respond to anti-inflammatory agents such as glucocorticoids.
  - Local irritations or burns in the treatment field generally resolve with time.
  - Close observation and treatment of any infections and palliation of symptoms, such as pain, dysphagia, dysuria, or diarrhea (depending on the site of treatment) are the mainstays of supportive care until healing has occurred.
- **Subacute and chronic toxicity**
  - Tends to be less amenable to therapy, as fibrosis and scarring are present.
  - Daily amifostine before head and neck radiation therapy decreases the incidence of xerostomia.[20]

Tumor Lysis Syndrome
- Tumor lysis syndrome occurs in patients with rapidly proliferating neoplasms that are highly sensitive to chemotherapy.
- Rapid tumor cell death releases intracellular contents and causes **hyperkalemia, hyperphosphatemia, and hyperuricemia.**
- Although reported in the treatment of a variety of malignancies, it is usually associated with **high-grade non-Hodgkin lymphoma and acute leukemia**.
- The diagnosis of tumor lysis syndrome is based on susceptibility, clinical suspicion, and close monitoring of laboratory data in patients at risk. Rapidly progressive hyperkalemia, hyperphosphatemia, and hyperuricemia as well as acutely worsening renal failure are the hallmarks.
- **Prophylaxis and pretreatment** are paramount in preventing tumor lysis syndrome.
- During induction chemotherapy, prophylactic measures typically include the following:
  - **Allopurinol,** 300 to 600 mg PO daily, and aggressive IV volume expansion (e.g., 3,000 mL/m^2/day).
  - The addition of **sodium bicarbonate,** 50 mEq/1,000 mL IV fluid, to alkalinize the urine may prevent uric acid nephropathy and acute renal failure, but should be avoided in hyperphosphatemia.
- **Rasburicase** is a recombinant urate oxidase enzyme that catalyzes the oxidation of uric acid into allantoin, a soluble metabolite. It can be used prophylactically or in the treatment of hyperuricemia.
- Despite these preventive measures, hemodialysis may be needed for hyperkalemia, hyperphosphatemia, acute renal failure, or fluid overload.

Hematologic Complications
- **Myelosuppression and febrile neutropenia**
  - A febrile neutropenic patient **should be presumed to be infected and must be evaluated and treated promptly in an inpatient setting.**
  - The risk of infection increases dramatically with neutropenia (defined as an absolute neutrophil count of <500/mm^3) and is directly related to the duration of the neutropenia.
  - Fever is defined as a single core temperature reading of >38.3°C orally or two readings of >38.0°C spanning 1 hour.
  - Other clinical signs of infection must be considered because the inflammatory response may be muted in the absence of neutrophils.

○ **Growth factors for myelosuppression**
- Growth factors include many cytokines that may ameliorate the myelosuppression associated with cytotoxic chemotherapy. They act on hematopoietic cells, stimulating proliferation, differentiation, commitment, and some functional activation.
- Because they can increase myelosuppression, they **should not be given within 24 hours of chemotherapy or radiation**.
- Filgrastim (**G-CSF**, given at an initial dose of 5 μg/kg SC/day or IV), and **pegfilgrastim** (a pegylated form of G-CSF 6 mg single dose), **beginning the day after the last dose of cytotoxic chemotherapy**, may reduce the incidence of febrile neutropenic events. Blood counts should be monitored twice a week during therapy. Bone pain is a common toxicity that can be managed with nonopiate analgesics.
- **Sargramostim** (**GM-CSF**) given subcutaneously at a dose of 250 μg/m^2/day beginning the day after the last dose of cytotoxic chemotherapy, shortens the period of neutropenia after stem cell transplant.

• **Anemia**
○ Anemia is a common side effect of multiple chemotherapeutic agents. Symptoms include fatigue, dyspnea, or lethargy.
○ RBC transfusions are indicated for patients who have symptoms of anemia, active bleeding, or a hemoglobin concentration below 7 to 8 g/dL. Because of anecdotal reports of graft versus host disease (GVHD) associated with transfusions, radiation of all blood products is generally recommended for immunosuppressed marrow transplant patients.
○ Recombinant **erythropoietin** (epoetin alfa) given at a starting dose of 150 U/kg SC three times a week or 40,000 U SC weekly has been shown to improve anemia and decrease transfusion requirements in cancer patients, particularly those in whom the anemia is predominantly caused by cytotoxic chemotherapy.[21]
○ **Darbepoetin alfa** is a recombinant erythropoietin with a longer half-life. It is started at 500 μg SC every 3 weeks.
○ Erythropoiesis-stimulating agents (ESA) such as epoetin and darbepoetin can only be administered with patient consent under a Risk Evaluation Mitigation Strategy (REMS) program. Hematocrit should be monitored weekly during therapy, and the dosage should be adjusted accordingly. ESAs should be discontinued when the chemotherapy is complete and the anemia has resolved. They should not be used when the patient is undergoing potentially curative therapy.

• **Thrombocytopenia**
○ Thrombocytopenia is another common side effect of chemotherapeutic agents toxic to the bone marrow. Symptoms include easy bruising and bleeding (e.g., epistaxis and gingival bleeding).
○ Thrombocytopenia <10,000/mm^3 which is the result of chemotherapy should be treated with platelet transfusions to minimize the risk of spontaneous hemorrhage.
○ Interleukin-11 was approved to reduce the duration and severity of thrombocytopenia after chemotherapy. However, limited efficacy and significant toxicity (fluid retention and atrial arrhythmias) have limited its use.
○ When prolonged thrombocytopenia is anticipated, histocompatibility testing should be performed before therapy so that HLA-matched single-donor platelets can be provided when alloimmunization makes the patient refractory to random-donor platelets.

Gastrointestinal Complications
• **Stomatitis**
○ The severity of stomatitis ranges from mild (oral discomfort) to severe (ulceration, impaired oral intake, and hemorrhage). Toxicity is more severe with simultaneous radiation therapy.
○ It is often the dose-limiting toxicity of methotrexate and 5-FU but can be an unpleasant consequence of many chemotherapeutic agents.

○ Healing generally occurs within 7 to 10 days of the development of symptoms.

○ For mild cases of stomatitis, oral rinses (chlorhexidine, 15 to 30 mL swish and spit tid, or a combination of equal parts diphenhydramine elixir, saline, and 3% hydrogen peroxide) may provide relief. Polyvinylpyrrolidone-sodium hyaluronate gel can also be used.

○ Palifermin, a keratinocyte growth factor analog, has been approved for use in chemotherapy-induced stomatitis.[22]

○ In severe cases, IV morphine is appropriate and IV fluids can be used to supplement oral intake as needed.

○ Patients with moderate or severe stomatitis may develop aspiration. Precautions should include elevation of the head of the bed and availability of a handheld suction apparatus.

○ In severe or prolonged episodes, superinfection with Candida or herpes simplex is possible and requires appropriate diagnosis and antimicrobial intervention.

• **Diarrhea**

○ In this context, diarrhea is the result of cytotoxicity to proliferating cells of the intestinal mucosa.

○ The use of oral opioid agents as antidiarrheals is commonly limited by abdominal cramping.

○ Severe diarrhea associated with 5-FU and LV may respond to octreotide, 150 to 500 µg SC tid.

○ Diarrhea, sometimes severe, is a common side effect of irinotecan and can be treated with loperamide, 4 mg PO, and then 2 mg every 2 hours while awake and 4 mg every 4 hours during the night.

○ In some cases, IV fluids are necessary to avoid intravascular volume depletion.

• **Nausea and vomiting**

○ Nausea and vomiting occur with varying degrees and frequency. The focus is on prevention.

○ Chemotherapy regimens are classified by emetic risk: high (>90%), moderate (30% to 90%), low (10% to 30%), and minimal (<10%) with recommendations for emesis prophylaxis dependent on level of risk. Suggestions for breakthrough antiemetic agent(s) are listed in Table 35-3.

TABLE 35-3 | **Recommendations for Breakthrough Antiemetic Therapy**

Phenothiazines
Prochlorperazine
Promethazine

Serotonin 5-HT$_3$ receptor antagonists
Granisetron
Ondansetron
Dolasetron

Benzodiazepines
Lorazepam

Steroids
Dexamethasone

Other
Haloperidol
Metoclopramide
Olanzapine
Scopolamine

Adapted from NCCN Guidelines® Version 1.2013 Antiemesis.

Other Specific Complications
- **Interstitial pneumonitis** may develop as a dose-related, cumulative toxicity, or as an idiosyncratic reaction.
  - The implicated agent should be discontinued.
  - The institution of glucocorticoids (e.g., prednisone, 1 mg/kg PO daily or equivalent) may be of some benefit. The long-term outcome, however, is unpredictable.
- **Hemorrhagic cystitis** may develop with either **cyclophosphamide or ifosfamide.**
  - Hemorrhagic cystitis is best anticipated and treated with prophylactic **mesna**.
  - Treatment consists of continuous bladder irrigation with isotonic saline and should continue until the hematuria resolves.

REFERENCES

1. Goldhirsch A, Glick JH, Gelber RD, et al. Meeting highlights: International Consensus Panel on the Treatment of Primary Breast Cancer. *J Natl Cancer Inst* 1998;90:1601–1688.
2. Piccart-Gebhart MJ, Procter M, Leyland-Jones B, et al. Trastuzumab after adjuvant chemotherapy in HER2-positive breast cancer. *N Engl J Med* 2005;353:1659–1672.
3. Slamon DJ, Leyland-Jones B, Shak S, et al. Use of chemotherapy plus a monoclonal antibody against HER2 for metastatic breast cancer that overexpresses HER2. *N Engl J Med* 2001;344:783–792.
4. Rosen LS, Gordon D, Kaminski M. Zoledronic acid versus pamidronate in the treatment of skeletal metastases in patients with breast cancer or osteolytic lesions of multiple myeloma: a phase III, double-blind, comparative trial. *Cancer J* 2001;7:377–387.
5. Auperin A, Arriagada R, Pignon JP, et al. Prophylactic cranial irradiation for patients with small-cell lung cancer in complete remission. Prophylactic Cranial Irradiation Overview Collaborative Group. *N Engl J Med* 1999;341:476–484.
6. Walsh TN, Noonan N, Hollywood D, et al. A comparison of multimodal therapy and surgery for esophageal adenocarcinoma. *N Engl J Med* 1996;335:462-467.
7. Macdonald JS, Smalley SR, Benedetti J, et al. Chemoradiotherapy after surgery compared with surgery alone for adenocarcinoma of the stomach or gastroesophageal junction. *N Engl J Med* 2001;345:725–730.
8. Fong Y, Cohen AM, Fortner JG, et al. Liver resection for colorectal metastases. *J Clin Oncol* 1997;15:938–946.
9. Martenson JA, Lipsitz SR, Lefkopoulou M, et al. Results of combined modality therapy for patients with anal cancer (E7283). *Cancer* 1995;76:1731–1736.
10. Kelly WK, Slovin S, Scher HI. Steroid hormone withdrawal syndromes. Pathophysiology and clinical significance. *Urol Clin North Am* 1997;24:421–431.
11. Einhorn LH. Treatment of testicular cancer: a new and improved model. *J Clin Oncol* 1990;8:1777–1781.
12. Keys HM, Bundy BN, Stehman FB. Cisplatin, radiation, and adjuvant hysterectomy compared with radiation and adjuvant hysterectomy for bulky stage IB cervical carcinoma. *N Engl J Med* 1999;340:1154–1161.
13. Calais G, Alfonsi M, Bardet E, et al. Randomized trial of radiation therapy versus concomitant chemotherapy and radiation therapy for advanced-stage oropharynx carcinoma. *J Natl Cancer Inst* 1999;91:2081–2086.
14. Gill PS, Wernz J, Scadden DT, et al. Randomized phase III trial of liposomal daunorubicin versus doxorubicin, bleomycin, and vincristine in AIDS-related Kaposi's sarcoma. *J Clin Oncol* 1996;14:2353–2364.
15. Ahmann FR. A reassessment of the clinical implications of the superior vena caval syndrome. *J Clin Oncol* 1984;2:961–969.

16. Riechelmann RP, Burman D, Tannock I, et al. Phase II trial of mirtazapine for cancer-related cachexia and anorexia. *Am J Hosp Palliat Care* 2010;27:106–110.
17. Sigurgeirsson B, Lindelof B, Edhag O, et al. Risk of cancer in patients with dermatomyositis or polymyositis. A population-based study. *N Engl J Med* 1992;326:363–367.
18. McEvoy KM, Windebank AJ, Daube JR, et al. 3,4-Diaminopyridine in the treatment of Lambert–Eaton myasthenic syndrome. *N Engl J Med* 1989;321:1567–1571.
19. Gould MK, Dembitzer AD, Doyle RL. Low-molecular-weight heparins compared with unfractionated heparin for treatment of acute deep venous thrombosis. A meta-analysis of randomized, controlled trials. *Ann Intern Med* 1999;130:800–809.
20. Kemp G, Rose P, Lurain J, et al. Amifostine pretreatment for protection against cyclophosphamide-induced and cisplatin-induced toxicities: results of a randomized control trial in patients with advanced ovarian cancer. *J Clin Oncol* 1996;14:2101–2112.
21. Crawford J. Recombinant human erythropoietin in cancer-related anemia. Review of clinical evidence. *Oncology (Williston Park)* 2002;16(9 suppl 10):41–53.
22. Hueber AJ, Leipe J, Roesler W. Palifermin as treatment in dose-intense conventional polychemotherapy induced mucositis. *Haematologica* 2006;91(8 suppl):ECR32.

36 Palliative Care and Hospice Medicine

Jonathan Byrd and Maria C. Dans

GENERAL PRINCIPLES

Over the course of the past century, how and where Americans die has changed greatly. Advancements in public health have led to increased life expectancy; some diseases, once rapidly fatal, have now become chronic illnesses. Although our ability to treat many diseases has improved, this evolution has created a new set of problems for patients, their families, and health care providers. The process of dying has lengthened, and in many cases, it has moved from homes to health care facilities. The palliative care and hospice movements arose in attempt to address these new challenges and to use the advancements of modern medicine to relieve suffering and to enhance quality of life.

Definition

- The World Health Organization defines palliative care as "the active total care of patients... Control of pain, of other symptoms, and of psychological, social, and spiritual problems...[in order to provide]...the best quality of life for patients and their families."[1]
- The National Consensus Project for Quality Palliative Care has broadened the definition:
  ○ The goal of palliative care is to prevent and relieve suffering and to support the best possible quality of life for patients and their families, regardless of the stage of the disease or the need for other therapies.
  ○ Palliative care is both a philosophy of care and an organized, highly structured system for delivering care.
  ○ Palliative care expands traditional disease-model medical treatments to include the goals of enhancing quality of life for patient and family, optimizing function, helping with decision making, and providing opportunities for personal growth.[2]
- Hospice is a specific type of palliative care designed for terminally ill patients who have a life expectancy of <6 months. Hospice agencies provide team-based services to patient, family, and caregivers in the home or an institution.

Epidemiology

- Over the past century, the most common causes of death in the United States have undergone a shift toward chronicity (e.g., congestive heart disease vs. acute myocardial infarction and chronic obstructive pulmonary disease vs. pneumonia).[3,4]
- As the technologic aspects of medicine have advanced, dying has been viewed more as a failure of therapy and less as a natural part of human existence. Diagnosis and cure may be considered more important targets of therapy than the relief of symptomatic distress and suffering.
- More people are very debilitated during the time before their death; increasingly, the care they need is provided not at home, but in institutions (Table 36-1).[5]
- Hospice use has been increasing: in 2010, 41.9% of Americans died while receiving hospice care compared to 11% in 1995. Hospice care, however, is still invoked late in the course of terminal illness—median length of hospice treatment was 20 days in 2010, with approximately 35.3% of people dying within 7 days of initiation of hospice care.[6]

TABLE 36-1	Percentage of Deaths by Location in the United States[a]

Location of death	Percentage
Hospital	57% (16% of these in emergency departments)
Residence	20%
Nursing home	17%
Other	6% (including those dead on arrival to hospital)

[a]Based on 1992 U.S. Vital Statistic Data published by the Institute of Medicine in 1997.
Data from Committee on Care at the End of Life, Institute of Medicine; Field MJ, et al., eds. *Approaching Death: Improving Care at the End of Life*. Washington, DC: National Academy Press; 1997.

- There has been a dramatic increase in medical care cost, especially at the end of life.
  - The cost of care provided during the last 6 months of life continues to be estimated at 10% of the total cost of health care.[7]
  - Much of this care is subsidized by the federal government. Medicare and Medicaid were not designed for care of the dying but provide approximately 50% of the funding.[8]
  - The rest of the financial burden falls mainly upon patients and their families, with up to 30% of families impoverished by a family member's death.[9]
- The modern hospice movement, and, subsequently, the specialty of palliative care developed as an attempt to improve care for dying patients and their families.
  - Saint Christopher's Hospice opened in London, UK, in 1967, and the first inpatient hospices were introduced in North America in the 1970s.
  - The Omnibus Budget Act of 1983 created the Medicare Hospice Benefit. It changed the delivery of hospice care in the United States by emphasizing care at home rather than at inpatient facilities.
  - The subspecialty of palliative care grew out of the modern hospice movement in the 1980s to address the needs of people with serious illness who might still be pursuing curative treatment. In 2006, the American Board of Medical Specialties approved the creation of Hospice and Palliative Medicine as an official subspecialty of 10 participating specialty boards (Anesthesiology, Emergency Medicine, Family Medicine, Internal Medicine, Pediatrics, Physical Medicine and Rehabilitation, Psychiatry and Neurology, Radiology, Surgery, and Obstetrics and Gynecology). Also in 2006, the Accreditation Council for Graduate Medical Education (ACGME) began the process of establishing standards for the creation of ACGME-accredited fellowships in Hospice and Palliative Medicine.

DIAGNOSIS

Palliative care and hospice services involve a multidisciplinary approach to address patient suffering.

Indications for Palliative and Hospice Care

While palliative care consults may be considered at any point during the course of a person's disease, national guidelines have been established to assist providers with determining **when to consider hospice** for specific life-limiting noncancer conditions.[10] These are detailed in Table 36-2.

Appropriate Timing

- Appropriate timing for palliative care and hospice interventions is presented in Figure 36-1.

TABLE 36-2 Possible Indications for Hospice Care

COPD:
- Oxygen dependent or unresponsive to bronchodilators
- Poor exercise capacity
- Unintentional weight loss
- Resting tachycardia
- Multiple acute care admissions per year

Cirrhosis/liver failure:
Mostly bed-bound with at least one of multiple comorbidities:
- Recurrent variceal bleeding
- Encephalopathy
- Refractory ascites
- Hepatorenal syndrome
- History of spontaneous bacterial peritonitis

Dementia:
- Bed-bound and unable to communicate verbally or ambulate without assistance.
- Progressive weight loss
- Fecal or urinary incontinence
- Presence of recurrent medical complications such as infections, dysphagia, or weight loss that require frequent acute care admissions

Congestive heart failure:
- NYHA Class IV failure
- Ejection fraction <20%
- Treatment optimized but still multiple acute care admissions per year

Renal failure:
- Chronic renal failure with creatinine >8.0 mg/dL, off dialysis

Acute phase of strokes/coma:
- Coma or persistent vegetative state secondary to stroke beyond 3 days' duration.
- Coma with any four of the following on day 3 of coma:
  ○ Abnormal brain stem response
  ○ Absent verbal response
  ○ Absent withdrawal response to pain
  ○ Serum creatinine >1.5 mg/dL
  ○ Age >70

Chronic phase of stroke/coma:
- Clear-cut predictors are not well established but may include the following:
- Poor functional or nutritional status
- Weight loss
- Significant dementia
- Serum albumin <2.5 mg/dL
- Recurrent medical complications requiring frequent acute care admissions.

NYHA, New York Heart Association. Data from Medical guidelines for determining prognosis in selected non-cancer diseases. *Hosp J* 1996;11:47–63.

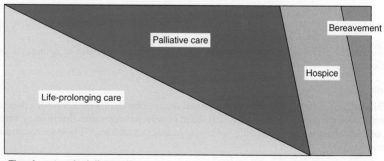

Figure 36-1 **Palliative and hospice care in the course of illness.** (Adapted from National Consensus Guidelines for Quality Palliative Care, 2002 and Stanford University Faculty Development Center End-of-Life Curriculum.)

- **Palliative care does not exclude the continuation of life-prolonging treatment** but rather complements curative therapy by helping clarify goals of care and improving symptomatic control.
- Based on Medicare guidelines, hospice eligibility requires a terminal diagnosis and a life expectancy of <6 months. Patients who live beyond 6 months must be reevaluated by their hospice agency, but may continue in hospice care as long as the conditions of their initial enrollment remain true.

Venues for Palliative and Hospice Interventions

- Palliative care and hospice care may be provided in either inpatient or outpatient settings.
- In the outpatient setting, palliative care may be performed:
  - By the primary care provider or treating specialists
  - In a palliative care subspecialty clinic by a board-certified palliative care provider and a multidisciplinary group that may involve social workers, chaplains, nurses, and therapists
- Outpatient hospice care can be arranged by a physician by contacting a local hospice organization that serves the patient's residential area. **Admission to hospice does not require a do not resuscitate order** and can be concurrent to other therapies.

Goal of Palliative Care

The goal of palliative care is to use the strengths of a multidisciplinary team to improve quality of life for both patient and family in the remaining time a patient has. Specific aims include the following:

- Clarifying patient, family, and care team goals, preferences, and choices
- Providing holistic care of patient and family
- Providing aggressive control of bothersome symptoms

TREATMENT

The principles of palliative care can assist in the following:

- Addressing bothersome symptoms such as pain, nausea, and dyspnea
- Sharing bad news
- Clarifying patient, family, and healthcare provider goals
- Identifying additional stakeholders
- Facilitating discussions to align the goals of care with the treatment plan

Assessing the Experience of the Suffering Patient

- Traditional medical practice views symptoms and signs as evidence of disease. This evidence should disappear once the appropriate diagnosis is made and therapeutic measures initiated.
- The palliative care approach complements traditional models by emphasizing that symptoms themselves are appropriate targets for therapy. It uses the clues that the disease process provides to understand and treat the symptoms.
- Symptoms have both physical and psychological components.
  - **Physical aspects** may be local (what is causing pain) or central (how pain is processed) components.
  - **Psychological components** include affective (how an illness is emotionally experienced), cognitive (what patients understand about their illness), and spiritual (how symptoms are organized by patients into a framework that allows them to understand their illness).

Steps to Sharing Bad News

- Many physicians have minimal formal training in sharing bad news during their preclinical years and few watch more experienced physicians model such conversations during their clinical rotations.[11]
- Discussions of bad news frequently involve raw emotion. They are difficult even under the best of circumstances and can be both personally and professionally challenging. Done skillfully, however, they can help patients, families, and health care providers move through difficult situations in a productive manner.
- Traditionally, effective communication has been viewed as something that physicians-in-training absorb through experience as a function of natural aptitude and not as a set of teachable skills. More recently, authors have emphasized that, regardless of affinity, there are several key steps to facilitating conversations about bad news.[12]
  - **Preparation** is extremely important and includes the following:
    - Understanding the medical condition and implications of available therapies and preparing resources if barriers exist.
    - Arranging an in-person meeting (if possible) to share the news, along with having a support person available.
    - Finding a quiet place and adequate time to sit and talk with minimal distractions. Turning pagers/cell phones to vibrate and instructing support staff not to interrupt, or when possible, including support staff who have a relationship with the patient may be helpful.
  - Next, **making a connection** with the person hearing the news is important. This begins with introductions of all parties involved, followed by an assessment of their immediate needs, comfort, and their understanding of the situation.
  - **Sharing the news** involves speaking slowly using clear and unambiguous language, prefacing the news with a statement, such as "I unfortunately have some bad news," and giving the news briefly.
  - After delivering the news, **assessment of the reaction is key**. A direct question about what the patient or family is thinking may prompt useful dialogue. Respond with brief, simple answers, and recognize that the emotional impact of the bad news may restrict the quantity of information that can be delivered. Follow-up is essential. If the recipient of the bad news is alone, ask whether someone should be called to provide additional support.
  - Finally, **transition to follow-up** by establishing a concrete plan for a future meeting to address additional questions. If a referral is necessary, identify whom that provider will be and how he or she will be contacted. Close the meeting with a **statement of concern and commitment to help**.
- It may be helpful after difficult discussions to debrief with other members of the health care team—pay attention to your feelings and needs as the provider who shares the bad news.

Goals of Care Discussions

Once the initial shock of bad news has subsided, it is important to establish clear goals for care in order to develop a rational therapeutic plan. One algorithm for addressing goals of care discussions is the GOOD acronym, developed as part of the Stanford End of Life Curriculum.[13]

Goals

- Before the discussion begins, it is essential to identify the stakeholders and assess their understanding of the current situation. The patient and his/her family are obvious stakeholders, but there are frequently many other people as well, including health care providers or members of the community.
- "Big picture goals" about the "who, what, when, and where" of living should be identified first because they provide the context. In addition, most "big picture" goals reveal underlying values that must be understood before moving onto specific aims.

Options
- Next, specific options are discussed by listing them and then narrowing them down by the requests of the involved stakeholders.
- Providers have an important role in discussing the benefits and burdens of the options available.
- Providers can help stakeholders understand the possible outcomes associated with available options.
- Values of the stakeholders are important because they help assign the relative importance of each outcome state.

Opinions
- Offer your opinion in a neutral manner, incorporating earlier data elucidated about patient and family views, clinician goals, benefits and burdens of care, probabilities of outcomes, and the values of the stakeholders involved.
- Many patients are interested to know what their caregivers' opinions are and, in fact, appreciate information provided along with a recommendation.

Document
- Finally, write a note that includes key information from the meeting including the names and relationships of the participants, decisions regarding the "big picture goals," the immediate care plan, and the care plan in the event of discussed scenarios.
- It is also helpful to include an assessment of the decision-making process, and whether it makes sense in light of the "big-picture goals."

Addressing End-of-Life Nutrition and Artificial Nutritional Support
- Many clinicians recommend for or against artificial nutrition on the basis of cultural or personal biases (e.g., fear of starving the patient) rather than medical evidence. A review of the published literature indicates the following:
  - Artificial nutrition can improve survival in acute catabolic states such as sepsis or in highly functional patients with advanced proximal gastrointestinal cancer, and in those with amyotrophic lateral sclerosis who desire nutrition.[14]
  - Tube feeding does not reduce the risk of aspiration pneumonia.[15,16]
  - Tube feeding does not prolong life in those with advanced cancer or dementia.[17]
  - Tube feeding may not improve quality of life and can decrease quality of life by depriving a patient of the pleasure of eating.[18]
  - Parenteral feeding carries risk of fluid overload, line infection, electrolyte imbalances, and hyperglycemia.
  - Most actively dying patients do not complain of hunger or thirst, though dry mouth is prevalent.[19]
  - Reduced appetite and weight loss are common in chronic disease.
- Knowing these facts and addressing a patient's nutritional preferences prior to the occurrence of cachexia or anorexia can reduce patient and family emotional stress and foster acceptance of the dying patient's altered eating habits.[20]
- It is important to differentiate between the provision of artificial nutrition and the acts of eating or feeding. Most people enjoy eating (even if only a few bites of their favorite food) and feeding a loved one who is sick can be a significant and pleasant nurturing activity for both patient and family.
- Appetite stimulants may be considered if prognosis is unclear and death not imminent.
  - Megestrol 400 to 800 mg/day, medroxyprogesterone 500 mg bid, or dexamethasone 2 to 4 mg bid have shown similar nonfluid weight gains but **have no effect on mortality and equivocal effects on quality of life.**[21]

- ○ Mirtazapine should be considered for concurrent cachexia and depression (common in end of life care) with one study showing an average weight gain of 3.9% body weight after 3 months of 30 mg/day; mirtazapine is not recommended in the absence of depression.[22,23]
- It is important to validate family members' concerns, especially in terms of their intent as those who love and care for the patient.
- Acknowledging the difficulty of the situation and the commitment of all concerned to the patient's well-being may help families make informed decisions regarding end of life nutritional preferences.

Assessing and Managing Nonpain Symptoms

Nausea and Vomiting
- Nausea and vomiting arise from the emetic center in the medulla, which receives input from, and is triggered by multiple sources including the following:
  - ○ Gastrointestinal tract (e.g., dysmotility, obstruction, or compression)
  - ○ Infection or inflammation (especially involving the gastrointestinal tract)
  - ○ Effects of medications that are sensed as toxins in the chemoreceptor trigger zone
  - ○ Vestibular instability
  - ○ Cognitive and affective components (e.g., environmental clues, underlying depression, or anxiety) that impact the cerebral cortex
- Understanding the origin of nausea can help to guide more specific and effective therapies based on relative receptor activity and drug targets (Table 36-3).[24]
- Though the mechanism is unclear, corticosteroids have good antiemetic properties. Steroids, marijuana/dronabinol, and the antidepressant mirtazapine through 5-HT$_3$ and 5-HT$_2$ blockade are used primarily in cancer and chemotherapy-related nausea (see Chapter 35).[25]
- If nausea or vomiting persists, an agent from a different class should be used rather than one with a similar mechanism of action to minimize side effects.

Dyspnea
- Dyspnea is the experience of shortness of breath. It is caused most commonly by a cardiac or pulmonary process, but it is also associated with debilitation, wasting syndrome, and progressive neurodegenerative diseases and can have a large affective component of panic and fear.

TABLE 36-3	Antiemetics for Specific Causes	
Cause of nausea	**Receptors involved**	**Useful drugs**
V Vestibular	H$_1$ histaminic M cholinergic	Scopolamine, promethazine
O Obstruction of the gastrointestinal tract	H$_1$ histaminic M cholinergic 5-HT$_3$ serotonergic	Senna products, dexamethasone, octreotide
M Dysmotility of the upper GI tract	H$_1$ histaminic M cholinergic	Metoclopramide
I Infection, inflammation	H$_1$ histaminic M cholinergic	Promethazine, prochlorperazine
T Toxins, such as opioids	D$_2$ dopaminergic 5-HT$_3$ serotonergic	Prochlorperazine, haloperidol, ondansetron

Modified from Hallenbeck J, Weissman D. Fast fact and concept #5: treatment of nausea and vomiting Center to Advance Palliative Care. www.capc.org. Last Accessed 1/12/15.

- Reversible causes including symptomatic pleural effusions, pneumonia, severe anemia, and ascites should be addressed with the patient's larger goals of care in mind.
- **Oxygen saturation, heart rate, arterial blood gases, and even respiratory rate can correlate poorly with the presence and severity of dyspnea.**
- **Opioids** are the best-studied medicines and current gold standard in the treatment of dyspnea with low-dose morphine (cumulative dose 10 to 30 mg/day) typically used.[26]
- Several studies have shown that opioid use for dyspnea when not increased too rapidly does not lead to respiratory depression, increased CO_2 retention, or early death.[27]
- Benzodiazepines are generally not helpful in relieving dyspnea, but may be used if there is a significant anxiety component related to the dyspnea.[28]
- Oxygen can also reduce dyspnea in those who are hypoxic but is no better than room air in patients without hypoxia.[29]
- Beneficial nonpharmacologic interventions including breathing training, gait aids, neuro-electrical muscle stimulation, and chest wall vibration were effective for relieving breathlessness while fan use, supportive music therapy, relaxation counseling, or psychotherapy were equivocal.[30]

Delirium
- Delirium involves acutely changing or fluctuating mental status. It is extremely common in terminally ill patients and is associated with agitated or hypoactive states.
- In elderly patients and patients with advanced cancer, **delirium is associated with worse survival and increased morbidity;** it should be treated aggressively to ensure patient comfort and safety.[31,32]
- Reversible causes should be identified and addressed promptly, including drug side effects, undertreated pain, urinary or bowel obstruction, and sensory deprivation (missing hearing aid, glasses, etc.).[32]
- Clinical guidelines suggest the following role of pharmacotherapy:
  ○ The initial focus should be to **reduce/discontinue any drug or intervention that is contributing to delirium** especially benzodiazepines, anticholinergics, and corticosteroids.
  ○ Secondary strategies include improving sleep hygiene through behavioral modifications (e.g., temporal clues such as turning TVs and lights off), reorientation, and if needed low-dose sedating antipsychotics at bedtime (haloperidol typically 0.5 to 1 mg PO, IM, or IV, chlorpromazine 10 to 25 mg PO or subcutaneously or olanzapine 5 mg PO).[33]

REFERRAL

Referral may be considered to other subspecialties, such as pain management (for invasive palliative anesthesia such as nerve or spinal blocks), radiation oncology (for palliative radiation therapy to improve pain), chaplaincy (for spiritual or existential distress), or psychiatry (for more complicated anxiety, depression, or associated psychosis).

MONITORING/FOLLOW-UP

A palliative care approach involves a multidisciplinary effort to support patients and families in clarifying and achieving their goals. This may involve frequent follow-up with various members of the team, including: nurses to facilitate patient care and coach families in new ways to nurture; physicians to develop and coordinate a medical plan for symptom control; social workers to provide grief counseling and address complex psychosocial issues; and chaplains to address spiritual aspects of end-of-life care.

ADDITIONAL RESOURCES

1. Growth House, run by the Inter-Institutional Collaborating Network on End-of-Life Care. http://www.growthhouse.org (last accessed 1/12/15).
2. Center to Advance Palliative Care. http://www.capc.org/ (last accessed 1/12/15).
3. The American Academy of Hospice and Palliative Medicine. http://www.aahpm.org (last accessed 1/12/15).
4. The National Hospice and Palliative Care Organization, including a search link for hospice and palliative care providers. http://www.nhpco.org (last accessed 1/12/15).

REFERENCES

1. Doyle DG, Hanks GWG, MacDonald N, eds. *Oxford Textbook of Palliative Medicine*, 2nd ed. Oxford, UK: Oxford University Press; 1998.
2. National Consensus Project for Quality Palliative Care. *Clinical Practice Guidelines for Quality Palliative Care*, 2nd ed. http://www.nationalconsensusproject.org. Last accessed 1/12/15.
3. Brim OG Jr, Friedman HE, Levine S, et al., eds. *The Dying Patient*. New York: Russell Sage Foundation; 1970.
4. Anderson RN. Deaths: leading causes for 1999. *Natl Vital Stat Rep* 2001;49:1–87.
5. Committee on Care at the End of Life, Institute of Medicine; Field MJ, et al., eds. *Approaching Death: Improving Care at the End of Life*. Washington, DC: National Academy Press; 1997.
6. NHPCO. *Facts and Figures: Hospice Care in America*. Alexandria, VA: National Hospice and Palliative Care Organization; 2012.
7. Cohen SB, Carlson BL, Potter DEB. Health care expenditures in the last six months of life. *Health Policy Rev (Am Stat Assoc Sect Health Policy)* 1995;1:1–13.
8. Gornick M, Warren JL, Eggers PW, et al. Thirty years of Medicare: impact on the covered population. *Health Care Finan Rev* 1996;18:179–237.
9. Covinsky KE, Landefeld CS, Teno J, et al. Is economic hardship on the families of the seriously ill associated with patient and surrogate care preferences? *Arch Intern Med* 1996;156:1737–1741.
10. Medical guidelines for determining prognosis in selected non-cancer diseases. *Hosp J* 1996;11:47–63.
11. American Association of Medical Colleges. *The Increasing Need for End of Life and Palliative Care Education. Contemporary Issues in Medical Education*. Washington, DC: American Association of Medical Colleges; 1999.
12. Buckman R. *How to Break Bad News*. Baltimore, MD: Johns Hopkins University Press; 1992.
13. Hallenback J. *Palliative Care Perspectives*. Oxford, UK: Oxford University Press; 1993.
14. Gibson S, Wenig BL. Percutaneous endoscopic gastrostomy in the management of head and neck carcinoma. *Laryngoscope* 1992;102:977–980.
15. Nakajoh K, Nakagawa T, Sekizawa K, et al. Relation between incidence of pneumonia and protective reflexes in post-stroke patients with oral or tube feeding. *J Int Med* 2000;247:39–42.
16. Croghan J, Burke EM, Caplan S, et al. Pilot study of 12-month outcomes of nursing home patients with aspiration on videofluoroscopy. *Dysphagia* 1994;9:141–146.
17. Meier DE, Ahronheim JC, Morris J, et al. High short-term mortality in hospitalized patients with advanced dementia: lack of benefit of tube feeding. *Arch Intern Med* 2001;161:594–599.
18. Callahan CM, Haag KM, Weinberger M, et al. Outcomes of percutaneous endoscopic gastrostomy among older adults in a community setting. *J Am Geriatr Soc* 2000;48:1048–1054.

19. Conill C, Verger E, Henríquez I, et al. Symptom prevalence in the last week of life. *J Pain Symptom Manage* 1997;14:328–331.
20. McMahon MM, Hurley DL, Kamath PS, et al. Medical and ethical aspects of long-term enteral tube feeding. *Mayo Clin Proc* 2005;80:1461–1476.
21. Lopinzi CL, Kugler JW, Sloan JA, et al. Randomized comparison of megesterol acetate versus dexamethasone versus fluoxymesterone for the treatment of cancer anorexia/cachexia. *J Clin Oncol* 1999;17:3299–3306.
22. Segers K, Surquin M. Can mirtazapine counteract the weight loss associated with Alzheimer's disease? A retrospective open label study. *Alzheimer Dis Assoc Disord* 2014;28:291-3.
23. Fox CB, Treadway AK, Blaszczyk AT, et al. Megestrol acetate and mirtazapine for the treatment of unplanned weight loss in the elderly. *Pharmacotherapy* 2009;29:383–397.
24. Hallenbeck J, Weissman D. Fast fact and concept #5: treatment of nausea and vomiting Center to Advance Palliative Care. www.capc.org. Last Accessed 1/12/15.
25. Wood GJ, Shega JW, Lynch B, et al. Management of intractable nausea and vomiting in patients at the end of life. *JAMA* 2007;298:1196–1207.
26. Abernathy AP, Currow DC, Frith PA, et al. Randomised, double blind, placebo controlled crossover trial of sustained release morphine for the management of refractory dyspnea. *BMJ* 2003;327:523–528.
27. Jennings AL, Davies AN, Higgins JP, et al. Opioids for the palliation of breathlessness in terminal illness. *Cochrane Database Syst Rev* 2012;(7):CD002066.
28. Simon ST, Higginson IJ, Booth S, et al. Benzodiazepines for the relief of breathlessness in advanced malignant and non-malignant diseases in adults. *Cochrane Database Syst Rev* 2010;(1):CD007354.
29. Abernathy AP, McDonald CF, Frith PA, et al. Effect of palliative oxygen versus room air in relief of breathlessness in patients with refractory dyspnea: a double-blind, randomized controlled trial. *Lancet* 2010;376:784–793.
30. Bausewein C, Booth S, Gysels M, et al. Non-pharmocological interventions for breathlessness in advanced stages of malignant and nonmalignant diseases. *Cochrane Database Syst Rev* 2008;(2):CD005623.
31. Witlox J, Eurelings LS, de Jonghe JF, et al. Delirium in elderly patients and the risk of postdischarge mortality, institutionalization, and dementia: a meta-analysis. *JAMA* 2010;304:443–451.
32. Lawlor PG, Gagnon B, Manicini IL, et al. Occurrence, causes, outcomes of delirium in patients with advanced cancer: a prospective study. *Arch Intern Med* 2000;160:786–794.
33. National Comprehensive Cancer Network. Palliative Care: Delirium. NCCN Clinical practice guidelines in oncology. Version 2.2 013. http://www.nccn.org. Last accessed 1/12/15.

Pain Management

Nusayba Bagegni, Amy Sheldahl, and Maria C. Dans

GENERAL PRINCIPLES

- Pain is one of the most common complaints evaluated by physicians. It is the presenting symptom of myriad medical conditions. Some of these conditions are curable, but in many cases, the role of the physician is not to cure the disease but to control the pain associated with it.
- Historically, treatment of pain has been limited by fears of addiction and dependence as well as societal conventions on the role of pain in character development and the dying process. Pain therapy has evolved as physicians have come to view treatment of pain as an essential component of patient care—a task as important as treatment of the disease itself.
- This chapter will discuss the general principles of pain management. While many of these concepts have been developed for the treatment of chronic cancer pain, they can be applied to patients experiencing pain associated with many other disease processes.

Definition

The International Association for the Study of Pain (IASP) defines pain as "an unpleasant sensory and emotional experience, associated with actual or potential tissue damage, or described in terms of such damage."[1] **Pain is extremely subjective by nature,** so a more clinically accessible definition might be that pain is whatever the patient says it is.

Classification

- Classification of pain into subsets based on mechanism and time course can guide therapy. Pain in a given patient often falls into several of these categories; all relevant categories should be addressed for adequate treatment.
- **Acute pain**
  - Acute pain is associated with a recent, often reversible etiology.
  - Examples include joint injuries, postoperative pain, and pain associated with acute infection or trauma.
- **Chronic pain**
  - Chronic pain results from irreversible or not easily reversible etiologies.
  - Examples include pain due to malignancy, some forms of low back pain (LBP), and severe degenerative joint disease.
- **Nociceptive pain**
  - Nociceptive pain is classically associated with acute pain and injury. Tissue damage via mechanical, chemical, or thermal processes triggers activation of nociceptive pain fibers.
  - Pain may be described as sharp, gnawing, or aching. It is usually well localized and often worse with movement.
- **Neuropathic pain**
  - Neuropathic pain (also referred to as neurogenic pain) is due to nerve injury in the central or peripheral nervous system. All pain is modulated by central pain processing pathways; in neuropathic pain, there is frequently an abnormality caused by tissue damage or disease in the processing pathways that contributes to the ongoing pain.
  - Pain may be described as burning or stinging and may be accompanied by numbness, tingling, allodynia (pain in response to a stimulus, i.e., normally innocuous), or hyperalgesia (increased sensitivity to pain).

- **Visceral pain**
  - Visceral pain is due to stretching, crushing, or ischemia of organs supplied by visceral nerve fibers.
  - Pain may be described as squeezing, cramping, dull, or aching. It is frequently poorly localized; occasionally referred to a cutaneous dermatome supplied by the same nerve roots; and often associated with autonomic symptoms including nausea and vomiting.

Epidemiology
- LBP accounts for one-fifth of visits to medical clinics and is second only to upper respiratory illnesses as a symptom-related reason for a visit.[2,3]
- Up to 75% of patients with advanced cancer report being in pain.[4]
- Up to 50% of patients with cancer or their surrogates reported moderate to severe pain in last 3 days of life.[5]
- Pain is one of the most feared symptoms of cancer, and cancer-related pain is more likely to be poorly controlled in the elderly (age >70), minorities, and patients with a good functional status.[6,7]

Pathophysiology
- Painful stimuli activate nociceptors in the skin, joints, organs, and other tissues. Nerves transmit these signals to the central nervous system.
- Synaptic transmission and central pain processing pathways modulate the transmission of pain signals, and pain is ultimately experienced via the central nervous system.
- Pain may be due to injury at any level of the pain pathway, including tissue damage that stimulates nociceptors, injury to nerves that carry or modulate pain signals, and damage to central nervous system neurons involved in pain processing.

DIAGNOSIS

Clinical Presentation
- A thorough history is paramount for the accurate diagnosis and treatment of pain. A history should include information regarding the patient's pain as presented in Table 37-1.
- Pain severity is best assessed by patient self-report and may be aided by visual analogue scales, numerical rated scales, and/or verbal rated scales.[8]
- Physical examination can aid in diagnosing some causes of acute pain, such as joint injury or infection.
- The physician should also assess for signs of a source of chronic pain, such as cancer or neuropathy.
- All patients should be assessed for signs of hemodynamic instability, peritonitis, or other causes of acute pain, which require emergent evaluation for stabilization.
- Acute pain is typically accompanied by physical signs, such as tachycardia, diaphoresis, hypertension, and obvious physical discomfort. **Patients with chronic pain often have few physical signs of pain.**
- **Pain may exist without physical manifestations**.

Diagnostic Testing
- **No diagnostic test is available to provide objective assessment of pain**.
- Diagnostic testing is indicated when the history and physical examination point toward sources of pain, which may be amenable to curative treatment.
- Additional testing is sometimes indicated for pain that may require specialized interventions such as surgery, although a discussion of this topic is beyond the scope of this text.

TABLE 37-1	Pain History

- **Location**
- **Radiation**
- **Quality**
  - ○ Somatic
  - ○ Visceral
  - ○ Neuropathic
- **Longitudinal course**
  - ○ Acute
  - ○ Chronic
  - ○ Breakthrough
  - ○ Episodic
  - ○ Diurnal variation
- **Aggravating/alleviating factors**
  - ○ Prior therapies and their efficacies
  - ○ Specific triggering activities
  - ○ Positional component

- **Associated symptoms**
  - ○ Dyspnea
  - ○ Nausea/vomiting
  - ○ Diaphoresis
- **Psychological state**
  - ○ Spiritual distress
  - ○ History of mood disorder
  - ○ History of substance abuse
- **Impact of pain on the patient's daily functioning**
  - ○ Self-care
  - ○ Work
  - ○ Hobbies
- **Severity, multiple scales available**
  - ○ Numerical scale: 0–10
  - ○ Visual analogue scale
  - ○ FACES scale by Wong-Baker for patients with limited cognition

TREATMENT

- A thorough history, physical examination, and diagnostic tests as indicated should identify potentially curable causes of pain. If treatable causes of pain are discovered, pain control should be pursued along with curative therapy.
- When no curable cause of pain is found, therapy should proceed with a combination of nonpharmacologic treatments, medications, and possibly targeted procedures, if applicable.
- All interventions and therapies should be tailored to meet the needs of each patient. **Complete relief of pain may not be possible;** satisfactory control of pain, however, may allow participation in important activities or other specific goals of the patient.

Historical Perspective

- The **World Health Organization (WHO) pain ladder,** developed in 1982, was the result of a public health initiative designed to provide a framework to improve pain control for patients with cancer worldwide. In this simple algorithm, treatment of pain is addressed in three steps. If pain persists at a given step, treatment is advanced to the next step. All steps recommend the use of adjuvant therapy, if indicated.
  - ○ **Step 1 (mild pain):** Nonopioid analgesic, such as acetaminophen or nonsteroidal anti-inflammatory drugs (NSAIDs).
  - ○ **Step 2 (moderate pain):** Weak opioid +/− nonopioid analgesic.
  - ○ **Step 3 (severe pain):** Strong opioid +/− nonopioid analgesic.
- The WHO ladder helped change attitudes toward pain management and heightened physician awareness of the importance of pain management.
- With rational pain management, addiction and tolerance are less likely to be clinical problems.[9]
- While most patients can achieve improved pain relief using this algorithm, **the WHO ladder does have limitations.**
  - ○ It does not include an assessment step.
  - ○ It does not take into account targeted therapy for neuropathic pain.

- It does not allow for nonpharmacologic strategies.
- While it is common practice to follow the WHO's recommendation to combine NSAIDs with opioids, **there is no evidence base to support a clinical difference in pain relief when opioids are given in combination with NSAIDs as compared with either drug alone.**[10]

Basic Pain Management Principles

- For acute self-limited pain, short-acting agents can be used as needed.
- Analgesics may be used before engaging in activities that provoke pain, for example, dressing changes or physical therapy.
- **For chronic pain,** adequate **analgesia is best obtained with a combination of long-acting basal pain medication and doses of short-acting medications as needed** for breakthrough pain.
  - Breakthrough doses should be 5% to 15% of total daily dose.
  - Basal dose should be increased in patients consistently requiring >2 to 3 breakthrough doses per day.
  - Dose escalation for inadequate pain control should increase the 24-hour dose by 30% to 50%.
- While neuropathic pain is responsive to opioid therapy, adjuvant therapy with antidepressants or anticonvulsants may confer additional benefit.[11]
- Start with the lowest effective dose of medication and titrate up as needed.
- Be careful to **avoid acetaminophen overdose** when using opioid/acetaminophen combination pills.

Medications

Nonopioid Analgesics

- **Nonsteroidal anti-inflammatory drugs**
  - NSAIDs exert antipyretic, analgesic, and anti-inflammatory effects via inhibition of cyclooxygenase isoenzymes (COX1 and/or COX2 depending on the agent), which leads to decreased production of thromboxane and prostaglandins via the arachidonic acid pathway.
  - NSAIDs are effective for mild pain, especially pain with an inflammatory component.
  - Most NSAIDs have an analgesic ceiling effect, a dose above which there is little improvement in analgesia, but increased risk of adverse effects.
  - These drugs are relatively contraindicated in patients with renal insufficiency or with a history of peptic ulcer disease.
  - Adverse effects of NSAIDs include gastrointestinal tract bleeding via gastritis or ulcer formation, platelet dysfunction, and renal insufficiency. Aspirin may precipitate bronchospasm in patients with severe asthma.
  - Gastrointestinal side effects may be reduced by using proton pump inhibitors or H2-blockers to suppress gastric acid production.
  - Details regarding commonly used NSAIDs are presented in Table 37-2.
- **Acetaminophen**
  - Acetaminophen exerts analgesic and antipyretic effects. Its exact mechanism of action is poorly understood.
  - Analgesic dosing is 325 to 650 mg PO every 4 to 6 hours or 1 g 3 to 4 times/day. **Maximum daily dose** should not exceed 4 g/day for patients with normal hepatic function; patients with liver disease should not take >2 g/day. The recommended maximum dose for patients >70 years of age is 3 g/day.
  - An analgesic ceiling effect likely occurs at doses of 1 g.[12]

TABLE 37-2	Commonly Used Nonsteroidal Anti-Inflammatory Drugs	
Drug	**Dose**	**Forms**
Aspirin	325–650 mg PO q4–6 hours up to 4 g/day	Tablets/caplets
	Ceiling effect on analgesia at 1,000 mg/day	Buffered caplets
		Enteric coated
		Chewable
		Gum (Aspergum)
		Rectal suppository
Ibuprofen	200–800 mg PO 3–4 times/day	Tablets/caplets
Diclofenac	50–150 mg/day in 2–3 divided doses	Immediate or extended-release tablet
		Gel for topical use with osteoarthritis (Voltaren Gel)
		Transdermal patch (Flector)
Naproxen	250–500 mg q12 hours	Tablet
	Ceiling effect on analgesia at 1,000 mg/day	Suspension
Celecoxib	100–200 mg q12–24 hours	Tablet
Indomethacin	20–50 mg PO tid	Short-acting or extended-release tablets
		Suppository
		Suspension

- The major adverse effect of acetaminophen is liver toxicity, ranging from mild transaminitis to fulminant hepatic failure. Patients with underlying liver disease or heavy alcohol use can experience liver damage at lower doses.
- Acetaminophen is available in tablet, oral liquid, intravenous, and suppository forms.

Opioids
- Opioids exert analgesic effects to alter pain perception via opioid receptors in both the central nervous system and the spinal cord.
- Unlike other classes of analgesics, opioids have a very large titration range. **The analgesic ceiling effect generally occurs only at extremely high doses of opioids.**
- Opioids offer flexibility in dosing routes that can be customized to a patient's needs.
- Doses can be given via oral, transdermal, sublingual, intravenous, rectal, subcutaneous, intrathecal, intraventricular, buccal, and epidural routes.
- Refer to Table 37-3 for commonly prescribed opioids and dosing.[13]
- Data comparing opioid efficacy are limited, and the results are largely equivocal. Opioid selection may be based on desired route of administration, availability, and individual patient tolerance for a given drug.
- **Meperidine**
  - Meperidine is **NOT recommended** for treatment of pain because of limited efficacy and a very short duration of analgesia with significant euphoria. Historically, it has been a significant prescription drug of abuse.
  - Its active metabolite **normeperidine accumulates in renal failure and can lower the seizure threshold.**

TABLE 37-3 Commonly Prescribed Opioids[a]

Drug	Generic or trade name(s) and formulations	Recommended dosing interval
Morphine		
Short acting	Morphine sulfate immediate-release tablet: 15, 30 mg	q2–4 hours[b]
	Morphine sulfate solution: 10 mg/5 mL, 20 mg/5 mL, 20 mg/mL	q2–4 hours[c]
	Roxanol solution: 10 mg/2.5 mL, 20 mg/mL, 100 mg/5 mL	q4 hours
	Morphine sulfate suppository: 5, 10, 20, 30 mg	q4 hours
Extended release	Morphine sulfate extended-release tablet: 15, 30, 60, 100, 200 mg	q8–12 hours
	Avinza: 30, 45, 60, 75, 90, 120 mg	q24 hours
	Kadian: 10, 20, 30, 40, 50, 60, 70, 80, 100, 130, 150, 200 mg	q12–24 hours
	MS Contin: 15, 30, 60, 100, 200 mg	q8–12 hours
Oxycodone		
Immediate release	Oxycodone tablet: 5, 10, 15, 20, 30 mg	q4–6 hours
	OxyIR: 5 mg	q4 hours
	ETH-oxydose solution: 20 mg/mL (berry flavor)	q4 hours
	OxyFast solution: 20 mg/mL	q4 hours
Sustained release	Oxycodone extended-release tablet: 10, 20, 40, 80 mg	q12 hours
	OxyContin: 10, 20, 40, 80 mg	q12 hours
Hydromorphone		
Tablet	Hydromorphone: 2, 4, 8 mg	q3–4 hours
	Dilaudid: 2, 4, 8 mg	q3–4 hours
Suppository	Hydromorphone suppository: 3 mg	q6–8 hours
	Dilaudid: 3 mg	q6–8 hours
Liquid	Dilaudid: 1 mg/mL	q3–4 hours
Fentanyl		
Transdermal	Fentanyl: 12,[d] 25, 50, 75, 100 µg/hour	q72 hours
	Duragesic: 12,[d] 25, 50, 75, 100 µg/hour	q72 hours
Transmucosal	Actiq: 200, 400, 600, 800, 1,200, 1,600 µg (berry flavored, also known as fentanyl lollipop)	May repeat 1× after initial dose if pain persists; maximum 4 units/day

[a]Opioids are generally administered intravenously only in the hospital setting, although occasionally they are given subcutaneously in the outpatient setting. This usually occurs in a home hospice setting, and dosing is equivalent to intravenous dosing. Intravenous administration of opioids will not be discussed in this outpatient care manual.
[b]Peak serum concentration of most short-acting oral morphine preparations occurs after 1 hour. Short-acting doses can be given as frequently as every 2 hours without stacking/overlapping doses. While relatively stable pain is appropriately treated with breakthrough doses every 4 hours as needed, out-of-control pain can be addressed by dosing short-acting opioids every 2 hours.
[c]Initial dosing of short-acting oral morphine for opioid-naïve patients is 5–10 mg every 4 hours as needed. For an opioid-naïve patient starting oral morphine, solution should be used, as short-acting tablets are only available in 15- and 30-mg formulations.
[d]Duragesic and fentanyl 12 µg/hour patches actually supply 12.5 µg/hour.
Drug information from Lexi-Comp Online Drug Database. 2015. http://www.lexi.com. Last accessed 1/12/15.

- **Tramadol**
  - Tramadol is both an opioid agonist and a centrally acting nonopioid analgesic that acts on pain processing pathways.
  - Dosing is 50 to 10 mg PO every 4 to 6 hours. Maximum daily dose is 400 mg/day.
  - Side effects include flushing, headache, dizziness, insomnia, somnolence, nausea, vomiting, constipation, dyspepsia, and pruritus. Dose titration starting with 25 mg and gradually increasing can improve tolerance.
  - Tramadol is **metabolized by the liver and excreted largely by the kidneys.** It is not dialyzable. **It has an active metabolite that can lower the seizure threshold,** particularly when taken in combination with some antidepressant medications. It should not be used in patients with known seizure disorders.
- **Codeine**
  - Codeine is an opioid prodrug with modest antitussive effects.
  - To exert analgesic effect, codeine must be metabolized to morphine by the liver. **Up to 10% of the US population lacks the appropriate enzyme for codeine metabolism.** In these patients, codeine will provide analgesia similar to acetaminophen, but with higher rates of constipation. Like morphine, its clearance is reduced in the setting of renal impairment.
- **Morphine**
  - Morphine is often the first-line opioid given its safety profile, ease of use, availability, and physician experience with its use.
  - Two **active metabolites** of morphine can accumulate in renal insufficiency, so alternate opioids may be considered for patients with renal impairment.
- **Oxycodone**
  - While a single meta-analysis found pain control to be slightly better with morphine than with oxycodone, dry mouth and drowsiness were less prevalent with oxycodone.[14]
  - Oxycodone has few renally cleared active metabolites.
- **Hydromorphone**
  - Available data suggest no significant difference in analgesia or side effects between hydromorphone and other opioids.[15]
  - Hydromorphone has few renally cleared active metabolites.
- **Methadone**
  - Methadone is an opioid agonist as well as an N-methyl-D-aspartic acid antagonist, producing analgesia with additional adjuvant effects for neuropathic pain.
  - The half-life of methadone is relatively long and varies significantly between patients. **The duration of methadone's analgesic effect is much shorter than its half-life.**
  - Methadone interacts with many common medications resulting in further **pharmacokinetic variability.**
  - Methadone has similar efficacy to morphine for cancer pain with similar side effects in short-term studies. However, in long-term studies, methadone side effects were more pronounced.[16] In addition, recent data suggest an increase in mortality in patients using methadone, and the Food and Drug Administration (FDA) has urged caution and careful titration of methadone in pain therapy.[17]
  - Methadone can be a very useful drug for chronic pain, but it is **best prescribed by physicians experienced with its use.** Close follow-up during dose titration is essential.
- **Fentanyl**
  - Fentanyl may cause less constipation than other opioids; however, the difference is likely to be small.[18,19]
  - Transdermal fentanyl is best used for stable pain syndromes.
  - Fentanyl has no renally cleared active metabolites.
  - Fentanyl patch absorption requires skin adhesion and subcutaneous fat. Response is less predictable in patients with cachexia, fever, or diaphoresis.

- **Alternative opioid formulations**
  - **Opioid combination pills** with acetaminophen or ibuprofen are available in a wide variety of doses, but dose titration is limited by the maximum daily dose of acetaminophen or ibuprofen. Commonly prescribed combination pills are presented in Table 37-4.
  - **Considerations for patients unable or unwilling to take oral analgesics.**
    - Transdermal fentanyl is useful if pain is stable.
    - **Extended-release formulations of any oral opioids must not be chewed or crushed.** Special coatings on the tablets or granules slow the medication's release; destroying the integrity of the coating can result in potentially fatal overdose.
    - Liquid formulations of short-acting opioids can be given at scheduled intervals to provide basal analgesia. For example, 10 mg liquid morphine sulfate every 6 hours as basal medication, with 5 mg liquid morphine every 4 hours as needed for breakthrough pain.
    - Kadian (morphine sulfate extended release) comes in a capsule that can be opened. The granules must not be crushed but may be sprinkled in water and administered via gastrostomy tube ($\geq$16 French).
- **Conversion between opioids**
  - Use caution when converting between opioids as equianalgesic doses are approximations only (refer to Table 37-5).

TABLE 37-4	Opioid Combination Preparations	
Drug	**Generic or trade name(s) and formulations**	**Recommended dosing interval**
Oxycodone + APAP	Dosage in mg oxycodone/mg APAP	q6 hours
Tablets	Oxycodone/APAP: 2.5/325, 5/325, 7.5/325, 7.5/500, 10/325, 10/650	
	Endocet: 5/325, 7.5/325, 7.5/500, 10/325, 10/650	
	Magnacet: 5/400, 7.5/400, 10/400	
	Percocet: 2.5/325, 5/325, 7.5/500, 10/650	
	Primalev: 2.5/300, 5/300, 7.5/300, 10/300	
	Roxicet: 5/500	
Solution	Roxicet: 5/325 per 5 mL	q6 hours
Hydrocodone + APAP	Dosage in mg hydrocodone/mg APAP	
Tablet	Hydrocodone/APAP: 2.5/325, 2.5/500, 5/325, 5/500, 5/650, 7.5/325, 7.5/500, 7.5/650, 7.5/750, 10/325, 10/500, 10/650, 10/660	q4–6 hours
	Lortab: 5/500, 7.5/500, 10/500	
	Norco: 5/325, 7.5/325, 10/325	
	Vicodin: 5/500, 7.5/750 ES, 10/660 HP	
Elixir	Hydrocodone: 7.5/500 per 15 mL	q4–6 hours
	Lortab: 7.5/500 per 15 mL	
Hydrocodone + ibuprofen	Dosage in mg hydrocodone/mg ibuprofen	
Tablet	Hydrocodone/ibuprofen: 7.5/200	q4–6 hours
	Vicoprofen: 7.5/200	

APAP, acetaminophen; ES, extra strength; HP, high potency.

TABLE 37-5	Equianalgesic Opioid Doses
Drugs	**Equianalgesic dose (mg)**
Morphine PO	30
Morphine IV	10
Oxycodone	20
Hydrocodone	30
Hydromorphone PO	7.5
Hydromorphone IV	1.5

Drug information from Lexi-Comp Online Drug Database. 2015. http://www.lexi.com. Last Accessed August 3, 2014.

- Calculate the 24-hour dose of the current drug.
- Convert this drug to the equivalent dose of the desired new drug with the following equation:

$$\left(\begin{array}{c}\text{24 - hour dose of}\\\text{current drug}\end{array}\right) \times \left(\dfrac{\begin{array}{c}\text{New drug equianalgesic}\\\text{equivalent}\end{array}}{\begin{array}{c}\text{Current drug equianalgesic}\\\text{equivalent}\end{array}}\right) = \text{New drug 24 - hour dose}$$

- Reduce dose by 25% to 35% of the calculated new drug equivalent dose to account for incomplete cross-tolerance between opioids.
- Divide the calculated new 24-hour dose by the number of doses planned per day. For example, divide by 2 for twice daily OxyContin or by 4 for doses of oxycodone given every 6 hours.
- If using a basal dose of analgesic, calculate breakthrough doses of the new drug as 5% to 15% of the total daily dose, given at a frequency based on drug half-life.
  ○ Ensure that the patient has adequate doses of breakthrough analgesia available when converting between opioids.
  ○ **The basal analgesic dose is intentionally reduced during opioid conversion to avoid risks of oversedation and respiratory depression with incomplete opioid cross-tolerance.** This means that a patient's pain may initially be undertreated with the new basal dose.
  ○ Short-acting opioids can be given as frequently as every 2 hours for breakthrough pain during opioid transitions to avoid pain crises in the setting of lowered basal analgesia.
  ○ Patients consistently requiring more than 2 to 3 doses of breakthrough pain medication per day may require an increase in their basal dose.
  ○ **Conversion to/from fentanyl**
    - Use Table 37-6 when converting between fentanyl transdermal patches and oral morphine.
    - Increase the dose of fentanyl patch on the basis of the amount of daily breakthrough opioid required.
    - Do not titrate patch dose more frequently than every 72 hours.
    - Patches may not be cut. The lowest dose fentanyl patch is 12.5 µg/hour.
    - **Converting to the fentanyl patch:** The fentanyl patch takes 8 to 12 hours to reach peak effect, so place the patch at the same time as the last dose of oral long-acting medication is given.
    - **Discontinuing the fentanyl patch:** Remove the patch and start the new extended-release opioid 12 hours later.
    - Short-acting oral opioids can be used as needed every 2 hours for breakthrough pain during transitions to and from fentanyl patches.

TABLE 37-6 Oral Morphine/Transdermal Fentanyl Conversions

24-Hour PO morphine dose (mg)	Transdermal fentanyl equivalent (μg/hour)
60	25
120	50
180	75
240	100
300	125
360	150
420	175
480	200

Adjuvant Drugs for Opioid Side Effects
- **Constipation**
  - Both pain relief and constipation are related to steady-state levels of opioids. All patients on opioids are at risk for constipation, and tolerance does not develop for this side effect.
  - There is limited evidence as to the most appropriate bowel regimen, but most patients on chronic opioids will require more than one anticonstipation drug. The combination of a **stool softener plus a stimulant laxative** is a reasonable starting point.
    - **Docusate** sodium is a detergent stool softener given in doses of 50 to 500 mg/day divided once to four times daily. **Sennosides** is a stimulant laxative given in doses of 8.6 to 51.6 mg/day divided two or three times daily (maximum dose 100 mg/day).
    - Docusate/sennosides combination tablets (50 mg/8.6 mg) are also available; however, it may be less expensive for the patient if docusate and sennosides are prescribed separately.
    - Encourage adequate fluid intake.
    - Lactulose 10 to 20 g/day (15 to 30 mL) can be added and titrated up to 40 g/day, if needed.
    - Polyethylene glycol is an osmotic agent that may also be added. Dosing is 17 g (about one heaping tablespoon) dissolved into 4 to 8 oz of water once daily. This agent has not been FDA approved for long-term use.
  - Titrate up the daily bowel regimen if no bowel movement occurs for 2 to 3 days.
  - If refractory constipation develops, rule out complete or partial bowel obstruction before advancing therapy.
  - PO **naloxone** can also be helpful for refractory opioid-induced constipation.
    - The dose is 0.4 mg PO every 2 to 4 hours as needed.
    - There is little systemic absorption of PO naloxone, so oral dosing should not interfere with pain control. Monitor closely, however, for increased pain.
  - Subcutaneous **methylnaltrexone** is useful for patients with opioid-induced constipation who cannot tolerate oral therapy. It is contraindicated in patients with partial or complete bowel obstruction. Dosing varies with patient weight.
- **Sedation**
  - Sedation is common with initiation or up-titration of opioids; tolerance usually develops over 2 to 3 days.
  - If sedation persists consider decreasing the basal opioid dose and using increased breakthrough doses when needed.
  - Switching opioids may help, if sedation is refractory.
- **Nausea**
  - There are two forms of nausea associated with opioids, early and late.

- **Early onset nausea** occurs within 15 to 30 minutes of drug administration, is related to changes in serum drug concentration and is more common with intravenous opioids. This type of nausea responds well to serotonin antagonists such as ondansetron 4 to 8 mg PO/IV or dopamine antagonists such as low-dose haloperidol (dose may be as low as 0.5 to 1 mg PO/IV; note, this use of haloperidol is not FDA approved).
- **Nausea that occurs later** in opioid therapy is usually due to insufficient treatment of constipation. This form of nausea responds to improved bowel regimen.
- **Respiratory depression**
  - Respiratory depression can occur with opioid administration, and is seen more frequently with initiation or up-titration of therapy. **Respiratory depression is usually preceded by sedation.**
  - Dosage should be started low and titrated up carefully in opioid-naïve patients.
  - IV naloxone can be used for life-threatening respiratory depression. Opioid reversal can result in a pain crisis, so naloxone should be diluted and titrated to effect.
- **Pruritus**
  - Pruritus occurs with opioid use due to **opioid-induced histamine release.**
  - This side effect is **classically associated with morphine** and may be less pronounced with other opioids, such as hydromorphone or oxycodone.
  - Antihistamines can be used as needed.
  - Tolerance usually develops, but if persistent, consider switching opioids.

Adjuvants for Neuropathic Pain

- Adjuvant analgesics have synergistic effects when combined with opioid medications and have been underused in the treatment of cancer pain.[20]
- Some medications may require titration over **days to weeks for maximal results.**
- Addition of adjuvant analgesics, however, can confer great benefits: adjuvant analgesics have been shown to increase the therapeutic index of opioids and reduce opioid side effects.[21]
- **Antidepressants**
  - One-third of patients with neuropathic pain achieve moderate or better pain relief with adjuvant therapy with **tricyclic antidepressants** (TCAs).
  - **Selective norepinephrine reuptake inhibitors** (SNRIs), including duloxetine and venlafaxine, have demonstrated similar efficacy to TCAs for treatment of neuropathic pain.[22] Duloxetine has also been approved for the treatment of diabetic neuropathy.[20]
  - Effective analgesic dose is often lower and onset of effect earlier than when treating depression.[6]
- **Anticonvulsants**
  - **Gabapentin** is frequently used to treat chronic neuropathic pain and there is strong evidence to support its use in the treatment of diabetic neuropathy, postherpetic neuralgia, and acute postoperative pain after craniotomy.[20]
    - Starting dose is generally 300 mg at bedtime. This may be titrated up to a maximum of 3,600 mg/day, given in divided doses every 8 hours.
    - Maximum dose is lower in patients with renal insufficiency.
    - Most patients will require at least 900 to 1,500 mg/day to achieve pain control.
    - Gabapentin can cause sedation, but this effect usually attenuates after 3 to 5 days. It is important to closely monitor for sedation especially when titrating gabapentin along with an opioid.
  - **Pregabalin** is a newer anticonvulsant, with a mechanism of action, efficacy, and range of adverse effects similar to gabapentin. The dose range is 100 to 600 mg/day divided into 2 or 3 doses.
  - **Carbamazepine** has some efficacy in neuropathic pain, such as trigeminal neuralgia and diabetic neuropathy.

- **Lamotrigine** has been used to treat trigeminal neuralgia, HIV neuropathy, and central poststroke pain. There are reports of good effect with the use of **levetiracetam** and **oxcarbazepine** in the treatment of chronic neuropathic pain. More studies are needed; the evidence is evolving.[23]
- **Other adjuvants**
  - **Local anesthetics** such as lidocaine transdermal patches may be effective for some localized pain due to strains, sprains, or tumor invasion of tissue. In order to prevent systemic absorption, they should be applied to intact skin for no more than 12 hours/day.
  - **Steroids** may be useful for patients with metastatic bone pain or nerve compression.[20] They can increase appetite and help with nausea.
  - **Bisphosphonates** can be helpful for refractory bone pain and for chronic regional pain syndrome.[8,21]
  - **Benzodiazepines and selective serotonin/norepinephrine reuptake inhibitors** may decrease anxiety and thus help patients cope with chronic pain.
  - **Neuroleptics** cannot be recommended for adjuvant pain therapy on the basis of current available data.[24]

Other Nonpharmacologic Therapies

- Psychotherapy, cognitive-behavioral therapy, mindfulness, and counseling can be useful adjuncts for patients with chronic pain.
- Physical and occupational therapy can help some patients increase functionality and independence.
- Acupuncture has also been used with success as a therapy in cancer-related pain.
- Massage may be helpful for some patients.
- Radiation therapy is indicated for cancer pain caused by metastatic disease to bone and brain and for radicular pain caused by tumors compressing neural structures.
- Transcutaneous electrical nerve stimulation is available for pain therapy, although there are currently insufficient data to support its use.[25–27]

REFERRAL

- If pain cannot be adequately controlled, referral to a pain specialist should be considered for more advanced medical management or specialized procedures.
- A full discussion of procedural interventions for pain syndromes is beyond the scope of this chapter.
- Available techniques include steroid injections, neurolytic blocks, and surgical procedures such as rhizotomy, cordotomy, and implantation of intrathecal or intraventricular opioid delivery systems.

MONITORING/FOLLOW-UP

- Treatment of pain is an iterative process; one of its most important components is close follow-up and frequent reevaluation of the therapeutic plan.
- If pain is not controlled, appropriate adjustments to the patient's regimen should be made.

REFERENCES

1. Pain terms: a list with definitions and notes on usage. Recommended by the IASP Subcommittee on Taxonomy. *Pain* 1979;6:249.
2. Hart LG, Deyo RA, Cherkin DC. Physician office visits for low back pain. Frequency, clinical evaluation, and treatment patterns from a U.S. National Survey. *Spine* 1995;20:11–19.

3. Deyo RA, Weinstein JN. Low back pain. *N Engl J Med* 2001;344:363–370.
4. Riechelmann RP, Krzyzanowska MK, O'Carroll A, et al. Symptom and medication profiles among cancer patients attending a palliative care clinic. *Support Care Cancer* 2007;15:1407–1412.
5. Teno JM, Hakim RB, Knaus WA, et al. Preferences for cardiopulmonary resuscitation: physician–patient agreement and hospital resource use. The SUPPORT Investigators. *J Gen Intern Med* 1995;10:179–186.
6. Swarm R, Abernethy AP, Anghelescu DL, et al. Adult cancer pain. *J Natl Compr Canc Netw* 2010;8:1046–1086.
7. Cleeland CS, Gonin R, Hatfield AK, et al. Pain and its treatment in outpatients with metastatic cancer. *N Engl J Med* 1994;330:592–596.
8. Jost L, Roila F. Management of cancer pain: ESMO clinical practice guidelines. *Ann Oncol* 2010;21:257–260.
9. Azevedo São Leão Ferreira K, Kimura M, Jacobsen Teixeira M. The WHO analgesic ladder for cancer pain control, twenty years of use. How much pain relief does one get from using it? *Support Care Cancer* 2006;14:1086–1093.
10. McNicol E, Strassels SA, Goudas L, et al. NSAIDS or paracetamol, alone or combined with opioids, for cancer pain. *Cochrane Database Syst Rev* 2005;(1):CD005180.
11. Eisenberg E, McNicol E, Carr DB. Opioids for neuropathic pain. *Cochrane Database Syst Rev* 2013;(8):CD006146.
12. Skoglund LA, Skjelbred P, Fyllingen G. Analgesic efficacy of acetaminophen 1000 mg, acetaminophen 2000 mg, and the combination of acetaminophen 1000 mg and codeine phosphate 60 mg versus placebo in acute postoperative pain. *Pharmacotherapy* 1991;11:364–369.
13. Lexi-Comp Online Drug Database. 2015. http://www.lexi.com. Last accessed 1/12/15.
14. Reid CM, Martin RM, Sterne JA, et al. Oxycodone for cancer-related pain: meta-analysis of randomized controlled trials. *Arch Intern Med* 2006;166:837–843.
15. Quigley C, Wiffen P. A systematic review of hydromorphone in acute and chronic pain. *J Pain Symptom Manage* 2003;25:169–178.
16. Nicholson AB. Methadone for cancer pain. *Cochrane Database Syst Rev* 2007;(4): CD003971.
17. FDA. *Methadone Hydrochloride Information-FDA ALERT [11/2006]: Death, Narcotic Overdose, and Serious Cardiac Arrhythmias.* http://www.fda.gov/Safety/MedWatch/ SafetyInformation/SafetyAlertsforHumanMedicalProducts/ucm150642.htm. Published November 2006. Last accessed 1/12/15.
18. Ahmedzai S, Brooks D. Transdermal fentanyl versus sustained-release oral morphine in cancer pain: preference, efficacy, and quality of life. The TTS-Fentanyl comparative trial group. *J Pain Symptom Manage* 1997;13:254–261.
19. Mercadante S, Porzio G, Ferrera P, et al. Sustained-release oral morphine versus trans-dermal fentanyl and oral methadone in cancer pain management. *Eur J Pain* 2008; 12:1040–1046.
20. Mitra R, Jones S. Adjuvant analgesics in cancer pain: a review. *Am J Hosp Palliat Care* 2012;29:70–79.
21. Khan MI, Walsh D, Brito-Dellan N. Opioid and adjuvant analgesics: compared and contrasted. *Am J Hosp Palliat Care* 2011;28:378–383.
22. Saarto T, Wiffen PJ. Antidepressants for neuropathic pain. *Cochrane Database Syst Rev* 2007;(4):CD005454.
23. Goodyear-Smith F, Halliwell J. Anticonvulsants for neuropathic pain: gaps in the evidence. *Clin J Pain* 2009;25:528–536.
24. Seidel S, Aigner M, Ossege M, et al. Antipsychotics for acute and chronic pain in adults. *Cochrane Database Syst Rev* 2013;(8):CD004844.

25. Nnoaham KE, Kumbang J. Transcutaneous electrical nerve stimulation (TENS) for chronic pain. *Cochrane Database Syst Rev* 2008;(3):CD003222.
26. Robb K, Oxberry SG, Bennett MI, et al. A Cochrane systematic review of transcutaneous electrical nerve stimulation for cancer pain. *J Pain Symptom Manage* 2009;37:746–753.
27. Walsh DM, Howe TE, Johnson MI, Sluka KA. Transcutaneous electrical nerve stimulation for acute pain. *Cochrane Database Syst Rev* 2009;(2):CD006142.

38 Geriatrics

Lauren M. Young and David B. Carr

Geriatrics

Primary care providers are frequently faced with an aging patient population in their practice. Many practitioners also work in hospital settings or skilled nursing centers that have an ever-increasing elderly population. Identifying and evaluating geriatric syndromes such as dementia and incontinence, addressing polypharmacy, preventing injury and disability, maintaining function, and discussing advance directives are just a few of the important priorities in providing appropriate care to older adults.

Preventing Disability and Maintaining Function

- The decision to screen for various diseases in the older adult is often complicated by limited life expectancy with advanced age, the presence of comorbid illnesses, the reluctance of the patient to undergo testing, and the paucity of literature that would demonstrate efficacy of screening in late life.
- However, it should be noted that **the average 85-year-old woman has a life expectancy well past 5 years,** which is often within the range of survival rates quoted for many cancer treatments.
- In addition, the common causes of morbidity and mortality in advanced age remain cardiac disease, pulmonary disease, cerebrovascular disease, dementia, diabetes, influenza or pneumonia, and unintentional injuries.
- The decision to perform screening and health maintenance in the older adult should be **individualized for each patient.**
- **Smoking cessation** has been found to be beneficial and bestow health benefits despite advanced age.
- **Primary prevention of hypercholesterolemia** in patients older than age 70 is now less controversial, and secondary prevention has been demonstrated to decrease rates of myocardial infarction and death in older adults.
- The benefits of **weight training and aerobic activity** in maintaining cognitive and physical health are well proven, and these interventions should be discussed and encouraged with elderly patients.

Geriatric Syndromes

- Common geriatric syndromes or disorders in the outpatient setting that should be identified include the following: dementia, depression, falls, urinary incontinence (UI), malnutrition, frailty, impotence, sensory deprivation, polypharmacy, and delirium.
- The clinician, patient, and/or family may identify these conditions. However, many of these syndromes are not identified or evaluated unless the primary care physician systematically screens for them.
- Clinicians should inquire about the presence of these syndromes with their older adult patients and caregivers during office visits.
- **Selected screening measures** should also be incorporated in yearly health examinations for patients >65 years of age. These may include the following:
  ○ Comprehensive medication review
  ○ Screening for hearing impairment (by questionnaire or handheld audiometry) and visual impairment (Snellen eye chart or Rosenbaum pocket chart)

○ Identifying the presence of or risk for falls or motor vehicle crashes
○ Screening for dementia (Table 38-1) and depression[1]
○ Discussing and documenting advance directives and identifying a surrogate decision maker
• In addition, many of these screens can serve as a baseline and can be repeated during future examinations to determine response to treatment.

Assessment of Function

• Many disorders come to the attention of the physician if they are impairing job performance or function at home.
• Diagnoses such as dementia require documentation of new-onset functional impairment, and improvements in functional status are often used as a marker of treatment success.
• In addition, a review of the activities of daily living can assist in targeting additional assistance that may be needed at home.

TABLE 38-1   Short Blessed Screening Test for Cognitive Impairment

Cognitive screen	Maximum error	Error score	× Weight	= Subscore
1. What year is it now? _____	1	_____	× 4	= _____
2. What month is it now? _____ Repeat this phrase after me and remember it: John Brown, 42 Market Street, Chicago Number of trials to learning: _____ (max 3)	1	_____	× 3	= _____
3. About what time is it without looking at your watch? (within 1 hour) Response: _____ Actual time: _____	1	_____	× 3	= _____
4. Count backward from 20 down to 1. Mark correctly sequenced numbers: 20 19 18 17 16 15 14 13 12 11 10 9 8 7 6 5 4 3 2 1	2[a]	_____	× 2	= _____
5. Say the months of the year in reverse. Circle the correct months: D N O S A JL JU MY AP M F J Time _____ sec.	2[a]	_____	× 2	= _____
6. Repeat the name and address I asked you to remember. Mark correct responses: <u>John Brown</u>, <u>42 Market Street</u>,[b] <u>Chicago</u> ___ ___, __ ___, ___	5	_____	× 2	= _____
Total weighted error score[c]				= _____

[a]Scoring: 0 = no errors; 1 = 1 error; 2 = ≥2 errors.
[b]An answer of either Market or Market Street is acceptable.
[c]A total weighted error score of ≥9 indicates a need for further assessment.
Modified from Katzman R, Brown T, Fuld P, et al. Validation of a short Orientation-Memory-Concentration Test of cognitive impairment. *Am J Psychiatry* 1983;140:734–739.

TABLE 38-2	Activities of Daily Living
Instrumental activities of daily living	**Basic activities of daily living**
Shopping	**D**ressing
Housework	**E**ating
Accounting	**A**mbulation
Food preparation	**T**oileting/incontinence
Transportation/driving	**H**ygiene/grooming

Modified from Fleming KC, Evans JM, Weber DC, et al. Practical functional assessment of elderly patients: a primary care approach. *Mayo Clin Proc* 1995;70:890–910.

- Clinicians should be prepared to quickly assess and document the presence of functional impairment due to any illness and should monitor for changes over time.
- Two mnemonics for basic and instrumental activities of daily living are listed in Table 38-2.[2]

Geriatric Assessment

- Geriatric assessment is a holistic approach to patient care and focuses on the physical, functional, social, and psychological health of the individual along with providing assistance to caregivers.
- Geriatric assessment can be practically performed in the outpatient setting by the primary care clinician in conjunction with a social worker or a gerontologic case manager, who can be consulted in difficult cases.
- The role of the social worker may include locating a chore worker to assist the caregiver, finding a durable power of attorney (DPOA), providing financial information, assisting with Medicare or Medicaid eligibility, management of caregiver stress, counseling, referral to state and local area agencies on aging, addressing advance directives, or recommending relocation to assisted living or long-term care centers.
- Geriatric evaluations should include the physical, functional, social, and psychological assessment of patients in the context of their current environment. These assessments can assist patients and their families regarding the myriad of issues that can affect the independence of frail older adults in the community.

Drug Prescribing in Older Adults

Factors That Affect Drug Metabolism

- The duration that a particular drug exerts its effect in any patient is based on the volume of distribution (V_d) of the drug, the metabolism of the drug (hepatic function), and the clearance (renal function), all of which can change with aging.
- The time for a drug to decline to one-half of its concentration is known as the drug's **biologic half-life.** The half-life is directly proportional to the V_d and inversely proportional to the clearance. V_d is determined by the degree of plasma protein binding and by the patient's body composition.

Age-Related Changes in Drug Metabolism

Changes in Body Composition

- The proportion of adipose tissue increases with aging. This increase results in a larger V_d and longer half-life, and therefore, lipophilic medications such as benzodiazepines have a longer duration of action.
- Total body water decreases by 15% in those >80 years of age. The V_d for hydrophilic drugs, such as lithium, cimetidine, and ethanol, is decreased, resulting in higher drug concentrations.

- On average, elderly persons have decreased lean body mass. Digoxin, which binds to muscle adenosine triphosphatase, may have a decreased V_d, resulting in toxicity at lower doses.
- The concentrations of plasma proteins such as albumin also tend to decline in older adults. This results in a reduced protein-bound form of many drugs and greater amount of free drug levels. Examples include digoxin, phenytoin, and warfarin. Most drug level determinations measure total (protein-bound and free levels) drug concentrations. Thus, total drug levels may not accurately reflect drug activity.

Changes in Hepatic and Renal Metabolism

- In general, there is a decrease in the number of hepatocytes and liver mass with age.
- Drugs that have a large first-pass effect in the liver, such as β-blockers, nitrates, calcium channel blockers, and tricyclic antidepressants (TCAs), may be effective at lower doses.
- Phase I (cytochrome P-450) oxidation declines on average with aging, and doses of medications such as benzodiazepines should be reduced. Knowledge about cytochrome P-450 drug interactions has grown and should be reviewed by all prescribing clinicians.
- Medications that are primarily excreted by the kidney often need to be adjusted by estimating creatinine clearance by age and body weight (see Chapter 23). Examples such as aminoglycosides, digoxin, atenolol, vancomycin, lithium, and acyclovir require dose reductions in older adults.

Changes in Pharmacodynamics

- End-organ responsiveness to a drug at the receptor level may change with age. Changes in receptor binding, a decrease in receptor number, or altered translation of a receptor-initiated cellular response into a biochemical reaction may be responsible.
- Consistent findings in the literature include the following:
  - Decreased response to β-blockers.
  - Increased sensitivity to benzodiazepines, opiates, warfarin, and anticholinergics.
  - Clinicians should be aware that dose adjustments in these drugs may be necessary.

Steps in Preventing Polypharmacy and Drug Toxicity

Reducing Medications

- The initial step in assessing polypharmacy is to identify all prescription and over-the-counter drugs.
- Older adults may be treated by several physicians and obtain their medications at several pharmacies.
- The patient and, if necessary, a family member should bring in all medications to each visit for review including over-the-counter medications and herbal products.
- All drugs should be recorded by generic name, and unnecessary medications should be discontinued. The clinical indication should be identified for all drugs.
- The side effect profiles should be reviewed and safer medications substituted. Side effects may not be reported by patients, so obtaining a careful history focused on drug side effects is very important.

Starting New Medications

- Before a new drug is started, risk factors for adverse drug reactions, such as advanced age, liver or kidney disease, or use of multiple medications, should be identified.
- Providers should review a patient's specific allergic reactions to medications, and drugs that have cross-reactivity should be identified.
- It is imperative to make a firm diagnosis before drug therapy is initiated.
- Attempts should be made to manage medical conditions (e.g., hypertension, diabetes) without drugs when possible.
- The clinician should establish a therapeutic goal and an appropriate time frame for treatment duration.

- Generic medications are generally preferred for their lower cost. However, this can be challenging when prescribing medications with a narrow therapeutic index. Significant variations may occur when changing between a name brand and generic or between different generic suppliers.
- Choosing a once-a-day drug, starting at a low dose, and titrating slowly are sound principles when prescribing to older adults.
- Avoid treating side effects of one drug with more drugs (e.g., treating edema from calcium channel blocker with furosemide).

Adherence

- The risk of medication errors increases dramatically with the number of medications taken by the patient.
- Several steps to improve adherence when ordering medications are suggested:
  ○ Drug regimens should be simple.
  ○ Use the same administration schedule with other drugs and time with a daily routine such as a meal.
  ○ Instruct relatives and caregivers on drug regimens and enlist others, such as home health nurses and pharmacists, to assist with education and appropriate delivery.
  ○ Be sure that the patient can afford the medication, has transportation to the pharmacy, can open the container, and read the label.
  ○ Encourage the use of aids, such as pillboxes, calendars, and an updated medication record.
  ○ Attempt to treat multiple problems with one medication.
- Reviewing patients' knowledge of the reason they take each medication and inquiring about adverse drug reactions on each visit are essential aspects of successful pharmacotherapeutic prescribing in the elderly.

Avoid Drugs with Anticholinergic Side Effects

- **Medications with anticholinergic side effects can contribute to falls, cognitive impairment, delirium, and urinary retention in elderly patients.** Physicians need to be aware of potential anticholinergic side effects of drugs.
- An anticholinergic risk scale (ARS) is available to estimate the extent to which an individual patient is at risk of anticholinergic side effects that may lead to cognitive impairment and delirium.[3]
  ○ Higher ARS scores have been associated with an increased risk of anticholinergic adverse effects in elderly patients. High-risk medications include early TCAs, first-generation antihistamines, early typical antipsychotics, and oxybutynin. Moderate-risk medications include desipramine, nortriptyline, selective antihistamines, tolterodine, loperamide, and cimetidine. Relatively lower-risk medications include metoclopramide, mirtazapine, paroxetine, ranitidine, quetiapine, and risperidone.[3]
  ○ Clinicians should be aware that even if an individual drug has weak anticholinergic activity (e.g., prednisone, furosemide), the combination of drugs may be cumulative and cause side effects.
- **Antibiotic overuse** is a concern in older adults, and geographic areas with high prescribing rates could benefit from targeted programs to reduce unnecessary prescription.[4]
- **High-risk drugs** include insulin, warfarin, digoxin, sulfonylureas, benzodiazepines, and antipsychotics. These drugs should be prescribed with caution, especially in frail older adults with complex comorbidities.[5]
- In general, drugs should usually be tapered down at the same rate at which they were titrated up when the drug therapy was initiated. Common drugs that may require tapering include opioids, β-blockers, clonidine, gabapentin, memantine, selective serotonin reuptake inhibitors (SSRIs), serotonin-norepinephrine reuptake inhibitors (SNRIs), TCAs, and benzodiazepines.[6]
- In 2012, the American Geriatrics Society updated the **Beers criteria** for medications that should be used with caution in the elderly. The Beers criteria include but are not

limited to first-generation antihistamines, antispasmodics, α_1-blockers, TCAs with high anticholinergic side effects, digoxin >0.125 mg a day, antipsychotics, anxiolytics, metoclopramide, nonsteroidal antiinflammatory drugs (NSAIDs), and skeletal muscle relaxants.[7]

- More recently, Screening Tool of Older Person's (potentially inappropriate) Prescriptions (**STOPP) criteria for potentially inappropriate prescriptions** (PIPs) were found to be more highly associated with adverse drug events that cause or contribute to urgent hospitalization when compared to Beers criteria.[8] By the STOPP criteria, the most commonly prescribed inappropriate medications include proton pump inhibitors (>8 weeks), aspirin, benzodiazepines, loop diuretics (as first-line antihypertensives), NSAIDs (long-term use), opiates, and neuroleptics.

Falls

GENERAL PRINCIPLES

- Accidents were the eighth leading cause of death in the older adult population in 2011. Common accidents in older adults include falls and motor vehicle crashes. Burns, accidental poisoning, smoke inhalation, and hypothermia in demented patients are not uncommon, especially in patients with cognitive impairment.
- Falls are the leading cause of injury among the elderly and are important to identify and prevent in older adults.[9]
- Compared with adults 65 to 74 years old who fall, individuals 75 years old and older with falls are four to five times as likely to be admitted to a long-term care facility for a year or longer.[10]
- Safety issues should be addressed for all older adults. Extrinsic factors contribute to 30% of falls. Thus, home safety assessments, such as those provided by occupational therapists, should be considered to modify the environment to prevent falls and injuries.
- Osteoporosis should be identified and, if present, treated. Adequate calcium intake and vitamin D should be assessed and provided to all individuals.
- A family history of fracture, patient history of fracture or falls, gait difficulties, balance impairment, and/or medications should be evaluated and addressed.

Risk Factors

- To prevent falls and subsequent injury, a thorough review of the patient and environment is needed to target recommendations.[11,12]
- Risk factors for falling as identified by the U.S. Preventative Services Task Force (USPSTF) are advanced age, history of mobility difficulties and falls, as well as poor performance on the up-and-go test (see below).
- Common intrinsic factors contributing to falls in older adults include the following:
  ○ Medical and neuropsychiatric conditions
  ○ Gait and balance disorders
  ○ Proximal muscle weakness
  ○ Visual or hearing impairment
  ○ Postural hypotension
  ○ Vertigo
- Common causes of these disorders include the following: dementia, Parkinson disease, diabetes, cerebrovascular accidents, peripheral neuropathy, deconditioning, arthritis, cataracts, glaucoma, foot abnormalities, and dehydration.
- Medications and human factors causing impaired cognition, delirium, and orthostatic hypotension contribute to falls. These include the following:
  ○ Hypnotics, sedatives, anxiolytics, psychotropics, antihypertensives, diuretics, systemic glucocorticoids, and hypoglycemics
  ○ Alcohol consumption and illicit drug use

- Syncope, seizures, vestibular dysfunction, acute illnesses, arrhythmia, subclavian steal, and carotid sinus hypersensitivity should be considered but are less common.
- Common extrinsic or environmental factors contributing to falls in older adults include the following:
  - Lack of or inappropriate use of assistive devices (e.g., walker, cane, grab bars, raised toilet seat, shower chair) or improper footwear
  - Environmental hazards such as low light, steps in poor repair, lack of railing, throw rugs, low-lying furniture, clutter, and pets.

Prevention

- Providing appropriate therapy for intrinsic risk factors and elimination or modification of extrinsic risk factors as described above are the first steps in prevention.
- A **home occupational therapy assessment** can assist with management of environmental risk factors.[13]
- **Physical therapy** is often helpful for gait and balance training, evaluation for an assistive device, and muscle strengthening when indicated.
- **Community engagement in classes that focus on balance** such as tai chi, group exercise classes, and home physiotherapy has shown a cumulative 13% decreased risk in falls in individuals at increased risk for falling.[13]
- **Vitamin D** supplementation, especially in individuals with low levels, has been shown to reduce the risk of falling.[13]
- There are mixed results on the use of hip protectors to prevent hip fractures from falls. A 2010 Cochrane review of randomized and quasi-randomized studies of hip protectors used in the community and nursing homes was unable to find significant benefit after eliminating several biased randomized controlled trials. However, hip protectors may reduce hip fractures in the frail elderly living in a nursing home setting if there is good compliance.[14]
- Vision correction is not associated with reduced risk of falling, but is associated with higher confidence of not falling.[13]

DIAGNOSIS

Clinical Presentation

- Careful history including thorough medication review, comprehensive review of symptoms (e.g., urinary frequency, nocturia), and evaluation for potential extrinsic as well as intrinsic factors should be completed.
- Screens that detect impairment in lower extremity muscle strength, gait, and balance appear to be a powerful predictor of disability in the older adult.[15]
  - A lower extremity mobility screen such as the **up-and-go test** should be considered for older adults.[16] Gait, balance, and strength are assessed during this test.
  - Lower extremity strength can be assessed with a **chair stand test** (i.e., standing up from a chair and sitting down as quickly as possible with arms crossed against the chest). There are several variations of this test. One measures the time to complete five chair stands with a cutoff score of ≥ 12 seconds requiring further evaluation, while another version measures the number of chair stands completed in 30 seconds. Patients requiring the use of hands and those who are slow likely have lower extremity weakness. Endurance is also evaluated in the 30-second test.
  - A **progressive Romberg test** may be used to evaluate balance.

Diagnostic Testing

- Laboratory testing and/or if indicated neuroimaging should be performed.
- Laboratory tests include complete blood count (CBC), basic metabolic profile (BMP), glucose, vitamin B_{12}, thyroid-stimulating hormone (TSH), and 25-hydroxyvitamin D.
- Bone density scan should be considered.

TREATMENT

- A thorough examination of the older adult for **occult fractures** on presentation after a fall is mandatory.
- A high clinical index of suspicion for a nondisplaced fracture should be maintained in older adults who have persistent joint pain and negative plain films. A low threshold should exist for obtaining a bone scan or MRI in these patients. Common occult fractures that are missed on plain films include pelvic insufficiency and hip fractures.
- CT scan of the head should be considered in a patient with a head injury. Anticoagulation status should be reviewed, and neurologic exam should be performed serially.
- Evaluate skin for hematomas. Clinical awareness for potential development of intramuscular or retroperitoneal hematomas is important, especially for patients on anticoagulation. Also refer to the Prevention section above.

Physical Activity

- Physical activity can be health enhancing. Inactivity has been associated with poor outcomes, and high levels of activity have been associated with improved morbidity, mortality, function, and quality of life. Data exist to indicate that physical activity reduces the risk for many diseases such as diabetes, stroke, cancer, osteoporosis, and depression. In older adults, exercise can promote weight loss, reduce falls and hip fractures, as well as reduce the risk of functional impairment and sarcopenia.
- Clinicians should counsel their patients on engaging in routine exercise. Patients should be provided with an activity prescription that emphasizes practical activity such as walking, gradual increase in activity over time, and referral to a supervised evidence-based program that can provide social support.
- 150 minutes a week (30 minutes 5 days a week) of moderate level of aerobic activity is recommended, if not limited for health reasons (e.g., cardiac, musculoskeletal).[17]
- Balance training, especially tai chi, has been associated with a reduction in fall risk.
- Resistance training is recommended three times a week for muscle strengthening, along with flexibility exercises.
- High-level intense activity such as running should be recommended with caution and close scrutiny, especially in those that have been extremely sedentary or have significant comorbid illnesses.
- Exercise can be part of a weight reduction program in older adults with elevated BMIs who are motivated to lose weight.
- Clinicians should consider adopting a brief assessment of the level of physical activity such as the **Rapid Assessment of Physical Activity.**[18]

Driving and Older Adults

GENERAL PRINCIPLES

- Driving issues in the older adult may come to the attention of the primary care physician due to concerns raised by the family or patient, the presence of comorbidities, or requests for referrals for fitness-to-drive evaluations from the Department of Motor Vehicles (DMV).
- Patients without dementia may have insight into their declining driving skills and may question their own ability to drive safely and/or avoid exposure to high-risk situations.
- Older adults are statistically the safest age group based on absolute crash risk per year, but are more vulnerable to injury than other age groups in motor vehicle crashes.
- The average older adult lives about 7 years without the ability to drive a car, and clinicians should assist transitions into driving retirement with community mobility counseling.

• There is no off-road test or group of tests that can provide a determination of who is fit to drive, but some tests have been associated with increased risk of a motor vehicle crash and/or impaired road performance.

DIAGNOSIS

Clinical Presentation

• The assessment should start with a history and physical examination as well as a functional assessment and some type of disease severity measure.[19]
• Inquiries about crashes, tickets, near misses, or becoming lost in previously familiar environments should be addressed to the patient and, if possible, a friend or family member. Information from an informant who has driven with the patient may be useful.
• A review of medications that have the potential to sedate the older adult should be sought, with efforts at drug reduction or substituting safer alternatives.
• A search for diseases that have the potential to increase crash risk should be pursued and may include, but are not limited to, dementia, psychiatric disorders, stroke, sleep apnea, arthritis, alcohol use, sensory deprivation, seizures, diabetes, or heart disease.
• Vision, hearing, attention, visuospatial skills, judgment, muscle strength, and flexibility should be assessed.

Diagnostic Testing

• The American Medical Association has recently recommended that office practitioners adopt a brief set of office tests that may identify older adults who are at risk for driving problems.[20]
• Referral to a subspecialist or neuropsychologist may be necessary if the primary care physician is unsure as to whether the patient is safe behind the wheel.
• Occupational therapists or **driving rehabilitation specialists** who have experience in assessing older drivers can be invaluable in the evaluation process with on-the-road tests or by recommending and implementing adaptive equipment.

TREATMENT

• Efforts should be made at stabilizing or improving comorbid illnesses or functional abilities when possible.
• Counseling older drivers to use safety restraints, refrain from drinking alcohol when driving, obey the speed limit, avoid cellular phones, and consider a refresher course for driving such as the American Association of Retired Persons (AARP) Driver Safety Program may be useful in reducing crash rates and injury.
• In the event that the clinician makes a recommendation to stop driving, this information should be communicated in a professional and sensitive manner and documented in the medical record.
• It is helpful to discuss alternate modes of transportation. If the clinician is not well versed in this area, referral to a social worker or gerontologic care manager may be in order.
• Patients may refuse to stop driving despite the advice of their physician or family or both.
• Demented drivers may lack insight into their own safety risk. Therefore, removing the car from the premises, hiding the car keys, changing the locks, filing down the ignition key, or disabling the battery cables may be necessary.
• Letters can be written to the DMV to reveal medical conditions and/or provide opinions on traffic safety and may be ethically appropriate. Some states have laws that grant physicians civil immunity from reporting unsafe drivers, and some have mandatory reporting requirements. **Physicians should be aware of state and local requirements for reporting and obtain legal advice before breaching confidentiality.**

Urinary Incontinence

GENERAL PRINCIPLES

- UI, **involuntary leakage of urine,** is a common problem for older adults. It is **not a normal condition of aging.**
- Women experience UI twice as frequently as men with its prevalence increasing with age. This may be due to a variety of factors including female urinary tract anatomy, childbirth, and/or menopause.[21]
- **Reversible causes** of UI can be remembered using the **DIAPERS** mnemonic: **d**rugs (e.g., diuretics), **i**nfection, **a**trophic vaginitis, **p**sychological (depression, delirium, dementia), **e**ndocrine (polyuria due to medical conditions such as hyperglycemia, hypercalcemia), **r**estricted mobility or **r**etention, and **s**tool impaction.
- **Anatomic causes** of UI include the following:
  - Nerve damage, spinal cord injury, and other neurologic disorders
  - Anatomic floor defects, such as vaginal prolapse
  - Enlarged prostate
  - Cancer

Types of Incontinence

- **Urge** incontinence is part of the overactive bladder syndrome and is presumed to be due to uninhibited bladder contractions or detrusor overactivity.
- **Stress** incontinence or stress leakage occurs when increases in intra-abdominal pressure overcome sphincter closure mechanisms in the absence of a bladder contraction. Stress UI is the most common cause of UI in younger women and the second most common cause in older women. It may occur in older men after transurethral or radical prostatectomy.
- **Mixed incontinence is the most common type of UI in women**. This is generally thought to represent the overlap of two mechanisms: detrusor overactivity and impaired urethral sphincter function.
- **Functional** incontinence occurs in individuals with medical problems that effect mobility and cognition, interfering with their ability to reach a toilet without assistance.
- The term **overflow incontinence** has been used to describe the dribbling and/or continuous leakage associated with incomplete bladder emptying due to impaired detrusor contractility and/or bladder outlet obstruction. Leakage typically is small volume, although its continual nature can lead to significant wetting.

DIAGNOSIS

Clinical Presentation

History
- Patients may be reluctant discussing UI with a physician, so all women who have had children, patients at increased risk for UI (i.e., diabetes, neurologic disease), and all patients >65 years of age should be asked specifically about incontinence symptoms.
- Patients should be asked about symptoms compatible with urinary tract infections (UTI) such as dysuria/burning, frequency, urgency, suprapubic pain, hematuria, back/flank pain, and fever.
- Vaginal symptoms (discharge, odor, dryness, pruritus, and dyspareunia) may suggest a gynecologic cause.
- **Urgency** is accepted as both a sensitive and specific symptom for detrusor overactivity, but published trials are lacking.
- Leakage with **stress** maneuvers (e.g., coughing, nose blowing, laughing, bending over, running, changing position) is highly sensitive for **stress UI.**

- With **overflow** incontinence, there may be a weak urinary stream, dribbling, intermittency, hesitancy, frequency, and nocturia. It is seen more frequently in men and can be caused by blockage of the urethra, such as by prostate enlargement, stone or neoplasm, or constipation.
- A bladder diary of fluid intake, measured voided volumes, activities, and occurrences of urinary leakage is helpful.
- Assessment of quality of life is important along with cognitive and physical status.

Physical Examination
- Unless the history and/or other portions of the physical examination are highly suggestive of a specific cause, a genital and rectal examination should be done.
- A cough test with a full bladder to assess for urinary leakage may be performed in the office. Immediate leakage is consistent with stress UI, and delayed leakage is associated with urge UI.

Diagnostic Testing
- A **urinalysis** with reflex culture should be done to evaluate for a UTI.
- **Postvoid residual** volume should be measured; elevated levels are associated with overflow incontinence.
- Patients with complicated incontinence-associated extensive pelvic surgery, pelvic radiation, hematuria, recurrent UTIs, pain, possible fistula, high postvoid residual, significant pelvic prolapse, or failure to improve within the scope of your practice require **referral to a urologist or urogynecologist for a more detailed evaluation** (e.g., urodynamic testing, cystoscopy).

TREATMENT

The first step in the management of UI is to **identify and/or treat reversible causes** by avoiding caffeine, alcohol, and excessive fluid intake and treating UTIs, uncontrolled diabetes, and so forth.

Medications
- Pharmacologic treatment of UI is widely used for urge and mixed incontinence if behavioral therapy alone is not successful.
- **Anticholinergics** with antimuscarinic effects are the most frequently prescribed medications for urge incontinence. Commonly used agents include the following:
  - **Oxybutynin** started at a low dose of 2.5 mg two to three times daily up to 20 mg/day in divided doses (immediate release) and 5 to 10 mg/day titrated by 5 mg/week to 30 mg/day maximum (extended release). It is also available in gel that can be applied to the shoulders, upper arms, abdomen, or thighs. It is also available over the counter as a transdermal patch.
  - **Tolterodine** 1 to 2 mg twice a day (immediate release) and 2 to 4 mg/day (extended release).
  - **Fesoterodine**, start 4 mg once daily, may increase to 8 mg once daily.
  - **Trospium** 20 mg twice daily dose needs to be decreased to 20 mg once daily in the elderly and those with renal impairment (immediate release) and 60 mg daily with renal and hepatic exclusions (extended release).
  - **Because of their anticholinergic actions, patients need to be monitored for side effects** (e.g., dry mouth, drowsiness, constipation, blurred vision, urinary retention).
- Agents like **solifenacin** and **darifenacin** are more selective for M_3 muscarinic acetylcholine receptors that are found in the bladder and gastrointestinal tract, but evidence for superior clinical efficacy and tolerability is not clear.

- **β-3 adrenergic receptor agonists** (selective, **mirabegron**) are extended-release antispasmodics, which relax bladder smooth muscle. This medication requires adjustment for both renal and hepatic disease.
- **α-Adrenergic antagonists** (nonselective: terazosin and doxazosin; selective: tamsulosin, alfuzosin, and silodosin) can be used in men with overflow incontinence due to benign prostatic hypertrophy (BPH).
- **5-α-reductase type I and II antagonists** (finasteride and dutasteride) block the conversion of testosterone to 5-α-dihydrotestosterone, which may help men with BPH and urinary symptoms through prostate shrinkage. Tadalafil, a phosphodiesterase type 5 inhibitor, is also Food and Drug Administration (FDA) approved for BPH.
- **Topical estrogen** may be tried in postmenopausal women with atrophic vaginitis.
- OnabotulinumtoxinA (Botox) injections into the bladder cause muscle relaxation through acetylcholine antagonism. This procedure is FDA approved for those who cannot tolerate or do not adequately respond to anticholinergic medications.

Other Nonpharmacologic Therapies

- One to two voidings per night is normal in older adults. Sleep disorders should be excluded such as obstructive sleep apnea.
- For nocturia, patients should **restrict fluid intake four hours before bedtime.**
- **Eliminate medications (e.g., alcohol, diuretics)** causing or exacerbating UI, if possible.
- Pessaries may be used in women with vaginal or uterine prolapse.
- **Nonpharmacologic behavioral interventions**
  - For stress and urge incontinence bladder retraining, regular voiding based on bladder diary and urgency control is recommended.
  - Pelvic muscle/Kegel exercises also help control UI.
  - Biofeedback can be used in combination with pelvic muscle exercises.
  - For cognitively impaired population, prompted toileting every 2–3 hours during the daytime is recommended.
- **Neuromodulation** is FDA approved for individuals with urge UI unresponsive to biofeedback and medications. Surgical placement is only completed if an external modulator yields a fifty percent reduction in symptoms.

Surgical Management

- Surgical treatment can be considered in stress UI when patients do not respond to medical treatment adequately.
- There are three main types of surgery for women with stress UI including retropubic suspension (Burch) and two types of sling procedures. Tension-free vaginal tape (TVT) is also being successfully used.
- Surgical treatments are available for men with UI due to nerve injury including artificial sphincter, male sling, and urinary diversion. Artificial sphincters can be created in women as well.
- Surgical treatment of BPH may also be indicated and effective but may result in postoperative incontinence due to prostatectomy itself.

SPECIAL CONSIDERATIONS

- For individuals unable to maintain adequate hygiene, pads or adult diapers should be encouraged along with routine disposal of soiled protective products and changing of soiled garments.
- **Avoid the use of urinary catheters** for UI or chronic urinary retention due to their increased risk of bacterial colonization. They may be considered in the treatment of nonhealing stage III or IV pressure ulcers or when requested by patient or family for comfort measures.

Pressure Ulcers

GENERAL PRINCIPLES

Definition
- The National Pressure Ulcer Advisory Panel (NPUAP) defines pressure ulcers (formerly called decubitus ulcers) as a localized injury to the skin and/or underlying tissue, usually over a bony prominence, as a result of pressure alone or in combination with shear.
- As a pressure ulcer heals, it should be described as healing of the deepest stage of that particular ulcer's history, regardless of the current depth of the ulcer.
- **Eschar** (necrotic tissue/scab) describes black, brown, or tan tissue adherent to the wound bed or ulcer edges.
- **Slough** is mucinous yellow or white tissue/dead cells found in the wound bed.
- **Granulation tissue** refers to pink or dark red tissue with a shiny, moist, granular appearance.
- **Epithelial tissue** is new pink or shiny white tissue (skin) that develops from the edges of the wound or as islands on the ulcer surface.
- **Closed/resurfaced** wounds are completely covered with epithelium.

Classification
- **Stage 1:** Skin intact but with nonblanchable redness for >1 hour after relief of pressure.
- **Stage 2:** Blister or other break in the dermis with partial thickness loss of dermis, with or without infection.
- **Stage 3:** Full-thickness tissue loss. Subcutaneous fat may be visible; destruction extends into muscle with or without infection. Undermining and tunneling may be present.
- **Stage 4:** Full-thickness skin loss with involvement of bone, tendon, or joint, with or without infection. Often includes undermining and tunneling.
- **Unstageable:** Tissue loss in which the depth of the ulcer is unable to be determined due partial or complete coverage by slough or eschar.
- **Suspected deep tissue injury**: Localized discoloration, purple or maroon in color, of intact skin or blister, indicating underlying soft tissue injury.

Risk Factors
- Risk factors include the following:
  - Malnutrition/obesity.
  - Immobility.
  - Vascular insufficiency.
  - Systemic illnesses/inflammatory states.
  - Wet, macerated or dry, desiccated skin, both of which promote breakdown of the skin.
  - Moisture from urinary or fecal incontinence and friction (pulling the patient across bed sheets).
  - Shearing forces (patients sliding down a bed with the head elevated) can combine to damage tissue further.
- Once the pressure on tissue exceeds intracapillary pressure (10 to 30 mm Hg), tissue ischemia can occur.

Prevention
- **Relieve pressure** by frequent position changes with scheduled repositioning of the patient while in bed, elevating heels off the bed and minimizing time in the seated position. Increasing patient mobility, exercise, massage, and/or physical therapy are also helpful.
- Keeping the skin dry, preventing friction, and avoiding shearing forces (lowering the head of the bed to <30 degrees) can assist in prevention and healing.

- Topical creams and lubricants can be helpful to treat dry skin, provide a skin barrier, and increase blood flow to the area of application (e.g., Extra Protective Cream).
- It is imperative to **protect patients who are incontinent** from being exposed to urine by frequently changing soiled garments and linens.

DIAGNOSIS

- The clinical diagnosis of pressure ulcers is relatively straightforward.
- The typical patient is elderly, but they also occur in patients with significant neurologic impairment and/or severe illness who spend considerable amounts of time sitting in a wheelchair or lying in bed.
- Typical locations include sacrum, ischial tuberosities, greater trochanters, lateral malleoli, and heels.
- Every ulcer should be staged and documented by a physician.
- It is worth noting that essentially all pressure ulcers are colonized with bacteria. **Clinically significant wound infection may be suggested by erythema, warmth, swelling, tenderness, and purulent discharge.**
- More deep-seated infections may present with symptoms and signs of cellulitis, osteomyelitis, and sepsis.
- Available testing modalities for osteomyelitis include plain radiography (limited sensitivity and specificity), MRI (high sensitivity but low specificity), CT, and nuclear imaging (operating characteristics very dependent on the clinical situation).
- Alternative or potentially coexistent conditions include venous insufficiency ulcers, arterial/ischemic ulcers, and diabetic neuropathic ulcers.

TREATMENT

- Treatment of pressure ulcers depends on the stage and severity of the ulcer. Providers should monitor closely for signs of infection as well as document the length, width, and presence of tunneling of the pressure ulcer using a validated scale for healing pressure ulcers. The **pressure ulcer scale for healing (PUSH) tool** is a research-validated tool and was developed by the NPUAP.[22]
- Adequate **nutrition** is critical for wound healing. Calorie, protein supplements, or both may be helpful adjuncts to promote healing of wounds.
- Recent data question the usefulness of vitamin C and zinc supplementation.
- Adequate pain control should be provided.
- A stage 1 ulcer is a warning that more serious tissue damage may follow if appropriate preventive measures are not instituted in a timely fashion. Preventive measures should be reviewed and intensified in this setting.
- A transparent film, adhesive, semipermeable polyurethane membrane can be used in stage 1 or 2 wounds to facilitate autolytic debridement.
- For stage 2 and 3 wounds, dressings and gels, such as **hydrocolloids** (e.g., DuoDERM, Tegasorb) and **hydrogels** (e.g., IntraSite, SoloSite), cover the wound bed facilitating autolytic debridement and provide a surface to which epithelial cells can migrate.
- **Wet-to-dry dressings** can be used for noninfected wounds. However, if not changed routinely, they simply remove migrating epithelial tissue and inhibit further healing.
- **Topical enzymatic debridement** agents with collagenase (e.g., Santyl ointment) and/ or **sharp mechanical debridement** can be used to remove black eschar, with the goal of promoting granulating tissue, which promotes healing.
- **Alginates** (e.g., Kaltostat) are seaweed-derived, absorbent dressings. They form a gel-fiber matrix when in contact with fluid and can be helpful in moderate-to-heavy exudative stage 3 or 4 ulcers. Because they are nonadhesive, they can be easily removed but require a secondary dressing.

- **Topical antibiotic creams** are generally not used for routine wound care unless the area is infected. Polysporin, silver sulfadiazine, or mupirocin (the latter for methicillin-resistant *Staphylococcus aureus*) can be helpful in reducing bacterial counts.
- **Systemic antibiotics** should be used in cellulitis, deep-seated infections, and/or sepsis.
- **Consultation with a general or plastic surgeon** may be necessary to assist with wound closure. Options include debridement, flap procedures, or both.

SPECIAL CONSIDERATIONS

- In **nonhealing wounds,** bacterial or fungal infections should be considered; a stellate fungal rash may be present on the surrounding skin. This should be treated with an antifungal agent.
- Rarely, a **temporary urinary catheter** may need to be considered to improve healing in refractory cases.
- **Support mattresses** that use foam, air, or water can also assist in prevention or healing. Deep wounds into the muscle or bone (stage IV) or multiple nonhealing wounds may benefit from an air-fluidized bed or low-air-loss bed. However, their cost and size may be prohibitive.
- **Weight distributing cushions** for wheelchairs that use air, foam, and gel are also available and can be individualized for a patient's specific needs. Donut-shaped devices should be avoided.

COMPLICATIONS

Osteomyelitis should be considered when bone is exposed or in nonhealing wounds that continue to drain or are exudative. Consultation for bone biopsy by a plastic surgeon or musculoskeletal radiologist should be considered for targeted antibiotic therapy. In chronic osteomyelitis, bone debridement may be necessary.

Malnutrition: Protein-Energy Undernutrition

GENERAL PRINCIPLES

- Weight loss due to decreased appetite or anorexia has a multitude of causes in the older adult and often is multifactorial. Causes may include but are not limited to the following:
  - Therapeutic diets, such as a salt-restricted, low-cholesterol, or diabetic diets.
  - Cachexia from advanced end-organ disease (e.g., congestive heart failure, chronic obstructive pulmonary disease [COPD]).
  - Malabsorption.
  - Cancer.
  - Thyroid disease.
  - Stress response from acute illness such as infection, trauma, or wounds.
  - Chronic illness/inflammatory states, alcoholism, pain, anxiety, medications, decreased physical activity, loss of appetite, nonconducive environment, poor food preparation, consistency, and presentation, as well as poverty.
  - Isolation, loneliness, depression, and cultural food preferences may also contribute.
  - Difficulty with feeding due to hand and upper extremity disability, cognitive impairment, mental illness or psychosis, oral or dental disease, ill-fitting dentures, or excessive aerobic activity is not uncommon.
  - Individuals living in nursing homes or in outpatient rehab are particularly at high risk.
- The mnemonic MEALS ON WHEELS may be helpful to the clinician in identifying reversible causes for protein-energy malnutrition (Table 38-3).[23]

TABLE 38-3	Reversible Causes for Protein-Energy Malnutrition

M: medications (e.g., antibiotics, antiarrhythmics, anticonvulsants, antineoplastics, colchicine, digoxin, NSAIDs, hormones, iron, laxatives, opiates, psychiatric drugs, and many others)

E: emotional problems (e.g., depression, bereavement), elder abuse

A: anorexia tardive (i.e., anorexia nervosa in the elderly), alcoholism

L: late-life paranoia/mania

S: swallowing problems (e.g., dysphagia, odynophagia, apraxia, globus hystericus), stones (i.e., cholelithiasis)

0: oral problems (e.g., poor dentition, ill-fitting dentures)

N: no money, no friends, nosocomial infection

W: wandering, continuous pacing, and other dementia-related behaviors

H: hyperthyroidism, hypercalcemia, hypoadrenalism

E: enteric problems (e.g., achalasia, chronic constipation, GERD, malabsorption, PUD)

E: eating problems (e.g., apraxia, lack of hand-feeding)

L: low-cholesterol and low-sodium diets

S: shopping and meal preparation problems

NSAIDs, nonsteroidal anti-inflammatory drugs; GERD, gastroesophageal reflux disease; PUD, peptic ulcer disease.
Modified from Morley J. Anorexia of aging: physiologic and pathologic. *Am J Clin Nutr* 1997;66:760–773.

- Negative consequences of malnutrition include the following:
  - Bone demineralization and fracture.
  - Poor wound healing/chronic infections.
  - Muscle wasting.
  - Peripheral edema in the absence of cardiovascular disease.
  - Cognitive and functional decline.
  - Death. The risk of death in individuals residing in a long-term care facility who lose 5% of their bodyweight over the course of a month is 10 times higher than those gaining weight during a month.[24,25]

DIAGNOSIS

- A simple method to identify protein-energy undernutrition in older adults is to follow **serial weights.** In general, weight loss is significant if there is **an unintentional 5% loss of body weight in 1 month, 7.5% loss in 3 months, or 10% loss in a 6-month** period of time. Weight loss >25% over a year is considered severe.
- **Albumin** (g/dL) **levels <3.5** are considered protein undernutrition. Levels between 2.8 and 3.5 are considered mild, 2.1 to 2.7 moderate, and <2.1 indicate severe loss of protein stores.
- **Prealbumin** has a shorter half-life of 48 to 96 hours, whereas albumin is 18 to 20 days and is a better tool for serial monitoring of nutritional improvement. Transferrin can also be used due to its shorter half-life of 7 to 10 days.
- **Older adults** in the community with a **BMI <22 kg/m²** are considered malnourished.
- In fact, a higher BMI has been associated with a lower risk of mortality in the elderly population.[26]

- The association of frailty and BMI in older adults is a U-shaped curve. In addition to low BMIs being associated with frailty, BMIs >30 kg/m^2 (obesity) are as well.[27,28]
- The proposed BMI for individuals between 65 and 70 years old is 24 to 28 kg/m^2 and 25 to 30 kg/m^2 for those older than 70 years.
- **Circumference** measurements of waist-to-hip ratio, midupper arm, forearm, and calf can be useful when a patient cannot be weighed. **Skinfold measurements** can also be used.
- Weight loss due to diuresis or volume status should not be included when determining nutritional status.
- Evaluation for etiology includes a careful history and physical exam as well as laboratory workup including CBC, erythrocyte sedimentation rate (ESR), and TSH.
- A more detailed general discussion of malnutrition and specific treatment guidelines may be found in Chapter 22.

TREATMENT

- If appropriate, remove all dietary restrictions.
- Meal consistency should be appropriate for a patient's dentitia and swallowing capabilities. Involvement of a speech-language pathologist may be beneficial if dysphagia (e.g., coughing during meals) or pocketing of food is present.
- Some patients may require verbal cueing or hand feeding. Communal meals can also improve intake.
- In the long-term care setting, weekly measurements of weight and frequent assessment by a dietician are appropriate.
- Any readily reversible causes should be addressed (e.g., depression, if present, should be treated).
- If patients are unable to sustain themselves from a nutritional standpoint after reversible causes of weight loss have been identified and treated, input from a dietitian and the judicious use of nutritional supplements may be in order. Supplements should be given between meals.
- Additionally, if physically able, a resistance-focused exercise program should be established to avoid loss of lean muscle mass and stimulate appetite.

Medications

- **Tetrahydrocannabinol/dronabinol** and **megestrol** have been effective in promoting weight gain in certain conditions (e.g., AIDS and cancer); although the data are limited, they may be of benefit in malnourished older adults. Confusion can be associated with dronabinol, while venous thrombophlebitis and adrenal suppression have been noted with megestrol.
- **Mirtazapine,** a mild antidepressant, can also stimulate appetite and cause weight gain. Starting dose is typically 7.5 mg and can be increased as high as 45 mg. Sedation is a common side effect, so it is typically prescribed at night.
- **Oxandrolone** is an anabolic steroid and can also be used in certain cases for weight gain. The dose is typically 2.5 to 5 mg twice a day. It is contraindicated in the setting of prostate cancer and liver disease. A course of therapy is about 2 to 4 weeks and can be used intermittently according to response of the patient.
- **Unfortunately, medications that promote weight gain can have serious side effects and must be carefully considered in the context of the potential benefits.**
- Anorexia is a common side effect of medications. For example, donepezil, which is commonly used in dementia, may contribute to weight loss by adverse gastrointestinal effects and anorexia. Medications should be carefully reviewed and adjusted or replaced if potential offenders are identified.

Other Nonpharmacologic Therapies

- Despite these efforts, the use of **artificial nutrition and hydration** may need to be addressed.
- Patients with significant chronic malnutrition are at risk for refeeding syndrome if nutrients are introduced too quickly or in too high volumes resulting in hypophosphatemia, hyperglycemia, hyperinsulinemia along with hypokalemia, hypomagnesemia, and fluid retention.
- Thiamine and other micronutrients should be initiated prior to initiating feedings and supplements.
- It is important that the risks and benefits of **tube feedings** (typically administered after pursuing surgical or percutaneous gastrostomy, although can be administered through a temporary Dobhoff tube via nasogastric or nasal-duodenal route) are discussed with the patient, surrogate decision maker, or both.
  - Gastrostomy feeding tubes are typically helpful in cases in which there is anticipated functional improvement (e.g., cerebrovascular accident).
  - Tube feedings can assist with providing adequate calories and hydration.
- Careful consideration of the patient's **goals of care** and overall assessment of the patient's medical conditions and identification of terminal illnesses is imperative.
  - If appropriate, **hospice eligibility** should be determined.
  - The **Karnofsky Performance Scale Index** is a tool used to quantify functional impairment. Low scores are associated with poor outcomes.
  - The **Morbidity Risk Index** is a tool that uses the minimum data set in the longer-term care setting and may be helpful in determining life expectancy and appropriateness of interventions in moderate to advanced dementia.[29]
- There are no data to indicate that gastrostomy feeding tubes prevent respiratory infection, improve morbidity or quality of life, prevent pressure sores, improve functional status, or delay mortality in the patient with advanced dementia.[30]

Physical Frailty

- Definitions of frailty are centered on the concept of decreased physiologic reserve or increased vulnerability to stress as measured by physical activity, weight loss, walking speed, and levels of fatigue/weakness. The pathophysiology of frailty is based on the accumulation of multiple chronic illnesses (e.g., COPD, cancer, heart failure [HF]) and/or the dysregulation of physiologic processes that result in a reduction in the ability to maintain homeostasis under stressful conditions.[31,32]
- Frailty occurs across a continuum with an initial period that is asymptomatic, thus providing a potential window for prevention.
- Resistance training to build strength and muscle mass as well as aerobic exercise to improve stamina and endurance appear to be the most effective prevention.[32]
- Following hospitalization, it may take a patient three times the length of stay to regain prior physicality.
- Depending on the patient's needs, admission to an acute rehabilitation center, skilled nursing facility with rehabilitation, or outpatient versus in-home physical and occupational therapy should be considered.
- In the advanced stages of physical frailty, older adults are at increased risk of adverse outcomes including hospitalization, falls, injuries, infections, functional impairment, and mortality.
- Specific domains frequently measured to identify someone with frailty include mobility or gait speed, level of physical activity, endurance, nutrition, weight loss, strength, and balance. Cognition is sometimes considered another contributing domain.
- Primary frailty occurs from intrinsic aging processes and likely is associated with chronic inflammation, sarcopenia, low hormone levels (e.g., testosterone, estrogen), increased insulin resistance, decreased physical activity, and possibly low levels of vitamins.

- Secondary frailty is typically due to a wasting disease such as advanced COPD, HIV/AIDS, and cancer.
- **Currently, there are no hormone replacement therapies or medications that can be recommended to reverse physical frailty.**
- Failure to thrive is a controversial term in geriatrics and likely represents the most advanced stages of physical and/or cognitive frailty, but still requires a thorough investigation for underlying causes such as medication-induced anorexia, depression, elder abuse, and/or occult malignancy.

Ethics

Advance Directives

- It is imperative that physicians in outpatient and long-term care settings discuss advance directives openly with older adults and their families.
- Many patients desire to avoid cardiopulmonary resuscitation, intubation, and/or ventilation, intensive care unit treatment, dialysis, or tube feedings on the basis of quality-of-life issues or futility of treatment.
- Some interventions such as tube feedings in advanced neurodegenerative disease such as Alzheimer disease have not been shown to prolong survival, improve functional outcomes, decrease pressure sore rates, or reduce infections.[30]
- Even if questions such as code status are not decided before an acute event, it is of the utmost importance to identify a surrogate decision maker for the patient. Usually, a family member or friend can be identified who can assist in making difficult decisions.
- A legal document such as a DPOA or health care proxy is preferred, because guardianship is often a lengthy process that is difficult to expedite.
- Many older adults with an early dementing illness may lack the capacity to handle their financial or medical affairs but can consistently identify a family member or friend who can be designated their legal DPOA or health care proxy.

Informed Consent and Decision-Making Capacity

- When discussing options or interventions with a patient, it is important to follow the steps of informed consent. This generally includes the nature and purpose of the test or procedure, the risk and benefits, the probable outcome of the intervention or refusal of the plan, and any additional alternatives to the diagnostic test or procedure.
- Decision-making capacity of the patient should be assessed because many individuals have cognitive impairment and lack insight into their limitations.
- A patient with capacity has the ability to communicate choices, understand and retain relevant information, appreciate the situation and its consequences, and manipulate information rationally.[33]

ADDITIONAL RESOURCES

A pocket card for Beers criteria is available for free on the American Geriatric Society website. http://geriatricscareonline.org/ProductStore/pocketcards/10/. Last accessed 1/12/15.

National Institutes of Health. Exercise and physical activity: your everyday guide from the national institute on aging. http://www.nia.nih.gov/health/publication/exercise-physical-activity/introduction. Last a accessed 1/12/15.

World Health Organization. Physical activity and older adults. http://www.who.int/dietphysicalactivity/factsheet_olderadults/en/. Last accessed 1/12/15.

REFERENCES

1. Katzman R, Brown T, Fuld P, et al. Validation of a short Orientation-Memory-Concentration Test of cognitive impairment. *Am J Psychiatry* 1983;140:734–739.
2. Fleming KC, Evans JM, Weber DC, et al. Practical functional assessment of elderly patients: a primary care approach. *Mayo Clin Proc* 1995;70:890–910.
3. Rudolph JL, Salow MJ, Angelini MC, et al. The anticholinergic risk scale and anticholinergic adverse effects in older persons. *Arch Intern Med* 2008;168:508–513.
4. Zhang Y, Steinman MA, Kaplan CM. Geographic variation in outpatient antibiotic prescribing among older adults. *Arch Intern Med* 2012;172:1465–1471.
5. Steinman MA, Hanlon JT. Managing medications in clinically complex elders: "There's got to be a happy medium." *JAMA* 2010;304:1592–1601.
6. Bain KT, Holmes HM, Beers MH, et al. Discontinuing medications: a novel approach for revising the prescribing stage of the medication-use process. *J Am Geriatr Soc* 2008;56:1946–1952.
7. The American Geriatric Society 2012 Beers Criterial Update Expert Panel. American Geriatrics Society updated Beers criteria for potentially inappropriate medication use in older adults. American Geriatric Society, 2012.
8. Lam MP, Cheung BM. The use of STOPP/START criteria as a screening tool for assessing the appropriateness of medications in the elderly population. *Expert Rev Clin Pharmacol* 2012;5:187–197.
9. United States. Centers for Disease Control and Prevention, National Center for Injury Prevention and Control. Web-based Inquiry Statistics Query and Reporting Systems (WISQARS). 2012. http://cdc.gov/injury/wisqars. Last accessed 1/12/15.
10. Hornbrook MC, Stevens VJ, Wingfield DJ, et al. Preventing falls among community-dwelling older persons: results from a randomized control trial. *Gerontologist* 1994;34:16–23.
11. Fuller GF. Falls in the elderly. *Am Fam Physician* 2000;61:2159–2168.
12. American Geriatrics Society, British Geriatrics Society, and American Academy of Orthopaedic Surgeons Panel on Falls Prevention. Guideline for the prevention of falls in older persons. *J Am Geriatr Soc* 2001;49:664–672.
13. Michael YL, Lin JS, Whitlock EP, et al. *Interventions to Prevent Falls in Older Adults: An Updated Systematic Review [Internet]*. Rockville, MD: Agency for Healthcare Research and Quality (US); 2010. (Evidence Syntheses, No. 80.) Available at: http://www.ncbi.nlm.nih.gov/books/NBK51685/. Last accessed 1/12/15.
14. Santesso N, Carrasco-Labra A, Brignardello-Petersen R. Hip protectors for preventing hip fractures in older people. *Cochrane Database Syst Rev* 2014;(3):CD001255.
15. Guralnik JM, Ferrucci L, Simonsick EM, et al. Lower-extremity function in persons over the age of 70 years as a predictor of subsequent disability. *N Engl J Med* 1995;332:556–561.
16. Podsiadlo D, Richardson S. The timed "Up & Go": a test of basic functional mobility for frail elderly persons. *J Am Geriatr Soc* 1991;39:142–148.
17. Centers for Disease Control and Prevention. Physical activity: how much physical activity do older adults need? http://www.cdc.gov/physicalactivity/everyone/guidelines/olderadults.html. Last accessed 1/12/15.
18. Topolski TD, LeGerfo JL, Patrick DL, et al. The rapid assessment of physical activity (RAPA) among older adults. *Prev Chronic Dis* 2006;3:A118.
19. Carr DB, Ott BR. The older driver with cognitive impairment: "It's a very frustrating life." *JAMA* 2010;303:1632–1641.
20. Carr DB, Schwartzberg JG, Manning L, et al. *Physicians guide to assessing and counseling older drivers*, 2nd ed. Washington, DC: National Highway Traffic Safety Administration; 2010. Available at: http://geriatricscareonline.org/ProductAbstract/physicians-guide-to-assessing-and-counseling-older-drivers/B013. Last accessed 1/12/15.

21. National Kidney and Urologic Diseases Information Clearinghouse (NKUDIC). National Institute of Health Publication No. 08-4132. Urinary incontinence in women. 2010. Available at: http://kidney.niddk.nih.gov/KUDiseases/pubs/uiwomen/index. aspx. Last accessed 1/12/15.

22. Gardner SE, Frantz RA, Bergquist S, et al. A prospective study of the pressure ulcer scale for healing (PUSH). *J Gerontol A Biol Sci Med Sci* 2005;60:93–97.

23. Morley J. Anorexia of aging: physiologic and pathologic. *Am J Clin Nutr* 1997;66:760–773.

24. Ryan C, Bryant E, Eleazer P, et al. Unintentional weight loss in long-term care: predictor of mortality in the elderly. *South Med J* 1995;88:721–724.

25. Sullivan DH, Johnson LE, Bopp MM, et al. Prognostic significance of monthly weight fluctuations among older nursing home residents. *J Gerontol A Biol Sci Med Sci* 2004;59:M633–M639.

26. Grabowski DC, Ellis JE. High body mass index does not predict mortality in older people: analysis of the Longitudinal Study of Aging. *J Am Geriatr Soc* 2001;49:968–979.

27. Blaum CS, Xue QL, Michelon E, et al. The association between obesity and the frailty syndrome in older women: the Women's Health and Aging Studies. *J Am Geriatr Soc* 2001;53:927–934.

28. Hubbard RE, Lang IA, Llewellyn DJ, et al. Frailty, body mass index, and abdominal obesity in older people. *J Gerontol A Biol Sci Med Sci* 2010;65:377–381.

29. Mitchell SL, Kiely DK, Hamel MB, et al. Estimating prognosis for nursing home residents with advanced dementia. *JAMA* 2004;291:2734–2740.

30. Finucane TE, Christmas C, Travis K. Tube feeding in patients with advanced dementia: a review of the evidence. *JAMA* 1999;282:1365–1370.

31. Fried LP, Tangen CM, Walston J, et al. Frailty in older adults: evidence for a phenotype. *J Gerontol A Biol Sci Med Sci* 2001;56:M146–M156.

32. Espinoza S, Walston JD. Frailty in older adults: insights and interventions. *Cleve Clin J Med* 2005;72:1105–1112.

33. Applebaum PS. Assessment of patients' competency to consent to treatment. *N Engl J Med* 2007;357:1834–1840.

39 Allergy and Immunology

Michael J. Tang, Parul J. Gor, and James A. Tarbox

ALLERGY

GENERAL PRINCIPLES

Epidemiology

- Allergy is highly prevalent in the US, affecting about 50 million people.
- Approximately 30 to 60 million people in the US have seasonal and perennial allergies.[1] Food allergies have been reported in up to 3% to 6% of the general population, while life-threatening reactions to insect stings have been reported in approximately 3% of adults and 0.6% to 0.8% of children.[2,3]
- Medication allergies are difficult to study and vary greatly among populations.

Classification

The classic **Gel and Coombs classification** is as follows:

- **Type I reaction** (immediate hypersensitivity): Immunoglobulin E (IgE)-mediated release of histamine and other mediators from mast cells and basophils. Allergic reactions further characterized in this section involve the type I reaction
- **Type II reaction** (cytotoxic hypersensitivity): Immunoglobulin G (IgG) or immunoglobulin M (IgM) antibodies bound to cell surface antigens, with subsequent complement fixation
- **Type III reaction** (immune complex hypersensitivity): Circulating antigen-antibody immune complexes that deposit in postcapillary venules, with subsequent complement fixation
- **Type IV reaction** (cell-mediated delayed hypersensitivity): Mediated by T cells

Pathophysiology

- For an allergic reaction to occur, **allergen-specific IgE** must be cross-linked on the surface of mast cells and basophils. Within minutes, there is an initial release of mediators known as the **early phase**. Lymphocytes and eosinophils arrive 4 to 72 hours later and drive the **late-phase** response. Often, symptoms subside or disappear completely after the early phase only to reappear with the late phase.
  - **Early phase:** Mast cells release histamine, cytokines, leukotrienes, prostaglandins, and tryptase. Because mast cells are the only cells in the body that release tryptase, **the serum level of tryptase is increased after a systemic allergic reaction.** Basophils also release histamine and various cytokines. Histamine mainly binds to the H_1 receptor, leading to increased vascular permeability and edema. Perturbation of nerve endings leads to increased mucus production and the sensation of itch.
  - **Late phase:** Lymphocytes are recruited to the site by the cytokines released in the early-phase response. These cells further exacerbate the reaction through the release of additional cytokines. The presence of certain cytokines and leukotrienes then attracts eosinophils, and they release additional leukotrienes, which can lead to bronchoconstriction. They also release several toxic proteins, including major basic protein, which leads to disruption of the airway epithelium.

- An **allergen** is a protein or carbohydrate against which the body can produce IgE. Allergens may be inhaled, ingested, or injected into the body, where they encounter IgE bound to mast cells or basophils. The first time that a person is exposed to a specific allergen, no allergic response can occur because this initial exposure is required for the immune system to make IgE against the allergen.
  - **Seasonal allergens** are certain airborne allergens that are more prevalent at specific times of the year. These seasonal allergens include tree, grass, and weed pollens (most often seen in the spring, early summer, and early fall, respectively).
  - **Perennial allergens** are present all year and include dust mites, cockroaches, and molds (although some molds have a seasonal increase in midsummer).
  - Other allergens are encountered only through specific exposures. These include medications, stinging insect venoms, animal danders, and foods.
- **Haptenation:** Most medications are too small to elicit an IgE response; however, the drug may bind to serum proteins, which then allow for sensitization. The IgE produced is directed against the medication, and subsequent exposure leads to binding of IgE to the drug alone.

DIAGNOSIS

Clinical Presentation

History
- **Symptoms:** Runny nose, sneezing, wheezing, conjunctivitis, rashes, or swelling that occurs year round (perennial) or restricted to specific exposures.
- **Exacerbating/alleviating factors:** Pets, smoke, perfume, change in air temperature, and certain seasons.
- **Environmental history:** Where does the patient work, live, and play? What exposures are present in each of these environments? Does the patient have a pet?
- **Family history:** Are there other members of the family with allergic diseases (including asthma)? A child with one parent with allergic disorders has a 40% chance of having allergies (and/or allergic asthma). Two parents increase the risk to 60% to 80%.
- **Psychosocial issues:** It is important to determine if any psychosocial issues exist that may interfere with the patient's care. For example, one should determine if the patient has appropriate social support. It is also helpful to determine the patient's goal for the visit.

Physical Examination
- **Appearance**
  - **Mouth breathing** due to nasal congestion may be present.
  - Because of edema in the nasal tissues, the draining veins under the eyes may be compressed, leading to pooling of blood and darkening of the region under the eyes, known as **allergic shiners.**
  - Patients may also have infraorbital folds or **Dennie-Morgan lines,** as well as a **nasal crease,** a transverse line across the lower portion of the nose.
  - Patients with the hyper-IgE syndrome have a coarse facies and may have recurrent "cold" soft tissue abscesses, which are abscesses that lack erythema.
- **Skin examination**
  - **Urticaria,** or hives, is a maculopapular erythematous, often pruritic, eruption in the cutaneous tissues.
  - **Angioedema** is edema in the subcutaneous (SC) tissues and is often painful but not pruritic.
  - **Dermatographism** (or dermographism) is the tendency to form wheal-and-flare responses (urticate) to firm pressure applied to the skin.

○ **Head, ears, eyes, nose, and throat:** The anatomy of the nose must be clearly evaluated, looking for the presence of swollen and edematous turbinates, pale- or blue-tinged nasal mucosa, polyps (whitish to clear sacs often hanging from the underside of the turbinates), and any septal deviation, ulceration, or perforation that may alter airflow.
- **Pulmonary:** A thorough lung examination is required; make note of wheezing or increased expiratory phase. In some patients, the use of a forced expiratory maneuver helps to expose wheezing that cannot be heard at rest.

Diagnostic Testing
- All testing modalities may have false positives, and therefore, correlation with the patient's symptoms and exposures is necessary.
- **Epicutaneous: This is the most specific test available and identifies most clinically significant allergens.** Although sensitivity to most allergens can be evaluated using epicutaneous or intradermal skin tests, food allergens should only be evaluated using epicutaneous methods.
- **Intradermal:** This type of skin test is more sensitive than epicutaneous testing but less specific. Irritant effects may cause many more false positives, and the risk of a systemic reaction is also increased with intradermal testing.
- **In vitro tests:** These tests evaluate for the presence of IgE in the patient's serum against specific allergens, which are usually immobilized on a disk or plastic plate. They only determine whether specific IgE exists in the blood and may give positives to allergens to which the patient is not being exposed or is not clinically allergic. In general, the sensitivity and specificity of in vitro tests are similar to those of intradermal skin testing alone.

TREATMENT

Medications
- Medications commonly used for allergic conditions are detailed in Table 39-1.
- Treatments for various specific allergic conditions are discussed in detail in following sections.

Corticosteroids
- Steroids inhibit the production of cytokines, which effectively prevents the late-phase response. Steroids do not block the immediate-phase response and are **not a contraindication to skin testing.**
- Long-term use of steroids is associated with side effects. The risk of side effects is much greater with systemic (oral) steroids than with topical (inhaled) steroids.
  ○ **Posterior capsular cataracts** are associated with prolonged use, and annual ophthalmologic examinations are recommended for patients on any continual steroid dose (inhaled or oral).
  ○ **Adrenal suppression** occurs with extended use of oral (any dose) or high-dose inhaled steroids. Short courses (less than a month) of oral steroids do not appear to have a significant effect on the hypothalamus-pituitary-adrenal axis.
  ○ **Osteoporosis** is a risk of corticosteroid use; patients should be encouraged to take supplemental calcium and may require bone density scans to evaluate their risk.

Immunotherapy
- Indications include allergic rhinitis, venom hypersensitivity, and atopic dermatitis if associated with aeroallergen sensitivity. The mechanisms of action are still under investigation.
- Treatment consists of initial SC injections that contain increasing doses of the allergen extracts to which the patient is sensitive. Once the buildup phase is completed, the patient is kept at a maintenance dose for several years. The recommended length of therapy is variable (usually at least 3 to 5 years). Immunotherapy **should be prescribed by an allergist only** after skin testing or, under special circumstances, based on the results of in vitro testing.

TABLE 39-1 Commonly Used Outpatient Medications in Allergy and Immunology

Medication	Class	Usual adult dosage	Indications	Major side effects	Other[a]
Chlorpheniramine	A-1st	4 mg q12 hours	AR, UR, ANA	Fatigue, drowsiness, impaired mental performance, dry mouth, urinary retention	Category B 72 hours[b]
Diphenhydramine	A-1st	25–50 mg q6–8 hours	AR, UR, ANA	Fatigue, drowsiness, impaired mental performance, dry mouth, urinary retention	Category B 72 hours[b]
Cetirizine	A-2nd	10 mg qd	AR, UR, ANA	Minimal sedation	Category B 7–10 days[b]
Levocetirizine	A-2nd	5 mg qd	AR, UR, ANA	Minimal sedation	Category B 7–10 days
Fexofenadine	A-2nd	60 mg bid 180 mg qd	AR, UR, ANA		Category C 5–7 days[b]
Loratadine	A-2nd	10 mg qd	AR, UR, ANA		Category B 7–10 days[b]
Azelastine	NA	137 μg/spray 1–2 sprays each nostril bid	AR	Dysgeusia, upper respiratory irritation/infection, sedation possible	Category B 7 days[b]
Olopatadine	NA/MS	665 μg/spray 2 sprays each nostril bid	AR	Dysgeusia, epistaxis, nasal ulceration	Category C 7 days[b]
	OA/MS	0.1% solution (Patanol) 1 drop each eye bid 0.2% solution (Pataday) 1 drop each eye qd	AC	Headache, ocular irritation, upper respiratory irritation	Category C
Bepotastine	OA	1.5% solution 1 drop each eye bid	AC	Taste abnormality, headache, ocular irritation, upper respiratory irritation/infection	Category C

Drug	Route	Dose	Indication	Side effects	Pregnancy category
Azelastine/ fluticasone	NA/NS	137/50 µg/spray 1 spray each nostril bid	AR	Dysgeusia, nausea/vomiting, upper respiratory irritation/infection, epistaxis, rare systemic steroid side effects	Category C
Beclomethasone	IS	40, 80 µg/inhalation 1–2 inhalations bid	AS	Headache, upper respiratory irritation/ infection, possible systemic steroid side effects	Category C
	NS	42 µg/spray (Beconase AQ) 1–2 sprays each nostril bid 80 µg/spray (Qnasl) 2 sprays each nostril qd	AR	Nasal irritation, epistaxis, pharyngitis, rare systemic steroid side effects	Category B
Budesonide	IS	90, 180 µg/inhalation 2 inhalations qd	AS	Headache, dyspepsia, dyspepsia, nausea, arthralgia, weakness, back pain, upper respiratory irritation/infection, possible systemic steroid side effects	Category C
	NS	32 µg/spray 1–2 sprays each nostril qd	AR	Nasal irritation, epistaxis, pharyngitis, rare systemic steroid side effects	Category B
Ciclesonide	IS	80, 160 µg/inhalation 1–2 inhalations bid	AS	Headache, upper respiratory irritation/ infection, possible systemic steroid side effects	Category C
	NS	37 µg/spray (Zetonna) 1 spray each nostril qd 50 µg/spray (Omnaris) 2 sprays each nostril qd	AR	Headache, upper respiratory irritation/ infection, epistaxis, rare systemic steroid side effects	Category C
Cromolyn	MS	5.2 mg/spray 1 spray each nostril 3–6x/day	AR	Headache, nasal irritation, cough, hoarseness, bad taste	Category B
	Ophth. MS	4% solution 1–2 drops each eye 4–6x/day	AC, VC	Eye irritation	Category B

(*Continued*)

TABLE 39-1 Commonly Used Outpatient Medications in Allergy and Immunology *(Continued)*

Medication	Class	Usual adult dosage	Indications	Major side effects	Other[a]
Flunisolide	IS	80 µg/inhalation 2–4 inhalations bid	AS	Headache, upper respiratory irritation/infection, dyspepsia, possible systemic steroid side effects	Category C
	NS	25 µg/spray 2 sprays each nostril bid–tid	AR	Nasal irritation, rare systemic steroid side effects	Category C
Fluticasone	IS	44, 110, 220 µg/inhalation (Flovent HFA) 2 inhalations bid 50, 100, 250 µg/inhalation (Flovent Diskus) 1–2 inhalations bid	AS	Headache, fatigue, malaise, oral thrush, upper respiratory irritation/infection, hoarseness, dysphonia, pain, rash, nausea/vomiting, possible systemic steroid side effects	Category C
	NS	27.5 µg/spray (Veramyst) 50 µg/spray (Flonase) 1–2 sprays each nostril qd	AR	Headache, nausea/vomiting, upper respiratory irritation/infection, epistaxis, rare systemic steroid side effects	Category C
Mometasone	IS	110, 220 µg/inhalation 1–2 inhalations qd–bid	AS	Headache, fatigue, pain, upper respiratory irritation/infection, oral thrush, dyspepsia, possible systemic steroid side effects	Category C
	NS	50 µg/spray 2 sprays each nostril qd	AR	Headache, upper respiratory irritation/infection, rare steroid side effects	Category C
Triamcinolone	NS	55 µg/spray 1–2 sprays each nostril qd	AR	Headache, upper respiratory irritation/infection, dysgeusia, dyspepsia, rare systemic steroid side effects	Category C
Mometasone/formoterol	IS/LABA	100/5 µg/inhalation 200/5 µg/inhalation 2 inhalations bid	AS	LABAs increase the risk of asthma-related death and should only be used in those not controlled with IS alone; headache, upper respiratory irritation/infection, possible systemic steroid side effects	Category C

Drug	Class	Dosing	Indication	Side effects	Pregnancy category
Fluticasone/salmeterol	IS/LABA	41, 115, 230/21 µg/inhalation (Advair HFA) 2 inhalations bid; 100, 250, 500/50 µg/inhalation (Advair Diskus) 1 inhalation qd	AS	LABAs increase the risk of asthma-related death and should only be used in those not controlled with IS alone; headache, upper respiratory irritation/infection, nausea vomiting, possible systemic steroid side effects	Category C
Salmeterol Diskus	LABA	50 µg/inhalation 1 inhalation bid	AS	LABAs increase the risk of asthma-related death and should only be used in those not controlled with IS alone	Category C
Albuterol	SABA	90 µg/inhalation 2 puffs inhalations q4-6 hours	AS	May make patient tremulous, nervous, anxious, tachycardic, etc.	Category C
Zafirlukast	LTA	20 mg bid	AS, AR	Headache, nausea	Category B
Montelukast	LTA	10 mg qhs	AS, AR	Headache	Category B
Zileuton	LTA	600 mg qid; 1,200 mg (extended release) bid	AS, AR	Headache, upper respiratory irritation/infection, dyspepsia, nausea, diarrhea, elevated transaminases (monitor)	Category C
Ipratropium bromide	IAC	17 µg/inhalation 2 inhalations 4-6x/day	AS	Headache, upper respiratory irritation/infection, dyspepsia, nausea	Category B
	NAC	21, 42 µg/spray 2 sprays each nostril bid-tid	NAR	Dry mouth, nasal mucosa, epistaxis	Category B

A-1st, first-generation antihistamine; A-2nd, second-generation antihistamine; AC, allergic conjunctivitis; ANA, anaphylaxis; AR, allergic rhinitis; AS, asthma; IAC, inhaled anticholinergic; IS, inhaled steroid; LABA, long-acting bronchodilator; LTA, leukotriene antagonist; MS, mast cell stabilizer; NA, intranasal antihistamine; NAC, intranasal anticholinergic; NAR, nonallergic rhinitis; NS, nasal steroid; OA, ocular antihistamine; SABA, short-acting bronchodilator; UR, urticaria; VC, vernal conjunctivitis.

[a]Includes pregnancy category: A, human studies show no risk; B, no evidence of risk in studies; C cannot rule out risk due to lack of studies; D, evidence of risk.
[b]Time before skin testing that antihistamine should be discontinued.

- Adverse reactions are usually mild, with only localized pruritus, erythema, and edema. However, some reactions can be severe and include asthmatic flares, diffuse urticaria, and even anaphylactic shock.
  - The highest risk of a reaction is during the initial buildup phase; however, **a reaction may occur at any dose.**
  - A physician and staff who are experienced in treating anaphylactic shock and an emergency cart **must** be immediately available.
  - The risk for a reaction from an injection is greatest up to 30 minutes following the shot (60 minutes for venom immunotherapy), and patients should not be allowed to leave the office until this period has passed.
  - Any time that a patient has had a significant reaction, immunotherapy should be held, pending discussion with an allergist.

Other Nonpharmacologic Therapies

Environmental control measures are the first and most important therapy for allergic disorders. These interventions limit or prevent exposure to allergens. Examples of appropriate control measures include the following:

- **Pets** (in particular pets with fur)
  - Keep pet out of home or at least out of the bedroom.
  - Remove carpeting.
  - Wash the pet regularly.
- **Dust mites**
  - Wash bedding in hot water ($\geq 130°F$) weekly.
  - Use synthetic pillows, blankets, and mattresses.
  - Encase the pillows and mattress in dust mite–proof encasings.
  - Maintain home humidity level at $<45\%$.

ANAPHYLAXIS

GENERAL PRINCIPLES

- Anaphylaxis represents the **rapid release of mast cell mediators.** The symptoms of anaphylaxis may be related to one or, more commonly, multiple organ systems and are among the most rapid and profound of the allergic reactions; without rapid treatment, they may prove to be fatal.
- Anaphylactic reactions are not rare. Lifetime prevalence is 0.05% to 2%.
  - Antibiotics and nonsteroidal anti-inflammatory drugs (NSAIDs) are the most common culprits in adults. Insect stings are another common cause.
  - Penicillin reactions occur in 1 to 5 per 10,000 patient courses of treatment, and fatalities can occur at 1 per 50,000 to 100,000 courses.
- Although the office management is essentially identical, anaphylaxis can be divided into two broad categories: IgE mediated and non–IgE-mediated (formerly known as anaphylactoid reactions).

Classification

- Anaphylactic reactions can be classified according to the severity of the reaction. The most common classification is shown in Table 39-2.
- Anaphylaxis may be monophasic, biphasic, or, in rare cases, prolonged. As noted previously, classic allergic reactions may have an early and a delayed or late phase. It is not uncommon to see a patient successfully treated for anaphylaxis has a second, often equally profound, reaction 4 to 12 hours following the initial anaphylactic reaction.

TABLE 39-2	Classification of Anaphylactic/Anaphylactoid Reactions According to Severity			
Grade	Skin	GI	Respiratory	Cardiovascular
I	Pruritus, urticaria, flushing, edema, etc.	None	None	None
II	Pruritus, urticaria, flushing, edema, etc.	Nausea	Dyspnea	Tachycardia Hypotension
III	Pruritus, urticaria, flushing, edema, etc.	Vomiting Diarrhea	Bronchospasm Cyanosis	Shock
IV	Pruritus, urticaria, flushing, edema, etc.	Vomiting Diarrhea	Respiratory arrest	Cardiac arrest

Pathophysiology

- The rapid release of vasoactive mediators results in a loss of vascular tone, resultant pooling in the splanchnic bed, and functional hypovolemia. Because of increased capillary permeability, fluid and colloid are lost into the extravascular space and the net effect is a profound decrease in blood pressure (BP).
- Other manifestations of anaphylaxis include bronchospasm, laryngeal edema, profuse nasal discharge, watery itchy eyes, marked postnasal drip, nausea, vomiting, diarrhea, abdominal cramping, uterine cramping, urticaria, angioedema, and rarely anaphylactic-induced pulmonary edema and acute heart failure.

Prevention

- Prevention is one of the most important aspects of management.
- Emphasis should include instructing the patient that **most severe reactions** (including those to food, drugs, stinging insects, and radiocontrast media) **rarely go away.** If these reactions are identified, the patient should be advised to avoid that agent in the future. Individuals who are food sensitive should read all labels for prepared food and inquire for the presence of that food at restaurants. The Food Allergy and Anaphylaxis Network (http://www.foodallergy.org, last accessed 1/13/15) can help individuals by identifying food that contains potent allergens and in designing meals that avoid those allergens.
- Every patient who has experienced anaphylaxis in the past should have a **self-injectable epinephrine prescribed and should carry it at all times.** A medical alert bracelet or necklace that identifies important allergens (especially drug allergy) is also an important preventive measure.

DIAGNOSIS

The diagnosis is likely when **one of the three following criteria** occurs:

- **Acute skin and/or mucosal symptoms** (e.g., hives, pruritus, flushing, and lip/tongue/uvula swelling) and one of the following:
  - Respiratory symptoms (e.g., wheezing, stridor, shortness of breath, hypoxia)
  - Hypotension or associated end-organ dysfunction (e.g., hypotonia, syncope, or incontinence)
- **Exposure to probable allergen and greater than or equal to 2 of the following:**
  - Skin-mucosal tissue involvement
  - Respiratory symptoms
  - Hypotension or end organ dysfunction
  - Persistent gastrointestinal symptoms (e.g., emesis, abdominal pain)

- **Decreased BP after exposure to a known allergen:** systolic BP <90 mm Hg or >30% decrease.[4]

TREATMENT

- Perhaps, the most important aspect of the treatment of anaphylaxis is the **early recognition** and treatment. **If anaphylaxis is suspected, treatment should be initiated without waiting to see if the reaction becomes worse.** True anaphylaxis rarely goes away without treatment.
- The cornerstone of treatment is placing the **patient in supine position** with rapid administration of **epinephrine** and **fluid.** Other therapies may be added later. Most studies of fatal anaphylaxis have demonstrated failure to introduce these measures as a major contributor to the adverse outcome.
- Patients with acute anaphylaxis are often hypoxic. Thus, the rapid establishment of an **adequate airway** is critical.
- The outpatient treatment of anaphylaxis should be directed toward stabilizing the patient to assure a patent airway and maintain an adequate BP. Once this has been established, the patent should be **rapidly transported to an emergency care facility.**

Basic Office Emergency Kit
This should include the following:

- Epinephrine: 1:1,000 aqueous for SC and IM use and 1:10,000 aqueous for IV use
- Racemic epinephrine: inhaler or nebulizer use
- IV fluids: colloid and crystalloid
- Large-bore IV catheter
- Tourniquet
- Oxygen with face mask or nasal prongs
- Ambu bag
- Additional medications: H_1 antihistamines, H_2 antihistamines, and corticosteroids

Medications
Adrenergic/Sympathomimetic Agents
- **The most important agent for the treatment of anaphylaxis is epinephrine,** which should be given as soon as the reaction is recognized. The usual doses for epinephrine are shown in Table 39-3. It is important to remember that in most cases, SC or IM epinephrine is adequate, with recent data suggesting that IM administration is preferred.
- **Intravenous epinephrine should always be given using 0.1 mg/mL or 1:10,000 aqueous.** Intermittent epinephrine can be repeated at 15- to 20-minute intervals and, after four doses, if necessary, can be followed by continuous intravenous therapy until the BP is stabilized.
- Other sympathomimetic agents that may be useful include terbutaline (given SC or IM), dopamine, dobutamine, and norepinephrine. In general, these agents are used in profound and prolonged anaphylactic reactions and are beyond the scope of this chapter.
- Aerosolized racemic epinephrine can be tried in patients who have laryngeal edema; however, if this is not available or is not rapidly effective, use of an endotracheal tube, cricothyroid puncture, or tracheotomy may be necessary to protect the airway. The establishment of an airway should be accompanied by the use of oxygen therapy.

Fluids
- Establishment of IV access and the institution of fluid replacement therapy should be accomplished as soon as epinephrine has been given.

TABLE 39-3	Doses for Epinephrine in the Treatment of Anaphylaxis
Manifestations	**Dose and route**
Grade I or II	0.3–0.5 mg (1:1,000) SC or IM adults 0.01 mg/kg (1:1,000) SC or IM children Repeat every 12–20 minutes × 4
Severe reaction—grade III	0.5–1.0 mg (1:1,000) SC or IM adults 0.01–0.02 mg/kg SC or IM children Repeat every 3 minutes × 4
Severe reaction—grade IV	0.1–1.0 mg (1:10,000) IV adults 0.01–0.02 mg (1:10,000) IV children
Continuous IV therapy, if intermittent therapy fails	0.1–1.0 µg/kg/min; titrate to maintain blood pressure
Upper respiratory compromise	1.0–4.0 mg (racemic) by inhalation (metered-dose inhaler or nebulizer)

- Two types of fluids are available for therapy, **colloid** (albumin, hydroxyethyl starch [hetastarch], pentastarch, dextrans, and blood and blood products) and **crystalloid** (dextrose, saline, and Ringer lactate).
- The choice between colloid and crystalloid has received significant attention. Colloid solutions have been associated with increased oxygen saturation and less increase in lung water than crystalloid solutions. **Some colloid solutions are associated with adverse side effects,** such as anaphylactoid reactions (dextrans) and potential for infectious diseases (blood and blood products). Of the colloid solutions, hydroxyethyl starch is the preferred solution. An initial infusion of 500 mL is followed by any crystalloid fluid with a goal of maintaining adequate BP.

Antihistamines
- Antihistamines are a useful **adjunct** (IV, IM, PO), particularly for patients who experience urticaria or generalized skin pruritus.
- However, **antihistamines are not a substitute for epinephrine and fluids.** One should not give an antihistaminic and then wait to see if it is effective, even in mild anaphylaxis.

Other Agents
- **Glucagon:** May be effective in patients taking β-blockers.
- **β-Agonists:** Patients who experience significant bronchospasm should receive a short-acting β-agonist.

VENOM HYPERSENSITIVITY

GENERAL PRINCIPLES

- Only insects with true stingers are included within the order hymenoptera. Some examples are yellow and bald-faced hornet, yellow jacket, paper wasp, honeybee, and fire ants.
- Venom protein includes many vasoactive amines, alkaloids, and species-specific proteins, such as hyaluronidase, acid phosphatase, and phospholipase A.
- Estimates suggest that 6% to 17% of the population in the US have specific IgE against hymenoptera venoms with a small predilection toward males.[5]
- Clinically significant hymenoptera venom allergic reactions occur in approximately 3% of adults and 0.6% to 0.8% of children.[3]

- **Local reactions** are characterized by induration, erythema, and pain at the sting site. The area involved can spread to regions of the body that are directly adjacent to the sting site, but as long as these sites are contiguous, the reaction is still considered local. These reactions are often quite dramatic and may last for up to a week, but they rarely progress and need no further evaluation.
- **Systemic reactions** include any reactions that occur away from the initial sting site.
  ○ Systemic reactions can include urticaria, bronchospasm, laryngeal edema, hypotension, and other symptoms of anaphylaxis.
  ○ Most patients who have a severe reaction have no history of venom-induced anaphylaxis.
  ○ In patients with a history of a systemic reaction, 60% have a similar reaction with a re-sting; without intervention, this risk decreases to 40% at 10 to 20 years since the previous sting.
- A prior sting sensitizes the individual to the hymenoptera venom, producing a specific IgE. Each subsequent sting can cause an increased likelihood of sensitization.

DIAGNOSIS

- **Type of insect:** It is important to identify the stinging insect, as this will guide skin testing and ultimate therapy. It is also helpful to determine if the patient was stung once or multiple times and by one or more insects.
- **Site of sting:** The location of the sting may be important in determining whether or not a systemic reaction occurred. It can also aid in identification of the insect involved. For example, honeybees usually sting only when they are stepped on. Yellow jackets, however, attack people when their food source is threatened. This usually happens in the late fall, when they can be found scavenging for food in garbage containers.
- Various concentrations of venoms are used to determine sensitivity to hymenoptera venoms. False-positive skin test results may be due to venom cross reactivity.
- **It is preferable to wait 3 to 6 weeks after having a reaction before skin testing to prevent false negatives.**

TREATMENT

- **Local reactions** require supportive care of ice, compression, and elevation. In severe local reactions, corticosteroids (usually 0.5 mg/kg prednisone) are sometimes prescribed to help decrease edema and irritation. Antihistamines can help alleviate the pruritus that is often associated with a sting.
- **Systemic reactions**
  ○ Acute treatment of a systemic reaction includes the liberal use of IM (preferable) or SC epinephrine (Table 39-3) to rapidly treat anaphylaxis.
  ○ β-Agonists are useful if bronchospasm develops from the sting (e.g., albuterol metered-dose inhaler or nebulizer).
  ○ Antihistamines are also helpful in the acute treatment to block the effects of histamine release.
  ○ Corticosteroids (0.5 to 1.0 mg/kg prednisone for 7 to 10 days) reduce edema as well as help prevent a late-phase response from occurring.
  ○ Long-term therapy involves initiation of venom immunotherapy, which has been shown to reduce the patient's risk of a systemic reaction from a subsequent sting to that of the general population. In addition to immunotherapy, any patient who has had a systemic reaction to a sting should have self-injectable epinephrine (EpiPen) prescribed and be taught how to use it appropriately. Besides epinephrine, these patients should have antihistamines with them at all times. Patients are also encouraged to wear a medical alert bracelet that identifies them as venom allergic.
  ○ **Immunotherapy**

- Once patients begin venom immunotherapy, they are protected from subsequent stings, even if they are in the buildup phase of the injections.
- The maintenance dose of the injections usually contains 100 μg venom proteins— roughly 1.5 to 2.0 times the amount in a single sting.
- The question of how long a patient should continue to receive immunotherapy is still under investigation. Some physicians treat for 5 years and then discontinue the shots, whereas others continue immunotherapy until the patient's skin test results become negative or at least a log-fold less reactive. The patient, primary care physician, and allergist should all be involved in the decision of when to discontinue immunotherapy.

URTICARIA AND ANGIOEDEMA

Approximately 15% to 24% of the US population will experience at least one episode of urticaria (hives), angioedema, or both in their lifetime.[6] Among those experiencing either angioedema or urticaria, approximately 50% will present with both conditions simultaneously, while about 10% experience chronic urticaria without angioedema.[7]

Urticaria

GENERAL PRINCIPLES

- Urticaria is an erythematous maculopapular eruption in the superficial layers of the dermis and is associated with pruritus.
- It can be further divided into acute and chronic lesions based on the temporal nature of the rash.
- **Acute urticaria** is any urticarial episode that lasts for <6 weeks.
- **Chronic urticaria** is when the episode lasts for >6 weeks. An urticarial episode consists of a period when hives are present daily or nearly daily. It should be noted that a given crop of hives will likely be present only for a short period, but the patient may have multiple crops of hives during the episode.

Etiology

- **Acute urticaria:** Most of the inciting agents that lead to acute urticaria can be easily identified because of the close temporal relationship between exposure and hive development. Often, the patient has already identified the responsible agent before seeking medical attention.
  - **Foods:** Milk, egg, fish, tree nuts, wheat, soy, peanuts, and shellfish are most common.
  - **Medications:** For example, penicillin.
  - **Infections:** Usually viral infections.
  - **Physical causes:**
    - Cold, heat, pressure, sun, water, vibration, cholinergic stimulation, and exercise.
    - In some patients, exercise is a trigger only when closely preceded by eating.
- **Chronic urticaria:**
  - The inciting agents that lead to chronic urticaria are much more difficult to identify because the temporal relationship is not as clear.
  - These patients tend to be more emotionally and physically affected by their disease and its chronicity.
  - Chronic urticaria has been attributed to the following:
    - **Medications:** for example, NSAIDs.
    - **Collagen vascular disease:** for example, systemic lupus erythematosus.
    - **Neoplasia.**

- **Autoimmune diseases:** most often associated is **thyroid disease.** Patients may be hypo-, hyper-, or even clinically euthyroid but usually have antithyroid peroxidase autoantibodies. In these patients (including the clinically euthyroid), treatment with physiologic doses of thyroid hormone often leads to resolution of the urticaria.
  - **Diet:** frequently eaten foods.
  ○ Patients with chronic urticaria who have autoantibodies directed against either IgE or the high-affinity IgE receptor (FcεRI) do not respond well to antihistamines alone and often require corticosteroids for relief of their hives. Further treatment options for these patients include cyclosporine.[8]
- **Idiopathic urticaria,** the largest set of urticarias, is a catch-all group that represents those cases in which no etiology for the urticaria can be discerned.

Pathophysiology

- Urticaria is dermal edema resulting from vascular dilatation and leakage of fluid into the skin in response to molecules (histamine, bradykinin, leukotriene C4, prostaglandin D_2, and other vasoactive substances) released from mast cells and basophils.[9]
- The prototypical lesion and pruritus are the result of H_1 histamine receptor activation on endothelial and smooth muscle cells leading to increased capillary permeability and H_2 histamine receptor activation leading to arteriolar and venule vasodilation.
- Urticaria can be classified as immunologic or nonimmunologic.
- **Immunologic urticaria:**
  ○ Includes processes mediated by antibodies and/or T cells that result in mast cell activation.
  ○ Urticaria may result from the binding of IgG autoantibodies to IgE and/or to the receptor for IgE molecules on mast cells, representing a type II hypersensitive reaction. These autoimmune urticarias represent 30% to 50% of patients with chronic urticaria. However, mast cell activation can also result from type I, type III, and type IV hypersensitivity reactions.
- **Nonimmunologic urticarias:** Result from mast cell activation through membrane receptors involved in innate immunity (e.g., complement, Toll-like, cytokine/chemokine, and opioid) or by direct toxicity of xenobiotics (haptens, drugs).
- Urticaria may result from different pathophysiologic mechanisms that explain the great heterogeneity of clinical symptoms and the variable responses to treatment.[10]

DIAGNOSIS

Clinical Presentation

- Determine whether the urticaria is acute or chronic.
- It is also important to determine whether the lesions are pruritic or painful. Because vasculitis may present with urticarial lesions, it is critical to determine whether the individual crops of hives **last for >24 hours** and whether they **resolve with scarring.** Both of these conditions are associated with **urticarial vasculitis,** not urticaria.
- Specifically, the physician should look for evidence of thyroid disease, collagen vascular disease, occult infection, or malignancy.
- Several types of urticaria can develop from physical causes. These physical urticarias can be diagnosed by using various maneuvers to reproduce them. For example, **cold urticaria** can be diagnosed by placing an ice cube on the forearm for 4 minutes. The cube is then removed and the arm observed for 10 minutes. A hive that develops at the same location where the ice cube was indicates a positive test result.

Diagnostic Testing

- Consider checking complete blood cell count, erythrocyte sedimentation rate, liver function tests, antithyroid peroxidase antibodies, and urinalysis.

- **Chronic urticaria index:** Commercially available test to detect presence of anti-FcεRI autoantibodies may be obtained. Autologous serum skin testing is another option.
- **Skin and in vitro testing:**
  - Although the specific antigens that are responsible for urticaria are often hard to discern, it may be helpful in some patients to perform skin or in vitro testing.
  - These tests tend to be more useful in patients with acute urticaria in whom a specific food or medication is believed to be the offending agent.
  - Skin testing is the preferred modality to evaluate for allergy; however, patients with severe urticaria may require in vitro testing.
- In addition to specific food allergens, urticaria can develop from sensitivity to food additives. The only reliable test for sensitivity to food additives is a double-blind placebo-controlled challenge. These are usually performed in an allergist's office and take several hours to complete.

TREATMENT

- The most important therapeutic intervention is to **avoid the inciting agent(s)** and/or **treat the underlying condition.**
- Medications include use of antihistamines often in escalating doses, to control the pruritus and urticarial flares (see Table 39-1 for medications and doses). Patients may benefit from the addition of an H_2 receptor antagonist (cimetidine, ranitidine, famotidine, etc.).
- **Tricyclic antidepressants,** such as doxepin (starting dose, approximately 10 to 25 mg daily), are often used because of their strong antihistaminic activity. Because these medications are often sedating, they should be given shortly before or at bedtime.
- **Corticosteroids** can be used (prednisone, 0.5 mg/kg daily) to alleviate urticarial flares, but the numerous side effects of chronic use limit their use in chronic urticaria.
- In patients with **chronic idiopathic urticaria,** it is helpful to control their urticaria with appropriate doses of medications and then withdraw the medications after a specified duration of time (6 weeks to 6 months) to evaluate for the continued presence of urticarial lesions. If the hives recur, restart the medications for another period of time.

Angioedema

GENERAL PRINCIPLES

- Angioedema consists of edema in the deep layers of the dermis and is usually characterized by pain rather than pruritus, as seen with urticaria. Angioedema without urticaria usually presents as a painful, nonpruritic swelling of the deep dermis.
- **Allergic angioedema** is due to an IgE-mediated hypersensitivity reaction to drugs, foods, environmental exposures, insect stings, or other substances resulting in histamine release from mast cells.[11] **Most cases, however, are idiopathic.**
- **Nonallergic angioedema** occurs mostly as a result of **increased bradykinin levels.**[12,13] It can be further classified into hereditary, drug induced, acquired, and miscellaneous.
- **Acquired angioedema:**
  - **Acute:** Allergic, IgE-mediated drugs (angiotensin-converting enzyme [ACE] inhibitors, NSAIDs, fibrinolytic agents, estrogen, narcotics, some antibiotics), foods, insect bites, pollens and fungi, contrast dyes/drugs, serum sickness, and necrotizing vasculitis
  - **Chronic:** Idiopathic, acquired C1 inhibitor deficiency, angioedema-eosinophilia syndrome, and vibratory angioedema
- **Hereditary angioedema** (HAE): The kallikrein-kinin system fails to be inhibited because of **C1 inhibitor (C1INH) absence/dysfunction** and leads to early-acting complement components C4 and C2 to be low.[14]

- ○ Type 1: C1INH deficient or absent due to mutation (80% to 85% of HAE patients)
- ○ Type 2: C1INH dysfunctional (15% to 20% of HAE patients)
- ○ Type 3: C1INH level normal. Occurs in X-linked dominant fashion and therefore affects mainly women[15]
- A deficiency in C1INH can also be acquired, often associated with a hematologic malignancy and the subsequent production of an autoantibody that blocks the function of otherwise normal C1INH.
- **In most cases, angioedema is due to either a drug** (such as an ACE inhibitor, an angiotensin receptor blocker [ARB], aspirin, an antibiotic, or an NSAID) **or C1INH.**
- Angioedema from an ACE inhibitor or ARB can occur **at any point during a course** of treatment and necessitates discontinuation of the drug, even if it is not the cause, because these drugs can enhance angioedema caused by other factors.
  - ○ Clearly, all drugs of the same class need to be avoided; however, it is less clear whether sensitivity to one class necessitates avoidance of the other. However, several case histories have been reported in which angioedema has developed in patients with ACE inhibitor–induced angioedema when treating with an ARB therapy.[16]
  - ○ Therefore, if possible, it is probably best to avoid both classes of medications if a patient develops sensitivity to one of them.

DIAGNOSIS

- The most commonly affected areas are the soles of the feet, palms of the hands (including the thenar eminence), buttocks, and face (including the larynx, lips, tongue, and periorbital regions).
- Attacks can occur after even minimal trauma and may progress around the body. The greatest danger with angioedema is that it may involve the larynx and can lead to complete obstruction of the airway.
- Evaluation of HAE:
  - ○ To evaluate for possible deficiency in C1INH, a C4 level can be obtained. This is low even between attacks in HAE.
  - ○ Further evaluation includes a quantitative C1INH level. If this is not significantly decreased, a functional C1INH level should be obtained. This is reduced in either acquired or hereditary forms.
  - ○ Finally, low C1q level combined with a low C1INH and C4 warrants a workup for acquired angioedema.
  - ○ Patients with known or suspected angioedema due to a complement deficiency should be evaluated by an allergist/immunologist.

TREATMENT

- **Avoidance** of the causative agent is the primary treatment in drug-induced angioedema. As mentioned above, a reaction to an ACE inhibitor or ARB may be the reason to avoid all drugs of both classes.
- In cases in which angioedema is secondary to a malignancy, **treatment of the underlying disease** leads to resolution of the angioedema.
- For the treatment of acute angioedema, antihistamines and corticosteroids are helpful. Epinephrine can be lifesaving for severe reactions.
- Treatment of **HAE should be managed by an allergist/immunologist.** The following is an overview of the current treatment options:
  - ○ Berinert (C1 esterase inhibitor [human]): Plasma-derived concentrate of C1 esterase inhibitor.[17]

- ○ Kalbitor (ecallantide): Reversible inhibitor of plasma kallikrein that has been shown to be effective for acute attacks of swelling in HAE.[18]
- ○ Epinephrine has often been used for HAE, but there is no data to support its efficacy.
- ○ **The use of antihistamines and corticosteroids is of little value.**
- ○ Cinryze (C1 esterase inhibitor [human]): FDA-approved C1 esterase inhibitor that helps prevent swelling and/or painful attacks in teenagers and adults with HAE.[19]
- ○ **Androgens** (usually stanozolol) increase the levels of C1INH and prevent attacks of angioedema.
- ○ **Supportive therapy** is always important. Laryngeal angioedema may develop, and therefore, it is always important to safeguard the airway. Some patients may even require intubation or tracheostomy during their attacks.

DRUG ALLERGIES

GENERAL PRINCIPLES

Epidemiology

- Allergic reactions to drugs represent a major contributor to the spectrum of adverse drug reactions (ADRs).
- Studies suggest that as many as 15.1% of hospitalized patients in the US experience an ADR with an incidence of 3.1% to 6.2% of hospital admissions due to an ADR.[20]

Classification

- **Reactions related to the pharmacologic properties of the drug** such as side effects, toxic reactions, and drug interactions. These reactions are based on the chemical properties of the drug and therefore occur in all patients if a sufficient amount of drug is given. In many cases, the reaction may be lessened by decreasing the dose of the drug.
- **Reactions due to toxic metabolites** may mimic immunologic reactions or side effects. In this case, the biotransformation product rather than the drug itself is the offending agent. The reaction to sulfa-containing drugs (mostly sulfamethoxazole in patients who are HIV positive) is an example of this reaction. These reactions are different from other side effects, and the method for abrogating the reaction differs from that of other types of ADRs.
- **Idiosyncratic reactions** are adverse effects with an unknown mechanism. They are seen in susceptible individuals, but the basis for the susceptibility is not known. **They can occur at any point during therapy.** The reactions may be mild, such as the facial dyskinesis that is seen with phenothiazines, or devastating, such as the aplastic anemia with chloramphenicol. **Idiosyncratic reactions almost invariably recur if the drug is reintroduced.**
- **Immunologic reactions:**
  - ○ Reactions due to the production of antibodies or cytotoxic T cells directed against the drug or a biotransformation of the drug.
  - ○ Examples include contact sensitivity of fixed drug reactions (type IV or cell-mediated reaction); tissue-specific reactions due to T-cell immunity, such as drug-induced hepatitis; tissue-specific damage due to IgG antibodies (type II or III); and drug allergy due to IgE antibodies (type I).
  - ○ Other reactions are believed to have an immunologic basis, but the exact mechanism has not been elucidated. Examples include drug fever and erythema multiforme minor and major (Stevens-Johnson syndrome) and toxic epidermal necrolysis.

Pathophysiology

- **Mechanism of drug allergy:**
  - ○ The majority of the therapeutic agents are low molecular weight organic compounds and are not capable of inducing the production of either antidrug antibodies or T-cell

proliferation. It is only when the drug (or its biotransformation products) reacts covalently with a tissue protein (or carbohydrate) that acts as a hapten that it is capable of inducing an immune response.

 ○ The actual immunogen may be the hapten itself, the hapten-protein conjugate, or a tissue protein that has been altered by interaction so that it is now recognized as a foreign body.

 ○ Because a chemical bond must occur between the drug and the tissue protein, the propensity of that drug to bind to protein determines the allergenic potential of that drug. Thus, β-lactam antibiotics are very reactive with tissue protein and are major allergens, whereas cardiac glycosides are very nonreactive, and true allergy to this class of drugs is rarely seen.

• **Route of administration** is important in the induction phase of drug allergy.

 ○ Parenteral administration of a drug has the highest potential for inducing an immunologic reaction.

 ○ Oral administration is much less likely to result in an immunologic reaction to a drug.

 ○ Application of a drug to the skin may result in a contact sensitivity (type IV) rather than the production of antidrug IgE.

• **In all but the rarest cases**, **the actual immunogen is not known.**

 ○ This is important because the development of in vivo tests (skin tests) or in vitro tests (ImmunoCAP) is based on a thorough knowledge of the chemical structure of the allergen.

 ○ For the first-generation β-lactam antibiotics, the immunogens are well described or are surmised from extensive skin testing. Seventy five percent of patients with a history of penicillin reaction have a positive skin test result to penicilloyl-polylysine (Pre-Pen).

 ○ Other drug classes are being investigated, but the causative allergen in most cases is not known. It is possible to use the native drug as an allergen in the hope that the drug or its metabolite will provide an appropriate allergenic structure; however, the predictive value of these tests is questionable.

DIAGNOSIS

Clinical Presentation

• The drug or drugs that the patient had been taking at the time of the reaction. If the reaction occurred in the past, a chart review may be necessary.

• The **type of reaction** and the potential for that reaction to be immunologic in nature. It is often helpful for the physician to make a list of the potential offending drugs and then to rank the drugs by allergenic potential.

• The **severity of reaction** is also very important, as it determines the steps that may have to be taken to abrogate a similar reaction. An anaphylactic reaction is much more significant than a minor skin rash.

• A **history of reactions** to drugs is very helpful. Several groups have demonstrated that **a patient who has reacted to one drug is more likely to react to another when compared to a patient who has never reacted.** For some patients, true reactions are seen to multiple drug classes and probably represent an increased ability to react to haptenated proteins. This has been referred to as the **multiple drug allergy syndrome.**

• A **family history** of drug allergy is also a predictive factor. The relative risk of a drug reaction is multifold higher if the patient's mother or father has also had a drug reaction.

• Finally, **the presence of concurrent illness** should be established to ensure that the reaction is due to a drug and not from the illness. For example, a facial rash in a patient with lupus erythematosus is most likely the result of the disease process and not a drug reaction.

Diagnostic Testing

• **In vivo or in vitro testing:**

 ○ Skin testing is the most important technique for the diagnosis of a true drug allergy. Referral to an allergist/immunologist is necessary for skin testing to be performed.

- ○ In the case of penicillin or the first-generation cephalosporins, skin testing is easily performed and highly predictive of an allergic reaction.
- ○ In vitro testing has the same drawback as skin testing, as it relies on knowledge of the allergen.
- ○ These tests are further compromised by the amount of time that is necessary for the test to be performed (usually >24 hours), and, thus, they are not helpful in the acute situation.
- ○ Evidence has demonstrated that skin testing may not be reliable within the first several weeks after a severe drug reaction, and this may be the one situation in which in vitro testing is necessary.
- **Provocative dose challenge:**
  - ○ A provocative dose challenge provides a method for determining a patient's sensitivity to a given drug or drug class and for initiating therapy. Indeed, in practice, this is performed only when a decision to start the patient on the drug has been made.
  - ○ The challenge begins with a small (1:100) dose of the drug and proceeds rapidly to higher doses. If the patient tolerates a low dose (0.1 to 1 mg), then increasing doses are given at 15- to 30-minute intervals.
  - ○ The provocative dose challenge should be performed in a medical setting, where appropriate resuscitative measures are available.

TREATMENT

Alternate Drug Class

- The most effective therapy for drug allergy is the selection of an alternative drug class.
- In most cases, an effective therapeutic agent exists that does not cross-react with the drug to which the patient is sensitive.
- In some cases, an alternative drug may be of the same drug class but lacks a reactive side chain.
  - ○ An example is the substitution of lisinopril or enalapril, which does not have a sulfonamide side chain, and of captopril, which contains a sulfonamide.
  - ○ Similarly, ethacrynic acid may substitute for furosemide.
  - ○ The substitution of an alternative antibiotic, which may differ only in a reactive side chain, is often very effective and precludes the need for skin testing and desensitization.
- The selection of an alternative modality is also effective in anaphylactoid reactions.

Provocative Dose Challenge

- This can often be effective when skin testing or in vitro testing is not available.
- The physician should choose the drug class that is least likely to give a positive reaction. For example, patients who have a history of a reaction to a local anesthetic (which almost never causes a true allergic reaction) can receive a provocative challenge with the least reactive group of agents (those that do not contain a paraaminobenzoic acid ester group).
- Because preservatives such as parabens or additional agents such as β-adrenergic agonists can cause reactions, we recommend that the provocative challenge be carried out using preservative-free solutions.
- These are available as obstetric preparations of most local anesthetics. If a small (1 mL) dose of the local anesthetic does not provoke a reaction, this anesthetic can be used without hesitation.

Pretreatment Protocols

Pretreatment protocols to prevent or temper a reaction are available for a number of drug classes that cause reactions by anaphylactic or anaphylactoid mechanisms. The protocol that is used in the reintroduction of radiocontrast media is presented in Table 39-4.

| TABLE 39-4 | Protocol for Pretreatment of Patients with a History of Radiocontrast Media Reactions |

| Time before | Drug and dose | | |
the procedure	Prednisone[a]	Cimetidine[b]	Diphenhydramine[c]
13 hours	50 mg PO or IV	300 mg PO or IV	
7 hours	50 mg PO or IV	300 mg PO or IV	
1 hour[d]	50 mg PO or IV	300 mg PO or IV	50 mg PO or IV

[a]Other agents include methylprednisolone, 40 mg IV.
[b]Other agents include ranitidine, 150 mg.
[c]Other agents include chlorpheniramine, 10–12 mg.
[d]Can also add ephedrine, 25 mg PO, 1 hour before procedure.

Drug Desensitization

- The purpose of desensitization is to prevent a potentially life-threatening reaction. The procedure does not prevent the appearance of mild skin reactions such as pruritus or urticaria.
- This **should only be performed under the supervision of an allergist/immunologist** and only in a location that is capable of treating significant and potentially prolonged anaphylaxis.
- The desensitization procedure involves the introduction of minute amounts of the drug and then slowly increasing the dose (usually by doubling) every 15 to 20 minutes until a full therapeutic dose is achieved.
- The potential for a reaction is much less when oral medication is used.
- Importantly, **the desensitized state lasts only as long as the drug is given.** Once the drug has been stopped, the patient becomes sensitive again in 8 to 48 hours. **If the patient misses taking the drug for >12 hours, the procedure has to be repeated.** If the physician foresees a need to retreat with the same medication in a short period of time, the drug should be continued (usually orally) to avoid having to undergo another desensitization.

FOOD ALLERGIES

GENERAL PRINCIPLES

- General sensitivity to foods is common, but **food allergy is a term reserved for an immunologic-mediated sensitivity** (i.e., IgE mediated, cell mediated, and mixed).
- Patients may present with a number of varying symptoms: urticaria/angioedema, asthmatic flares, abdominal cramping, diarrhea, rhinoconjunctivitis, and anaphylaxis.
- Food allergy is thought to occur in <3% to 4% of adults. The overall prevalence is growing, particularly in developed countries.
- **IgE mediated:** Acute onset of symptoms including urticaria/angioedema, oral allergy syndrome (pruritus and mild edema confined to oral cavity), rhinitis, asthma, anaphylaxis, and food-dependent/exercise-induced anaphylaxis (food triggers anaphylaxis only if ingestion is followed by exercise).
- **Cell mediated:** Delayed onset with possible chronic clinical picture with symptoms of atopic dermatitis and/or eosinophilic gastroenteropathies (varying degrees of dysphagia or odynophagia).
- **Mixed IgE and cell mediated:** Delayed onset with dietary protein enterocolitis as well as dietary protein proctitis giving mucus-laden bloody stools in infants.[21,22]

- **Nonimmunologically mediated** mechanisms fall into the categories of enzymatic or transport deficiencies (e.g., lactase deficiency or glucose/galactose malabsorption, respectively).
- The mechanisms of allergy and tolerance have been under investigation, with the breakdown of gastrointestinal barrier and nonoral exposure (via respiratory sensitization and skin sensitization) as possible contributors to food allergies.[23-25]
- Proteins easily degraded by heat and chemicals are less likely to cause severe reactions in contrast to stable proteins as found in nuts and seeds.[26]
- Genetic influences have also been identified, as peanut allergy is much more likely in a child whose sibling has a known peanut allergy.[27]
- Hygiene theory postulates that decreased exposures to bacteria and infections may influence immune function with a more atopic clinical picture and an immune deviation toward a Th2 response, where interleukin (IL)-4, IL-5, and IL-13 induce IgE and eosinophilic inflammation, leading to disease.[28,29]

DIAGNOSIS

Clinical Presentation

- IgE-mediated food allergy:
  - Determine the timing of the reaction after ingestion of the suspected food.
  - Most allergic reactions occur within 15 to 30 minutes of ingestion. Reactions that occur hours after eating are much less likely to represent an allergic response.
  - In adults, the most often offending agents are peanuts, tree nuts, and shellfish. In children, the common offending foods also include milk, wheat, soy, and egg.
- Non–IgE-mediated food allergy:
  - Non–IgE-mediated food allergies can also present as food intolerance as described above.
  - **Eosinophilic gastroenteritis** is a disorder that is characterized by eosinophilic infiltration of the gastrointestinal wall and peripheral eosinophilia. These patients often present with malabsorption and usually have allergic diseases as well. They should be evaluated and treated by a specialist.

Diagnostic Testing

- The following tests should be performed in an allergist/immunologist's office. Any positive result on testing must be correlated with the patient's symptoms.
- Skin testing for the various food allergens is often performed. Because of the irritant nature of many food allergen preparations and the possibility of systemic reactions, only epicutaneous and not intradermal testing should be performed.
- In vitro testing allows for the determination of specific IgE against various food allergens.
- **The gold standard for diagnosing food allergy is the double-blind placebo-controlled food challenge.** These challenges can be dangerous and should be performed by allergists either in their clinic or in the hospital. If a food challenge does not show sensitivity to the suspected food, an open-label challenge with the food is usually performed.

TREATMENT

- **Avoid the offending food.**
- Educate the patient and family members/friends about how allergic reactions to foods occur, how to avoid these reactions, and how to treat when a reaction occurs.
- To treat episodes, the patient (and caregivers) should always have immediately available self-injectable epinephrine.

- ○ Any patients for whom self-injectable epinephrine is prescribed should have the proper use of the injector demonstrated to them in the physician's office and be able to replicate this for the physician prior to leaving.
  - ○ They should also be aware that whenever they have used their epinephrine, they should seek immediate medical attention.
- The risk of death from food allergies is increased when patients have asthma (see Chapter 16) and are unaware that they have ingested an allergen, when they are away from home or from a primary caregiver when the reaction occurs, and when the time to epinephrine injection is >30 minutes.[30]
- **Allergen-specific immunotherapeutics** are designed to present the allergen in a context that stimulates a Th1 immune response (e.g., interferon [IFN]-γ) or generates T regulatory cells that result in down-regulation of Th2 responses.
- **Anti-IgE antibodies** (omalizumab) as well as cytokine/anticytokine medications are considered not allergen specific and designed to modulate or interrupt the allergic responses.

RHINITIS AND RHINOCONJUNCTIVITIS

GENERAL PRINCIPLES

- Allergic rhinitis is inflammation of the nasal mucosa, and allergic rhinoconjunctivitis is the combination of inflammation of nasal mucosa and conjunctiva due to allergies.
- The disease tends to occur predominantly in childhood, and the onset is usually before puberty.
- Untreated, rhinoconjunctivitis can lead to several other diseases, including sinusitis, otitis media, and asthma.
- Nearly one-fifth of the general population has a form of seasonal or perennial allergic rhinoconjunctivitis, or both. In the US, approximately 30 to 60 million people are affected, 10% to 30% of adults and up to 40% of children.[1]
- **Inflammatory rhinitis/rhinoconjunctivitis**
  - ○ **Allergic:** Rhinitis due to the presence of specific IgE against seasonal or perennial allergens, or both. Inhaled allergens are recognized and processed by dendritic cells (antigen-presenting cells). The allergen is presented to CD4+ T cells, which produce cytokines that influence basophil proliferation (IL-13), B-cell class switching to IgE synthesis (IL-4), eosinophil proliferation (IL-5), and mast cell proliferation (IL-9).[31]
  - ○ **Infectious:** Often associated with viral upper respiratory infections (URI).
  - ○ **Nonallergic rhinitis with eosinophilia syndrome:** A poorly characterized syndrome consisting of nasal eosinophilia in a patient with rhinitis and no evidence of allergic sensitization.
  - ○ **Atrophic:** More common in elderly patients; occurs as a result of thinning of the nasal mucosa.
- **Noninflammatory rhinitis/rhinoconjunctivitis**
  - ○ **Vasomotor/gustatory:** Occurs within minutes of exposure to cold or foods, or both (or even with the thought of eating)
  - ○ **Rhinitis medicamentosa:** The result of overuse of an intranasal decongestant
  - ○ **Hormonal:** Seen in pregnancy and thyroid disease; resolves with treatment of the thyroid disease or conclusion of the pregnancy
- **Structural rhinitis/rhinoconjunctivitis**
  - ○ **Foreign body:** Usually a unilateral rhinitis.
  - ○ **Tumor/granuloma/hypertrophic sinuses:** Often unilateral rhinitis (except with hypertrophic sinuses).
  - ○ **Cerebrospinal fluid leak:** Unilateral rhinorrhea that contains glucose (nasal discharges have no glucose, but cerebrospinal fluid does).

○ **Ciliary dysfunction:** Diagnosed by an abnormally increased sugar transit time (saccharin test) from the anterior nares to the pharynx or by abnormal ciliary anatomy identified by electron microscopy of nasal mucosa biopsies.

DIAGNOSIS

- Assess symptoms including nasal discharge, nasal pruritus, sneezing, headaches, and unilateral or bilateral nares involvement. It is important to determine whether other organ systems are involved (such as the lungs or eyes).
- Determine seasonality of the patient's symptoms. Allergic sensitivity to tree, grass, and weed pollens tends to occur in the spring, summer, and fall, respectively, whereas allergies to dust mites, molds, and pets generally do not have a seasonal distribution.
- Obtain a history of aggravating and alleviating factors. Often, patients know that their symptoms are worse when they visit a friend with a cat or, perhaps, when they dust or go outside. They might note that they are better in less humid environments, for example.
- The physical exam findings are discussed above in the "Allergy" section.
- To identify the allergens to which a patient is sensitive, either skin testing (epicutaneous and intradermal) or in vitro testing can be performed. However, it is important that any positive results be correlated with the patient's symptoms.

TREATMENT

Environmental control measures are the most important therapeutic intervention. See the "Allergy" section above for a list of environmental control measures. Surgery is reserved for those patients who have chronic sinusitis and in whom no other therapy is able to control their rhinitis (see Chapter 40, Otolaryngology).

Medications
- **Antihistamines**
  ○ Once environmental control measures have been undertaken, a nonsedating antihistamine to block the symptoms associated with histamine release can be used.
  ○ Loratadine, fexofenadine, and levocetirizine are nonsedating antihistamines, because their incidence of net sedation is <2%.
  ○ Other second-generation antihistamines with very low sedation are cetirizine (oral preparation; net sedation approximately 7%) and azelastine (nasal spray preparation only; net sedation approximately 6%).
- **Anti-inflammatory agents**
  ○ Intranasal nonsteroidal anti-inflammatory medications, such as cromolyn sodium, are the safest agents to use and are now available over the counter. Unfortunately, for maximum effectiveness, cromolyn sodium (2 squirts/nostril) needs to be used four times per day.
  ○ **The most effective anti-inflammatory medications for rhinitis** (not just allergic but any inflammatory etiology) **are intranasal corticosteroids** (refer to Table 39-1 for doses).
  ○ Improvement may occur within 24 to 48 hours of starting the medication but **often takes up to a week before a full therapeutic effect** is reached.
  ○ The doses given are much lower than those used in asthma and, therefore, risks of systemic side effects from intranasal steroids are much lower.
  ○ The major side effect is epistaxis. If this occurs, the patient should stop using the nasal spray for several days until the bleeding stops (they can use intranasal saline during this period), and then they can restart the steroid spray.

- **Decongestants**
  - ○ **Oral** decongestants (such as pseudoephedrine) are useful in treating nonallergic rhinitis, especially in patients whose major symptom is nasal congestion.
  - ○ **Nasal** decongestants (β-adrenergic medications), although available over the counter, should be avoided if possible.
    - These medications provide immediate relief of nasal congestion; however, tachyphylaxis develops quickly.
    - Withdrawal of the drug leads to a rebound hyperemia with worsening nasal congestion; therefore, patients become habitual users of these medications by the time they see a physician (a condition known as rhinitis medicamentosa).
    - If patients must use an intranasal decongestant, they should use it for **no more than 3 days** at a time.
    - Habitual users often require a short course of systemic corticosteroid therapy to get them off the decongestant. Once the systemic corticosteroids have been started, patients should stop using their nasal decongestant and start an intranasal corticosteroid regimen.
- **Intranasal anticholinergics** are useful in patients with noninflammatory rhinitis. An intranasal anticholinergic (ipratropium bromide 0.03%, 1 to 2 sprays/nostril) can be used 10 to 15 minutes before each meal to help alleviate gustatory rhinorrhea.
- **Intranasal antihistamines** are also useful in patients with noninflammatory rhinitis. They may also be given in combination with intranasal steroids and have shown benefit in inflammatory rhinitis.
- **Immunotherapy** (see "Allergy" section above) is quite helpful in allergic rhinitis and can be thought of as a corticosteroid-sparing anti-inflammatory agent.
- Antibiotics are **not usually indicated** in rhinitis unless there is reason to believe that the patient may have an underlying bacterial sinusitis. In these cases, an antibiotic that has good sinus penetration and is active against *Streptococcus pneumoniae*, *Haemophilus influenzae*, and *Moraxella catarrhalis* is indicated (see Chapter 26).

ADDITIONAL RESOURCES

National Institute of Allergy and Infectious Diseases. (http://www.niaid.nih.gov), Last accessed 1/13/15.

National Heart, Lung, and Blood Institute Information Center. (http://www.nhlbi.nih.gov), Last accessed 1/13/15.

American Academy of Allergy, Asthma, & Immunology. (http://www.aaaai.org), Last accessed 1/13/15.

American College of Allergy, Asthma & Immunology. (http://www.acaai.org), Last accessed 1/13/15.

Food Allergy and Anaphylaxis Network. (http://www.foodallergy.org), Last accessed 1/13/15.

Asthma and Allergy Foundation of America. (http://www.aafa.org), Last accessed 1/13/15.

REFERENCES

1. Wallace DV, Dykewicz MS, Bernstein DI, et al. The diagnosis and management of rhinitis: an updated practice parameter. *J Allergy Clin Immunol* 2008;122:S1–S84.
2. Sicherer SH. Epidemiology of food allergy. *J Allergy Clin Immunol* 2011;127:594–602.
3. Golden DB, Moffitt J, Nicklas RA, et al. Stinging insect hypersensitivity: a practice parameter update 2011. *J Allergy Clin Immunol* 2011;127:e1–e23.

4. Sampson HA, Muñoz-Furlong A, Campbell RL, et al. Second symposium on the definition and management of anaphylaxis: summary report. *J Allergy Clin Immunol* 2006;117:391–397.

5. Golden DB. Epidemiology of insect venom sensitivity. *JAMA* 1989:262:240–244.

6. Yates C. Parameters for the treatment of urticaria and angioedema. *J Am Acad Nurse Pract* 2002;14:478–483.

7. Fox RW. Chronic urticaria and/or angioedema. *Clin Rev Allergy Immunol* 2002; 23:143–145.

8. Hollander SM, Joo SS, Wedner HJ. Factors that predict the success of cyclosporine treatment for chronic urticaria. *Ann Allergy Asthma Immunol* 2011;107:523–528.

9. Zuberbier T, Maurer M. Urticaria: current opinions about etiology, diagnosis and therapy. *Acta Derm Venereol* 2007;87:196–205.

10. Hennino A. Pathophysiology of urticaria. *Clin Rev Allergy Immunol* 2006;30:3–11.

11. Kulthanan K, Jiamton S, Boochangkool K, Jongjarearnprasert K. Angioedema: clinical and etiological aspects. *Clin Dev Immunol* 2007;2007:26438.

12. Bas M, Adams V, Suvorava T, et al. Nonallergic angioedema: role of bradykinin. *Allergy* 2007;62:842–856.

13. Agostoni A, Aygören-Pürsün E, Binkley K, et al. Hereditary and acquired angioedema: problems and progress: proceedings of the third C1 esterase inhibitor deficiency workshop and beyond. *J Allergy Clin Immunol* 2004;114:S51–S131.

14. Waytes AT, Rosen FS, Frank MM. Treatment of hereditary angioedema with a vaporheated C1 inhibitor concentrate. *N Engl J Med* 1996;334:1630–1634.

15. Cichon S, Martin L, Hennies HC, et al. Increased activity of coagulation factor XII (Hageman factor) causes hereditary angioedema type III. *Am J Hum Genet* 2006;79:1098–1104.

16. Cha YJ, Pearson VE. Angiooedema due to losartan. *Ann Pharmacother* 1999;33:936–938.

17. Craig TJ, Levy RJ, Wasserman RL, et al. Efficacy of human C1 esterase inhibitor concentrate compared with placebo in acute hereditary angioedema attacks. *J Allergy Clin Immunol* 2009;124:801–804.

18. Sheffer AL, Campion M, Levy RJ, et al. Ecallantide (DX-88) for acute hereditary angioedema attacks: integrated analysis of two double-blind, phase 3 studies. *J Allergy Clin Immunol* 2007;128:153–159.

19. Zuraw BL, Busse PJ, White M, et al. Nanofiltered C1 inhibitor concentrate for treatment of hereditary angioedema. *N Engl J Med* 2010;363:513–522.

20. Lazarou J, Pomeranz BH, Corey PN. Incidence of adverse drug reactions in hospitalized patients: a meta-analysis of prospective studies. *JAMA* 1998;279:1200–1205.

21. Sicherer SH, Sampson HA. Food allergy: recent advances in pathophysiology and treatment. *Annu Rev Med* 2009;60:261–277.

22. Sampson HA. Food allergy. Part 1: Immunopathogenesis and clinical disorders. *J Allergy Clin Immunol* 1999;103:717–728.

23. Chehade M, Mayer L. Oral tolerance and its relation to food hypersensitivities. *J Allergy Clin Immunol* 2005;115:3–12.

24. Fernandez-Rivas M, Bolhaar S, Gonzalez-Mancebo E, et al. Apple allergy across Europe: how allergen sensitization profiles determine the clinical expression of allergies to plant foods. *J Allergy Clin Immunol* 2006;118:481–488.

25. Strid J, Thomson M, Hourihane J, et al. A novel model of sensitization and oral tolerance to peanut protein. *Immunology* 2004;113:293–303.

26. Steckelbroeck S, Ballmer-Weber BK, Vieths S. Potential, pitfalls, and prospects of food allergy diagnostics using recombinant allergens or synthetic sequential epitopes. *J Allergy Clin Immunol* 2008;121:1323–1330.

27. Sicherer SH, Furlong TJ, Maes HH, et al. Genetics of peanut allergy: a twin study. *J Allergy Clin Immunol* 2000;106:53–56.

28. Voelker R. The world in medicine: the hygiene hypothesis. *JAMA* 2000;283:1282.
29. Lynch NR, Goldblatt J, LeSouef PN. Parasitic infections and risk of asthma and atopy. *Thorax* 1999;54:659–660.
30. Sampson HA, Mendelson L, Rosen JP. Fatal and near-fatal anaphylactic reactions to food in children and adolescents. *N Engl J Med* 1992;327:380–384.
31. Broide D. The pathophysiology of allergic rhinoconjunctivitis. *Allergy Asthma Proc* 2007;28:398–403.

Cerumen Impaction

GENERAL PRINCIPLES

- Cerumen is composed of desquamated skin and adnexal gland lipid secretions (sebaceous and apocrine sweat glands) in the external auditory canal (EAC). It functions to clean, protect, and lubricate the EAC.
- Risk factors for cerumen accumulation/impaction include age >60 years, cognitive impairment, obstruction of the EAC by hair proliferation or narrowing (e.g., scarring from chronic infection or in Down syndrome), foreign bodies (e.g., hearing aids or earplugs), the use of cotton-tipped swabs, skin conditions that affect the EAC, genetic factors, and impairment of self-migration of cerumen out of the EAC.
- Cerumen impaction may cause hearing loss, otalgia, fullness, itching, tinnitus, and cough, but it is mostly asymptomatic.

DIAGNOSIS

Diagnosis is made by direct visualization during otoscopy of cerumen, which ranges widely in texture (soft and liquid to hard and dry) and color.

TREATMENT

- The bony portion of the EAC can be quite sensitive and is easily abraded or lacerated.
- Home use of cotton swabs, aural jet irrigators, and ear candling is strongly discouraged.[1]
- **Removal of cerumen is recommended when accumulation/impaction causes symptoms or prevents adequate and necessary examination.**[1]
- Cerumen disimpaction may be achieved via **irrigation**, **cerumenolytics**, or **manual removal other than irrigation.**[1]
- **Irrigation**
  - This consists of flushing cerumen from the ear canal with a large syringe of water, hydrogen peroxide, or 50% solution of white vinegar with the patient sitting up.
  - The irrigant should be approximately body temperature and directed toward the superior wall of the EAC (rather than at the tympanic membrane [TM]) until the cerumen is extruded.
  - Irrigation is **contraindicated** when a history of perforation exists, infection is present, or the patient has had a prior ear surgery/mastoidectomy.
  - Excessive force induces pain and may result in EAC lacerations or TM perforation, but the latter is a rare complication.
  - Irrigation with plain tap water may be associated with otitis externa (OE) in diabetics. Otorrhea and/or otalgia should be reported promptly to the physician.
- **Cerumenolytics**
  - This entails instilling substances into the EAC, resulting in thinning or lubrication of the cerumen and promoting its egress from the EAC.
  - There are three types of topical agents used as cerumenolytics.

- **Water based,** such as plain water/saline, 3% hydrogen peroxide, 2% acetic acid (Acetasol), docusate 1% liquid (Colace), 10% sodium bicarbonate, and 10% triethanolamine polypeptide oleate condensate (Cerumenex, no longer available in the US due to ototoxicity concerns).
- **Oil based,** including olive oil, almond oil, mineral oil, and arachis (peanut) oil.
- **Non–water, non–oil-based** product available in the US is 6.5% carbamide peroxide (urea hydrogen peroxide) (Debrox, Murine).
  - Cerumenolytics are superior to no treatment for clearing cerumen and avoiding irrigation, but no particular agent has been found to be consistently better than the others or saline.[2,3]
  - The effectiveness of cerumenolytics increases with the number of days they are used.
  - All cerumenolytics may also be used prior to irrigation to increase the chance of success.
  - Use of cerumenolytics is contraindicated in patients with OE, otitis media (OM), and TM perforation.
- **Manual removal other than irrigation**
  - Manual removal requires clinician skill, adequate illumination, and the proper equipment.
  - Typically, a metal or plastic loop or spoon is used with direct visualization through a handheld otoscope.
  - Potential harms include pain, laceration of the EAC, perforation of the TM, and infection.
- Referral to an otolaryngologist is appropriate for use of a binocular microscope and otologic instruments when the cerumen is severely impacted or when other attempts have failed.
- Other factors that make referral appropriate include TM perforation, a history of TM or mastoid surgery, radiation to the EAC, EAC stenosis, or pain with other attempts at removal.

Otitis Externa

GENERAL PRINCIPLES

- OE is defined as inflammation of the EAC, which can be acute or chronic, bacterial or fungal, and limited to the EAC or extending to the surrounding skin, the auricle, or the skull base.
- **Bacteria account for 98% of acute otitis externa** (AOE), and cultures of purulent secretions typically reveal *Pseudomonas aeruginosa* and *Staphylococcus aureus*.
- Otomycosis is a superficial infection of the EAC caused by fungi such as *Aspergillus niger* and *Candida albicans*. Risk factors include recent antibiotic or steroid ear drops.
- **Necrotizing (malignant)** OE is a severe complication of AOE seen most commonly in the elderly, diabetics, and the immunocompromised. Infection aggressively spreads to the surrounding tissue including cartilage, temporal bone, and skull base; it can be viewed as an osteomyelitis of the temporal bone. It is most often caused by *P. aeruginosa*.

DIAGNOSIS

- Symptoms include unilateral itching or pain (which can be severe), hearing loss, and/or fetid drainage.
- Risk factors include water exposure such as swimming (swimmer's ear), local trauma with a foreign body, excess cleaning/scratching of the EAC, high humidity (tropical ear), warm temperatures, and hearing aid/ear plug use.
- Physical examination of an ear with AOE reveals a normal auricle but tenderness with tragal manipulation. The EAC skin is erythematous and edematous, with the lumen (which can occlude from the edema) containing moist desquamated debris, serum, or seropurulent secretions. In severe cases, the infection can extend beyond the EAC to the surrounding tissue, producing cellulitis of the periauricular skin and perichondritis of the auricle.

TABLE 40-1 Differential Diagnosis of Otitis Externa

Cerumen accumulation/impaction
Dermatitides of the EAC (e.g., allergic, atopic, and seborrheic) of the EAC
Furuncles of the EAC
Perichondritis (painful inflammation of the auricle)
Herpes zoster oticus (pain usually precedes the development of vesicles; facial
  nerve paresis confirms the Ramsay Hunt syndrome)
Suppurative OM with TM rupture
Cholesteatoma
Carcinoma of the EAC

EAC, external auditory canal; OM, otitis media; TM, tympanic membrane.

- The differential diagnosis of OE is presented in Table 40-1.
- The symptoms of otomycosis are similar to bacterial OE, but there is usually more itching and less pain. Exam shows a swollen and erythematous EAC with white, yellow, or black fluffy, spore-like fungal elements.
- Exam findings of necrotizing OE include pain out of proportion to exam, granulation tissue at the bony-cartilaginous junction, high fever, significant otorrhea, and cranial nerve palsies (most commonly facial nerve). CT, MRI, bone scanning, and erythrocyte sedimentation rate (ESR) can help confirm this diagnosis.

TREATMENT

- The EAC should be carefully cleaned by flushing out excess cerumen, desquamated skin, purulent material, and any foreign body, thereby allowing topical treatments to reach the affected skin.
- In advanced cases, proper cleansing may require referral to an otolaryngologist for the use of a binocular microscope and otologic instruments.
- There are a large number of topical otic preparations for treatment: acidifying agents, antiseptics, antibiotics, and corticosteroids, individually or in combination. All appear to have similar efficacy, but antibiotics with or without steroids are most commonly used.[4,5]
- The most common **topical otic antibiotics**
  - **Polymyxin B and neomycin** (with 1% hydrocortisone, previously sold under the brand name Cortisporin Otic, now generic, dosed tid to qid). With prolonged use, neomycin may actually cause chronic OE secondary to allergic dermatitis.
  - **Ciprofloxacin** 0.2% (with 1% hydrocortisone, Cipro HC Otic, dosed bid) and 0.3% (with 0.1% dexamethasone, Ciprodex Otic, dosed bid).
  - **Ofloxacin** 0.3% (Floxin Otic, dosed bid).
- Initial duration of therapy is 7 to 10 days, but that can be extended if the infection is not resolved. To deliver drops, another person should fill the EAC with drops while the patient lies with the infected ear up, and some gentle tragal manipulation can help the drops disperse throughout the EAC.
- **Antibiotics are clearly better than placebo,** and no single antibiotic has been clearly shown to be superior to any other. However, those treated with a quinolone may improve somewhat faster than those treated with a nonquinolone.[4,5]
- The addition of oral antibiotics is usually unnecessary except in patients with diabetes, immunodeficiency, or infection beyond the EAC.
- The addition of topical steroids to topical antibiotics does not seem to substantially improve clinical cure rates, though they may speed pain relief.

- When there is a suspected or known TM rupture, ototoxic agents (alcohol, acidifiers, Cortisporin, and aminoglycosides) should not be used. Ofloxacin and ciprofloxacin/dexamethasone are approved for middle ear use.[4]
- If the EAC is significantly narrowed because of edema, topical therapy may be difficult to deliver and a wick (Otowick, Merocel, or ribbon gauze) should be placed. The wick should be gently inserted into the EAC to provide a conduit for the antibiotic drops. As the edema recedes, the wick can be removed, usually after 24 to 72 hours.
- Otomycosis treatment is with acidifying drops such as 50% white vinegar solution, aluminum sulfate-calcium acetate (Domeboro), or antifungals solutions (clotrimazole, Lotrimin).
- Necrotizing OE requires hospital admission with otolaryngology consultation, topical and intravenous high-dose antipseudomonal antibiotic therapy, and ear cleaning, and occasionally, surgical debridement is required.

Otitis Media

GENERAL PRINCIPLES

- OM is inflammation of the middle ear.
- **Acute otitis media (AOM)** is defined by the presence of middle ear effusion with acute symptoms and signs of illness and middle ear inflammation.[6] It is an infectious process caused by viruses or bacteria and is **far more common in young children than adults,** but it does occur in adults.
  - The most common viruses are rhinoviruses, influenza viruses, adenoviruses, and respiratory syncytial virus.
  - The most common bacteria are *Streptococcus pneumoniae*, *Haemophilus influenzae*, and *Moraxella catarrhalis*.[7]
  - AOM is generally thought to be preceded by inflammation of the upper respiratory tract (e.g., a viral infection or allergic) resulting in obstruction of the isthmus of the eustachian tube (ET). Fluid accumulates in the middle ear due to negative pressure, with subsequent growth of microorganisms.
- **Otitis media with effusion** (OME, otherwise known as serous otitis) is a chronic form of middle ear inflammation with a persistent effusion without acute signs of infection.
- The ET, which is responsible for ventilation of the middle ear, is normally closed at rest, but opens during swallowing or autoinsufflation (Valsalva maneuver). Apart from AOM and OME, difficulty opening the ET, termed **eustachian tube dysfunction (ETD)**, can result in long-term negative middle ear pressure, causing thinning and inward collapse (atelectasis) of the TM, hearing impairment, difficulty with pressure changes (flying or scuba diving), and potentially cholesteatoma.[8] Causes and risk factors for ETD are presented in Table 40-2.

TABLE 40-2	Causes and Risk Factors for Eustachian Tube Dysfunction
Viral URIs	
Allergic rhinosinusitis	
Chronic sinusitis	
Gastropharyngeal reflux	
Ciliary dyskinesia	
Tobacco smoke	
XRT to the head and neck	
Adenoid hypertrophy	
Nasopharyngeal polyps	

URI, upper respiratory infection; XRT, radiation therapy.

DIAGNOSIS

- The most common symptoms of AOM are abrupt onset of otalgia, hearing loss, and occasionally fever.
- OME typically presents with ear fullness and hearing loss. Symptoms of acute infection like pain are absent.
- Otorrhea may develop if there is a TM perforation, which can be caused by excessive middle ear pressure.
- Otoscopy during AOM will show a bulging, sometimes erythematous, opaque TM with decreased mobility on pneumatic otoscopy. Normal middle ear landmarks, like the incudostapedial joint, will be obscured. Yellow purulent fluid is present behind the TM. Viral infection can display vesicles or bullae on the TM (bullous myringitis).
- Otoscopy during OME will show an opaque TM with decreased mobility, loss of middle ear landmarks, possibly air-fluid level or bubbles, or a TM with a radially injected vascular pattern. A clear effusion in the middle ear can be harder to visualize than a colored effusion (typically amber).

TREATMENT

- **Acute otitis media**
  - There are no evidence-based treatment recommendations specifically for adults with AOM. The recommendations here are based on those for pediatric patients.[6]
  - Observation of otherwise healthy patients with mild-to-moderate uncomplicated AOM for 2 to 3 days is appropriate.[6]
  - Antibiotic therapy may be helpful for those who are initially severely symptomatic or for those with persistent symptoms after 2 to 3 days.
  - **Amoxicillin** 500 mg tid for 5 to 10 days is a reasonable first-line choice for the majority of patients.[6]
  - Alternative first-line antibiotics include trimethoprim-sulfamethoxazole DS, 1 bid; azithromycin, 500 mg qd; or clarithromycin, 500 mg bid.
  - When patients fail to respond to first-line treatment or when there are significant concerns regarding resistance, amoxicillin-clavulanate, 875 mg bid, or cefuroxime axetil, 500 mg bid, may be used.
  - **Tympanocentesis,** performed by an otolaryngologist, for culture is rarely necessary but may be helpful in immunocompromised patients, patients whose symptoms fail to respond, or patients in whom complications of AOM, such as intracranial infection, develop.
- **Otitis media with effusion**
  - Because OME is not itself an infectious process, **antibiotic therapy is usually not indicated.**
  - Autoinsufflation (Valsalva maneuver), where air is forced up the ET by exhaling against a closed mouth and pinched nostrils, may be beneficial.[9]
  - Watchful waiting is a reasonable approach in the majority of adults. Referral to an otolaryngologist if persistent effusion after 2 to 3 months is reasonable for examination of the nasopharynx for an anatomic obstruction, like a tumor, and to consider ear tube placement.
  - Antihistamines, decongestants, and nasal corticosteroids are of uncertain efficacy with regard to OME.[10,11]
- The treatment of ETD most often involves treatment of the underlying cause (Table 40-2), including decongestants and antihistamines.[8] There is no evidence in humans that systemic steroids are effective; however, topical nasal steroids would be appropriate for ETD thought due to allergic rhinitis. Surgical treatments are possible but uncommonly used.

Tinnitus

GENERAL PRINCIPLES

- Tinnitus is a very common and oftentimes very bothersome complaint and is defined as the perception of sound that is not related to any external source. It can affect one or both ears and can be intermittent or continuous.
- **Objective tinnitus** refers to sounds arising from within the body that an examiner can also perceive. It is usually secondary to turbulent blood flow through vessels near the ear and is often pulsatile. Rarely, it can be caused by myoclonus of palatal or middle ear muscles, producing a clicking sound.
- **Subjective tinnitus,** on the other hand, is the perception of sound in the absence of an actual acoustic stimulus (internal or external). Subjective tinnitus is much more common than objective tinnitus.
- Prevalence of tinnitus increases with age. Tinnitus is **often associated with hearing loss.**
- There are many potential etiologies, some of them quite serious, but the cause is benign in the overwhelming majority of patients (Table 40-3).[12]

DIAGNOSIS

- Tinnitus may be described by patients in many ways including pulsing, humming, rushing, whooshing, clicking, cricket-like ringing, buzzing, hissing, whining, whistling, and high or low pitched.
- Particular attention should be paid to the otologic history including hearing loss, noise exposure, history of ear infections or ear surgery, cerumen impaction, vertigo, focal neurologic deficits, and exposure to ototoxins.
- Some patients with bothersome tinnitus have significant quality of life impairment, including sleep disturbance, impaired concentration, and mood alterations; they may require more aggressive treatment.
- Perform a head and neck exam, including otoscopy, neurologic exam including the cranial nerves, auscultation around the ear and of the carotid artery, and cardiac auscultation. Glomus tumors, which can cause pulsatile tinnitus, can be seen as reddish masses present inferiorly in the middle ear space.
- **Audiometry will be indicated for most patients**.
- In patients with a straightforward cause for the tinnitus (e.g., symmetric high-frequency hearing loss in a patient with noise exposure), no further workup is required. Referral to an otolaryngologist is appropriate when other abnormalities are seen on audiogram or there is evidence of objective tinnitus not clearly due to carotid stenosis, heart murmur, or a high flow state.
- Imaging of the brain should be undertaken in patients with focal neurologic signs.

TREATMENT

- Objective tinnitus, while much less common, may be amenable to specific therapies, such as surgery, to correct the underlying cause.
- Competing environmental sounds can mask the tinnitus. Common choices for masking include background noise including music, television, or a room fan. This strategy is especially useful for patients with difficulty sleeping.
- **Masking devices** are sometimes used to provide relief from intractable tinnitus. These are essentially sound generators worn like a hearing aid that produce low-level broadband noise and are available from audiologists. There are limited data on their effectiveness.[13]

TABLE 40-3 Causes of Tinnitus

Objective	Subjective
Pulsatile/vascular	**Otologic**
Arterial bruits (e.g., carotid stenosis)	Sensorineural hearing loss (e.g., presbycusis, noise induced, and other causes of sudden sensorineural hearing loss)
Valvular disease (e.g., aortic stenosis and other causes of a heart murmur)	
High cardiac output (e.g., systemic AVFs, hyperthyroidism, anemia, drug toxicity)	Conductive hearing loss (e.g., otosclerosis, cerumen, OE, AOM, OME, ETD, TM perforation, and cholesteatoma)
Cranial/cervical AVMs/AVFs (e.g., dural AVFs)	Autoimmune hearing loss (e.g., rheumatoid arthritis, lupus, Cogan syndrome, and others)
Venous hum (thought to be caused by turbulent blood flow in the internal jugular veins)	Multiple other causes of hearing loss (e.g., ischemia/infarct, endocrine, and metabolic)
Vascular tumors (e.g., paraganglioma/glomus tumor of the jugular bulb or middle ear)	Ménière disease
	Barotrauma (middle and/or inner ear)
Neuromuscular/anatomic	Ototoxic medications (e.g., aminoglycosides, vancomycin, and loop diuretics, salicylates/NSAIDs, cisplatin, antimalarials, and many others)
Palatal myoclonus	
Stapedial muscle spasm	
Tensor tympani spasm	
Patulous eustachian tube	**Neurologic**
	Acoustic neuroma (vestibular schwannoma)
Spontaneous	Other tumors in the cerebellopontine angle
Spontaneous otoacoustic emissions	Chiari malformations
	Multiple sclerosis
	Head injury
	Infectious
	OE/AOM
	Meningitis
	Viral cochleitis (e.g., herpesviruses, influenza, mumps, measles, rubella, HIV, and others)
	Lyme disease
	Syphilis

AOM, acute otitis media; AVF, arteriovenous fistula; AVM, arteriovenous malformation; ETD, eustachian tube dysfunction; HIV, human immunodeficiency virus; NSAID, nonsteroidal antiinflammatory drug; OE, otitis externa; OME, otitis media with effusion; TM, tympanic membrane. Data from Lockwood AH, Salvi RJ, Burkard RF. Tinnitus. *N Engl J Med* 2002;347:904–10.

- Drugs that are known to cause tinnitus, such as aspirin, nonsteroidal antiinflammatory drugs (NSAIDs), aminoglycosides, and heterocyclic antidepressants, should be discontinued, if possible. In addition, stimulants like caffeine, nicotine, and decongestants should be avoided.
- Many medications have been studied as treatments for tinnitus, including benzodiazepines, gabapentin, melatonin, and antidepressants.[14–16] While none have been clearly shown to be effective in eliminating tinnitus, in some patients, they do provide some benefit. Of those, melatonin has minimal side effects and is a reasonable option for patients with sleep disturbance from tinnitus.

- Tinnitus retraining therapy, which includes counseling and sound therapy several hours a day, may be helpful. The goal is to habituate the patient to the sound and to decrease its negative associations.[17]
- Cognitive-behavioral therapy may be helpful as well, especially in patients with underlying psychiatric disease.[18]

Vertigo

GENERAL PRINCIPLES

- **Dizziness** is a nonspecific term, and further characterization as vertigo, presyncope, or disequilibrium is helpful.
- Characteristics of vertigo help distinguish between central or peripheral causes.
- The most common peripheral causes of vertigo include benign paroxysmal positional vertigo (BPPV), Ménière disease, and vestibular neuritis.
  - **BPPV** is caused by loose particles (otoliths) in the semicircular canals (usually posterior canal).
  - **Ménière disease** is thought to be caused by elevated fluid pressures in the inner ear (endolymphatic hydrops).
  - **Vestibular neuritis** is thought to be caused by inflammation of the vestibular nerve.

DIAGNOSIS

Clinical Presentation

History
- Try to determine whether the dizziness is vertigo (the illusion of movement of self or environment), disequilibrium (general imbalance), or presyncope (patient feeling like he or she is going to pass out).
- If the patient has vertigo, ask about onset, triggers, duration of each episode, frequency of episodes, and associated symptoms (headaches, hearing loss, tinnitus, ear fullness, otalgia, postural instability).
- Look for red flags such as focal neurologic signs that may suggest stroke or brain lesion.
- Table 40-4 lists causes of vertigo, and Table 40-5 lists characteristics of each.[19]
  - **BPPV:** Sudden, intense vertigo lasting for *seconds* triggered by laying head back to one side or looking up.[20]
  - **Ménière disease:** Intermittent vertigo lasting *minutes to hours*, without a clear trigger, typically associated with unilateral aural fullness, tinnitus, and *fluctuating* hearing loss.
  - **Vestibular neuritis:** Severe sudden vertigo lasting for *days* associated with nausea and vomiting. If this is accompanied by sudden hearing loss, it is classified as **labyrinthitis**.

Physical Examination
- The goal of the exam is to determine whether the vertigo is peripheral (inner ear) or central (brain) (Table 40-6). The exam should include a full cranial nerve exam, otoscopy, and careful evaluation of the eyes for nystagmus in the following situations: looking straight ahead, gazing 30 degrees left and right, and while performing the Dix-Hallpike maneuver (Fig. 40-1).[20]
- In **BPPV,** rotary nystagmus may be observed with the head turned toward the affected side during the Dix-Hallpike maneuver.
- In **Ménière disease,** the physical exam is often normal with the exception of possible hearing loss.
- In **vestibular neuritis,** there is a mostly horizontal nystagmus that beats away from the affected ear.
- Table 40-5 provides additional details along with findings seen with stroke and migraine.[19]

TABLE 40-4   Causes of Dizziness and Vertigo

Vertigo	Disequilibrium
Peripheral	Peripheral neuropathy
Benign positional vertigo	Musculoskeletal problems affecting gait
Vestibular neuronitis	(e.g., arthritis and muscular weakness)
Labyrinthitis	Poor vision
Ménière disease (endolymphatic	Parkinson disease
hydrops)	Cerebellar atrophy
Herpes zoster oticus (Ramsay	Medications (e.g., antiepileptics, sedative
Hunt syndrome)	hypnotics)
Perilymphatic fistula	Vestibular disorders
Otitis media	
Cholesteatoma	**Presyncope**
Labyrinthine concussion	Orthostatic hypotension
Ototoxic medications	Vasovagal
Cogan syndrome	Arrhythmia
Recurrent vestibulopathy	Carotid sinus hypersensitivity
Acoustic neuroma (vestibular	Other causes of reduced cardiac output
schwannoma)	(e.g., aortic stenosis, hypertrophic
	obstructive cardiomyopathy)
Central	Vertebrobasilar insufficiency
Brainstem ischemia/infarction	
(e.g., Wallenberg syndrome)	**Nonspecific dizziness/light-headedness**
Cerebellar ischemia/infarction/	Hyperventilation
hemorrhage	Hypoglycemia
Migraine-associated vertigo	Medications
Basilar migraine	Depression
Multiple sclerosis	Anxiety
Chiari malformation	Panic disorder
	Somatization disorder
	Vestibular disorders

Diagnostic Testing

- **Audiometry** is indicated for patients with auditory symptoms.
- **Brain CT scan or MRI** may be helpful in workup of central vertigo.
- Vestibular testing is usually not indicated in the workup of peripheral vertigo.

TREATMENT

- **Benign paroxysmal positional vertigo:** Otolith repositioning with the **Epley maneuver** is successful in the vast majority of patients (Fig. 40-2).[20] Referral to an otolaryngologist for possible surgical intervention (e.g., canal plugging) is indicated for refractory cases.
- **Vestibular neuritis:** Vestibular suppressants (meclizine, benzodiazepines) and antinausea medications (promethazine) should be used to treat symptoms. Vestibular suppressants should not be used for more than a few days. **A short course of high-dose steroids is widely prescribed, though a recent meta-analysis did not support its use.**[21]
- Ménière disease: Acutely, vestibular suppressants and antiemetics are recommended. Chronically, diet modification (avoidance of salt, caffeine, and alcohol), trigger avoidance (nicotine, stress, fatigue, allergy), and diuretics.[22] Refractory cases may benefit from intratympanic gentamicin, intratympanic steroids, or surgery.

TABLE 40-5 Clinical Features of Common Causes of Vertigo						
Condition	Onset and time course of vertigo	Typical scenario	Auditory symptoms	Associated CNS symptoms and signs	Nystagmus	Vestibular exam findings
Benign paroxysmal positional vertigo (BPPV)	Recurrent episodes that last seconds to a few minutes	Most common cause of vertigo Distinctly caused by change in position often while in bed, looking up, and bending forward Sometimes associated with nausea and vomiting	No	No	Positionally provoked with rotatory and upward components (prototypical posterior canal involvement) Latency 3–5 seconds, duration 5–15 seconds Fatigable	Typical nystagmus provoked by the Dix-Hallpike maneuver
Vestibular neuritis	Abrupt onset over a few hours Resolves after a few days May be followed by months of vague dizziness	May have viral prodrome Severe vertigo worsened by head movement Often with severe nausea and vomiting Gait instability but able to walk, sway toward the side of the lesion	No	No	Spontaneous, unidirectional, usually horizontal/torsional May be suppressed by visual fixation	Positive head thrust test
Labyrinthitis	Same as vestibular neuritis	Same as vestibular neuritis	Unilateral sensorineural hearing loss	No	Same as vestibular neuronitis	Same as vestibular neuronitis

Ménière disease	Episodic over years with prolonged remissions Episodes may occur in clusters. Episodes minutes to hours duration	Triad of episodic vertigo, tinnitus, and hearing loss May be secondary to other inner ear disorders Some patients have relatively less vertigo and more hearing problems.	Low-pitched tinnitus Sensorineural hearing loss, fluctuating but progressive and permanent over years duration Ear fullness Otalgia Usually no	No	During episodes unidirectional, usually horizontal/torsional	May have positive head thrust sign
Migraine-associated vertigo	Recurrent spontaneous or positional episodes that last minutes to hours to days Severity is variable Some may report episodes of disequilibrium, imbalance, unsteadiness, or light-headedness rather than true vertigo Some may have more chronic dizziness and/or motion sensitivity	History of migraines Vertigo with migraine headache May be precipitated by typical migraine triggers Some feel this is an underappreciated. Very common cause of episodic vertigo	Headache with or following vertigo Headache may not always occur with episodes of vertigo and vice versa. Typical migrainous features often present (e.g., aura, unilateral, pulsating, photophobia, phonophobia, other visual symptoms, phonophobia, nausea, vomiting)	Nystagmus during episodes may have central or peripheral features.	Usually normal

(Continued)

TABLE 40-5 Clinical Features of Common Causes of Vertigo (*Continued*)

Condition	Onset and time course of vertigo	Typical scenario	Auditory symptoms	Associated CNS symptoms and signs	Nystagmus	Vestibular exam findings
Brainstem infarction	Abrupt onset, sometimes very severe	Older patients with vascular risk factors. Nausea and vomiting may be prominent. Severe gait instability, may fall when attempting to walk	No	Other findings of brainstem infarction including dysphagia, dysarthria, diplopia, Horner syndrome, deficits in pain and temperature sensation	Spontaneous nystagmus, may have any trajectory but usually horizontal/rotatory. Not fatigable. Not affected by visual fixation	Can have nystagmus, not fatigable. May change direction with head position change
Cerebellar infarction or hemorrhage	Same as brainstem infarction. Vertigo is not always present	Same as brainstem infarction. Headache may occur	No	Findings depend on area and degree of cerebellar involvement. Gait ataxia, truncal lateropulsion, limb incoordination. May be accompanied by medullary infarction with the findings as above	Same as brainstem infarction	Same as brainstem infarction

TABLE 40-6	Distinguishing Peripheral and Central Vertigo	
	Peripheral	Central
Vertigo	Often severe	Less severe
Nystagmus type	Positional[a] or spontaneous[b]	Spontaneous
Nystagmus direction	Horizontal with rotatory component or vertical with a torsional component (never exclusively vertical or rotatory)	Horizontal, vertical, or rotatory, including exclusively vertical or rotatory (which does not occur with peripheral causes)
	Unidirectional	May change direction with gaze
Effect of visual fixation	Inhibited	Not inhibited
Postural/gait instability	Mild to moderate, usually able to walk, sway toward side of lesion	Often severe, may not be able to walk without falling
Hearing loss/tinnitus	Sometimes[c]	Usually not
Other neurologic findings	No	Often
Head thrust test	Often abnormal,[b] eyes pulled off target and saccade back to target	Usually normal, eyes remain on target

[a]Benign paroxysmal positional vertigo (BPPV), Ménière disease, and migraine-associated vertigo.
[b]Vestibular neuritis, labyrinthitis.
[c]Labyrinthitis, Ménière disease.
Modified from Goebel JA. *Practical Management of the Dizzy Patient*, 2nd ed. Philadelphia, PA: Lippincott Williams & Wilkins; 2008.

Hearing Loss

GENERAL PRINCIPLES

- **Conductive hearing loss (CHL)** is caused by impaired sound transmission through external and middle ears. Examples include cerumen impaction, middle ear effusion, otosclerosis, and cholesteatoma.
- **Sensorineural hearing loss (SNHL)** is caused by dysfunction at the level of the inner ear, auditory nerve, or brain. Examples include presbycusis, noise-induced hearing loss, vestibular schwannoma (formerly known as acoustic neuroma), and Ménière disease.
- **Sudden sensorineural hearing loss** is an emergency that requires immediate treatment.

DIAGNOSIS

Clinical Presentation

- Table 40-7 includes a list of causes of hearing loss.[23,24] It is important to note side, age at onset, course of hearing loss (e.g., sudden, progressive, or fluctuating), associated symptoms (tinnitus, vertigo, aural fullness, otalgia, or otorrhea), and history of ear disease.
- Check for risk factors such as meningitis, head trauma, noise exposure, and ototoxic medications (chemotherapy, aminoglycosides).
- Check EAC for obstruction (e.g., cerumen, foreign body, infection, lesions). Look at the tympanic membrane for perforation, scarring, or retraction. Look for middle ear fluid or masses.

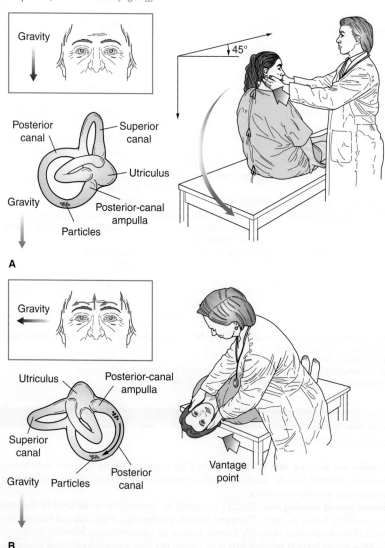

Figure 40-1 Dix-Hallpike maneuver. (From Furman JM, Cass SP. Benign paroxysmal positional vertigo. *N Engl J Med* 1999;341:1590–1596, with permission.)

- Perform a tuning fork test (512 Hz):
  ○ The **Weber** test: Place the vibrating tuning fork on the midline forehead between the eyebrows or one of the maxillary incisor teeth. The sound is perceived as louder in the ear with conductive loss or in the better-hearing ear with SNHL.
  ○ The **Rinne** test: Place the vibrating tuning fork on the mastoid process and then over but not touching the EAC. The sound is louder with the fork on the mastoid with CHL and louder over the EAC when conductive loss is not present.

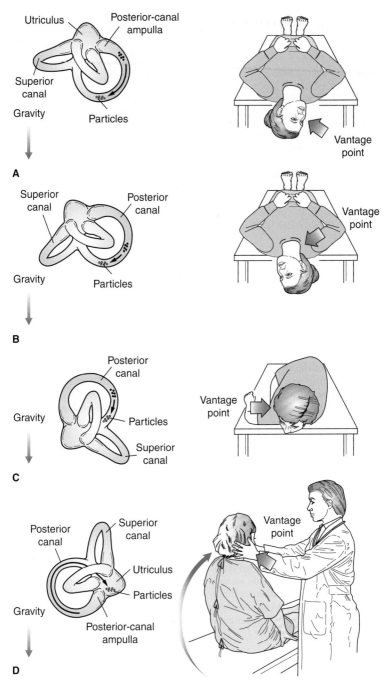

A

B

C

D

Figure 40-2 **Epley maneuver.** (From Furman JM, Cass SP. Benign paroxysmal positional vertigo. *N Engl J Med* 1999;341:1590–1596, with permission.)

TABLE 40-7	Causes of Hearing Loss

Conductive	Sensorineural
Congenital malformations	Congenital/hereditary
Cerumen impaction	Presbycusis
Foreign body in the EAC	Ménière disease
Otitis externa	Acoustic neuroma
Trauma to the EAC	Meningioma
Tumors of the EAC (e.g., squamous cell carcinoma and basal cell carcinoma)	Ototoxins (e.g., aminoglycosides, loop diuretics, antimetabolites, salicylates)
	Autoimmune inner ear disease
Bony tumors impinging on the EAC (e.g., osteoma and exostosis)	Perilymphatic fistula
Barotrauma	Barotrauma
Tympanic membrane perforation	Infections
Eustachian tube dysfunction	Meningitis
Otitis media	Syphilis
Cholesteatoma	Viral cochleitis
Otosclerosis	Multiple sclerosis
Glomus tumor	Stroke
	Trauma
	Idiopathic

EAC, external auditory canal.

Diagnostic Testing

- **Pure tone audiometry** allows for classification as conductive, sensorineural, or mixed. Other aspects of the audiogram provide useful information: speech discrimination suggests abnormalities in cochlear nerve; tympanometry is used to evaluate middle ear status.
- **Temporal bone CT and MRI** are used in select cases.
- **Lab testing** is rarely useful but can evaluate syphilis and autoimmune hearing loss.

TREATMENT

- **Sudden SNHL:** After confirmation by immediate audiogram, typical treatment is prednisone, 1 mg/kg/day up to 60 mg/day × 1 week, and then tapered over 14 days, with repeat audiometry 2 weeks into treatment. Intratympanic steroid injections are also commonly used. Treatment should ideally be started within 48 hours of onset. It is important to note that **studies on this point have come to contradictory conclusions.**[25–27] Urgent ENT consultation is recommended for workup and treatment.
- **Ménière disease:** Refer to vertigo section for treatment. Hearing loss is addressed with amplification.
- **Vestibular schwannoma:** Benign cranial nerve VIII tumor that is associated with unilateral SNHL, tinnitus. Treatment includes observation, surgery, or stereotactic radiation.
- **Autoimmune inner ear disease:** Bilateral, symmetric, rapidly progressive or fluctuating SNHL. Treatment consists of prednisone (1 mg/kg/day to a maximum of 60 mg/day) for 4 weeks, followed by a repeat audiogram. Responders are continued until recovery plateaus and then are decreased to 10 mg/day for 6 months. Nonresponders are tapered off prednisone over 14 days.[24]
- **Presbycusis:** Bilateral, symmetric, slowly progressive SNHL associated with aging and noise exposure. Treatment is ear protection in noise, hearing amplification, and cochlear implantation.
- **Otosclerosis:** Autosomal dominant inherited unilateral or asymmetric CHL or mixed hearing loss is seen in younger adults and more frequently in women. Otosclerosis is due to fixation of the stapes footplate. Treatment is hearing amplification or surgery.

- **Cholesteatoma:** Keratin cyst of the middle ear and/or mastoid. Recurrent infection and otorrhea is common. The cholesteatoma can erode bony structures of the middle ear, including the ossicles. Treatment is surgical resection with reconstruction of the ossicular chain when indicated.
- **Noise-induced hearing loss:** Prevention is by hearing protection. Occupational Safety and Health Administration (OSHA) publishes guidelines for maximum noise level and duration of noise exposure.

Epistaxis

GENERAL PRINCIPLES

- The location of epistaxis is anterior and thus easily visible in the front of the nasal cavity >80% of the time. This usually involves an area of the anterior nasal septum known as **Kiesselbach plexus,** where multiple vessels anastomose.
- In posterior epistaxis, the source of bleeding cannot be seen on anterior rhinoscopy and is more difficult to control.
- Dry nasal mucosa is a factor in many cases of epistaxis and occurs with increased frequency in winter months.
- The location and severity of the bleed will determine the algorithm for management.

DIAGNOSIS

- Refer to Table 40-8 for causes of epistaxis. Relevant history includes triggers (including trauma, manual manipulation), severity, location, duration, and frequency of bleeding.

TABLE 40-8	Causes of Epistaxis

Environmental factors	**Systemic/secondary causes**
Low humidity	Hypertension
Low air temperature	Atherosclerosis
Airborne irritants (including smoking)	Coagulopathies (e.g., von Willebrand
Toxic chemicals	disease, hemophilia)
Local causes	Thrombocytopenia or reduced platelet function
Trauma	Vascular disorders (e.g., HHT, scurvy,
Excessive picking	vasculitides)
Forceful/excessive nose blowing	Endocrine disorders (e.g., pheochro-
Accidents with facial trauma	mocytoma, glucocorticoid excess,
Foreign bodies	pregnancy)
Nasal septal deviation	Endometriosis
Acute URIs	
Allergic rhinitis	**Medications**
Nasal polyps	NSAIDs
Aneurysms	Warfarin
Neoplasms of the nose, sinuses, or	Aspirin
nasopharynx (e.g., squamous cell	Nasal/oral steroids
carcinoma, adenoid cystic carcinoma,	
inverted papilloma, melanoma)	
Cocaine snorting	

HHT, hereditary hemorrhagic telangiectasia; NSAID, nonsteroidal anti-inflammatory drug; URI, upper respiratory infection.

- Consider predisposing medical conditions (hypertension, liver disease, kidney disease, coagulopathy, thrombocytopenia), medications (anticoagulants, NSAIDs, steroid nasal sprays), intranasal cocaine use, and nasal cannula and nonhumidified continuous positive-airway pressure (CPAP) use.
- Hypertension itself typically is not the immediate cause of epistaxis. On the other hand, patients with significant epistaxis are frequently quite anxious and, therefore, likely to be hypertensive to some degree.
- Symptoms suggestive of underlying malignancy include unilateral nasal obstruction, severe unilateral bleeding, cheek numbness, and visual changes.
- Check for family history of epistaxis.
- Evaluate for risk factors, such as hypertension, and degree of blood loss as evidenced by hypotension and tachycardia. Anterior rhinoscopy involves use of a nasal speculum and headlight to visualize the anterior portion of the nose, mainly the Kiesselbach plexus. This area can also be visualized with an otoscope inside the nasal cavity. Look for predisposing conditions on exam such as deviated septum, septal perforation, and telangiectasias (suggestive of Osler-Weber-Rendu disease). For further evaluation, refer to otolaryngology for nasal fiberoptic endoscopy.
- Laboratory testing is appropriate to assess the severity of blood loss or coagulopathy.
- CT or MRI may be indicated to evaluate for neoplasms.

TREATMENT

- **All epistaxis:** Begin with fluid resuscitation and stabilization. Patient should lean forward to have blood run out of the nose rather than down the throat. Systemic coagulopathies should be reversed. Hypertension should be controlled, but precipitous drops in blood pressure are not necessary and may be injurious.
- **Anterior epistaxis:** Start by spraying nasal decongestant spray (oxymetazoline or phenylephrine) followed by pinching nose shut against the nasal septum using index and thumb for 15 continuous minutes. If the bleeding persists, spray again followed by another 15 minutes of continuous pressure. If the bleeding continues to be refractory, the patient may require nasal cauterization (typically with localized silver nitrate), nasal packing, or other maneuvers to control the bleeding. In these circumstances, emergency department evaluation may be warranted.
- **Posterior epistaxis:** Nasal packing is usually required using commercially available nasal packing. Nasal packing may require hospital admission for pain control and to monitor for persistent bleeding and reflex bradycardia. If packing fails to control the treatment, the patient will require either endoscopic surgery (cautery, arterial ligation) or neurointerventional arterial embolization via transfemoral catheter.
- **Posttreatment:** Nasal packs are usually kept in place for 3 to 5 days, and patients are given cephalexin (or other anti-*Staphylococcus* antibiotics) for toxic shock syndrome prophylaxis. All patients must use saline nasal spray and humidifier to decrease risk of recurrence. Nasal decongestant sprays can be used in cases of slight oozing but should not be used for more than 3 consecutive days due to rebound congestion. Finally, patients should avoid nose blowing, nose picking, straining, and anticoagulants, if possible. Predisposing conditions should be managed as indicated.
- Recurrent epistaxis should be referred to an otolaryngologist to rule out underlying pathology and to evaluate for possible surgical intervention.

Hoarseness

GENERAL PRINCIPLES

- Normal voice depends on passive vibration of the vocal cords in the adducted position during exhalation. Hoarseness (dysphonia) is a symptom of abnormal voice due to vocal cord pathology.

TABLE 40-9 Causes of Hoarseness

Infectious	**Neurologic**
Acute viral laryngitis	Neuromuscular disorders (e.g.,
Acute/chronic sinusitis	multiple sclerosis, myasthenia
Acute bronchitis	gravis, Parkinson disease)
	Spasmodic dysphonia
Inflammatory/irritant	Stroke
Acute/chronic vocal abuse	Vocal cord paralysis (e.g., postsurgical,
Alcohol	mass/tumor related)
Chemical fumes	
Chronic cough	**Systemic diseases**
Postnasal drip	Acromegaly
Habitual throat clearing	Amyloidosis
Inhaled corticosteroids	Hypothyroidism
Laryngopharyngeal reflux	Lupus
Smoking	Relapsing polychondritis
	Rheumatoid arthritis
Vocal fold lesions	Sarcoidosis
Direct trauma (e.g., intubation)	
Laryngeal papillomatosis	**Psychogenic**
Vocal fold bowing (presbylarynges)	Functional/conversion aphonia
Vocal fold/laryngeal malignancy	
Vocal fold nodules	**Others**
Vocal fold polyps	Muscle tension dysphonia

- Risk factors for hoarseness include smoking, voice abuse, laryngopharyngeal reflux (LPR), and impaired vocal cord motion.[28,29]
- See Table 40-9 for list of causes of hoarseness.

DIAGNOSIS

- Check for history of vocal overuse, smoking, alcohol use, gastroesophageal reflux, cough, neurologic disorders, neck trauma, postnasal drip, neck or chest surgery (which can cause recurrent laryngeal nerve injury resulting in vocal cord paralysis), and radiation. Worrisome symptoms include progressive disease, stridor, pain, hemoptysis, weight loss, and aspiration.
- This should include a thorough head and neck exam with particular attention paid to cranial nerves, oral cavity, oropharynx, and neck.
- Referral to ENT for transnasal flexible fiberoptic exam or transoral mirror exam to assess for vocal cord pathology is usually necessary for hoarseness that persists beyond 3 weeks. Further evaluations may be warranted, including imaging or biopsy. **Stridor is an indication for urgent referral to ENT.**
- A video laryngoscopic exam performed by a speech pathologist uses high-resolution video and strobe light to evaluate the mucosal wave of the vocal cords, which is necessary for the normal production of voice.
- If reflux is suspected, pH probe testing can be used to evaluate for LPR, but, most commonly, clinical response to a trial of proton pump inhibitors is used to confirm diagnosis.

TREATMENT

- **Acute laryngitis:** The most common cause of acute hoarseness, due to viral upper respiratory infection (URI). Typically resolves within 2 weeks. Treatment is hydration, humidification, and voice rest. Antibiotics are rarely indicated in adults.

- **Chronic laryngitis:** Often due to smoking, reflux, or postnasal drip. Treatment is hydration and elimination of the source of irritation.[29]
- **Vocal cord nodules:** Bilateral calluses on the vocal cords due to excessive or harsh voice use. Speech therapy helps the patient eliminate abusive voice patterns. If refractory, surgery can remove the nodules.
- **Vocal cord polyps:** Due to voice abuse or smoking. Smoking cessation and voice therapy are the mainstay of therapy. If persistent, transoral microsurgery can excise the polyps.
- **Laryngeal papilloma:** Due to human papillomavirus (HPV) type 6 or 11. Treatment is designed to decrease symptoms by excision of papillomata using a transoral approach. Papillomas frequently recur, and close surveillance is necessary.
- **Malignancy:** Usually seen in chronic smokers and drinkers. Tracheostomy may be required if the airway is obstructed. Treatment depends on histology, stage, and exact location. Uni- or multimodality treatment including surgery, radiation, and chemotherapy is used.
- **Vocal cord paralysis:** Paralysis can be unilateral or bilateral and is thought to be due to injury or inflammation of the vagus nerve or its recurrent laryngeal nerve branch, from iatrogenic (neck or chest surgery) injury, trauma, stroke, neoplasm, or idiopathic. In addition to hoarseness, vocal cord paralysis can lead to aspiration, due to inability to protect the airway during swallow or from oral secretions. Surgery to medialize the vocal cord, temporarily or long term, can address both problems. Bilateral vocal cord paralysis can cause airway obstruction and may need to urgently be addressed.
- **Vocal cord bowing (presbylarynx):** Due to vocalis muscle atrophy, which is more pronounced with advanced age. Patients tend to be soft spoken and have difficulty projecting voice. Speech therapy may be beneficial. In more severe cases, surgery can be considered to augment the vocal cords.
- **Spasmodic dysphonia:** A focal dystonia affecting either abductors or adductors of the vocal cords resulting in sudden choked-off speech or sudden breathy gaps in speech. Speech therapy is the treatment of choice. Botox may be used in refractory cases.

Sialolithiasis

GENERAL PRINCIPLES

- There are three pairs of major salivary glands: parotid, submandibular, and sublingual. Salivary gland duct stones (**sialolithiasis**) can result in blockage of the gland's secretions resulting in subsequent inflammation and, possibly, secondary bacterial infection (acute **sialadenitis**).[30]
- The Wharton duct, which drains the submandibular gland into the anterior floor of mouth, is the most common site for sialolithiasis.
- The pathophysiology of stone formation is not well understood, although relative stagnation of saliva in the setting of obstruction is thought to be contributory.
- Risk factors for the development of sialolithiasis include dehydration, medications causing dry mouth (anticholinergics, diuretics), trauma, gout, and smoking. Systemic hypercalcemia is not thought to be related.

DIAGNOSIS

- Although some salivary stones are asymptomatic, patients most often present with pain and swelling of the involved gland. Symptoms usually involve one gland at a time, although multiple stones can be present. Swelling can be episodic or persistent, oftentimes aggravated by eating.
- Physical exam findings will include swelling and tenderness of the involved gland, and purulent saliva may be expressed out of the papilla of the Wharton duct (anterior floor

of mouth) or the Stensen duct (buccal mucosa opposite second maxillary molar). A stone may be palpable in the floor of the mouth.

- Long-term obstruction can result in a firm, chronically inflamed gland.
- The differential diagnosis of symptomatic sialolithiasis includes viral sialadenitis (e.g., mumps, HIV, coxsackievirus, influenza, parainfluenza, herpes), bacterial sialadenitis (which can occur in the absence of stones), salivary gland tumors (benign or malignant), Sjögren syndrome, sarcoidosis, malnutrition/alcoholism, or radiation.
- CT scans can usually identify stones but also demonstrate abscess formation or underlying neoplastic process. Ultrasound can also detect up to 90% of stones >2 mm.[31] MRI and sialography are rarely indicated for diagnosis of sialolithiasis.[32]

TREATMENT

- In general, treatment is conservative and includes aggressive hydration, sialogogues (sour candy or lemon wedges), massaging the gland/duct, warm compresses, and eliminating any drugs that cause dry mouth. Most stones smaller than 2 mm will pass without any interventional procedure.
- Bacterial sialadenitis is treated with dicloxacillin or cephalexin for 7 to 10 days. *S. aureus* is the most common pathogen. When there is surrounding cellulitis or concern for local abscess formation, inpatient admission for IV antibiotics should be considered.
- Persistent, severe, and recurrent symptoms as well as a persistent mass despite antibiotic therapy should prompt referral to an otolaryngologist.
- Interventional procedures are usually avoided in the acute infectious period but may be pursued for persistent or recurrent symptoms. Stones may be amenable to removal with wire basket under fluoroscopic guidance or sialendoscopic visualization or through intraoral approach. Parotidectomy or submandibular gland excision may be required if gland-preserving approaches are not successful.

Neck Mass

GENERAL PRINCIPLES

- The neck can be divided into lateral and central compartments. The lateral compartment is further divided by the sternocleidomastoid muscle into anterior and posterior triangles.
- Age of the patient often is helpful in guiding workup and management. Masses in patients <40 years old are more likely to be benign and congenital in origin. **A persistent neck mass in an adult >40 should be considered neoplastic until proven otherwise.**
- The most common malignant neck mass in an adult is metastatic squamous cell carcinoma from the upper aerodigestive tract. Risk factors include smoking and drinking history.

DIAGNOSIS

Clinical Presentation

- A thorough history including duration of symptoms, growth pattern, and presence of pain should be obtained. Other important symptoms include unintentional weight loss, dysphagia, hoarseness, otalgia (oropharyngeal and laryngeal tumors often present with referred pain to the ear), or shortness of breath.
- A detailed physical exam is essential in establishing a proper diagnosis. Characteristics of the neck mass including the location, size, shape, mobility, and tenderness all give important clues. Physical exam should also include a very thorough head and neck exam

including examining the overlying skin for any lesions, exam of the cranial nerves, palpation of the thyroid gland, otoscopic exam, nasal exam, and a thorough exam of the oral cavity and oropharynx with special attention paid to any asymmetry of the tissues.

- **Reactive lymphadenitis** (e.g., from a recent URI or skin infection) is usually **tender, mobile, and rubbery** firm but not distinctly hard.
- **Congenital neck masses** (e.g., branchial cleft cysts, thyroglossal duct cysts) are usually softer, compressible, mobile, and not tender unless acutely infected. A midline neck mass that elevates with swallowing should raise suspicion of thyroglossal duct cyst.
- **Malignant tumors** (e.g., metastatic squamous cell carcinoma) are usually nontender and hard and can be fixed to underlying structures. Some tumors, like lymphoma, can grow rapidly.

Diagnostic Testing

- Further workup should be obtained in patients who have a neck mass lasting longer than 3 weeks despite a trial of antibiotic therapy.
- Laboratory testing can be helpful if there has been exposure to tuberculosis, brucellosis, *Bartonella*, or *Toxoplasma*. In patients with diffuse adenopathy, consider Epstein-Barr virus (EBV), cytomegalovirus (CMV), HIV, erythrocyte sedimentation rate (ESR), and/or C-reactive protein (CRP) testing.
- Initial imaging of a newly diagnosed neck mass should be CT of the neck with contrast, unless a thyroid mass is suspected, in which case ultrasound is recommended. MRI and PET scans are not indicated for first-line evaluation of a new neck mass.
- Fine-needle aspiration and/or core biopsy is the procedure of choice for obtaining tissue diagnosis, unless imaging suggests a highly vascular lesion. **Incisional and excisional biopsies are rarely indicated for initial diagnosis since they can impair surgical treatment of malignant tumors.**

TREATMENT

Treatment depends on the underlying cause. Patients with persistent neck mass longer than 3 weeks require referral to an otolaryngologist for further evaluation and treatment.

REFERENCES

1. Roland PS, Smith TL, Schwartz SR. Clinical practice guideline: cerumen impaction. *Otolaryngol Head Neck Surg* 2008;139:S1–S21.
2. Hand C, Harvey I. The effectiveness of topical preparation for the treatment of earwax: a systematic review. *Br J Gen Pract* 2004;54:862–867.
3. Burton MJ, Dorée CJ. Ear drops for the removal of ear wax. *Cochrane Database Syst Rev* 2009;(1):CD004326.
4. Rosenfeld RM, Brown L, Cannon CR, et al.; American Academy of Otolaryngology—Head and Neck Surgery Foundation. Clinical practice guideline: acute otitis externa. *Otolaryngol Head Neck Surg* 2006;134:S4–S23.
5. Rosenfeld RM, Singer M, Wasserman JM, et al. Systematic review of topical antimicrobial therapy for acute otitis externa. *Otolaryngol Head Neck Surg* 2006;134:S24–S48.
6. Lieberthal AS, Carroll AE, Chonmaitree T, et al. The diagnosis and management of acute otitis media. *Pediatrics* 2013;131:e964–e999.
7. Celin SE, Bluestone CD, Stephenson J, et al. Bacteriology of acute otitis media in adults. *JAMA* 1991;266:2249–2252.
8. Sproat R, Burgess C, Lnacaster T, et al. Eustachian tube dysfunction in adults. *BMJ* 2014;348:g1647.
9. Perera R, Glasziou PP, Heneghan CJ, et al. Autoinflation for hearing loss associated with otitis media with effusion. *Cochrane Database Syst Rev* 2013;(5):CD006285.

10. Tracy JM, Demain JG, Hoffman KM, et al. Intranasal beclomethasone as an adjunct to treatment of chronic middle ear effusion. *Ann Allergy Asthma Immunol* 1998;80:198–206.

11. Gluth MB, McDonald DR, Weaver AL, et al. Management of eustachian tube dysfunction with nasal steroid spray: a prospective, randomized, placebo-controlled trial. *Arch Otolaryngol Head Neck Surg* 2011;137:449–455.

12. Lockwood AH, Salvi RJ, Burkard RF. Tinnitus. *N Engl J Med* 2002;347:904–910.

13. Hobson J, Chisholm E, El Refaie A. Sound therapy (masking) in the management of tinnitus in adults. *Cochrane Database Syst Rev* 2012;(11):CD006371.

14. Robinson SK, Viirre ES, Stein MD. Antidepressant therapy in tinnitus. *Hear Res* 2007;226:221–231.

15. Piccirillo JF, Finnell J, Vlahiotis A, et al. Relief of idiopathic subjective tinnitus: is gabapentin effective? *Arch Otolaryngol Head Neck Surg* 2007;133:390–397.

16. Megwalu UC, Finnell JE, Piccirillo JF. The effects of melatonin on tinnitus and sleep. *Otolaryngol Head Neck Surg* 2006;134: 210–213.

17. Herraiz C, Hernandez FJ, Plaza G, et al. Long-term clinical trial of tinnitus retraining therapy. *Otolaryngol Head Neck Surg* 2005;133:774–779.

18. Martinez-Devesa P, Perera R, Theodoulou M, et al. Cognitive behavioural therapy for tinnitus. *Cochrane Database Syst Rev* 2010;(9):CD005233.

19. Goebel JA. *Practical Management of the Dizzy Patient*, 2nd ed. Philadelphia, PA: Lippincott Williams & Wilkins; 2008.

20. Furman JM, Cass SP. Benign paroxysmal positional vertigo. *N Engl J Med* 1999;341:1590–1596.

21. Fischman JM, Burgess C, Waddell A. Corticosteroids for the treatment of idiopathic acute vestibular dysfunction (vestibular neuritis). *Cochrane Database Syst Rev* 2011;(5):CD008607.

22. Coelho DH, Lalwani AK. Medical management of Meniere's disease. *Laryngoscope* 2008;118:1099–1108.

23. Nadol JB Jr. Hearing loss. *N Engl J Med* 1993;329:1092–1102.

24. Ruckenstein MJ. Autoimmune inner ear disease. *Curr Opin Otolaryngol Head Neck Surg* 2004;12:426–430.

25. Conlin AE, Parnes LS. Treatment of sudden sensorineural hearing loss: I. A systematic review. *Arch Otolaryngol Head Neck Surg* 2007;133(6):573–581.

26. Conlin AE, Parnes LS. Treatment of sudden sensorineural hearing loss: II. A meta-analysis. *Arch Otolaryngol Head Neck Surg* 2007;133:582–586.

27. Wei BP, Stathopoulos D, O'Leary S. Steroids for idiopathic sudden sensorineural hearing loss. *Cochrane Database Syst Rev* 2013;(7):CD003998.

28. Gupta R. Sataloff RT. Laryngopharyngeal reflux: current concepts and questions. *Curr Opin Otolaryngol Head Neck Surg* 2009;17:143–148.

29. Syed I, Daniels E, Bleach NR. Hoarse voice in adults: an evidence-based approach to the 12 minute consultation. *Clin Otolaryngol* 2009;34:54–58.

30. McQuone SJ. Acute viral and bacterial infections of the salivary glands. *Otolaryngol Clin North Am* 1999;32:793–811.

31. Alyas F, Lewis K, Williams M, et al. Diseases of the submandibular gland as demonstrated using high resolution ultrasound. *Br J Radiol* 2005;78:362–369.

32. Marchal F, Dulguerov P, Becker M, et al. Specificity of parotid sialoendoscopy. *Laryngoscope* 2001;111:264–271.

OVERVIEW

- Compromise to the skin and its functions can lead to disfigurement, discomfort, and disability. In the United States, one in three visits to a primary care physician involves at least one skin complaint.[1] Cutaneous findings may be valuable diagnostic and prognostic markers of internal disease that often precede other signs.[2]
- Skin disorders can cause significant psychological and emotional distress.[3] Support foundations for patients with skin disorders can be accessed through the American Academy of Dermatology (http://www.aad.org).
- Skin cancer is the most common type of cancer. The American Cancer Society recommends that everyone practice monthly skin checks and have regular total body skin examinations performed by a physician every 3 years from age 20 to 40 and yearly after age 40 (http://cancer.org).

Dermatologic History and Physical Examination

The elements of the dermatologic history are presented in Table 41-1.

MEDICAL HISTORY

- Many conditions may be associated with skin disease:
  - Autoimmune disease (lupus, dermatomyositis)
  - Endocrinopathy (diabetes mellitus, thyroid disease)
  - Hepatic dysfunction
  - Genetic disorders (neurofibromatosis, Down syndrome)
  - Immunosuppression (HIV/AIDS, transplant recipients)
  - Malignancy
  - Renal dysfunction
- Systemic medications are a frequent cause of rash and other skin complaints. All oral medications (especially new medications and antibiotics, antihypertensives, and antiepileptics), herbal supplements, and topical medications should be noted.
- Family history of primary skin diseases such as psoriasis, eczema, and skin cancer should be noted. Family history of autoimmune disorders or allergies may also be important.
- Occupational exposures, living conditions, and sexual history can be contributory.

PHYSICAL EXAMINATION

- Examine the entire skin surface as well as the palms and soles, genitals, oropharynx, and eyes. If there is a concern for or history of melanoma, examine the neck, axillae, and groin for lymphadenopathy.
- If a lesion is identified, classify it (see Table 41-2).

TABLE 41-1 Elements of the Dermatologic History

Subjective skin complaints
Pruritus
Pain
Crusting
Discharge
Redness
Scaling

Timing
Acute (hours)
Subacute (days)
Chronic (weeks to months)

Severity
Transient vs. constant
Subjective rating of discomfort

Constitutional symptoms
Fevers
Abdominal pain
Weakness

Prior skin history
Trauma
Previous surgery
Allergic reactions
Skin cancer

Prior treatment
Topical preparations
Antihistamines
Steroids
UV light treatment

Dermatologic Therapies

Skin disorders are characterized by pruritus, inflammation, alterations in hydration, and pain. Identification and treatment of specific underlying conditions should always be attempted.

DRY SKIN CARE

- Almost all itchy skin conditions are improved by the following regimen:
- Take short, cool baths or showers (<5 minutes).
- Use mild, nondrying soaps (e.g., Dove, Oil of Olay, or Cetaphil). Scrubbing or the use of washcloths and loofahs should be discouraged. Limiting the use of soap to the axilla and groin may be necessary.
- After bathing, pat dry and apply thick moisturizers such as petroleum jelly or other thick lubricants (e.g., Eucerin or Cetaphil creams). In general, ointments and creams are more

TABLE 41-2 Classification of Lesions

Primary lesions are induced by disease

Macule	<1-cm area of circumscribed color change, not palpable
Patch	>1-cm area of circumscribed color change, not palpable
Papule	<1-cm palpable mass
Plaque	>1-cm palpable mass
Nodule	>1-cm spherical papule
Vesicle	<1-cm fluid-filled papule
Bulla	>1-cm fluid-filled papule
Pustule	Pus-filled papule
Wheal	Edematous papule or plaque

Secondary lesions are induced by the patient

Excoriation	Linear erosions
Lichenification	Skin thickening, hyperpigmentation, and accentuated skin markings

effective than lotions. Patients may be instructed that moisturizers that come in a jar are generally more effective than those that come in a pump dispenser. Moisturizers should be applied while the skin is still damp and may be safely reapplied as often as needed.

WET SKIN CARE

Excessive moisture in intertriginous areas can lead to bacterial or yeast overgrowth and infection.

- Dry the affected area and apply powder or dry dressing of absorptive material. Use of a fan or hair dryer may be helpful prior to application of powder.
- Separate skin surfaces with absorptive materials.

ANTIPRURITICS

- Pruritus and burning can lead to uncontrolled scratching and can perpetuate an underlying condition.
- Topical agents can be used to control symptoms.
  - Camphor 1% to 3% and menthol provide a cooling sensation and may be stored in the refrigerator.
  - Phenol 0.25% to 2% causes local hypoesthesia but should not be used on raw or ulcerated skin.
  - Topical anesthetics (benzocaine), antihistamines (diphenhydramine), and neomycin are best avoided because of a high rate of contact dermatitis.
- Systemic antihistamines (H_1 receptor antagonists) are most useful in the treatment of urticaria but are also helpful in other pruritic skin disorders. First-generation antihistamines (diphenhydramine, hydroxyzine) are particularly useful in the evening due to their sedative effect. Second-generation antihistamines (cetirizine, loratadine) may be easier to tolerate during the day as they are nonsedating.[4]
- Gabapentin and other neuroleptic medications have shown efficacy in neuropathic pruritus as well as idiopathic itch.[5]

PROTECTION

- Cotton and rubber gloves can be used to avoid excessive contact with water or chemical irritants. Cotton absorbs palmar sweat and should be cleaned or changed frequently.
- Barrier creams and ointments may prevent contact with irritating chemicals but are not substitutes for mechanical barriers.

TOPICAL STEROIDS

- Topical steroids are first-line therapy for many dermatologic conditions (Table 41-3). Topical steroids are effective, but can have significant side effects including skin atrophy, striae, acne, infection, and even suppression of the pituitary-adrenal axis.[6] Side effects tend to occur with repeated application or application to the face, thin-skinned areas (neck, antecubital/popliteal fossae), or occluded areas (axillae, groin, inframammary folds). Patients should be reminded that a topical steroid should not be used as if it were a moisturizer. Topical steroids should be used on the affected areas of skin and never on normal skin.
- Several factors are important in determining the optimal steroid for a particular condition. Accurate diagnosis obviates the need for combination agents such as a weak azole antifungal and a high-strength topical steroid.

TABLE 41-3	Topical Steroids

Low strength
Hydrocortisone 1%, 2.5% (class 7)
Desonide 0.05% (class 6)

Medium strength
Fluocinolone acetonide 0.025% (class 5)
Triamcinolone acetonide 0.1% (class 4)

High strength
Fluocinonide 0.05% (class 2)

Highest strength
Betamethasone dipropionate 0.05% (class 1)
Clobetasol propionate 0.05% (class 1)

Note: Classes 6 and 7 are indicated for intermittent facial use. Classes 1 and 2 are indicated for palmar/plantar areas or severe/resistant lesions.

- **Base or vehicle:**
  - Ointments are more lubricating as well as more occlusive, making them more potent. A lubricating ointment is best for dry dermatitis.
  - Creams are less lubricating than ointments, but more so than gels, lotions, and solutions. A cream would be more appropriate for a weeping dermatitis. Creams are more likely than ointments to have additives that may irritate skin. If a patient complains of burning or stinging with a cream, it may be appropriate to switch to a comparable ointment.
  - Lotions, gels, foams, and solutions are easier to use in hair-bearing areas and are most often used in dermatitis of the scalp. Gels may also be appropriate for the oropharynx.
- **Strength:**
  - Higher-strength (classes 1 and 2) topical steroids are used for palmar/plantar areas or for severe or resistant lesions. They should never be used on the face.
  - Midstrength (classes 3 through 5) topical steroids may be used on most parts of the body, but should generally be avoided on the face, genital areas, or skin folds.
  - Lower-strength (classes 6 and 7) topical steroids may be safely used intermittently on the face.
- **Dosage:** Applications should generally be performed twice daily. When a cream or ointment is used, 1 g covers the face and 30 g covers the body of an adult (for 1 day).
- **Occlusion:** Occlusion with plastic wrap or gloves increases the potency of the steroid but should be reserved for severe, resistant lesions. A limited time course for occlusion should be specified. Occlusion increases both potency and risk of side effects.

SKIN NEOPLASMS

Basal cell carcinoma (BCC) and squamous cell carcinoma (SCC) of the skin, which are sometimes grouped together as nonmelanoma skin cancer (NMSC), are the most common types of cancer diagnosed in the United States.[7] Melanoma is much less common than NMSC, but the incidence of melanoma has been on the rise for several decades, especially among younger patients.[8]

SKIN CANCER PREVENTION

- Patients should be advised to avoid sun exposure between 10 AM and 3 PM.
- Clothing (including hats and swimwear) with sun protection factor (SPF) can be purchased online and in many activewear stores.

- Sunscreens are useful adjuncts to long sleeves and wide-brimmed hats for fair-skinned people or patients with dermatoses induced by ultraviolet light. A daily moisturizer with broad-spectrum (ultraviolet A [UVA] and ultraviolet B [UVB]) coverage, preferably with at least SPF 30, is appropriate for most fair-skinned individuals.
  - For certain light-sensitive disorders (e.g., systemic lupus erythematosus [SLE]) and photosensitizing drugs (e.g., tetracycline, sulfonamides, thiazides, quinolones), broad-spectrum sunscreens are necessary.
  - All sunscreens should be applied 30 minutes before exposure and should be reapplied at least every 90 minutes and after bathing, swimming, or excessive sweating.
  - Allergic and photosensitivity reactions occur to paraaminobenzoic acid, especially in patients who are sensitive to benzocaine, procaine, thiazides, and sulfonamides.
  - Titanium dioxide and zinc oxide are opaque sunscreens that shield against UVA and UVB by providing a physical block. They are particularly useful on the nose and lips.
- Patients should perform skin self-examinations monthly. Encourage patients to use the ABCDEs when examining their own skin. Lesions with the following traits are more likely to be malignant and should be evaluated by a physician.[9]
  - **Asymmetry:** If a line is drawn through the lesion, the two sides do not match.
  - **Border:** Irregular, notched, or scalloped borders are worrisome for melanoma.
  - **Colors:** Melanoma may have different shades of brown, tan, or black within one lesion. Red, blue, and white areas may also be present.
  - **Diameter:** A diameter of >6 mm is concerning for melanoma.
  - **Evolution:** Any change in size, shape, color, or other characteristic is more likely to be present in a malignant lesion, and this factor is often the most significant of the five when considering the likelihood of malignancy. Development of pain, pruritus, or bleeding of the lesion is also concerning for skin cancer.

SEBORRHEIC KERATOSIS

- Seborrheic keratoses are hyperkeratotic epidermal papules commonly found in middle-aged and elderly patients.
- Seborrheic keratoses are benign skin neoplasms that can be confused with skin cancer. They have no malignant potential.
- On exam, they have a waxy, stuck-on appearance and may be tan, yellow, dark brown, or black in color. White horn cysts may be visible on close inspection. There is always a well-defined border. They usually appear on the face, chest, and back.
- **Stucco keratoses** are a variant consisting of small white papules on the lower legs.
- **Dermatosis papulosa nigra** is a form of seborrheic keratosis that appears as multiple small, darkly pigmented, possibly pedunculated papules on the cheeks and periorbital areas of Black, Hispanic, and Asian patients.
- If symptomatic, seborrheic keratoses may be removed using laser, cryosurgery (liquid nitrogen), curettage, or excision. Most seborrheic keratoses, however, do not require treatment or are treated for cosmetic reasons. If a clinician is not certain of the diagnosis, manipulation must be avoided as the differential of pigmented lesions includes melanoma.

ACROCHORDON

Also called acrochordons, skin tags are pedunculated skin-colored to brown papules commonly occurring on skin experiencing friction, specifically the neck, axillae, and groin. Treatment options for irritated or cosmetically troubling lesions include snipping with scissors and, less commonly, electrodessication or cryosurgery.

KERATINOUS CYST

Cysts on the skin present as firm subcutaneous nodules often with a central black punctum. They are freely mobile. **Pilar cysts** frequently occur on the scalp. Inflamed cysts may be treated with corticosteroid injection or, if necessary, incision and drainage. Once inflammation has subsided, definitive treatment consists of excision. The entire epithelial lining surrounding the cyst must be removed to prevent recurrence.

LIPOMA

Lipomas present as rubbery subcutaneous tumors. They are freely mobile. Lipomas are benign lesions. Treatment consists of excision, but is generally reserved for changing, symptomatic, or cosmetically undesirable lesions.

MELANOCYTIC NEVUS

- By definition, a melanocytic nevus is a **benign skin neoplasm.** Nevi are common growths and usually appear from birth through ages 35 to 40.
- **Melanocytic nevi** present as circumscribed papules or macules and may be flesh colored or darkly pigmented. They present on any area of the skin but often are concentrated in sun-exposed areas.
- Unlike melanoma, nevi are symmetric with well-defined borders and uniform color. They are usually <6 mm in diameter.
- **Dysplastic nevi** may have many of the characteristics of melanoma. Dysplastic nevi are controversial, but it is generally agreed that patients with a large number of nevi, particularly irregular or dysplastic nevi, are at higher risk for developing melanoma and should be examined more frequently.

SOLAR LENTIGO

Solar lentigines are **benign** pigmented lesions caused by chronic sun exposure. On examination, they appear as tan to dark brown macules often on the face and dorsal hands. Special attention should be paid to lesions that violate the ABCDEs as the differential includes lentiginous-type melanoma. Biopsy of the entire clinical lesion is preferred to avoid sampling bias.

CHERRY ANGIOMA

Cherry angiomas are benign collections of blood vessels appearing as round, red papules. No treatment is necessary unless lesions become irritated or bleed.

ACTINIC KERATOSIS

- Actinic keratosis (AK) is a **premalignant lesion** caused by chronic sun exposure. If left untreated, a small percentage of AKs may develop into SCC.[10]
- On examination, AKs appear as erythematous, raised papules with a firm scaly texture. On palpation, they have a sandpaper feel and are often easier to palpate than see.
- Typically, actinic keratoses are treated with cryosurgery. Other therapeutic options for patients with persistent or widespread lesions include curettage, topical 5-fluorouracil, topical imiquimod, or photodynamic therapy.

Basal Cell Carcinoma

GENERAL PRINCIPLES

- BCC is common and associated with chronic sun exposure. Fair-skinned individuals are at the highest risk.
- Patients with a history of one BCC have a 50% risk of developing a second primary within 5 years.[11] There is a very low metastatic potential, but BCCs can cause significant local tissue destruction.
- Patients with a history of BCC should be examined every 6 to 12 months.

DIAGNOSIS

- BCC presents most commonly as a pearly, telangiectatic papule on the face or trunk.
- Superficial BCC may occur on the trunk and extremities and appear as a scaly plaque with raised borders. Ulceration is common.
- Diagnosis is made by shave or punch biopsy.

TREATMENT

- Surgical options include excision, electrodessication and curettage, or Mohs micrographic surgery if the BCC is located in a functionally or cosmetically sensitive area.
- Medical therapies include imiquimod and 5-fluorouracil for superficial BCCs.
- Radiation may be used to treat BCC in some instances when surgery is not an option.
- Vismodegib, a hedgehog inhibitor, has recently been approved by the FDA in the treatment of metastatic or locally advanced BCC.[12]

Squamous Cell Carcinoma

- SCC is caused by chronic sun exposure. SCC may also arise in chronic ulcers (Marjolin ulcer) or other chronic skin lesions.
- **People with fair skin and a history of actinic keratoses are at higher risk of developing SCC.** The risk of SCC is significantly increased in patients who are being treated with immunosuppressive medications, including patients with solid organ or allogeneic stem cell transplantation, inflammatory bowel disease, HIV, connective tissue disease, and myelodysplasia.[13]
- Patients with a history of one SCC are at higher risk of developing a second primary lesion. Metastasis is possible but uncommon, occurring in <5% of cases. Risk factors for metastasis include location (e.g., lips, ears, and genitalia), immunosuppression, and carcinomas arising from non-UV causes (e.g., long-standing discoid lupus or burns).[14]
- Patients with a history of SCC should be followed closely, and lymph node examination is recommended.
- SCC is characterized by a red scaly papule, plaque, or nodule, more commonly in a sun-exposed area. Lesions may have a verrucous appearance.
- Diagnosis is made by shave or punch biopsy.
- Surgical options include excision with at least 4-mm margins, Mohs micrographic surgery, or possibly electrodessication and curettage if histology is not aggressive.

Melanoma

GENERAL PRINCIPLES

- Melanoma can develop anywhere on the body. In Caucasian men, the back is the most common location, whereas in Caucasian women, the legs are most common.[15] Melanomas occur more often on the palms, soles, and nail beds in Asians, Hispanics, and African Americans.

- People with a family history of melanoma are at increased risk for developing melanoma; however, most melanomas are diagnosed in patients with no family history of melanoma.
- Unlike BCC and SCC, melanoma has a **high potential for metastasis**.
- Patients with melanoma should be examined for lymphadenopathy. Sentinel node biopsy may also be performed for cancer staging.

DIAGNOSIS

- On examination, asymmetry, irregular borders, multiple colors, and a diameter >6 mm are worrisome signs for a malignant lesion.
- Excisional biopsy should be performed on any concerning or changing lesion. It is preferable not to sample a portion of the lesion but to provide the entire clinical lesion for pathologic examination, as the melanoma may be present in only a portion of the clinical lesion. Additionally, the tumor thickness (Breslow thickness), which provides important prognostic information, may be lost if only a portion of a lesion is removed.

TREATMENT

- Wide local excision is the definitive treatment for melanoma. Excisional margins and need for sentinel lymph node biopsy are based on the Breslow thickness of the lesion.
- The role of complete lymphadenectomy in the surgical treatment of patients with positive sentinel nodes remains controversial.
- Metastatic melanoma may be treated with immunotherapy (interferon, IL-2, ipilimumab, vaccine therapy), chemotherapy, and the recently introduced targeted agent, vemurafenib, but prognosis remains generally poor.[16]

DERMATITIDES

Contact Dermatitis

GENERAL PRINCIPLES

- **Irritant contact dermatitis** is a nonallergic reaction of the skin to chemical or physical agents. Mild irritants require repeated or prolonged contact to cause dermatitis (e.g., soaps, detergents, and solvents). Strong irritants can cause dermatitis following a single exposure (e.g., strong acids or alkali).
- **Allergic contact dermatitis** is a form of delayed hypersensitivity (type IV reaction) that develops only in previously sensitized individuals. The distribution and pattern of the dermatitis may suggest a specific allergen. Patch testing may be necessary to identify the offending allergen. Common allergens include the following:
  - **Plants** (e.g., Rhus dermatitis, otherwise known as **poison ivy, oak, and sumac**): characterized by linear, vesicular lesions
  - **Metals** (e.g., nickel, chrome): commonly diagnosed on skin that touches jewelry and fasteners, especially the earlobes and the periumbilical area
  - **Rubber/latex:** affects skin in contact with gloves, condoms, and elastic
  - **Topical medications:** specifically neomycin, benzocaine, additives in creams, and other vehicles
  - **Cosmetics:** preservatives in makeup, perfume, and hair dye

DIAGNOSIS

- Acute dermatitis is characterized by erythema, weeping/oozing, crusting, and vesiculation. Poison ivy often produces linear vesicles. Severe lesions may demonstrate edema, ulceration, and large bullae.
- Chronic dermatitis is characterized by scale, dryness, and eventually thickening and hyperlinearity (lichenification) of the skin.
- The diagnosis is made largely by history of exposure to irritants or allergens.
- Skin examination may reveal a particular pattern associated with a type of dermatitis.

TREATMENT

- Mild dermatitis is treated with topical steroids, topical or systemic antipruritics, and avoidance of the offending agent.
- Severe blistering reactions are treated with oral prednisone, 0.5 to 1 mg/kg tapered over 14 to 21 days; antipruritics; and drying agents.

Atopic Dermatitis (Eczema)

- In contrast to contact dermatitis, atopic dermatitis is not caused by a specific irritant or allergen, although irritants and allergens can exacerbate eczema.
- Atopic dermatitis presents as erythematous, scaly plaques that may demonstrate lichenification and pigment alteration (hyper- or hypopigmentation).
- **Dyshidrotic eczema** is characterized by vesiculation. Scratching or rubbing worsens the condition.
- Commonly affected areas include skin flexures, hands, and feet.
- Effective therapy includes emollients, dry skin care, topical steroids, and antihistamines for reduction of pruritus. Choice of topical steroid depends on the location and severity of the lesion as well as the age of the patient.
- Recalcitrant cases may be treated with UV light therapy or immunosuppressants.
- Superinfection is common and should be treated with antibiotics targeting staph and strep.

Stasis Dermatitis

Stasis dermatitis is characterized by bilateral erythema, hyperpigmentation, and scaling that is most prominent on the lower legs. It may be mistaken for cellulitis, which is almost always unilateral. Successful treatment of stasis dermatitis requires reduction of lower extremity edema with compression stockings. Triamcinolone 0.1% ointment applied bid is an appropriate topical steroid.

Keratosis Pilaris

Keratosis pilaris is a common chronic papular eruption that occurs on the proximal extensor surfaces of the extremities and cheeks throughout life. The rash is characterized by scaly follicular papules and is usually asymptomatic. Treatment is often unsatisfactory and includes emollients, keratolytics, and topical retinoids.

Seborrheic Dermatitis

- Seborrheic dermatitis is a very common, usually mild dermatitis in adults. However, it can be quite severe in patients with HIV or Parkinson disease.[17]

- In adults, erythema with fine white or greasy scale is seen on the scalp (dandruff), eyebrows, eyelids, nasolabial folds, ears, sternal area, axillae, inframammary folds, and perineum.
- Antiseborrheic shampoos, such as selenium sulfide, zinc pyrithione, tar, or 2% ketoconazole are used at least every other day for 10 to 15 minutes. For the face or trunk, ketoconazole cream or 1% to 2.5% hydrocortisone cream bid is used.

Psoriasis

GENERAL PRINCIPLES

- Psoriasis is a chronic recurring condition with varying degrees of severity. While some patients suffer from widespread disease, others may have only a few small patches of involvement. Psoriatic arthritis involves the joints and may cause significant disfigurement and disability. Ten to twenty percent of patients with psoriasis will develop psoriatic arthritis.
- Psoriasis has been associated with high rates of cardiovascular disease.[18]
- Psoriasis is frequently associated with significant emotional distress and depression.[19]
- Stress, smoking, alcohol consumption, and certain medications (e.g., lithium, beta-blockers) can aggravate the disease. There may also be severe worsening of psoriasis after treatment with systemic steroids, and for this reason, **systemic steroids should not be used to treat psoriasis.**

DIAGNOSIS

- Examination reveals erythematous plaques with silvery scale on the elbows, knees, scalp, and trunk. Nail changes including pitting and "oil spots" may also be present. Psoriasis can progress to generalized erythroderma (psoriasis involving >90% body surface area [BSA]).
- **Guttate ("drop-like") psoriasis** is characterized by small, erythematous papules on the trunk and may be associated with streptococcal pharyngitis.

TREATMENT

- **Mild-to-moderate psoriasis** is treated topically with topical steroids, vitamin D_3 analogs (calcipotriene), retinoids (tazarotene), tar derivatives, natural sunlight, or narrowband UVB radiation. Calcipotriene and tazarotene are more expensive than topical steroids but less likely to cause skin atrophy. Calcipotriene can cause hypercalcemia if it is used on >10% of the body. Tazarotene can cause burning, erythema, and desquamation. Sunlight and UVB radiation can cause burning and increase the long-term risk of skin cancer.
- **Severe psoriasis** (>30% BSA) may require phototherapy or systemic agents (e.g., methotrexate, acitretin, cyclosporine, etanercept, adalimumab, infliximab, ustekinumab). These therapies must be closely monitored. Some biologic agents increase the risk of infection, especially reactivation of tuberculosis. Tuberculosis tests (purified protein derivative [PPD] or interferon-gamma release assay) must be checked yearly. Systemic therapies are for patients who are incapacitated by their disease and resistant to less toxic forms of treatment. They are the only therapies effective for psoriatic arthritis.
- **Scalp psoriasis** is treated topically with tar shampoo and steroid solutions. Prominent scale must be removed before topical treatments will work.
- **Guttate psoriasis** may respond to penicillin or amoxicillin if there is an underlying streptococcal infection. Phototherapy is also particularly effective for guttate psoriasis.
- **Inverse psoriasis** affects the axillae, inframammary folds, and groin. Topical steroids, often in combination with topical antifungals, are appropriate for these locations.

Pityriasis Rosea

- Pityriasis rosea is characterized by pink, oval papules with minimal peripheral scale. The papules align parallel to lines of skin cleavage, often resulting in a Christmas tree distribution on the trunk. The herald patch is a larger pink plaque that precedes the more diffuse rash.
- Pityriasis rosea may be mildly pruritic and is self-limiting, usually resolving in 6 to 12 weeks.
- Treatment is often frustrating, but sunlight, phototherapy, topical steroids, erythromycin, and antipruritics have all been reported to be effective.
- The rash of secondary syphilis can closely mimic pityriasis rosea. If there is any clinical suspicion, serologic testing for syphilis should be pursued.

Lichen Planus

- Lichen planus is characterized by pruritic, purple, polygonal papules that favor the volar wrists, ankles, and genitals. Lesions have lacy white scale (Wickham striae). Oral lesions are common and appear as lacy white plaques or erosions, often on the buccal mucosa.
- Lichen planus has been associated with chronic hepatitis, particularly in populations with a high incidence of hepatitis C.[20] Lichen planus may also be induced by systemic medications, most commonly ACE inhibitors and thiazide diuretics.
- Treatment is with topical steroids, emolliation, and antipruritics. Severe, generalized cases may require oral prednisone or phototherapy.

Thermal Burns

- Dermatitis of varying intensity may be caused by excessive heat on the skin.
- **First-degree burns** congest superficial blood vessels, causing erythema that may be followed by desquamation (e.g., sunburn). Treatment includes prompt cold application and emolliation.
- **Second-degree burns** cause edema, vesicles, and severe pain. Treatment includes prompt cold application and emolliation. Vesicles should not be opened unless they are tense and painful. When required, drainage under aseptic technique is recommended.
- **Third-degree burns** cause full-thickness necrosis of the skin and anesthesia. Severe second- and third-degree burns benefit from specialized teams of physicians.

ACNE

Acne Vulgaris

GENERAL PRINCIPLES

- Acne vulgaris often develops around puberty and persists long into adulthood.
- Acne is an inflammatory condition with an infectious component and is characterized by open comedones (blackheads) and closed comedones (whiteheads).
- Treatments require at least 2 months of regular use to show significant improvement. Therapies should be continued for at least this long before changing treatment course.
- Acne may be improved by the use of oral contraceptives (OCPs) but is often worsened by medroxyprogesterone (Depo-Provera).
- **Inflammatory acne** is characterized by erythematous papules and pustules.
- **Nodulocystic acne** is characterized by larger nodules and results in scarring and should be treated aggressively.

TREATMENT

- **Comedolytics** are the first-line therapy for acne.
  - **Benzoyl peroxide,** 2.5%, 5%, or 10%, is available as a wash or gel. Higher concentrations and gels may be used in patients with oily skin. Unlike topical antibiotics, benzoyl peroxide does not promote antibiotic resistance. Patients should be warned that benzoyl peroxide bleaches clothes.
  - **Topical retinoids** (tretinoin, adapalene, tazarotene) are available in creams and gels. They should be used in small quantities (a pea-sized amount covers the entire face) on clean, dry skin. Higher-concentration creams and gels can be drying and can predispose to photosensitivity. Less frequent application may be necessary if irritation is significant.
- **Topical antibiotics** can be used in inflammatory acne and are most helpful when used in combination with benzoyl peroxide or a topical retinoid.
  - **Clindamycin** solution, lotion, or pledget one to two times daily
  - **Erythromycin** solution or pledget one to two times daily
- **Systemic antibiotics** are often used in moderate-to-severe inflammatory acne and in nodulocystic acne. They should be tapered after several months of therapy. An inability to discontinue oral antibiotics without acne flare may be an indication for referral to a dermatologist for oral isotretinoin therapy.
  - Doxycycline, tetracycline, and minocycline are most commonly prescribed. Side effects include stomach upset and photosensitivity. Blue discoloration of the skin has been described with chronic use of minocycline.
  - Erythromycin may also be used. Allergies and side effects may limit antibiotic choices in a given patient.
- **Oral isotretinoin** is used in severe nodulocystic acne or acne vulgaris unresponsive to the therapies listed above. Isotretinoin, 1 mg/kg/day, is prescribed for 5 to 6 months. All other acne therapies should be discontinued prior to starting isotretinoin.
  - Because of the teratogenicity of the drug, isotretinoin is regulated by the government. Patients must register through an online monitoring system (iPLEDGE) and answer questions before filling a prescription. Furthermore, women of childbearing potential on isotretinoin are required to use two forms of birth control and have monthly pregnancy tests.
  - Isotretinoin is generally well tolerated, but side effects include liver function abnormalities, elevated triglycerides, photosensitivity, and severe dryness of the lips and skin. There is also a controversial association with depression and suicidality.
  - For patient safety and medicolegal reasons, isotretinoin should only be prescribed by a physician familiar with its use.

Hidradenitis Suppurativa

- Hidradenitis suppurativa presents as recurrent painful cysts and nodules of the axillae, groin, and buttocks. Sinus tract formation is common.
- While secondary infection may complicate hidradenitis, it is not a primarily infectious condition.
- Treatment ranges from topical and systemic antibiotics to intralesional corticosteroid injection to systemic retinoids and biologics. Surgical excision is the definitive therapy in the axillae, but is not always possible in the groin.

Acne Rosacea

GENERAL PRINCIPLES

- Acne rosacea usually affects patients between 30 and 60 years of age. It is more common in fair-skinned individuals.

- Rosacea is a chronic condition with intermittent exacerbations and remissions.
- There are several subtypes: erythematotelangiectatic, papulopustular, phymatous, glandular, and ocular.

DIAGNOSIS

- On examination, erythema and telangiectasias on the cheeks and nose are the most common findings. Inflammatory papules and pustules may be present on the face, particularly in a perioral distribution.
- Rhinophyma may be present in long-standing rosacea and is more common in men.
- Ocular changes, including dryness, irritation, conjunctivitis, blepharitis, and rarely keratitis may occur.
- Flushing of the cheeks is common and may be exacerbated by alcohol, heat, sun exposure, strenuous exercise, stress, medications, and certain foods (e.g., spicy, hot beverages, red wine).

TREATMENT

- Rosacea typically does not respond to comedolytics.
- Sunscreen is a first-line therapy for all patients. Sunlight, spicy foods, and hot beverages should be minimized if they are triggers.
- Topical antibiotics such as metronidazole gel or lotion and clindamycin are commonly used for papules and pustules.
- Sodium sulfacetamide wash or lotion may also be effective.
- Systemic antibiotics (doxycycline, 50 to 100 mg bid) may be effective for moderate-to-severe papulopustular rosacea.
- Laser therapy can be particularly effective for the redness and telangiectasias of rosacea, which typically does not respond well to medical treatments.

ULCERS

- Ninety percent of lower extremity ulcers are due to venous insufficiency, 5% result from arterial disease, and 5% are due to miscellaneous causes, including diabetic microangiopathy, pyoderma gangrenosum (PG), malignancy, vasculitis, and infection.
- Definitive diagnosis is often made by skin biopsy, but biopsy sites on the legs often heal poorly over a period of weeks to months, so they should be avoided if possible.
- **Venous ulcers** tend to occur on the lower medial aspect of the legs in areas of stasis dermatitis. Treatment aims to improve venous return with compression hose. Wet-to-dry dressings provide excellent debridement for 2 to 3 days, but longer use can interfere with wound healing. Most wounds improve if kept covered and moist. This is best achieved with occlusive dressings. Unna wraps may be particularly effective in severe cases. Surgery to correct venous return may be employed for patients with extensive venous hypertension or venous reflux disease.
- **Pyoderma gangrenosum** (PG) is a neutrophilic dermatosis that typically presents as an eroded nodule or pustule on the lower extremities, although it may occur anywhere on the body. PG is frequently associated with an underlying medical condition, most commonly inflammatory bowel disease.[21] Infection must be ruled out prior to making the diagnosis of PG, often necessitating a biopsy and culture. Treatment is typically initiated with topical and systemic steroids, with gradual transition to steroid-sparing agents.

BLISTERING DISORDERS

Pemphigus Vulgaris

- Pemphigus vulgaris is characterized by flaccid bullae that break easily, leaving denuded areas that increase in size with progressive peripheral detachment. Oral lesions are common.
- Prior to the introduction of systemic corticosteroids, the mortality of pemphigus was very high.
- **Pemphigus foliaceus** is characterized by more superficial flaccid bullae that may accumulate thick scale. Oral lesions are uncommon. Pemphigus foliaceus has a better prognosis than pemphigus vulgaris.
- Physical examination reveals flaccid bullae and erosions. Nikolsky sign (creation of blister with application of horizontal, tangential pressure to the skin) is present.
- Diagnosis is confirmed by skin biopsy with routine histologic examination and direct immunofluorescence. Patient serum can also be submitted for indirect immunofluorescence to follow autoantibody titers.
- **High-dose prednisone,** 1 to 2 mg/kg/day, is effective in controlling the disease. There is mounting evidence that early use of rituximab can decrease the need for systemic steroids and lead to long-term remission.[22]
- Supportive care in a hospital setting may be required if large areas of skin are denuded or mucosal involvement is severe.

Bullous Pemphigoid

- Bullous pemphigoid (BP) is characterized by large tense bullae on an erythematous base. It is most commonly seen in elderly patients.
- BP has a better prognosis than pemphigus.
- Physical examination reveals tense bullae. At its earliest stage, BP presents as urticarial plaques. It is less commonly seen on mucosal surfaces.
- Diagnosis is confirmed by biopsy for routine histologic examination and direct immunofluorescence.
- Localized disease may be treated with high-potency topical steroids.
- Generalized or persistent BP is treated with high-dose prednisone, 1 to 2 mg/kg/day, or steroid-sparing immunosuppressants such as gold, cyclophosphamide, azathioprine, or mycophenolate mofetil.

Dermatitis Herpetiformis

- Dermatitis herpetiformis usually presents in the second or third decade of life.
- It may be associated with gluten-sensitive enteropathy (celiac disease), but many patients deny gastrointestinal symptoms.
- Physical examination reveals eroded and crusted papules and rare vesicles that are symmetrically distributed on the extensor elbows, knees, and buttocks.
- Patients usually complain of intense pruritus.
- Diagnosis is confirmed by skin biopsy of lesional skin for routine histologic examination and perilesional skin for direct immunofluorescence. Laboratory tests for markers of celiac disease may also be useful in the diagnosis.
- Gluten-free diet is often helpful, but strict adherence is required.
- Dapsone, 50 to 150 mg/day, is highly effective.
- Antipruritics can be prescribed for symptomatic relief of the intense pruritus.

Erythema Multiforme

- Erythema multiforme is an acute, self-limited, often recurrent eruption characterized by "targetoid" lesions. The degree of severity varies widely.
- Lesions on the palms and soles are characteristic, but they may become more generalized.
- **Erythema multiforme minor** is localized to the skin, does not involve the mucosa, and has minimal to no prodromal symptoms.
- **Erythema multiforme major** is often preceded by a prodromal phase, and mucosal involvement is notable and may be severe.
- The clinical distinction between erythema multiforme major and Stevens-Johnson syndrome (SJS) may be challenging.
- Erythema multiforme is strongly associated with herpes simplex infection. Other infectious agents, such as *Streptococcus* and *Mycoplasma*, have also been reported as causes.[23]

Stevens-Johnson Syndrome and Toxic Epidermolysis Necrosis

GENERAL PRINCIPLES

- SJS and toxic epidermolysis necrosis (TEN) both present with a febrile, flu-like prodrome that rapidly progresses to skin pain, exanthem or targetoid lesions, and skin sloughing.
- Mucous membranes are always involved and consist of erosions of the mouth, eyes, genitalia, and lips with hemorrhagic crusts.
- SJS and TEN are a spectrum of disease; categorization depends on the BSA involved. SJS involves <10% BSA, TEN involves >30% BSA, and SJS/TEN overlap involves 10% to 30% BSA.
- Medications are the most common cause of SJS/TEN, most significantly penicillins, sulfonamides (e.g., trimethoprim-sulfamethoxazole), anticonvulsants (e.g., phenytoin, carbamazepine, lamotrigine), allopurinol, and nonsteroidal anti-inflammatory drugs (NSAIDs, e.g., piroxicam). However, up to 50% of cases are idiopathic.[24]
- Mortality of SJS is 1% to 5%, whereas mortality of TEN can be as high as 35%.

DIAGNOSIS

- Generalized skin sloughing is often seen on examination. The oral and genital mucosa should be examined; mucosal involvement presents with erosions and hemorrhagic crusts.
- Painful skin should be considered a serious warning sign.
- The Nikolsky sign is usually present.
- Diagnosis is confirmed by skin biopsy for routine histologic examination.

TREATMENT

- Treatment largely consists of symptomatic and supportive care. Admission to an intensive care unit, preferably a burn unit, is necessary if a significant area of skin is denuded. Intubation may be necessary. Any unnecessary medications should be held.
- Intravenous immunoglobulin (IVIG) is emerging as the treatment of choice in SJS/TEN. Systemic steroids are controversial and should probably be avoided unless they are administered before significant skin sloughing has occurred.[25]
- Antimicrobial silver impregnated dressings can be used to prevent secondary infection and can help limit painful dressing changes.

Drug Reaction with Eosinophilia and Systemic Symptoms

- Drug reactions in general and urticarial are covered in more detail in Chapter 39, Allergy and Immunology.
- Drug reaction with eosinophilia and systemic symptoms (DRESS) syndrome is a serious hypersensitivity syndrome that causes rash with fever and multiorgan involvement.
- The rash associated with DRESS is frequently maculopapular or morbilliform and usually resembles a typical drug rash. However, in contrast to a less serious drug eruption, patients with DRESS present with fever, lethargy, and lymphadenopathy, which may be confused with infection.
- Patients with DRESS frequently have abnormal liver function tests and peripheral eosinophilia or atypical lymphocytosis on complete blood count.[26] Less commonly, there can be lung involvement or myocarditis.
- A large number of medications have been reported to cause DRESS. The most commonly implicated are carbamazepine, allopurinol, phenobarbital, and minocycline.
- Early recognition of DRESS and discontinuation of all possible inciting medications are the key to treatment. Systemic steroids are usually necessary in serious cases of DRESS and should be slowly tapered off over several weeks. End-organ damage may present several months after the initial onset of DRESS, so patients should be followed closely, with particular attention to thyroid function.[27]

ARTHROPOD BITES/STINGS

GENERAL PRINCIPLES

Reactions to insect bites are usually triggered by a toxin or an allergen injected into skin by the offending arthropod.

DIAGNOSIS

- Elements of the history that may be helpful include history of working in a basement, activity in densely wooded areas, and recent travel.
- Diagnosis is largely based on examination of the bite. If a tick bite is suspected, inspect the skin for presence of the tick, which often goes unnoticed by the patient.
  - **Bee, wasp, and yellow jacket** stings consist of a painful red wheal with central punctum; the wheal fades in hours. A persistent local reaction with intense swelling around the sting area may arise and does not indicate a systemic allergy. In individuals with immediate systemic allergy, anaphylaxis may develop. Rarely, affected persons may manifest a delayed systemic allergic reaction that presents as urticaria, polyarthritis, and lymphadenopathy.
  - **Fire ant** stings produce wheals with two hemorrhagic puncta. These usually evolve into pustules within hours.
  - **Mosquito** bites appear as pruritic wheals developing within hours. Patients with blood dyscrasias or malignancies may display exuberant bullous reactions to bites.
  - **Flea** bites produce grouped urticarial papules, some with puncta, frequently on the legs.
  - **Tick** bites usually do not produce a wheal on the skin but may result in fevers, migratory rashes, joint pain, and other systemic symptoms.
  - **Spider** bites are usually not serious. However, brown recluse bites may cause painful necrotic ulcers, and black widow bites can cause systemic sequelae.

TREATMENT

- If insects are attached to the skin, they should be flicked or carefully removed (not squeezed) from the skin.

- Ticks are best removed with a steady upward pull after grasping them as close to the skin as possible with forceps. It is important to confirm that the head has been removed. Clean the wound with soap, water, or mild disinfectant solution.
- Ice, cold compresses, and phenolated calamine lotion are soothing agents. Topical steroids and oral antihistamines may be useful for itching and inflammation.
- Necrotic spider bites from a brown recluse or black widow may become superinfected and require antibiotics. Surgical debridement is generally contraindicated.
- Anaphylactic reactions require emergency treatment (see Chapter 39).

ALOPECIA

Alopecias are divided into two major categories: nonscarring and scarring. Careful examination of the scalp for areas of regrowth and presence of follicular openings is important in distinguishing nonscarring from scarring alopecia. Nonscarring alopecia has the potential for regrowth, whereas scarring alopecia does not.

Nonscarring Alopecia

- **Androgenetic alopecia** has a genetic predisposition and is caused by circulating androgens interacting with androgen receptors in hair follicles. In men, androgenetic alopecia affects 25% of men >25 years of age and 50% of men >50 years of age.[28] Male pattern usually begins with bitemporal recession. Female pattern is usually more diffuse, with sparing of the frontal hairline. Men can be treated with 5% minoxidil bid or 1 mg finasteride daily. These agents cause some hair regrowth but are more effective at preventing further hair loss. Finasteride is not indicated for women, but minoxidil bid may be of benefit.
- **Alopecia areata** is characterized by rapid, complete hair loss in one or more oval patches. The scalp is most often affected, but any hair-bearing area may be involved. Alopecia areata totalis and alopecia areata universalis involve all the hair of the head or entire body, respectively. Alopecia areata is considered to be an autoimmune disorder and may occasionally be associated with other autoimmune disorders, most commonly thyroid disease. Spontaneous regrowth often occurs within 6 months, but recurrence is common. Intralesional triamcinolone is used for persistent or rapidly enlarging patches.
- **Telogen effluvium** is characterized by abrupt, diffuse hair loss over the entire scalp that results in decreased hair density. Anagen hairs (growing phase) are prematurely pushed into the telogen phase (resting) of the hair cycle, usually 2 to 4 months after the inciting event. Hair loss can continue for a subsequent 4 months prior to regrowth occurring. Inciting events include pregnancy, febrile illness, surgery, crash diets, systemic anticoagulant therapy, or any stressful life episode. Treatment consists of reassurance and should be directed at eliminating the underlying cause.
- **Anagen effluvium** is a widespread loss of anagen hair from actively growing follicles due to arrest of cell division. It manifests as acute, severe hair loss. Causes include cytotoxic agents for cancer chemotherapy, thallium, boron, and radiation therapy.
- **Trichotillomania** is excessive and repeated manipulation of hair by the patient that results in hair breakage. It typically produces a well-circumscribed area of broken hairs and alopecia. Treatment should be directed at discussing the nature of the problem with the patient, who may unknowingly persist in manipulating his or her hair. Recalcitrant cases may require psychiatric evaluation and medication. Excessive traction on hair in certain hairstyles can cause hair loss through a similar mechanism. Although trichotillomania and traction alopecia are considered nonscarring, prolonged trauma to hair follicles may lead to permanent hair loss.
- Other causes of nonscarring alopecia include the following:
  - Endocrinologic abnormalities, most commonly thyroid disease.

○ OCPs may initiate androgenic alopecia in predisposed women, and telogen effluvium may develop 2 to 4 months after anovulatory agents are discontinued.

○ Nutritional causes include kwashiorkor, marasmus, zinc deficiency, essential fatty acid deficiency, and malabsorption.

Scarring Alopecia

• When hair follicles are scarred, hair loss is permanent. On physical examination, the follicular openings are no longer seen.

• Causes:

○ Long-standing infections, either bacterial and fungal (e.g., tinea capitis)

○ Neoplasm, either primary or metastatic

○ Physical and chemical agents

○ Autoimmune disorders, including discoid lupus erythematosus (DLE) and lichen planopilaris

○ Neutrophilic scalp dermatoses (dissecting scalp cellulitis and folliculitis decalvans)

NAIL DISORDERS

• Nail disorders are associated with systemic disease or congenital conditions or can be the result of infection, injury, or trauma.

• **Beau lines** are characterized by a transverse depression spanning the nail plate that is associated with any systemic stressor (e.g., chemotherapy, sepsis) that causes a temporary cessation of nail growth. The insult can be dated by measuring the distance between the proximal nail fold and the leading edge of the depression (fingernails grow 0.1 to 0.15 mm/day).

• **Onycholysis** is distal separation of the nail plate from the nail bed. Common causes include trauma, drug reactions, contact dermatitis, and psoriasis.

• **Onychomycosis** is discussed under the section "Fungal Skin Infections."

• Paronychia is localized infection at the nail margin. It may be acute (usually following trauma) or chronic (through occupational exposure). Cultures are frequently positive for *Staphylococcus aureus* in cases of acute paronychia. Treatment is based on the underlying cause. In acute paronychia, saline soaks and topical antibiotics can be prescribed. If an abscess is present, drainage and antibiotic treatment are indicated. In the case of chronic paronychia, steroid ointment is usually required, sometimes with the addition of a topical antifungal cream.[29]

PIGMENT DISORDERS

• Any inflammation of the skin may result in **postinflammatory pigment alteration**. Postinflammatory hyperpigmentation is especially common in darker skin types. Treatment is not necessary, and pigment will often revert to baseline over weeks to months. Areas of pigment alteration should not be treated as primary lesions. For example, patients treating eczematous rashes should be advised to taper topical steroids when redness, scale, and itching have resolved, not when pigment has normalized.

• **Vitiligo** is characterized by depigmented patches, often symmetric, around the eyes, nose, mouth, ears, genitals, and dorsal hands. It can be segmental or become generalized. It often has significant psychosocial effects, particularly in patients with darker skin. It is rarely associated with other autoimmune diseases. Recommendations include broad-spectrum sunscreens and observation for cutaneous malignancies in depigmented patches. Treatment is often difficult and includes topical steroids, phototherapy, and controlled exposure to sunlight. In severe cases, permanent depigmentation may be considered.

• **Melasma** is characterized by pigmented patches on the forehead, cheeks, lips, and extensor forearms. It is commonly seen with OCP use and pregnancy. Changing OCPs has little effect on disease course. Regular use of broad-spectrum sunscreen and vigorous photoprotection are most important in halting the progression of melasma. Topical hydroquinones, tretinoin, and laser may be used to treat existing melasma.

FUNGAL SKIN INFECTIONS
Candidiasis

Candidiasis is discussed in detail in Chapter 26, General Infectious Diseases.

Tinea Versicolor

• Tinea versicolor is a superficial cutaneous infection caused by the dimorphic organism *Malassezia*. In yeast form, these are normal skin flora, but conversion to the hyphal form is associated with the clinical condition. The rash is frequently seasonal, as high heat and humidity seem to facilitate the transformation to hyphal form.
• In immunocompromised patients, *Malassezia* may cause more serious infections including folliculitis, catheter-related fungemia, and focal infections.
• On physical examination, there are thin scaly papules and plaques on the trunk, extremities, and face. Papules and plaques may be hypo- or hyperpigmented. Lesions often are more pronounced after sun exposure.
• KOH examination reveals spores and pseudohyphae (macaroni and meatballs). Tinea versicolor is not amenable to culture.
• Selenium sulfide 2.5% shampoo is used every day for 15 minutes for 7 days, weekly thereafter, and more often if needed. Over-the-counter dandruff shampoos contain less selenium sulfide and require more frequent use. Any topical azole antifungal cream can be used twice daily for 2 weeks.
• Systemic antifungal therapy: a single dose of fluconazole 400 mg is effective, although the rate of relapse may be as high as 35%.[30]

Tinea Capitis

• Tinea capitis (scalp ringworm) is very rarely seen in patients >15 years of age. It is most often caused by *Trichophyton tonsurans*. It may be confused with other more common scalp dermatoses in adults, such as psoriasis or seborrheic dermatitis.
• Physical examination reveals scaling alopecia with broken hairs. Posterior cervical lymphadenopathy often develops.
• Differential diagnosis includes alopecia areata and seborrheic dermatitis. However, alopecia areata has no scaling, and seborrheic dermatitis has no alopecia.
• KOH examination of scale reveals hyphae; microscopic examination of broken hairs reveals endospores or ectospores. Fungal culture should be performed.
• **Griseofulvin**, 5 to 20 mg/kg/day for 4 to 8 weeks. It should be taken with a fatty meal and may cause photosensitivity. **Terbinafine, itraconazole, and fluconazole** have also been used successfully. Systemic therapy is required but can be supplemented with topical therapy to decrease the chance of spreading the disease; 2.5% selenium sulfide or 2% ketoconazole shampoo every other day is recommended.
• Children are no longer infectious once on treatment and can return to school.

Onychomycosis

- Onychomycosis refers to any fungal infection of the nail, with toenail infection much more common than fingernail. **Tinea unguium** specifically refers to nail infections caused by dermatophytes. Onychomycosis of the fingernail is more often due to the yeast *Candida albicans*. Onychomycosis is often of significant cosmetic concern to patients.
- Onychomycosis is typified by flaky, thickened, yellow finger or toenails. There are several patterns of onychomycosis: distal/lateral subungual (the most common type), proximal subungual (uncommon and characteristically occurring in immunocompromised patients), and white superficial.
- Examination of subungual debris or fragments of the thickened nail plate with KOH preparation should reveal hyphae. Culture and biopsy may also be used to confirm the diagnosis if necessary.
- Topical treatment (topical azoles, ciclopirox 8% solution) is usually not curative as monotherapy but may be of some benefit in mild onychomycosis that does not involve the lunula.
- **Terbinafine,** 250 mg PO daily, is often effective. Fingernail infections should be treated for 6 weeks and toenails for 12 weeks. Liver function tests must be monitored during therapy. Recurrence is common after cessation of therapy.[31]
- Patients should be reminded that nails will not look "normal" during or immediately after treatment. It takes several months (6 to 12 for fingernails, 12 to 18 for toenails) after initiation of therapy before a healthy appearing nail is seen.

Other Tinea Infections

GENERAL PRINCIPLES

- **Tinea corporis** (ringworm) is a dermatophytic infection of the skin, excluding the scalp, hands, feet, nails, and groin. It is most often caused by *Trichophyton rubrum*.
- **Tinea pedis** (athletes' foot) is usually caused by *Trichophyton mentagrophytes* in the acute form; the chronic form is commonly caused by *T. rubrum*. Both are contagious.
- **Tinea cruris** (jock itch) is most often caused by *T. rubrum*. It is much more common in men than in women. Obesity, perspiration, humidity, and autoinoculation from other sites of dermatophytic infection (e.g., tinea pedis, unguium) are contributing factors.

DIAGNOSIS

- In tinea corporis, examination reveals scaly, annular, slightly raised erythematous plaques. The plaques may be pustular at the margins and hypopigmented centrally.
- Tinea pedis is characterized by interdigital scaling and maceration. If soles are involved, the scaling is often in a "moccasin" distribution. Localized blisters can develop on the arch of the foot.
- Tinea cruris resembles tinea corporis and presents in the groin folds and bilateral buttocks, but never involves the penis or scrotum. Differential diagnosis includes intertrigo, candidiasis, and erythrasma. Candidiasis often involves the scrotum and presents with satellite pustules and bright red plaques. Erythrasma, a rare condition, is characterized by a hyperpigmented patch with fine scale and exhibits coral red fluorescence on Wood lamp examination.
- In all forms of tinea, skin scraping with KOH preparation shows branched hyphae.

TREATMENT

- In all forms of tinea, involved areas should be kept clean and dry, with use of drying powders as needed (particularly in the case of tinea cruris).

- Initial topical therapy includes antifungal creams such as **ketoconazole** 1% bid for up to 1 month. In severe cases, treatment with an oral antifungal agent may be required.
- For patients with recurrent, severe, or unresolving tinea infection, referral to a dermatologist may be necessary. Consider diabetes mellitus, HIV, or other immunocompromising condition in an adult with this diagnosis.

BACTERIAL SKIN INFECTIONS

Bacterial skin infections are discussed in detail in Chapter 26, General Infectious Diseases.

VIRAL SKIN INFECTIONS

Varicella-zoster virus and herpes simplex virus are discussed in Chapters 26 (General infectious Diseases) and 27 (Human Immunodeficiency Virus Infection and Sexually Transmitted Diseases), respectively.

Warts

- Warts are intraepidermal tumors caused by infection with the human papillomavirus.
- **Verruca vulgaris,** or common warts, are flesh- to brown-colored hyperkeratotic papules. Acral areas are most frequently affected, but any skin or mucous membrane may be involved.
- **Filiform warts** are finger-like slender projections that arise particularly on the face or neck.
- Flat warts **(verruca plana)** are small, 1- to 3-mm flesh- to tan-colored papules on the face, neck, extensor upper extremities, and extensor lower extremities.
- **Plantar warts** are common warts that involve the thick skin of the sole.
- **Condyloma acuminata** are anogenital warts and are the most common sexually transmitted infection.
- Warts may resolve spontaneously or recur after apparent cure. Treatments often need to be repeated.
- Topical agents include keratolytic preparations, such as salicylic acid as well as tretinoin or podophyllum. Imiquimod is effective for genital warts.[32]
- Surgical destruction involves cryosurgery using liquid nitrogen, electrodessication and curettage, excision, or laser therapy.

Molluscum Contagiosum

- Mollusca are grouped umbilicated papules caused by the molluscum contagiosum virus.
- They are very common in children and spread easily through physical contact. Mollusca can be transmitted through sexual contact and is most often seen as a sexually transmitted infection in adults. If widespread mollusca are seen in adults, HIV should be suspected.
- Mollusca appear as small (1 to 5 mm), discrete flesh-colored or pearly white waxy papules with central umbilication. They are commonly found on the face and flexures in children and on the genital area, lower abdomen, and thighs in adults. Lesions may become inflamed in children who pick or scratch them.
- Spontaneous resolution usually occurs in immunocompetent individuals.
- If treatment is desired, cryotherapy or topical cantharidin can be used.
- HIV patients often require more aggressive therapy, and referral to a dermatologist is appropriate.

SKIN INFESTATIONS

Scabies

- The causative agent is the mite *Sarcoptes scabiei.*
- Patients give a history of intense pruritus on the hands, feet, and genitalia. Multiple family members are often afflicted.
- Immunosuppressed or debilitated patients may develop crusted scabies, where mites are so numerous that the skin takes on a crusted appearance.
- Careful examination of the web spaces of the hands will often reveal the characteristic burrow made by a female mite. Scraping these burrows will produce the highest yield on KOH preparations.
- **Permethrin** 5% cream is applied over the entire body from the neck down and left on overnight. All persons living in the home should also be treated. The treatment should be repeated in 1 week.
- Bedding and exposed clothing must be washed, and items that cannot be easily washed should be placed in a sealed bag for 1 week.

Pediculosis

- The causative agent is the louse (*Pediculus* spp.). Different varieties infest different areas of the body.
- Commonly affected areas include the scalp (including eyelashes in children), body hair, and pubic hair.
- Lice lay eggs on hair shafts that can be seen as white ovals (nits).
- Some diseases, such as epidemic typhus, are transmitted between humans via louse vectors.
- Infestations may be asymptomatic or cause pruritus.
- **Permethrin** 1% rinse is the first-line therapy. Resistant cases may require permethrin 5% cream or lindane shampoo. Removal of all nits with a fine comb is essential to treatment success. Family members are often treated as well.

SKIN SIGNS OF AUTOIMMUNE DISEASE

Lupus Erythematosus

- LE is a multisystem disorder. It can range from a relatively benign but bothersome cutaneous eruption with no internal involvement to a severe systemic disease that is potentially fatal (see Chapter 33, Rheumatologic Diseases).
- **Chronic cutaneous lupus erythematosus** is also known as DLE. It is characterized by erythema, scaling, hypopigmentation, follicular plugging, scarring, and telangiectasias. DLE may be localized or widespread. Widespread discoid lesions occur above and below the neck. Systemic LE will develop in only 5% of DLE patients.[33]
- **Subacute cutaneous lupus erythematosus** is nonscarring with prominent photosensitivity. Most patients are antinuclear antibody positive and anti-Ro/SS-A positive. Of patients with subacute cutaneous lupus erythematosus, 50% meet clinical criteria for SLE, although they usually have a mild systemic disease if present.[34]
- **Acute cutaneous lupus erythematosus** is characterized by malar rash, DLE lesions, photosensitivity, and oral ulcers.
- Diagnosis can often be made from clinical exam. Distribution of lesions and presence of scars should be noted. History of worsening of symptoms with sun exposure is important.

- Biopsy of active lesions is helpful in confirming the diagnosis. Biopsy for direct immuno-fluorescence (lupus band) has largely been supplanted by serologic testing in SLE. Direct immunofluorescence may be beneficial in cases of suspected DLE.
- Serum tests for common markers of autoimmune disease, such as antinuclear antibody and anti-Ro/SS-A antibodies, may be useful.
- Cutaneous lupus often responds to antimalarials (e.g., hydroxychloroquine) and topical steroids. Sun protection is important, even in darker skin types.

Dermatomyositis

- Dermatomyositis combines an inflammatory myopathy with characteristic cutaneous findings (see Chapter 33, Rheumatologic Diseases). Dermatomyositis sine myositis has characteristic skin findings without evidence of myopathy.
- Dermatomyositis may be associated with an underlying malignancy, particularly ovarian cancer. Newly diagnosed patients should have all age-appropriate cancer screenings performed, and imaging may be considered in select cases.[35]
- Pathognomonic signs on examination include a heliotrope rash, which is a violaceous hue over the eyelids, and Gottron papules, which are erythematous papules over the knuckles.
- Other cutaneous findings include periungual telangiectasias, photosensitivity, rash on the neck and upper chest (shawl sign), calcinosis cutis (more common in children), cuticular hypertrophy, and splinter hemorrhages.
- Laboratory findings include elevated muscle enzymes, the presence of myositis antibodies, and a pauci-inflammatory interface dermatitis on biopsy.
- The cutaneous disease often responds to therapy for the systemic disease, such as antimalarials, systemic steroids, and methotrexate.

Scleroderma

- Scleroderma is characterized by thickening or hardening of the skin associated with increased dermal or subcutaneous sclerosis, or both. Localized cutaneous disease can occur, which includes morphea, linear scleroderma, and facial hemiatrophy.
- Systemic disease is further classified into two conditions:
  - **Limited scleroderma (CREST):** calcinosis, Raynaud phenomenon, esophageal dysmotility, sclerodactyly, and telangiectasia
  - **Diffuse scleroderma,** or progressive systemic sclerosis
- **Nephrogenic systemic fibrosis** is a scleroderma-like illness that presents in patients with renal failure and has been strongly linked to use of specific gadolinium MRI contrast media.[36] Typically, nephrogenic systemic fibrosis starts distally on the extremities and progresses proximally.
- Cutaneous manifestations include generalized sclerosis, acrosclerosis/sclerodactyly, calcinosis cutis, pruritus, nail fold capillary changes, mat-like telangiectasias, Raynaud phenomenon, taut facies, and salt-and-pepper dyspigmentation.
- Skin biopsy for routine histologic examination confirms the diagnosis.
- Cutaneous sclerosis and pruritus often responds to psoralen (a light sensitizer) combined with UVA therapy, though treatment is difficult and the disease is usually progressive.[37]

Vasculitis

GENERAL PRINCIPLES

- Cutaneous vasculitis most commonly presents as **palpable purpura**. Most cases are caused by skin-limited **small vessel leukocytoclastic vasculitis**, but cutaneous vasculitis may also be associated with the systemic vasculitides.

- Fifty percent of cases are idiopathic, but potential causes include the following:
  - Infection: hepatitis, *Streptococcus*, upper respiratory viruses.
  - Drugs: antibiotics, barbiturates, amphetamines, propylthiouracil.
  - Autoimmune disease: SLE, rheumatoid arthritis.
  - Other causes include cryoglobulinemia, Henoch-Schönlein purpura (IgA-related vasculitis), antineutrophil cytoplasmic antibody (ANCA)-associated vasculitides, and Churg-Strauss syndrome.

DIAGNOSIS

- Screening for a history of autoimmune disorder, infection, or new medication is important.
- Skin biopsy for routine histologic examination confirms the diagnosis. Biopsy for direct immunofluorescence is useful in cases of suspected IgA-related vasculitis.
- Laboratory work to be considered in the appropriate clinical setting includes urinalysis, stool guaiac, complete blood count, erythrocyte sedimentation rate (ESR), chest radiography, hepatitis panel, antinuclear antibodies (ANA), ANCA, and cryoglobulins.

TREATMENT

- Most cases of cutaneous-only small-vessel leukocytoclastic vasculitis are self-limited. Treatment should be aimed at underlying causes.
- Prednisone improves the cutaneous disease but does not change the overall course.
- Appropriate treatment for most patients includes rest and NSAID medications.

Erythema Nodosum

GENERAL PRINCIPLES

- Erythema nodosum commonly presents in young women.
- Fifty percent of cases are idiopathic, but potential causes include the following:
  - **Streptococcal pharyngitis** and other upper respiratory tract infections
  - **Medications:** OCPs, sulfonamides, trimethoprim-sulfamethoxazole, salicylates, phenacetin, iodides, bromides
  - **Inflammatory bowel disease:** ulcerative colitis, Crohn disease, infectious colitis
  - **Pulmonary disease:** tuberculosis, sarcoidosis (Löfgren syndrome), coccidioidomycosis, histoplasmosis, blastomycosis, lymphoma
  - Behçet disease

DIAGNOSIS

- Physical examination reveals tender subcutaneous nodules, commonly on the shins.
- Skin biopsy can confirm the diagnosis, but erythema nodosum is generally a clinical diagnosis.
- Appropriate evaluation includes complete blood count, PPD, and chest x-ray. If an obvious disease trigger is not apparent, effort should be made to identify the underlying cause.

TREATMENT

- Most cases are self-limited, lasting 3 to 6 weeks. Treatment is aimed at removing the offending agent or treating the underlying disease.
- Initial therapy is NSAIDs.

• Alternate therapies include oral potassium iodide, indomethacin, or colchicine. Steroids, intralesional, or systemic should only be considered once infections have been excluded or for recalcitrant cases.

SKIN SIGNS OF INTERNAL MALIGNANCY

Cutaneous Metastases

• The overall incidence of metastasis to skin is low.
• Metastatic carcinoma appears as firm subcutaneous nodules. The trunk and scalp are the most frequently affected sites.
• Melanoma is the most common cancer to metastasize to the skin. Solid organ cancers that may metastasize to the skin include the lung, breast, gastrointestinal tract, ovary, and kidney.

Lymphoreticular and Hematologic Malignancies

• Metastasis or paraneoplastic phenomena may affect the skin.
• Leukemia cutis or lymphoma cutis can resemble carcinomatous skin metastasis and appear as firm papules, nodules, or plaques. They are more likely to be hemorrhagic.
• Gingival hypertrophy and bleeding are common with leukemia.
• **Sweet syndrome** (acute febrile neutrophilic dermatosis) is associated with hematologic malignancies in at least 10% of cases, most commonly acute myelogenous leukemia.[38] Sweet syndrome presents as a febrile illness with characteristic "juicy" red nodules and plaques. Biopsy for routine histologic examination and for tissue culture (to rule out infection) confirms the diagnosis.
• **Cutaneous T-cell lymphoma** is frequently referred to as its most common subtype, mycosis fungoides; cutaneous T-cell lymphoma may present with erythematous patches, plaques, nodules, tumors, generalized erythroderma, or its leukemic variant Sézary syndrome. Diagnosis is made with skin biopsy. Treatment is dictated by disease stage and may range from topical steroids and UV light treatment to chemotherapy.

SKIN SIGNS OF ENDOCRINOLOGIC DISORDERS

Thyroid Disorders

• **Hyperthyroidism** is associated with fine thin hair that may progress to diffuse alopecia, velvety skin with increased warmth and sweating, palmar erythema, and diffuse hyperpigmentation.
• **Graves disease** is associated with ophthalmopathy (exophthalmos, lid puffiness, and proptosis), pretibial myxedema, thyroid acropachy (characterized by digital clubbing), and soft tissue swelling of the hands and feet.
• **Hypothyroidism** is associated with congenital hypothyroidism, generalized myxedema, xerosis, keratoderma, cold pale skin, carotenemia, brittle hair that may progress to alopecia, loss of lateral third of eyebrows, and brittle, slow-growing nails.

Diabetes Mellitus

• **Diabetic dermopathy** appears as atrophic hyperpigmented patches on the shins.
• **Necrobiosis lipoidica diabeticorum** is characterized by well-circumscribed, yellow-brown, shiny plaques with pronounced epidermal atrophy and telangiectasia, commonly seen on the shins.

Lipoprotein Disorders

- **Eruptive xanthomas** arise in groups and exhibit an inflammatory acneiform appearance. They may be mistaken for pustules. Patients are at risk for acute pancreatitis. Plasma triglycerides are markedly increased, but cholesterol is often normal. Etiologic factors include genetic lipoprotein lipase deficiency, ethanol abuse, estrogens, or retinoids.
- **Tendon xanthomas** are subcutaneous nodules that affect the tendons with normal-appearing overlying skin. They may be mistaken for rheumatoid nodules. If plasma cholesterol is increased, the most likely cause is familial hypercholesterolemia. Patients are at risk for atherosclerosis and coronary disease.
- **Xanthelasma** is the most common but least specific type of xanthoma. It arises in the periocular area, especially on the eyelids; 50% of patients have increased serum cholesterol.[39]

REFERENCES

1. Lowell BA, Froelich CW, Federman DG, et al. Dermatology in primary care: prevalence and patient disposition. *J Am Acad Dermatol* 2001;45:250–255.
2. Nahass GT, Meyer AJ, Campbell SF, et al. Prevalence of cutaneous findings in hospitalized medical patients. *J Am Acad Dermatol* 1995;33:207–211.
3. Wakkee M, Nijsten T. Comorbidities in dermatology. *Dermatol Clin* 2009;27:137–147.
4. Lee EE, Maibach HI. Treatment of urticaria. An evidence-based evaluation of antihistamines. *Am J Clin Dermatol* 2001;2:27–32.
5. Winhoven SM, Coulson IH, Bottomley WW. Brachioradial pruritus: response to treatment with gabapentin. *Br J Dermatol* 2004;150:786–787.
6. Walsh P, Aeling JL, Huff L, et al. Hypothalamus-pituitary-adrenal axis suppression by superpotent topical steroids. *J Am Acad Dermatol* 1993;29:501–503.
7. Stern RS. Prevalence of a history of skin cancer in 2007: results of an incidence-based model. *Arch Dermatol* 2010;146:279–282.
8. Reed KB, Brewer JD, Lohse CM, et al. Increasing incidence of melanoma among young adults: an epidemiological study in Olmsted County, Minnesota. *Mayo Clin Proc* 2012;87:328–334.
9. Shenenberger DW. Cutaneous malignant melanoma: a primary care perspective. *Am Fam Physician* 2012;85:161–168.
10. Criscione VD, Weinstock MA, Naylor MF, et al. Actinic keratoses: natural history and risk of malignant transformation in the Veterans Affairs Topical Tretinoin Chemoprevention Trial. *Cancer* 2009;115:2523–2530.
11. Karagas MR, Stukel TA, Greenberg ER, et al. Risk of subsequent basal cell carcinoma and squamous cell carcinoma of the skin among patients with prior skin cancer. Skin Cancer Prevention Study Group. *JAMA* 1992;267:3305–3310.
12. Sekulic A, Migden MR, Oro AE, et al. Efficacy and safety of vismodegib in advanced basal-cell carcinoma. *N Engl J Med* 2012;366:2171–2179.
13. Glover MT, Deeks JJ, Raftery MJ, et al. Immunosuppression and risk of non-melanoma skin cancer in renal transplant recipients. *Lancet* 1997;349:398.
14. Rowe DE, Carroll RJ, Day CL. Prognostic factors for local recurrence, metastasis, and survival rates in squamous cell carcinoma of the skin, ear, and lip. Implications for treatment modality selection. *J Am Acad Dermatol* 1992;26:976–990.
15. Clark LN, Shin DB, Troxel AB, et al. Association between the anatomic distribution of melanoma and sex. *J Am Acad Dermatol* 2007;56:768–773.
16. Chapman PB, Hauschild A, Robert C, et al. Improved survival with vemurafenib in melanoma with BRAF V600E mutation. *N Engl J Med* 2011;364:2507–2516.
17. Sindrup JH, Lisby G, Weismann K, et al. Skin manifestations in AIDS, HIV infection, and AIDS-related complex. *Int J Dermatol* 1987;26:267–272.

18. Gelfand JM, Neimann AL, Shin DB, et al. Risk of myocardial infarction in patients with psoriasis. *JAMA* 2006;296:1735–1741.

19. Bhutani T, Patel T, Koo B, et al. A prospective, interventional assessment of psoriasis quality of life using a nonskin-specific validated instrument that allows comparison with other major medical conditions. *J Am Acad Dermatol* 2012;69:e79–e88.

20. Shengyuan L, Songpo Y, Wen W, et al. Hepatitis C virus and lichen planus: a reciprocal association determined by a meta-analysis. *Arch Dermatol* 2009;145:1040–1047.

21. Binus AM, Qureshi AA, Li VW, et al. Pyoderma gangrenosum: a retrospective review of patient characteristics, comorbidities and therapy in 103 patients. *Br J Dermatol* 2011;165:1244–1250.

22. Cianchini G, Lupi F, Masini C, et al. Therapy with rituximab for autoimmune pemphigus: results from a single-center observational study on 42 cases with long-term follow-up. *J Am Acad Dermatol* 2012;67:617–622.

23. Atkinson TP, Boppana S, Theos A, et al. Stevens-Johnson syndrome in a boy with macrolide-resistant Mycoplasma pneumoniae pneumonia. *Pediatrics* 2011;127:e1605–e1609.

24. Harr T, French LE. Toxic epidermal necrolysis and Stevens-Johnson syndrome. *Orphanet J Rare Dis* 2010;5:39.

25. Huang YC, Li YC, Chen TJ. The efficacy of intravenous immunoglobulin for the treatment of toxic epidermal necrolysis: a systematic review and meta-analysis. *Br J Dermatol* 2012;167:424–432.

26. Cacoub P, Musette P, Descamps V, et al. The DRESS syndrome: a literature review. *Am J Med* 2011;124:588–597.

27. Chen YC, Chang CY, Cho YT, et al. Long-term sequelae of drug reaction with eosinophilia and systemic symptoms: a retrospective cohort study from Taiwan. *J Am Acad Dermatol* 2013;68:459–465.

28. Ellis JA, Sinclair R, Harrap SB. Androgenetic alopecia: pathogenesis and potential for therapy. *Expert Rev Mol Med* 2002;4:1–11.

29. Tosti A, Piraccini BM, Ghetti E, et al. Topical steroids versus systemic antifungals in the treatment of chronic paronychia: an open, randomized double-blind and double dummy study. *J Am Acad Dermatol* 2002;47:73–76.

30. Partap R, Kaur I, Chakrabarti A, et al. Single-dose fluconazole versus itraconazole in pityriasis versicolor. *Dermatology* 2004;208:55–59.

31. Sigurgeirsson B, Olafsson JH, Steinsson JB, et al. Long-term effectiveness of treatment with terbinafine vs itraconazole in onychomycosis: a 5-year blinded prospective follow-up study. *Arch Dermatol* 2002;138:353–357.

32. Schöfer H. Evaluation of imiquimod for the therapy of external genital and anal warts in comparison with destructive therapies. *Br J Dermatol* 2007;157:52–55.

33. Healy E, Kieran E, Rogers S. Cutaneous lupus erythematosus—a study of clinical and laboratory prognostic factors in 65 patients. *Ir J Med Sci* 1995;164:113–115.

34. Sontheimer RD, Thomas JR, Gilliam JN. Subacute cutaneous lupus erythematosus: a cutaneous marker for a distinct lupus erythematosus subset. *Arch Dermatol* 1979;115:1409–1415.

35. Sigurgeirsson B, Lindelöf B, Edhag O, et al. Risk of cancer in patients with dermatomyositis or polymyositis. A population-based study. *N Engl J Med* 1992;326:363–367.

36. Zou Z, Zhang HL, Roditi GH, et al. Nephrogenic systemic fibrosis: review of 370 biopsy-confirmed cases. *JACC Cardiovasc Imaging* 2011;4:1206–1216.

37. Kroft EB, Berkhof NJ, van de Kerkhof PC, et al. Ultraviolet A phototherapy for sclerotic skin diseases: a systematic review. *J Am Acad Dermatol* 2008;59:1017–1030.

38. Cohen PR, Kurzrock R. Sweet's syndrome and cancer. *Clin Dermatol* 1993;11:149–157.

39. Bergman R. The pathogenesis and clinical significance of xanthelasma palpebrarum. *J Am Acad Dermatol* 1994;30:236–242.

42 Psychiatry
Luigi R. Cardella and Luis A. Giuffra

OVERVIEW

- Psychiatric disorders include a heterogeneous collection of conditions related to behavior, mood, interpersonal interactions, cognition, and personal identity. All cause **impairment in personal well-being and meaningful function.**
- Internists are integral in the care of patients with mental illness. Primary care physicians provide the sole mental health care for 60% to 70% of patients in the US with psychiatric disorders.[1]
- Denial or the fear of social stigma induces many patients with psychiatric symptoms to seek help from a primary care physician rather than a psychiatrist. Alternatively, such patients may present with somatic or nonspecific complaints.

Epidemiology

- **Approximately one in four American adults suffers from a diagnosable mental disorder annually.** Mental illness is widespread across the population, and approximately 6% suffer from serious mental illness. Psychiatric disorders are the leading causes of disability for ages 15 to 44 in the US and Canada.
- Nearly half of patients with mental illness suffer from two or more psychiatric disorders at a single time. Symptoms may also overlap between several conditions. Disease severity sharply increases for coexisting mental illnesses.

Associated Conditions

- Several neurogenetic syndromes (e.g., Turner syndrome, Down syndrome, fragile X syndrome, Prader-Willi syndrome) and medical diseases have associated psychiatric manifestations.
- Socioeconomic, environmental, and cultural stressors contribute to the pathogenesis and definition of psychiatric diseases. The effective treatment and management of mental disorders therefore requires a biopsychosocial approach.

Relationships between Psychiatric and Medical Illnesses

- **Psychiatric illnesses are intimately intertwined with medical illnesses.** Underlying medical ailments (including endocrine disorders, cardiovascular disease, and respiratory conditions) are associated with increased rates of mental health disorders. Conversely, patients with significant psychiatric conditions have an increased risk for many medical disease categories.
- The severity of psychiatric illness is directly correlated to poor disease control and morbidity in conditions, such as diabetes and heart failure. For example, depression predicts an increased incidence of stroke in hypertensive patients.
- Studies suggest that successful treatment of psychiatric symptoms is associated with significant improvement in physical health and medical outcomes, including mortality.
- Medical illness is a risk factor for the development or exacerbation of depression, and depression is itself a risk factor for medical illness.[2]

Evaluation

- Patients with one psychiatric disorder should be screened for other coexisting psychiatric disorders.
- Patients should also undergo a thorough mental status examination, with **objective** evaluation of the following[3]:
  - ○ **Appearance and general behavior** (e.g., dress, grooming, hygiene, level of distress, degree of eye contact, attitude toward the interviewer [including evaluation of cooperativity])
  - ○ **Motor activity** (e.g., psychomotor agitation, tremors, dyskinesias, akathisia, mannerisms, tics, catatonic posturing, echopraxia, apparent responses to hallucinations, gait/neurologic defects)
  - ○ **Speech characteristics** including rate, rhythm, volume, amount, latency, tone, inflection, and articulation
  - ○ **Mood** (internal/subjective emotional state) and **affect** (the range, stability, and appropriateness of emotional expression)
  - ○ **Flow of thought** (e.g., logicality, sequentiality, goal directedness)
  - ○ **Thought content** including ideas of reference, overvalued ideas, ruminations, obsessions, compulsions, phobias, and delusions (e.g., erotomania, delusions of persecution, infidelity, infestation, somatic illness, guilt, worthlessness, thought insertion, thought withdrawal, thought broadcasting)
  - ○ **Thoughts or impulses of harm to self or others** (e.g., intensity, specificity of plans, when they occur, what prevents the patient from acting on them)
  - ○ **Perceptual disturbances** including hallucinations (a perception in the absence of a stimulus), illusions (an erroneous perception in the presence of a stimulus), and depersonalization (feeling detached from oneself)
  - ○ **Sensorium/cognition** (e.g., level of consciousness, orientation, attention, concentration, memory)
  - ○ **Insight** (e.g., understanding of current problems, motivation to change health risk behaviors)
  - ○ **Judgment** (i.e., appropriate decision-making abilities)

DEPRESSION

GENERAL PRINCIPLES

Classification

- Mood disorders form a phenotypic spectrum of abnormally altered emotional state.
- Mood disorders are subdivided into those with
  - ○ Only abnormally low mood (unipolar depression syndromes)
  - ○ Cycling between abnormally elevated and abnormally depressed moods (bipolar syndromes)
  - ○ Simultaneous depression and mania (mixed mood syndromes)[4]
- Mood disorders present with a **heterogeneous range of symptom severity and functional impairment**.
- Given the complexity of the diagnosis and management of bipolar disorder, a discussion of this illness is beyond the scope of this chapter. **If you suspect your patient to have bipolar illness, referral to a psychiatrist is indicated.** If your patient is exhibiting signs of mania (see "Clinical Presentation"), psychiatric hospitalization may be indicated and the patient should be referred to the nearest emergency department.

Epidemiology

- Depression is **extremely common** worldwide. Nearly 10% of American adults suffer from a mood disorder annually, and the lifetime prevalence of depressive illness is approximately 17% in the US.

- The median age of onset for mood disorders is 25 to 35 years of age.
- Depressive disorders are more common in women, especially postmenopausal women.[5]

Etiology/Pathophysiology

- Mood disorders stem from incompletely understood interactions between psychophysiologic stressors and alterations in neurohormonal pathways. Multiple different pathophysiologic changes can cause similar phenotypes.
- Serotonin- and norepinephrine-dependent pathways in the limbic system may play a key role in depression. Glutamate and gamma-aminobutyric acid (GABA) levels in the prefrontal cortex have also been shown to have a role in depression.[6] Additional changes in the hypothalamus-pituitary-adrenal axis are also likely involved.[7]
- Major depression exhibits complex inheritance patterns, likely involving multiple genes. Genetic predisposition is stronger in bipolar disorders and in recurrent depression.[7]

Risk Factors

- Depression syndromes are more likely in those with a history of depression, anxiety, and/or substance abuse; chronic medical illness; family history of major depression; domestic abuse/violence; stressful life events (e.g., death of a loved one, divorce, job change, motor vehicle accident); recent myocardial infarction or stroke; or recent pregnancy.[8]
- Patients should be evaluated for depression if they exhibit work or relationship dysfunction, changes in interpersonal relationships, worsening performance in activities of daily living, poor follow-through with prior treatment recommendations, multiple unexplained symptoms or frequent medical visits, dampened affect, unintended weight gain or loss, sleep disturbances or chronic fatigue, dementia or memory impairment, irritable bowel syndrome, or fibromyalgia syndrome, and if they volunteer complaints of stress or mood disturbances.[8,9]

Associated Conditions

- **Anxiety disorders and substance abuse frequently co-occur with depressive disorders**.[5]
- Significant medical, psychological, or environmental stressors precipitate the first episode of major depression in 40% to 60% of patients.[8]

Depression and Medical Illnesses

- Depression has a complex interdependent relationship with medical illness. Medical illnesses may
  - Be a direct biologic cause of depression (e.g., thyroid disorder, stroke)
  - Contribute to psychological stressors
  - Predispose to depression though changes in neurohormonal signaling
  - Mimic signs and symptoms of depression (e.g., anemia)[10,11]
- **Overwhelming evidence suggests that depression is associated with worse outcomes, impaired control, and increased risk of complications in diseases such as diabetes mellitus, stroke, myocardial infarction, and congestive heart failure**.[10]
- Poor control of medical illnesses may also contribute to worsened outcomes in depression.
- Treatment of associated medical illnesses may improve depression and vice versa, though data are limited.

DIAGNOSIS

Clinical Presentation

- Compared with nonpathologic normal sadness, depression exhibits a greater intensity, a longer duration, associated neurovegetative symptoms, and a **significant impact on patients' function**.
- **Major depression is characterized by at least 2 weeks of persistently decreased mood and/or anhedonia** (a significant loss of interest in previously interesting activities).

Patients also exhibit associated psychophysiologic changes in sleep, appetite, thought patterns, motivation, and overall function.[4] The Diagnostic and Statistical Manual of Mental Disorders-IV-Text Revision (DSM-IV-TR) and DSM-5 criteria are minimally different.[4,12]

- **Subsyndromal depression** patients meet two to three symptom criteria, rather than the three or more necessary to diagnose major depression.
- In **bipolar depression**, patients present with episodes similar to major depression but also have a history of manic or hypomanic episodes (abnormally and persistently elevated/expansive/irritable mood with distractibility, insomnia, grandiosity, flight of ideas/feelings, racing thoughts, agitation/increased goal-directed activity, increased/pressured speech, and/or risk taking/hedonism).
- **Mixed mood syndromes** manifest symptoms of both mania and depression during the same episode.[4]
- The Two-Question Screen is sensitive but not specific for depression[9,13]:
  - Over the past month, have you been bothered by little interest or pleasure in doing things?
  - Over the past month, have you been bothered by feeling down, depressed, or hopeless?
  - **If the patient answers yes to either screening question, evaluation should be performed using a quantitative standardized instrument** (e.g., the PHQ-9, Beck Depression Inventory, or Hamilton Depression Rating Scale).[8]
- Initial evaluation should also include the following:
  - Screening for suicidality or self-harm (see "Deliberate Self-Harm and Suicidality" section)
  - Assessment of depression severity
  - Evaluation for bipolar and mixed mood disorders
  - Screening for concurrent psychiatric issues including substance abuse

Differential Diagnosis

- A great many medical conditions are strongly associated with or contribute to mood disorders including cardiac, endocrine, infectious, metabolic, neoplastic, and neurologic disorders as well as effects due to medications, toxins, and illicit substances.
- Depression must be distinguished from other psychiatric conditions (Table 42-1).[4,14]
- Appropriate laboratory and radiographic testing should be performed to evaluate for medical conditions contributing to the patient's depression.

TREATMENT

- Depression treatment consists of three phases[15,16]:
  - **Acute therapy** (usually 6 to 12 weeks)
  - **Continuation** (4 to 9 months), which targets prevention of relapse
  - **Maintenance** (6 months to years), which targets prevention of a new distinct episode of major depression
- **Bipolar and mixed mood syndromes require mood stabilizers (e.g., atypical antipsychotics, anticonvulsants, lithium) before antidepressant treatment to prevent triggering mania.**
- Bipolar disorder eventually manifests in up to 10% of patients initially thought to have unipolar depression.
- Strongly consider treatment of patients with low mood who do not strictly meet criteria for depression but exhibit significant functional impairment.

Acute Therapy

- Patients and family members should be educated that
  - Depression is a medical illness, not a sign of weak character.
  - Depression can be effectively treated.
  - Patients improve with treatment.
  - Depression can recur, and patients should seek treatment early if symptoms return.[8]

TABLE 42-1 Psychiatric Differential Diagnosis for Major Depression[5,8]

	Similarities to major depression	Differences from major depression
Bipolar disorders	• Depressive episodes may be clinically similar to unipolar depression	• History of at least one manic or hypomanic episode • Antidepressant treatment of depression in bipolar disorder can precipitate a manic episode
Seasonal affective disorder	• Symptoms identical to depression during episodes	• Depressive episodes show a seasonal pattern (typically a fall or winter predominance) • Episodes regress completely as the season changes
Dysthymia (now referred to as persistent depressive disorder by DSM-5)	• Low mood and affect • Chronic, recurrent course • Associated changes in sleep, energy, concentration, and appetite • May predispose to major depression	• Lesser symptom severity, without anhedonia • Depressed mood, more days than not, for at least 2 years • Lesser risk of self-harm or suicide
Adjustment disorder	• Low mood and affect • Precipitated by life stressors • High rates of coexistent anxiety	• Lesser symptom severity, without anhedonia • Symptoms resolve with resolution of the stressor • Lesser feelings of guilt/worthlessness • Lesser changes in appetite, sleep, or energy • Lesser risk of self-harm or suicide
Bereavement	• Low mood and affect • Impaired function • Precipitated by loss of loved one • Potential hallucinations and illusions • May progress to major depression	• Symptoms last <2 months • Less severe impairment • Lesser feelings of guilt or suicidal ideation
Psychotic disorders (e.g., schizophrenia, schizoaffective disorder)	• May include symptoms of depression or mania • Hallucinations or delusions may resemble psychosis in mania or depression • May occur in concurrence with depression or mania	• Mood symptoms brief relative to the total duration of the psychotic disturbance • Significant negative symptoms (i.e., flattened affect, disorganized speech/behavior)

(Continued)

TABLE 42-1	Psychiatric Differential Diagnosis for Major Depression[5,8] (*Continued*)

	Similarities to major depression	Differences from major depression
Dementia	• Cognitive symptoms similar to depression in elderly patients • Decreased motivation and function • Associated with physical symptoms including sleep dysfunction • May predispose to concurrent major depression	• Premorbid history of declining cognitive function • Variable rate of decline (e.g., rapid to subacute to chronic) depending on underlying etiology
Medical disorders (e.g., endocrine, neurologic)	• Overlap in signs and symptoms with depression • May predispose to depression	• Symptoms improve with treatment of the underlying condition alone
Substance related (e.g., withdrawal, intoxication, pharmaceutical)	• Overlap in signs and symptoms with depression • Substance abuse may predispose to depression	• Symptoms improve with treatment of the underlying condition alone

- Acute therapy should target symptom remission and not merely improvement.[8,11,16] Response to treatment is defined as a ≥50% reduction in symptomatology.[8]
- **Depression-specific psychotherapies and antidepressant medications** have similar response rates for **mild** depression. Both are acceptable initial approaches.
- **Antidepressants** should be started in patients with **moderate or severe** major depression. Adjuvant psychotherapy may improve response, especially in severe, recurrent, or chronic depression.[8,11,16–20]
- **Depression with psychotic features** should be treated with a combination of an antidepressant and an antipsychotic medication and/or electroconvulsive therapy (ECT).[2]
- Patients may require ≥6 weeks to achieve full symptom remission after treatment begins.[8,21]
- If a patient experiences a symptom reduction of ≥25% 4 to 6 weeks after treatment initiation but is not yet in remission, continue current therapy with medication uptitration if tolerated.[8]
- If there is <25% reduction of symptoms after 6 weeks of **appropriate** therapy, either adding or switching to another treatment are both effective.[8]
- Patients who do not respond to an initial selective serotonin reuptake inhibitor (SSRI) have a modestly better chance of response, if changed to a non-SSRI rather than a different SSRI.[8,11,21]
- Augmentation may include the addition of serotonin-norepinephrine reuptake inhibitors (SNRIs), tricyclic antidepressants (TCAs), bupropion, mirtazapine, and/or adjuvant nonpharmacologic interventions. Other strategies may require the assistance of a psychiatrist.

- Figure 42-1 provides a recommended schema for acute treatment with antidepressant medications. Other well-validated algorithms can be used, including the algorithms used in the STAR-D study for depression and the STEP-BD study for bipolar disorder.[22–24]
- Medications should be tapered when discontinued or added, with vigilance for drug-drug interactions, overlapping side effect profiles, and withdrawal phenomena.
- Patients should be routinely **monitored for suicide risk** throughout therapy.

Duration of Treatment

- Treatment should be continued for **at least 4 to 9 months after remission of symptoms** (the continuation phase).[25] Recurrent episodes imply the need for longer medication maintenance.
  - First episode: continue medication for 6 to 12 months, withdraw gradually.
  - Second episode: continue medication for 3 years, withdraw gradually.
  - Three episodes or more: continue medication indefinitely.
- When antidepressants are discontinued, it is commonly recommended that the medications be tapered over 2 to 4 weeks to minimize withdrawal.[8]

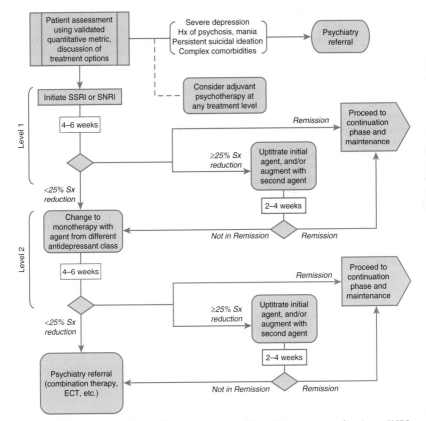

Figure 42-1 Suggested schema for acute therapy with antidepressant medications. SNRI, serotonin-norepinephrine reuptake inhibitor; SSRI, selective serotonin reuptake inhibitor.

Medications

- Data suggest **minimal difference in efficacy among antidepressants for the acute treatment** of depression.[26,27]
- While data are limited, **it appears that most medications are also equally effective in preventing relapse.** Side effect profiles and cost considerations should guide treatment choices (see Table 42-2).
- Adherence to medication, even after symptom improvement, is key. Premature discontinuation of antidepressant treatment is associated with a 77% increase in the risk of relapse or symptom recurrence.[8]
- Risks for premature self-discontinuation include younger age, lower educational status, and higher self-perceived mental health.[21]
- **SSRIs and SNRIs are considered first-line agents given their side effect profiles.** There appears to be minimal within-class differences in efficacy.
- **TCAs** are effective but should be used cautiously given **cardiac side effects and risk for lethal overdose.** Higher doses of TCAs may be more effective in those who partially respond to lower doses.
- Monoamine oxidase inhibitors (MAOIs) should be restricted to patients unresponsive to other medications because of their potential for **drug interactions, serious side effects, and the necessity of dietary restrictions.** Psychiatric consultation is strongly recommended if an MAOI is considered.
- Psychostimulants (e.g., dextroamphetamine, methylphenidate, and methylamphetamine) are useful adjuvant treatments for depression but have not been adequately studied for use as monotherapy. Psychiatric consultation is strongly recommended if stimulants are considered.
- St. John's wort and S-adenosyl methionine (SAM-e) are sometimes self-prescribed as natural antidepressants. Studies show mixed results regarding efficacy of these as antidepressants and serious drug-drug interactions as well as the heterogeneity of commercially available preparations argue against use.[8,18,28] Other herbals and dietary supplements, such as kava-kava, omega-3 fatty acid (docosahexaenoic acid), and valerian root, have not been proven effective for the treatment of depression.[8,28]

Other Nonpharmacologic Therapies

- **Several psychotherapy modalities are effective in the treatment of depression.**[19] Such interventions should be performed by therapists specifically trained in these techniques.
- **Combined therapy using both pharmacologic and psychological therapy may be more effective than either intervention alone.**[8,19]
- **ECT** may benefit patients with refractory depression, depression with psychotic features, and geriatric patients.
- Other neuromodulation techniques (e.g., repetitive transcranial magnetic stimulation, deep brain stimulation, and vagus nerve stimulation) have shown some promise in treating resistant depression but require psychiatric evaluation.
- Depression that is worse in winter (i.e., seasonality) often improves with phototherapy using broad-spectrum bright light (typically 10,000 lux).[29] Such therapy should be initiated only by clinicians trained in prescribing phototherapy.
- Aerobic exercise may be of adjuvant benefit in reducing depressive symptoms.[8,18,30] Patients should aim for 30 minutes of moderate-intensity exercise, 3 to 5 days per week.

REFERRAL

- Multiple trials demonstrate the benefit of a collaborative care model with the close integration of physicians, mental health professionals, and case managers.[8] While both general medicine and psychiatric specialty settings yield good initial outcomes, therapeutic alliance with mental health specialists should be strongly considered.[21]

TABLE 42-2   Antidepressant Medications

	Usual starting dose (mg/day)	Usual total therapeutic dose (mg/day)	Side effects (SFx) and clinical notes	Qualitative frequency of common side effects								
				Headache	Insomnia or agitation	Sedation	Nausea	Diarrhea	Dry mouth	Weight loss	Weight gain	Anti-cholinergic effects
Selective serotonin reuptake inhibitors (SSRIs)			Sexual side-effects. Headache and jitteriness often subside after first 4–7 days. Risk of birth malformations. Risk seizures at very high doses. Risk serotonin syndrome if given with MAOIs.									
Citalopram (Celexa)	10–20	20–60	Less Rx-Rx interactions than other SSRIs.	+	+	– –	+++	+	++	+	+	– –
Escitalopram (Lexapro)	10	10–20	Single isomer formulation of citalopram, similar SFx profile.	+++	+	– –	++	+	+	– –	+	– –
Fluoxetine (Prozac)	5–10	20–60	CYP2D6 inhib. Take in morning to reduce insomnia. Active metabolites (long half-life, avail. in once-weekly formulation). Transiently decreases appetite.	++	++	– –	+++	++	+	+	– –	– –
Fluvoxamine (Luvox)	25	50–300	Affects multiple CYP isoforms. Increased risk Rx-Rx interact vs. other SSRIs.	+++	+	+	+++	++	++	+	+	– –
Paroxetine (Paxil)	5–10	20–60	CYP2D6 inhib. Higher rates of extrapyramidal SFx and withdrawal SFx vs. other SSRIs. Less GI SFx if taken with food.	++	+	+	+++	++	++	+	++	+

(Continued)

TABLE 42-2 Antidepressant Medications (*Continued*)

	Usual starting dose (mg/day)	Usual total therapeutic dose (mg/day)	Side effects (SFx) and clinical notes	Qualitative frequency of common side effects								
				Headache	Insomnia or agitation	Sedation	Nausea	Diarrhea	Dry mouth	Weight loss	Weight gain	Anticholinergic effects
Sertraline (Zoloft)	25–50	50–200	CYP2D6 inhib. but less potent inhib. than fluoxetine. Very sedating, best taken at night.	+++	++	– –	+++	++	++	– –	+	– –
Serotonin-norepinephrine reuptake inhibitors (SNRIs)												
Duloxetine (Cymbalta)	30	60–120	Contraind. if signif. renal/hepatic disease. May impair glycemic control in DM. Possible addition benefits in chronic pain control.	++	++	–	++	++	++	+	– –	– –
Venlafaxine (Effexor), Venlafaxine XR (Effexor XR)	37.5	75–300	CYP2D6 inhib.: incr. SFx if switching from CYP2D6-metabol. agents. High risk of withdrawal SFx. HTN, MI at high doses.	++	+++	–	++	+	++	+	–	–
Desvenlafaxine (Pristiq)	50	50	Active metabolite of venlafaxine: similar SFx but does not interact with CYP2D6. May increase LDL	– –	++	–	++	++	++	+	– –	–
Noradrenergic agonist-specific serotonergic antagonist												

Drug	Starting dose (mg)	Dose range (mg/d)	Comments									
Mirtazapine (Remeron)	15	15–45	Neurotransmitters affected are dose related. SFx may be greater at lower doses. Lower risk sexual SFx than SSRI. Risk bone marrow toxicity.	++	--	+++	+	+	+	+++	--	+++	+
Dopamine-norepinephrine reuptake inhibitors													
Bupropion (Wellbutrin)	75–150	300–450	Risk of seizure. Mild stimulating properties. May be beneficial in treating SSRI-related sexual SFx. Caution in hepatic impairment.	+++	++	--	+	+	+	--	++	--	--
Bupropion SR/XL (Wellbutrin SR/XL)	150	300–400		+++	+	--	+	+	+	--	++	--	--
Serotonin modulators													
Nefazodone (Serzone)	50	300–600	Potent CYP3A4 inhib. Increases REM sleep. Less sexual SFx than other antidepressants. Risk QTc prolong if given with cisapride. Risk hepatotoxicity, Stevens–Johnson synd. Not available in the United States	+++	+	++	++	++	+	++	--	+	+
Trazodone (Desyrel)	50	75–200	Postural hypotension and nausea. Risk priapism, arrhythmias. Used as hypnotic; no longer used at antidepressant doses.	++	--	+++	+++	+	+	+++	--	+	--

(Continued)

TABLE 42-2 Antidepressant Medications (Continued)

	Usual starting dose (mg/day)	Usual total therapeutic dose (mg/day)	Side effects (SFx) and clinical notes	Qualitative frequency of common side effects								
				Headache	Insomnia or agitation	Sedation	Nausea	Diarrhea	Dry mouth	Weight loss	Weight gain	Anti-cholinergic effects
Vilazodone (Viibryd)	10	40	Strong CYP3A4 inhib. Bioavailability reduced with fasting. Extensive protein binding.	+	++	--	+++	+++	+	--	--	--
Tricyclics and tetracyclics (TCAs)			Affect multiple neurotransmitter systems. Risk of QTc prolongation, arrhythmia, MI. Anticholinergic effects incl. orthostasis, sexual dysfunction. Rare bone marrow and hepatic toxicity. Lower seizure threshold. Levels increased by concomitant SSRI. Potentially fatal at overdose.									
Amitriptyline (Elavil)	25–50	100–300	Metabol. to nortriptyline by liver.	++	--	+++	+	+	+++	--	+++	+++
Amoxapine (Asendin)	50	100–400		+	++	++	+	--	++	--	+	+
Clomipramine (Anafranil)	25	100–250		+++	++	+++	++	+	+++	--	+++	+++
Desipramine (Norpramin)	25–50	150–200		+	+	+++	+	+	+	+	+	+
Doxepin (Adapin, Sinequan)	25–50	100–300		+	--	+++	+	+	++	--	+++	++

Drug	Starting Dose (mg)	Dose Range (mg)	Comments									
Imipramine (Tofranil)	25–50	150–300	Metabol. to desipramine by liver. Incr. orthostasis and arrhythmia vs. other TCAs.	+	++	+	+	+	+++	+	+++	++
Maprotiline (Ludiomil)	50	100–225		+	+++	+	+	++	– –	– –	++	+
Nortriptyline (Pamelor)	25	75–100	Lower rates of orthostasis and arrhythmias vs. other TCAs.	+	++	+	+	+	+	+	+	++
Protriptyline (Vivactil)	10	15–60		+	+	+	+	++	– –	– –	– –	+
Trimipramine (Surmontil)	25–50	100–300	Risk serotonin syndrome if given with or close to discontinuation of SSRIs.	+	+++	+	+	+	– –	– –	+++	+++
Monoamine oxidase inhibitors (MAOIs)												
Isocarboxazid (Marplan)	20	40–60	Dose-related hypotension, sexual SFx, sleep disturbance. Need low tyramine diet.	++	+	+	+	+	– –	+	+	– –
Phenelzine (Nardil)	15	15–90	Dose-related hypotension, sexual SFx, sleep disturbance. Rare hepatotoxicity. Need low tyramine diet.	++	+	+	+	+	– –	+	++	– –
Selegiline (Emsam)	6 (Patch)	6–12		++	– –	++	++	++	– –	– –	– –	– –
Tranylcypromine (Parnate)	10	30–60	Dose-related hypotension, sexual SFx, sleep disturbance. May cause transient hypertension for 3–4 hours after doses. Need low tyramine diet.	++	++	+	+	+	– –	++	++	– –

Contraind., contraindicated; CYP, cytochrome-P450; DM, diabetes mellitus; HTN, hypertension; immed, immediate; inhib, inhibition; LDL, low density lipoprotein; metabol., metabolized; MI, myocardial infarction; Rx-Rx interact., drug-drug interaction; signif., significant; SFx, side effects; QTc, corrected QT interval; – –, rare; +, seldom; ++, common; +++, frequent.
Modified from Clinical Pharmacology. 2014. http://www.clinicalpharmacology-ip.com. Last accessed 2/1/15. Depression Guideline Panel. U.S. Department of Health and Human Services. Agency for Health Care Policy and Research. *Depression in Primary Care: Treatment of Major Depression.* AHCPR Publication No. 93-0551. Rockville, MD: AHCPR; 1993; Gartlehner G, Hansen RA, Thieda P, et al.; U.S. Department of Health and Human Services. Agency for Healthcare Research and Quality. *Comparative Effectiveness of Second-Generation Antidepressants in the Pharmacologic Treatment of Adult Depression.* AHRQ Publication No. 07-EHC007-EF. Bethesda, MD: AHRQ; 2007.

- Psychotherapy should be administered by a skilled therapist. Data suggest that the success of psychotherapy may be linked to the experience level of practitioners.
- Strongly consider **psychiatrist or mental health specialist referral** if there is intolerance or minimal benefit with first-line agents; signs of psychosis or suicidal ideation; severe symptoms or functional impairment; comorbid medical, psychiatric, or substance abuse disorders; symptoms or history suggestive of mania/bipolar disease or seasonal affective disorder; plans for psychotherapy; need for frequent or close follow-up; and/or patient requests for specialist treatment.
- Consider **hospitalization** if the patient poses a serious risk for harm to self or others (involuntary hospitalization may be necessary), is severely ill and lacks adequate social supports, has not responded adequately to outpatient treatment, or has significant comorbid psychiatric or medical conditions.[16]

MONITORING/FOLLOW-UP

Expert opinion recommends patients should be

- Seen within 2 weeks after starting any medications to evaluate for tolerability, effectiveness, and appropriate dosage
- Followed at least every 2 weeks until significant symptom improvement
- Followed at least every 3 months after symptom remission.[25]

OUTCOME/PROGNOSIS

- Depression is a heterogeneous disorder with a highly variable course.[7]
- In most patients, major depression is a relapsing-remitting illness with a >40% risk of recurrence within 2 years after the first depressive episode.[14]
- Repetitive episodes increase the risk of future recurrence.
- Relapse prevention with pharmacologic and nonpharmacologic modalities diminishes but does not completely prevent relapse.[19] Clinicians should be mindful to monitor for depression recurrence.

DELIBERATE SELF-HARM AND SUICIDALITY

GENERAL PRINCIPLES

- Deliberate self-harm commonly involves self-cutting, self-poisoning, or intentional medication overdose.[31]
- Suicide is an act of self-harm with a fatal outcome, consciously initiated and performed with the expectation of death.[31]
- Individual self-harm acts vary in their associated suicidal intent, degree of planning (e.g., meticulous vs. impulsive, precautions against rescue), and lethality of method (e.g., violent vs. passive).

Epidemiology

- About 3% to 5% of the population has made an attempt at deliberate self-harm at some time during their lives.[31]
- Approximately one quarter of those with one self-harm attempt will reattempt self-harm within 4 years, with a long-term suicide risk of 3% to 7%.[5]
- The median mortality from suicide after an act of deliberate self-harm is 1.8% within the first year, 3.0% within 1 to 4 years, 3.4% within 5 to 10 years, and 6.7% within 9 years or longer.[31]

- Younger adults are more likely to attempt nonfatal self-harm, whereas older adults are more likely to complete suicide.
- Women attempt suicide two to three times as often as men, but men are four times as likely to die by suicide.[5]
- The highest suicide rates in the United States are found in white men >85 years of age.[5]
- >90% of those who commit suicide suffered from a mental illness, most commonly a mood or a substance abuse disorder.[5]

Etiology/Pathophysiology

- Evidence suggests that genetic predisposition, biologic changes, and psychosocial factors all contribute to deliberate self-harm.[31]
- Reduced serotonin function and lowered cerebrospinal 5-hydroxyindoleacetic acid levels in the central nervous system may underpin the pathophysiologic changes of self-harm.
- Patients who deliberately self-harm also show personality traits of impulsiveness, aggression, inflexibility, and impaired judgment.

Risk Factors

- A large number of risk factors have been associated with suicide attempts including the following[8,31,32]:
  - Suicidal thoughts, **past attempts**, specific/lethal plans, access to **firearms**
  - Psychiatric illness (depression, bipolar disorder, schizophrenia, substance abuse)
  - Psychological features (shame, low self-esteem, impulsiveness, aggression, hopelessness, severe anxiety)
  - Significant burden of medical illness
  - Socioeconomic factors (lack of support, unemployment, recent stressful events)
  - Demographics (women/younger more likely to attempt; men/older more likely to succeed; widowed/divorced/single)
- Studies have not found racial predispositions for attempting suicide.[8,14]
- Factors with a protective effect include positive social support, children at home, responsibility to family, pregnancy (in the absence of peripartum depression), religious beliefs, life satisfaction, and good judgment/problem-solving skills/coping skills.[32]
- **Antidepressants, including SSRIs and TCAs, may increase risk of suicidality during the initial treatment of psychiatric illness when compared with placebo.** The U.S. Food and Drug Administration issued a warning about the risks of suicidal thinking and behavior in adults aged 18 to 24 years during the first 1 to 2 months of treatment for major depression.[33]

DIAGNOSIS

- At-risk patients should be assessed for thoughts of causing deliberate harm to themselves or others.[8,32]
- Useful questions include the following:
  - Do you feel that life is worth living?
  - Do you wish you were dead?
  - Have you thought about hurting yourself or ending your life?
    - If so, how often have those thoughts occurred?
    - Have you gone so far as to think about how you would do so?
    - Do you have access to a way to carry out your plan?
- What keeps you from harming yourself?
- Do you feel that others are responsible for your problems? If so, have you thought about harming or punishing them?

TREATMENT

- **Immediate hospitalization with close observation should strongly be considered for patients who are deemed high risk for harm to self or others**; evidence psychosis or command hallucinations; have current impulsive behavior, severe agitation, or poor judgment; have a specific suicide plan with persistent intent/ideation; have made precautions against discovery or rescue; have previously attempted suicide using means with high lethality; have significant comorbid psychiatric illness (including depression or substance abuse); and are male and >45 years of age.[32]
- Causes of suicidality or homicidality (e.g., substance withdrawal or intoxication, psychiatric illness, depression) should be identified and treated appropriately.
- Pharmacologic and psychotherapeutic interventions may be beneficial for the treatment of those without underlying reversible causes, though data are limited and inconsistent.

Medications

- **Antidepressant medications** (e.g., SSRIs, SNRIs, TCAs) should be used to treat depressed patients with suicidal ideation (see Table 42-2).[32]
- Lithium reduces the risk of both suicide and suicide attempts when used as long-term maintenance for recurring bipolar disorder and major depressive disorder.
- Anticonvulsant agents used as mood stabilizers (e.g., valproate, carbamazepine, lamotrigine) have not been shown to reduce risk of suicidal behavior.
- Benzodiazepines may ameliorate the suicide risk in an agitated patient because of anxiolytic effects but should be used cautiously as they also disinhibit behavior and enhance impulsivity, particularly in patients with borderline personality disorder.
- **No pharmaceutical treatments have clearly shown usefulness for reducing recurrent self-harm not associated with underlying psychiatric illness.**[31]

Other Nonpharmacologic Therapies

- Clinical consensus suggests skilled psychosocial interventions and specific psychotherapeutic techniques (e.g., cognitive behavioral therapy [CBT] and dialectical behavior therapy) be used in preventing recurrent self-harm.[31,32]
- ECT may provide short-term reduction in suicidal ideation, especially in cases of severe depression.[32,34]
- While recommended, intensive follow-up plus outreach, nurse-led management, emergency contact cards, and hospital admission have not consistently been shown to reduce recurrent self-harm compared with usual care.[31,34]

REFERRAL

Patients with recurrent or persistent suicidal ideation or self-harm attempts should be cared for in collaboration with psychiatrists and other mental health professionals.

FOLLOW-UP

- Patients who have attempted deliberate self-harm are at risk for future attempts. Repetition is more likely in patients aged 25 to 49 years; unemployed or socioeconomically disadvantaged; divorced, living alone, or with unstable living situations; who have a criminal record; who have a history of stressful traumatic life events or come from a so-called broken home; who have a history of substance abuse, depression, or personality disorder; and who have recurrent feelings of hopelessness or powerlessness.[31]
- Patients should be routinely monitored by clinicians and family members for evidence of suicidal ideation or recurrent self-harm behaviors. Repeat or long-term hospitalization may be necessary if the patients are persistently a threat to themselves or others.

ANXIETY DISORDERS

- Anxiety disorders are the most common mental health illnesses, affecting nearly one in five American adults.[3] The disorders are **typified by increased agitation, nervousness, and autonomic tone that disrupt general well-being and function.**
- Anxiety disorders include panic disorder, obsessive-compulsive disorder, posttraumatic stress disorder, generalized anxiety disorder (GAD), and phobias (see Table 42-3).[4,14]
- Anxiety disorders frequently coexist with depressive disorders or substance abuse. In addition, most people with one anxiety disorder also have another anxiety disorder.[5]
- Medical issues such as hypoglycemia, hyperthyroidism, respiratory disease, gastrointestinal disease, and medication side effects all predispose to anxiety disorders. Improvement in these conditions may improve psychiatric issues.

Generalized Anxiety Disorder

GENERAL PRINCIPLES

GAD is characterized by **unreasonably excessive concern** about common issues, such as finances, family, or work. In GAD, worries become so exaggerated that there is difficulty in performing day-to-day tasks. Other anxiety disorders should be ruled out. DSM-IV-TR and DSM-5 criteria are essentially the same.[4,12]

Epidemiology

- About 3% of American adults suffer from GAD.[3] However, studies suggest that GAD may be more prevalent in primary care settings, and suggest that GAD is the anxiety disorder most often seen by general internists.[35]
- GAD develops gradually and may present at any age, though the median age of onset is about 30 years.
- Similar to other anxiety disorders, GAD is more common in women than in men.[5]

Etiology/Pathophysiology

- GAD develops from a combination of biologic and psychosocial factors.
- Multiple neurotransmitter and endocrine pathways, including the hypothalamic-pituitary-adrenal axis, have been implicated.[36] Medical disorders such as chronic pain, endocrine diseases, and pulmonary conditions may predispose to generalized anxiety.
- Social and environmental stressors, including recent unfavorable events, also likely contribute to GAD.[37]
- **Maladaptive cognitive strategies play a prominent role in GAD.** Worry subjectively increases preparedness for feared events but also causes distress over them. GAD patients subconsciously overvalue the worry process and, over time, develop a cycle of worry proneness.[35]
- Predisposition to GAD appears modestly inheritable but incompletely understood.[36,37]

Associated Conditions

- Patients with GAD may exhibit worsening job performance, changes in interpersonal relationships, multiple unexplained symptoms or frequent medical visits, concentration difficulties, sleep disturbances or chronic fatigue, and increasing alcohol/tobacco use.
- Patients with GAD are at high risk for developing another anxiety disorder or major depression.[37,38]
- More than one-third of GAD patients abuse alcohol or illicit drugs.[35]

TABLE 42-3 Characteristics of Common Anxiety Disorders[5,8]

	Defining characteristics	Additional features
Panic disorder	• Recurrent unexpected short-lived episodes of marked autonomic arousal (e.g., tachycardia, palpitations, sweating, shortness of breath) and catastrophic thinking (e.g., fear of fainting, dying, "depersonalization"). • Attacks are abrupt in onset, unprovoked, and unexplained.	• Impairment stems from worry about potential future panic episodes. • Possible evolution into avoidance of places or situations associated with past panic episodes (a.k.a., agoraphobia). • Panic episodes may awaken patient from sleep during non-REM states. • Symptoms may fluctuate in intensity.
Generalized anxiety disorder (GAD)	• Excessive worry about multiple foci of concern for more days than not with significant disruption of daily life.	• Association with nonspecific somatic complaints including fatigue, insomnia, and muscle tension. • Related concentration difficulties, irritability, or restlessness. • Episodes peak in 5–10 minutes, last 15–20 minutes.
Post-traumatic stress disorder (PTSD)	• Intense fear, helplessness, and "flashbacks" following an extreme traumatic stressor with perceived risk of death or serious injury. • Patients avoid reminders of the trauma and experience hyperarousal (i.e., easy startle, irritability, difficulty concentrating, insomnia).	• Possible traumas may include violent or sexual assault, kidnapping, incarceration, natural disasters, or severe accidents. • Patients may also experience PTSD from witnessed events or events experienced by a family member or loved one.
Phobias	• Unreasonably excessive and persistent fear triggered by the presence or anticipation of a specific stimulus. • Phobias cause significant impairments in function due to avoidance behaviors.	• Common phobias include animals (e.g., dogs, insects, spiders); environmental features (e.g., closed spaces, heights, darkness); and social situations (e.g., public speaking, eating in public).
Obsessive-compulsive disorder (OCD)	• Presence of either obsessions (repetitive intrusive anxiety-provoking thoughts) or compulsions (repetitive anxiety-relieving behaviors or mental acts designed to neutralize obsessions).	• Patients often recognize the irrationality of their obsessions. • The nature of the patients' obsessions and compulsions may change over time.

- **GAD is a chronic condition but can be improved or controlled with treatment.** Twenty-five percent of adults with GAD will be in full remission after 2 years, and 38% will have a remission after 5 years.[37]
- However, nearly one-third of patients in full remission will have a clinically significant relapse within 5 years; the rate is even higher for those with only partial remission.[37]

DIAGNOSIS

Clinical Presentation

- The hallmark of GAD is **excessive and difficult-to-control worry about multiple issues,** often despite insight that the anxiety is more intense than warranted.[36]
- Unlike other anxiety disorders, worry in GAD is **not limited to a specific trigger or social situation** (e.g., phobias). GAD patients may experience discrete panic attacks but their anxiousness is **persistent, pervasive, and focused on multiple components** of normal daily living.
- In addition to excessive worry, patients may exhibit other nonspecific signs including irritability or fatigue, difficulty concentrating, increased startle responses, and/or sleep disturbances including insomnia.[38]
- Patients with GAD frequently have associated **somatic symptoms** including headaches, muscle tension and myalgias, difficulty swallowing (i.e., globus hystericus), nausea, tremor or tics, sweating, lightheadedness or dyspnea, frequent urination, and/or hot flashes.[35,36,38]
- Symptom severity fluctuates over time and is often worse during periods of increased stress.[36]
- GAD patients often seek medical care for their somatic symptoms, but do not necessarily volunteer concerns about their psychological ones.[35,36]
- Screening can be performed using the 7-item Anxiety Scale (GAD-7), which has reasonable reliability, sensitivity, and specificity.[39]
- Further assessment should be made through a validated quantitative measure such as the Generalized Anxiety Disorder Questionnaire IV (GAD-Q-IV).[40]
- Initial evaluation should include the following:
  - Screening for suicidality or self-harm
  - Assessment of anxiety severity and impact
  - Screening for concurrent psychiatric issues including depression and substance abuse
- Appropriate laboratory and radiographic testing should be performed if there are potentially treatable medical conditions contributing to the patient's symptomatology.

Differential Diagnosis

- Many medical conditions are associated with or contribute to anxiety disorders including cardiac, endocrine, infectious, metabolic, neoplastic, and neurologic disorders as well as effects due to medications, diet, toxins, and illicit substances.
- GAD must be distinguished from other psychiatric conditions (Table 42-3).[4,14]

TREATMENT

- Both medications and nonpharmacologic treatments benefit GAD, but it is uncertain which is more effective. At least one study involving a pediatric population has shown that sertraline in combination with CBT is more effective than either treatment alone.[41]
- Strongly consider **psychiatrist or mental health specialist referral** if there are severe symptoms or functional impairment; signs of psychosis or suicidal ideation; comorbid medical, psychiatric, or substance abuse disorders; plans for psychotherapy; need for frequent or close follow-up; and/or patient requests for specialist treatment.[38]

Medications

- The **SSRIs and SNRIs** have all shown benefit over placebo in treating GAD and should be considered first-line agents (Table 42-3).[35,37,42]
  - Although data are limited, there appears to be minimal efficacy and tolerability differences amongst these medications.[37]
  - **Patients typically require at least 4 to 6 weeks of therapy with SSRIs before symptoms improve**.
- **Imipramine** has demonstrated benefit for GAD; other TCAs are less well studied.[35,37,42] However, the side effect profile of imipramine suggests that it should be considered a second-line agent.
- **Benzodiazepines** have proven utility in the **temporary** mitigation of GAD (Table 42-4).[37,43]
  - Short-term adjuvant therapy with long-acting benzodiazepines may benefit some patients during the initial phase of treatment with SSRIs or SNRIs.
  - Trials have not shown benefit over other agents when used for long-term anxiety control. The prolonged use of benzodiazepines in GAD also increases risk for dependence, sedation, and traffic accidents.[37]
  - These agents should be limited to use for breakthrough anxiety.
  - There does not appear to be significant within-class efficacy differences among the long-acting benzodiazepines.[37]
- Hydroxyzine (a first-generation antihistamine) has been successfully used as an anxiolytic in GAD.[37] Data regarding its efficacy have been mixed, however, and sedating side effects may limit its usefulness.

Other Nonpharmacologic Therapies

- Psychotherapy is an effective treatment for GAD.[44]
- **CBT** focused on insight, education, and coping strategies reduces anxiety symptoms and is beneficial as both short- and long-term treatment.[35,36,39]
  - CBT is more effective than other psychological therapies.[45]
  - CBT should be administered by a skilled therapist. Data suggest that the success of psychotherapy is linked to the experience level of practitioners, though some patients may benefit from nonspecialist delivered supportive psychotherapy alone.[35]
- Relaxation training had historically been used in treating GAD but has not been well studied in clinical trials.[35] Related methods such as applied relaxation and mindful meditation appear to have some efficacy.[37]
- Aerobic exercise and exercise training likely have general anxiety-lowering benefits but have not been well-studied in the treatment of GAD.[30]

Panic Disorder and Agoraphobia

GENERAL PRINCIPLES

- Panic attacks are discrete sudden periods of intensive apprehension or terror, often accompanied by physiologic symptoms (e.g., palpitations, chest pain, shortness of breath, dizziness) and feelings of impending doom DSM-IV-TR and DSM-5 criteria are essentially the same.[4,12]
- Panic disorder is diagnosed, however, only when recurrent unpredictable panic attacks are followed by at least 1 month of persistent concern about having another panic attack or significant behavioral changes related to the attacks.[4,14]
- Agoraphobia (an irrational fear of public places, crowds, or being outside the home) may also develop in the setting of recurrent panic attacks.

TABLE 42-4 Frequently Used Benzodiazepines

Drug	Onset of action	Half-life	Relative potency	Usual total dose (mg/day)	Usual dosing frequency	Notes
Alprazolam (Xanax)	Medium	Interm.	4	0.5–4	tid	High-potency: increased risk withdrawal
Alprazolam XR (Xanax XR)	Varies	Long	4	0.5–6	once daily	Absorption rate affected by food, time of day of administration
Chlordiazepoxide (Librium)	Medium	Long	0.1	15–30	tid	Active metabolites with long half-life of elimination
Clonazepam (Klonopin)	Medium	Long	2	0.5–2	bid	Total doses >1 mg/day not shown to be more effective for symptom control
Clorazepate (Gen-Xene)	Rapid	Short	0.1	15–60	bid to qid	
Diazepam (Valium)	Rapid	Long	0.2	4–20	bid to qid	
Estazolam (Prosom)	Rapid	Interm.	3	1–2	hs	High-potency. Usually used to treat insomnia
Flurazepam (Dalmane)	Rapid	Short	0.2	15–30	hs	Usually used to treat insomnia
Lorazepam (Ativan)	Medium	Interm.	1	0.5–6	bid to tid	
Oxazepam (Serax)	Slow	Interm.	0.7	30–120	tid to qid	
Quazepam (Doral)	Rapid	Long	0.2	7.5–15	hs	Usually used to treat insomnia
Temazepam (Restoril)	Medium	Interm.	0.2	7.5–30	hs	Usually used to treat insomnia
Triazolam (Halcion)	Rapid	Short	3.3	0.125–0.25	hs	Usually used to treat insomnia

Short, <6 hours; interm., 6–20 hours; long, >20 hours; bid, twice daily; tid, three times daily; qid, four times daily; hs, at bedtime.

Higher relative potency designates more potent agents (i.e., inverse of dose equivalents). All benzodiazepines have longer-lasting and more potent effects in patients with hepatic impairment. CYP-450 interactions change the metabolism of many benzodiazepines. Patients with panic disorder may need higher total doses than those with GAD for symptom relief.

Modified from Sadock BJ, Sadock VA. *Concise Textbook of Clinical Psychiatry*, 3rd ed. Philadelphia, PA: Lippincott Williams & Wilkins; 2008.

Epidemiology

- Approximately 3% of American adults have panic disorder; of these, one in three develops agoraphobia. Panic disorder is twice as common in women, and moderately heritable.[5,46]
- Panic disorder typically first manifests in late adolescence or early adulthood, but the age of onset extends throughout adulthood.[5,38,46]

Etiology/Pathophysiology

- The underpinnings of panic disorder and agoraphobia are multifactorial and incompletely understood. Dysfunction of serotonin-, norepinephrine-, and GABA-mediated central nervous system pathways may be implicated. In addition, patients may have idiosyncratic changes in autonomic system regulation.
- Panic disorder also appears to have an important cognitive-behavioral aspect, and its onset is often preceded by stressful life events.[35,38,46]

Associated Conditions

- Patients with panic disorder may exhibit worsening job performance, changes in interpersonal relationships, multiple unexplained symptoms or frequent medical visits, concentration difficulties, sleep disturbances or chronic fatigue, and/or increasing alcohol/tobacco use.
- Patients with panic disorder are at high risk for developing another anxiety disorder, depression, or substance abuse.
- The risk of suicide and attempted suicide is markedly higher in patients with panic disorder.[46]
- Panic disorder is an independent risk factor for coronary heart disease.[35]
- If untreated, panic disorder chronically recurs with an unpredictable waxing and waning course. Patients may experience residual symptoms, including agoraphobia and somatization, even during periods when actual panic attacks are quiescent.

DIAGNOSIS

Clinical Presentation

- Not all patients who experience panic attacks will develop panic disorder.[38] The impact of panic disorder stems mainly from worry about future panic attacks or the possible implications of physical symptoms.
- Panic attacks may feel truly life threatening. Patients are often consumed by recurrent "what if?" worries related to the perceived dangerousness of panic attacks and may persistently seek medical consultations despite reassurance.
- Patients with panic disorder typically first present to emergency or primary care settings with unexplained symptoms rather than direct concerns about panic attacks. Complaints commonly include the following: noncardiac chest pain, palpitations, unexplained faintness, unexplained vertigo and dizziness, irritable bowel symptoms, dyspnea or tachypnea, feelings of impending doom or depersonalization, and nocturnal awakenings from panic attacks.[35,38]
- **Agoraphobia** sufferers typically have more severe impairment and panic symptomatology but are more likely to seek treatment than other panic disorder patients.[35]
- Screening with two questions from the Anxiety and Depression Detector yields a high sensitivity and moderate specificity for panic disorder[35,47]:
  - In the past 3 months, did you ever have a spell or an attack when all of a sudden you felt frightened, anxious, or very uneasy?
  - In the past 3 months, would you say that you have been bothered by nerves or feeling anxious or on edge?
  - If the patient answers "yes" to either screening question, further evaluation should be performed using a quantitative standardized instrument.

- Initial evaluation should include the following:
  - Screening for suicidality or self-harm
  - Assessment of panic disorder severity
  - Screening for concurrent psychiatric issues including substance abuse
- Appropriate laboratory and radiographic testing should be performed if there are potentially treatable medical conditions (e.g., hyperglycemia, hyperthyroidism, or a pheochromocytoma) contributing to the patient's symptomatology.

Differential Diagnosis

- As noted, many medical conditions are associated with or contribute to anxiety disorders.
- Panic disorder must be distinguished from other psychiatric conditions (Table 42-4).[4,14]

TREATMENT

- **Panic disorder is highly treatable** and the majority of patients receive benefit with appropriate therapy.[38]
- Strongly consider **psychiatrist or mental health specialist referral** if there are severe symptoms or functional impairment; agoraphobia; recurrent panic attacks despite treatment; signs of psychosis or suicidal ideation; comorbid medical, psychiatric, or substance abuse disorders; plans for psychotherapy; need for frequent or close follow-up; and/or patient requests for specialist treatment.[38]

Medications

- Medications improve anxiety and decrease the frequency of panic attacks.[35,38,46]
- **SSRIs** are considered the drugs of choice in treating panic disorder (Table 42-3). Efficacy appears similar among the SSRIs. Data also suggest comparable efficacy for venlafaxine.[35,46]
- **Benzodiazepines** are beneficial in acutely reducing the symptoms of panic attacks but have a high potential for abuse, dependence, and tolerance (Table 42-4).[35,38,46] Short-term adjuvant therapy with long-acting benzodiazepines may benefit some patients during the initial phase of other therapies.
- Bupropion has not been adequately studied to support its use for panic disorder, especially as many patients report that its activating effects actually worsen panic symptoms.[35]
- β-blockers may help some patients control physical symptoms, though they have not shown effectiveness for panic disorder in controlled trials.[35,38]
- Gabapentin may exhibit anxiolytic benefit in panic disorder, though data are mixed.[48]
- **Side effects that mimic panic attack symptoms may occur during either initiation or discontinuation of medications.** Antidepressants should be started at half the usual initial dose and gradually titrated when increased or withdrawn. Frequent reassurance may aid patient compliance.

Nonpharmacologic Therapies

- **CBT** is effective for treating panic disorder and is supported by robust clinical trial data.
  - It is unclear whether CBT is superior to pharmacotherapy but some data suggest that the benefits of CBT may be long lasting.[35,46]
  - Combined treatment with CBT and antidepressants may be more beneficial than with either modality alone for short-term symptom reduction.[46]
  - More than one-third of patients with panic disorder either cannot tolerate or do not respond to appropriate SSRI or venlafaxine therapy. Many patients who do not respond to medication will, however, respond to CBT.
  - CBT should be administered by a skilled therapist. Data suggest that the success of psychotherapy is linked to the experience level of practitioners.

- Aerobic exercise, breathing techniques, and relaxation/biofeedback exercises may indirectly improve panic disorder through lowering hyperreactivity to bodily sensations, though few studies have evaluated their use.[30,35,46] Similarly, yoga and meditation have theoretical benefit but have been formally evaluated only on a limited basis.[49]

PSYCHOSIS AND SCHIZOPHRENIA

GENERAL PRINCIPLES

- Psychosis denotes a **disturbed perception of reality** including hallucination, delusion, or thought disorganization.
- Psychotic states are associated with increased agitation, aggression, impulsivity, and behavioral dysfunction.
- Psychosis may be due to
  ○ Underlying psychiatric illness (e.g., schizophrenia, mania)
  ○ Substance abuse (e.g., cocaine intoxication, alcohol withdrawal)
  ○ Medication side effects (e.g., corticosteroids)
  ○ Medical illnesses (e.g., delirium, encephalitis)
- Patients have variable insight into their psychosis and may or may not recognize the derangements in their thought processes.[14,50]

Epidemiology

- Approximately 1% of the American adult population has schizophrenia and it is equally frequent in men and women.
- Schizophrenia typically first manifests in men during their late teens or early 20s; women usually exhibit symptoms in their 20s or early 30s.[5]
- Schizoaffective and mood disorder-associated psychosis may be more common in women.
- Approximately 80% of untreated manic patients develop psychotic symptoms. Psychotic symptoms in the context of mania or depression are often, but not always, congruent with mood (e.g., grandiose delusions).

Etiology/Pathophysiology

- The pathophysiology of schizophrenia is poorly understood. Some studies demonstrate abnormally elevated dopaminergic activity, altered neural network activation patterns, and anatomic atrophy in the central nervous system of patients with schizophrenia.[51,52]
- These changes likely result from complex interactions between multiple genes and environmental factors.[51]

Associated Conditions

- A total of 40% to 50% of patients with schizophrenia suffer from **substance abuse issues** with tobacco, alcohol, or illicit drugs.[8]
- Schizophrenic patients are also predisposed to be victims of violence and are at higher risk of suicide, depression, homelessness, and unemployment.

DIAGNOSIS

Clinical Presentation

- Types of psychotic symptoms include the following:
  ○ **Hallucinations** are false perceptions in one of the sensory modalities (e.g., auditory, visual, tactile, olfactory, gustatory). Auditory hallucinations are more common in psychoses due to a primary psychiatric disorder such as schizophrenia. While present in primary psychotic disorders, visual hallucinations should be treated as organic until proven otherwise.

○ **Delusions** are false beliefs that are firmly held despite obvious evidence to the contrary. Delusions are distinct from ideas typical of the patient's background cultural, religious, or familial belief system. Common delusions include thoughts of persecution, thoughts of grandiosity or superhuman abilities, and thoughts of hyperreligiosity. Delusions are characterized as bizarre or nonbizarre on the basis of their degree of plausibility.

○ **Delusions of reference** are a common type of delusion in which a patient believes that neutral information refers specifically to him or her. Patients may believe in the receipt of special messages transmitted from the television, radio, newspaper, or psychic communications.

○ **Illogical thought processes** are evidenced by nonsensical speech and loose associations, with accompanying functional impairment, bizarre behaviors, and agitation or aggression.

○ **Agitation** can manifest as both heightened emotional arousal and increased motor activity. Agitation is not exclusive to psychosis but frequently accompanies it.

• **Schizophrenia** is a severe, chronic disorder characterized by periods of active psychosis and an insidious deterioration of social, occupational, and personal functioning. Symptoms are typically subcategorized as follows:

○ **Positive symptoms**, including psychosis with hallucinations, delusions, and thought disorganization

○ **Negative symptoms**, including blunted affect, loss of social interest, decreased motivation, anhedonia, and decreased verbal communication

○ **Cognitive symptoms**, including deficits in memory, attention, verbal processing, and executive function

○ **Affective symptoms**, such as bizarre or inappropriate affect and predisposition for major depression

• Psychotic patients should undergo a complete mental status examination.

• Patients should be specifically questioned about hearing voices; seeing things others do not see; sensations of things touching or crawling on the skin; experiencing odd smells or tastes; fears that others are following, spying on, or wish to cause them harm; thought reading; special messages from television or radio; unusual religious experiences; and special powers or abilities.

Diagnostic Criteria/Differential Diagnosis

• Schizophrenia is characterized by abnormalities of thought (e.g., delusion, hallucinations, and language disorganization) for at least 6 months. These abnormalities significantly affect social functioning. The DSM-5 criteria are essentially the same as the prior DSM-IV-TR criteria.[4,12]

• Schizophrenia must be distinguished from other psychotic conditions (Table 42-5).[4,14]

• Many medical illnesses and certain drug intoxications are associated with psychotic symptoms.

TREATMENT

• The treatment of psychosis and schizophrenia is complex and **should be done in conjunction with a psychiatrist or similarly qualified healthcare professional**.

• Treatment for psychosis should be voluntary whenever possible but the nature of the illness may lead patients to fear or avoid treatment. Such patients may benefit from involuntary treatment, especially if they exhibit a high risk for harm to self or others.

• Symptomatic treatment of psychosis is appropriate, even if diagnostic evaluation is still in progress.

• **Goals for the acute treatment** of schizophrenia include the following[50,52,53]:

○ Preventing self-harm

○ Controlling disturbed behavior

TABLE 42-5 Psychiatric Differential Diagnosis of Psychosis[5,8]

	Defining characteristics	Additional features
Schizophrenia	• Combination of positive and negative symptoms, social withdrawal, and psychosis • Psychotic symptoms last for 1 month or longer	• May occur in conjunction with mania or depression but mood symptoms are brief relative to the total duration of the illness
Brief psychotic disorder	• Characterized by a total duration of < 1 month	• May be associated with borderline personality disorder (if so, symptoms usually last <1 day)
Schizoaffective disorder	• Features of both schizo-phrenia and mood disorder • Mood symptoms present for a substantial portion of the total duration of illness	• Psychosis persists even after mood improvements
Mood disorder with psychotic features	• Psychotic symptoms that occur exclusively during a manic or depressive episode (i.e., in unipolar or bipolar depression)	• Delusions often mood congruent (i.e., grandiosity in mania, somatic illness in depression) • Psychosis remits when mood improves
Delusional disorder	• Nonbizarre delusions occurring in the absence of other significant psychi-atric symptoms	• Common delusions include thoughts of erotomania, grandiosity, jealousy, persecution, or somatic illness
Delirium-associated	• Characterized by impaired judgment, orientation, mem-ory, affect, and concentra-tion, in association with a known medical illness	• Possible medical illnesses include trauma, infection, tumor, metabolic, endo-crine, intoxication (psy-choactive substance use), epilepsy, withdrawal state
Substance-induced psychosis	• Due to substance abuse or withdrawal • May persist beyond acute intoxication (i.e., flashbacks) • May signal life-threatening withdrawal syndromes (e.g., delirium tremens)	
Medication-induced psychosis	• Symptoms directly attribut-able to known medication side effects	• Commonly seen with corti-costeroids, L-DOPA
Dementia-associated psychosis	• Dementia (with decline in cognitive function) typically present before psychosis	• Prominent in Lewy body and end-stage dementia
Ethnic/familial/societal belief system	• May contain ideas or con-cepts that are acceptable in the cultural context • Not considered psychosis	

- Reducing the severity of psychosis and associated symptoms (e.g., agitation, aggression, negative symptoms, affective symptoms)
- Addressing factors that precipitated the acute psychotic episode
- Connecting the patient and family with appropriate support
- **Assess the patient for risk factors for suicide or self-harm** including prior self-harm attempts, depressed mood, hopelessness, anxiety, suicidal ideation, presence of command hallucinations, extrapyramidal side effects, and alcohol or other substance use.
- When compared with the general population, schizophrenic patients have a significantly higher prevalence of diseases including diabetes mellitus, metabolic syndrome, coronary heart disease, and chronic obstructive pulmonary disease.[54] Both antipsychotic medication side effects and sequelae of the primary disease seem to contribute. Such patients should undergo routine screening for such illnesses, with emphasis on early interventions and preventative measures.

Medications

- In schizophrenia, antipsychotic medications are **primarily effective for control of positive symptoms.** Negative symptoms show a modest response to antipsychotics, affective symptoms respond in about half of patients, and cognitive symptoms respond minimally.[50,52,53]
- Antipsychotic medications are often classified as first generation (i.e., conventional, typical) or second generation (i.e., atypical). **The nonspecific effect on agitation begins early; antipsychotic effect may take longer.** Common antipsychotics are presented in Table 42-6.[50]

TABLE 42-6 Commonly Used Antipsychotic Medications

	Typical dose range (mg/day)	Chlorpromazine equivalents (mg/day)	Half-life (hours)
First-generation agents (conventional antipsychotics)			
Phenothiazines			
Chlorpromazine	300–1,000	100	6
Fluphenazine	5–20	2	33
Perphenazine	16–64	10	10
Thioridazine	300–800	100	24
Trifluoperazine	15–50	5	24
Butyrophenone			
Haloperidol	5–20	2	21
Others			
Loxapine	30–100	10	4
Thiothixene	15–50	5	34
Second-generation agents (atypical antipsychotics)			
Aripiprazole (Abilify)	10–30	—	75
Asenapine (Saphris)	10–20	—	24
Clozapine (Clozaril)	150–600	—	12
Iloperidone (Fanapt)	12–24	—	18
Lurasidone (Latuda)	40–120	—	29
Olanzapine (Zyprexa)	10–30	—	33
Paliperidone (Invega)	6–12	—	23
Quetiapine (Seroquel)	300–800	—	6
Risperidone (Risperdal)	2–8	—	24
Ziprasidone (Geodon)	120–200	—	7

Data from American Psychiatric Association. Practice guideline for the treatment of patients with schizophrenia, second edition. *Am J Psychiatry* 2004;161:1–56; Clinical Pharmacology. 2014. http://www.clinicalpharmacology-ip.com. Last accessed 2/1/15.

TABLE 42-7 Qualitative Frequency of Antipsychotic Side Effects

Drug	EPS, tardive dyskinesia	Prolactin elevation	Weight gain	Glucose abnormalities	Lipid abnormalities	QTc prolongation	Sedation
Haloperidol (Haldol)	+++	+++	+	+	+	+	++
Aripiprazole (Abilify)	+	—	+	—	—	—	+
Asenapine (Saphris)	+	++	+	+	—	+	++
Clozapine (Clozaril)	—	—	+++	+++	+++	+	+++
Iloperidone (Fanapt)	+	—	++	++	++	++	+
Lurasidone (Latuda)	+	+	+	+	—	—	++
Olanzapine (Zyprexa)	+	+	+++	+++	+++	+	++
Paliperidone (Invega)	++	+++	++	++	++	++	+
Quetiapine (Seroquel)	—	—	++	+	+	++	++
Risperidone (Risperdal)	++	+++	++	+	+	+	+
Ziprasidone (Geodon)	+	+	—	—	—	++	+

EPS, extrapyramidal side effects (akathisia, parkinsonism, dystonia); —, rare; +, seldom; ++, common; +++, frequent.
Data from Lehman AF, Lieberman JA, Dixon LB, et al.; American Psychiatric Association. Practice guideline for the treatment of patients with schizophrenia, second edition. *Am J Psychiatry* 2004;161:1–56; Dixon L, Perkins D, Calmes C; American Psychiatric Association. *Guideline Watch (September 2009): Practice Guideline for the Treatment of Patients with Schizophrenia.* American Psychiatric Association; 2009; Drugs for psychotic disorders. *Treat Guidel Med Lett* 2010;8:61–64.

- Atypical antipsychotics are a heterogeneous group of medications with respect to efficacy and side effect profile (Table 42-7).[50,53,55–57]
  - Atypical agents may be less likely to induce extrapyramidal side effects than high-potency conventional medications but have an increased risk for other adverse effects including weight gain.[55]
  - Atypical antipsychotics are no more beneficial for the control of symptoms than first-generation agents with the exception of clozapine, which was demonstrated in the CATIE trial.[58]
  - Clozapine decreases the rate of suicide and self-harm attempts in schizophrenia.[59]
- Antipsychotic medications should be chosen based on side effect profile and patient comorbidities.
- Expert opinion recommends low-dose risperidone, quetiapine, olanzapine, or aripiprazole for psychosis in elderly patients.[60]
- Adverse effects from antipsychotic medications include the following:
  - Hyperprolactinemia (galactorrhea, amenorrhea, loss of libido)
  - Weight gain, dyslipidemia, hyperglycemia
  - QTc prolongation (arrhythmia, sudden cardiac death)
  - Acute dystonia (acute muscular rigidity, laryngospasm)
  - Parkinsonism (masked facies, stooped posture, tremor, rigidity)
  - Akathisia (intense restlessness)
  - Tardive dyskinesia (involuntary movements)
  - Neuroleptic malignant syndrome (rigidity, tremor, autonomic instability, mental status changes, potential for death)
- Diphenhydramine or benztropine are helpful in treating extrapyramidal effects (i.e., dystonia, akathisia, parkinsonism).[53] Propranolol or other β-blockers may be helpful in treating akathisia.
- A sizable minority of schizophrenic patients do not achieve complete symptom remission despite appropriate antipsychotic medications. Adjuvant treatments including lamotrigine, lithium, carbamazepine, benzodiazepines, β-blockers, valproate, and ECT have been used in schizophrenics whose psychoses did not respond to traditional therapy.[61,62]

Other Nonpharmacologic Therapies

- ECT may be useful for the treatment of psychosis refractory to antipsychotic medications, those with prominent catatonic features, or those with comorbid depression or suicidality.[50,52,53]
- Psychological therapy techniques may be effective adjuvants for psychosis, though data are limited.
- Multiple psychosocial interventions, including vocational training programs and case managers, seem to be beneficial in assisting those with schizophrenia.[50,53]

OUTCOME/PROGNOSIS

- Schizophrenic patients have a **chronic illness with a fluctuating course.**
- More than 70% of first-episode patients achieve a full remission of psychotic signs and symptoms within 3 to 4 months and >80% achieve stable remission at the end of 1 year.[50]
- Predictors of poor treatment response include male gender, pre- or perinatal injury, severe hallucinations and delusions, attentional impairments, poor premorbid function, longer duration of untreated psychosis, and distressing emotional climate (e.g., hostile and critical attitudes and overprotection by others in one's living situation or high levels of expressed emotion).[50]
- There is significant unexplained heterogeneity in the long-term outcomes of schizophrenic patients. Poor outcome occurs in <50% of patients, but, frustratingly, good outcome also occurs in <50% of patients.[52] Importantly, 20% to 40% attempt suicide and 7% will die of it.[50]

SPECIAL CONSIDERATIONS IN GERIATRIC PATIENTS

GENERAL PRINCIPLES

- **Depression and anxiety are not part of the normal aging process.** These illnesses have considerable negative influence on elderly patients' quality of life.
- Older adults who require recurrent hospitalizations or long-term nursing home care have increased rates of mental health illnesses compared with their peers.
- Some psychiatric disorders in geriatric patients seem to derive from pathophysiology dissimilar to younger adults and may involve subacute neurologic degeneration or ischemia.[2,5,20,63]
- **Underlying medical conditions** (such as advanced cardiac, pulmonary, or neurologic illness) predispose to depression and anxiety. The causality of such associations is complex and likely involves both physiologic changes as well as psychosocial stressors.
- **Medical diseases common in the geriatric population may present with psychiatric symptoms.** Older adults with psychiatric symptoms should be screened for conditions including thyroid and adrenal dysfunction; diabetes mellitus; cardiac arrhythmia or ischemia; nutritional deficiencies; malignancy, including pancreatic cancer; stroke, Parkinson disease, or neurologic disorders; chronic pain; sleep disorders; occult infections; and medication side effects.
- Elderly patients with mental health disorders **often present atypically,** emphasizing somatic manifestations of their illness rather than psychiatric ones. Practitioners should exercise high levels of vigilance when evaluating older patients and avoid the mistake of simply treating symptoms without addressing possible underlying mental health issues.
- Geriatric patients are **prone to medication side effects and drug-drug interactions.** Medications should be initiated at lower doses than in younger patients and titrated slowly. Medical comorbidities should be considered when selecting therapeutic modalities and medications.
- **Referral to a psychiatrist** or other mental health professional should be considered for all elderly adults with mental health disorders given the complexity of care in this population.

DEPRESSION IN OLDER ADULTS

- **Depression can be subtle in older adults**. Rather than endorsing sadness or feeling depressed, older patients will often manifest depression as[47,64]:
  - Apathy or decreased interest in previous hobbies
  - Feelings of ill health with vague somatic symptoms
  - Lack of energy
  - Psychomotor slowing or agitation
  - Worsening control of comorbid medical illnesses and medical noncompliance
  - Sleep disturbances or early morning awakenings
  - Cognitive impairment including memory deficits and slowed information/visuospatial processing
  - Delusions of guilt and worthlessness
  - Auditory/visual hallucinations
- Geriatric patients are at **increased risk for completed suicide** compared with younger adults.[5]
- Patients with symptoms of depression or a positive Two Question Screen should be evaluated using a **geriatric-specific metric,** such as the Geriatric Depression Scale.[65,66]

- Even subsyndromal depression is associated with worsened function, increased mortality, and increased risk of suicide in older adults. Treatment should strongly be considered in such cases given the favorable response rate and benefit of intervention.
- **Antidepressant medications should be considered for all geriatric patients with depression.**[2]
- Skilled psychotherapy augments rates of response to medications and may alone be sufficient in mild depression if pharmacologic therapy is contraindicated.[11,63,67,68]
- Data support the efficacy and tolerance of multiple classes of antidepressants in the elderly.[2,11,67] **SSRIs or nonselective serotonin agonists (e.g., mirtazapine, bupropion, and SNRIs) should be used as first-line agents** for geriatric depression given a more benign side effect profile compared with TCAs (Table 42-3).[2,11,20,67] However, these agents may cause falls, sleep disturbances, anorexia, sinus bradycardia, and hyponatremia in the elderly.
- **Highly anticholinergic mediations,** including amitriptyline and imipramine, are **relatively contraindicated** in older adults because of risk of arrhythmia, narrow angle glaucoma, urinary retention, delirium, and orthostasis. Older adults also have an increased risk for cardiovascular complications from TCAs and antipsychotics.[64]
- ECT is generally safe in geriatric patients and may be especially useful for those with severe symptoms including suicidality, catatonia, and psychosis.[2,64,69]
- Remission of depression progresses more slowly in the elderly. More than half of geriatric patients treated with antidepressants eventually experience treatment response within 2 months.[2,67] If symptoms persist after 6 to 8 weeks, additional or alternative treatment options should be considered.
- Assessing therapeutic response should include evaluation of overall quality of life, performance of activities of daily living, and control of comorbid illnesses.[68]
- Maintenance treatment with antidepressants or ECT should continue for at least 12 months in older adults with moderate or severe depression to reduce the risk of recurrence. Continuance for even longer durations may be worthwhile in such patients.[2,70,71] Skilled psychotherapy is a helpful adjuvant in preventing recurrence of moderate or severe geriatric depression but should not be used alone.[67,70,71]

ANXIETY IN OLDER ADULTS

- Anxiety problems, including GAD, are common in geriatric populations.[67,72,73]
- Practitioners must differentiate whether an older patient's symptoms are due to a primary anxiety disorder or secondary to other causes. Cardiac diseases, respiratory illnesses, and medication side effects disproportionately affect older adults and are significantly anxiogenic if not well controlled.
- Agitation (the physical manifestations of hyperactivity) subtly differs from anxiety but should be distinguished as it may require alternate treatment. Elderly adults with agitation do not typically experience the sense of dread or impending doom characteristic of anxiety. Agitation without clear anxiety is also frequent in patients with dementia or delirium.
- Rather than endorsing worry, geriatric patients with anxiety disorders are **more likely to present with nonspecific complaints** including the following[72,73]:
  - Concentration or memory difficulties
  - Restlessness or irritability
  - Muscle tension
  - Vague visceral discomfort
  - Recurrent cardiovascular or gastrointestinal symptoms without clear medical explanations
  - Continued medical complaints despite negative workup
  - Fatigue

- ○ Decreased physical activity and functional independence
- ○ Low mood or depression
- ○ Increased feelings of loneliness
- ○ Avoidance of certain situations, tasks, or locations
- Anxiety prominently affects sleep in older adults; data suggest that 90% of older adults with GAD report dissatisfaction with sleep.[74]
- Anxiety disorders are frequently associated with depression in older populations.[72,73] The co-occurrence of both disorders increases the risk for suicidality and substance abuse.
- It is unclear which metrics are best to screen older adults for anxiety disorders. The Generalized Anxiety Disorder Severity Scale (GADSS) may help in evaluating for either GAD or panic disorder in elderly patients.[75,76]
- Despite the prevalence of anxiety disorders in geriatric populations, few potential treatment options have been rigorously studied.[67,72,73]
- **SSRIs** appear useful for treating geriatric anxiety disorders (Table 42-3). Both citalopram and escitalopram have shown benefit in the treatment of GAD and panic disorder in small trials.[77,78] Minor side effects are relatively frequent in older patients using SSRIs for anxiety and include fatigue, sleep disturbances, and urinary symptoms. More serious adverse reactions, including hyponatremia, may also occur.
- **Venlafaxine** may also be used to treat older adults with GAD, with an efficacy, safety, and tolerability similar to that in younger patients.[79]
- **Benzodiazepines** are the most frequently prescribed anxiolytics for older patients (Table 42-6).[67,72,80] Compared with placebo, these medicines seem to decrease anxiety symptoms.[72] However, benzodiazepines **increase the risk for falls and cognitive impairment** in the elderly and should be used cautiously. Geriatric patients have decreased rates of drug metabolism and may tolerate intermediate-acting agents better than long-acting ones. Trials have not yet directly compared benzodiazepines with other treatments for geriatric anxiety.
- **CBT** has consistently shown promise for the management of geriatric anxiety disorders.[67,72,81,82] The benign side effects of CBT suggest that it should be considered in all elderly anxiety patients. Other psychological techniques may also be effective but have not yet been adequately evaluated.[67,72,81]

PSYCHOSIS IN OLDER ADULTS

- Psychotic symptoms are widespread in the elderly, with prevalence estimates ranging from approximately 1% to 5% in community-based cohorts to as high as 10% to 63% in nursing home populations.[69]
- Psychosis in elderly patients may be due to schizophrenia/schizoaffective disorder, mood disorders (e.g., depression or mania), dementia (e.g., Alzheimer disease, Lewy body dementia), delirium, delusional disorders, substance-induced disorders, Parkinson disease, and medication side effects.
- **The most statistically frequent causes of geriatric psychosis are Alzheimer dementia, depression, and delirium**; these conditions should be considered when evaluating any geriatric patient with psychosis.[69] Treatment choices should be based on the etiology of the patient's psychosis.
- Up to 40% of hospitalized geriatric patients with depression manifest psychosis.[69] **All elderly adults with psychosis should be assessed for depression.** Hallucinations and delusions in patients with depression or mania are often (but not necessarily) mood congruent.
- **Both ECT and antipsychotics** appear to be useful adjuvants for treating depression with psychotic features in older adults who do not respond to antidepressant medications alone.[2,60,64,69]

- Consensus statements support multidisciplinary psychosocial interventions for both older patients with chronic psychotic illnesses and their families.[67] Useful interventions include vocational/social skills training and community support programs.
- Expert opinion, consensus statements, and the few available studies all concur that antipsychotic medications are effective for psychosis or schizophrenia in older patients.[60,67,69] **Atypical antipsychotics are generally preferred** for most geriatric psychotic disorders and typically used at lower doses than in younger patients.[60] Commonly used antipsychotics are presented in Table 42-6.
- Pharmacologic treatment of psychosis in the elderly should be managed in conjunction with a psychiatrist or similarly qualified mental health specialist. Special attention should be given to patients' age-related issues including pharmacokinetics, comorbid illnesses, and polypharmacy.
- **Older patients are particularly susceptible to adverse reactions from antipsychotic medications** including (Table 42-7) parkinsonism (i.e., bradykinesia, tremor, cogwheeling rigidity, masked facies), dystonia (involuntary muscle spasms that may be painful), akathisia (feelings of increased agitation and restlessness), Tardive dyskinesia (repetitive purposeless, involuntary movements), weight gain, dyslipidemia, hyperglycemia, cardiac arrhythmias, QTc prolongation, and sudden death.[53,56,57,67,69]
- In younger patients, extrapyramidal side effects (including parkinsonism, dystonia, and akathisia) are often treated with diphenhydramine or benztropine. However, these **anticholinergic agents frequently cause problems, such as cognitive impairment, constipation, and orthostasis in the elderly and must be used with caution**.
- The development of extrapyramidal symptoms or Tardive dyskinesia in the elderly is more frequent with use of conventional antipsychotics (e.g., haloperidol) than atypical ones.[76]
- **Antipsychotic medication therapy has been associated with an increased mortality in geriatric patients with dementia,** especially from cardiovascular or infectious etiologies. As such, atypical antipsychotic medicines carry an FDA boxed warning regarding their use in dementia-related psychosis. Mortality risk in the elderly may be higher with conventional antipsychotic agents compared with atypical antipsychotics.[69]

ADDITIONAL RESOURCES

- MedLine Plus. Mental health. http://www.nlm.nih.gov/medlineplus/mentalhealth.html. Last accessed: 2/1/15.
- National Institutes of Mental Health. Mental health topics. http://www.nimh.nih.gov/health/topics/index.shtml. Last accessed: 2/1/15.
- PsychCentral. Mental health & psychology resources online. http://psychcentral.com/resources/. Last accessed: 2/1/15.

REFERENCES

1. Stiebel V, Schwartz CE. Physicians at the medicine/psychiatric interface: what do internist/psychiatrists do? *Psychosomatics* 2001;42:377–381.
2. Shanmugham B, Karp J, Drayer R, et al. Evidence-based pharmacologic interventions for geriatric depression. *Psychiatr Clin North Am* 2005;28:821–835.
3. American Psychiatric Association. Psychiatric evaluation of adults, second edition. *Am J Psychiatry* 2006;163:3–36.
4. American Psychiatric Association. *Diagnostic and Statistical Manual of Mental Disorders (DSM-IV-TR). Text Revision*, 4th ed. Arlington, VA: American Psychiatric Publishing, Inc.; 2000.

5. National Institute of Mental Health. The numbers count: mental disorders in America. http://www.nimh.nih.gov/health/publications/the-numbers-count-mental-disorders-in-america/index.shtml. Last accessed 2/1/15.

6. Hasler G, van der Veen JW, Tumonis T, et al. Reduced prefrontal glutamate/glutamine and gamma-aminobutyric acid levels in major depression determined using proton magnetic resonance spectroscopy. *Arch Gen Psychiatry* 2007;64:193–200.

7. Belmaker RH, Agam G. Major depressive disorder. *N Engl J Med* 2008;358:55–68.

8. Institute for Clinical Systems Improvement (ICSI). *Major Depression in Adults in Primary Care*. Bloomington, MN: ICSI; 2008.

9. U.S. Preventive Services Task Force. Screening for depression: recommendations and rationale. *Ann Intern Med* 2002;136:760–764.

10. Egede LE. Disease-focused or integrated treatment: diabetes and depression. *Med Clin North Am* 2006;90:627–646.

11. Fochtmann IJ, Gelenberg AJ. *Guideline Watch: Practice Guideline for the Treatment of Patients with Major Depressive Disorder*, 2nd ed. Arlington, VA: American Psychiatric Association; 2005.

12. American Psychiatric Association. *Diagnostic and Statistical Manual of Mental Disorders*, 5th ed. Arlington, VA: American Psychiatric Publishing, Inc.; 2013.

13. Whooley MA, Avins AL, Miranda J, et al. Case-finding instruments for depression: two questions are as good as many. *J Gen Intern Med* 1997;12:439–445.

14. First MB, Frances A, Pincus HA. *DSM-IV-TR Handbook of Differential Diagnosis*. Arlington, VA: American Psychiatric Publishing, Inc.; 2002.

15. American Psychiatric Association. Practice guideline for the treatment of patients with major depressive disorder (revision). *Am J Psychiatry* 2000;157:1–45.

16. American Psychiatric Association. *Practice Guideline for the Treatment of Patients with Major Depressive Disorder*, 3rd ed. Arlington, VA: American Psychiatric Association; 2010. Available at: http://psychiatryonline.org/guidelines.aspx. Last accessed 2/1/15.

17. King V, Robinson S, Bianco T, et al.; U.S. Department of Health and Human Services, Agency for Healthcare Research and Quality. *Choosing Antidepressants for Adults*. AHRQ Pub. No. 07-EHC007-3. Rockville, MD: Agency for Healthcare Research and Quality; 2007.

18. Barbui C, Butler R, Cipriani A, et al. Depression in adults (drug and other physical treatments). *BMJ Clin Evid* 2007;06:1003.

19. Butler R, Hatcher S, Price J, et al. Depression in adults: psychological treatments and care pathways. *BMJ Clin Evid* 2007;08:1016.

20. Lawhorne L. Depression in the older adult. *Prim Care* 2005;32:777–792.

21. Cain RA. Navigating the sequenced treatment alternatives to relieve depression (STAR*D) study: practical outcomes and implications for depression treatment in primary care. *Prim Care* 2007;34:505–519.

22. Rush AJ, Trivedi M, Fava M. Depression, IV: STAR*D treatment trial for depression. *Am J Psychiatry* 2003;160:237.

23. Simon NM, Otto MW, Weiss RD, et al. Pharmacotherapy for bipolar disorder and comorbid conditions: baseline data from STEP-BD. *J Clin Psychopharmacol* 2004;24:512–520.

24. Perlis RH, Ostacher MJ, Patel JK, et al. Predictors of recurrence in bipolar disorder: primary outcomes from the Systematic Treatment Enhancement Program for Bipolar Disorder (STEP-BD). *Am J Psychiatry* 2006;163:217–224.

25. Qaseem A, Snow V, Denberg TD, et al. Using second-generation antidepressants to treat depressive disorders: a clinical practice guideline from the American College of Physicians. *Ann Intern Med* 2008;149:725–733.

26. Schatzberg AF, Cole JO, DeBattista C. *Manual of Clinical Psychopharmacology*, 6th ed. Arlington, VA: American Psychiatric Publishing, Inc.; 2007.

27. Gartlehner G, Hansen RA, Thieda P, et al.; U.S. Department of Health and Human Services, Agency for Healthcare Research and Quality. *Comparative Effectiveness of Second-Generation Antidepressants in the Pharmacologic Treatment of Adult Depression.* AHRQ Publication No. 07-EHC007-EF. Bethesda, MD: Agency for Healthcare Research and Quality; 2007.
28. Crone CC, Gabriel G. Herbal and nonherbal supplements in medical-psychiatric patient populations. *Psychiatr Clin North Am* 2002;25:211–230.
29. Terman M, Terman JS, Ross DC. A controlled trial of timed bright light and negative air ionization for treatment of winter depression. *Arch Gen Psychiatry* 1998;55:875–882.
30. Ströhle A. Physical activity, exercise, depression and anxiety disorders. *J Neural Transm* 2009;116:777–784.
31. Soomro GM. Deliberate self-harm (and attempted suicide). *BMJ Clin Evid* 2008;12:1012.
32. American Psychiatric Association. Practice guideline for the assessment and treatment of patients with suicidal behaviors. *Am J Psychiatry* 2003;160:1–60.
33. U.S. Food and Drug Administration. Antidepressant use in children, adolescents, and adults. http://www.fda.gov/cder/drug/antidepressants/default.htm. Last accessed 2/1/15.
34. Hawton K, Townsend E, Arensman E, et al. Psychosocial and pharmacological treatments for deliberate self harm. *Cochrane Database Syst Rev* 2000;(2):CD001764.
35. Shearer SL. Recent advances in the understanding and treatment of anxiety disorders. *Prim Care* 2007;34:475–504.
36. National Institute of Mental Health, U.S. Department of Health and Human Services. *Anxiety Disorders.* NIH Publication No. 07-4677. Bethesda, MD: National Institute of Mental Health; 2007.
37. Gale C, Millichamp J. Generalised anxiety disorder. *BMJ Clin Evid* 2007;11:1002.
38. National Institute of Mental Health. U.S. Department of Health and Human Services. *Anxiety Disorders.* NIH Publication No. 09-3879. Bethesda, MD: National Institute of Mental Health; 2009.
39. Spitzer RL, Kroenke K, Williams JB, et al. A brief measure for assessing generalized anxiety disorder: the gad-7. *Arch Intern Med* 2006;166:1092–1097.
40. Newman MG, Zuellig AR, Kachin KE, et al. Preliminary reliability and validity of the Generalized Anxiety Disorder Questionnaire-IV: a revised self-report diagnostic measure of generalized anxiety disorder. *Behav Ther* 2002;33:215–233.
41. Walkup JT, Albano AM, Piacentini J, et al. Cognitive behavioral therapy, sertraline, or a combination in childhood anxiety. *N Engl J Med* 2008;359:2753–2766.
42. Kapczinski F, Lima MS, Souza JS, et al. Antidepressants for generalized anxiety disorder. *Cochrane Database Syst Rev* 2003;(2):CD003592.
43. Martin JL, Sainz-Pardo M, Furukawa TA, et al. Benzodiazepines in generalized anxiety disorder: heterogeneity of outcomes based on a systematic review and meta-analysis of clinical trials. *J Psychopharmacol* 2007;21:774–782.
44. Hunot V, Churchill R, Silva de Lima M, et al. Psychological therapies for generalised anxiety disorder. *Cochrane Database Syst Rev* 2007;(1):CD001848.
45. Leichsenring F, Salzer S, Jaeger U, et al. Short-term psychodynamic psychotherapy and cognitive-behavioral therapy in generalized anxiety disorder: a randomized, controlled trial. *Am J Psychiatry* 2009;166:875–881.
46. Kumar S, Malone D. Panic disorder. *BMJ Clin Evid* 2008;12:1010.
47. Means-Christensen AJ, Sherbourne CD, Roy-Byrne PP, et al. Using five questions to screen for five common mental disorders in primary care: diagnostic accuracy of the anxiety and depression detector. *Gen Hosp Psychiatry* 2006;28:108–118.
48. Mula M, Pini S, Cassano G. The role of anticonvulsant drugs in anxiety disorders: a critical review of the evidence. *J Clin Psychopharmacol* 2007;3:263–272.

49. Krisanaprakornkit T, Sriraj W, Piyavhatkul N, et al. Meditation therapy for anxiety disorders. *Cochrane Database Syst Rev* 2006;(1):CD004998.

50. American Psychiatric Association. Practice guideline for the treatment of patients with schizophrenia, second edition. *Am J Psychiatry* 2004;161:1–56.

51. Jindal RD, Keshavan MS. Neurobiology of the early course of schizophrenia. *Expert Rev Neurother* 2008;8:1093–1100.

52. van Os J, Kapur S. Schizophrenia. *Lancet* 2009;374:635–645.

53. Lehman AF, Buchanan RW, Dickerson FB, et al. Evidence-based treatment for schizophrenia. *Psychiatr Clin North Am* 2003;26:939–954.

54. Oud MJ, Meyboom-de Jong B. Somatic diseases in patients with schizophrenia in general practice: their prevalence and health care. *BMC Fam Pract* 2009;10:32.

55. Leucht S, Corves C, Arbter D, et al. Second-generation versus first-generation antipsychotic drugs for schizophrenia: a meta-analysis. *Lancet* 2009;373:31–41.

56. Lehman AF, Lieberman JA, Dixon LB, et al.; American Psychiatric Association. Practice guideline for the treatment of patients with schizophrenia, second edition. *Am J Psychiatry* 2004;161:1–56.

57. Dixon L, Perkins D, Calmes C; American Psychiatric Association. *Guideline Watch (September 2009): Practice Guideline for the Treatment of Patients with Schizophrenia.* American Psychiatric Association; 2009. http://psychiatryonline.org/pb/assets/raw/sitewide/practice_guidelines/guidelines/schizophrenia-watch.pdf. Last accessed January 30, 2015.

58. McEvoy JP, Lieberman JA, Stroup TS, et al. Effectiveness of clozapine versus olanzapine, quetiapine, and risperidone in patients with chronic schizophrenia who did not respond to prior atypical antipsychotic treatment. *Am J Psychiatry* 2006;163:600–610.

59. Meltzer HY, Alphs L, Green AI, et al. Clozapine treatment for suicidality in schizophrenia: International Suicide Prevention Trial (InterSePT). *Arch Gen Psychiatry* 2003;60:82–91.

60. Alexopoulos GS, Streim J, Carpenter D, et al. Using antipsychotic agents in older patients. *J Clin Psychiatry* 2004;65:5–99.

61. Schwarz C, Volz A, Li C, et al. Valproate for schizophrenia. *Cochrane Database Syst Rev* 2008;(3):CD004028.

62. Dold M, Li C, Tardy M, et al. Benzodiazepines for schizophrenia. *Cochrane Database Syst Rev* 2012;(11):CD006391.

63. Wilson KC, Mottram PG, Vassilas CA. Psychotherapeutic treatments for older depressed people. *Cochrane Database Syst Rev* 2008;CD004853.

64. Stek ML, Van der Wurff FB, Hoogendijk WL, et al. Electroconvulsive therapy for the depressed elderly. *Cochrane Database Syst Rev* 2003;(2):CD003593.

65. Holroyd S, Clayton AH. Measuring depression in the elderly: which scale is best? *MedGenMed* 2000;2. http://www.medscape.com/viewarticle/430554. Last accessed 2/1/18.

66. Sheikh JI, Yesavage JA. Geriatric depression scale (GDS): recent evidence and development of a shorter version. In: Brink TL, ed. *Clinical Gerontology: A Guide to Assessment and Intervention.* New York, NY: The Haworth Press; 1986:165–173.

67. Bartels SJ, Dums AR, Oxman TE, et al. Evidence-based practices in geriatric mental health care: an overview of systematic reviews and meta-analyses. *Psychiatr Clin North Am* 2003;26:971–990.

68. Mackin RS, Arean PA. Evidence-based psychotherapeutic interventions for geriatric depression. *Psychiatr Clin North Am* 2005;28:805–820.

69. Broadway J, Mintzer J. The many faces of psychosis in the elderly. *Curr Opin Psychiatry* 2007;20:551–558.

70. Reynolds CF, Frank E, Perel JM, et al. Nortriptyline and interpersonal psychotherapy as maintenance therapies for recurrent major depression: a randomized controlled trial in patients >59 years. *JAMA* 1999;281:39–45.

71. Reynolds CF, Dew MA, Pollock BG, et al. Maintenance treatment of major depression in old age. *N Engl J Med* 2006;354:1130–1138.

72. Wetherell JL, Lenze EJ, Stanley MA. Evidence-based treatment of geriatric anxiety disorders. *Psychiatr Clin North Am* 2005;28:871–896.

73. Blazer DG, Steffens DC. *The American Psychiatric Publishing Textbook of Geriatric Psychiatry*, 4th ed. Arlington, VA: American Psychiatric Publishing, Inc.; 2009.

74. Brenes GA, Miller ME, Stanley MA, et al. Insomnia in older adults with generalized anxiety disorder. *Am J Geriatr Psychiatry* 2009;17:465–472.

75. Weiss BJ, Calleo J, Rhoades HM, et al. The utility of the Generalized Anxiety Disorder Severity Scale (GADSS) with older adults in primary care. *Depress Anxiety* 2009;26:E10–E15.

76. Andreescu C, Belnap BH, Rollman BL, et al. Generalized Anxiety Disorder Severity Scale validation in older adults. *Am J Geriatr Psychiatry* 2008;16:813–818.

77. Blank S, Lenze EJ, Mulsant BH, et al. Outcomes of late-life anxiety disorders during 32 weeks of citalopram treatment. *J Clin Psychiatry* 2006;67:468–472.

78. Lenze EJ, Rollman BL, Shear MK, et al. Escitalopram for older adults with generalized anxiety disorder: a randomized controlled trial. *JAMA* 2009;301:295–303.

79. Katz IR, Reynolds CF III, Alexopoulos GS, et al. Venlafaxine ER as a treatment for generalized anxiety disorder in older adults: pooled analysis of five randomized placebo-controlled clinical trials. *J Am Geriatr Soc* 2002;50:18–25.

80. Benitez CI, Smith K, Vasile RG, et al. Use of benzodiazepines and selective serotonin reuptake inhibitors in middle-aged and older adults with anxiety disorders: a longitudinal and prospective study. *Am J Geriatr Psychiatry* 2008;16:5–13.

81. Ayers CR, Sorrell JT, Thorp SR, et al. Evidence-based psychological treatments for late-life anxiety. *Psychol Aging* 2007;22:8–17.

82. Stanley MA, Wilson NL, Novy DM, et al. Cognitive behavior therapy for generalized anxiety disorder among older adults in primary care: a randomized clinical trial. *JAMA* 2009;301:1460–1467.

Neurologic Disorders

Scott A. Norris, Enrique Alvarez, and Sylvia Awadalla

Headache

GENERAL PRINCIPLES

- Primary headache disorders account for 20% of neurology outpatient visits. Lifetime prevalence of tension-type headache is 78% and migraine is 16%.[1]
- Most patients who seek medical care for headache have migraine; two-thirds seek medical care in a primary care physician's office.[2,3]
- Headaches may herald life-threatening conditions suggested by red flags (Table 43-1).

DIAGNOSIS

Headaches are divided into primary and secondary types.

- **Primary headache syndromes** are not associated with other diseases and include migraine, tension-type, and cluster headaches.
- **Secondary headaches** are common manifestations of other diseases (Table 43-2).

Clinical Presentation

- Headache diagnosis relies on a detailed medical history (e.g., frequency, duration, location, severity, photophobia, phonophobia, nausea, vomiting, autonomic signs).
- Red flags (Table 43-1) increase the suspicion for secondary headache disorders.
- Abnormal neurologic signs suggest secondary headache disorders.
- General and neurologic examination may include funduscopy, palpation of temporal arteries, auscultation for carotid bruits, palpation of the temporomandibular joint, and examination of neck and shoulder muscles.

Diagnostic Criteria
Migraine
- Divided into two major subtypes:
  - Without aura (common migraine). See Table 43-3 for detailed diagnostic criteria.[4]
  - With aura (classical migraine; approximately one-third of patients).
- Auras are recurrent attacks of reversible focal neurologic symptoms that develop over 5 to 20 minutes, last for <60 minutes, and are often associated with a migraine headache.[4]
  - Visual auras are most common and can include fortification spectra and scotoma.
  - Less common aura symptoms may include paresthesias, numbness, weakness, gait instability, speech change, and others.

Tension-Type Headache
- Most common type of primary headache.
- See diagnostic criteria for tension-type headaches in Table 43-4.[4]

Cluster Headache
- Most common trigeminal autonomic headache characterized by brief (15 to 180 minutes), severe, unilateral pain. See diagnostic criteria in Table 43-5.[4]

TABLE 43-1	Headache Red Flags

New headaches
Beginning after the age of 50
Significant change in headache patterns or characteristics (e.g., increasing frequency or severity)
Worrisome associated features (e.g., impaired consciousness, focal weakness)
Systemic illness (e.g., cancer, HIV, other immunosuppression)
Systemic symptoms (e.g., fever, stiff, neck, weight loss)
Rapid onset of headache (i.e., thunderclap headache)
Headache secondary to head trauma

- Cluster headaches are more common in men than in women.
- Unlike migraine, patients are often restless during cluster headaches.

Medication Overuse Headache
- A secondary headache type defined as an interaction between a medication used excessively in a susceptible patient.[4]
- Most common cause of headache occurring on more than 15 days/month in the setting of analgesic overuse (>15 days/month for >3 months).[4]
- Can develop with analgesic overuse in patients with tension, migraine, or cluster headaches.
- **Acetaminophen, aspirin, opiates, and combinations of caffeine and butalbital** (e.g., Fiorinal, Fioricet, and Esgic) **are frequently implicated**.

Diagnostic Testing
- No testing is warranted with a typical history, no red flags, and a normal examination.
- Testing may include the following if history and exam suggest secondary headache:
  - Head CT
  - MRI of the brain with and without contrast
  - Angiography (magnetic resonance angiography [MRA], computed tomography angiography [CTA], carotid ultrasound, or conventional catheter)

TABLE 43-2	Secondary Headache Differential Diagnosis

Vasculitis (e.g., temporal arteritis, primary central nervous system angiitis)
Infection (e.g., meningitis, encephalitis, abscess)
Cerebral venous sinus thrombosis
Intracranial hypotension (i.e., cerebrospinal fluid leak)
Hydrocephalus
Idiopathic intracranial hypertension (i.e., pseudotumor cerebri)
Hemorrhage (intracerebral, subarachnoid, subdural)
Mass lesion (e.g., tumor, infection/abscess, hematoma)
Systemic illness (e.g., fever, infection, severe hypertension)
Medication side effect
Upper cervical spine disease
Acute sinusitis
Temporomandibular joint dysfunction
Many others

TABLE 43-3	Migraine Without Aura Diagnostic Criteria

≥5 attacks lasting 4–72 hours
≥2 of the following:
- Unilateral location
- Pulsating/throbbing
- Moderate or severe in intensity
- Made worse by routine physical activity

≥1 of the following:
- Nausea and/or vomiting
- Photophobia and phonophobia

Data from Headache Classification Subcommittee of the International Headache Society. The International Classification of Headache Disorders: 2nd edition. *Cephalalgia* 2004;24:9–160.

- Blood tests (e.g., erythrocyte sedimentation rate [ESR])
- Cervical spine imaging
- Lumbar puncture (LP)

TREATMENT

- Patient and family **education**
  - The most effective treatment for headaches is **prevention**.
  - **Headache hygiene:** recognition and avoidance of migraine triggers including emotional stress, hormonal fluctuation, missed meals, caffeine withdrawal, weather changes, sleep disturbance, muscular tension, alcohol, heat, dehydration, and certain foods. A headache diary may be helpful in elucidating triggers in individual patients.
  - Discuss limiting acute treatments to minimize medication overuse headaches.
- **Stop analgesic overuse**
  - Cessation of the offending acute medications may be difficult for many patients.
    - Headache transformation is likely to occur with 5 days of butalbital, 8 days of opioid, 10 days of triptan, and 10 to 15 days of NSAID use per month.[5]
    - Acute migraine treatment should be limited to 2 or fewer days per week.
    - **Opioids and butalbital should be avoided**.
  - Following cessation, **headaches may temporarily get worse**.
  - Multiple strategies can be employed based on individual circumstances: stop or taper acute medications, steroid taper, hospitalization for rescue medication (e.g., dihydroergotamine [DHE], prochlorperazine, droperidol), and/or initiation of prophylactic medication.

TABLE 43-4	Tension-Type Headache Diagnostic Criteria

Headache lasting from 30 minutes to 7 days
Headache has at least two of the following characteristics:
- Bilateral location
- Pressing/tightening (nonpulsating) quality
- Mild or moderate intensity
- Not made worse by routine physical activity

Both of the following:
- No nausea or vomiting
- Not >1 of photophobia or phonophobia

Data from Headache Classification Subcommittee of the International Headache Society. The International Classification of Headache Disorders: 2nd edition. *Cephalalgia* 2004;24:9–160.

TABLE 43-5 Cluster Headache Diagnostic Criteria

Severe, unilateral orbital, supraorbital, and/or temporal pain lasting 15–180 minutes untreated

Headache associated with at least one of the following ipsilateral to the pain:
- Conjunctival injection
- Lacrimation
- Nasal congestion
- Rhinorrhea
- Forehead and facial sweating
- Miosis
- Ptosis
- Eyelid edema

Frequency of attacks from 1 every other day to 8 per day

Data from Headache Classification Subcommittee of the International Headache Society. The International Classification of Headache Disorders: 2nd edition. *Cephalalgia* 2004;24:9–160.

Medications

Acute Headache Treatment (Migraine and Tension Type)

- The following medications used to treat acute headaches are most effective when taken at headache onset and may be used in combination.
- Use of butalbital-containing medications (e.g., Fioricet, Fiorinal, and Esgic) should be approached with caution.
- Over-the-counter (OTC) analgesics: **NSAIDs, acetaminophen, aspirin, and caffeine** are often effective as a first-line therapy and may be combined for better effect.
- **Antiemetics:**
  - Commonly used to treat migraine pain, particularly if headaches are accompanied by nausea/vomiting.
  - Examples include **metoclopramide** (Reglan) 10 mg IV and **prochlorperazine** (Compazine) 10 mg IV/IM/PR.[6,7] Droperidol has also been shown to be effective; however, there is an FDA boxed warning regarding QT prolongation and torsades de pointes with IV administration. A 12-lead ECG must be obtained prior to administration of droperidol and the patient monitored for arrhythmias afterwards. Promethazine (Phenergan) should not be given IV/SC due to the risk of severe tissue necrosis/gangrene with extravasation (FDA boxed warning).
  - Side effects include sedation, akathisia, and QT prolongation. Diphenhydramine (12.5 mg IV) may be given concomitantly to prevent akathisia and dystonic reactions.
- **Triptans**
  - Triptans are serotonin receptor 1b/1d agonists that are thought to be relatively specific in their effectiveness for migraine headache. Multiple studies have demonstrated effectiveness.[8] All are most effective when used early.
  - Multiple triptans exist (e.g., almotriptan, eletriptan, frovatriptan, naratriptan, rizatriptan, sumatriptan, and zolmitriptan) and differ in half-life, route of administration, and cost. Common regimens include the following:
    - **Sumatriptan** 25 to 100 mg **PO** ×1, may repeat after 2 hours, maximum dose 200 mg/24 hours.[9] Sumatriptan 4 to 6 mg **SC** ×1, may repeat after 1 hour, maximum dose 12 mg/24 hours.[10] SC administration is faster in onset but associated with more side effects. Sumatriptan 5 to 20 mg **intranasal** ×1, may repeat after 2 hours, maximum dose 40 mg/24 hours.[11]
    - **Eletriptan** 20 to 40 mg ×1, may repeat after 2 hours, maximum dose 80 mg/24 hours.
    - **Rizatriptan** 5 to 10 mg ×1, may repeat after 2 hours, maximum dose 30 mg/24 hours.

- **Almotriptan** 6.25 to 12.5 mg ×1, may repeat after 2 hours, maximum dose 25 mg/24 hours.
- **Zolmitriptan** 1.25 to 2.5 mg PO ×1, may repeat after 2 hours, maximum dose 10 mg/24 hours. Zolmitriptan 2.5 to 5 mg intranasal ×1, maximum dose 10 mg/24 hours.
  - All available oral triptans appear to be relatively equally effective.[12]
  - **Contraindications** exist due to the vasoconstrictive effects and include ischemic heart disease, coronary artery vasospasm, peripheral arterial disease, uncontrolled hypertension, headaches associated with weakness, and concurrent (or within 2 weeks) monoamine oxidase inhibitor (MAOI) use.
  - Monitor for symptoms of serotonin syndrome, which could arise with monotherapy or coadministration with a selective serotonin reuptake inhibitor (SSRI) or serotonin norepinephrine reuptake inhibitor (SNRI), necessitating discontinuation of drug and supportive care.
- **Dihydroergotamine**
  - DHE is an agonist of multiple serotonin receptor subtypes, including 1b/1d, dopamine receptors, and is also a nonselective α-adrenergic blocker. It may be used for acute migraine treatment and is often used **to break status migrainosus** (debilitating migraine lasting >72 hours).
  - Alone, DHE may be less effective than a triptan or an antiemetic, but when combined with an antiemetic it is superior to ketorolac and meperidine. DHE may also be more effective at preventing recurrences.[8,13]
  - Parenteral DHE is usually given in combination with an IV antiemetic (prochlorperazine or metoclopramide) due to the fairly high rate of DHE-induced nausea.
  - For acute migraine treatment
    - DHE 1 mg **IM or SC**, may repeat q1 hour to a maximum dose of 3 mg/day.
    - DHE 1 mg **IV**, may repeat q1 hour to a maximum dose of 2 mg/day.
    - DHE **nasal** 0.5 mg (1 spray) **each nostril**, may repeat in 15 minutes, maximum 2 mg (4 sprays)/attack or 3 mg (6 sprays)/day.
  - DHE for intractable migraine is an off-label usage but has been found to be effective if several trials.[14–16] The typical protocol starts with IV metoclopramide 10 mg over 30 minutes. A 0.5 test dose of DHE is then given. Those with persistent headache are given 1 mg DHE IV with 10 mg metoclopramide every 8 hours, typically over 2 to 3 days.
  - Contraindications are similar to that of triptans. Serotonin syndrome may occur when DHE is administered with an SSRI. Coadministration with CYP3A4 inhibitors (e.g., protease inhibitors, macrolides, and azole antifungals) is also contraindicated.

Prophylactic Treatment (Migraine and Tension Type)
- The decision to treat with prophylactic medications is based upon the frequency and duration of headaches, amount of disability caused, and response to acute headache medicines.[17]
- Nonpharmacologic therapies include physical therapy and behavioral therapy (e.g., biofeedback and relaxation training).
- **Anticonvulsants**[17–19]:
  - **Topiramate**: start at 25 mg daily and increase to 50 mg bid, maximum dose 200 mg/day.[20] Central nervous system (CNS) side effects are relatively common including paresthesia, fatigue, drowsiness, dizziness, nervousness, memory and language difficulty, and poor concentration. Anorexia, nausea, dysgeusia, diarrhea, and weight loss are also fairly common. Side effects are more common with higher doses.
  - **Valproic acid/divalproex**: start at 250 mg bid and increase to a maximum of 500 mg bid.[21] Extended release divalproex may be given 200 to 1,000 mg daily. There is an FDA boxed warning for hepatotoxicity and teratogenicity. Common side effects include nausea/vomiting, weight changes, hair loss, drowsiness, insomnia, tremor, and thrombocytopenia.
  - **Gabapentin** is most likely not effective.[22]

- **Antihypertensives**[17–19]
  - β**-Blockers**
    - **Propranolol**: start at 80 mg/day divided tid/qid, increase to a maximum of 160 to 240 mg divided tid/qid, or use long-acting propranolol.
    - **Metoprolol**: start at 50 mg bid, may increase to a maximum of 200 mg/day.
  - Calcium channel blockers do not have nearly as convincing evidence for migraine prophylaxis, but they are frequently used. Verapamil is most common, starting at 120 mg divided tid increased to a maximum of 480 mg divided tid, or extended release verapamil.
  - Angiotensin-converting enzyme (ACE) inhibitors and angiotensin receptor blockers (ARB) may also have some prophylactic efficacy.
- **Antidepressants**[17–19]
  - **Tricyclic antidepressants** (TCAs): amitriptyline 10 to 150 mg at bedtime.[23] Common side effects include dry mouth, drowsiness, and weight gain.
  - SSRIs and SNRIs may also be effective. A small randomized trial showed that venlafaxine XR 150 mg was effective for migraine prophylaxis.[24]
- **NSAIDs** such as ibuprofen and naproxen may be beneficial for migraine prophylaxis but they can also be medication overuse headaches.
- **OTC agents**: probably/possibly effective agents include butterbur (*Petasites hybridus*) extract 50 to 75 mg bid, riboflavin (200 mg bid), magnesium (300 to 600 mg/day), feverfew extract (MIG-99) 6.25 mg tid, and Co-Q10 (100 mg tid).[17,19,25]
- **Botulinum toxin** is probably ineffective for intermittent migraine prophylaxis.[19] It may, however, be effective for chronic, refractory headaches.[26]

Cluster Headache Treatment
- Prevention includes avoidance of triggers including alcohol and nitrates.
- Abortive therapies include inhaled oxygen by mask (high flow), triptans (SC or nasal), and DHE (see above).[16,27,28]
- Prophylaxis can be attempted with verapamil, lithium, valproate, corticosteroids, and melatonin.[29]

Seizures

GENERAL PRINCIPLES

- A seizure is a transient occurrence of signs and/or symptoms due to abnormal excessive or synchronous neuronal activity in the brain.[30]
- Epilepsy is a disorder of the brain characterized by an enduring predisposition to generate epileptic seizures.[30] The occurrence of a single seizure does not necessitate the diagnosis of epilepsy.
- An unprovoked seizure occurs without a precipitant, thus excluding those associated with acute CNS insult or metabolic/toxic disturbance including alcohol withdrawal.
- Seizures affect almost 2 million Americans. The age-adjusted prevalence of epilepsy is 6.8/1,000 population.[31] The cumulative incidence of having an unprovoked seizure is 4.1% and the cumulative incidence of epilepsy is 3.1%.[32]
- Table 43-6 presents a list of the more common causes of seizures.
- **Focal seizures** arise from epileptogenic foci in a localized region of one cerebral hemisphere and are further classified based upon level of consciousness.[33] Focal seizures include simple partial seizures and complex partial seizures.
- **Generalized seizures** involve widespread regions in both brain hemispheres with impairment of consciousness and include nonconvulsive (absence) and convulsive (myoclonic, clonic, tonic, tonic-clonic, and atonic) seizures.

TABLE 43-6 Etiology of Seizures

Idiopathic	Nonstructural/metabolic
Presumed genetic origin	Medications that lower seizure threshold (β-lactams, alcohol, meperidine, neuroleptics, antidepressants [including bupropion])
Structural	Drug withdrawal (benzodiazepines, alcohol, antiepileptic drugs)
Cerebrovascular	Electrolyte abnormalities (hyper/hyponatremia, hyper/hypocalcemia, hyper/hypoglycemia, hypomagnesemia, hypophosphatemia)
Congenital	
Trauma	
Neoplasm	
Degenerative neurologic disorder	Uremia
Infection	Hypoxia/anoxia
	Acute febrile illnesses
	Drug intoxication (cocaine, phencyclidine, theophylline)

- **Simple partial seizures**
  - Involve **no impairment of consciousness**.
  - **Usually brief**, lasting approximately 15 seconds to 2 minutes.
  - Can manifest as stereotypic motor movements, abnormal somatosensory symptoms (e.g., paresthesias), special sensory symptoms (e.g., visual, auditory, olfactory, gustatory, or vertigo), neuropsychiatric symptoms (e.g., emotion, memory, cognition, or perceptions), and autonomic symptoms (e.g., epigastric rising, pallor, flushing, or piloerection).
- **Complex partial seizures**
  - Stereotyped partial seizures **with impaired consciousness**.
  - May include motionless staring, behavioral arrest, unresponsiveness, oral or limb automatisms, focal limb posturing, or clonus.
  - Usually last 30 seconds to 3 minutes and are often followed by postictal confusion.
- **Secondarily generalized tonic-clonic seizures**
  - Secondary generalization is caused by the spread of ictal discharge from a localized focus to involve both hemispheres symmetrically.
  - Tonic and/or clonic movements are usually asymmetric.
  - Often accompanied by postictal confusion.
- **Typical absence seizure**
  - Characterized by **sudden behavioral arrest**, loss of awareness, and blank staring.
  - **Brief**, lasting 5 to 30 seconds with immediate return to baseline consciousness.
- **Generalized tonic-clonic seizures**
  - Generalized tonic-clonic seizures are characterized by tonic stiffening of axial and limb muscles lasting 10 to 15 seconds.
  - The clonic phase involves clonic jerking that increases in frequency and amplitude with bilateral upper extremity flexion and bilateral lower extremity extension.
  - Tonic and/or clonic movements are usually symmetric and last 1 to 2 minutes.
  - Consciousness recovers in minutes but **postictal confusion** may last for hours.
- **Psychogenic nonepileptic seizures (PNES)**
  - PNESs are paroxysmal changes in behavior that superficially resemble epilepsy but have a psychological rather than a medical cause.[34]
  - 12% to 20% of patients seen in epilepsy clinics have PNES but 10% to 30% of PNES patients also have epilepsy.
  - Treatment consists of psychological intervention and weaning off antiepileptic medications.

DIAGNOSIS

Clinical Presentation

- The goal of the history is to identify possible triggers of provoked seizures and to distinguish seizures from other paroxysmal events, such as syncope, episodic movement disorders, PNES, narcolepsy/cataplexy, and transient ischemic attacks (TIAs).
- A reliable description of the seizure should be obtained (preferably from a bystander when consciousness is impaired). However, bystander reports of seizure duration are often unreliable.
- The purpose of a detailed neurologic examination is to elicit focal findings suggestive of a structural lesion.

Diagnostic Testing

- The purpose of diagnostic testing is to distinguish provoked seizure from unprovoked seizure, and to determine the risk of recurrence.
- **Electroencephalogram** (EEG)
  - A normal EEG does not rule out epilepsy.
  - 30% to 40% of first EEGs show abnormalities. Early EEGs within 24 hours have a higher yield (51%) than after 24 hours (34%).[35]
  - Epileptiform abnormalities may confirm a diagnosis of epileptic seizures and distinguish partial seizures from generalized seizures.
  - An abnormal EEG approximately doubles the risk of seizure recurrence.[36]
  - Extended video-EEG (e.g., 24-hour monitoring) is helpful in evaluating seizure types (including PNES) and in localizing seizure origins for possible surgical intervention.
  - Ambulatory EEG is often less useful due to artifacts in the record and difficulty correlating unmonitored clinical events with the EEG tracing.
- **Brain MRI**: workup of a seizure should include brain MRI with and without contrast to evaluate for structural lesions (e.g., mesial temporal sclerosis) that may benefit from surgical resection.
- **LP**: used to rule out CNS infections or carcinomatosis if there is clinical suspicion.

TREATMENT

- **First seizures generally do not require antiepileptic drug (AED) treatment**.
  - Recurrence risk for a second unprovoked seizure is 34% at 5 years.
  - The probability of achieving seizure control with AED treatment is the same for those treated immediately versus those treated after the second seizure.[37]
- The goal for the management of epilepsy is to minimize seizure frequency and medication side effects.
  - Titrate medication dosage to find the lowest dose necessary to control seizures.
  - Decrease modifiable triggers such as sleep deprivation, alcohol intake, caffeine, and stress.
  - Implement seizure calendars to monitor seizure frequency.
- Patients with intractable epilepsy, despite sufficient trials of multiple AEDs, may be candidates for resective epilepsy surgery and should be referred to an epilepsy center.

Medications

First-Generation AEDs

- These include phenytoin, carbamazepine, phenobarbital, and valproic acid (see Table 43-7).
- Advantages of use include ease of monitoring therapeutic serum levels.
- Carbamazepine has been associated with an increased risk of Stevens-Johnson in certain Asian populations carrying the HLA-B*1502 allele.

- Valproic acid can increase free phenytoin levels and inhibit the metabolism of other drugs.
- Drug-drug interactions of enzyme-inducing first generation AEDs (carbamazepine, phenytoin, and phenobarbital) are common, which result in the following:
  ○ Increased metabolism of oral contraceptive pills and reduced hormone levels
  ○ Increased metabolism of warfarin and reduced anticoagulant activity
  ○ Increased TCA levels while TCAs increase AED levels
  ○ Decreased levels of valproic acid
- Enzyme-inducing first-generation agents cause vitamin D deficiency. Supplementation with calcium and vitamin D helps prevent osteopenia and osteoporosis.

Second-Generation AEDs

- These include levetiracetam, topiramate, zonisamide, lamotrigine, oxcarbazepine, gabapentin, pregabalin, and lacosamide (Table 43-7).
- Generally, they have better side-effect profiles, little to no need for serum monitoring, less frequent dosing, and fewer drug interactions.
- Rashes with mucosal involvement and systemic symptoms require immediate attention, as the rashes can represent potentially fatal reactions, such as **toxic epidermal necrolysis or Stevens-Johnson syndrome**.[38]

Benzodiazepines

- Used in the **acute treatment of seizures**; typically lorazepam 1 to 2 mg intramuscularly or intravenously, repeated as needed every 3 to 5 minutes while carefully monitoring for respiratory depression.
- Clonazepam is occasionally used long-term in patients with generalized epilepsy, particularly myoclonus, that is, refractory to multiple other medications. However, tolerance can develop necessitating escalating doses for seizure control.
- Side effects include sedation, irritability, ataxia, and respiratory depression.

Discontinuation of AEDs

- **Unless specified by state laws or guidelines, physicians need to come to an agreement with their patients regarding prudent seizure precautions during the withdrawal period**.
- Recurrence of seizures is unpredictable and influenced by the duration of active disease and seizure-free period.
- Tapering of AEDs should be slow (over 2 to 3 months) to avoid triggering a seizure.
- Taper one drug at a time for patients on polytherapy.

SPECIAL CONSIDERATIONS

Driving

- Longer seizure-free intervals (>6 to 12 months) are associated with reduced risk of motor vehicle accidents.
- Each state determines the required seizure-free interval, requirements for physician reporting, liability for driving recommendations, and whether mitigating factors are considered. Rules can be found at the Epilepsy Foundation website: http://www.epilepsy.com/learn/seizures-youth/about-teens-epilepsy/driving-and-transportation (last accessed 1/29/15).

Pregnancy

- All women of childbearing age on AEDs should be supplemented with folic acid 1 mg daily or 4 mg/day if taking valproic acid or carbamazepine.
- **All AEDs are associated with teratogenic potential**. Valproic acid is most associated with teratogenicity in the first trimester.[39]

Seizures | **915**

TABLE 43-7 Antiepileptic Drugs

Drug	Indication	Dosing^a	Therapeutic range (µg/mL)	Side effects	Notes
Phenytoin	Partial epilepsy SGTC	300 mg/day or 5–6 mg/kg/day in divided doses; can load with fosphenytoin IV 15–20 mg/kg	10–20	Gingival hyperplasia, vitamin D and folate deficiency	Propensity for toxicity due to zero-order kinetics Signs of toxicity: sedation, incoordination, nystagmus
Phenobarbital	Partial epilepsy PGTC SGTC	Typical dose: 60 mg bid to tid	10–40	Sedation, vitamin D deficiency, memory loss, depression	Sign of toxicity: sedation
Carbamazepine	Partial epilepsy PGTC SGTC	Start: 200 mg bid Typical dose: 800–1,200 mg/day	4–12	Vitamin D deficiency, leukopenia, hyponatremia	Autoinduction of metabolism Signs of toxicity: ataxia, nausea, vision changes
Valproic acid	Partial epilepsy SGTC PG	Start: 10–15 mg/kg/day or load IV; increase by 5–10 mg/kg/day as needed	50–100	Weight gain, tremor, hair loss	Teratogenic, hepatotoxic Signs of toxicity: sedation, nausea/vomiting
Levetiracetam	Partial epilepsy Adjunct for PGTC Adjunct for SGTC	Start: 500 mg bid or can load IV up to 2,000 mg. Maximum: 3,000 mg/day		Irritability, headache, depression, psychosis	Few drug interactions, dose must be adjusted for reduced renal function
Lacosamide	Adjunct for partial epilepsy	Start: 50 mg bid; increase by 100 mg/week to 200–400 mg/day		Headache, dizziness, diplopia, nausea	Few drug interactions, dose must be adjusted for reduced renal function

(*Continued*)

TABLE 43-7 Antiepileptic Drugs (*Continued*)

Drug	Indication	Dosing[a]	Therapeutic range (µg/mL)	Side effects	Notes
Topiramate	Partial epilepsy PGTC SGTC	Start: 25 mg/day Recommended dose: 200–400 mg/day		Nephrolithiasis, paresthesias, psychomotor slowing	Improves headaches, associated with weight loss
Zonisamide	Partial epilepsy Adjunct for PGTC SGTC	Start: 100 mg/day; increase by 100 mg/week to 300–600 mg/day		Nephrolithiasis, Stevens-Johnson syndrome, dizziness	Long half-life, improves headaches, weight loss, contraindicated with sulfa allergy
Lamotrigine	Partial epilepsy PGTC SGTC	Start: 25 mg/day Follow titration to 250 mg bid		Tremor, rash, Stevens-Johnson syndrome (use long titration)	Drug of choice in pregnancy and if coexistent mood disorder
Oxcarbazepine	Partial epilepsy PGTC SGTC	Start: 300 mg bid Follow titration to 1,200–2,400 mg/day		Somnolence, dizziness, rash, headache	Less frequent side effect compared with carbamazepine
Gabapentin	Partial epilepsy SGTC	Start: 300 mg/day Maximum: 1,200 mg tid		Sedation, weight gain	Few drug interactions, dose must be adjusted for reduced renal function
Pregabalin	Adjunct for partial epilepsy	Start: 75 mg bid; increase to 300–600 mg/day		Dizziness, sedation	Few drug interactions, dose must be adjusted for reduced renal function

[a]These doses only represent guidelines and actual dosing may require lower or higher doses.
PG, primary generalized; PGTC, primary generalized tonic-clonic; SGTC, secondary generalized tonic-clonic.

Alcohol Withdrawal Seizures

- Alcohol withdrawal seizures are associated with relative or absolute withdrawal of ethanol.[40]
- They typically occur between 7 and 48 hours after cessation of drinking (peak 12 to 24 hours).
- Seizures are usually generalized tonic-clonic.
- Most patients (>60%) experience more than one seizure, and about 33% go on to develop delirium tremens, which continues to have a relatively high in-hospital mortality.
- Treatment involves IV benzodiazepines or the resumption of alcohol. Administer thiamine prior to providing glucose-containing fluids.
- **There is no role for long-term AEDs unless there is an underlying epileptic disorder**.

Multiple Sclerosis

GENERAL PRINCIPLES

- The incidence of MS is influenced by environmental and genetic factors. Prevalence in the United States is approximately 1/1,000. This increases to 1% with a first-degree relative, 5% in dizygotic twins, and 25% in monozygotic twins.
- Typically, multiple sclerosis (MS) is diagnosed in early adulthood and is more common in women (3:1).
- Patients may present with a relapsing or progressive course but must demonstrate dissemination in time and space.
- MS is an autoimmune-mediated process characterized by demyelinating plaques with predilection for periventricular white matter, corpus callosum, optic nerves, brainstem, cerebellum, and cervical spinal cord white matter.[41] Gray matter (cortical) lesions are increasingly identified, but are poorly visualized on MRI.[42]

DIAGNOSIS

Clinical Presentation

- Relapsing-remitting MS (RRMS): 85% of MS patients begin with relapses (also called attacks or exacerbations) of worsening neurologic functioning followed by periods with partial or complete recovery.
- Secondary progressive MS (SPMS): 50% of RRMS patients may transform to a SPMS stage where deficits gradually worsen in-between relapses.
- Primary progressive MS (PPMS): patients have a gradual progressive disease course from onset with no specific relapses.
- Attacks typically evolve over a period of days, plateau, and then improve over weeks.
- Patients may present with a myriad of symptoms and signs including focal weakness, focal sensory complaints, Lhermitte sign (electric shock sensation down trunk and limbs induced by neck flexion), fatigue, unilateral loss of vision, diplopia, ataxia, or bladder complaints.
- A detailed neurologic examination is important to identify deficits related to demyelinating plaques and to monitor progression of disease.

Diagnostic Testing

- **McDonald diagnostic criteria** (2010 revision) are used for diagnosis to establish dissemination in time and space (see Table 43-8).[43]
- Brain and/or cervical spine MRI is used to identify and monitor lesions especially since some brain lesions can be clinically silent.
- Cerebrospinal fluid (CSF) often shows intrathecal antibody production (requires concurrent serum sample). **Elevated CSF restricted oligoclonal bands are identified in >95% of MS patients**.
- Visual-evoked potentials may identify optic nerve lesions.

TABLE 43-8	Diagnostic Criteria for Multiple Sclerosis (2010 Revised McDonald Criteria)	

Clinical attacks[a] (history)	Lesions[a] (exam or MRI)	Additional evident to make diagnosis (evidence must be consistent with MS)
≥2	≥2 OR 1+ a reasonable historical attack	None—meets criteria for MS
≥2	1	Dissemination in space (DIS) • Await lesion • OR clinical attack
1	≥2	Dissemination in time (DIT) • Asymptomatic enhancing and nonenhancing lesions • OR new lesion on follow-up MRI • OR second clinical attack
1	1	Meet DIS AND DIT as described above
0 (Progressive MS)	1 year of progressive symptoms and at least two of the following: • Positive brain MRI (≥1 T2 lesion) • Positive spinal cord MRI (≥2 T2 lesions) • Positive IgG index OR CSF-restricted oligoclonal bands	

[a]DIS requires lesions in at least two of the following four CNS areas: periventricular, juxtacortical, infratentorial, and spinal cord.
Data from Polman CH, Reingold SC, Banwell B, et al. Diagnostic criteria for multiple sclerosis: 2010 revisions to the McDonald criteria. *Ann Neurol* 2011;69:292–302.

- Other conditions may mimic MS and depending on the associated symptoms, it may be useful to check vitamin B_{12}, thyroid-stimulating hormone (TSH), serum rapid plasma reagin (RPR), HIV, antinuclear antibodies (ANA), and extractable nuclear antigens (ENA).
- Evaluation for **neuromyelitis optica** (NMO) with an NMO-IgG should be considered if patient presents with recurrent optic neuritis and longitudinally extensive transverse myelitis on MRI (>3 vertebral segments).[44] One-third of NMO patients are seronegative.
- Infections and metabolic disturbances must be considered as they can mimic relapses and cause pseudoexacerbations.

TREATMENT

Acute Treatment

- IV methylprednisolone has been shown to hasten return to neurologic baseline. Typical dosing is 1 g daily, which can be divided, for 3 to 5 days. IV steroids may be followed by an oral prednisone taper over 4 weeks.[45,46]
- Plasma exchange is an option for severe relapses or if unresponsive/intolerant to steroids.[47]
- Physical therapy and occupational therapy can help address functional needs.

Disease-Modifying Therapy

- Consider referral to neurologist or dedicated MS center for long-term management.
- Immunomodulatory treatments aim to prevent further relapses, but do little to repair existing damage.
- Treatment of a clinically isolated syndrome, or a single monophasic attack, with immunomodulatory therapy may delay progression to clinically definite MS.[48,49]

- FDA-approved treatments for RRMS include interferon-β, glatiramer acetate, fingolimod, teriflunomide (active compound of leflunomide), and natalizumab.[50]
  - Many of these medications (with the exception of glatiramer acetate) can cause leukopenias and liver enzyme abnormalities that must be monitored.
  - These medications should not be used during pregnancy, although glatiramer acetate appears to be safe and is pregnancy category B.
- **Natalizumab** is a monoclonal antibody, which has been associated with **progressive multifocal leukoencephalopathy (PML)**. Risk factors include length of treatment, prior treatment with immunosuppressant medications, and prior exposure to the JC virus.[51]
- There are no FDA-approved treatments for PPMS, although some patients may benefit from treatment particularly if they are younger or an MRI shows new lesions.[52]

Treatment of Related Symptoms
- Depression is common and is responsive to SSRIs or bupropion.
- Pain and spasms are common and may respond to medications, such as gabapentin, carbamazepine, duloxetine, tricyclics, and muscle relaxants.
- Urinary symptoms (spasticity, incontinence) may improve with treatment and warrant consideration of urologic consultation.
- Fatigue may respond to amantadine or modafinil.

Neuropathy

GENERAL PRINCIPLES

- **Diabetes is the most common etiology** of neuropathy in the US, while leprosy is the most common cause in undeveloped countries.
- Characterization of neuropathy is crucial to guide the differential diagnosis and includes temporal profile (onset and duration), family history, and anatomic classification including
  - Fiber type (motor vs. sensory, large vs. small, somatic vs. autonomic)
  - Axonal versus demyelinating
  - Distribution affected (e.g., length dependent, specific dermatome, multifocal)

DIAGNOSIS

Clinical Presentation
History
- Common complaints are paresthesias, numbness, pain, weakness, and autonomic symptoms.
- Questions should focus on duration, course, and distribution of complaints.
- Consider relationship to other medical conditions and medications; chemotherapeutic agents and antiretrovirals commonly cause neuropathy.
- Family history may identify hereditary neuropathies.
- Social history should include occupation (toxin exposure), sexual history (HIV, hepatitis C), recreational drug use (vasculitis secondary to cocaine), smoking (paraneoplastic disease), and excessive alcohol intake or dietary habits (vitamin deficiencies).

Physical Examination
- Evaluate patterns of sensory loss in specific dermatomal or nerve distributions.
  - Diabetic polyneuropathy typically is symmetric in a stocking-glove distribution.
  - Large fiber involvement causes vibratory and proprioceptive loss.
  - Phalen maneuver (flexing wrists for 60 seconds) or Tinel sign (tapping the median nerve at the wrist) may elicit carpal tunnel syndrome symptoms.[53] But both have limited sensitivity and specificity.[54]

- Evaluate for patterns of weakness and atrophy.
  - Toe extension and ankle dorsiflexion weakness may be seen in polyneuropathy.
  - Isolated weakness is typical of mononeuropathies and if more generalized may suggest a myopathy.
  - If the symptoms of weakness and/or numbness are primarily in the hands, cervical myelopathy should be excluded.
- Deep tendon reflexes are typically depressed or lost in large fiber neuropathy (ankle jerk lost first), and is more prominent in demyelinating neuropathies.
- Evaluate orthostatic blood pressure to assess for autonomic involvement.
- Gait may be affected in severe neuropathy.
- Signs of upper motor neuron disease are typically absent; if present, they may represent amyotrophic lateral sclerosis or spinal cord disease.

Differential Diagnosis

Many conditions can affect the peripheral nerves (see Table 43-9), and about 25% of cases of chronic polyneuropathy remain unknown. The most common presentations are described below.

Diabetic Neuropathy
- Over 30% of diabetic patients have a length-dependent peripheral neuropathy.
- Burning and pain are common symptoms suggesting a small fiber neuropathy, which may progress over months to years.

TABLE 43-9 | Causes of Peripheral Neuropathy

Systemic disease
Diabetic neuropathy
Renal insufficiency
Hypothyroidism
Chronic liver disease
Celiac disease
Critical illness

Vasculitic
Systemic lupus erythematous
Scleroderma
Rheumatoid arthritis
Polyarteritis nodosa
Granulomatosis with polyangiitis
Churg-Strauss syndrome
CREST
Cryoglobulinemia
Vasculitis restricted to peripheral nerves

Infiltrative
Sarcoidosis
Amyloidosis
Neoplastic

Infectious
HIV
Lyme disease
Leprosy

Nutritional
Vitamin B_{12} deficiency
Vitamin B_1 deficiency
Vitamin E deficiency
Vitamin B_6 intoxication

Immune mediated
CIDP
Guillain-Barré syndrome
Paraneoplastic
Multifocal motor neuropathy
Sulfatide antibody related
MAG antibody related

Hereditary
Charcot-Marie-Tooth disease
Hereditary liability to pressure palsies
Hereditary sensory autonomic

Physical
Trauma
Focal compression
Entrapment

Miscellaneous
Idiopathic
Chronic alcoholism
Drugs
Toxins and heavy metals

CIDP, chronic inflammatory demyelinating polyneuropathy; CREST, calcinosis, Raynaud phenomenon, esophageal motility disorders, sclerodactyly, and telangiectasia; MAG, myelin-associated glycoprotein.

- Electrodiagnostic studies may be normal early or demonstrate an axonal sensory-motor polyneuropathy that may have autonomic involvement.
- Skin biopsies may show a decrease in nerve fibers distally.

Entrapment Neuropathies

- Systemic diseases like thyroid disease, diabetes, or amyloidosis increase susceptibility to entrapment neuropathies.
- **Carpal tunnel syndrome** (CTS) is caused by increased pressure within the carpal tunnel producing **median nerve** ischemia.[53]
  - There is sensation loss in thumb, second, and third digits, lateral half of fourth digit, and the adjacent palmar surface.
  - Thenar muscle atrophy can eventually occur.
  - Median nerve conduction delay is evident across the wrist on nerve conduction studies (NCS).
- The **ulnar nerve** may become compressed in the retrocondylar groove near the elbow, which becomes more exposed with a flexed elbow and commonly occurs during sleep. Sensory loss occurs in the medial half of the fourth digit, entire fifth digit, and the adjacent palmar surface. Weakness is seen in the first dorsal interosseous muscle.
- **Radial nerve** entrapment in the radial groove of the forearm results in wrist drop.
- **Meralgia paresthetica** produces lateral thigh sensory complaints as a result of lateral femoral cutaneous compression at the pelvic brim by obesity and tight-fitting garments.

Trigeminal Neuralgia

- Classic trigeminal neuralgia is generally thought to be due to trigeminal nerve root compression by an overlying blood vessel resulting in demyelination of sensory fibers.
- When bilateral, consider other etiologies such as multiple sclerosis.
- Patients suffer from lancinating pain in distribution of the fifth cranial nerve (third, second, and first divisions in order of most commonly affected).

Bell Palsy

- Bell palsy is a unilateral peripheral facial nerve cranial mononeuropathy causing upper and lower facial weakness with possible alteration of taste and hearing (hyperacusis).
- It is often idiopathic, but etiologies such as Lyme disease, sarcoid, and syphilis should be considered, especially if recurrent or bilateral.

Vasculitic Neuropathy

- Vasculitis neuropathy is a subacute progressive painful sensorimotor axonal neuropathy.
- It classically presents as **mononeuritis multiplex** but may present as symmetric polyneuropathy.
- It is usually associated with systemic vasculitic disorders but may be confined to the peripheral nerves, causing peripheral nerve infarction secondary to vascular occlusion by inflammation and fibrinoid necrosis.[55]
- Nerve biopsy may show epineural inflammation, vessel wall pathology, and axonal loss.

Guillain-Barré Syndrome

- Guillain-Barré syndrome (GBS) presents as a rapidly progressive ascending weakness with areflexia and variable sensory involvement. Symptoms peak within 4 weeks.[56]
- *Campylobacter jejuni* or cytomegalovirus (CMV) infection may precede the neuropathy.
- Respiratory muscles are often involved; 25% of patients require ventilator support.
- Electrodiagnostic studies may not reveal the typical demyelination for 2 weeks.
- Increased CSF protein is present in approximately 80% of patients.

Chronic Inflammatory Demyelinating Polyneuropathy

- Chronic inflammatory demyelinating polyneuropathy (CIDP) is **the most common type of acquired chronic demyelinating polyneuropathy.**[57]
- It affects motor nerves more than sensory nerves.
- The course may be relapsing or progressive, evolving over ≥2 months.
- Electrodiagnostic studies demonstrate reduced conduction velocity and conduction block in multiple nerves indicating demyelination.
- CSF protein is typically moderately elevated.
- Nerve biopsy is considered if there is a high clinical suspicion for CIDP, as electrodiagnostic testing is often nondiagnostic.

HIV Neuropathy

- Distal sensory polyneuropathy is the most common neurologic manifestation of HIV.
- This neuropathy affects >50% of HIV patients.[58]
- Evidence for axonal sensory neuropathy is demonstrated on electrodiagnostic studies.
- HIV neuropathy remains prevalent despite advent of highly active antiretroviral therapy.

Diagnostic Testing

Laboratories

- Initial laboratory work includes complete blood cell count (CBC), complete metabolic panel (CMP), vitamin B_{12}, folate, TSH, hemoglobin A1C, ESR, and serum protein electrophoresis (SPEP) with immunofixation.
- Additional laboratory work should be considered depending upon the clinical scenario. This includes ANAs, ENAs, rheumatoid factor (RF), urine protein electrophoresis (UPEP), cryoglobulins, quantitative immunoglobulins, HIV, copper, vitamin E, anti-GM1 ganglioside antibodies, anti-sulfatide antibodies, anti–myelin-associated glycoprotein antibodies, and paraneoplastic antibody panel.

Diagnostic Procedures

- **Electromyography** (EMG) and NCSs are often recommended.
  - They can help differentiate axonal versus demyelinating neuropathies.
  - The distribution of involvement can be confirmed: mononeuropathy, polyneuropathy, mononeuropathy multiplex, plexopathy, or radiculopathy.
- If radiculopathy or myelopathy (spinal cord disease) is suspected, MRI of the appropriate level of the spine is recommended.
- **Nerve and muscle biopsy** may be useful in identifying immune-mediated (e.g., CIDP), inflammatory (e.g., vasculitis), or infiltrative (e.g., amyloidosis) causes of neuropathy.
- Genetic testing is pertinent if a hereditary neuropathy is suspected.

TREATMENT

- If secondary to another disease, **aggressive treatment of the underlying etiology** (e.g., diabetes, hypothyroidism, vitamin B_{12} deficiency, and renal insufficiency) may stabilize or improve neuropathic symptoms.
- Physical and occupational therapy can lessen disability. Ankle foot orthotics aid ambulation in patients with foot drop. Weight loss and proper foot care is encouraged, especially if obese and/or diabetic.
- For **CTS**, wrist splinting, keeping the wrist in a neutral position, is often helpful. Compression often occurs while sleeping and is not limited to overuse. Carpal tunnel release may be indicated with axonal loss or prolonged symptoms.
- Patients with compressive **ulnar neuropathy** at the elbow should avoid prolonged elbow flexion and leaning on the involved elbow. Nerve transposition may be considered for cases refractory to splinting.

- Treatment of **trigeminal neuralgia:**
  - First-line therapy includes carbamazepine (starting at 200 mg twice daily titrating up to effect). Oxcarbazepine, baclofen, and lamotrigine may also be useful.[59]
  - Microvascular decompression of the nerve should be considered in patients with refractory symptoms.
- Treatment of **Bell palsy:**
  - Corneal protection may be necessary (e.g., Lacri-Lube and an eye patch at night).
  - Treatment with oral steroids is beneficial, particularly if started within 3 days of symptom onset.[60,61] Consider the addition of acyclovir, valacyclovir, or famciclovir in patients with evidence of herpes infections and severe palsy.[62,63]
  - More than 90% of patients achieve full recovery with good prognostic indicators including incomplete paralysis, early improvement, young age, and preservation of taste. Electrical stimulation of the facial nerve does not hasten the recovery.
- **Vasculitic neuropathy** is treated with corticosteroids or immunosuppression.
- **GBS** typically requires hospital admission for intravenous immunoglobulins (IVIG) or plasma exchange.[56]
- **CIDP** is treated with IVIG, plasma exchange, or corticosteroids.[57]
- **Symptomatic treatment of neuropathic pain**[64]
  - Nonopiate agents remain the mainstay of therapy. Tramadol, a partial opioid agonist, and opiates must be prescribed with caution, if needed, given the potential for addiction and abuse.[65]
  - **Antiepileptics** such as gabapentin, pregabalin, carbamazepine are first-line agents.[66–69]
    - **Gabapentin** is typically started at 300 mg tid and can be slowly titrated up to 1,200 mg tid (maximum dose 3,600 mg/day). Gabapentin is thought to act via the $\alpha_2\delta$ subunit of voltage-dependent calcium channels thereby decreasing the release of neurotransmitters. If side effects are a concern gabapentin can be started at 100 mg tid. Dosage and frequency should be decreased in patients with chronic kidney disease. Side effects include fatigue, drowsiness, dizziness, ataxia, tremor, nystagmus, headache, and edema. Data supporting the use of gabapentin specifically for diabetic peripheral neuropathy are conflicting.
    - **Pregabalin** is usually started at 50 mg bid and slowly titrated to a maximum of 150 mg bid, alternatively 100 mg tid. This drug is also thought to act by binding the $\alpha_2\delta$ subunit. Relatively frequent side effects include fatigue, somnolence, dizziness, confusion, ataxia, headache, tremor, diplopia, and edema.
    - **Carbamazepine** immediate release is started at 100 mg bid and can be increased in 200 mg/day increments to a maximum of 1,200 mg/day. There are FDA boxed warnings for severe skin reactions in patients with the HLA-B*1502 (most often seen in Asians) allele and for agranulocytosis/aplastic anemia. The leukocyte count should be monitored. Adverse reactions also include somnolence, weakness, dizziness, headache, ataxia, rash, and nausea/vomiting.
  - **Antidepressants** such as TCAs (amitriptyline, nortriptyline) and SNRIs (duloxetine, venlafaxine) are other first- or second-line agents.[70,71]
    - **Amitriptyline** is started at 25 to 50 mg at bedtime and can be titrated up to a maximum of 150 mg/day. Nortriptyline likely has less anticholinergic side effects and is started at 10 to 25 mg at bedtime up to a maximum of 75 mg/day. Desipramine is another reasonable option.
    - **Duloxetine** has an FDA-approved indication for diabetic neuropathy; the starting dose is 30 mg/day, and then increased to 60 mg/day. Higher doses are not additionally effective.
    - **Venlafaxine**, like duloxetine, is an SNRI and is presumed to be effective at a dosage range between 75 and 225 mg/day (if immediate release, in 2 or 3 divided doses).
    - SSRIs are not known to useful for neuropathic pain.
  - Topical lidocaine and capsaicin may provide additional pain control.

Dystonia

- Dystonias are characterized by involuntary, sustained, patterned, and often repetitive muscle contractions leading to repetitive twisting movements and abnormal postures of the trunk, neck, face, or arms and legs.[72]
- Dystonias can be triggered by certain actions and relieved by so-called sensory tricks (e.g., touching the side of one's face), leading to the erroneous impression that the disorder is psychogenic.
- **Early-onset** (<25 years) forms of dystonia typically begin focally and gradually spread to involve other body regions, becoming progressively debilitating. **Adult-onset** (>25 years) forms usually begin within craniofacial or cervical musculature and do not migrate or progress significantly over time.
- Common focal dystonias include blepharospasm, task-specific limb dystonias (e.g., writer's cramp), cervical dystonia (e.g., spasmodic torticollis), vocal cord dystonia (e.g., spasmodic dysphonia), and oromandibular dystonia.[72]
- Patients with early onset dystonia should be tried on carbidopa/levodopa to evaluate for dopa-responsive dystonia, a rare genetic form of dystonia. Anticholinergics, benzodiazepines, baclofen, dopaminergic agents, dopamine-depleting agents, and tetrabenazine a vesicular monoamine transporter 2 inhibitor) may result in some benefit.
- Botulinum toxin injection to affected muscles is the treatment of choice for focal dystonias.

Essential Tremor

GENERAL PRINCIPLES

- Essential tremor is the most common neurologic cause of postural (e.g., maintaining posture with hands outstretched) or action (e.g., intentionally touching nose with index finger) tremor.
- Severe essential tremor may have a rest component.
- Essential tremor may begin on one side but eventually becomes bilateral/symmetrical.
- Approximately 50% have an autosomal dominant pattern of inheritance.

CLINICAL PRESENTATION

- Patients may report improvement of essential tremor following alcohol intake.
- Postural or action tremors have a broad differential. Worsening of tremor despite therapeutic trials or development of bradykinesia, rigidity, and postural instability should prompt further evaluation and referral to a movement disorder clinic.
- Patients with Parkinson disease (PD) may have a postural/action tremor.
- Exaggerated physiologic tremor is a commonly observed postural tremor in anxiety, stimulants (e.g., nicotine, caffeine), thyrotoxicosis, and drug or alcohol toxicity or withdrawal.
- Medication-induced tremor is common in the setting of antidepressants, β-agonists, steroids, valproate, lithium, neuroleptics, metoclopramide, theophylline, and levothyroxine.[73]
- Wilson disease should be considered in any patient under the age of 40 with tremor or other involuntary movements or postures (check serum ceruloplasmin).
- Screening for endocrine and toxic causes should include hyperthyroidism, hypoglycemia, caffeine consumption, nicotine use, chronic alcohol consumption, and medications.

TREATMENT

- **Propranolol** (immediate or sustained release): titrate to effect (usually 160 to 320 mg).[74]
- **Primidone**: begin 62.5 mg daily and titrate to effect, usually 62.5 to 1,000 mg daily.[74]

- Second-line medications include gabapentin, topiramate, and clonazepam.
- **Deep brain stimulation** is highly effective for medically refractory cases.

Parkinson Disease and Related Conditions

GENERAL PRINCIPLES

- **Parkinsonism** is a syndrome characterized by tremor, bradykinesia, rigidity, and postural instability. **PD** is the most common cause of parkinsonism.
- PD is a common neurodegenerative disease associated with progressive loss of dopaminergic neurons in substantia nigra of the brainstem and presence of Lewy bodies.
  - Dementia is a common feature of PD. PD can coexist with other dementias (e.g., Alzheimer disease, vascular dementia).
  - If dementia begins early in the course, consider other forms of parkinsonism.
  - Typical age of onset is around 60, but there is considerable variability.[75]
  - About 10% of cases are genetic; this is more common in early-onset patients.
- **Secondary parkinsonism** may result from agents with dopamine-blocking properties (e.g., antipsychotics and antiemetics).
  - Ninety percent begin within 3 months of starting the offending agent.[76]
  - Offending agents should be withdrawn gradually to avoid reemergent dyskinesia.
- Other neurodegenerative forms of parkinsonism (so-called Parkinson-plus syndromes) are rarer and less likely to respond to dopaminergic drugs.[77]
  - These include **dementia with Lewy bodies**, **progressive supranuclear palsy**, **multiple system atrophy**, and **corticobasal degeneration**.
  - Early and severe postural instability and/or dementia are clues for these syndromes; there is extensive clinical overlap between these and PD.
- **Normal pressure hydrocephalus** may also mimic parkinsonism. The clinical triad consists of dementia, urinary incontinence, and a magnetic gait.

DIAGNOSIS

- History and examination should focus on clinical features of parkinsonism.
  - Tremor occurs predominantly at rest.
  - Bradykinesia.
  - Rigidity is often described as lead pipe.
  - Postural instability can contribute to falls.
- Symptoms in PD often begin on one side and remain asymmetric until later in the disease. Consider other etiologies of parkinsonism if clinical features are symmetric.
- Other common motor findings include shuffling gait, stooped posture, loss of facial expression, decreased blinking, decreased arm swing, and occasional freezing of gait.
- Common nonmotor symptoms include cognitive dysfunction/dementia, psychosis and hallucinations, mood disorders, depression, anxiety, apathy and abulia, sleep disorders, excessive daytime somnolence, fatigue, autonomic dysfunction, olfactory dysfunction, sensory complaints, and seborrhea.[78]

TREATMENT

- **Carbidopa/levodopa is the most effective symptomatic therapy.**[79,80]
  - Other dopaminergic agents such as **MAOI and catechol-O-methyl transferase (COMT) inhibitors** are also used.[81]
  - Early treatment of PD with levodopa does not accelerate the course of the disease and may even slow it down.[82]

- Dopamine agonists (e.g., pramipexole, ropinirole) may be associated with less dyskinesia but may increase risk of peripheral edema, somnolence/sudden sleep, constipation, hallucinations, nausea, and impulse control disorders.[83]
- PD is progressive, requiring gradual increases in medication over time.
- Treatment complications include dyskinesias and motor fluctuations. Other common side effects include somnolence, orthostatic hypotension, hallucinations, psychosis, anorexia, and nausea.
- Dopamine antagonists (antiemetics, antipsychotics, etc.) and anticholinergics can worsen parkinsonism.
  - Ondansetron should be used for nausea. Domperidone, which is not available in the US, can be used in refractory cases.
  - Low-dose quetiapine (starting 12.5 to 25 mg at night) should be reserved for refractory psychosis.
- Medically refractory cases of PD may be treated with deep brain stimulation.[84]

Dementia

GENERAL PRINCIPLES

- 10% of persons over age 65 and up to 50% over 85 have dementia.
- **Dementia** is a deterioration in cognitive, reasoning, and language abilities of sufficient severity to **interfere with activities of daily living**.
- **Mild cognitive impairment** (MCI) is mild memory loss that may be evident on standardized testing but **causes minimal impairment of activities of daily living**. Between 6% and 25% of patients with MCI progress to dementia each year.
- **Delirium** is an acute impairment in awareness and orientation with disturbances of perception (i.e., hallucinations) in which symptoms typically wax and wane. In contrast, dementia has a more chronic steady decline in memory with clear sensorium.
- Dementia **commonly results from a primary degenerative process** resulting in accumulation of abnormal proteins in the brain. **Alzheimer disease is the most common form**.

DIAGNOSIS

Clinical Presentation
History
- The newly released Diagnostic and Statistical Manual (DSM) V now defines criteria for major and mild neurocognitive disorders.[85]
- **Major neurocognitive disorder** must meet the following criteria[85]:
  - Evidence of a **significant cognitive decline from prior** performance in at least one cognitive domain (learning/memory, language, complex attention, executive function, and social cognition). Ideally this should be confirmed with neuropsychologic testing or some other quantified clinical assessment.
  - Cognitive deficits **interfere with typical activities** (at least requiring assistance with executive functioning tasks).
  - Cognitive deficits are **not exclusively due to delirium**.
  - Cognitive deficits not better explained by another mental disorder.
- **Mild neurocognitive disorder** must meet these criteria[85]:
  - Evidence of **modest cognitive decline** from prior performance (learning/memory, language, complex attention, executive function, and social cognition).
  - Cognitive deficits **do not interfere with independent activities of daily living**.

○ Cognitive deficits are **not exclusively due to delirium**.

○ Cognitive deficits not better explained by another mental disorder.

• Interview both the patient and a collateral source.

• Review prescription and nonprescription medications as possible etiologies.

Physical Examination

• Cognitive screening instruments (short blessed, AD8, mini mental status examination, or Montreal Cognitive Assessment) are easy to administer and follow over time.[86,87]

• **Cardinal features of Alzheimer disease** on mental status examination include amnestic memory loss, language deterioration, and visual-spatial impairment.[88] Motor, sensory, and gait deficits can be seen in later stages.

• Evaluate the signs of parkinsonism (resting tremor, rigidity, bradykinesia, postural instability), which may suggest a Parkinson-plus syndrome (see "Parkinson Disease" section).

• Primitive reflexes called frontal release signs may reemerge (e.g., palmomental, glabellar, grasp, snout, and suck).

Differential Diagnosis

• Table 43-10 presents the differential diagnosis of dementia.

• **Alzheimer disease** is the most common progressive neurodegenerative disorder with prominent memory, cognitive, and visual-spatial deficits.

• **Dementia related to parkinsonism** has a clinical and pathologic overlap with Alzheimer disease and PD. In addition to memory and cognitive difficulties, patients exhibit signs of parkinsonism with rigidity, bradykinesia, postural instability, and tremor. Visual hallucinations may be prevalent.

• **Frontotemporal dementia** is commonly misdiagnosed as Alzheimer disease. It tends to present with prominent behavioral (e.g., disinhibition, impulsivity, apathy, and loss of insight) or language abnormalities (e.g., nonfluent or fluent aphasias).[89]

TABLE 43-10 Causes of Dementia

Alzheimer disease
Parkinsonian dementias
  • Parkinson disease with dementia
  • Dementia associated with Lewy bodies
  • Multiple system atrophy (MSA)
  • Progressive supranuclear palsy (PSP)
  • Corticobasal degeneration
Frontotemporal dementia
Vascular dementia
Creutzfeldt-Jakob disease (CJD)
HIV dementia complex
Other infectious causes (e.g., neurosyphilis)
Alcoholic dementia
Posttraumatic dementia
Depression presenting as dementia (pseudodementia)
Multiple sclerosis
Normal pressure hydrocephalus (NPH)
Neoplasms
Paraneoplastic limbic encephalitis
Metabolic causes of dementia
Medication effects

- **Vascular dementia** classically involves a step-like progression of symptoms with evidence of multiple strokes on brain imaging.
- **Creutzfeldt-Jakob disease** is a rapidly progressive dementing disease often accompanied by myoclonus. It is a **prion** disease with familial and sporadic forms. Definitive diagnosis can only be made by brain biopsy or at autopsy, but LP, MRI (diffusion imaging), and EEG findings can be helpful.[90]

Diagnostic Testing

- Check CBC, CMP, TSH, vitamin B_{12}, and brain imaging to evaluate potential reversible causes of dementia (<10%). ESR, HIV, RPR, and heavy metal screening may be evaluated if there are historical or clinical indications.
- In most cases, head CT with contrast is adequate to evaluate for structural etiologies. Brain MRI may provide more sensitivity in differentiating subtypes of dementia.
- If the clinical scenario is suggestive, LP can help evaluate for indolent CSF infection or metastatic cancer.
- Rapidly progressive dementia (weeks to months) warrants diffusion-weighed MRI and LP to evaluate for elevated 14-3-3 and tau protein in Creutzfeldt-Jakob disease.

TREATMENT

- The patient and family should be informed early on of diagnosis, degree of disability, and prognosis, to allow for initiation of appropriate care.
- Legal issues, such as identifying a durable power of attorney, should be pursued early in the course, along with a discussion of advance directives.
- Social and psychological needs of the caregiver should be assessed.
  - Family and caregivers must often make decisions regarding finances and safety issues, such as driving and adequacy of living situations.[88]
  - Organizations such as the Alzheimer's Association, American Parkinson disease Association may provide family support and respite care services.

Medications

- **Cholinesterase inhibitors**
  - Donepezil, rivastigmine, galantamine, and tacrine work by reversibly binding and inactivating acetylcholinesterase (cholinesterase inhibitors). Tacrine can cause hepatotoxicity and is rarely used.
  - The choice between agents is largely based upon cost, individual patient tolerability, and physician experience, as efficacy appears to be similar.
  - Use has demonstrated modest improvements in cognitive and global assessments, but cost-effectiveness is debated.[91]
  - Transdermal preparations of rivastigmine may provide similar efficacy in a preferred mode of delivery.[92]
  - Common side effects include nausea, vomiting, and diarrhea.
  - Possible indications for withdrawing or substituting cholinesterase inhibitors include allergic reactions, unmanageable side effects, continued cognitive decline despite a 6-month trial of the medication, and family choice.[88]
- **N-methyl-D-aspartate (NMDA) receptor antagonists**
  - Memantine is a low-moderate affinity NMDA receptor antagonist.
  - In a randomized controlled trial, combination therapy of memantine added to donepezil benefited cognition, behavior, and functional outcomes in moderate to severe Alzheimer disease.[93]
- **Antipsychotics**
  - Psychosis, aggression, and agitation have been treated with atypical antipsychotics.

TABLE 43-11	Environmental and Behavioral Interventions for Managing Difficult Behaviors in Dementia

Educate about dementia and agitation
Talk to patients/distract attention
Identify specific precipitants to behavior
Experiment with targeted changes to schedule
Separate disruptive and noisy persons from quieter persons
Control door access; use safety latches to prevent egress
Provide reassurance and verbal efforts to calm
Reduce isolation
Encourage joining support groups
Provide a predictable routine for the patient
Structure the environment
Provide orienting stimuli
Provide bright daytime lighting
Use a night light in bedroom during sleep

- In a randomized controlled trial, the overall effectiveness of antipsychotic medications in patients with Alzheimer disease was limited by side effects and intolerability.[94] Meta-analyses have suggested that there may be an associated increase in mortality as well.[95]
- Extended antipsychotic use in demented patients should be reserved for those who exhibit clinically appreciable benefits with minimal side effects.

Other Nonpharmacologic Therapies

Maintaining general health care, exercise, proper nutrition, and social interaction are vital to overall well-being. Refer to Table 43-11 for potential environmental and behavioral interventions.

Stroke

GENERAL PRINCIPLES

- Stroke is defined as a sudden-onset, focal deficit in neurologic function due to **ischemic infarction** (85%) or **intracerebral hemorrhage** (15%).
- Stroke is subdivided into several types based on presumed mechanism and associated risk factors (see Table 43-12).

TABLE 43-12	Stroke Subtypes and Associated Modifiable Risk Factors

Stroke subtypes	Modifiable risk factors
Ischemic • Large vessel atherosclerotic • Cardioembolic • Small vessel/lacunar • Cryptogenic	Hypertension Diabetes mellitus Cigarette smoking Carotid stenosis Atrial fibrillation Heart failure
Hemorrhagic • Subarachnoid • Intraparenchymal	Hypertension Alcohol abuse Trauma

- Early rehabilitation is important as most improvement occurs within the first 6 months.
- Secondary stroke prevention involves long-term management of stroke risk factors.
- **TIA** is a transient (<24 hours) neurologic deficit caused by focal ischemia without acute infarction.[96] Stroke risk is highest in the few weeks following a TIA.[97] Similar management principles apply to stroke and TIA patients.

DIAGNOSIS

Clinical Presentation

- **Sudden** onset of focal **neurologic deficits** representing a specific **vascular territory**.
- Typical stroke symptoms include hemiparesis, dysarthria, aphasia, diplopia, hemi- or quadrantanopia, vertigo, numbness, and ataxia.
- **Abrupt loss of consciousness is a relatively infrequent presentation of ischemic stroke** and more likely represents syncope, seizure, or toxic/metabolic conditions.
- Examination should focus on identifying focal neurologic deficits.

Differential Diagnosis

- **Seizure** can be followed by a focal neurologic deficit (Todd paralysis).
- **Complex migraine** can present with neurologic deficits prior to development of a headache.
- **Metabolic disturbances** including electrolyte abnormalities, infections, toxins, and hypoglycemia can result in focal neurologic deficits.
- **Brain tumors** may occasionally present with acute focal deficits resembling stroke.
- **Peripheral vertigo** can mimic posterior circulation strokes.

Diagnostic Testing

- **Noncontrast head CT** identifies hemorrhagic stroke reliably but is limited in acute ischemic strokes and those involving the cerebellum and brainstem.
- **MRI** with diffusion sequences is the gold standard test for ischemic stroke.
- **Carotid duplex ultrasound** is indicated to assess for carotid stenosis in patients with suspected anterior circulation strokes.
- **ECG** should be obtained in all patients to screen for structural abnormalities and arrhythmias that can increase stroke risk. Long-term monitoring with event recorder may be required if the patient is at risk for paroxysmal atrial fibrillation.
- **Echocardiography** can complement ECG in identifying cardiac sources of thrombus.
- Conventional **angiography** remains the gold standard to evaluate the cranial vasculature and is generally used prior to endarterectomy or stenting and for evaluating vasospasm after nontraumatic subarachnoid hemorrhage. MR and CT angiography are noninvasive alternatives that may help identify stroke etiology.

TREATMENT

Acute Stroke Treatment

Patients should be referred without delay to the nearest emergency room for possible thrombolytic therapy and monitoring.

Primary and Secondary Stroke Prevention

- **Antihypertensive therapy**
  - Hypertension is a risk factor for all stroke subtypes. Blood pressure control is a cornerstone in stroke prevention, and may decrease recurrent stroke risk by 20% to 25%.[98]
  - Goal of therapy should be <140/90.[99]
  - In the immediate poststroke setting, a cautious approach to the treatment of arterial hypertension may be advisable to promote cerebral perfusion.

- ○ An individualized approach is recommended, taking into account a given patient's particular medical problems and other circumstances.[98]
- ○ Hypertension management is discussed in detail in Chapter 6.
- **Antiplatelet therapy**
  - ○ Antiplatelet therapy reduces the risk of recurrent ischemic stroke in patients with **noncardioembolic** stroke or TIA.
  - ○ **Aspirin** (81 to 325 mg/day), **clopidogrel** (75 mg/day), and **aspirin with extended-release dipyridamole** are considered acceptable first-line therapies.
    - ▪ Aspirin is currently far less expensive and thus is preferable for most patients. There is no difference in efficacy between 81 and 325 mg.
    - ▪ Clopidogrel (75 mg/day) is an acceptable alternative for patients allergic to aspirin.
    - ▪ The combination of aspirin and clopidogrel provides a minor additional stroke benefit but increases the risk of hemorrhage.[100]
  - ○ **Warfarin** is generally indicated for cardioembolic stroke, but does not provide superior protection against noncardioembolic stroke and increases hemorrhage risk.[101]
- **Atrial fibrillation**
  - ○ Risk of stroke from atrial fibrillation can be calculated using the **CHADS2** criteria, where one point is given for **C**ongestive heart failure, **H**ypertension >140/90, **A**ge ≥75, and **D**iabetes mellitus and two points for prior **S**troke/TIA/thromboembolism.[102]
  - ○ **Warfarin** (goal INR 2 to 3) has been shown to reduce relative stroke risk by up to 70% in patients with paroxysmal or persistent atrial fibrillation.
  - ○ **Dabigatran** (150 mg twice daily), **apixaban** (5 mg twice daily), and **rivaroxaban** (20 mg daily) are all approved for the prevention of stroke in patients with **nonvalvular** atrial fibrillation with at least one additional risk factor. Adjust doses for renal impairment.
  - ○ Aspirin (325 mg/day) reduces stroke risk by only one-half that of warfarin, but may be used on low-risk patients who are unable to tolerate warfarin.
  - ○ The major complication with this therapy is increased bleeding risk. Prior nontraumatic intracranial hemorrhage is a contraindication to anticoagulation, and recent or recurrent hemorrhage from other sites (e.g., gastrointestinal) is a relative contraindication to anticoagulation.
  - ○ See Chapter 14 for more information on anticoagulation and Chapter 10 regarding atrial fibrillation.
- **Valvular heart disease and prosthetic heart valves**
  - ○ A history of valvular heart disease places a patient at increased risk of embolic stroke.
  - ○ Management of valvular disease is discussed in Chapter 9.
- **Carotid stenosis**
  - ○ Patients with **symptomatic** carotid stenosis of >70% with a reasonable life expectancy are likely to benefit from **carotid endarterectomy,** if performed in center with a perioperative stroke and death rate of <3%.[99,103]
  - ○ Some patients with 50% to 69% stenosis will also benefit depending upon age, gender, and other risk factors, and should be referred to an experienced neurologist or vascular surgeon if symptomatic.
  - ○ **Carotid endarterectomy** is recommended within 2 weeks in patients with TIA, but may require a longer interval in patients with (larger) strokes.
  - ○ Carotid artery stenting has yet to be as rigorously investigated as endarterectomy and is generally reserved for patients who are deemed to be high-risk surgical candidates.[98]
- **Diabetes mellitus**
  - ○ Diabetes is clearly a risk factor for first stroke and is probably a risk factor for recurrent stroke.[98]
  - ○ Treating to reasonable glycemic goals likely decreases risk. On the other hand, intensive glycemic control (HbA$_{1c}$ <6% to 6.5%) has not been shown to be of added benefit over standard care.[98,99,104–106]

- ○ The American Diabetes Association recommends a target or <7%, but therapy must obviously be individualized.[107]
- ○ Diabetes management is discussed in detail in Chapter 20.
- **Lipid-lowering therapy**
  - ○ Observational studies suggest that hyperlipidemia is less of a risk factor for stroke than for ischemic heart disease. Patients with ischemic heart disease, however, do experience a reduction in primary stroke risk when taking either pravastatin or simvastatin.
  - ○ Atorvastatin showed secondary stroke reduction in patients with noncardioembolic stroke or TIA with a low-density lipoprotein of 100 to 190 mg/dL who had no history of ischemic heart disease, although there was a slight increase in hemorrhagic stroke risk.[108]
  - ○ Most stroke patients will have one or more identifiable vascular risk factors and thus will benefit overall from the use of a statin or other lipid-lowering agent (see Chapter 11).
- **Smoking cessation**
  - ○ Smoking cessation is universally recommended in patients surviving stroke and is discussed in detail in Chapter 45.[98,99]
  - ○ Cigarette smoking doubles the risk of ischemic stroke.
  - ○ This increased risk disappears within 5 years of smoking cessation.
- **Lifestyle (exercise and diet):** Patients should be counseled on modifiable risk factors including diet, physical activity, obesity, body fat distribution, metabolic syndrome, excessive alcohol consumption, and drug abuse.

Concussion and Traumatic Brain Injury

GENERAL PRINCIPLES

- **Mild traumatic brain injury** (TBI) occurs with head injury due to contact and/or acceleration/deceleration forces.
- **Concussion** includes less severe TBI resulting in an alteration in mental status, which does not necessarily involve a loss of consciousness.
- **Second impact syndrome** is when a second concussion occurs before resolution of symptoms from the first, which can be associated with cerebral edema and catastrophic effects.
- The most frequent causes of concussion in children are sports and bicycle accidents, while falls and motor vehicle accidents are the main causes in adults.

DIAGNOSIS

Clinical Presentation

History
- TBI can range in spectrum and commonly is mild (see Table 43-13 for concussion grades).
- Confusion and amnesia are common in concussion; loss of consciousness is not required.
- **Postconcussive syndrome** includes headache, nausea, dizziness, and impairment of concentration and memory. It can last **days to months** following the concussive event.
- Concussion may be associated with a single brief seizure. This does not predispose to epilepsy and does not require anticonvulsant treatment.[109]
- The long-term effects of multiple concussions include cognitive decline, such as dementia pugilistica in boxers.

Physical Examination
- Mental status examination to evaluate the level of consciousness and memory.
- Evaluate for signs of basilar skull fracture including hemotympanum, CSF otorrhea or rhinorrhea, raccoon eyes (periorbital ecchymosis), and Battle sign (mastoid ecchymosis).

TABLE 43-13	Grades of Concussions and Time to Return to Play

Grade	Time until return to play[a]
Grade 1: Transient confusion lasting <15 minutes with no loss of consciousness	
• Single	15 minutes
• Multiple	1 week
Grade 2: Transient confusion lasting >15 minutes with no loss of consciousness	
• Single	1 week
• Multiple	2 weeks
Grade 3: Any loss of consciousness	
• Brief loss of consciousness (seconds)	1 week
• Prolonged loss of consciousness (minutes)	2 weeks
• Multiple	≥1 month, based on clinical decision of evaluating physician

[a]Only after being asymptomatic with normal neurologic assessment at rest and with exercise.

- Evaluate for any accompanying neurologic signs including aphasia, weakness, sensory deficits, and ataxia.

Diagnostic Testing
- Patients with moderate or severe headache, nausea, vomiting, or any neurologic deficit after a TBI, including concussion, should be evaluated with a head CT to detect subdural and epidural hematomas.[110]
- A brain MRI should be considered in patients who present later in follow-up.

TREATMENT

- Nonopioid analgesics are used to treat headaches.
- Vestibular suppressants may be indicated if vertigo is present.
- Cognitive rehabilitation may be beneficial.
- Guidelines exist for preventing **second impact syndrome** (Table 43-13).[111] There is a movement toward more conservative management recommending a **"no same day return to play."** Thereafter, players should not return to play until the day after all symptoms have resolved.[112,113]

Central Vertigo

GENERAL PRINCIPLES

- **Vertigo** is defined as an inappropriate sensation of motion due to dysfunction of the vestibular system involving either the peripheral or central nervous system.
- "Dizziness" can describe a variety of sensations including vertigo, but also ataxia, orthostatic hypotension, cardiac arrhythmias including symptomatic bradycardia, drug-induced symptoms, anxiety disorders, hyperventilation, and sensory disturbances. The history and physical exam are imperative to distinguish these very different entities.
- Vertigo is divided into central and peripheral causes (see Chapter 40). This section focuses on central vertigo.

DIAGNOSIS

- **Vertiginous migraine**
  - Vertiginous symptoms of variable duration proceed or are accompanied by migraine headache, but vertigo may occur in headache-free interval.
  - Often associated with typical migraine features, such as photophobia, phonophobia, and osmophobia (see "Headache" section).
- **Vertebrobasilar ischemia/stroke**
  - TIA and stroke are a medical emergency (see "Stroke" section).
  - Vertigo can result from ischemia to the brainstem and cerebellum (vertebrobasilar insufficiency) that may occur in isolation or with other focal neurologic deficits.
  - Accompanying brainstem signs may include diplopia, gaze palsies, facial weakness, dysarthria, or dysphagia along with cerebellar signs of limb or gait ataxia.
  - Brain MRI with stroke protocol sequences can aid in diagnosis, while additional consideration should be given to evaluation of the posterior circulation with CT angiogram, MR angiogram, or conventional angiogram.
- **Other common causes include** trauma, multiple sclerosis can rarely present with isolated vertigo, brainstem or cerebellar tumors, and tumors of the 8th cranial nerve (schwannomas [e.g., with neurofibromatosis type II], dermoid, epidermoid, and metastatic).

TREATMENT

The treatment of central vertigo is the treatment of the specific cause. See Chapter 40 for treatment of peripheral vertigo.

REFERENCES

1. Rasmussen BK, Jensen R, Schroll M, et al. Epidemiology of headache in a general population—a prevalence study. *J Clin Epidemiol* 1991;44:1147–1157.
2. Lipton RB, Dodick D, Sadovsky R, et al. ID Migraine validation study. A self-administered screener for migraine in primary care: the ID Migraine validation study. *Neurology* 2003;61:375–382.
3. Lipton RB, Stewart WF, Simon D. Medical consultation for migraine: results from the American Migraine Study. *Headache* 1998;38:87–96.
4. Headache Classification Subcommittee of the International Headache Society. The International Classification of Headache Disorders: 2nd edition. *Cephalalgia* 2004;24:9–160.
5. Bigal ME, Serrano D, Buse D, et al. Acute migraine medications and evolution from episodic to chronic migraine: a longitudinal population-based study. *Headache* 2008;48:1157–1168.
6. Kelly AM, Walcynski T, Gunn B. The relative efficacy of phenothiazines for the treatment of acute migraine: a meta-analysis. *Headache* 2009;49:1324–1332.
7. Kelley NE, Tepper DE. Rescue therapy for acute migraine, part 2: neuroleptics, antihistamines, and others. *Headache* 2012;52:292–306.
8. Kelley NE, Tepper DE. Rescue therapy for acute migraine, part 1: triptans, dihydroergotamine, and magnesium. *Headache* 2012;52:114–128.
9. Derry CJ, Derry S, Moore RA. Sumatriptan (oral route of administration) for acute migraine attacks in adults. *Cochrane Database Syst Rev* 2012;(2):CD008615.
10. Derry CJ, Derry S, Moore RA. Sumatriptan (subcutaneous route of administration) for acute migraine attacks in adults. *Cochrane Database Syst Rev* 2012;(2):CD009665.
11. Derry CJ, Derry S, Moore RA. Sumatriptan (intranasal route of administration) for acute migraine attacks in adults. *Cochrane Database Syst Rev* 2012;(2):CD009663.

12. Ferrari MD, Roon KI, Lipton RB, et al. Oral triptans (serotonin 5-HT(1B/1D) agonists) in acute migraine treatment: a meta-analysis of 53 trials. *Lancet* 2001;358:1668–1675.

13. Colman I, Brown MD, Innes GD, et al. Parenteral dihydroergotamine for acute migraine headache: a systematic review of the literature. *Ann Emerg Med* 2005;45:393–401.

14. Raskin NH. Repetitive intravenous dihydroergotamine as therapy for intractable migraine. *Neurology* 1986;36:995–997.

15. Silberstein SD, Schulman EA, Hopkins MM. Repetitive intravenous DHE in the treatment of refractory headache. *Headache* 1990;30:334–339.

16. Nagy AJ, Gandhi S, Bhola R, et al. Intravenous dihydroergotamine for inpatient management of refractory primary headaches. *Neurology* 2011;77:1829–1832.

17. Silberstein SD. Practice parameter: evidence-based guidelines for migraine headache (an evidence-based review): report of the Quality Standards Subcommittee of American Academy of Neurology. *Neurology* 2000;55:754–762.

18. Silberstein SD, Holland S, Freitag F, et al. Evidence-based guideline update: pharmacologic treatment for episodic migraine prevention in adults: report of the Quality Standards Subcommittee of the American Academy of Neurology and the American Headache Society. *Neurology* 2012;78:1337–1345.

19. Pringsheim T, Davenport WJ, Becker WJ. Prophylaxis of migraine headache. *CMAJ* 2010;182:E269–E276.

20. Linde M, Mulleners WM, Chronicle EP, et al. Topiramate for the prophylaxis of episodic migraine in adults. *Cochrane Database Syst Rev* 2013;(6):CD010610.

21. Linde M, Mulleners WM, Chronicle EP, et al. Valproate (valproic acid or sodium valproate or a combination of the two) for the prophylaxis of episodic migraine in adults. *Cochrane Database Syst Rev* 2013;(6):CD010611.

22. Linde M, Mulleners WM, Chronicle EP, et al. Gabapentin or pregabalin for the prophylaxis of episodic migraine in adults. *Cochrane Database Syst Rev* 2013;(6):CD010609.

23. Jackson JL, Shimeall W, Sessums L, et al. Tricyclic antidepressants and headaches: systematic review and meta-analysis. *BMJ* 2010;341:c5222.

24. Ozyalcin SN, Talu GK, Kiziltan E, et al. The efficacy and safety of venlafaxine in the prophylaxis of migraine. *Headache* 2005;45:144–152.

25. Holland S, Silberstein SD, Freitag F, et al. Evidence-based guideline update: NSAIDs and other complementary treatments for episodic migraine prevention in adults: report of the Quality Standards Subcommittee of the American Academy of Neurology and the American Headache Society. *Neurology* 2012;78:1346–1353.

26. Dodick DW, Turkel CC, DeGryse RE, et al. OnabotulinumtoxinA for treatment of chronic migraine: pooled results from the double-blind, randomized, placebo-controlled phases of the PREEMPT clinical program. *Headache* 2010;50:921–936.

27. Law S, Derry S, Moore RA. Triptans for acute cluster headache. *Cochrane Database Syst Rev* 2013;(7):CD008042.

28. Magnoux E, Zlotnik G. Outpatient intravenous dihydroergotamine for refractory cluster headache. *Headache* 2004;44:249–255.

29. Leone M, D'Amico D, Frediani F, et al. Verapamil in the prophylaxis of episodic cluster headache: a double-blind study versus placebo. *Neurology* 2000;54:1352–1355.

30. Fisher RS, van Emde Boas W, Blume W, et al. Epileptic seizures and epilepsy: definitions proposed by the International League Against Epilepsy (ILAE) and the International Bureau for Epilepsy (IBE). *Epilepsia* 2005;46:470–472.

31. Hauser WA, Annegers JF, Kurland LT. Prevalence of epilepsy in Rochester, Minnesota: 1940–1980. *Epilepsia* 1991;32:429–445.

32. Hauser WA, Annegers JF, Kurland LT. Incidence of epilepsy and unprovoked seizures in Rochester, Minnesota: 1935–1984. *Epilepsia* 1993;34:453–468.

33. Commission on Classification and Terminology of the ILAE. Proposal for revised clinical and electroencephalographic classification of epileptic seizures. *Epilepsia* 1981;22:489–501.

34. Goldstein LH, Mellers JD. Recent developments in our understanding of the semiology and treatment of psychogenic nonepileptic seizures. *Curr Neurol Neurosci Rep* 2012;12:436–444.

35. King MA, Newton MR, Jackson GD, et al. Epileptology of the first-seizure presentation: a clinical, electroencephalographic, and magnetic resonance imaging study of 300 consecutive patients. *Lancet* 1998;352:1007–1011.

36. van Donselaar CA, Schimsheimer RJ, Geerts AT, et al. Value of the electroencephalogram in adult patients with untreated idiopathic first seizures. *Arch Neurol* 1992;49:231–237.

37. Musicco M, Beghi E, Solari A, et al. Treatment of first tonic-clonic seizure does not improve the prognosis of epilepsy. First Seizure Trial Group (FIRST Group). *Neurology* 1997;49:991–998.

38. Roujeau JC, Stern RS. Severe adverse cutaneous reactions to drugs. *N Engl J Med* 1994;331:1272–1285.

39. Wyszynski DF, Nambisan M, Surve T, et al. Increased rate of major malformations in offspring exposed to valproate during pregnancy. *Neurology* 2005;64:961–965.

40. Victor M, Brausch C. The role of abstinence in the genesis of alcoholic epilepsy. *Epilepsia* 1967;8:1–20.

41. Noseworthy JH, Lucchinetti C, Rodriguez M, et al. Multiple sclerosis. *N Engl J Med* 2000;343:938–952.

42. Calabrese M, Filippi M, Gallo P. Cortical lesions in multiple sclerosis. *Nat Rev Neurol* 2010;6:438–444.

43. Polman CH, Reingold SC, Banwell B, et al. Diagnostic criteria for multiple sclerosis: 2010 revisions to the McDonald criteria. *Ann Neurol* 2011;69:292–302.

44. Wingerchuk DM, Lennon VA, Pittock SJ, et al. Revised diagnostic criteria for neuromyelitis optica. *Neurology* 2006;66:1485–1489.

45. Filippini G, Brusaferri F, Sibley WA, et al. Corticosteroids or ACTH for acute exacerbations in multiple sclerosis. *Cochrane Database Syst Rev* 2000;(4):CD001331.

46. Burton JM, O'Connor PW, Hohol M, et al. Oral versus intravenous steroids for treatment of relapses in multiple sclerosis. *Cochrane Database Syst Rev* 2012;(12):CD006921.

47. Cortese I, Chaudhry V, So YT, et al. Evidence-based guideline update: plasmapheresis in neurologic disorders: report of the Therapeutics and Technology Assessment Subcommittee of the American Academy of Neurology. *Neurology* 2011;76:294–300.

48. Kappos L, Freedman MS, Polman CH, et al.; BENEFIT Study Group. Effect of early versus delayed interferon β-1b treatment on disability after a first clinical event suggestive of multiple sclerosis: a 3-year follow-up analysis of the BENEFIT study. *Lancet* 2007;370:389–397.

49. Pittock SJ, Weinshenker BG, Noseworthy JH, et al. Not every patient with multiple sclerosis should be treated at time of diagnosis. *Arch Neurol* 2006;63:611–614.

50. Harrison DM. Multiple sclerosis. *Ann Intern Med* 2014;160:ITC4-2–ITC4-18.

51. Bloomgren G, Richman S, Hotermans C, et al. Risk of natalizumab-associated progressive multifocal leukoencephalopathy. *N Engl J Med* 2012;366:1870–1880.

52. Hawker K, O'Connor PP, Freedman MS, et al. Rituximab in patients with primary progressive multiple sclerosis: results of a randomized double-blind placebo-controlled multicenter trial. *Ann Neurol* 2009;66:460–471.

53. Katz JN, Simmons BP. Clinical practice. Carpal tunnel syndrome. *N Engl J Med* 2002;346:1807–1812.

54. D'Arcy CA, McGee S. Does this patient have carpal tunnel syndrome? *JAMA* 2000;283:3110–3117.

55. Gorson KC. Vasculitic neuropathies: an update. *Neurologist* 2007;13:12–19.

56. Hughes RA, Cornblath DR. Guillain-Barré syndrome. *Lancet* 2005;366:1653–1666.

57. Köller H, Kieseier BC, Jander S, et al. Chronic inflammatory demyelinating polyneuropathy. *N Engl J Med* 2005;352:1343–1356.

58. Simpson DM, Kitch D, Evans SR, et al.; ACTG A5117 Study Group. HIV neuropathy natural history cohort study: assessment measures and risk factors. *Neurology* 2006;66:1679–1687.

59. Gronseth G, Cruccu G, Alksne J, et al. Practice parameter: the diagnostic evaluation and treatment of trigeminal neuralgia (an evidence-based review): report of the Quality Standards Subcommittee of the American Academy of Neurology and the European Federation of Neurological Societies. *Neurology* 2008;71:1183–1190.

60. Sullivan FM, Swan IR, Donnan PT, et al. Early treatment with prednisolone or acyclovir in Bell's palsy. *N Engl J Med* 2007;357:1598–1607.

61. Engström M, Berg T, Stjernquist-Desatnik A, et al. Prednisolone and valaciclovir in Bell's palsy: a randomised, double-blind, placebo-controlled, multicentre trial. *Lancet Neurol* 2008;7:993–1000.

62. Hato N, Yamada H, Kohno H, et al. Valacyclovir and prednisolone treatment for Bell's palsy: a multicenter, randomized, placebo-controlled study. *Otol Neurotol* 2007;28:408–413.

63. Minnerop M, Herbst M, Fimmers R, et al. Bell's palsy: combined treatment of famciclovir and prednisone is superior to prednisone alone. *J Neurol* 2008;255:1726–1730.

64. Mendell JR, Sahenk Z. Clinical practice. Painful sensory neuropathy. *N Engl J Med* 2003;348:1243–1255.

65. de leon-Casasola OA. Opioids for chronic pain: new evidence, new strategies, safe prescribing. *Am J Med* 2013;126:S3–S11.

66. Moore RA, Wiffen PJ, Derry S, et al. Gabapentin for chronic neuropathic pain and fibromyalgia in adults. *Cochrane Database Syst Rev* 2011;(3):CD007938.

67. Moore RA, Staube S, Wiffen PJ, et al. Pregabalin for acute and chronic pain in adults. *Cochrane Database Syst Rev* 2009;(3):CD007076.

68. Wiff PJ, McQuay HJ, Moore RA. Carbamazepine for acute and chronic pain. *Cochrane Database Syst Rev* 2005;(3):CD005451.

69. Zhou M, Chen N, He L, et al. Oxcarbazepine for neuropathic pain. *Cochrane Database Syst Rev* 2013;(3):CD007963.

70. Lunn MP, Hughes RA, Wiffen PJ. Duloxetine for treating painful neuropathy, chronic pain or fibromyalgia. *Cochrane Database Syst Rev* 2014;(1):CD007115.

71. Moore RA, Derry WS, Aldington D, et al. Amitriptyline for neuropathic pain and fibromyalgia in adults. *Cochrane Database Syst Rev* 2012;(12):CD008242.

72. Tarsy D, Simon DK. Dystonia. *N Engl J Med* 2006;355:818–829.

73. Morgan JC, Sethi KD. Drug-induced tremors. *Lancet Neurol* 2005;4:866–876.

74. Louis E. Essential tremor. *Lancet Neurol* 2005;4:100–110.

75. Lang AE, Lozano AM. Parkinson's disease: first of two parts. *N Engl J Med* 1998;339:1044–1053.

76. van Gerpen JA. Drug-induced parkinsonism. *Neurologist* 2002;8:363–370.

77. Poewe W, Wenning G. The differential diagnosis of Parkinson's disease. *Eur J Neurol.* 2002;9(suppl 3):23–30.

78. Fahn S. Description of Parkinson's disease as a clinical syndrome. *Ann N Y Acad Sci* 2003;991:1–14.

79. Miyasaki JM, Martin W, Suchowersky O, et al. Practice parameter: initiation of treatment for Parkinson's disease: an evidence-based review: report of the Quality Standards Subcommittee of the American Academy of Neurology. *Neurology* 2002;58:11–17.

80. Nutt JG, Wooten, GF. Clinical practice. Diagnosis and initial management of Parkinson's disease. *N Engl J Med* 2005;353:1021–1027.

81. Zesiewicz TA, Hauser RA. Medical treatment of motor and nonmotor features of Parkinson's disease. *Continuum* 2007;13:12–38.

82. Fahn S, Oakes D, Shoulson I, et al.; The Parkinson Study Group. Levodopa and the progression of Parkinson's disease. *N Engl J Med* 2004;351:2498–2508.

83. Dodd ML, Klos KJ, Bower JH, et al. Pathological gambling caused by drugs used to treat Parkinson disease. *Arch Neurol* 2005;62:1377–1381.

84. Siddiqui MS, Okun MS. Deep brain stimulation in Parkinson's disease. *Continuum* 2007;13:39–57.

85. American Psychiatric Association. *Diagnostic and Statistical Manual of Mental Disorders: DSM-5.* Washington, DC: American Psychiatric Association; 2013

86. Galvin JE, Roe CM, Powlishta KK, et al. The AD8: a brief informant interview to detect dementia. *Neurology* 2005;65:559–564.

87. Galvin JE, Roe CM, Xiong C, et al. Validity and reliability of the AD8 informant interview in dementia. *Neurology* 2006;67:1942–1948.

88. Cummings JL. Alzheimer's disease. *N Engl J Med* 2004;351:56–67.

89. Liscic RM, Storandt M, Cairns NJ, et al. Clinical and psychometric distinction of frontotemporal and Alzheimer dementias. *Arch Neurol* 2007;64:535–540.

90. Wang LH, Bucelli RC, Patrick E, et al. Role of magnetic resonance imaging, cerebrospinal fluid, and electroencephalogram in diagnosis of sporadic Creutzfeldt-Jakob disease. *J Neurol* 2013;260:498–506.

91. Crome P, Lendon C, Shaw H, et al.; AD2000 Collaborative Group. Long-term donepezil treatment in 565 patients with Alzheimer's disease (AD2000): randomised double-blind trial. *Lancet* 2004;363:2105–2115.

92. Winblad B, Grossberg G, Frölich L, et al. IDEAL: a 6-month, double-blind, placebo-controlled study of the first skin patch for Alzheimer disease. *Neurology* 2007;69:S14–S22.

93. Tariot PN, Farlow MR, Grossberg GT, et al.; Memantine Study Group. Memantine treatment in patients with moderate to severe Alzheimer disease already receiving donepezil: a randomized controlled trial. *JAMA* 2004;291:317–324.

94. Schneider LS, Tariot PN, Dagerman KS, et al.; CATIE-AD Study Group. Effectiveness of atypical antipsychotic drugs in patients with Alzheimer's disease. *N Engl J Med* 2006;355:1525–1538.

95. Schneider LS, Dagerman KS, Insel P. Risk of death with atypical antipsychotic drug treatment for dementia: meta-analysis of randomized placebo-controlled trials. *JAMA* 2005;294:1934–1943.

96. Easton JD, Saver JL, Albers GW, et al. Definition and evaluation of transient ischemic attack: a scientific statement for healthcare professionals. *Stroke* 2009;40:2276–2293.

97. Giles MF, Rothwell PM. Prognosis and management in the first few days after a transient ischemic attack or minor ischaemic stroke. *Int J Stroke* 2006;1:65–73.

98. Kernan WN, Ovbiagele B, Black HR, et al. Guidelines for the prevention of stroke in patients with stroke and transient ischemic attack: a guideline for healthcare professionals from the American Heart Association/American Stroke Association. *Stroke* 2014;45:2160–2236.

99. Goldstein LB, Bushnell CD, Adams RJ, et al. Guidelines for the primary prevention of stroke: a guideline for healthcare professionals from the American Heart Association/American Stroke Association. *Stroke* 2011;42:517–584.

100. Diener HC, Bogousslavsky J, Brass LM, et al.; MATCH Investigators. Aspirin and clopidogrel compared with clopidogrel alone after recent ischaemic stroke or transient ischaemic attack in high-risk patients (MATCH): randomised, double-blind, placebo-controlled trial. *Lancet* 2004;364:331–337.

101. Chimowitz MI, Lynn MJ, Howlett-Smith H, et al.; Warfarin-Aspirin Symptomatic Intracranial Disease Trial Investigators. Comparison of warfarin and aspirin for symptomatic intracranial arterial stenosis. *N Engl J Med* 2005;352:1305–1316.

102. Gage BF, van Walraven C, Pearce L, et al. Selecting patients with atrial fibrillation for anticoagulation: stroke risk stratification in patients taking aspirin. *Circulation* 2004;110:2287–2292.

103. North American Symptomatic Carotid Endarterectomy Trial (NASCET) Collaborators. Beneficial effect of carotid endarterectomy in symptomatic patients with high-grade carotid stenosis. *N Engl J Med* 1991;325:445–453.

104. Ismail-Beigi F, Craven T, Banerji MA, et al.; ACCORD Trial Group. Effect of intensive treatment of hyperglycaemia on microvascular outcomes in type 2 diabetes: an analysis of the ACCORD randomised trial. *Lancet* 2010;376:419–430.

105. Advance Collaborative Group; Patel A, MacMahon S, et al. Intensive blood glucose control and vascular outcomes in patients with type 2 diabetes. *N Engl J Med* 2008;358:2560–2572.

106. Duckworth W, Abraira C, Moritz T, et al.; VADT Investigators. Glucose control and vascular complications in veterans with type 2 diabetes. *N Engl J Med* 2009;360:129–139.

107. American Diabetes Association. Standards of medical care in diabetes—2014. *Diabetes Care* 2014;37:S14–S80.

108. Amarenco P, Bogousslavsky J, Callahan A III, et al.; Stroke Prevention by Aggressive Reduction in Cholesterol Levels (SPARCL) Investigators. High-dose atorvastatin after stroke or transient ischemic attack. *N Engl J Med* 2006;355:549–559.

109. Ropper AH, Gorson KC. Clinical practice. Concussion. *N Engl J Med* 2007;356:166–172.

110. Haydel MJ, Preston CA, Mills TJ, et al. Indications for computed tomography in patients with minor head injury. *N Engl J Med* 2000;343:100–105.

111. Practice parameter: the management of concussion in sports (summary statement). Report of the Quality Standards Subcommittee. *Neurology* 1997;48:581–585.

112. American Academy of Neurology. *Position Statement: Sports Concussion.* American Academy of Neurology; 2013. https://www.aan.com/go/about/position. Last accessed 2/1/15.

113. Harmon KG, Drezner J, Gammons M, et al. American medical society for sports medicine position statement: concussion in sport. *Clin J Sport Med* 2013;23:1–18.

44 Ophthalmology

Ian Pitha, Arsham Sheybani, and Linda Tsai

Introduction

Patients suffering from eye symptoms often initially present to their primary care provider. Therefore, it is important for primary care providers to feel comfortable evaluating and triaging these patients. The goal of this chapter is to familiarize primary care providers with the basics of taking an ocular history and performing a targeted ophthalmologic exam and to provide the tools needed to identify entities that can be managed in a primary care setting and those that require urgent or emergent ophthalmologic evaluation. Following a brief discussion of the ocular history and physical exam, as well as current screening recommendations, this chapter will then be organized primarily by the patient's presenting symptom(s) and will cover etiology, symptoms, and management of each entity (see Fig. 44-1).

OCULAR HISTORY AND PHYSICAL EXAM

Careful history and examination are essential for correct diagnosis, triage (Table 44-1), and treatment of ocular conditions.

History

- Correct diagnosis depends on a carefully taken, complete medical history, including past medical history, medications, family history, social history, and occupational history.
- Key elements of the ocular history are presented in Table 44-2.
- An essential initial step is to determine whether symptoms presented acutely, subacutely, or chronically.

Physical Examination

- **Visual acuity**
  - Obtaining an accurate, best-corrected visual acuity is the most important component of the physical exam.
  - Visual acuity should be tested in each eye while the patient is wearing glasses. Ideally a distance chart should be used; however, a near card can yield useful information as well.
  - If formal vision charts are not available, have the patient attempt to read newspaper print or your name badge.
  - If the patient cannot read the largest font on the chart, halve the distance between the patient and the chart and document the vision with "10" in the numerator (e.g., 10/200). If the patient still cannot read the chart check their ability to count fingers, or perceive hand motion or light.
  - If patients do not have their glasses with them, their visual acuity when looking through a pinhole can be checked. Pinholing may resolve refractive error and is useful in the patient who cannot be optimally corrected.
- **Pupillary exam**
  - Compare the size and shape of the pupils in light and dark conditions.
  - Check for an afferent pupillary defect (APD) using the swinging flashlight test. When a light is directed from one eye to the other while the patient focuses on a distant target, the pupils should remain symmetrically constricted owing to the consensual light

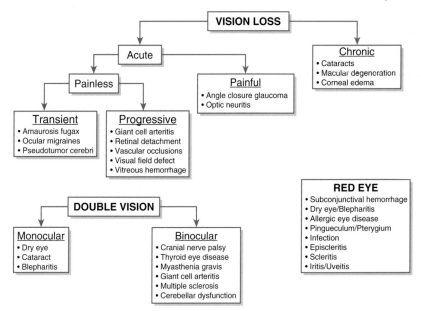

Figure 44-1 Rapid evaluation of ophthalmologic problems.

response. If the pupils dilate when the light is moved from the right to the left eye, then there is an APD of the left eye.

○ Presence of an APD is evidence of optic nerve disease or significant retinal damage and should be evaluated in every patient presenting with vision loss.

TABLE 44-1 Ophthalmology Referral Guide

See immediately or send to emergency department (EMERGENCY)
Chemical burns
Acute decrease of visual acuity to ≤20/100 with suspicion of central retinal artery
    occlusion or temporal arteritis
Severe pain
Evidence of orbital cellulitis
Evidence or suspicion of penetrating injury to the globe, eyelid laceration, and
    orbital fracture

See ophthalmologist within 24 hours (ACUTE)
Corneal abrasion/contact lens
Acute decrease in vision
Mild-to-moderate pain
Preseptal (periorbital) cellulitis
Conjunctival or corneal foreign body
Hyphema
Acute visual filed loss
Flashes of light or floaters

See ophthalmologist with 1 week (SUBACUTE)
Red eye with no vision loss
Red eye with no pain

TABLE 44-2 Elements of the Ophthalmologic History

Subjective ocular complaints
Differentiate between eyelid and eyeball complaints if possible
Change in vision
Pain
Diplopia
Flashes or floaters
Crusting
Discharge
Tearing
Redness
Photophobia

Timing
Acute (hours)
Subacute (days)
Chronic (weeks to months)

Severity
Transient vs. constant
Monocular versus binocular
Subjective rating of discomfort
"Wakes me up from sleep"

Constitutional symptoms
Nausea
Vomiting
Headache
Weakness
Numbness
Dizziness

Prior ocular history
Prior trauma
Previous eye surgery
Amblyopia (lazy eye)
Cataract
Glaucoma
Age-related macular degeneration (ARMD)
High myopia
Dry eye
Blepharitis (eyelid disease)

- **Ocular motility:** The alignment of each eye in primary gaze, the ability of each eye to move in all directions of gaze, and the presence of nystagmus should be noted. The location of the corneal light reflex can be used to detect subtle deviations of eye position.
- **Visual fields**
  - Have the patient cover one eye, and, while making eye contact with the patient, hold your fingers out into the four main quadrants.
  - Minor field defects can be detected and documented by further visual field testing in the eye professional's office.
- **Intraocular pressure**
  - Intraocular pressure (IOP) is quantitatively measured in the eye professional's office by tonometry.
  - Extremely elevated IOPs, as occurs in angle-closure glaucoma, can occasionally be assessed qualitatively by palpation.
- **External exam:** Although most of the external exam is ideally performed using a slit lamp microscope, a penlight is useful as an initial screening tool.
- **Eyelid examination**
  - Examine for evidence of erythema, edema, trauma, or eyelid lesions.
  - Ptosis can be assessed by measuring the distance in millimeters between the corneal light reflex and the margin of the upper eyelid.
  - Assess for proptosis (prominent eyes) or enophthalmos (recession of the eyeball into the orbit).
  - Basal cell carcinomas affecting the eyelid most commonly develop on the lower eyelid.[1]
- **Anterior segment examination**
  - The **conjunctiva** is the clear vascularized tissue overlying the sclera. Injection of the conjunctiva can occur in many conditions including viral and bacterial conjunctivitis.

- The **cornea** is the transparent, anterior wall of the outer eye. Assess the clarity of the cornea; any opacity should be characterized as diffuse or focal. Central focal opacities are more detrimental to vision than peripheral opacities.
  - The **anterior chamber** is the fluid-filled space in between the cornea and the iris. White blood cells (hypopyon) or blood (hyphema) in the anterior chamber will obstruct the view of the iris.
  - Irregularities in the shape of the **iris** should be noted.
  - The **lens** lies posterior to the iris and can appear yellow or opaque if a cataract is present. Patients who have had previous cataract surgery could have a shimmering, reflective quality to their lens.
- **Fundus examination**
  - Most examinations in the office setting do not require dilation. Dilated fundus examinations are performed to assess retinal vascular health or to rule out findings, such as papilledema or vitreous hemorrhage.
  - Pharmacologic dilation is usually performed in adults with phenylephrine hydrochloride 2.5% or tropicamide 1%, or both, and causes decreased accommodation for 4 to 6 hours.
  - The patient should not be dilated without the direction of an ophthalmologist in the following circumstances: suggestion of a shallow anterior chamber, patient undergoing neurologic observation, and any question of an APD.

OPHTHALMIC SCREENING

- Patients with specific medical conditions or who are taking certain medications should undergo periodic examinations by an ophthalmologist (Table 44-3).
- Other groups of patients should ideally be specifically asked about ocular complaints (Table 44-3).
- The definition of legal blindness in the U.S. is central visual acuity of 20/200 or less in the better eye with the use of a correcting lens. An eye with a visual field that extends <20 degrees is considered to have a visual acuity of <20/200 regardless of the measured acuity.
- Visual requirements for obtaining a driver's license are determined by each state.

TABLE 44-3	Indications for Ophthalmic Screening

Patients who should have ophthalmic exams
Age over 40 years
Past retinal detachment
Past serious ocular trauma
Diabetes mellitus
Hypertension
Sickle cell disease
Family history of glaucoma
Family history of other ocular conditions
Plaquenil use

Patients who should be questioned about ocular complaints
Graves or thyroid disease
Autoimmune disease
Patients with frequent falls/accidents

Symptom-Based Approach

VISION LOSS

Acute vision loss should be evaluated immediately in order to rule out processes that have systemic or devastating sequelae, such as giant cell arteritis, acute angle-closure glaucoma, optic neuritis, endophthalmitis, retinal detachment, and posttraumatic processes (ruptured globe, hyphema).

Acute Painless Vision Loss
Is the process transient or is it present for more than 24 hours?

Transient Vision Loss
- **Amaurosis fugax**
  - **Etiology:** Amaurosis fugax is **transient monocular vision loss** due to retinal arterial occlusion. The occlusion is usually caused by a cholesterol or platelet embolus but can result from vasospasm. The **most common sources of an atheroma resulting in amaurosis fugax are the carotid arteries**. Evidence of a **Hollenhorst plaque** (refractile cholesterol plaque visible in the retinal vasculature) may be seen on physical examination.
  - **Symptoms:** Often described as a **shade or curtain coming over the vision** that lasts a few minutes, it is most common in patients >50 years or those with a history of vascular disease. A full ophthalmologic examination must be performed by an ophthalmologist to rule out impending vascular occlusion.
  - **Management:** Medical evaluation, including carotid Dopplers, cardiac echocardiography, and basic hematologic workup, should be performed to rule out systemic disease, even in the absence of Hollenhorst plaques. Patients should be sent to an ophthalmologist immediately if the vision loss has not recovered.
- **Ophthalmic migraines**
  - **Etiology:** A history of migraine may or may not be present. Ophthalmic migraines cause transient episodes that usually lead to at least 5 to 15 minutes of obscuration of vision.
  - **Symptoms:** Fortification (jagged lightning bolts) and scintillating scotomas (blind spot centrally with hazy edges) are characteristic. Colored lights and other visual symptoms can occur. Visual acuity should return to baseline after the episode but headache or mild nausea may follow.
  - **Management:** Careful history should be taken to rule out concomitant neurologic symptoms. Both eyes are usually affected, although it may be sufficiently asymmetric as to appear to be monocular. If truly monocular, then prompt referral to an ophthalmologist is necessary to rule out retinal pathology.
- **Pseudotumor cerebri**
  - **Etiology:** Pseudotumor cerebri typically occurs in overweight young women and is more common in pregnancy. It is usually idiopathic but may be caused by vitamin A toxicity (>100,000 U/day), cyclosporine, tetracycline, oral contraceptives, or systemic steroid withdrawal.
  - **Symptoms:** Patients will describe **headache**, **transient visual obscurations** often associated with changes in posture, **diplopia**, **tinnitus**, dizziness, and nausea.
  - **Management:** If disc edema is seen, then a mass or venous thrombosis should be ruled out by an MRI and MR venography. Elevated opening pressure on lumbar puncture with normal cerebrospinal fluid (CSF) composition will confirm the diagnosis. Send patient to an ophthalmologist who can follow visual fields in order to monitor for vision loss and response to therapy. Counsel the patient on weight loss if overweight. Discontinue any causative medications. Medical treatment is achieved with acetazolamide 250 mg PO qid initially, increasing to 500 mg PO qid if tolerated and necessary. Surgery can be considered if medical options fail however this will require input from an ophthalmologist.

Progressive/Stable Vision Loss

- **Giant cell arteritis (GCA) or temporal arteritis (ischemic optic neuropathies)**
  - **Symptoms:** This potentially life-threatening disease should always be considered when sudden painless vision loss develops in a patient over 50 years old.[2,3] Concomitant symptoms of malaise, weight loss, anorexia, scalp tenderness, jaw claudication, or shoulder/limb girdle weakness should be documented.
  - **Management:** Because this is a systemic disease that may lead to bilateral blindness within a few days, **early diagnosis and a high level of suspicion are required**. Referral emergently to an ophthalmologist is needed to differentiate between causes of sudden painless vision loss that are associated with GCA versus those that have no association or risk of vision loss in the other eye. If there is a high index of suspicion, consider an immediate dose of **oral steroids** prior to a patient going for blood work (complete blood count [CBC], erythrocyte sedimentation rate [ESR], C-reactive protein [CRP]) on their way to the ophthalmologist, or presenting to an emergency room. A temporal artery biopsy should be done within 2 weeks of starting steroids in any patient in whom the clinical suspicion is high.

- **Retinal detachment**
  - **Etiology:** As the vitreous body pulls away from the retina, it can pull the retina off with it. Patients are at higher risk with increasing age and if they are very near-sighted, postsurgical, or posttrauma. Similar symptoms of acute onset of floaters and occasional flashes but no vision loss may be seen with acute **posterior vitreous detachment**; however, a dilated exam by an ophthalmologist is still needed to rule out a retinal detachment.
  - **Symptoms:** Presents with constant photopsia (flashing lights), floaters, and sometimes a shade over the part of the vision in one eye. Partial detachments may not affect central visual acuity dramatically, but those that involve the central macular area with significantly decreased visual acuity can be associated with an APD.
  - **Management:** These patients need an emergent extensive dilated retinal examination by an ophthalmologist.

- **Vascular occlusions: central retinal artery and vein occlusion (CRAO/CRVO) or branch artery and vein occlusions**
  - **Etiology:** This is often seen in people with previously diagnosed vascular disease; it may also occur in younger patients and requires evaluation for embolic (for arterial occlusion) or thrombotic (for venous occlusion) disease. On funduscopic examination, there may be evidence of pallor, vascular **box-carring**, and a **cherry-red spot**. Optic nerve swelling, venous engorgement, retinal hemorrhage, and cotton-wool spots, are often collectively described as **blood and thunder (CRVO)**.
  - **Symptoms:** Severe painless vision loss generally to the point of counting-fingers vision or worse. Many will awaken with poor vision or describe the very moment at which the vision was affected. As above, **patients must be screened for GCA symptoms** if over 50 years old.
  - **Management:** Irreversible damage has been shown to occur after 90 minutes of occlusion and, therefore, patients should be sent to the emergency room or for referral immediately.[4]
    - If the patient is diagnosed quickly enough with a CRAO, interventional radiologists may be able to treat the patient with catheterization of the ophthalmic artery and injection with thrombolytics, although this is not commonly indicated.[5]
    - After the acute event, the patient requires a workup for embolic disease and follow-up for late ocular complications including neovascularization and its resultant complications. Follow-up with an ophthalmologist is imperative to treat ocular complications common with these processes.

- **Visual field defects**
  - **Etiology:** Visual field defects may occur from retinal and optic nerve disease but may also indicate intracranial disease. Lesions anterior to the optic chiasm (e.g., retina,

glaucoma, and optic neuritis) produce lesions in one eye only. Pituitary adenomas at the optic chiasm may produce bitemporal field loss. Retrochiasmal (e.g., damage to the optic tracts, radiations, or the occipital cortex) lesions produce homonymous hemianopsias or other homonymous defects. Stroke is the most common cause of homonymous hemianopsia.

- ○ **Symptoms:** Patients will describe areas in the visual field that are black or missing.
- ○ **Management:** Generally bilateral visual field loss needs neurologic evaluation and imaging. An ophthalmologist can perform formal visual fields in the office to more precisely determine the pattern of field loss that can help in localization of the pathology.
- **Vitreous hemorrhage**
  - ○ **Etiology:** Vitreous hemorrhage is often seen in those with diabetes, vein occlusions, and retinal holes or breaks. Vitreous hemorrhage may occur after trauma or with any condition that causes abnormal retinal neovascularization. **Terson syndrome** is vitreous and retinal hemorrhage in association with subarachnoid hemorrhage (SAH).
  - ○ **Symptoms:** Patients will describe sudden onset of **floaters**, **veils**, spider webs, or looking through red (blood). Vision can be moderately or severely impaired depending on the amount of bleeding.
  - ○ **Management:** Have the patient maintain an upright posture with the head of bed elevated while sleeping so that the blood may settle. Refer to an ophthalmologist to monitor progression and treat any retinal pathology. Unresolved hemorrhage may eventually require surgical removal. Stopping anticoagulation should only be considered if there is no risk of systemic complications of discontinuing therapy. Discussion with the ophthalmologist regarding the etiology of the bleed may reveal that discontinuing anticoagulation may be of little therapeutic value.

Acute Painful Vision Loss

- **Angle-closure glaucoma**
  - ○ **Etiology:** Angle-closure glaucoma is a rare disorder that occurs when the anterior chamber is anatomically narrow and the dilated iris closes off the outflow of aqueous humor causing an acute rise in IOP.[6] This event can cause an extremely elevated IOP (possibly up to the 70s), and patients are at risk for vascular occlusions and glaucomatous damage to the optic nerve.
  - ○ **Symptoms: Severe pain**, decreased vision, colored halos, corneal edema, and **headache/eye pain**. Nausea, vomiting, and abdominal pain may also occur. The **pupil is usually fixed** and does not react to light.
  - ○ **Management: Send to an ophthalmologist** to manage the IOP initially with medications. But the definitive treatment is a laser peripheral iridotomy, which should be performed as soon as possible; this procedure is also done on the unaffected eye for prophylaxis.[6]
- **Optic neuritis**
  - ○ **Etiology:** Optic neuritis is an inflammation of the optic nerve that may involve the optic disc (with hyperemia and optic disc swelling). It may alternatively be retrobulbar (with no apparent optic disc changes but more pain on extraocular motions). **Demyelinating disease (multiple sclerosis) is the most common etiology** in the proper demographic but is often idiopathic.[7,8] Atypical optic neuritis should be worked-up in conjunction with an ophthalmologist/neurologist or neuroophthalmologist.
  - ○ **Symptoms:** Sudden vision loss associated with **pain with eye movements** and significantly reduced acuity.
  - ○ **Management:** These patients should be followed by an ophthalmologist and referred to a neurologist for imaging to look for demyelinating disease. Autoimmune disease should be investigated should the MRI demonstrate atypical findings or an absence of demyelinating lesions. Treatment consists of either parenteral steroids or supportive care.

Oral steroids have not been shown to be effective and may even be deleterious. If the MRI reveals two or more characteristic demyelinating lesions, the patient may benefit from treatment with intravenous (IV) interferon-β within 28 days of symptom onset to decrease the rate of progression to definitive **multiple sclerosis.**[9]

Chronic Vision Loss

- **Cataract** is an opacification of the lens that occurs with aging or secondarily after trauma, chronic inflammation or steroid use, among other causes.
  - **Etiology:** Cataracts are a normal part of aging. They are the most common cause of media opacity and are usually gradual in onset (over months to years). Changes in the lens thickness occur with cataract development and initially can be corrected by a change in glasses.
  - **Symptoms:** As the lens opacifies, patients may note **decreased night vision,** difficulty with glare, **difficulty with reading,** and decreased distance acuity. Rarely, patients complain of double vision and decreased color vision and brightness in the affected eye.
  - **Management:** The **indication for elective surgical cataract removal** is that the cataract affects activities of daily living. Rarely, the cataract may need to be removed if it causes a secondary glaucoma or if it interferes with monitoring other ocular diseases, such as macular degeneration, diabetes, or glaucoma. Elective cataract surgery is performed under local or topical anesthetic as an outpatient and can be offered to any patient who is visually impaired and in stable medical health.
  - **Anticoagulants** required for medical care generally do not need to be discontinued. A recent history and physical examination are required but excessive laboratory testing is not typically indicated.[10–13]
- **Age-related macular degeneration (ARMD) is a disease of the retina that can cause significant visual impairment.**
  - **Etiology:** ARMD is a chronic, often progressive disease that affects central vision. It is often bilateral but may be asymmetric. ARMD may be dry (atrophic) or wet (exudative or neovascular). **Risk factors** include increased age, cigarette smoking, family history, and race (white).[14]
  - **Symptoms:** Progression is usually slow but sudden profound **central vision loss** occurs if a subretinal neovascular membrane develops with hemorrhage and scarring.
  - **Management:** Referral to an ophthalmologist to monitor disease is essential. Home monitoring with an **Amsler grid** is recommended for early detection of central distortion. The Age-Related Eye Disease Study demonstrated that in patients with moderate-to-severe ARMD treatment with vitamins and antioxidants reduced the rate of progression to severe vision loss.[15] Injections of anti-VEGF (vascular endothelial growth factor) agents for exudative or wet-type macular degeneration have improved the outcome for this ocular disease.[16]
- **Glaucoma** is a neurodegenerative disease that targets the optic nerve. Although glaucoma can be associated with an elevated IOP, this finding is not required for diagnosis.
  - **Etiology:** Glaucoma is **a leading cause of blindness** in the US. African Americans affected by glaucoma are particularly susceptible to vision loss.[17] Patients with a family history of glaucoma should be examined by an ophthalmologist to determine if regular follow-up is indicated.
  - **Symptoms:** Most patients with glaucoma are **asymptomatic.** Many lose significant peripheral vision before having any visual symptoms. Patients with a history of prior glaucoma surgery are at risk of endophthalmitis. **Any patient with prior glaucoma surgery with an acute red eye or pain should be seen immediately by an ophthalmologist.**
  - **Management:** These patients need frequent follow-up with an ophthalmologist. Frequency of visits is dictated by the IOP control and the severity of disease. General

follow-up is usually every 6 months, with visual field testing every year. Monitoring of optic cup enlargement, especially with concomitant IOP monitoring, is a way to quantify the severity of the progression of glaucoma. Treatment involves medical, laser, or surgical interventions aimed at lowering the IOP.

- **Corneal edema**
  - **Etiology:** If gradual, it may be due to underlying corneal disease, prior ocular surgery, or trauma. Patients with keratoconus can have acute episodes of corneal edema. Acutely, it may be secondary to increased IOP as in angle-closure glaucoma or rubeosis irides. Inflammation, infection, or opacity of the cornea may be difficult to differentiate from corneal edema with penlight examination.
  - **Symptoms:** Corneal edema is usually associated with **pain**. There is a **hazy appearance of the cornea** and decreased vision.
  - **Management:** Referral to an ophthalmologist based on symptom onset and severity.

RED EYE

- Referring to hyperemia or bleeding of the superficial vessels of the conjunctiva, episclera, or sclera, the red eye may or may not be associated with pain.[18–20] However, it does not usually cause significantly decreased visual acuity. **Contact lens wearers with poor contact lens hygiene presenting with red eye are at high risk for corneal ulcers and should be referred immediately.**
- **Subconjunctival hemorrhage**
  - **Etiology:** A subconjunctival hemorrhage consists of blood over the white sclera and under the clear conjunctiva. The patient should be questioned about other bleeding episodes or bruising, use of anticoagulants and aspirin, and hypertension.
  - **Symptoms:** Although these can be quite dramatic in appearance and alarming to the patient, they are self-limited, do not affect vision, and are generally painless. It may be seen after inadvertent trauma or straining.
  - **Management:** Patients may have mild eye irritation due to increased corneal dryness. Treatment involves cool compresses and artificial tears as needed. If the vision is reduced especially in the setting of trauma, refer to an ophthalmologist. Anticoagulants do not need to be discontinued for an isolated subconjunctival hemorrhage. If multiple episodes occur or if other systemic symptoms are present, a hematologic workup may be indicated.
- **Dry eye and blepharitis**
  - **Etiology:** Dry eyes are very common, especially in cases of lagophthalmos (incomplete closure) with Bell palsy, thyroid disease, rheumatologic diseases, contact lens wear, and age. Often a decrease in the protein or oil component of the tears due to eyelid disease (rosacea, **blepharitis**, or meibomianitis) leads to a decrease in the quality, not quantity, of tears. Symptoms of dryness may be worsened by some systemic medications (antihistamines, antidepressants, or hormone replacement). Abnormal contour of the ocular surface can also produce irregularity in the tear film (see pterygium/pinguecula).
  - **Symptoms:** Usually burning, irritation, mildly decreased vision, and foreign body sensation.[21] Patients may even complain of overflow tearing with extreme sensitivity to air, light, and prolonged usage of eyes, especially with near vision.
  - **Management:** A trial of **artificial tears** with carboxymethylcellulose along with eyelid scrubs is often recommended. Referral to an ophthalmologist more acutely if the patient has poor contact lens hygiene (prolonged wear and lack of cleaning) or mechanical cause of dryness (e.g., inability to close the eye due to a seventh nerve palsy).
- **Seasonal allergies**
  - **Etiology:** Patients with a history of allergies are commonly affected. Frequently, localized allergy to ophthalmic drops can occur and present in a similar fashion. Seasonal allergies are a very common cause of red eyes.

- ○ **Symptoms:** Itching, redness, tearing, foreign body sensation.
- ○ **Management:** For occasional use, over-the-counter antihistamines are reasonable, but for chronic use, an ophthalmologist can prescribe more effective medications.
- **Injected pterygium and pinguecula**
  - ○ These are two types of conjunctival degeneration/abnormal growth on the conjunctiva that can become inflamed. They can contribute to corneal dryness as well.
  - ○ Treatment is initially with artificial tears, surgical treatment is needed in some cases (see Dry Eye).
- **Infections**
  - ○ **Etiology:** Infections are a common cause of the red eye. **Blepharitis** is caused by a mild eyelid infection, which can lead to a foreign body sensation (especially in the morning) and dry eye. **Herpes simplex keratitis** can lead to corneal ulceration and scarring and should be referred to an ophthalmologist.
  - ○ **Symptoms: Viral and bacterial conjunctivitis** are associated with redness, mucous discharge, crusting, and tearing. In patients with **contact lens use** and associated redness, prompt referral to an ophthalmologist to rule out corneal ulceration is paramount.
  - ○ **Management:** Although topical antibiotics are useful, **topical corticosteroids should not be used without consultation by an ophthalmologist**. If symptoms are progressive on treatment or the patient wears contact lenses, prompt referral to an ophthalmologist is necessary.
- **Episcleritis and scleritis**
  - ○ **Etiology:** Episcleritis is localized inflammation of the episclera. Scleritis is an inflammatory disorder of deeper sclera and can be vision threatening. Scleritis may indicate a serious systemic disease such as a collagen vascular disorder or other autoimmune disease.
  - ○ **Symptoms:** Redness, **pain especially to touch**. Vision is usually unaffected unless scleritis is posterior or associated with corneal thinning. Episcleral redness blanches with phenylephrine; redness from scleritis does not.
  - ○ **Management:** Patients need to be monitored carefully for the development of scleral thinning and possible perforation. Scleritis is typically treated with systemic steroids; however, evaluation by an ophthalmologist prior to initiating therapy is advised.
- **Iritis**
  - ○ **Etiology:** Iritis is caused by inflammation of the iris, ciliary body, or both. It can be associated with systemic or localized ocular autoimmune disease. As such, recurrent episodes require a medical evaluation guided by the patient's history and presentation. This may include CBC, antinuclear antibodies (ANA), rheumatoid factor (RF), syphilis testing, antineutrophil cytoplasmic antibodies (ANCA), human leukocyte antigen-B27, tuberculosis testing, angiotensin-converting enzyme (ACE) level, and/or chest radiography.
  - ○ **Symptoms:** Redness, pain, decreased vision, and **light sensitivity**. A perilimbal distribution of redness is often present. It can be unilateral or bilateral.
  - ○ **Management:** If suspected, evaluation by an ophthalmologist is indicated.

EYE PAIN

See entries for dry eye, episcleritis/scleritis, corneal abrasion, iritis, angle-closure glaucoma, infections, optic neuritis, corneal edema, and trauma.

OCULAR TRAUMA

- If there is significant (360 degrees) subconjunctival hemorrhage with swelling of the conjunctiva (chemosis), severely decreased vision, eyelid laceration, or a concerning history, referral to an emergency room is warranted to rule out a ruptured globe. An **orbital CT** with coronal cuts is the preferred study to rule out posterior globe rupture and/or intraocular foreign body. A visual acuity assessment should be attempted by gently lifting even a swollen lid and having a patient read a near-card as this is the "vital sign" of the eye and can guide the physician in triaging the patient.

- **If a globe rupture is suspected**[22]
  - Keep the eye covered with an eye shield or by taping a disposable cup over it, making sure the rim rests on the bony orbit and not the eye.
  - Keep the patient NPO.
  - Consider tetanus prophylaxis.
  - Administer antiemetics to prevent Valsalva that can expulse the contents of the eye, particularly if the patient must travel a distance to reach the emergency department.
- **Chemical burn**
  - **Etiology:** Alkaline substances penetrate and saponify tissues and cause severe injury—these include ammonia, sodium hydroxide (lye), calcium hydroxide (lime), magnesium hydroxide, potassium hydroxide, and cement. Acids coagulate the conjunctival surface, and, therefore, penetrate the eye much less. Causative acids include hydrochloric, hydrofluoric, acetic, nitrous, sulfuric, and sulfurous.
  - **Symptoms:** Eye may be red, photophobic, painful, and have epithelial defects detectable with fluorescein and a cobalt blue light/Woods lamp. **It may also be white—an ominous sign of complete ischemia.**
  - **Management: Irrigate, irrigate, irrigate!** Immediate flushing of the eye with water or normal saline for at least 10 minutes. This can be performed while the patient is **transferred to an emergency department**.
    - Begin flushing with any neutral fluid that is available.
    - If a Morgan lens is not available, an IV bag connected to nasal cannula placed over the bridge of the nose is effective.
    - Be sure to irrigate the fornices (under the lids) to wash out any particles. Evert the eyelids if necessary.
    - **Do not attempt to neutralize** the chemical with acidic or basic fluids.
  - pH paper should be used to measure the pH of the eye; the pH should be taken a few minutes after the eye has been flushed, before instilling any ophthalmic drops, and it should be 7.0 (if pH paper is not available, the pH square of a urinalysis strip works).
  - Rarely, a retained foreign body causes continued release of the chemical and needs to be removed. This is more common with alkali burns.
  - **Refer** to an ophthalmologist when the patient's condition is stable for evaluation and treatment of chemical damage.
- **Corneal abrasion**
  - **Symptoms:** Corneal abrasions are common and often present with significant redness, pain, photophobia, or lid swelling after trauma. A topical anesthetic is often used in the office to increase patient comfort. Evaluation can be aided with fluorescein staining and observation with cobalt blue-filtered light. **If the history involves grinding metal or projectiles (small or large) refer to an ophthalmologist as there may be a foreign body or a ruptured globe.**
  - **Topical anesthetics** aid greatly in examination of the eye but **should never be used for treatment**, as they may cause epithelial toxicity, decreased healing, and a neurotrophic ulcer.
  - **Management:** Treatment should include antibiotic eye drops (usually sulfacetamide 10%, 1 drop qid for 1 week, or tobramycin 0.3%, 1 drop qid for 1 week) or antibiotic ointment (polymyxin B sulfate [Polysporin Ophthalmic], 1/8-inch strip bid, or erythromycin, 1/8-inch strip bid). If it is certain that the injury has recently occurred (within a few hours), there is no evidence of infection, there is no retained foreign body, and the patient is not a contact lens wearer, the eye may be patched however this is not generally recommended.

- Any corneal haze or evidence of nonhealing abrasion (**no improvement in 24 to 36 hours**) should be reevaluated by an ophthalmologist.
- **Orbital fractures**
  - **Symptoms:** Orbital fractures are often seen due to blunt trauma. Patients can be asymptomatic or they can have **diplopia** at baseline or with extreme gaze. The eyelids are generally swollen—slowly elevate the lid to obtain a visual acuity with a near-card. There may be **decreased sensation** inferior to the orbit or **numbness** in the upper teeth on the affected side.
  - **Management:** Referral to an emergency department may be warranted. Orbital CT with axial and coronal cuts is the study of choice. Secondary ocular injuries should be highly suspected when motility is abnormal or vision is markedly decreased. Fractures should be treated with cephalexin 250 mg PO qid for 10 days. Emphasis on **no nose blowing** and oxymetazoline tid for 3 days aids in decreasing the risk of extension of sinus disease into the orbit and limits orbital emphysema. While many fractures need no surgical repair, referral to a surgeon should be expedited should there be diplopia in primary gaze and/or significant enophthalmos (recession of the eyeball into the orbit).
- **Foreign body/rust ring**
  - **Symptoms:** pain, redness, decreased vision with a history of working around grinding metal, a dirty environment, or other environmental factors that can lead to small particles becoming lodged in the anterior surface of the eye.
  - **Management:** Foreign bodies can be carefully removed with either a wet cotton tip or needle under direct visualization using a slit lamp. A burr drill is occasionally used to remove rust rings. After the foreign body is removed, the eye should be treated with topical antibiotic (see the "Corneal Abrasions" section). Eversion of the eyelid should be performed to rule out retained foreign bodies under the eyelid. Generally, the patient should be referred to an ophthalmologist.
- **Traumatic iritis and hyphema**
  - **Etiology:** Traumatic iritis must be differentiated from bleeding (microhyphema) and infection. Hyphema is blood in the anterior eye chamber and may lead to decreased vision, photophobia, and a dull achiness around the eye. Usually, it is a result of direct trauma to the eye, but it can be caused by abnormal blood vessels (secondary to tumors, diabetes, chronic inflammation, intraocular surgery, etc.).
  - **Symptoms:** Traumatic iritis is common 2 to 3 days after blunt trauma and may present with decreased vision, photophobia, and dull pain. A hyphema presents more acutely posttrauma with decreased vision; however, both need to be seen and treated by an ophthalmologist.
  - **Management:** Pain and decreased vision after trauma should be evaluated and followed by an ophthalmologist to rule out additional ocular involvement and manage possible complications such as rebleeding in the eye, increased IOP, and corneal blood staining. Hyphema is often treated with dilation, light activity, rigid shield, and topical steroid medication, but may require surgical washout if medical management is insufficient. The status of **sickle cell disease/trait should be noted**, as it affects the clearance of red blood cells from the anterior chamber through the trabecular meshwork and may lead to complications.

DOUBLE VISION

- Monocular diplopia is refractive in nature and should be evaluated by an ophthalmologist usually on a routine basis unless in the setting of trauma.
- Binocular diplopia has a larger differential.[23,24] Asking if the double vision resolves by closing either eye is a good way to differentiate monocular versus binocular diplopia. If the patient notes resolution of diplopia after covering either eye, then it is likely binocular

diplopia. The essential job of the clinician is to examine the patient's eye movements and evaluate the cranial nerves (CN).

- **Abnormal motility**
  - Abnormalities of eye motility may suggest an acute or chronic CN palsy (III, IV, or VI) or extraocular muscle disorder.
  - Acute abnormalities are usually accompanied by complaints of diplopia, which may be horizontal or vertical in nature.
  - Chronic motility defects may be asymptomatic.
  - Medical conditions such as thyroid eye disease (especially **Graves disease**), idiopathic inflammatory pseudotumor (ocular myositis), myasthenia gravis (MG), giant cell arteritis, demyelinating disease (multiple sclerosis), and cerebellar dysfunction may manifest with abnormal eye movements.

- **Ocular myasthenia gravis**
  - **Etiology:** MG is an autoimmune-mediated disease or rarely myasthenia-like from medications like penicillamine or aminoglycosides. Patients may have an associated thymoma or Graves disease.
  - **Symptoms:** Drooping of eyelids worse at the end of the day or with fatigue, intermittent binocular double vision especially if **worse with fatigue**.[25] Additional symptoms include difficulty swallowing, breathing, and proximal limb weakness.
  - **Management:** By far the most common cause of ptosis is levator dehiscence; however, MG should always be included in the differential. In the office, one can have the patient look up at your finger for 1 minute to assess fatigability of the ptosis. If it worsens with prolonged up-gaze, one should entertain the possibility of MG. It may then be prudent to refer the patient to a neurologist for more testing while ordering MG antibodies (anti-ACHr, anti-MuSK, striational/titan antibodies) and thyroid function tests (including thyroid-stimulating antibody [TSI]).

- **Thyroid disease/Graves disease**
  - **Etiology: The most common cause of unilateral AND bilateral proptosis is thyroid eye disease.** Graves disease is an autoimmune disease associated with hyperthyroidism. However, thyroid eye disease may appear or progress in patients who are clinically euthyroid or hypothyroid. Tobacco usage has been associated with higher incidence of ocular complications.
  - **Symptoms:** The most common manifestations include **eyelid retraction, double vision, proptosis, and corneal dryness**.
  - **Management:** Referral to an ophthalmologist with an orbital CT with axial and coronal cuts in conjunction with thyroid testing (thyroid stimulating hormone [TSH], free thyroxine [T4], TSI) is critical. Smoking cessation is essential for managing these patients.

- **Intracranial aneurysm**
  - Rarely intracranial aneurysms may present with ocular CN defects.
  - Involvement of CN III–VI should suggest cavernous sinus pathology.
  - Pupil-involving CN III defects can be seen in posterior communicating artery aneurysms, and MR angiography may be helpful in diagnosis.
  - Diabetic or microvascular ischemic third nerve palsy usually spares the pupil and recovers spontaneously.

EYELID DISORDERS

- These problems can overlap with the red eye entities. For example, eyelid crusting, especially in the mornings with foreign body sensation and mild blurred vision especially in a patient with acne rosacea is most like blepharitis-associated dry eye.
- Keep in mind that **malignant eyelid lesions** include basal cell, squamous cell, and sebaceous cell carcinomas, and **can mask as chronic eyelid disease**.[26]

- **Chalazion/hordeolum**
  - **Etiology:** A chalazion is a chronic lipogranulomatous inflammatory lesion due to an obstructed meibomian gland in the eyelid. A hordeolum, or stye, is an acute, painful inflammatory lesion of eyelid glands, and is typically caused by a staphylococcal infection.
  - **Symptoms:** Each may initially present with acute inflammatory signs while a chalazion develops into a relatively painless nodule, a hordeolum can incite a localized cellulitis.
  - **Management: Mainstays of treatment are hot compresses with gentle massage along with topical or oral antibiotics if indicated.** If the lesion has not completely resolved and is no longer actively inflamed, surgical incision and drainage may be recommended. Rarely, a chalazion may be mistaken for a malignant lesion and vice versa so referral to an ophthalmologist is warranted especially if the lesion does not resolve in 4 weeks.
- **Cellulitis**
  - **Etiology:** Preseptal cellulitis is usually secondary to localized trauma or skin defect (scratch, cut, rash) while orbital cellulitis is secondary to sinus disease in an overwhelming majority of cases.
  - **Symptoms:** Swelling of the eyelids with pain, warmth, and tenderness to touch without motility or visual disturbances is **preseptal**. If there is difficulty with eye motility or decreased vision then the process affects the **postseptal** orbit and can threaten the globe or cavernous sinus.
  - **Management:** Preseptal cellulitis can be managed conservatively with oral antibiotics (amoxicillin/clavulanate 875/125 mg PO bid for adults or trimethoprim/sulfamethoxazole 160/800 mg, one tablet tid to two tablets bid in those allergic to penicillin). Worsening preseptal cellulitis while on oral antibiotics or orbital cellulitis needs admission for IV antibiotics along with an orbital CT scan. Rarely orbital inflammatory disease can manifest as orbital cellulitis especially if there is no sinus disease on orbital CT scans. Consultation by an oculoplastic surgeon in these cases is advised.
- **Herpes zoster ophthalmicus (HZO)**
  - **Etiology:** Varicella-zoster virus.
  - **Symptoms:** Dermatomal skin rash with pain, paresthesias, and vesicles (later in the disease). Sometimes eye redness, decreased vision, and eye pain occur. Hutchinson sign (rash on the tip of the nose) is associated with intraocular involvement. HZO is almost always unilateral and does not cross the midline.
  - **Management:** If <40 years old, consider testing for HIV. Oral acyclovir 800 mg PO 5×/day or valacyclovir 1,000 mg tid for 7 to 10 days when the patient presents within the first week of symptoms. Erythromycin ointment to skin lesions. If there is any eye pain, referral to an ophthalmologist within a few days is advised. If there are signs of **motility abnormalities, an APD, or concern for orbital involvement**, then admission for IV acyclovir should be initiated.
- **Ptosis and dermatochalasis**
  - **Etiology:** Ptosis is a common condition that may occur from congenital disease, neurologic disease, or involutional changes with aging. Dermatochalasis is excess eyelid skin that may cause symptoms similar to those of ptosis.
  - **Symptoms:** Eyelid drooping or excess skin obstructing the vision. See the section on Myasthenia Gravis above.
  - **Management:** If the upper eyelid appears to interfere with the superior field of vision, or if the patient is symptomatic, surgical intervention is possible. Blepharoplasty is the treatment for symptomatic dermatochalasis. If there is any suspicion of a mass occupying the orbit or neurologic disease (both of which can present with eyelid droop), referral to an ophthalmologist can aid in the diagnostic evaluation.
- **Dacryocystitis**
  - **Etiology:** Dacryocystitis is an infection of the tear sac from inadequate drainage of tear.

- **Symptoms:** Dacryocystitis presents with redness, pain, and swelling in the inferomedial part of the lower eyelid.
- **Management:** Acutely, oral antibiotics are necessary (cephalexin, 250 mg PO qid for 10 days). Surgical **dacryocystorhinostomy** is usually required after the inflammation has resolved because recurrences are likely. An ophthalmologist or oculoplastic surgeon can aid in the management of this condition as other entities including chalazion/hordeolum, canaliculitis, and lacrimal sac tumors can have similar presentations.

REFERENCES

1. Payne JW, Duke JR, Butner R, et al. Basal cell carcinoma of the eyelids. A long-term follow-up study. *Arch Ophthalmol* 1969;81:553–558.
2. Weyand CM, Goronzy JJ. Giant-cell arteritis and polymyalgia rheumatica. *Ann Intern Med* 2003;139:505–515.
3. Waldman CW, Waldman SD, Waldman RA. Giant cell arteritis. *Med Clin North Am* 2013;97:329–335.
4. Hayreh SS, Zimmerman MB, Kimura A, et al. Central retinal artery occlusion. Retinal survival time. *Exp Eye Res* 2004;78:723–736.
5. Schumacher M, Schmidt D, Jurklies B, et al. Central retinal artery occlusion: local intra-arterial fibrinolysis versus conservative treatment, a multicenter randomized trial. *Ophthalmology* 2010;117:1367–1375.
6. Lam DSC, Tham CCY, Lai JSM, et al. Current approaches to the management of acute primary angle closure. *Curr Opin Ophthalmol* 2007;18:146–151.
7. Balcer LJ. Clinical practice. Optic neuritis. *N Engl J Med* 2006;354:1273–80.
8. Chen L, Gordon LK. Ocular manifestations of multiple sclerosis. *Curr Opin Ophthalmol* 2005;16:315–320.
9. CHAMPS Study Group. Interferon beta-1a for optic neuritis patients at high risk for multiple sclerosis. *Am J Ophthalmol* 2001;132:463–471.
10. Cavallini GM, Saccarola P, D'Amico R, et al. Impact of preoperative testing on ophthalmologic and systemic outcomes in cataract surgery. *Eur J Ophthalmol* 2004;14:369–374.
11. Keay L, Lindsley K, Tielsch J, et al. Routine preoperative medical testing for cataract surgery. *Cochrane Database Syst Rev* 2012;(3):CD007293.
12. Schein O, Katz J, Bass EB, et al. The value of routine preoperative medical testing before cataract surgery. Study of Medical Testing for Cataract Surgery. *N Engl J Med* 2000;342:168–175.
13. Guirguis-Blake J. Preoperative testing for patients undergoing cataract surgery. *Am Fam Physician* 2009;80:1228.
14. de Jong PT. Age-related macular degeneration. *N Engl J Med* 2006;355:1474–1485.
15. Chew EY, Clemons TE, Agrón E, et al. Long-term effects of vitamins C and E, β-carotene, and zinc on age-related macular degeneration: AREDS report no. 35. *Ophthalmology* 2013;120:1604–1611.
16. Cheung CMG, Wong TY. Treatment of age-related macular degeneration. *Lancet* 2013;382:1230–1232.
17. Bourne R, Price H, Stevens G; GBD Vision Loss Expert Group. Global burden of visual impairment and blindness. *Arch Ophthalmol* 2012;130:645–647.
18. Cronau H, Kankanala RR, Mauger T. Diagnosis and management of red eye in primary care. *Am Fam Physician* 2010;81:137–144.
19. Wirbelauer C. Management of the red eye for the primary care physician. *Am J Med* 2006;119:302–306.
20. Leibowitz HM. The red eye. *N Engl J Med* 2000;343:345–351.
21. Bernardes TF, Bonfioli AA. Blepharitis. *Semin Ophthalmol* 2010;25:79–83.

22. Romaniuk VM. Ocular trauma and other catastrophes. *Emerg Med Clin North Am* 2013;31:399–411.

23. Friedman DI. Pearls: diplopia. *Semin Neurol* 2010;30:54–65.

24. Rucker JC, Tomsak RL. Binocular diplopia. A practical approach. *Neurologist* 2005;11:98–110.

25. Vaphiades MS, Bhatti MT, Lesser RL. Ocular myasthenia gravis. *Curr Opin Ophthalmol* 2012;23:537–542.

26. Zucker JL. The eyelids: some common disorders seen in everyday practice. *Geriatrics* 2009;64:14–19, 28.

Smoking Cessation
Megan E. Wren

GENERAL PRINCIPLES

Smokers Can Quit

- Since the publication of the first Surgeon General's Report on Smoking and Health in 1965, the rate of smoking among adult Americans has gradually decreased from 42% down to 19%.[1]
- Over time, the average number of cigarettes smoked per day has declined to 15; now, fewer than 10% smoke 30 or more cigarettes per day (one pack contains 20 cigarettes).[1]
- Among current smokers, more than two-thirds report that they want to quit and just over half have made a quit attempt in the past year.[2]
- Smokers wanting to quit have to overcome both a strong habit and a physiologic addiction to nicotine.
  - Nicotine from cigarette smoke reaches the brain in <10 seconds.[3] This rapid delivery to the mesolimbic reward system makes smoking very addicting. Because nicotine has a half-life of just 30 minutes, the smoker soon craves another cigarette.
  - Smoking is also a conditioned behavior—the act of smoking is quickly rewarded with pleasurable feelings—the satisfaction of smoking. This conditioning is also tied to cues in the environment: certain places, times, or events are strong triggers for a desire to smoke.
- Since tobacco use is both a learned behavior and a physical addiction to nicotine for the majority of smokers, the combination of counseling and pharmacologic therapies can produce higher quit rates than either one alone.
- The clinician should recognize **tobacco dependence as a chronic disease**, subject to periods of remission and relapse, and requiring ongoing counseling. Fortunately, effective interventions are now available that may increase abstinence rates to 20% to 30%.[4]
- Although individual quit attempts have a low success rate, many people can be successful with repeated attempts. In fact, **of all Americans who have smoked, half have successfully quit.**[2]

Guidelines

- Multiple organizations partnered to develop a clinical practice guideline summarizing evidence-based recommendations on the treatment of tobacco use. It was published as a U.S. Public Health Service (PHS) Report and is available online at http://www.ahrq.gov/professionals/clinicians-providers/guidelines-recommendations/tobacco/clinicians/update/index.html (last accessed 1/14/15).
- Key recommendations of the PHS guideline include the following:
  - Tobacco dependence is a chronic condition that often requires repeated intervention and multiple attempts to quit. Effective treatments exist that can significantly increase rates of long-term abstinence.
  - It is essential to consistently identify and document tobacco use status and treat every tobacco user seen in a health care setting.
  - Tobacco dependence treatments are effective. Clinicians should encourage every patient willing to make a quit attempt to use the counseling treatments and medications recommended in this guideline.

○ Even brief tobacco dependence treatment is effective and should be offered to every patient who uses tobacco.
○ Individual, group, and telephone counseling is effective; their effectiveness increases with treatment intensity (time). Two components of counseling are especially effective:
  ▪ Practical counseling (problem solving/skills training)
  ▪ Social support delivered as part of treatment
○ Numerous effective pharmacotherapies for smoking cessation now exist. Except in the presence of contraindications, these should be used with all patients attempting to quit smoking.
○ The combination of counseling and medication is more effective than either alone. Clinicians should encourage all individuals making a quit attempt to use both counseling and medication.
○ If a tobacco user is unwilling to make a quit attempt, clinicians should use motivational treatments shown to be effective in increasing future quit attempts.
○ Telephone quitline counseling is effective with diverse populations and has broad reach.

Counseling for Behavior Change

• Brief counseling should be provided to all smokers at every visit. Interventions as short as 3 minutes can increase quit rate significantly.
• The five As technique for brief office counseling of smokers is familiar to many clinicians. A brief summary is provided below; more detail is available in the PHS Report, pages 37 to 43.[4]
  ○ **ASK**: Ask about smoking... every patient, every visit. Make it one of the vital signs so it isn't forgotten.
  ○ **ADVISE**: Advise all smokers to quit. Physicians' advice is a strong incentive to attempt smoking cessation.
    ▪ Be empathetic, not confrontational.
    ▪ Use a clear, strong message such as, "Quitting smoking is the most important thing you can do to protect your health now and in the future. I can help you."
    ▪ Personalize the message by stressing the relevance to the patient's current medical problems and symptoms. Most smokers are unaware of smoking's connection with a wide array of problems from acid reflux to osteoporosis to macular degeneration, as well as vascular disease and many cancers.
  ○ **ASSESS**: Assess the smoker's willingness to make a serious quit attempt in the next 30 days (see "Readiness for Change" below).
  ○ **ASSIST**: Assist in the quit attempt. If the patient is ready to make a serious attempt to quit, then make smoking cessation the focus of the visit. Three elements of successful smoking cessation treatment strategies include social support, pharmacologic therapy, and skills training or problem-solving techniques.
    ▪ Help the patient set a **specific quit date** in the next couple of weeks. Write it in the chart and on a prescription pad to make it an official commitment.
    ▪ Review prior quit attempts. What worked? What didn't work and may have contributed to relapse?
    ▪ The patient should enlist the aid of family and friends.
    ▪ Discuss anticipated triggers and challenges, and strategies to cope with them (see "Challenges and Strategies" below). Anticipate nicotine withdrawal symptoms, cues to smoking, and danger situations.
    ▪ Before the quit date, he/she should start to break the habit by avoiding smoking in the usual places. Make the home and car smoke free.
    ▪ Provide educational materials. Offer referrals to classes, websites such as www.smoke-free.gov, or a telephone quitline (1-800-QUIT-NOW) for additional counseling.
    ▪ **Recommend pharmacotherapy, unless contraindicated**.

○ **ARRANGE**: Arrange follow-up in person or by phone within the first week and again within the first month.
  ▪ Successful quitters should be congratulated and reminded to be on guard against tempting situations and cravings, which can persist for months to years.
  ▪ Those who did not try to quit should be assessed for willingness to change and encouraged to again set a quit date when ready.
  ▪ Those who quit and have relapsed should be encouraged to learn from the experience.
  ▪ Focus on the positive (congratulate for the days or weeks of abstinence).
  ▪ Educate that "a lapse is not a relapse"; encourage the patient to try again.
  ▪ Help the patient feel empowered to try again by discussing strategies to cope with challenging situations.
• **Readiness for change**: The Prochaska model of stages of change provides a useful framework for targeting interventions to the smoker's willingness to attempt to quit. Knowing the patient's readiness for change can guide the physician's time allotment to counseling in each visit. See Chapter 46 for a more detailed overview of the stages of change.

Challenges and Strategies

• **Practical counseling should be provided**.
  ○ Review past quit attempts including identification of what helped during the quit attempt and what factors contributed to relapse.
  ○ Tobacco users who have failed in previous quit attempts should be told that most people make repeated quit attempts before they are successful.
  ○ Discuss challenges/triggers and how the patient will successfully overcome them. Advise the removal of all tobacco from home, car, and work environment.
  ○ Because alcohol can cause relapse, the patient should consider limiting/abstaining from alcohol while quitting.
  ○ Quitting is more difficult when there is another smoker in the household. Patients should encourage housemates to quit with them or not smoke in their presence.
• **Strategies to help with lifestyle changes include**:
  ○ Counterconditioning—substitute other activities or experiences when tempted by cravings or stress.
  ○ Stimulus control—avoid situations that are likely to produce temptation or pressure.
  ○ Reinforcement management—reward small successes.
• **Withdrawal symptoms** include irritability, dysphoria, restlessness, anxiety, difficulty concentrating, headache, insomnia, and increased appetite. Educate the patient that the withdrawal symptoms will abate over a few weeks. Smoking cessation also triggers cravings for cigarettes, which can last for months to years. Cravings, although intense, are usually brief. A few minutes of distraction can help the patient ride out the craving—deep breathing, exercise, or a change in activity can all be helpful.
• **Delayed quitting** can occur. In a study with over 2,000 participants on varenicline, bupropion, or placebo, the authors found that about 60% of successful quitters were continuously abstinent by week 2, while about 40% were "delayed quitters" who smoked during 1 or more weeks in weeks 2 to 8.[5] This suggests that smokers who are motivated to quit should continue treatment despite lack of early success.
• **Weight gain** is a concern for many patients contemplating smoking cessation.
  ○ Often cited as 2 to 3 kg, the actual weight gain is quite variable. A recent meta-analysis found a mean weight gain of 4 to 5 kg after a year of abstinence, but roughly one-third gained <5 kg, one-third gained 5 to 10 kg, and 14% gained >10 kg. Of note, 16% to 21% actually lost weight.[6]
  ○ **Exercise** has been shown in some studies to reduce cigarette cravings and tobacco withdrawal symptoms.[7]
  ○ **Pharmacologic therapy** with nicotine, bupropion, or varenicline attenuated weight gain in the short term but not at 1 year postcessation.[8]

- **Coughing** may temporarily increase in the weeks following smoking cessation as cough reflex sensitivity is restored.[9]
- **Depression and anxiety** may be exacerbated in patients with a history of psychiatric illness. Those patients should be offered counseling and/or medications.
- **Cost** is an issue for many patients; smoking cessation products are expensive, and insurance coverage is variable.
  - Since bupropion is an antidepressant, it is more likely to be covered by insurance plans.
  - Some smoking cessation products are available through quitlines or community clinics.
  - Smoking cessation products are often less expensive than smoking, but cigarette prices vary considerably: from $4.41/pack in North Dakota to $10.05/pack in New York for monthly costs of $132.00 to $301.00 for 1 pack/day.[10]

For Patients Unwilling to Quit

- Patients may be unwilling to attempt to quit smoking for many reasons: lack of knowledge, lack of money or health insurance, or fears or concerns about quitting, or they may be demoralized because of previous relapses. Such patients may respond to brief interventions based on principles of **motivational interviewing** (MI), a patient-centered counseling technique.[11]
- **Clinician lectures or arguments for quitting tend to increase the patient's resistance to change**. MI techniques help patients find their own reasons for change.
- MI techniques focus on exploring the smoker's feelings, beliefs, and values in an effort to uncover any ambivalence about using tobacco. Once ambivalence is uncovered, the clinician selectively elicits, supports, and strengthens the patient's "change talk" (e.g., reasons, ideas, and need for eliminating tobacco use) and "commitment language" (e.g., intentions to take action to change smoking behavior, such as not smoking in the home). See Table 45-1 for details.[4]

MEDICATIONS

Recommendations

- Pharmacologic therapy can **approximately double the quit rate** as compared to placebo and should be offered to all patients except in the presence of limited special circumstances (see below).
- First-line treatments include nicotine replacement therapy (NRT), sustained-release bupropion (bupropion SR), and varenicline (see Table 45-2).

Nicotine Replacement Therapy

- NRT provides an alternative source of nicotine to ease withdrawal symptoms while the patient learns new nonsmoking behaviors. Many studies have documented that the use of NRT can increase long-term success rates 1.5-fold (nicotine replacement gum) to 2-fold (other NRT) compared to placebo.[4]
- NRT is most effective when combined with counseling. The effectiveness of counseling increases with the intensity of treatment, but even brief interventions are of benefit.
- Some experts advocate so-called harm reduction—the use of NRT for as long as it takes to keep patients from smoking.[12]

Safety of Nicotine Replacement Therapy

- Smokers smoke in order to get nicotine, but **essentially all of the adverse health effects of smoking stem from other constituents in tobacco and its smoke**. Thus, a cigarette is a contaminated drug delivery device. Cigarette smoke contains over 4,000 chemical compounds (the tar), ranging from carbon monoxide to hydrogen cyanide, and 69 of which are known carcinogens, including arsenic, benzene, and polonium 210.[13]

TABLE 45-1	General Principles of Motivational Interviewing and Examples of Language to Use
1. Express empathy	• Use open-ended questions to explore concerns and benefits of quitting: ○ "How important do you think it is for you to quit smoking?" ○ "What might happen if you quit?" • Use reflective listening: reflect words or meaning, and summarize: ○ "So you think smoking helps you to maintain your weight." ○ "What I have heard so far is that smoking is something you enjoy. On the other hand, your boyfriend hates your smoking, and you are worried you might develop a serious disease." • Normalize feelings and concerns: ○ "Many people worry about managing without cigarettes." • Support the patient's autonomy and right to choose or reject change: ○ "I hear you saying you are not ready to quit smoking right now. I'm here to help you when you are ready."
2. Develop discrepancy	• Highlight the discrepancy between the patient's present behavior and expressed priorities, values, and goals: ○ "It sounds like you are very devoted to your family. How do you think your smoking is affecting your children?" • Reinforce and support "change talk" and "commitment" language: ○ "So, you realize how smoking is affecting your breathing and making it hard to keep up with your kids." ○ "It's great that you are going to quit when you get through this busy time at work." • Build and deepen commitment to change: ○ "There are effective treatments that will ease the pain of quitting, including counseling and many medication options." ○ "We would like to help you avoid a stroke like the one your father had."
3. Roll with resistance	• Back off and use reflection when the patient expresses resistance: ○ "Sounds like you are feeling pressured about your smoking." • Express empathy: ○ "You are worried about how you would manage withdrawal symptoms." • Ask permission to provide information: ○ "Would you like to hear about some strategies that can help you address that concern when you quit?"
4. Support self-efficacy	• Help the patient to identify and build on past successes: ○ "So you were fairly successful the last time you tried to quit." • Offer options for achievable small steps toward change: ○ Call the quit line (1-800-QUIT-NOW) for advice and information. ○ Read about quitting benefits and strategies. ○ Change smoking patterns (e.g., no smoking in the home). ○ Ask the patient to share his or her ideas about quitting strategies.

TABLE 45-1	General Principles of Motivational Interviewing and Examples of Language to Use (*Continued*)

Content Areas To Be Addressed: The Five Rs

Relevance	Encourage the patient to indicate why quitting is personally relevant, being as specific as possible.
Risks	Ask the patient to identify potential negative consequences of tobacco use. Suggest or highlight those that seem most relevant to the patient. (Emphasize that low-tar/low-nicotine cigarettes or use of other forms of tobacco will not eliminate these risks.)
Rewards	Ask the patient to identify potential benefits of stopping tobacco use. Suggest and highlight those that seem most relevant to the patient (feeling better, looking better, saving money, setting a good example, etc.).
Roadblocks	Ask the patient to identify barriers to quitting. Provide treatment to address barriers (see "Challenges and Strategies" above).
Repetition	The MI counseling should be repeated every time an unmotivated patient visits the clinic setting.
	Tobacco users who have failed in previous quit attempts should be told that most people make repeated quit attempts before they are successful.

Modified from Fiore MC, Jaen CR, Baker TB, et al. *Clinical Practice Guideline. Treating Tobacco Use and Dependence: 2008 Update*. Rockville, MD: U.S. Department of Health and Human Services, Public Health Service; 2008. http://www.ahrq.gov/professionals/clinicians-providers/guidelines-recommendations/tobacco/clinicians/update/index.html. Last accessed 1/14/15.

- The dose-response relation for nicotine is flat making the effects of smoking plus NRT similar to smoking alone.
- NRT is a safe alternative to cigarettes and **does not cause heart attacks, lung cancer, or asthma**, as some have claimed.[14]
- The most common side effect of nicotine is local irritation, such as a rash under a nicotine patch or throat irritation from inhaled nicotine.
- Overuse of nicotine, whether from smoking or from NRT, can cause symptoms of nausea, vomiting, dizziness, sweating, palpitations, or anxiety.
- Massive overdose can cause seizures and cardiovascular collapse. All nicotine-containing products should be disposed of out of reach of small children and pets to avoid accidental poisoning. NRT is unlikely to cause addiction due to the low level of nicotine (<half that of smoking) and the slow delivery to the brain.

Safety of NRT in Patients with Cardiovascular Disease

- Oxidizing chemicals in smoke likely contribute to an increased risk of thrombotic complications and reduction in nitric oxide availability.[4] Unlike cigarette smoking, **NRT does not cause platelet aggregation or thrombotic complications**.[15]
- Transdermal nicotine in smokers with known coronary artery disease (CAD) has been shown to cause no significant differences in heart rate, in blood pressure, or in duration or frequency of ischemic episodes on ambulatory ECG monitoring.[16]
- NRT use was not associated with an increased risk of adverse cardiovascular events in the first year after acute coronary syndrome (ACS).[17]
- The use of nicotine gum did not increase cardiovascular deaths or hospitalizations, even in patients who smoked while using NRT and/or used NRT for more than a year.[18]
- Stress testing in smokers with known CAD showed that addition of a nicotine patch improved exercise tolerance and decreased ischemia, despite continued smoking and

TABLE 45-2 Medications to Aid Smoking Cessation

Products and brands	Dosage	Side effects and precautions	Approximate cost/month[a]
First-Line Pharmacotherapies			
Nicotine gum Nicorette, generics (OTC)	2 mg/piece (smoke <1 ppd) 4 mg/piece (smoke >1 ppd) Use at least 9 pieces/day; max 24 pieces	Mouth soreness Dyspepsia	$90–$150 (10 doses/day)
Nicotine lozenge Commit, generics (OTC)	2 mg/piece (TTFC <30 minutes) 4 mg/piece (TTFC >30 minutes) Use at least 9 pieces/day; max 24 pieces	Mouth soreness Dyspepsia	$120–$160 (10 doses/day)
Nicotine inhaler Nicotrol Inhaler (Rx)	6–16 cartridges/day	Irritation of mouth and throat	$210 (8 doses/day)
Nicotine nasal spray Nicotrol NS (Rx)	8–40 doses/day	Nasal irritation	$210 (10 doses/day)
Nicotine patch Nicoderm CQ, Nicotrol (OTC) Generics (OTC) Habitrol, ProStep (Rx)	21, 14, or 7 mg/24 hours 15, 10, or 5 mg/16 hours Use each strength for 2–4 weeks.	Local skin reaction Insomnia, vivid dreams	$60–$170

Medication	Dosage	Adverse Effects / Cautions	Price[a]
Bupropion SR Zyban or Wellbutrin SR (Rx) Generic (Rx)	150 mg q A.M. × 3 days, then 150 mg bid Start 1 week before quit date; continue 3–6 months.	Insomnia, dry mouth, nausea Neuropsychiatric changes Many drug interactions CONTRAINDICATED if history of or risk of seizures (see text) CAUTION if renal or hepatic dysfunction	$60–$230
Varenicline Chantix (Rx)	0.5 mg q A.M. × 3 days, then 0.5 mg bid × 4 days, then 1 mg bid Start 1 week before quit date; continue 3–6 months.	Nausea, insomnia, headache Neuropsychiatric changes Possible increase in CV events CAUTION if renal dysfunction	$180–$220
Second-Line Pharmacotherapies[b]			
Clonidine Catapres or Catapres patch (Rx) Generic	0.1–0.3 mg bid	Sedation, constipation Hypotension Risk of rebound hypertension	$15–$150
Nortriptyline Pamelor (Rx) Generic (Rx)	75–100 mg/day	Sedation, dry mouth, constipation	$15–$500

[a]Informal survey of prices in several pharmacies in the St. Louis, MO area, January, 2013.

[b]Not FDA approved for smoking cessation.

OTC, over the counter; ppd, pack per day; Rx, by prescription only; TTFC, time to first cigarette after waking.

increased serum nicotine levels. The reduction in ischemia correlated with reduced exhaled carbon monoxide levels, as the subjects spontaneously reduced their smoking while wearing the nicotine patches.[19,20] This clearly shows that **smoking while wearing a nicotine patch is not dangerous**.

- NRT use in high-risk smokers hospitalized with ACS or decompensated heart failure was safe and was associated with a decrease in readmissions and a decrease in all-cause mortality.[21]
- The American Heart Association and the American College of Cardiology support the use of NRT to aid in smoking cessation in patients with atherosclerotic vascular disease.[22–24]

Assessing Nicotine Dependence

- An estimate of a person's dependence on nicotine can guide dosing of NRT. Plasma levels of nicotine and cotinine vary from person to person, and only weakly correlate with the number of cigarettes smoked per day. A study in regular smokers found that among 1 pack per day (ppd) smokers, plasma cotinine levels varied 74-fold.[25]
  - Highly dependent persons smoke within 30 minutes of waking and typically smoke >one-half ppd.
  - Persons with low nicotine dependence wait more than 30 minutes for the first cigarette of the day and usually smoke <1 ppd.
- On an adequate dose of NRT, the patient will still have cravings but should feel relatively comfortable between cravings. If the NRT dose is too low, the patient will experience ongoing withdrawal symptoms and strong cravings. If the dose is too high, the patient will experience symptoms of nicotine overdose.

Specific Products

- **Nicotine gum** (polacrilex) is available over the counter in 2-mg and 4-mg strengths; the 4-mg strength is recommended for those who smoke more than 1 ppd and/or smoke within 30 minutes of awakening.
  - The nicotine is absorbed only through the buccal mucosa, and absorption is decreased by acidic beverages, so the patient should be instructed not to eat or drink while chewing the gum or 15 minutes before. Eating or drinking or rapid chewing will cause the nicotine to be swallowed, and it will cause heartburn, hiccups, or dyspepsia.
  - The gum should be chewed slowly until a peppery taste emerges, then left between the cheek and gum for buccal absorption. The gum should be chewed slowly and intermittently for approximately 30 minutes or until the taste dissipates.
  - It takes several minutes for the nicotine to reach the bloodstream, so there will not be the immediate satisfaction of smoking.
  - Patients will be more successful if they use at least 9 pieces a day.[26,27] They should use it on a fixed schedule, one piece every 1 to 2 hours for at least 1 to 3 months, then start to slowly taper the number of pieces per day (one piece per day every 4 to 7 days). The maximum daily dose is 24 pieces. Common side effects include mouth soreness, dyspepsia, and hiccups.
- **Nicotine lozenges** are available over the counter in 2-mg and 4-mg strengths; the 4-mg strength is recommended for those who smoke within 30 minutes of awakening.
  - Similar to the nicotine gum, the nicotine is absorbed through the buccal mucosa, so patients must not eat or drink while using it.
  - Patients will be more successful if they use at least 9 pieces a day: 1 piece every 1 to 2 hours for at least 1 to 3 months, then taper off. The maximum daily dose is 24 pieces. Side effects include mouth soreness, dyspepsia, and hiccups.
- **Nicotine patches** are available over the counter in several strengths, typically 21, 14, or 7 mg/day.
  - Most patients should start with the strongest patch, unless they smoke <10 cigarettes/day and wait more than 30 minutes to smoke after awakening. The highest strength

patch is used for 2 to 6 weeks, then the intermediate strength for 2 weeks, and then the lowest strength for 2 weeks.

- Highly dependent smokers may need 2 or more full-strength patches for adequate replacement therapy.
- Each morning, a patch should be placed on a relatively hairless location on the trunk or upper arm (hair may be shaved). Locations should be rotated to minimize skin irritation. Hands should be washed after handling patches. The used patch should be folded in half and thrown away out of reach of children and pets.
- Patches either may be used overnight to minimize morning cravings or may be taken off at bedtime to minimize insomnia and vivid dreams. If the patch is not worn overnight, morning withdrawal symptoms may be treated with a faster-acting form of nicotine.
- The most common side effects include insomnia and skin irritation. It is common to feel tingling under the patch for the first hour.
- **Nicotine nasal spray** is available by prescription only and is less popular with patients (expensive and awkward to use).
  - The spray has a faster onset of action than the gum or patch and therefore has greater potential for dependence.
  - The most common side effect is nasal irritation, which can be minimized by avoiding sniffing or inhaling while administering.
  - Patients should use one spray in each nostril (for a total dose of 1 mg) and should use 1 to 2 doses/hour with a maximum of 40 doses/day.
- **Nicotine inhalers** are available by prescription only and are also less popular with patients (expensive and awkward to use).
  - Each cartridge delivers 4 mg nicotine over 80 inhalations. Patients should use 6 to 16 cartridges daily for up to 6 months. The vapor is absorbed in the mouth and throat and has a fairly fast onset of action. The inhaler is puffed frequently for 20 minutes (much more frequently than a cigarette).
  - Because the nicotine is absorbed only through the buccal mucosa and absorption is decreased by acidic beverages, the patient should be instructed not to eat or drink while using the inhaler or 15 minutes before.
  - The most common side effects are irritation of the mouth and throat, coughing, dyspepsia, and rhinitis.

Nonnicotine Medications

Bupropion

- Bupropion SR is thought to work by enhancing dopaminergic activity in the central nervous system.
- In randomized controlled trials, subjects treated with bupropion SR had **abstinence rates of about twice that of the placebo group**.[28] Efficacy is independent of a history of depression.
- Bupropion SR should be started 1 to 2 weeks before the quit date at 150 mg each morning for 3 days, then 150 mg twice daily for 7 to 12 weeks. Evening dosing may lead to insomnia so the second dose should be in the late afternoon. A lower dose of 150 mg once daily may be as effective as twice-daily dosing.[29]
- Studies have used bupropion for 7 to 52 weeks. Longer duration was associated with delay and attenuation of relapse and weight gain.[30]
- The most common side effects are insomnia (about 20%), dry mouth, and nausea.
- Due to a risk of seizures (approximately 1 in 1,000), bupropion SR should not be used in patients with a history of seizure, head trauma, and brain tumor; in those with anorexia/bulimia and hepatic failure; or in those using drugs that may increase the risk of seizures (theophylline, systemic steroids, antipsychotics, antidepressants, hypoglycemics/insulin, or abuse of alcohol or stimulants).
- Bupropion SR is contraindicated in patients with use of a monoamine oxidase inhibitor within 14 days.

- In 2008, the U.S. Food and Drug Administration (FDA) warned of neuropsychiatric symptoms and **suicidal events**, even in individuals with no history of psychiatric disease, based on postmarketing reports.[31] Patients should be monitored for changes in behavior, hostility, agitation, depressed mood, or suicidal ideation.

Varenicline

- The newest medication approved for smoking cessation is varenicline, a partial nicotine agonist. It binds to the α4β2-nicotinic acetylcholine receptors, stimulating dopamine release to reduce craving and withdrawal symptoms while also blocking binding of nicotine to reduce the reinforcing effects of smoking (satisfaction).
- Varenicline has been shown to **more than double the placebo quit rate** and may be more effective than bupropion.[4,32,33]
- Varenicline should be started at least a week prior to the patient's quit date at 0.5 mg once daily for 3 days, then 0.5 mg twice daily for 4 days, and then 1 mg twice daily. Varenicline should be continued for 12 weeks; successful quitters may be continued for an additional 12 weeks to reduce relapses.
- The most common adverse effects of varenicline were nausea (in more than one-quarter patients), headache, vomiting, flatulence, insomnia, abnormal dreams, and dysgeusia. Nausea is reduced when varenicline is taken with food and a glass of water.
- The FDA has warned of neuropsychiatric symptoms and **suicidal events**, even in individuals with no history of psychiatric disease, based on postmarketing reports.[31] Patients should be monitored for changes in behavior, hostility, agitation, depressed mood, or suicidal ideation. The FDA also warned that patients taking varenicline may experience impairment of the ability to drive or operate heavy machinery.[34]
- In 2011, the FDA warned that varenicline may increase the risk of adverse cardiovascular events in patients with known cardiovascular (CV) disease.[35] This was based on a trial that showed a nonsignificant increase in CV events.[36] A 2011 meta-analysis showed a statistically significant increase in CV events, while a 2012 meta-analysis showed no statistically significant difference in rates of CV events with varenicline.[37,38] A large prospective cohort study published in 2012 showed no increase in the risk of major cardiovascular events in varenicline users versus bupropion.[39]

Other Medications

- **Nortriptyline** is considered a second-line agent.
  - It is not FDA approved for smoking cessation, but there have been several published reports that demonstrate efficacy in smoking cessation that exceeds placebo but is less than bupropion.[40]
  - As with other tricyclic antidepressants, nortriptyline often causes dry mouth, constipation, and sedation.
  - An advantage of nortriptyline is its affordability.
- **Clonidine** is considered a second-line agent.
  - Clonidine **can approximately double the quit rate** and is inexpensive. However, it is rarely used for smoking cessation due to troublesome side effects including dry mouth, sedation, and orthostatic hypotension. Abrupt cessation of high-dose clonidine can cause rebound hypertension.
  - For smoking cessation, clonidine is usually used at low doses, 0.1 to 0.2 mg twice daily.
- Benzodiazepines and selective serotonin reuptake inhibitors (SSRIs) are **not** effective for smoking cessation.

Combination Therapy

- Combination therapy with the nicotine patch and a faster-acting form (gum, lozenge, spray, inhaler) has been shown to be more effective than with either alone.[4,41]
- Bupropion combined with NRT is more effective than with either alone.[4,21,42]

Special Circumstances

Pregnancy and Lactation

- Clinicians should provide intensive counseling to help pregnant and lactating women quit smoking.
- Nicotine gum is rated category C, and the patches are rated category D, but the circulating nicotine levels are only about half those seen in pack-a-day smokers, and NRT lacks the carbon monoxide and toxic chemicals of tobacco smoke.
  ○ It has been suggested that NRT be considered if prior attempts to quit have been unsuccessful and the patient continues to smoke while pregnant.[43]
  ○ The American Congress of Obstetricians and Gynecologists (ACOG) opinion states that NRT "must be used under close medical supervision and only after weighing the known risks of smoking against the possible risks of the NRT during pregnancy."[44]
  ○ Each patient should be informed about the presumed risks and benefits.
- Bupropion is rated as category C. ACOG reviewed the literature on the use of antidepressants during pregnancy and concluded that the limited data available do not suggest an increased risk of fetal anomalies or adverse pregnancy events with bupropion.[45]
- Varenicline is rated as category C. There are no studies of its use in pregnancy.

Cardiovascular Disease

- NRT has been extensively studied and has been found to be **safe for patients with stable coronary artery disease** and to actually decrease myocardial ischemia (see above section on "Safety of NRT in Patients with Cardiovascular Disease").
- Bupropion has been found to be safe and effective in a study of patients hospitalized with ACS or decompensated heart failure.[21] The intervention group received counseling plus bupropion and/or NRT (47% used bupropion with or without NRT). Over the 2-year follow-up period, the intervention patients had less than half as many readmissions and only one-quarter of the mortality rate; the absolute risk reduction in mortality was 9.2% with a number needed to treat of 11.
- Bupropion overdose can cause tachycardia, conduction delays, and arrhythmias.
- The studies to date on varenicline in CV patients have had mixed results (see "Varenicline" section above).

REFERENCES

1. Current cigarette smoking among adults—United States, 2011. *MMWR* 2012;61(44): 889–894.
2. CDC. Quitting smoking among adults—United States, 2001–2010. *MMWR* 2011;60: 1513–1519.
3. Jarvis MJ. ABC of smoking cessation: why people smoke. *BMJ* 2004;328(7434):277–9.
4. Fiore MC, Jaen CR, Baker TB, et al. *Clinical Practice Guideline. Treating Tobacco Use and Dependence: 2008 Update*. Rockville, MD: U.S. Department of Health and Human Services, Public Health Service; 2008. http://www.ahrq.gov/professionals/clinicians-providers/guide-lines-recommendations/tobacco/clinicians/update/index.html. Last accessed 1/15/15.
5. Gonzales D, Jorenby DE, Brandon TH, et al. Immediate versus delayed quitting and rates of relapse among smokers treated successfully with varenicline, bupropion SR or placebo. *Addiction* 2010;105:2002–13.
6. Aubin HJ, Farley A, Lycett D, et al. Weight gain in smokers after quitting cigarettes: meta-analysis. *BMJ* 2012;345:e4439.
7. Roberts V, Maddison R, Simpson C, et al. The acute effects of exercise on cigarette cravings, withdrawal symptoms, affect, and smoking behaviour: systematic review update and meta-analysis. *Psychopharmacology (Berl)* 2012;222:1–15.
8. Farley AC, Hajek P, Lycett D, et al. Interventions for preventing weight gain after smoking cessation. *Cochrane Database Syst Rev* 2012;(1):CD006219.

9. Dicpinigaitis PV, Sitkauskiene B, Stravinskaite K, et al. Effect of smoking cessation on cough reflex sensitivity. *Eur Respir J* 2006;28:786–90.

10. Tobacco Free Kids. *State Cigarette Tax Rates & Rank, Date of Last Increase, Annual Pack Sales & Revenues, and Related Data.* Washington DC: Tobacco Free Kids. Available at: www.tobaccofreekids.org/research/factsheets/pdf/0099.pdf. Last accessed 1/14/15.

11. Miller WR, Rollnick S. *Motivational Interviewing: Preparing People for Change,* 2nd ed. New York: Guilford Press; 2002.

12. Royal College of Physicians. *Harm Reduction in Nicotine Addiction: Helping People Who Can't Quit. A Report by the Tobacco Advisory Group of the Royal College of Physicians.* London: Royal College of Physicians, 2007. Available at: http://www.rcplondon.ac.uk/sites/default/files/documents/harm-reduction-nicotine-addiction.pdf. Last accessed 1/14/15.

13. U.S. Department of Health and Human Services. *The Health Consequences of Involuntary Exposure to Tobacco Smoke: A Report of the Surgeon General. Secondhand Smoke What It Means to You.* U.S. Department of Health and Human Services, Centers for Disease Control and Prevention, Coordinating Center for Health Promotion, National Center for Chronic Disease Prevention and Health Promotion, Office on Smoking and Health, 2006. Available: http://www.surgeongeneral.gov/library/reports/. Last accessed 1/15/15.

14. Bobak A. Perceived safety of nicotine replacement products among general practitioners and current smokers in the UK: impact on utilization. UK National Smoking Cessation Conference, 2005. Available at: www.uknscc.org/2005_UKNSCC/speakers/alex_bobak.html. Last accessed 1/15/15.

15. Blann AD, Steele C, McCollum CN. The influence of smoking and of oral and transdermal nicotine on blood pressure, and haematology and coagulation indices. *Thromb Haemost* 1997;78:1093–1096.

16. Tzivoni D, Keren A, Meyler S, et al. Cardiovascular safety of transdermal nicotine patches in patients with coronary artery disease who try to quit smoking. *Cardiovasc Drugs Ther* 1998;12:239–244.

17. Woolf KJ, Zabad MN, Post JM, et al. Effect of nicotine replacement therapy on cardiovascular outcomes after acute coronary syndromes. *Am J Cardiol* 2012;110;968–970.

18. Murray RP, Bailey WC, Daniels K, et al. Safety of nicotine polacrilex gum used by 3,094 participants in the Lung Health Study. Lung Health Study Research Group. *Chest* 1996;109:438–445.

19. Mahmarian JJ, Moyé LA, Nasser GA, et al. Nicotine patch therapy in smoking cessation reduces the extent of exercise-induced myocardial ischemia. *J Am Coll Cardiol* 1997;30:125–130.

20. Leja M. Nicotine patches are safe to use in patients with coronary artery disease and stress induced myocardial ischemia. *J Am Coll Cardiol* 2007;49(9S1):209A.

21. Mohiuddin SM, Mooss AN, Hunter CB, et al. Intensive smoking cessation intervention reduces mortality in high-risk smokers with cardiovascular disease. *Chest* 2007;131:446–452.

22. Ockene IS, Miller NH. Cigarette smoking, cardiovascular disease, and stroke: a statement for healthcare professionals from the American Heart Association. American Heart Association Task Force on Risk Reduction. *Circulation* 1997;96:3243–3247.

23. Smith SC Jr, Benjamin EJ, Bonow RO, et al. AHA/ACCF secondary prevention and risk reduction therapy for patients with coronary and other atherosclerotic vascular disease: 2011 update. *J Am Coll Cardiol* 2011;58:2432–2446.

24. Rooke TW, Hirsch AT, Sanjay Misra S, et al. 2011 ACCF/AHA focused update of the guideline for the management of patients with peripheral artery disease (updating the 2005 guideline). *J Am Coll Cardiol* 2011;58:2020–2045.

25. Muscat JE, Stellman SD, Caraballo RS, et al. Time to first cigarette after waking predicts cotinine levels. *Cancer Epidemiol Biomarkers Prev* 2009;18:3415–3420.

26. Garvey AJ, Kinnunen T, Nordstrom BL, et al. Effects of nicotine gum dose by level of nicotine dependence. *Nicotine Tob Res* 2000;2:53–63.

27. Sachs DP. Effectiveness of the 4-mg dose of nicotine polacrilex for the initial treatment of high-dependent smokers. *Arch Intern Med* 1995;155:1973–1980.

28. Hughes JR, Stead LF, Lancaster T. Antidepressants for smoking cessation. *Cochrane Database Syst Rev* 2014;(2):CD000031.

29. Hurt RD, Sachs DP, Glover ED, et al. A comparison of sustained-release bupropion and placebo for smoking cessation. *N Engl J Med* 1997;337:1195–1202.

30. Hays JT, Hurt RD, Rigotti NA, et al. Sustained-release bupropion for pharmacologic relapse prevention after smoking cessation. A randomized, controlled trial. *Ann Intern Med* 2001;135:423–433.

31. U.S. Food and Drug Administration. *Information for Healthcare Professionals: Varenicline (marketed as Chantix) and Bupropion (marketed as Zyban, Wellbutrin, and generics).* U.S. Department of Health and Human Services; 2009. Available at: http://www.fda.gov/Drugs/DrugSafety/PostmarketDrugSafetyInformationforPatientsandProviders/DrugSafetyInformationforHeathcareProfessionals/ucm169986.htm. Last accessed 1/15/15.

32. Gonzales D, Rennard SI, Nides M, et al. Varenicline, an alpha4beta2 nicotinic acetylcholine receptor partial agonist, vs sustained-release bupropion and placebo for smoking cessation: a randomized controlled trial. *JAMA* 2006;296:47–55.

33. Jorenby DE, Hays JT, Rigotti NA, et al. Efficacy of varenicline, an alpha4beta2 nicotinic acetylcholine receptor partial agonist, vs placebo or sustained-release bupropion for smoking cessation: a randomized controlled trial. *JAMA* 2006;296:56–63.

34. U.S. Food and Drug Administration. *Public Health Advisory: Important Information on Chantix (varenicline).* U.S. Department of Health and Human Services; 2008. Available at: www.fda.gov/Drugs/DrugSafety/PostmarketDrugSafetyInformationfor PatientsandProviders/DrugSafetyInformationforHeathcareProfessionals/PublicHealth Advisories/ucm051136.htm. Last accessed 1/15/15.

35. U.S. Food and Drug Administration. *FDA Drug Safety Communication: Chantix (varenicline) may Increase the Risk of Certain Cardiovascular Adverse Events in Patients with Cardiovascular Disease.* U.S. Department of Health and Human Services, 2011. Available at: http://www.fda.gov/Drugs/DrugSafety/ucm259161.htm. Last accessed 1/15/15.

36. Rigotti NA, Pipe AL, Benowitz NL, et al. Efficacy and safety of varenicline for smoking cessation in patients with cardiovascular disease: a randomized trial. *Circulation* 2010;121:221–229.

37. Singh S, Loke YK, Spangler JG, et al. Risk of serious adverse cardiovascular events associated with varenicline: a systematic review and meta-analysis. *CMAJ* 2011;183:1359–1366.

38. Prochaska JJ, Hilton JF. Risk of cardiovascular serious adverse events associated with varenicline use for tobacco cessation: systematic review and meta-analysis. *BMJ* 2012;344:e2856.

39. Svanström H, Pasternak B, Hviid A. Use of varenicline for smoking cessation and risk of serious cardiovascular events: nationwide cohort study. *BMJ* 2012;345:e7176.

40. Hughes JR, Stead LF, Lancaster T. Nortriptyline for smoking cessation: a review. *Nicotine Tob Res* 2005;7:491–499.

41. Smith SS, McCarthy DE, Japuntich SJ, et al. Comparative effectiveness of 5 smoking cessation pharmacotherapies in primary care clinics. *Arch Intern Med* 2009;169:2148–2155.

42. Stead LF, Perera R, Bullen C, et al. Nicotine replacement therapy for smoking cessation. *Cochrane Database Syst Rev* 2012;(11):CD000146.

43. Benowitz N, Dempsey D. Pharmacotherapy for smoking cessation during pregnancy. *Nicotine Tob Res* 2004;6(suppl 2):S189–S202.

44. American College of Obstetricians and Gynecologists. Committee Opinion No. 471: smoking cessation during pregnancy. *Obstet Gynecol* 2010;116:1241–1244.

45. American College of Obstetricians and Gynecologists. Use of psychiatric medications during pregnancy and lactation. ACOG Practice Bulletin No. 92. *Obstet Gynecol* 2008;111:1001–1020.

46 Alcohol Abuse and Dependence

Luigi R. Cardella and Luis A. Giuffra

GENERAL PRINCIPLES

Alcohol use disorders (AUDs) are commonly encountered in primary care. Although modest alcohol use has proven cardioprotective benefits, abuse of alcohol can have detrimental physical, mental, emotional, and social effects. Alcohol-related health problems are numerous, including hepatic cirrhosis, pancreatitis, hypertension, cardiomyopathy, numerous cancers, dementia, and gastrointestinal bleeding. Fetal alcohol syndrome is the number one known cause of intellectual disability. Alcohol abuse and dependence have a heavy burden on society as a whole, as alcohol has been cited in half of all homicides and traffic fatalities. Patients of all ages, races, and socioeconomic status can suffer from alcoholism, and physicians should screen patients for alcohol use and abuse in each patient encounter.

Definitions

- **Alcohol abuse** is defined by the Diagnostic and Statistical Manual (**DSM**) **IV** as a maladaptive pattern of use associated with one or more of the following:
  - Failure to fulfill work, school, or social obligations
  - Recurrent substance use in physically hazardous situations
  - Recurrent legal problems related to substance use
  - Continued use despite alcohol-related social or interpersonal problems
- **Alcohol dependence (DSM IV)** is a maladaptive pattern of use associated with three of the following seven behaviors over a 12-month interval:
  - Tolerance.
  - Evidence of withdrawal.
  - Alcohol ingested in larger quantity than intended.
  - Significant time spent obtaining or using alcohol.
  - Persistent desire to cut back or discontinue alcohol use.
  - Alcohol use continues despite physical and psychological distress.
  - Social or occupational tasks are harmed.
- Of note, while 50% of patients with alcohol abuse will persistently have alcohol problems, only 10% will actually go on to develop dependence.
- The new **DSM V** combines alcohol abuse and dependence under **alcohol use disorder** (AUD). Anyone meeting any 2 of the 11 following criteria over the preceding 12 months may be diagnosed with AUD. The presence of 2 to 3 criteria is mild AUD, 4 to 5 moderate, and ≥6 severe.
  - Alcohol is taken in larger amounts or over a longer time than intended
  - Persistent desire or unsuccessful attempts to control or reduce alcohol consumption
  - A significant time spent in activities to obtain alcohol, use alcohol, or recover from its effects
  - Craving, urge, or strong desire to drink
  - Recurrent drinking causing failure to fulfill obligations at work, school, or home
  - Continued drinking in spite of recurrent or persistent social or interpersonal problems caused or exacerbated by alcohol

- ○ Reducing or giving up important social, occupational, or recreational activities due to drinking
- ○ Recurrent drinking when it is physically hazardous
- ○ Continued drinking in spite of knowing that alcohol is causing or exacerbating a persistent or recurrent physical or psychological problem
- ○ Tolerance
  - ▪ Need for increased amounts of alcohol to achieve the same effect
  - ▪ Reduced effect with continued use of the same amount of alcohol
- ○ Withdrawal
  - ▪ Characteristic withdrawal symptoms
  - ▪ Alcohol or another substance used to avoid or relieve withdrawal symptoms
- The National Institute of Alcohol Abuse and Alcoholism defines so-called at-risk drinking as follows:
  - ○ Men, >14 drinks per week or >4 drinks per occasion
  - ○ Women, >7 drinks per week or >3 drinks per occasion
  - ○ Those who habitually drink above these levels are at risk for alcoholism and alcohol-related problems

Epidemiology

- At some point in their lifetime, over 90% of the US population has had an alcoholic drink, and 80% of all high school seniors have had a drink by graduation.
- A recent study showed the lifetime prevalence of alcohol abuse to be 17.8% and the lifetime prevalence of alcohol dependence to be 12.5%.[1]
- After smoking and obesity, alcoholism is the third leading cause of preventable death in the US.
- Approximately 85,000 deaths a year in the US are attributed to alcohol, and the estimated costs attributed to alcohol are $185 billion yearly.[2]
- Binge drinking, defined as >5 drinks in a sitting for men and >4 drinks in a sitting for women, is prevalent among teens and college students. It contributes to high levels of risky sexual behavior, drunk driving, and poor academic performance in this patient population.
- It should be noted that patients with AUDs come from all walks of life. Physicians should not refrain from asking patients about alcohol use because they do not fit the stereotype of a typical alcoholic. **All patients should be screened for possible alcohol use.**

Risk Factors

- Rates of alcohol abuse are higher in young males, single patients, those with lower income, and those from Native American or Caucasian descent. The prevalence of alcoholism is twice as high in men as in women.
- Studies have shown that those who begin drinking at an earlier age are much more likely to develop alcoholism than those who start after age 21.
- Recent evidence has shown that genetic factors can play a role in the development of alcoholism. Identical twins have been found to have a higher concordance of alcohol use than fraternal twins.

Associated Conditions

- AUDs are associated with numerous conditions, including depression, anxiety, and other substance use disorders.
- Patients who present with AUDs should be screened for **coexisting substance abuse or psychiatric disorders**.
- Data from 1998 show that 30% of smokers are alcoholics and 80% of alcoholics are smokers.[3]

DIAGNOSIS

- See the "Definitions" section for precise definitions of alcohol abuse/dependence and AUD.
- In this context, **screening may be a more appropriate term**.
- It should be noted in the definitions of alcohol abuse and dependence that the amount of alcohol consumed is not important. Although the consumption of higher amounts of alcohol may put someone at an elevated risk for an AUD, **the amount itself does not diagnose someone as having a disorder**.

Clinical Presentation

- As alcoholism can affect patients from all walks of life, physicians must **maintain a high index of suspicion** and should question patients about alcohol consumption at each encounter.
- **Screening should be done with validated tests** such as the CAGE or AUDIT (Alcohol Use Disorder Identification Test) questionnaires (see the "Diagnostic Testing" section).
- Physicians should be nonconfrontational and use nonjudgmental language when questioning patients about alcohol use.
- **Patients frequently deny alcohol problems** for a variety of reasons, including refusing to acknowledge the disease, shame or embarrassment, social stigma of being an alcoholic, and fear of being reported to employers or family members.
- Although physicians should be firm in discussing alcohol abuse with patients, they must also be empathic and should listen to what patients have to say about their disease.
- A mental status examination should be documented even if the patient is suspected to be intoxicated. However, a repeat examination is compulsory when the patient is no longer intoxicated.
- Unless patients are intoxicated at the time of examination, the physical exam is not of great help in diagnosing alcohol disorders.
- Signs of chronic alcohol use include testicular atrophy, gynecomastia, spider angiomata, enlarged spleen, and shrunken or enlarged liver.

Differential Diagnosis

Conditions which may be associated, or confused, with alcohol disorders include depression, anxiety disorder, bipolar disorder, insomnia, and dysthymic disorder.

Diagnostic Testing

- The older CAGE questionnaire is the best-studied screening test for AUDs and is presented in Table 46-1.[4]
  - Patients who answer yes to any of the CAGE questions require further assessment and intervention. **Patients who answer yes to two out of the four questions are seven times more likely to have alcohol dependence** than the general population.
  - The sensitivity and specificity of two affirmative responses to the CAGE questionnaire is 77% and 79%, respectively; these values decrease for unhealthy alcohol use.[5] Critics point out that it fails to identify binge drinkers and it does not distinguish current from

TABLE 46-1 CAGE Questionnaire

Have you ever felt the need to **CUT** down your drinking?
Have people **ANNOYED** you by criticizing your drinking?
Have you ever felt **GUILTY** about your drinking?
Have you ever had an **EYE-OPENER** to steady your nerves or to rid yourself of a hangover in the morning?

TABLE 46-2 Alcohol Use Disorders Identification Test

1. How often do you have a drink containing alcohol?
   (0) Never (skip   (1) ≤Monthly   (2) 2–4 times/   (3) 2–3 times/   (4) ≥4 times/
     to questions   month   week   week
     9 and 10)

2. How many drinks containing alcohol do you have on a typical day when you are drinking?
   (0) 1–2   (1) 3–4   (2) 5–6   (3) 7–9   (4) ≥10

3. How often do you have six or more drinks on one occasion?
   (0) Never   (1)<Monthly   (2) Monthly   (3) 2–3 times/   (4) ≥4 times/
                                                     week   week

Skip to questions 9 and 10 if total for questions 2 and 3 = 0

4. How often during the last year have you found that you were not able to stop drinking once you had started?
   (0) Never   (1)<Monthly   (2) Monthly   (3) 2–3 times/   (4) ≥4 times/
                                                     week   week

5. How often during the last year have you failed to do what was normally expected from you because of drinking?
   (0) Never   (1) <Monthly   (2) Monthly   (3) 2–3 times/   (4) ≥4 times/
                                                     week   week

6. How often during the last year have you needed a first drink in the morning to get yourself going after a heavy drinking session?
   (0) Never   (1) <Monthly   (2) Monthly   (3) 2–3 times/   (4) ≥4 times/
                                                     week   week

7. How often during the last year have you had a feeling of guilt or remorse after drinking?
   (0) Never   (1) <Monthly   (2) Monthly   (3) 2–3 times/   (4) ≥4 times/
                                                     week   week

8. How often during the last year have you been unable to remember what happened the night before because you had been drinking?
   (0) Never   (1) <Monthly   (2) Monthly   (3) 2–3 times/   (4) ≥4 times/
                                                     week   week

9. Have you or someone else been injured as a result of your drinking?
   (0) No   (2) Yes, but   (4) Yes, during
                                            not in the   the last
                                            last year   year

10. Has a relative or friend or a doctor or other health worker been concerned about your drinking or suggested you cut down?
    (0) No   (2) Yes, but   (4) Yes, during
                                             not in the   the last
                                             last year   year

Total score ≥8 indicates hazardous and harmful alcohol use, as well as possible alcohol dependence (≥7 for women and men >65 years).
Modified from Babor TF, Higgins-Biddle JC, Saunders JB, et al. *AUDIT. The Alcohol Use Disorders Identification Test: Guidelines for Use in Primary Care*, 2nd ed. Geneva, Switzerland: World Health Organization Department of Mental Health and Substance Dependence; 2001.

past alcohol use. Although it may have its flaws, **it remains a reasonable tool to screen patients** and is quick, easy to use, and easy to remember.
- Another screening tool is the AUDIT questionnaire (Table 46-2).[6–9]
  - **Studies have shown that the AUDIT to be superior to the CAGE questionnaire in patients with active alcohol abuse or dependence.**[10] It has also been found to have a higher sensitivity in populations with low rates of alcohol use.

TABLE 46-3 | **AUDIT-C Questionnaire**

1. How often do you have a drink containing alcohol?

   (0) Never   (1) ≤Monthly   (2) 2–4 times/   (3) 2–3 times/   (4) ≥4 times/

                                                       month   week   week

2. How many drinks containing alcohol do you have on a typical day when you are drinking?

   (0) 1–2   (1) 3–4   (2) 5–6   (3) 7–9   (4) ≥10

3. How often do you have six or more drinks on one occasion?

   (0) Never   (1) <Monthly   (2) Monthly   (3) Weekly   (4) Daily or

                                                                            almost

                                                                            daily

Scoring: ≥4 points for men or ≥3 points for women constitutes a positive screen.

- ○ The abbreviated three-item AUDIT-C questionnaire may also be an effective screening tool in primary care settings (Table 46-3).[8,11–14]
- **Perhaps, easiest of all in primary care is single question screening:** "How many times in the past year have you had 5 (4 for women) or more drinks containing alcohol?" One or more heavy drinking days constitutes a positive screen.[8,15]
- **Laboratory testing** does not have a prominent role in diagnosing AUDs.
  - ○ Although tests such as γ-glutamyltransferase (GGT), liver function tests, and mean corpuscular volume can be abnormal in patients with chronic alcohol use, their sensitivity does not approach 50%, and they **should not be used as screening laboratories**. They can be checked, however, when evaluating patients with chronic alcohol use to help manage patients.
  - ○ Blood alcohol levels may be useful in patients who appear to be intoxicated.
  - ○ Ethyl glucuronide (EtG) can be detected in various body fluids, tissue, and hair up to 80 hours after the complete elimination of alcohol from the body. This marker has a serum sensitivity of 92% and specificity of 91%.[16]

TREATMENT

- The first step in treating patients with alcohol abuse and dependence is making the patient aware that they have a disease. This should be done in an empathic and nonjudgmental manner.
- Patients must be willing to change. The physician must listen to the patient and assess their readiness and willingness to change.
- Involving family members and friends is a good strategy to ensure that the patient has a strong support network when they leave the office. This should not be done without approval of the patient.
- **Brief interventions have been shown to reduce alcohol consumption.**[17]
- Physicians should remember the Five As when conducting a brief intervention[8,18]:
  - ○ **Ask**: Ask about alcohol use (see the "Diagnosis" section).
  - ○ **Advise**: Advise patients that their drinking puts them at high risk for alcoholism and alcohol-related problems. The specific effects of high-risk drinking should be explained.
  - ○ **Assess**: Assess the patient's readiness to change and advise accordingly (see below).
  - ○ **Assist**: Provide specific self-help information.
  - ○ **Arrange**: Arrange follow-up.
- Although not without critics, the Prochaska **transtheoretical model of stages of change** is relatively well known to many clinicians, and may serve to provide some very general

guidelines regarding how much and what type of effort to invest.[19,20] To some extent, the dividing lines between stages are arbitrary, individuals may not progress in a sequential manner between the stages, and the stages may not be mutually exclusive.

- **Precontemplation stage:** The person is unaware or underaware of the problem and has no intention of changing the behavior. The physician's role is to advise the patient about the need to reduce alcohol consumption and the hazards of drinking. The counseling can be quite brief, just a minute or two, but should be repeated at every visit.
- **Contemplation stage:** The patient is aware that a problem exists but is not yet ready to make a full commitment to take action. This stage may last for long periods of time. The physician's role is to continue stressing the hazards of drinking and the benefits of behavior change. How to choose a goal can also be discussed.
- **Preparation stage:** The patient intends to take action in the next few months; this may be a brief stage. The physician should increase the intensity and specificity of counseling and help the patient choose a goal and give advice and encouragement. When a patient is really ready to commit to change, this should be the main focus of the office visit.
- **Action stage:** This is the most visible stage in which the addictive behavior is altered (for 1 day to 6 months). Review specific advice and continue to provide encouragement.
- **Maintenance stage:** The patient maintains the change and works to prevent relapse. This stage extends beyond 6 months and may last a lifetime. The physician should provide follow-up and continued encouragement.
- **Relapse stage:** This can also be termed recycle because the patient again moves through the cycle and may achieve long-term success on subsequent cycles. The physician should assist the patient in renewing the process.

- Patients should be encouraged to avoid bars and social gatherings which may strongly encourage the patient to drink, and to seek help when relapse is near. Patients must learn how to cope with stress and anxiety once they abstain from alcohol.
- Constant follow-up is an integral part of treating patients. Unfortunately, **<25% of patients will stay abstinent after a year.** Given this high relapse rate, physicians and patients may find treatment difficult and frustrating. Nevertheless, continued and consistent interaction with the patient is key to successful recovery.

Medications

- **Disulfiram**, an inhibitor of the enzyme aldehyde dehydrogenase, has been used to treat patients with AUDs once they become abstinent. Consumption of alcohol results in the accumulation of acetaldehyde and the development of symptoms including tachycardia, dyspnea, flushing, nausea, vomiting, headache, hypotension, and dizziness. Data supporting the use of disulfiram is equivocal.[21,22] It may be more effective when compliance is monitored.[8]
- **Naltrexone**, an opiate antagonist, has been used in alcoholics to decrease use. Several reviews have generally supported the use of naltrexone.[8,23–27] The COMBINE study found better outcomes with the addition of naltrexone to medical management.[28]
- **Acamprosate** is a structural analog of γ-amino butyric acid but its mechanism of action is not fully understood. Reviews also support its use.[8,23,25,27,29] However, in the COMBINE study, acamprosate was not more effective than placebo.[27,28]
- Benzodiazepines, β-blockers, clonidine, and anticonvulsants have all been used to treat alcohol withdrawal.

Other Nonpharmacologic Therapies

- Brief interventions are 10 to 15 minutes patient encounters where counseling, feedback, goal setting, and follow-up are discussed. Numerous trials have shown these encounters to be effective in reducing drinking and increasing abstinence.[17]

- The COMBINE study also demonstrated that cognitive behavior therapy was a helpful addition to medical management.[28]
- Alcoholics Anonymous and other support groups are effective community resources for patients. Physicians should have information about these resources in their office for patients who are willing to use them.

Lifestyle/Risk Modification

- Patients should be educated that abstinence is the most effective method of preventing relapse. Patients should adjust their lifestyle as much as possible to optimize their chance of remaining abstinent.
- This includes avoiding bars and other social gatherings where the pressure to drink may be significant.
- In addition, patients should be aware of relapse triggers and should have numbers to call if they are in a situation where they may falter.
- Patients with AUDs are prone to poor nutrition and may benefit from vitamin supplementation, especially folic acid.
- Patients with alcohol abuse and dependence should be warned against driving and operating machinery when intoxicated.

SPECIAL CONSIDERATIONS

Patients who are withdrawing from alcohol, have delirium tremens or hallucinations, or have significant psychiatric comorbidity should be considered for inpatient treatment. Detailed discussion of these disorders is beyond the scope of this chapter.

COMPLICATIONS

- Patients who continue to abuse alcohol are predisposed to numerous health conditions. These include cirrhosis, dementia, Wernicke-Korsakoff syndrome, heart disease, malnutrition, pancreatitis, and numerous cancers.
- Women should especially be cautious when pregnant, as even small amounts of alcohol use have been shown to have negative effects on the growing fetus.

REFERRAL

Referrals to a psychiatrist can be helpful in patients with comorbid psychiatric disease such as depression or bipolar disorder.

REFERENCES

1. Hasin DS, Stinson FS, Ogburn E, et al. Prevalence, correlates, disability, and comorbidity of DSM-IV alcohol abuse and dependence in the United States: results from the National Epidemiologic Survey on Alcohol and Related Conditions. *Arch Gen Psychiatry* 2007;64:830–842.
2. Saitz R. Clinical practice. Unhealthy alcohol use. *N Engl J Med* 2005;352:596–607.
3. Miller NS, Gold MS. Comorbid cigarette and alcohol addiction: epidemiology and treatment. *J Addict Dis* 1998;17:55–66.
4. Mayfield D, McLeod G, Hall P. *Am J Psychiatry* 1974;131:1121–1123.
5. Maisto SA, Saitz R. Alcohol use disorders: screening and diagnosis. *Am J Addict* 2003;12(suppl 1):S12–S25.

6. Saunders JB, Aasland OG, Babor TF, et al. Development of the Alcohol Use Disorders Identification Test (AUDIT): WHO Collaborative Project on early detection of persons with harmful alcohol consumption—II. *Addiction* 1993;88:791–804.

7. Babor TF, Higgins-Biddle JC, Saunders JB, et al. *AUDIT. The Alcohol Use Disorders Identification Test: Guidelines for Use in Primary Care*, 2nd ed. Geneva, Switzerland: World Health Organization Department of Mental Health and Substance Dependence; 2001.

8. National Institute on Alcohol Abuse and Alcoholism. *Helping Patients Who Drink Too Much: A Clinician's Guide. Updated 2005 Edition*. NIH Publication No. 07-3769. Washington, DC: National Institute on Alcohol Abuse and Alcoholism; 2007.

9. Berner MM, Kriston L, Bentele M, et al. The alcohol use disorders identification test for detecting at-risk drinking: a systematic review and meta-analysis. *J Stud Alcohol Drugs* 2007;68:461–473.

10. Bradley KA, Bush KR, McDonell MB, et al.; The Ambulatory Care Quality Improvement Project (ACQUIP). Screening for problem drinking: Comparison of CAGE and AUDIT. *J Gen Intern Med* 1998;13:379–388.

11. Taj N, Devera-Sales A, Vinson DC. Screening for problem drinking: does a single question work? *J Fam Pract* 1998;46:328–335.

12. Williams R, Vinson DC. Validation of a single screening question for problem drinking. *J Fam Pract* 2001;50:307–312.

13. Seale JP, Boltri JM, Shellenberger S, et al. Primary care validation of a single screening question for drinkers. *J Stud Alcohol* 2006;67:778–784.

14. Kriston L, Hölzel L, Weiser AK, et al. Meta-analysis: are 3 questions enough to detect unhealthy alcohol use? *Ann Intern Med* 2008;149:879–888.

15. Smith PC, Schmidt SM, Allensworth-Davies D, et al. Primary care validation of a single-question alcohol screening test. *J Gen Intern Med* 2009;24:783–788.

16. Zimmer H, Schmitt G, Aderjan R. Preliminary immunochemical test for the determination of ethyl glucuronide in serum and urine: comparison of screening method results with gas chromatography-mass spectrometry. *J Anal Toxicol* 2002;26:11–16.

17. Kaner EF, Beyer F, Dickinson HO, et al. Effectiveness of brief alcohol interventions in primary care populations. *Cochrane Database Syst Rev* 2007;(2):CD004148.

18. Babor TF, Higgins-Biddle JC. *Brief Intervention for Hazardous and Harmful Drinking: A Manual for Use in Primary Care*. Geneva, Switzerland: World Health Organization Department of Mental Health and Substance Dependence; 2001.

19. Riemsma RP, Pattenden J, Bridle C, et al. Systematic review of the effectiveness of stage based interventions to promote smoking cessation. *BMJ* 2003;326:1175–1177.

20. Bridle C, Piemsma RP, Pattenden J, et al. Systematic review of the effectiveness of health behavior interventions based on the transtheoretical mode. *Psychol Health* 2005;20:283–301.

21. Hughes JC, Cook CC. The efficacy of disulfiram: a review of outcome studies. *Addiction* 1997;92:381–395.

22. West SL, Garbutt JC, Carey, TS, et al. *Pharmacotherapy for alcohol dependence. Evidence Report Number 3*. (Contract 290-97-0011 to Research Triangle Institute, University of North Carolina, Chapel Hill). AHCPR Publication No. 99-E004. Rockville, MD: Agency for Health Care Policy and Research; 1999.

23. Bouza C, Angeles M, Munoz A, et al. Efficacy and safety of naltrexone and acamprosate in the treatment of alcohol dependence: a systematic review. *Addiction* 2004;99:811–828.

24. Srisurapanont M, Jarusuraisin N. Opioid antagonists for alcohol dependence. *Cochrane Database Syst Rev* 2010;(12):CD001867.

25. Buonopane A, Petrakis IL. Pharmacotherapy of alcohol use disorders. *Subst Use Misuse* 2005;40:2001–2020, 2043–2048.

26. Pettinati HM, O'Brien CP, Rabinowitz AR, et al. The status of naltrexone in the treatment of alcohol dependence: specific effects on heavy drinking. *J Clin Psychopharmacol* 2006;26:610–625.

27. Jonas DE, Amick HR, Feltner C, et al. Pharmacotherapy for adults with alcohol use disorders in outpatient settings: a systematic review and meta-analysis. *JAMA* 2014;311:1889–1900.

28. Anton RF, O'Malley SS, Ciraulo DA, et al. Combined pharmacotherapies and behavioral interventions for alcohol dependence: the COMBINE study: a randomized controlled trial. *JAMA* 2006;295:2003–2017.

29. Overman GP, Teter CJ, Guthrie SK. Acamprosate for the adjunctive treatment of alcohol dependence. *Ann Pharmacother* 2003;37:1090–1099.

Index

Note: Italicized *f* and *t* refer to figures and tables

12-lead electrocardiogram 18
5-α-reductase inhibitors 75

A

Abatacept 669
Abciximab 276
Abdominal aortic aneurysm, screening for 100
Abdominal pain 590–594. *See also*
    Gastrointestinal complaints
  causes of 591–592*t*
  clinical presentation 590, 591*t*, 592–593, 592*t*
  diagnostic testing 594
  general principles 590
  history of 590, 591*t*, 592*t*, 593
  location of 590, 591*t*
  physical examination 593
Abnormal liver chemistries 601–605
  causes of 603*t*
  clinical presentation 601–602
  diagnostic testing 602, 604–605
  differential diagnosis 602
  general principles 601
  treatment of 605
Abscesses 538
Acamprosate 975
ACE inhibitors 141–142
Acesulfame K 460*t*
Acetaminophen 665, 696, 761
Acetaminophen hepatotoxicity 627–628
Achilles tendonitis 716
Acid-base disorders 491
Acne 852–854
  acne rosacea 853–854
  acne vulgaris 852–853
  hidradenitis suppurativa 853
  nodulocystic 852
Acne rosacea 853–854
Acne vulgaris 852–853
Acquired inhibitors of coagulation factors 281
Acrochordons 846
Actinic keratosis 847
Activated partial thromboplastin time (aPTT)
    266, 267*t*
Acupuncture 690, 698
Acute chest syndrome 298, 299
Acute flexion-hypertension injury 687
Acute kidney injury (AKI) 488–506
  clinical presentation 489–490
  definition of 488
  diagnostic testing 490–491
  dialytic therapy for 492
  endogenous toxins 489*t*

etiology/pathophysiology of 488
  exogenous toxins 489*t*
  intrinsic renal causes of 488
  nondialytic therapy for 491–492
  postrenal failure 488
  prerenal azotemia 488
Acute tubular necrosis (ATN) 488
Acyclovir 569
Adalimumab 669
Adenosine 169, 223*t*
Adequate index (AI) 456
Adherence 7–8
Adhesive capsulitis 700
Adjustment disorder 873*t*
Adjuvant chemotherapy 725, 734
Adrenal crisis 441
Adrenal failure 440–442
  clinical presentation 440–441
  diagnostic testing 441
  general principles 440
  primary 440
  secondary 440
  treatment of 441–442
    adrenal crisis 441
    outpatient maintenance therapy 441–442
Adrenal nodules, incidental 443–444
Adrenergic agents 802
  α-adrenergic antagonists 783
  β-adrenergic antagonists 436
  α₁-adrenergic blockers 74, 78
  β-adrenergic receptor blockers 191*t*
Age-related muscular degeneration (ARMD) 947
Agitation 893
  α-agonists 20
  β-agonists 803, 804
  β₂-agonists 358*t*
Agoraphobia 888, 890–892. *See also* Anxiety
    disorders
  associated conditions 890
  definition of 888
  diagnosis of 890–891
  epidemiology of 890
  etiology/pathophysiology of 890
  general principles 888
  treatment of 891–892
Agranulocytosis 437
Albumin 604
Albuterol 346*t*
Alcohol 459, 636
Alcohol abuse 970–976
  associated conditions 971
  complications 976
  definition of 970–971

Alcohol abuse (*Continued*)
  diagnosis 972–974
  epidemiology of 971
  identification test 973*t*
  lifestyle/risk modification 976
  medications 975
  referral 976
  risk factors 971
  screening for 102
  treatment 974–976
Alcohol cessation 636
Alcohol consumption
  chronic pancreatitis and 637
  colorectal cancer 94
  macronutrients and 459
  medications for 394, 394*t*
  psoriasis and 851
  reduce of 145*t*
Alcohol dependence 970
Alcohol use disorder identification test
    (AUDIT) questionnaire 972, 974*t*
Alcohol use disorders (AUDs) 970
Alcohol-induced liver disease 626–627
Aldosterone antagonists 175, 192*t*
Alendronate 50
Alfuzosin 75
Alginates 785
Alkaline phosphatase (ALP) 604
Alkaloids 730*t*
Alkylating agents 729*t*
Allergens 794
Allergy 793–816
  anaphylaxis 800–803
  angioedema 807–809
  classification of 793
  clinical presentation 794–795
  diagnostic testing 795
  drug allergies 809–812. *See also* Drug allergies
  epidemiology of 793
  food allergies 812–814
  outpatient medications 796–799*t*
  pathophysiology of 793–794
  rhinitis 814–816
  rhinoconjunctivitis 814–816
  treatment of 795–800
    environmental control 800
    medications 795–800
  urticaria 805–807
  venom hypersensitivity 803–805
Alli 476
Alloantibodies 281
Allopurinol 673, 743
Almotriptan 910
Alopecia 858–859
  androgenetic 85, 858
  areata 858
  nonscarring 858–859
  scarring 859

Alosetron 655
Alpha-1 antitrypsin (α1AT) deficiency 624
Alternative medicine 464, 473–474*t*
Alzheimer disease 926
Amaurosis fugax 944
Ambulatory blood pressure monitoring
    (ABPM) 133
Ambulatory pH monitoring 610–611
American Urological Association Symptom
    Index (AUA-SI) 71, 73*t*
Aminosalicylates 647
Aminotransferases 604
Amiodarone 222*t*, 225
Amitriptyline 923
Amlodipine 174*t*
Amoxicillin 518, 823
Amphotericin B 555, 556, 571
Amylase 404
Amylin agonists 419
Amyloidosis 305, 498
Anagen effluvium 858
Anakinra 669
Anal cancer 734
Anal fissure 600
Analgesia 636
Anaphylaxis 800–803. *See also* Allergy
  classification of 800–801
  diagnosis 801–802
  general principles 800
  pathophysiology 801
  prevention 801
  treatment 802–803
Anaplasma phagocytophilum 559
Anaplasmosis 560
Androgen steroid therapy 629
Androgenetic alopecia 85
Androgens 809
Anemia 285–288
  aplastic 295
  autoimmune hemolytic 296–297
  of chronic disease 294–295
  chronic kidney disease and 503–504
  classification of 284
  clinical presentation 284
  Cooley 288
  definition of 284
  diagnostic testing 285
  drug-induced hemolytic 297
  general principles 284
  hemolytic 295–296
  iron deficiency 285–288
  macrocytic 290–292
  microangiopathic hemolytic 297
  microcytic 285–290
  normocytic 294–302
Anesthesia
  general 299
  general *vs.* regional 13

local 299
regional 13, 299
Angina 163–164
classification of 164*t*
differential diagnosis of 165*t*
Angioedema 807–809
acquired 807
allergic 807
diagnosis 808
general principles 807–808
hereditary 807–808
nonallergic 807
treatment of 808–809
Angiotensin receptor blockers (ARBs) 142, 190*t*, 424, 503
Angiotensin-converting enzyme inhibitors (ACEI) 141–142, 175, 189*t*, 332, 503
Angle-closure glaucoma 946
Animal bite wounds 540–541
Ankle pain 715–716
Ankle-brachial index (ABI) 161, 426
Ankylosing spondylitis 644, 677
Anorectal disorders 600–601. *See also* Gastrointestinal complaints
clinical presentation 600
diagnostic testing of 600–601
differential diagnosis 600
treatment of 601
Anorectal manometry 599
Anorexia 741
Anoscopy 600
Antiarrhythmics 270*t*
Antibiotics 270*t*, 816
for acne 853
aerosolized 364
for cystic fibrosis 363
for inflammatory bowel diseases 647
macrolide 364
topical 853
Anticentromere antibodies 661, 679
Anticholinergic agents 597, 655
Anticholinergic risk scale (ARS) 776
Anticholinergics 782, 816
Anticoagulant therapy 31, 270*t*
apixaban 316
artificial heart valves in 317*t*
dabigatran 316–317
follow-up 323
fondaparinux 314
inferior vena cava filters 318
low molecular weight heparins 315
oral direct Xa inhibitors 316
risk management and complications 320–323
rivaroxaban 316
unfractionated heparins 315
warfarin 317–318
Anticoagulation 198, 216–217
and antiplatelet therapy 198

duration of 318–319
Anticoagulation management, perioperative 30–31
Anticonvulsants 33, 270*t*, 697, 768–669, 910
Antidepressants 697, 768, 874, 877–881*t*, 923
Antiemetics 754*t*, 909
Antiepileptics 915–916*t*, 923
Antigenic drift 521
Antigenic shift 521
Antihistamines 270*t*, 803, 804, 815
for angioedema 809
Antihypertensives 270*t*, 911, 930–931
Anti-IgE antibodies 814
Anti-inflammatory drugs 270*t*
Anti–Jo-1 antibodies 661
Antimetabolites 729*t*
Antimicrobial agents 547
Antimitochondrial antibodies 622
Antineutrophil cytoplasmic antibody (ANCA) 661
Antinuclear antibody (ANA) 621, 661
Antiphospholipid antibody (APA) syndrome 310
Antiphospholipid syndrome (APS) 675
Antiplatelet agents 30–31
Antiplatelet management, perioperative 30–31
Antiplatelet therapy 171–173, 198, 422–423, 931
Antipruritics 844
Antipsychotics 33, 895, 895*t*, 928–929
Anti–Scl-70 antibodies 661, 679
Anti–Sm 675
Anti–smooth muscle antibodies (ASMA) 621
Antispasmodic agents 655
Antitumor necrosis factor agents 648
Anxiety disorders 885–892
characteristics of 886*t*
generalized anxiety disorder 885–888
in older adults 889–901
panic disorder 888–892
Aortic coarctation 136*t*
Aortic regurgitation (AR) 209–210
Aortic stenosis
clinical presentation 206–207
diagnostic testing 207–208
general principles 206
history 206–207
pathophysiology of 206
physical examination 207
treatment of
medications 208
percutaneous management 208
surgical management 208
Apatite deposition disease 674
Aphthous ulcers 644
Apixaban 316
Aplastic anemia (AA) 295
Aplastic crisis 298, 300
Apley scratch test 701

Apprehension sign 701
  posterior 702
Arformoterol tartrate 346*t*
Aromatase inhibitors 732
Arrhythmias
  antiarrhythmic medications 221–223*t*
  atrial fibrillation 224–227
  atrial flutter 227
  atrial tachycardia 229
  bradyarrhythmias 237–240
  classification of 218–219, 219*f*
  congenital arrhythmias 240–241
  diagnostic tools 218
  general approach to 218
  implantable cardiac defibrillator 246–248
  multifocal atrial tachycardia 230, 230*f*
  narrow-complex tachycardia 219–230
  pacemakers 242–246, 243*t*, 244*t*
  reentrant supraventricular tachycardia
    227–229, 228*f*
  sinus tachycardia 220, 224
  syncope 241–242
  tachyarrhythmias 219
  ventricular arrhythmias 232–235
  wide-complex tachycardias 230–232
Arrhythmogenic right ventricular dysplasia
  240–241
Arterial blood gas (ABG) 26
Arthritis 658–663
  diagnostic testing 661, 663
  evaluation of 659*f*
  general principles 658
  history 658
  physical examination 658–660
Arthropod bites/stings 857–858
Artificial heart valves 9*t*, 319
Artificial sweeteners 459, 460*t*
Artificial tears 948
Ascites 186, 602, 632–633
  malignant 741
Aspart 419
Aspartame 460*t*
Aspirin 171, 276, 301, 302, 762*t*, 931
Asthma 351–360. *See also* Chronic obstructive
    pulmonary disease (COPD)
  vs. chronic obstructive pulmonary disease 341
  classification of severity 352*t*
  clinical presentation 353–354
  common mimics of 355*t*
  diagnostic testing of 354–356
  differential diagnosis of 354
  epidemiology of 352
  gastroesophageal reflux disease and 608
  general principles 351–352
  history 353–354
  pathophysiology of 353
  physical examination 354
  stepwise management in adults 357*t*
  treatment of 356–360

Atenolol 222*t*
Atherosclerosis 250
Atopic dermatitis 550
Atorvastatin 256*t*
Atovaquone 547*t*, 561
Atrial fibrillation 224–227. *See also*
    Arrhythmias; Narrow-complex tachycardia
  ablation 225
  diagnosis of 224, 224*f*
  general principles 224
  perioperative 226
  preexcitation 226
  sinus rhythm 225
  thromboembolic risk 226
  treatment of 224–227
  ventricular rate control 225
Atrial flutter 227
Atrial septostomy 385
Atrial tachycardia 229
Autoimmune conditions 636
Autoimmune disease 159, 863–866
  dermatomyositis 864
  erythema nodosum 865–866
  lupus erythematosus 863–864
  scleroderma 864
  vasculitis 864–865
Autoimmune hemolytic anemia (AIHA)
  296–297
Autoimmune hepatitis 621–622
Autonomic neuropathy 425–426
Autotitrating positive airway pressure
  (APAP) 391
AV nodal reentrant tachycardia (AVNRT) 227
AV reentrant tachycardia (AVRT) 227
Avascular necrosis (AVN) 298, 709
Azelastine 816
Azithromycin 524, 547, 561, 578

B

β_2-adrenergic agonists 491
β_3-adrenergic receptor agonists 783
Babesia microti 560
Babesiosis 560–561
Back pain, low 691–698
  clinical presentation 693–695
  diagnostic testing 695–696
  epidemiology of 691
  etiology of 691–692
  nonspecific musculoskeletal 691
  treatment of 696–698
    injection therapies 697
    medications 696–697
    nonpharmacologic therapies 697–698
    surgical management 698
Bacterial vaginosis 59–60, 575
Bacteriuria 483, 534–535
Bacteriuria, asymptomatic 534–535
Baker cyst 712, 713

Baldness 85
Bariatric surgery 421
Barium enema 599
Barium swallow 586
Barrett esophagus 610, 613–614
Basal cell carcinoma 848
Basal metabolic rate (BMR) 457
Basophils 793
Beau lines 859
Beers criteria 776–777
Bell palsy 921
Benign paroxysmal positional vertigo (BPPV) 826, 827
Benign prostatic hyperplasia 71–76
  clinical presentation 71–72
  diagnostic testing 72, 74
  general principles 71
  treatment 74–76
Benign skin neoplasm 847
Benzodiazepines 33, 745t, 755, 769, 888, 889t, 891, 897, 914
Benzoyl peroxide 853
Bereavement 873t
Beta-thalassemia 288
Bevacizumab 734
Bicipital tendonitis 699
Bifidobacterium spp., 472t
Bile acid sequestrant resins 259
Bile duct 637
Biliary disease 635
Bilirubin 602
Binge drinking 971
Biotin 463t
Bipolar disorders 873t
Bisphosphonates 49–50, 769
Bites
  animal 540–541
  human 540–541
  spider 541–542
Bladder cancer 724
Blastomyces dermatitidis 555
Blastomycosis 555–556
Bleeding time (BT) 265
Blepharitis 948
Blistering disorders 855–857
  bullous pemphigoid 855
  dermatitis herpetiformis 855
  drug reaction with eosinophilia and systemic symptoms 857
  erythema multiforme 856
  pemphigus vulgaris 855
  Stevens-Johnson syndrome 856
  toxic epidermolysis necrosis 856
α₁-blockers 143–144
β-blockers 19–20, 137, 138, 143, 173, 225, 891, 911
Blood pressure 133
BODE index 350, 350t
Body mass index (BMI) 455, 457t

Bone densitometry 48
Bone marrow (BM)
  aspiration 286
  biopsy 285, 305
Bone metastases 741
Bone mineral density (BMD) 46
Bone scintigraphy 696
Borrelia burgdorferi 558
Bortezomib 739
Botanical dietary supplements 473–474t
Botulinum toxin 586, 911
Bradyarrhythmias 237–240
  conduction abnormalities 237–240, 239t
  sinus node dysfunction 237, 238t
Branch artery and vein occlusions 945
Breast cancer. *See also* Cancer
  diagnosis of 726–727
  metastasis 732
  screening for 92–93
  treatment of 732–733
Breast masses 58–59
Breastfeeding, adult immunizations and 124
β-receptors 143
Bromocriptine 418–419, 448
Bronchiectasis 362
Bronchitis 341
  acute 519–521
  chronic 341
Bronchoalveolar lavage (BAL) 377
Bronchodilators 343
  long-acting 345
  short-acting 344–345
Bronchoscopy 334, 375
Brugada syndrome 240
B-type natriuretic peptide (BNP) 159, 186
Bullectomy 348
Bullous pemphigoid 855
Bunion 717
Bupropion 891, 965–966
Burkholderia cepacia 366
Burns
  chemical 950
  first-degree 852
  second-degree 852
  thermal 852
  third-degree 852
Bursitis 712
  olecranon 704
  pes anserine 713
  prepatellar 715
  septic 670–671
  subacromial 699

C

Cabergoline 448
Cachexia 741

CAGE questionnaire 972*t*
Calcific tendonitis 699
Calcineurin inhibitors (CNI) 635
Calcitonin 51–52
Calcium 465*t*
Calcium channel blockers 137, 142–143, 174, 225, 383, 911
Calcium gluconate 491
Calcium stones 512, 515
Calcium supplements 53
Campylobacter jejuni 921
Cancer 725–746
  breast cancer 732–733
  chemotherapy 728–731
  complications, treatment-related 742–746
    gastrointestinal complications 744–745
    hematologic complications 743–744
    radiation therapy complications 743
    tumor lysis syndrome 743
  complications, tumor-related 739–742
    bone metastases 741
    brain metastasis 739–740
    malignant ascites 741
    malignant pericardial effusions 740
    malignant pleural effusions 741
    paraneoplastic syndromes 741–742
    spinal cord compression 740
    superior vena cava obstruction 740
  diagnosis of 726–728
    breast cancer 726–727
    cancer of unknown primary site 727
    leukemia 727–728
    lymphoma 727
    multiple myeloma 728
  gastrointestinal malignancies 733–734
    anal cancer 734
    colon cancer 734
    esophageal cancer 733–734
    gastric cancer 734
  genitourinary malignancies 734–735
    bladder cancer 734
    prostate cancer 734–735
    renal cell cancer 735
    testicular cancer 735
  grade of tumor 725
  gynecologic malignancies 735–736
    cervical cancer 735–736
    endometrial cancer 736
    ovarian cancer 736
  head and neck cancer 736
  leukemia 738–739
  liquid malignancies 725
  lung cancer 733
  lymphoma 737–738
  malignant melanoma 736
  sarcomas 736–737
  screening 4
  solid malignances 725
  stages of 725
Cancer of unknown primary site 737
Cancer screening 92–99
  breast cancer 92–93
  cervical cancer 93–94
  colorectal cancer 94–96
  lung cancer 96
  ovarian cancer 98
  prostate cancer 96–97
  recommendations 4
  testicular cancer 98
Cancer treatment 728–739
  for breast cancer 732–733
  chemotherapeutic medications 729–731*t*
  for gastrointestinal malignancies 733–734
  general principles 731, 738
  for genitourinary malignancies 734–735
  for gynecologic malignancies 735–736
  for head and neck cancer 736
  leukemia 738–739
  for lung cancer 733
  lymphoma 737–738
  malignant melanoma 736
  sarcomas 736–737
Cancer-related anorexia and cachexia (CRCA) 741
Candida albicans 61
Candidal infections 553–554
Candidal vaginitis 554
Candidiasis 554, 571, 860
Candiduria 554
Capnocytophaga canimorsus 540
Capsaicin 665
Carbamazepine 768, 915*t*, 923
Carbidopa/levodopa 925
Carbohydrates 457–458
Carbuncles 538
Cardiac resynchronization therapy 197
Cardiac tamponade 203
Cardiomyopathy
  hypertrophic 200–201
  restrictive 201–202
Cardiopulmonary exam 134
Cardiovascular disease 967
Cardiovascular risk assessment, preoperative 13–21
  algorithm for 17*f*
  clinical presentation in 14–17
  congestive heart failure 23
  diagnostic criteria 17–18
  diagnostic testing 18–19
  hypertension 21
  implantable cardioverter defibrillators 22–23
  metabolic equivalents 16*t*
  pacemakers 22–23
  physical examination in 14–17
  revised cardiac risk index 15*t*
  treatment 19–21

medications 19–20
revascularization 20–21
valvular heart disease 22
Cardioversion, direct current 225
Carotid endarterectomy 931
Carotid stenosis 931
Carpal tunnel syndrome 706, 921
Carvedilol 143, 222*t*
Cataracts 947
Catecholaminergic ventricular tachycardia 241
Catheter-associated upper extremity DVT 318
Cation exchange resins 491
Cauda equina syndrome 693, 694
Ceftriaxone 574, 578, 582
Celecoxib 762*t*
Celiac plexus nerve block 636
Cellulitis 535–537, 953
Central retinal artery occlusion 945
Central retinal vein occlusion 945
Central vertigo 831*t*, 933–934
Centrally acting adrenergic agonists 144
Centrally acting agents 655–656
Cerumen impaction 819–820
    diagnosis 819
    general principles 819
    treatment 819–820
Cerumenolytics 819–820
Cervical cancer 735–736
Cervical cancer screening 56–57, 93–94
Cervical disc disease 687
Cervical intraepithelial neoplasias 57
Cervical radiculopathy 687, 689*t*
Cervical spine 658
Cervicitis 574–575
Cetirizine 815
Chalazion 953
Chancroid 578
Chelation therapy 289
Chemopreventive agents 731*t*
Chemotherapy 725–726
    intra-arterial 731
    intracavitary 731
    maintenance 725
    myelodysplastic syndrome 294
    neoadjuvant 425
    pleural effusion 406
Cherry angioma 847
Chest pain, noncardiac 334–335
    chest wall disorders 334
    definition 334
    diagnosis of 335
    in gastroesophageal reflux disease 608
    general principles 334
    pleural disorders 334
    treatment of 334
Chest radiography (CXR) 166, 186, 374–375, 401, 407
Chest wall deformities 328

Chest wall disorders 334
Chicken pox, vaccination for 117–118
Chlamydia 574–575
Chloroquinone 547*t*
Cholangiocarcinoma 631
Cholecystectomy 636
Cholelithiasis 298, 300, 635
Cholesteatoma 835
Cholesterol 458–459
    low-HDL 257
    non-HDL 257
Cholesterol stones 635
Cholestyramine 260, 597, 654
Choline 463*t*
Cholinesterase inhibitors 928
Chondroitin 471*t*
Chromium 466*t*
Chronic bronchitis 341
Chronic inflammatory demyelinating polyneuropathy (CIDP) 922
Chronic kidney disease (CKD) 28
    classification of 501, 501*t*
    definition of 501
    diagnosis of 502
    general principles 500–501
    hypertension and 139
    referral 506
    treatment of 28, 503–505
        anemia 503–504
        diabetes mellitus 503
        dyslipidemia 503
        hypertension 503
        metabolic acidosis 505
        nutrition 505
        secondary hyperparathyroidism 504–505
Chronic obstructive pulmonary disease (COPD) 341–366
    acute exacerbations of 351
    BODE index 350, 350*t*
    classification of 341
    clinical presentation 342–343
    definition of 341
    epidemiology of 341
    health maintenance 350
    laboratory tests for 343
    physical examination 342–343
    risk factors 341, 342*t*
    severity of 343*t*
    symptoms of 342
    therapy at each stage of 345*f*
    treatment of 344–350
        medications 344–348
        nonpharmacologic therapy 348
        patient education 350
        pulmonary rehabilitation 349
        smoking cessation 349
        surgical management 348–349
Churg-Strauss vasculitis 681

Chylomicronemia syndrome 253*t*
Cigarette smoking 162. *See also* Smoking cessation
C1INH 807–808
Ciprofloxacin 547, 570, 578, 821
Cirrhosis 630. *See also* Hepatobiliary diseases
  ascites 632–633
  diagnosis 631
  esophageal and gastric varices 632
  general principles 631
  hepatopulmonary syndrome 633
  hepatorenal syndrome 633–634
  portal hypertension 631–632
  portosystemic encephalopathy 633
  spontaneous bacterial peritonitis 632–633
Clavulanic acid 518
Clindamycin 60, 561, 572, 573, 853
Clonidine 144, 966
Clopidogrel 172, 931
Clostridium difficile infection (CDI)
  diagnosis of 552
  general principles 551–552
  treatment of 552
Clotrimazole 554
Cluster headache 906–907
Coagulation disorders, inherited
  hemophilia A 277–278
  hemophilia B 278
  von Willebrand disease 278–280
Coagulation factors, acquired inhibitors of 281
Coagulation studies 12
Cobalamin 462*t*
Cocaine abuse 159
Coccidioides immitis 556
Coccidioidomycosis 556, 572
Cockroft-Gault formulation 484
Codeine 764
Coenzyme Q10, 470*t*
Cognitive-behavioral therapy (CBT) 656, 888, 891
Colchicine 672
Cold agglutinin disease 296
Cold-antibody AIHA (CAIHA) 296
Colesevelam 260, 418
Colestipol 260
Colon cancer 734
Colonoscopy 599, 600, 653
Colorado tick fever 557
Colorectal cancer screening 94–96
Combined hyperlipidemia 251*t*
Comedolytics 853
Community-acquired methicillin-resistant *Staphylococcus aureus* (CA-MRSA) 535
Community-acquired pneumonia 523–525
Concussion 932–933
  clinical presentation 932–933
  diagnostic testing 933
  general principles 932

  grades of 933*t*
  treatment of 933
Conductive hearing loss (CHL) 831
Condyloma acuminata 862
Congenital arrhythmias 240–241. *See also* Arrhythmias
  arrhythmogenic right ventricular dysplasia 240–241
  Brugada syndrome 240
  familiar polymorphic ventricular tachycardia 241
  long QT syndrome 240
  short QT syndrome 240
Conjunctiva 942
Conjunctivitis 949
Consolidation chemotherapy 725
Consolidation therapy 738
Constipation 597–600. *See also* Gastrointestinal complaints
  clinical presentation 598
  diagnostic testing of 598–599
  differential diagnosis 598
  general principles 597–598
  opioid side effects 767
  treatment of 599–600
Constrictive pericarditis 202–203
Contact dermatitis 849–850
Continuous positive airway pressure (CPAP) 391
Cooley anemia 288
Copper 466*t*
Copper-chelating agents 626
Cornea 943
Corneal abrasions 950–951
Corneal edema 948
Coronary angiography 19, 169–170, 187
Coronary artery bypass graft (CABG) 170, 172, 176
Coronary artery disease (CAD)
  angina in 163–164
  diabetes mellitus and 158
  heart failure 184
  screening for 100
Coronary artery vasospasm 679
Coronary vasospasm 165
Corticosteroid management, perioperative 31–33
  diagnosis 32
  etiology/pathophysiology 32
  treatment 32–33
Corticosteroids 634
  for allergy 795
  for angioedema 809
  for asthma 358*t*
  for chronic obstructive pulmonary disease 347
  for inflammatory bowel diseases 647
  osteoporosis and 53

for rheumatoid arthritis 668
urticaria 807
for venom hypersensitivity 804
Cosyntropin stimulation test 441
Cough 330–332
    causes of 331*t*
    diagnosis of 330–332
    general principles 330
    treatment of 332
Courvoisier sign 602
Crackles 328
C-reactive protein (CRP) 158–159, 661
Creatinine 72, 470*t*, 484
Creatinine clearance (CrCl) 484
Creutzfeldt-Jakob disease 928
Crohn disease 642–643, 677
Cromolyn sodium 815
Cryoglobulinemia 681
Cryptococcosis 556–557, 571–572
Cryptococcus neoformans 556, 571
Cryptogenic organizing pneumonia (COP)
    377, 378
Cryptosporidiosis 573
Cryptosporidium spp., 573
Crystalline arthropathies 700
Crystals 483
Cubital tunnel syndrome 704
Cushing syndrome 136*t*, 442–443
Cutaneous metastases 866
Cutaneous T-cell lymphoma 866
Cutaneous vasculitis 681
Cyanocobalamin 292
Cyclooxygenase-2 (COX-2) inhibitors 276
Cyclophosphamide 746
Cyclospora cayetanensis 573
Cystatin C 485
Cystic fibrosis (CF) 360–366, 636
    acute exacerbations of 365–366
    Burkholderia cepacia complex 366
    clinical presentation 361–362
    diagnosis of 361
    diagnostic testing 362–363
    differential diagnosis of 362
    extrapulmonary manifestations 361–362
    general principles 360–366
    hemoptysis in 366
    monitoring of 366
    pathophysiology of 360–361
    pulmonary manifestations 361
    survival rate 360
    treatment of 363–366
        lung transplantation 365
        medications 363–365
        nonpharmacologic 365
        pancreatic enzyme supplementations 365
        pharmacologic 363–365
        vitamin supplementation 365
Cystine stones 515

D

Cytology 404
Cytomegalovirus (CMV) esophagitis 609
Cytomegalovirus (CMV) reactivation
    568–569
Cytomegalovirus (CMV) retinitis 568
Cytoplasmic antineutrophilic cytoplasmic
    antibody (cANCA) 377

Dabigatran 316–317, 321–322, 931
Dacryocystitis 953–954
Dapsone 572
Darbepoetin alfa 744
Darifenacin 782
DASH dietary pattern 145–146, 145*t*
D-dimers 267, 311
De Quervain tenosynovitis 706
Debridement 785
Decongestants 518
    nasal 816
Decreasing caloric intake 476
Deep vein thrombosis (DVT) 309
    anatomic location of 309
    diagnostic testing 311–314
    etiology/pathophysiology of 309
Dehydration 299
Delirium 755, 926
Delusions 893
Dementia 926–929
    causes of 927*t*
    clinical presentation 926–927
    diagnostic testing 928
    differential diagnosis 927–928
    frontotemporal 927
    general principles 926
    vs. major depression 874
    treatment
        medications 928–929
        nonpharmacologic therapies 929
Denosumab 52
Depression 870–884. *See also* Psychiatric
    disorders
    associated conditions 869
    bipolar 872
    classification of 870
    clinical presentation 871–872
    differential diagnosis 872, 873–874*t*
    epidemiology 870–871
    etiology/pathophysiology 871
    medical illness and 869, 871
    mixed mood syndrome 872
    monitoring/follow-up 882
    in older adults 898–899
    outcome/prognosis 882
    referral 876, 882
    risk factors 871
    subsyndromal 872

Depression (*Continued*)
  treatment 872–876
    acute therapy 872, 874–875, 875*f*
    duration of 875
    medications 876
    nonpharmacologic therapies 876
Dermatitides 849–852
  atopic dermatitis 850
  contact dermatitis 849–850
  keratosis pilaris 850
  lichen planus 852
  pityriasis rosea 852
  psoriasis 851
  seborrheic dermatitis 850–851
  stasis dermatitis 850
  thermal burns 852
Dermatitis herpetiformis 855
Dermatochalasis 953
Dermatology
  medical history 842, 843*t*
  physical examination 842
  therapies
    antipruritics 844
    dry skin care 843–844
    protection 844
    topical steroids 844–845, 845*t*
    wet skin care 844
Dermatomyositis 683–684, 741, 864
Dermatosis papulosa nigra 846
Detemir 420
Dexamethasone 443, 740
Diabetes mellitus (DM) 28–30, 412–426
  chronic kidney disease and 503
  criteria for 6*t*
  diagnosis of 414–415
  drug- or chemical-induced 413
  endocrinopathies 413
  exocrine pancreas, diseases of 413
  general principles 412
  gestational 413, 415
  heart failure 184
  hypertension and 138
  ischemic heart disease and 158
  monogenetic 413
  prevention/management of complications
      422–426
    autonomic neuropathy 425–426
    cardiovascular disease 422–424
    dyslipidemia 423–424
    foot care 426
    hypertension 423
    nephropathy 424
    neuropathy 425–426
    peripheral neuropathy 425
    retinopathy 425
    smoking cessation 424
  screening for 5, 99–100, 424
  stroke and 931

target glucose levels 29
treatment of 29, 415–422
  bariatric surgery 421
  diet 421–422
  exercise 422
  glycemic control 415–416
  hemoglobin A_{1C}, 416
  hypoglycemia 416–417
  immunizations 422
  insulin 419
  medications 417–420
  nonpharmacologic therapy 421
  psychosocial assessment 422
  self-monitoring of capillary blood glucose 416
  type 1, 29, 412, 420
  type 2, 29–30, 412–413, 420
Diabetic dermopathy 866
Diabetic neuropathy 920–921
Diarrhea 548–552, 594–597.
    See also Gastrointestinal complaints
  bacterial 549*t*, 570
  in cancer patients 745
  causes of 595*t*
  clinical presentation 594
  Clostridium difficile infection 551–552
  diagnosis of 548
  diagnostic testing 596–597
  differential diagnosis 596
  general principles 548, 594
  HIV infection and 570
  predominant 654–655
  traveler's 546–547
  treatment of 548, 551, 597
    empiric 551
    rehydration 548, 551
Diclofenac 762*t*
Diet 145–146, 162
Dietary guidelines 455–457
Dietary reference intakes 455–456
Dietary supplements 464
Digital rectal examination 70
Digoxin 193*t*, 202, 223*t*, 225, 383
Dihydroergotamine 910
Dihydropyridines 142, 174*t*
Diltiazem 223*t*
Dipeptidyl peptidase-4 inhibitors 418
Diphtheria vaccines 108–110, 109*f*
Dipyridamole 169, 276
Direct renin inhibitors 142
Direct thrombin inhibitor, oral 316–317
Direct Xa inhibitors, oral 316
Disc herniation 693
Disequilibrium 826
Disopyramide 221*t*
Disseminated intravascular coagulation 281
Disulfiram 975
Diuretics 140–141, 195*t*, 383, 491
Divalproex 910

Dix-Hallpike maneuver 826, 832*f*
Dizziness 826, 827*t. See also* Headache
Dobutamine 169
Doctor-patient interactions 8–9
Dofetilide 223*t*
Donovan bodies 579
Dopamine norepinephrine reuptake
    inhibitors 879*t*
Doxazosin 74
Doxorubicin 737
Doxycycline 518, 547*t*, 558–560, 559, 560,
    579, 582
Drawer test, anterior 713
Driving issues, in old adults 779–780
Drop arm sign 701
Drug allergies 809–812
    classification of 809
    clinical presentation 810
    diagnostic testing 810–811
    epidemiology 809
    pathophysiology 809–810
    treatment 811–812
        alternate drug class 811
        drug desensitization 812
        pretreatment protocols 811–812
        provocative dose challenge 811
Drug metabolism
    affecting factors 774
    age-related changes in 774–775
    drug toxicity 775–777
    polypharmacy prevention 775–777
Drug reaction with eosinophilia and systemic
    symptoms (DRESS) syndrome 857
Drug toxicity 775–777
Drug-induced hemolytic anemia 297
Drug-induced liver injury (DILI) 627
Drug-nutrient interactions 464, 468–469*t*
Dry skin care 843
Duke treadmill score 168
Duloxetine 923
Duodenal obstruction 637
Dupuytren contracture 706
Dust mites 800
Dutasteride 75
Dyshidrotic eczema 850
Dyskinesia 362
Dyslipidemia 250–261
    atherosclerosis 250
    chronic kidney disease and 503
    clinical dyslipoproteinemias 250
    diabetes and 423–424
    differential diagnosis 251*t*
    general principles 250
    genetic 252–253*t*
    lipoproteins 250
    risk assessment 254
    screening for 5, 99, 250
    standard care for 250

    treatment of 254–261
        clinical ASCVD 255
        with diabetes 256
        hypertriglyceridemia 257, 260–261
        low HDL cholesterol 257
        low-density lipoprotein 255–256
        starting and monitoring therapy 258–259
        statin therapy 256*t*
        therapeutic lifestyle change 254, 255*t*
        without diabetes 256
Dyslipoproteinemias 250
Dyspepsia 492–494. *See also* Gastrointestinal
    complaints
    clinical presentation of 493
    diagnostic testing 494
    general principles 492
    treatment of 494
Dysphagia 584–589. *See also* Gastrointestinal
    complaints
    causes of 585*t*
    clinical presentation 584–585
    diagnostic testing of 585–586
    differential diagnosis of 585
    general principles 584
    treatment of 586
Dysplasia 614
Dysplastic nevi 847
Dyspnea 328–330, 754–755
    clinical presentation 329
    diagnostic testing 330
    general principles 328–329
    Medical Research Council scale 350*t*
    pulmonary diseases 328
    treatment of 330
Dysthymia 873*t*
Dystonia 924

E

Ecchymoses 265
Ectoparasitic infections 581
Eczema 850
Ehrlichia chaffeensis 560
Ehrlichiosis 560
Elbow pain 703–706
    clinical presentation 704–705
    diagnostic testing 705
    general principles 703–704
    treatment of 705–706
Electrocardiography
    aortic regurgitation 209
    aortic stenosis 207
    heart failure 186
    functional mitral regurgitation 214
    12-lead 18
    mitral stenosis 211
    mitral regurgitation, 213
    stroke, 930

Electroencephalogram (EEG) 913
Electrophysiology (EP)
  atrial tachycardia 229
  low back pain 696
Emollient laxatives 599
Emphysema 341
Empyema 405
Endocarditis
  nonbacterial 742
  prophylaxis 34, 37–38, 215–216
Endometrial cancer 736
Endomyocardial biopsy 187, 202
Endoscopic retrograde cholangiopancreatogra-
  phy (ERCP) 604, 637
Endoscopic variceal ligation (EVL) 632
Endothelin receptor antagonists (EARs)
  383, 384*t*
Enemas 600
Energy requirements 457*t*
Entrapment neuropathies 921
Eosinophilic gastroenteritis 813
Eosinophilic lung diseases 377
Eosinophilic pneumonia, chronic 378
Epicondylitis 704
Epidural steroid injections 698
Epilepsy 911
Epinephrine 802, 803*t*, 809
Episcleritis 645, 949
Episodic hemolysis 300
Epistaxis 835–836
  anterior 836
  causes of 835*t*
  diagnosis 835–836
  general principles 835
  posterior 836
  treatment of 835–837
Epithelial cells 483
Eplerenone 141, 175
Epley maneuver 827, 833*f*
Epstein-Barr virus 569
Eptifibatide 276
Erectile dysfunction 78–82
  clinical presentation 78–79
  definition 78
  diagnostic testing 79
  referral 82
  risk factors 79*t*
  treatment 80–81
Erlotinib 733
Eruptive xanthomas 867
Erysipelas 535–537
Erythema multiforme 856
Erythema nodosum (EN) 644, 865–866
Erythrocyte sedimentation rate (ESR) 661
Erythrocytosis 742
Erythromycin 853
Erythropoietin, recombinant 744
Esmolol 222*t*

Esophageal cancer 733–734
Esophageal manometry 586, 611
Esophageal varices 632
Esophagitis
  candidal 609
  eosinophilic 608–609
  pill 609
Essential hypertension 131
Essential nutrients 455
Essential thrombocythemia (ET) 302
Essential tremor 924
Estrogen replacement therapy (ERT) 52
Estrogen therapy (ET) 55–56
Estrogen, topical 783
Etanercept 669
Ethambutol 527, 527*t*
Eustachian tube dysfunction (ETD)
  causes and risk factors for 822*t*
  general principles 822
  treatment of 823
Event monitor 218
Everolimus (EVL) 635
Exenatide 419
Exercise 145, 145*t*, 187, 196, 422
Eyelid, examination of 942
Ezetimibe 260

F

FABERE sign 710
Facet joint injection 697–698
Falls
  clinical presentation 778
  diagnostic testing 778–779
  general principles 777
  prevention of 778
  risk factors 777–778
  treatment of 779
Famciclovir 569
Familial combined hyperlipidemia (FCH) 252*t*
Familial defective apolipoprotein B-100, 251*t*
Familial dysbetalipoproteinemia 252*t*
Familial hypercholesterolemia 252*t*
Familial hyperchylomicronemia 253*t*
Familial polymorphic ventricular
  tachycardia 241
Familial thrombocytopenia 275
Fasting plasma glucose (FPG) 414
Fat 458
  dietary sources of 459*t*
  trans fat 458
Fat malabsorption 637
Fat replacements 459
Fat-soluble vitamins 462–463*t*
Fatty casts 483
Febrile neutropenia 743
Fecal incontinence 600
Felons 707

Felty syndrome 666
Fenofibrate 260
Fentanyl 764, 766
Ferric gluconate 287*t*
Ferritin 286
Ferrous fumarate 287*t*
Ferrous gluconate 287*t*
Ferrous sulfate 286, 287*t*
Ferumoxytol 287*t*
Fever, tick-borne 557
Fever of unknown origin (FUO) 561–562
Feverfew 34
Fiber 458
Fibrinogen 159, 267
Fibromyalgia 684
Filiform warts 862
Finasteride 75, 85
Flat feet 717
Flat warts 862
Flavivirus family 620
Flecainide 222*t*
Fluconazole 61, 554, 556, 557, 572, 609, 860
5-fluoracil 734
Fluoride 467*t*
Fluorodeoxyglucose positron emission
        tomography (¹⁸F-FDG PET) 408
Fluoroquinolones 534
Fluticasone propionate 346*t*
Fluvastatin 256*t*
Focal nodular hyperplasia (FNH) 629–630
Focal segmental glomerulosclerosis (FSGS)
        494–495
Focal seizures 911
Folate deficiency 290
Folic acid 299, 463*t*
Folinic acid 573
Fondaparinux 314–316, 321
Food allergies 812–814
    clinical presentation 813
    diagnostic testing 813
    general principles 812–813
    IgE-mediated 812
    non-IgE-mediated 813
    treatment of 813–814
Food guide pyramid 456
Foot care, in diabetic patients 426
Forefoot pain 621–622, 717–718
Formoterol 346*t*
Frailty 789–790
Frontotemporal dementia 927
Frozen shoulder 699
Funduscopic exam 134, 943
Fungal infections 554–557, 571–572
    blastomycosis 555–556
    coccidioidomycosis 556
    cryptococcosis 556–557
    histoplasmosis 554–555
    onychomycosis 553

oral candidiasis 554
    sporotrichosis 553
    superficial 553–554
    tinea 553
Fungal skin infections 860–862
    candidiasis 860
    onychomycosis 861
    tinea capitis 860
    tinea corporis 861
    tinea cruris 861
    tinea pedis 861
    tinea versicolor 860
Furosemide 446
Furuncles 538

G

Gabapentin 56, 768, 891, 910, 916*t*, 923
Gait 658
Gallstones 635, 645
Ganciclovir 569
Gastric cancer 734
Gastric varices 632
Gastroesophageal reflux disease (GERD)
        607–614
    clinical presentation 608
    complications 613–614
        Barrett esophagus 613–614
        extraesophageal complications 614
        mucosal erosion/strictures 613
    definition of 607
    diagnostic testing 609–611
    differential diagnosis 608–609
    scleroderma and 679
    treatment of 611–613
Gastrointestinal complaints 584–605
    abdominal pain 590–594
    abnormal liver chemistries 601–605
    anorectal disorders 600–601
    constipation 597–600
    diarrhea 594–597
    dyspepsia 589–590
    nausea 586–589
    vomiting 586–589
Gastrointestinal malignancies 733–734
Gel and Coombs classification 793
Gemfibrozil 260
Generalized anxiety disorder 885–888.
        See also Psychiatric disorders
    associated conditions 885, 887
    characteristics of 886*t*
    diagnosis of 887
    epidemiology of 885
    etiology/pathophysiology of 885
    general principles 885
    treatment of 887–888
Generalized seizures 911–912
Genetic testing 362

Genital ulcer syndromes 575–579
  chancroid 578
  granuloma inguinale 579
  herpes 577–578
  lymphogranuloma venereum 578–579
  syphilis 575–577
Genitourinary malignancies 734–735
Genitourinary symptoms 56
Geriatrics 772–790
  activities of daily living in 774t
  decision-making capacity and 790
  driving 779–780
  drug prescription 774–777
  ethics in 790
  falls 777–779
  functional assessment 773–774
  geriatric assessment 774
  informed consent in 790
  maintaining functions in 772
  malnutrition 786–789
  physical activity 779
  physical frailty 789–790
  pressure ulcers 784
  preventing disability in 772
  screening test 773t
  syndromes 772–773
  urinary incontinence 781–783
Gestational diabetes mellitus 413, 415
Gestational hypertension 149
Gestational thrombocytopenia 275
Giant cell arteritis (GCA) 681, 682, 945
Ginger 34
Gingko 34
Glargine 420
Glaucoma 647, 946–948
Glenohumeral joint 699
Glenoid labrum 699
Glinides 417
Globus 584
Glomerular filtration rate (GFR) 484
Glomerulonephritis 492–500
  asymptomatic 492
  chronic 493
  diagnosis of 498–499
  differential diagnosis of 494–498
  focal segmental 494–495
  general principles 492
  hematuria 493
  membranoproliferative 495–496
  nephritic syndrome 493
  nephrotic syndrome 493
  poststreptococcal 497
  proteinuria 492–493
  rapidly progressive 493
  treatment of 500
Glucagon 803
Glucagon-like peptide-1 (GLP-1) agonists 419
Glucocorticoids 272, 364, 447, 668

Glucosamine 470t
Glucose intolerance 637
Glucose-6-phosphate dehydrogenase
    deficiency 300
α-glucosidase inhibitors 418
Glulisine 420
Goiter
  multinodular 439
  toxic multinodal goiter (MNG) 435
Golfer's elbow 704
Gonorrhea 574
Goodpasture disease 497
Gout 717
  diagnosis of 672
  general principles 671
  treatment of 672–673
Granular casts 483
Granulocyte macrophage colony–stimulating
    factor (GM-CSF) 377
Granulocytosis 742
Granuloma inguinale 579
Granulomatosis with polyangiitis (GPA)
    377, 378
Graves disease 435, 952
Griseofulvin 860
Growth factors 744
Guanadrel 144
Guanethidine 144
Guillain-Barré syndrome (GBS) 921
Guttate psoriasis 881
Gynecologic malignancies 735–736

H

Hairy cell leukemia 728, 739
Hallucinations 892
Hallux rigidus 717
Hallux valgus 717
Hand and wrist pain 706–708
  clinical presentation 707–708
  diagnostic testing 708
  general principles 706–707
  treatment of 708
Haptenation 794
Haptoglobin 295
Harris-Benedict equation 457
Hashimoto disease 432
Head and neck cancer 736
Headache 906–911
  clinical presentation 906
  cluster 911
  diagnostic criteria for 906–907
  diagnostic testing 907–908
  differential diagnosis for 907t
  general principles 906
  medication overuse 907
  migraine with aura 908t
  migraine without aura 908t

red flags 907*t*
tension-type 909–911
treatment of 908–911
Hearing loss 831–832, 834–835
  causes of 834*t*
  clinical presentation 831–832
  conductive 831
  diagnostic testing 834
  general principles 831
  noise-induced 835
  sensorineural 831
  sudden sensorineural 831
  treatment of 831–835
Heart failure (HF)
  acute decompensated 198–199
  advanced 197–198
  causes of 184*t*
  chest radiography in 186–187
  chronic 187–198
  classification of 182, 183*f*
  clinical presentation 185–186
  definition 182
  diagnostic procedure
    coronary angiography 187
    CT 187
    endomyocardial biopsy 187
    magnetic resonance angiography 187
    myocardial perfusion imaging 187
  electrocardiography 186
  epidemiology of 182, 184
  etiology of 182, 184, 184*t*
  general principles 182–185
  history 185
  hypertension and 138–139
  laboratory testing 186
  outcome/prognosis 199–200
  pathophysiology 184, 185
  perioperative considerations for 23
  physical examination 185–186
  with preserved ejection fraction 182
  with preserved systolic function 184*t*
  risk factors 184
  treatment of 187
  volume status assessment 186
Heart murmurs, evaluation of 207*f*
Heartburn 609
Heel pain 716–717
Hemangioma 629
Hematologic diseases 284–306
  amyloidosis 305
  anemia 285–288
    aplastic 295
    autoimmune hemolytic 296–297
    of chronic disease 294–295
    classification of 284
    clinical presentation 284
    cooley 288
    definition of 284

    diagnostic testing 285
    drug-induced hemolytic 297
    general principles 284
    hemolytic 295–296
    iron deficiency 285–288
    macrocytic 290–292
    microangiopathic hemolytic 297
    microcytic 285–290
    normocytic 294–302
  leukocytosis 303–304
  leukopenia 304
  monoclonal gammopathies 304–305
  multiple myeloma 305
  myelodysplastic syndrome 292–294
  polycythemia 301
  red cell enzyme deficiencies 300
  sickle cell disease 297–300
  thrombocytosis 302
  white blood cell disorders 303–305
Hematologic malignancies 866
Hematuria 508–516. *See also* Nephrolithiasis
  causes of 509*t*
  classification of 508
  clinical presentation 510
  definition of 508
  diagnostic testing 510–512
  etiology of 508
  evaluation of 511*f*
  microscopic 508, 511*f*
  nephritic syndrome and 493
  risk factors 509*t*
  treatment of 512
Hemochromatosis, hereditary 624–625
Hemoglobin A1C
  diabetes mellitus 416, 503
  goals of 163
  glycemic goals 415
  monitoring/follow-up 366
Hemoglobin H disease 289
Hemoglobin, in urine 482
Hemolysis, chronic 298, 300
Hemolytic anemia 295–296
  autoimmune 296–297
  drug-induced 297
  microangiopathic 297
Hemolytic-uremic syndrome (HUS) 272–273
Hemophilia A 277–278
Hemophilia B 278
Hemoptysis 332–334
  in cystic fibrosis 366
  diagnosis of 333–334
  general principles 332–333
  treatment of 334
Hemorrhagic cystitis 746
Hemorrhoids, external 600
Hemostasis
  acquired coagulation disorders 280–281
  chemotherapy-induced thrombocytopenia 275

Hemostasis (*Continued*)
  clinical presentation 265
  diagnostic testing 265–267
    laboratory testing 265
    primary hemostasis testing 265–266
    secondary hemostasis testing 266–267
  drug-induced thrombocytopenia 270–271
  ecchymoses in 265
  familial thrombocytopenia 275
  general principles 265
  gestational thrombocytopenia 275
  hemolytic-uremic syndrome 272–273
  heparin-induced thrombocytopenia 273–274
  history 265
  immune thrombocytopenic purpura 268–269
  inherited coagulation disorders
    hemophilia A 277–278
    hemophilia B 278
    von Willebrand disease 278–280
  laboratory teste 265
  liver disease and 275
  petechiae in 265
  physical examination 265
  platelet disorders 267–268, 268*t*
  posttransfusion purpura 274–275
  primary 265
  qualitative platelet disorders 276
  secondary 265
  thrombocytopenia 267–268, 268*t*
  thrombotic thrombocytopenic purpura
    271–272
Henoch-Schönlein purpura 496
Heparin
  low molecular weight 315
  unfractionated 315
Heparin-induced thrombocytopenia (HIT)
    273–274, 310
Hepatic artery thrombosis 635
Hepatitis A virus (HAV) 617
  vaccination for 113–114
Hepatitis B, chronic 620
Hepatitis B virus (HBV) 583, 618, 619*t*, 620
  vaccination for 114–117, 117*t*
Hepatitis C, chronic 621
Hepatitis C virus (HCV) 620–621
Hepatobiliary diseases 645
  acetaminophen hepatotoxicity 627–628
  alcohol-induced liver disease 626–627
  cirrhosis 631–634
  drug-induced liver injury 627
  immune-mediated liver disease
    autoimmune hepatitis 621–622
    primary biliary cirrhosis 622–623
    primary sclerosing cholangitis 622–623
  liver transplantation 634–635
  metabolic liver disease
    alpha-1 antitrypsin 624
    hereditary hemochromatosis 624–625

    nonalcoholic fatty liver disease 624
    Wilson disease 625–626
  outpatient biliary 635–637
  pancreatic diseases 635–637
  tumors of liver
    adenoma 629
    cholangiocarcinoma 631
    focal nodular hyperplasia 629–630
    hemangioma 629
    hepatocellular carcinoma 630
  viral hepatitis
    hepatitis A 617
    hepatitis B 618, 619*t*, 620
    hepatitis C 620–621
Hepatocellular carcinoma (HCC) 630
Hepatomegaly 186, 602
Hepatopulmonary syndrome 633
Hepatorenal syndrome (HRS) 633–634
Herbal dietary supplements 473–474*t*
Herbal medications 34
Herceptin 732
Hereditary angioedema (HAE) 807–808
Hereditary hemochromatosis 624–625
Hereditary pancreatitis 636
Herpes 577–578
Herpes esophagitis 609
Herpes simplex keratitis 949
Herpes simplex virus-2 (HSV-2) 569
Herpes zoster
  skin and soft tissue infections 543
  vaccination for 118–119
Herpes zoster ophthalmicus (HZO) 953
Heterozygous factor V Leiden 319
Hidradenitis suppurativa 853
High-density lipoprotein cholesterol (HDL-C)
    161, 261
Hip fractures 710
Hip pain 708–711. *See also* Musculoskeletal
    complaints
  clinical presentation 709–710
  general principles 708–709
  treatment 710–711
Hirsutism 452–453
  diagnosis of 452
  etiology of 452
  general principles 452
  treatment of 452–453
Histamine 793
Histamine-2 receptor antagonists 611
Histoplasma capsulatum 554, 572
Histoplasmosis 554–555, 572
HIV neuropathy 922
Hoarseness 380, 836–838
  causes of 837*t*
  diagnosis 837
  general principles 836–837
  treatment of 837–838
Hodgkin disease 727, 737

Holter monitor 218
Homocysteine 159
Homocystinuria 310
Hordeolum 953
Hormonal agents 730t
Hormone therapy 732
Hospice care 748–756
  appropriate timing 749–751
  epidemiology of 748–749
  indications for 749, 750t
  venues for 751
Hot flashes 55–56
Human bite wounds 540–541
Human immunodeficiency virus (HIV)
      infection 159, 566–573
  clinical presentation 566–567
  complications of 568–573
    bacterial infections 570
    fungal infections 571–572
    metabolic complications 573
    mycobacterial infections 571
    neoplasms 573
    protozoal infections 572–573
    viral infections 568–570
  diagnostic testing 567
  general principles 566
  treatment of 567–568
Human papillomavirus (HPV) 56,
      580, 735
Hyaline casts 483
Hyaluronic acid analog injections 665–666
Hydralazine 144, 194t
Hydrocele 82, 83
Hydrocolloids 785
Hydrogels 785
Hydromorphone 764
Hydroxychloroquine 668
Hydroxymethylglutaryl-coenzyme A eductase
      inhibitors (statins) 250
Hydroxyurea 299, 301
Hydroxyzine 888
Hyoscyamine 655
Hyperaldosteronism, primary 135t, 148
Hypercalcemia 444–447, 741
  causes of 445t
  clinical presentation 445–446
  diagnostic testing 446
  general principles 444–445
  in paraneoplastic syndromes 741
  treatment of 446–447
Hypercalciuria 515
Hypercholesterolemia 251t
Hypercoagulability testing 312
Hypercoagulable states 310
Hyperkalemia 491
Hyperlipidemia 250
Hyperosmolar agents 599
Hyperoxaluria 515

Hyperparathyroidism 444, 447, 502
  secondary 502, 504–505
Hyperprolactinemia 447–449
  causes of 448t
  diagnosis of 488
  general principles 447
  treatment of 448–449
    macroadenomas 449
    microadenomas 448–449
Hypersensitivity pneumonitis (HP) 377, 378
Hypertension 130–150
  causes of, secondary 135–136t
  chronic kidney disease and 503
  classification of 130, 131t
  definition of 130
  diagnosis of 131–134
    ambulatory blood pressure monitoring 133
    blood pressure 133
    history 131–132
    physical examination 133–134
  epidemiology of 130–131
  epistaxis and 836
  essential/primary 131
  etiology of 131
  gestational 149
  heart failure 184
  ischemic heart disease and 162
  lifestyle modifications 145t
  perioperative considerations for 21
  pregnancy and 149
  prevalence of 130
  refractory 146
  resistant 146–147
  screening for 4–5, 99, 99t, 131
  secondary 131, 132, 147–149
  treatment of 134, 137–146
    medications 134, 137–144
    nonpharmacologic therapy 144–146
Hypertension, pulmonary 378–386
  classification of 379t, 383t
  clinical presentation 380
  diagnostic tests 380–381
  evaluation of 382f
  general principles 378–380
  right heart catheterization 381
  treatment of 381–386
Hypertensive urgencies and emergencies 149–150
Hyperthyroidism 435–439
  causes of 438
  clinical presentation 435
  diagnostic testing of 435–436
  differential diagnosis of 436t
  general principles 435
  in pregnancy 439
  skin signs of 866
  treatment of 436–439
    radioactive iodine therapy 437–438
    subtotal thyroidectomy 438

Hyperthyroidism (*Continued*)
  symptomatic therapy 436
    thionamides 436–437
  urgent therapy 439
Hypertonic saline 363
Hypertriglyceridemia 251*t*, 257, 260–261
Hypertrophic cardiomyopathy (HCM) 200–201
Hyperuricemia 673
Hyperuricosuria 515
Hyphema 951
Hypocitraturia 515
Hypoglycemia 416–417
Hypogonadism 449–451
  causes of androgen deficiency 450*t*
  etiology of 450–451
  general principles 449–450
  testicular disorders 450
Hypopyon 943
Hypothalamic pituitary dysfunction 450–451
Hypothyroidism 432–435
  clinical presentation 433
  diagnostic testing 433
  general principles 432
  iatrogenic 432
  pregnancy and 434
  primary 432
  secondary 432
  skin signs of 866
  subclinical 434
  T4 requirements 434
  treatment of 433–435
    follow-up/dose adjustment 434
    thyroid hormone replacement 433–434

I

Ibandronate 50
Ibuprofen 762*t*
Idiopathic interstitial pneumonias 376*t*
Idiopathic pancreatitis 636
Idiopathic pulmonary fibrosis (IPF) 375,
    375*t*, 376*t*
Ifosfamide 746
IgA nephropathy 496
IgE-mediated food allergy 812
Imidazole 61
Imipramine 888
Immune thrombocytopenic purpura (ITP).
    See also Hemostasis
  clinical presentation 268–269
  diagnostic testing 269
  drugs implicated in 270*t*
  general principles 268
  treatment of 269
Immune-mediated liver disease
  autoimmune hepatitis 621–622
  primary biliary cirrhosis 622–623
  primary sclerosing cholangitis 622–623

Immunizations, adult 102–123
  in diabetic patients 422
  documentation of prior vaccinations 104
  dosage and schedule 105–106*t*
  general principles 102, 103*t*
  hypersensitivity to vaccine components 104
  legal responsibilities of provider 103–104
  patient groups 123–126
    health care workers 126
    immunosuppressed patients 124–125
    persons with acute illness 125
    persons with chronic illness 125
    pregnant women 124
    travelers 126
  resources for information 102–103
  timing of administration 104
  vaccines 107–123
    Haemophilus influenzae type B 121
    hepatitis A 113–114
    hepatitis B 114–117, 117*t*
    herpes zoster 118–119
    human papillomavirus 120–121
    influenza 110–111
    measles, mumps, and rubella 107–108
    meningococcal 119–120
    pneumococcal 111–113, 113*t*
    polio 121
    rabies 122–123
    tetanus, diphtheria, and pertussis vaccines
      108–110, 109*f*
    tetanus/diphtheria toxoid with acellular
      pertussis 108–109
    varicella 117–118
Immunodeficiencies 562–563
  antibody production 562–563
  B cell function 562–563
Immunomodulators 648
Immunosuppression 562–563
  antitumor necrosis factor agents 562
  primary immunodeficiencies 562–563
Immunotherapy 795, 816
Impetigo 539
Impingement sign 701
Implantable cardioverter defibrillators (ICDs)
    196, 246–248
  cardioversion/defibrillation 248
  complications and malfunction of 247
  electromagnetic interference 248
  magnet application 247
  management of 246–247
  MRI imaging and 247
  perioperative considerations for 22–23
  perioperative management 247
  physical activity and 248
  radiation therapy and 247–248
Implantable event monitor 218
Incontinence
  functional 781

mixed 781
overflow 781
stress 781
urge 781
Indomethacin 762*t*
Induction chemotherapy 725
Infectious arthritis 670–671
Infectious diseases 517–563
  Clostridium difficile infection 551–552
  deep fungal infections 554–557
  diarrheal illness 548–552
  fever of unknown origin 561–562
  immunosuppression 562–563
  respiratory tract infections 517–529
    acute bronchitis 519–521
    acute rhinosinusitis 517–518
    community-acquired pneumonia 523–525
    influenza 521–522
    latent tuberculosis 528–529
    pharyngitis 518–519
    tuberculosis 526–528
  skin and soft tissue infections 535–543
    abscesses 538
    animal and human bite wounds 540–541
    carbuncles 538
    cellulitis 535–537
    erysipelas 535–537
    furuncles 538
    herpes zoster 543
    impetigo 539
    necrotizing fasciitis 539–540
    spider bites 541–542
  superficial fungal infections 553–554
  tick-borne disease 557–561
    anaplasmosis 560
    babesiosis 560–561
    ehrlichiosis 560
    Lyme disease 558–559
    Rocky Mountain spotted fever 559
  travel medicine 544–547
    malaria 547
    pretravel consultation 544
    returning traveler 544–546
    traveler's diarrhea 546–547
  urinary tract infections 530–535
Infective endocarditis (IE) 215
Inferior vena cava (IVC) filters 318
Inflammatory acne 852
Inflammatory bowel diseases (IBDs) 642–649
  cancer surveillance 649
  Crohn disease 642–643
  diagnostic testing 645–647
  differential diagnosis for 646*t*
  epidemiology of 644
  extraintestinal manifestations of 644
  general principles 642–644
  incidence rates 644
  risk factors of 644

Infliximab 669
Influenza 521–522
  vaccination 196
  vaccines 110–111, 175
Inherited coagulation disorders
  hemophilia A 277–278
  hemophilia B 278
  von Willebrand disease 278–280
Insect sting 804
Insoluble fiber 458
Insomnia 393–396
  causes and associated characteristics 393*t*
  diagnosis of 393–394
  general principles 393
  lifestyle/risk modification 396
  medications for 394–395*t*
  nonpharmacologic therapy for 396
Insulin 30, 419, 491
Internal hemorrhoids 600
Interstitial lung diseases (ILDs)
  blood/urine test for 374*t*
  classification scheme for 372*t*
  clinical presentation 371–373
  diagnosis of 373*f*
  differential diagnosis 375–378
  general principles 371
  high-resolution computed tomography for 374–375
  history 371–373
  hypersensitivity pneumonitis 377, 378
  laboratory tests 373
  lung biopsy 375
  physical examination 373
  plain chest radiography for 374
  prevalence of 371
  pulmonary function tests 375
  sarcoidosis 377, 378
  treatment of 378
Interstitial pneumonitis 746
Intra-articular steroids 665
Intracranial aneurysm 952
Intraocular pressure 942
Intrathecal chemotherapy 731
Inverse psoriasis 851
Iodine 467*t*
Ipratropium bromide 346*t*
Iris 943
Iritis 949
Iron 466*t*
Iron deficiency anemia 285–288
  clinical presentation of 285
  diagnostic testing of 286–287
  general principles 285
  history 285
  physical examination 285
  treatment of 286–288
Iron dextran 287*t*, 288
Iron sucrose 287*t*

Iron sulfate elixir 286
Irrigation
  for cerumen impaction 819
Irritable bowel syndrome (IBS) 650–656
  classification of 650, 651*t*
  clinical presentation 652
  constipation-predominant 653–654
  diagnostic testing 652–653
  diarrhea-predominant 654–655
  epidemiology of 650
  general principles 650, 651*t*
  pathophysiology of 650, 652
  treatment of 653–656
    medications 653–656
    nonpharmacologic therapies 656
Ischemic heart disease 138, 158–177
  aldosterone antagonists 175
  angina in 163–164
  angiotensin-converting enzyme inhibitors 175
  antiischemic therapy for 173–175
    beta-blockers 173
    calcium channel blockers 174
    nitrates 174
    ranolazine 175
  antiplatelet therapy for 171–173
  autoimmune diseases and 159
  clinical presentation of 163–165
  cocaine abuse and 159
  diagnostic procedures
    coronary angiography 169–170
    exercise treadmill testing 168
    pharmacologic stress testing 168–169
    stress testing 166–167
    stress tests with imaging 169
  differential diagnosis of 165–166, 165*t*
  epidemiology of 158
  history 163–164
  human immunodeficiency virus and 159
  imaging of 166
  nonpharmacologic therapies 175–176
  peripheral arterial disease 158
  physical examination of 164–165
  prevention of 160–163
    aerobic exercise 162
    age 161
    cigarette smoking 162
    diabetes care 163
    diet 162
    hypertension 162
    lipids 161
    metabolic syndrome 163
    obesity 162–163
  revascularization in 176
  risk factor 158–159
  statin therapy 175
Isoniazid 527, 527*t*
Isospora belli 573
Isosporiasis 573
Isotretinoin 853

Isradipine 174*t*
Itraconazole 555, 556, 572, 860

J

JAK2 V617F mutation 301, 302
JC virus 569
Joint injections 665–666
Jugular venous distention (JVD) 186

K

Kallmann syndrome 451
Kaposi sarcoma 737
Karnofsky performance scale index 789
Keratinous cyst 847
Keratoconjunctivitis sicca 622
Keratosis pilaris 850
Ketoacidosis 413
Ketoconazole 862
Kiesselbach plexus 835
Klinefelter syndrome 450
Knee, examination of 660
Knee pain 711–715. *See also* Musculoskeletal
    complaints
  clinical presentation 712–713
  diagnostic testing 714
  general principles 711–712
  treatment of 714–715

L

Labetalol 143
Laboratory testing, preoperative 11–13
  coagulation studies 12
  complete blood count 12
  renal function tests 12
  serum electrolytes 12
  urinalysis 12–13
Lachman test 713
Lacosamide 915*t*
Lactation 290
Lactobacillus spp., 472*t*
Lambert-Eaton myasthenic syndrome
    741–742
Lamotrigine 769, 916*t*
Laryngeal papilloma 838
Laryngitis 837–838
Laryngoscopy 586
Latent tuberculosis 528–529
Laxatives, stimulant 599
Leflunomide 668–669
Left bundle branch block (LBBB) 169
Leg ulcers 298, 300
Lenalidomide 739
Leukemia 727–728, 738–739
  acute 727–728, 738
  chronic 728, 738–739
  chronic lymphocytic 728, 738–739

chronic myelogenous 728, 739
hairy cell 739
testicular masses and 82
Leukocyte esterase 482
Leukocytosis 303–304
Leukopenia 304
Leukotriene modifiers 359*t*
Leukotrienes 793
Levalbuterol 346*t*
Levetiracetam 915*t*
Levodopa 925
Levothyroxine 433
Lice 863
Lichen planus 852
Lidocaine 221*t*, 665
Lifestyle counseling 6–7
Lifto-ff test 701
Linaclotide 654
Lintigo, solar, 736–737
Lipids 161
Lipoic acid 471*t*
Lipoma 847
Lipoprotein 159, 250, 251*t*
disorders 867
Lispro 420
Listeria monocytogenes 549*t*
Lithium 34
Liver disease 27–28
alcohol-induced 626–627
diagnosis of 27
drug-induced 627–628
hemostasis and 280
metabolic
alpha-1 antitrypsin 624
hereditary hemochromatosis 624–625
nonalcoholic fatty liver disease 624
Wilson disease 625–626
treatment of 27–28
viral
hepatitis A 617
hepatitis B 618, 619*t*, 620
hepatitis C 620–621
Liver transplantation 630, 634–635
Long QT syndrome 240
Loop diuretics 141, 188*t*
Loop recorder 218
Loperamide 547, 551, 654
Lorcaserin 476
Lovastatin 256*t*
Low back pain (LBP) 691–698. *See also*
Musculoskeletal complaints
clinical presentation 693–695
diagnostic testing 695–696
epidemiology of 691
etiology of 691–692
nonspecific musculoskeletal 691
treatment of 696–698
injection therapies 697
medications 696–697

nonpharmacologic therapies 697, 698
surgical management 698
Low HDL 251*t*
Low molecular weight heparin (LMWH) 314, 315
Low-density lipoprotein (LDL) 159, 161, 258–260
Lower esophageal sphincter (LES) 607
Low-oxalate diet 515
Low-protein diet 515
Low-salt diet 196
Lubiprostone 654
Lung cancer
screening for 96
small-cell 733
treatment of 733
Lung sounds 328
Lung volume reduction surgery 349
Lungs
biopsy 375
nonrespiratory functions 327
respiratory functions 327
transplantation 349
Lupus erythematosus 863–864
acute cutaneous 863
chronic cutaneous 863
cutaneous, subacute 863
Lupus nephritis 496, 497*t*
Lyme disease 558–559
Lymph adenopathy, cervical 727
Lymphangioleiomyomatosis (LAM) 377, 378
Lymphocytes 793
Lymphocytosis 403
Lymphogranuloma venereum 578–579
Lymphoma 82, 727, 737–738
Lymphoreticular malignancies 866

M

Ma huang 34
Macroadenomas 449
Macroalbuminuria 502
Macrocytic anemia 290–292
clinical presentation of 291
diagnostic testing 291–292
etiology of 290–291
general principles 290
history 291
megaloblastic 290–291
nonmegaloblastic 291
physical examination 291
treatment of 292
Macrolide antibiotics 364
Macronutrient substitutes 459
Macronutrients 455
Magnesium 465*t*
Magnetic resonance angiography (MRA) 187, 313

Magnetic resonance cholangiopancreatography (MRCP) 604
Major depression 871
Malaria 547
Malassezia spp., 860
Male hypogonadism 449–451
  causes of androgen deficiency 450*t*
  etiology of 450–451
  general principles 449–450
  testicular disorders 450
Male pattern hair loss 85
Malignant transformation 629
Malnutrition 786–789
  causes of 787*t*
  definition of 455
  diagnosis 787–788
  general principles 786–787
  treatment of 788–789
Manganese 467*t*
Marjolin ulcer 848
Massage 697
Mast cells 793
McMurray test 713
Mean corpuscular volume (MCV) 974
Measles 107–108
Meclizine 827
Mediastinal radiotherapy 406
Mediastinum, midline mass in 727
Medical Research Council dyspnea scale 350*t*
Medicare Hospice Benefit 749
Medication overuse headache 907
Mefloquine 547*t*
Megestrol 788
Meibomianitis 948
Melanocytic nevus 847
Melanoma 848–849
  malignant 736
Melasma 860
Memantine 928
Membranoproliferative glomerulonephritis 495–496
Ménière disease 826, 827, 834
Meningeal carcinomatosis 740
Meningococcal, vaccination for 119–120
Meniscal tears 711
Menopause 54–56
  clinical presentation 54–55
  diagnostic testing 55
  general principles 54
  treatment 55–56
Men's health
  androgenetic alopecia 85
  benign prostatic hyperplasia 71–76
  erectile dysfunction 78–82
  priapism 84–85
  prostate cancer screening 69–71
  prostatitis 76–78
  testicular masses 82–84

Meperidine 762
Meralgia paresthetica 710, 921
Mesothelial cells 403
Metabolic acidosis 502, 505
Metabolic equivalents (METs) 16*t*
Metabolic liver disease 624–626.
    See also Hepatobiliary diseases
  alpha-1 antitrypsin 624
  hereditary hemochromatosis 624–625
  nonalcoholic fatty liver disease 624
  Wilson disease 625–626
Metabolic syndrome 163
Metastases
  bone 741
  brain 739–740
Metatarsalgia 717
Metered-dose inhalers (MDIs) 344
Metformin 417, 453
Methadone 764
Methimazole 436
Methotrexate 668
Methyldopa 149
Methylnaltrexone 767
Methylprednisolone 272, 918
Methylxanthines 347
Metoclopramide 612
Metoprolol 222*t*
Metronidazole 60, 61, 582
Mexiletine 222*t*
Microadenomas 448–449
Microalbuminuria 493, 502
Microangiopathic hemolytic anemia (MAHA) 271, 297
Microcytic anemia 285–290
  iron deficiency 285–288
  thalassemia 288–290
Micronutrients 455
Midfoot pain 717–718
Migraine 906
  with aura 908*t*
  without aura 908*t*
  ophthalmic 944
Mild cognitive impairment (MCI) 926
Minerals 465–467*t*
Minimal change disease (MCD) 494
Minoxidil 85, 144
Mirtazapine 788
Mite 863
Mitral regurgitation (MR)
  degenerative
    clinical presentation 212–213
    diagnostic testing 213
    etiology of 212
    general principles 212–213
    pathophysiology of 212
    treatment of 213–214
  functional
    clinical presentation 214

diagnostic testing 214
  general principles 214
  treatment of 215
Mitral stenosis 210–212
  clinical presentation 211
  diagnostic testing 211
  etiology of 210
  general principles 210–211
  pathophysiology of 210–211
  treatment of 211–212
Mitral valve prolapse 212
Mitral valve repair 214
Mixed mood syndrome 872
Model for end-stage liver disease (MELD)
  score 634
Modified barium swallow 586
Molluscum contagiosum 580–581, 862
Molybdenum 467t
Monoamine oxidase inhibitors (MAOIs)
  33, 881t
Monoclonal gammopathies 304
  amyloidosis 305
  multiple myeloma 305
  of unknown significance 304–305
  Waldenström macroglobulinemia 304
Morbidity risk index 789
Morphine 299, 764
Morton neuroma 718
mTOR inhibitors 635
Mucopurulent cervicitis (MPC) 575
Multidisciplinary biopsychosocial therapy 698
Multinodular goiter 439
Multiple myeloma (MM) 305, 728, 739
Multiple sclerosis 917–919
  clinical presentation 917
  diagnostic criteria for 918t
  diagnostic testing 917–918
  general principles 917
  treatment of 918–919
Mumps 107–108
Murphy sign 602
Muscle relaxants 696
Musculoskeletal complaints 335, 644, 687–718
  ankle pain 715–716
  elbow pain 703–706
  heel pain 716–717
  hip pain 708–711
  knee pain 711–715
  low back pain 691–698
  mid- and forefoot pain 717–718
  neck pain 687–690
  shoulder pain 699–703
  wrist and hand pain 706–708
Mycobacterial infections 571
Mycobacterium avium complex (MAC) 571
Mycobacterium avium-intracellulare 366
Mycobacterium tuberculosis 526
Mycophenolate mofetil 635

Myelodysplastic syndrome (MDS) 292–294
  classification of 292–293
  clinical presentation 293
  diagnostic testing 293
  epidemiology 293
  general principles 292
  laboratory testing 293
  risk factors 293
  treatment of 293–294
    chemotherapy 294
    elderly 294
    hematopoietic stem cell transplantation 294
    supportive treatment 293
Myelography 696
Myelopathy 688, 690
Myelosuppression 743
Myocardial bridging 166
Myocardial infarction (MI) 158
Myocardial perfusion imaging (MPI) 187

N

Nadolol 173t
NaHCO₃, 491
Nail disorders 859
Naloxone 767
Naltrexone 975
Naproxen 762t
Narrow-complex tachycardia 219–230
  atrial fibrillation 224–227
  atrial flutter 227
  atrial tachycardia 229
  multifocal atrial tachycardia 230, 230f
  reentrant supraventricular tachycardia
    227–229, 228f
  sinus tachycardia 220, 224
Nasal decongestants 816
Nasal potential difference 363
Natalizumab 919
Nausea 586–589. See also Gastrointestinal
    complaints
  in cancer patients 745
  causes of 588t, 754
  clinical presentation 586–587
  diagnostic testing 587
  in palliative care 754
  treatment of 587, 589
Neck mass 839–840
  clinical presentation 839–840
  congenital 840
  diagnostic testing 840
  general principles 839
  treatment of 840
Neck pain 687–690
  clinical presentation 688–689
  diagnostic testing 689–690
  general principles 687–688
  treatment 690

Necrobiosis lipoidica diabeticorum 866
Necrotizing fasciitis 539–540
Necrotizing otitis externa 820
Nedocromil 359t
Neer impingement sign 701
Neomycin 821
Neotame 460t
Nephritic syndrome 493
Nephrogenic systemic fibrosis 864
Nephrolithiasis 512–516. See also Hematuria
  calcium stones 512, 515
  clinical presentation 513
  cystine stones 515
  diagnostic testing 513–514
  prevalence of 512
  risk factors 513
  struvite stones 513
  treatment of 514–516
    acute management 514
    chronic management 515–516
    dietary modification 514–515
  uric acid stones 512, 515
Nephrotic syndrome 493
Nephrotoxicity 665
Neuroleptics 759
Neurologic exam 134
Neurologic pain 335
Neuropathic pain 758
Neuropathy 425–426, 919–923
  causes of 920t
  clinical presentation 919–920
  diagnostic testing 922
  differential diagnosis 920–922
  general principles 919
  treatment of 922–923
Neurosyphilis 575
Neutrophil count 403
Niacin 259, 462t
Nicotine replacement therapy (NRT) 965–966
  cardiovascular disease and 967
  inhaler 965
  lactation and 967
  lozenges 964
  nasal spray 965
  patches 964–965
  pregnancy and 967
  safety of 959, 961
Nicotinic acid 259
Nifedipine 174
Nipple discharge 57-58
Nisoldipine 174t
Nitrates 174, 194t
Nitroglycerin 174
N-methyl-D-aspartate (NMDA) receptor
    antagonists 928
Nociceptive pain 758
Nodulocystic acne 852
Nonalcoholic fatty liver disease (NAFLD) 624

Nonalcoholic steatohepatitis (NASH) 631
Nondihydropyridines 174, 174t
Nongonococcal urethritis (NGU) 575
Non-Hodgkin lymphoma 737–738
Nonselective β-blockers 632
Nonspecific interstitial pneumonitis (NSIP)
    376t, 377, 378
Non-steroidal anti-inflammatory drugs
    (NSAIDs) 276, 665, 672, 678, 696,
    761, 911
Noradrenergic agonist-specific serotonergic
    antagonist 877–878t
Normocytic anemia 294–302
  anemia of chronic disease 294–295
  aplastic anemia 295
  autoimmune hemolytic anemia 296–297
  drug-induced hemolytic anemia 297
  hemolytic anemia 295–296
  microangiopathic hemolytic anemia 297
  polycythemia 301
  red cell enzyme deficiencies 300
  sickle cell diseases 297–300
  thrombocytosis 302
Norovirus 546
Nortriptyline 966
Nutrition 455–464
  chronic kidney disease and 505
  dietary guidelines 455–457
  dietary supplements 464
  drug-nutrient interactions 464, 468–469t
  macronutrient 457–459
  micronutrients 459, 461–463t
  obesity 464–477
Nystatin 554, 609

O

Obesity 464, 475–477
  bariatric surgery for 476
  clinical presentation 464, 475
  definition of 455
  diagnostic testing 475
  general principles 464
  ischemic heart disease and 162–163
  lifestyle modification and 476–477
  medications for 475–476
  screening for 5, 101
  treatment of 475–477
Obsessive-compulsive disorder, characteristics
    of 886t
Obstructive sleep apnea (OSA)
  classification of 389
  clinical presentation 390
  definition of 389
  diagnostic testing 391
  differential diagnosis 390
  epidemiology 389
  hypertension and 135t, 148

pathophysiology 389
prevention 390
risk factors 389
treatment 391–392
lifestyle/risk modificatin 392
medications 391
nonpharmacologic therapy 391–392
surgical management 392
Occupational therapy 669
Octreotide 636
Ocular 645
Ocular motility 942
Ocular myasthenia gravis 952
Ocular trauma 949–951
chemical burn 950
corneal abrasions 950–951
foreign body/rust ring 951
hyphema 951
orbital fractures 951
ruptured globe 950
traumatic iris 951
Odynophagia 584–586
Ofloxacin 821
Olanzapine 897
Omega-3 fatty acids 471t
Onycholysis 859
Onychomycosis 859, 861
Ophthalmic migraines 944
Ophthalmology 940–954
Opiates 696–697
Opioids 762–767
adjuvants for neuropathic pain 768
adjuvants for side effects 767–768
combination preparations 765t
conversion between 765–766
treatment of dyspnea with 755
Optic neuritis 946–947
Optic neuropathies, ischemic 945
Oral candidiasis 554
Oral contraceptive (OC) 453, 629
Oral direct thrombin inhibitor 316–317, 316–318, 322
Oral direct Xa inhibitors 316
Oral glucose tolerance test (OGTT) 414
Orbital fractures 951
Orlistat 475–476
Orthodeoxia 633
Orthostatic proteinuria 486
Oseltamivir 522
Osgood-Schlatter disease 712
Osler-Weber-Rendu disease 836
Osmotic laxatives 654
Osteoarthritis 663, 665–666
diagnosis of 663
general principles 663
glenohumeral joint and 699
hip pain 711
knee pain 711

neck pain in 687
treatment of 665–666
joint injections 665–666
medications 665, 703
nonpharmacologic measures 666
surgery 666
wrist and hand pain 707
Osteogenic sarcoma 737
Osteomyelitis 786
Osteonecrosis 709
Osteoporosis
clinical presentation 46, 47
corticosteroid-induced 53
definition 46
diagnostic testing 47–49, 48t, 49t
general principles 46
inflammatory bowel diseases and 644
in men 53
patient education 54
risk factors 46, 47t
screening for 101
treatment 49–53
diet therapy 53
exercise 53
fall prevention 54
medications 49–52
Otitis externa (OE) 820–822
diagnosis 820–821, 821t
general principles 820
necrotizing 820
treatment of, 821–822
Otitis media (OM) 822–823
acute 822, 823
diagnosis 823
general principles 822
treatment 823
Otitis media with effusion (OME) 822, 823
Otitis, serous 822
Otomycosis 822
Otosclerosis 834
Ottawa knee rules 714, 714t
Oval fat bodies 483
Ovarian cancer 736
screening 98
Overflow incontinenc 781
Overnutrition 464, 475–477
Oxaliplatin 734
Oxandrolone 788
Oxcarbazepine 769, 916t
Oxybutynin 782
Oxycodone 764
Oxygen concentrators 348
Oxygen therapy 348, 383, 386

P

Pacemaker mediated tachycardia (PMT) 245
Pacemaker syndrome 245

Pacemakers 242–246
  biventricular 243
  complications and malfunction of 245–246
  dual chamber 243
  general principles 242
  management of 245
  modes 244t, 245
  perioperative considerations for 22–23
  single chamber 243
Pain 636, 758
  acute 758
  chronic 758
  definition of 758
  diagnosis of 759–760
  epidemiology of 759
  history 760t
  monitoring/follow-up 769
  neuropathic 758
  nociceptive 758
  pathophysiology of 759
  referral 769
  treatment of 760–769
    medications 761–762
    nonpharmacologic therapies 769
    WHO pain ladder 760
  visceral 758
Palifermin 745
Palliative care 748–756
  appropriate timing 749–751
  cost of 749
  definition of 748
  epidemiology of 748–749
  goals of 752–753
  indications for 749
  monitoring/follow-up 755
  patient assessment in 751
  referral 755
  treatment in 751–755
    artificial nutrition support 753–754
    end-of-life nutrition 753–754
    nonpain symptoms 754–755
    sharing bad news 752
    venues for 751
Palliative therapy 732
Pancreatic ascites 637
Pancreatic calcification 636
Pancreatic cancer 637
Pancreatic endocrine dysfunction 365
Pancreatic enzyme supplementation 365, 636
Pancreatitis 335
  chronic 636–637
  hereditary 636
  idiopathic 636
  tropical 636
Panic disorder 888, 890–892. *See also* Anxiety
    disorders
  associated conditions 890
  characteristics of 886t

definition of 888
diagnosis of 890–891
epidemiology of 890
etiology/pathophysiology of 890
general principles 888
treatment of 891–892
Pantothenic acid 463t
Paraneoplastic syndromes 741
Parapneumonic effusions 405
Parathyroid hormone (PTH) 52
Parathyroidectomy 447
Parkinson disease 925
Parkinsonism 925, 927
Paronychia 707
Pasteurella spp., 540
Patellar compression test 713
Patellofemoral pain syndrome (PFPS) 711
Patrick test 710
Peak exploratory flow rate (PEFR) 355
Pediculosis 863
Pediculosis pubis 581
Pelvic inflammatory disease (PID) 582
Pemphigus foliaceus 855
Pemphigus vulgaris 855
Penicillins 216
Pentamidine 572
Pentoxifylline 626–627
Percutaneous coronary intervention (PCI) 21, 172
Perennial allergens 794
Pericardial effusions, malignant 740
Pericarditis 676
Periodic health examination 1–2
  adolescents/young adults 1–2
  midlife adults 2
  older adults 2
Peripheral arterial disease (PAD)
  ischemic heart disease and 158
  screening for 100
Peripheral neuropathy 425
Peripheral smear 291
Perirectal fistula 600
Permethrin 863
Pertussis vaccines 108–110, 109f
Pes planus 717
Petechiae 265
PFA-100, 266
Pharyngitis 518–519
  group a streptococcal (GAS) pharyngitis
    518–519
Phenobarbital 915t
Phenothiazines 745t
Phentermine 476
Phenytoin 915t
Pheochromocytoma 136t
Phlebotomy 301
Phobias, characteristics of 886t
Phosphodiesterase inhibitors 74, 80–81, 383, 384t
Phosphorus 465t, 504

Physical examination 133–134
Physical therapy 669
Picornavirus 617
Pigment disorders 859–860
Pigment stones 635
  black 635
  brown 635
Pilar cysts 847
Pindolol 84*t*
Pitavastatin 256*t*
Pityriasis rosea 852
Plantar fasciitis 716
Plantar warts 862
Plasma cells 403
Plasma exchange (PEX) 272
Platelet
  count 265
  disorders 267–268, 268*t*
  inhibitors 270*t*
  pheresis 302
  reduction therapy 302
Platinum-containing agents 730*t*
Platypnea 633
Pleural, biopsy 404
Pleural disorders 334
Pleural effusion 400–406
  clinical presentation 400–401
  closed pleural biopsy 404
  definition of 400
  diagnostic testing 401–404
  empyema 405
  etiology of 400
  evaluation of 402*f*
  exudative 400, 404
  fluid appearance 402
  malignant 741
  parapneumonic 405
  transudative 400, 404
  treatment of 405–406
Pleurectomy 405
Pleuritic pain 335
Pleuritis 676
Pleurodesis 405
Pneumococcal pneumonia 196
Pneumococcal vaccine 111–113, 113*t*, 299
Pneumocystis jiroveci pneumonia (PCP) 523, 568, 572
Pneumonia 298
  bacterial 570
  community-acquired 523–525
  cryptogenic organizing 377, 378
  pneumococcal 196
  Pneumocystis jiroveci 568, 572
Pneumothorax 366
Podagra 717
Podophyllin 580
Polio vaccination 121
Polyarteritis nodosa 681

Polyarthralgia 660*f*
Polycystic ovary syndrome 452
Polycythemia vera (PV) 301
Polymyalgia rheumatica 682
Polymyositis 683–684
Polymyxin B 821
Polypharmacy 775–777
Polysaccharideiron complex 287*t*
Popeye sign 702
Portal hypertension 631–632
Portosystemic encephalopathy (PSE) 633
Postconcussive syndrome 932
Postexposure prophylaxis 617, 618
Postnasal drip 332
Poststreptococcal glomerulonephritis 497
Posttransfusion purpura (PTP) 274–275
Posttransplant complications 635
Post-traumatic stress disorder (PTSD), characteristics of 886*t*
Postviral bronchial hyperreactivity 332
Potassium 465*t*
Potassium-sparing agents 141
Potassium-sparing diuretics 188*t*
Pouchitis 648
Pramlintide 419
Pravastatin 256*t*
Prednisone 272, 441–442, 572, 855
Preeclampsia 149
Preexposure prophylaxis 617, 618
Pregabalin 768, 916*t*, 923
Pregnancy 290
  adult immunizations and 124
  hypertension and 149
  hyperthyroidism in 439
  nicotine replacement therapy and 967
  in sickle cell patient 298
Premature ventricular contraction (PVC) 232
Preoperative laboratory testing 11–13
  coagulation studies 12
  complete blood count 12
  renal function tests 12
  serum electrolytes 12
  urinalysis 12–13
Presbycusis 834
Pressure ulcers 784–786
  classification of 784
  complications 786
  definition of 784
  diagnosis 785
  prevention 784–785
  risk factors 784
  treatment of 785–786
Presyncope 826
Priapism 84–85, 299
Primaquine 572
Primary biliary cirrhosis (PBC) 622–623
Primary ciliary dyskinesia 362
Primary hyperaldosteronism 135*t*, 148

Primary sclerosing cholangitis (PSC)
    622–623, 645
Probenecid 673
Probiotics 472*t*
Procainamide 221*t*
Prochlorperazine 909
Proctalgia fugax 600
Proctoscopy 599
Progressive multifocal leukoencephalopathy
    569
Proguanil 547*t*
Prolotherapy 698
Promethazine 587, 827
Promotility agents 612
Propafenone 222*t*
Prophylaxis 617, 618
Propylthiouracil 436
Prostacyclin analogues 383, 384*t*
Prostanoids 383, 384*t*
Prostate cancer 734–735
Prostate cancer screening 96–97
  algorithm for 72*f*
  digital rectal examination 70
  general principles 69
  prostate-specific antigen 70–71, 70*t*
Prostate-specific antigen (PSA) 70–71, 70*t*
Prostatitis 76-78
  acute 76
  chronic 76-78, 77*t*
  general principles 76
  treatment 77–78
Protamine 315, 320
Protease inhibitors 159
Proteinuria 485-487, 493
Prothrombin time (PT) 266, 267*t*, 604
Proton pump inhibitors (PPIs) 586, 609–610
Protozoal infections 572–573
Pruritus 768
Pruritus ani 600
Pseudoclaudication 693
Pseudocysts 657
Pseudogout 673-674, 717
Pseudoresistance 146
Pseudotumor cerebri 944
Psoriasis, scalp 851
Psoriatic arthritis 677
Psychiatric disorders 971
Psychogenic nonepileptic seizures (PNES) 912
Psychosis 892-897
  associated conditions 892
  definition of 892
  diagnosis of 892-893
  differential diagnosis of 893, 894*t*
  DSM-IV-TR criteria 893
  epidemiology of 892
  etiology/pathophysiology of 892
  in older adults 900–901
  outcome/prognosis of 897
  treatment of 895-897

  medications 895, 895*t*, 897
  nonpharmacologic therapies 897
  types of 892–893
Psychotic disorders 873*t*
Ptosis 953
Pulmonary alveolar proteinosis (PAP)
    377, 378
Pulmonary angiography 313
Pulmonary arterial hypertension (PAH) 379*t*,
    380–386, 385*f*
Pulmonary complaints 327–339
  auscultated pulmonary sounds 328
  cough 330–332
  dyspnea 328–330
  hemoptysis 332–334
  lung functions and 327
  noncardiac chest pain 334–335
  pulmonary function tests 336–339
  pulmonary physical examination 327
  radiographic studies 339*t*
Pulmonary embolism (PE) 309
  anatomic location of 309
  diagnostic testing 311–314
  etiology/pathophysiology of 309
Pulmonary evaluation, preoperative
  clinical presentation 23–24
  diagnostic criteria for 24–25
  diagnostic testing 25–26
  history 23–24
  overview 23
  postoperative pneumonia risk index 24*t*
  treatment 26–27
    obstructive lung disease therapy 26
    smoking cessation 26
Pulmonary function test (PFT) 336–339
  for chronic obstructive pulmonary disease
    343, 344*t*
  initial evaluation of 337*f*
  interpretation of 336, 337*f*, 338*t*
  for interstitial lung diseases 375
  ordering appropriate tests 336
  predicted values 336
Pulmonary hypertension (PH) 378–386
  classification of 379*t*, 383*t*
  clinical presentation 380
  diagnostic tests 380–381
  evaluation of 382*f*
  general principles 378–380
  right heart catheterization 381
  treatment of 381–386
Pulmonary Langerhans cell histiocytosis
    (PLCH) 378
Pulmonary mass 406
Pulmonary nodule, solitary 406–409
  clinical presentation 407
  definition of 406
  diagnostic testing 407–409
  differential diagnosis of 406*t*
  etiology of 407

pulmonary mass 406
survival rate 406
Pulmonary physical examination 327–328
Pulmonary rehabilitation 365
Pulmonary venous hypertension (PVH) 380
Pulsus alternan 186
Pupillary exam 940, 941
Pyoderma gangrenosum (PG) 644, 854
Pyrazinamide 527, 527*t*
Pyridoxine 462*t*
Pyrimethamine 573

Q

Qualitative platelet disorders 276
Quinidine 221*t*
Quinolone 574

R

Rabies 122–123
Radial nerve entrapment 921
Radiation therapy 732, 737
Radioactive iodine therapy 437–438
Radiocontrast agents 488
Raloxifene 51
Ramsay Hunt syndrome 543
Ranolazine 175
Rapid plasma reagin (RPR) 576
Rapidly progressive glomerulonephritis
(RPGN) 493
Rasburicase 743
Raynaud phenomena 679
RBC casts 483
Reactive arthritis 677
Recombinant erythropoietin 744
Recommended dietary allowance (RDA) 455
Rectal cancer 734
Rectal prolapse 600
Rectosigmoid intussusception 600
Red blood cells 482
Red cell enzyme deficiency 300
Red cell fragmentation 296
Red eye 948–949
blepharitis 948
dry eye 948
episcleritis 949
infections 949
iritis 949
scleritis 949
seasonal allergies 948–949
subconjunctival hemorrhage 948
Reentrant supraventricular tachycardia.
See also Arrhythmias; Narrow-complex
tachycardia
antidromic 229
atypical 229
diagnosis of 228–229
ECG features of 228, 228*f*

forms of 228
general principles 227–228
orthodromic 229
treatment of 229
typical 228–229
Refractory hypertension 146
Rehydration 548, 551
Rejection, chronic 635
Renal cell cancer 735
Renal medullary infarction 298
Renal parenchymal disease 135*t*, 148
Renal tubular defects 298
Renal tubular epithelial cells 483
Renovascular disease 135*t*, 148
Reserpine 144
Resistant hypertension 146–147
Respiratory depression 768
Respiratory tract infections 517–529
acute bronchitis 519–521
acute rhinosinusitis 517–518
community-acquired pneumonia 523–525
influenza 521–522
latent tuberculosis 528–529
pharyngitis 518–519
tuberculosis 526–528
Restless legs syndrome 396–397
Restrictive cardiomyopathy 201–202
Restrictive ventilatory defect 375
Reticulocyte count 285
Reticulocyte index (RI) 285
Reticulocytosis 291
Retinal detachment 945
Retinoids 853
Retinopathy 425
Retroperitoneum, midline mass in 727
Revascularization 20–21
Rhabdomyolysis 260
Rheumatoid arthritis 666–669
criteria for 667*t*
diagnosis of 666–667
general principles 666
treatment of 667–669
medications 668–669
nonpharmacologic therapies 669
surgical management 669
Rheumatoid factor (RF) 661
Rhinitis 814–816
diagnosis 815
general principles 814–815
inflammatory 814
noninflammatory 814
structural 814
treatment 815–816
antihistamines 815
anti-inflammatory agents 815
decongestants 816
immunotherapy 816
intranasal anticholinergics 816
intranasal antihistamines 816

Rhinitis medicamentosa 814
Rhinoconjunctivitis 814–816
Rhinosinusitis, acute 517–518
Riboflavin 462*t*
Rickettsia rickettsii 559
Rifampin 527, 527*t*
Rifaximin 546
Rimantadine 522
Rinne test, for hearing loss 832
Risedronate 50
Rituximab 272, 669
Rivaroxaban 316
Rivastigmine 928
RNA virus 617, 620
Rocky Mountain spotted fever 559
Rosuvastatin 256*t*, 259
Rotator cuff tears 699
Rotator cuff tendonitis 699
Rotavirus 549*t*
Rubella 107–108
Ruptured globe 950

S

S3 heart sound 186
Saccharin 460*t*
Sacroiliitis 644
Saline diuresis 446
Salmeterol 346*t*
Salmonella sp., 570
Sarcoidosis 377, 378
Sarcomas, soft tissue 736–737
Sarcoptes scabiei 863
Saw palmetto 75
Scabies 581, 863
Schatzki ring 584
Schistocytes 271
Sciatica 693–694, 694*t*
Scleritis 949
Scleroderma 678–679, 864
Scleroderma renal crisis 679
Screening for disease 89–102
    abdominal aortic aneurysm 100
    alcohol abuse and dependence 102
    cancer screening 4, 92–99
        breast cancer 92–93
        cervical cancer 93–94
        colorectal cancer 94–96
        lung cancer 96
        ovarian cancer 98
        prostate cancer 96–97
        testicular cancer 98
    coronary heart disease 100
    diabetes mellitus 5, 6*t*, 99–100
    dyslipidemia 5, 99
    general principles 89, 90–91*t*
    hepatitis C 102
    hypertension 4–5, 99, 99*t*
    obesity 5, 101

        osteoporosis 101
        peripheral arterial disease 100
        schedule 90–91*t*
        sexually transmitted diseases 101
        thyroid disease 100
        tobacco abuse 6
Seasonal affective disorder (SAD) 873*t*
Seasonal allergens 794
Seasonal allergy 948–949
Seborrheic dermatitis 850–851
Seborrheic keratosis 846
Sedation 767
Seizures 911–919
    diagnosis 913
    etiology of 912*t*
    focal 911
    general principles 911–912
    generalized 911
    treatment of 913–917
Selective serotonin reuptake inhibitors (SSRIs)
        33, 656, 874, 877–878*t*
Selenium 466*t*
Selenium sulfide 860
Self-harm and suicidality 882–884
Self-monitoring of capillary blood glucose
        (SMBG) 416
Sensorineural hearing loss (SNHL) 831
Sentinel lymph node 732
Seronegative spondyloarthropathies 676–678
    clinical presentation 677
    diagnostic testing 678
    general principles 676–677
    treatment of 678
Serotonin 5-HT$_3$ receptor agonists 745*t*
Serotonin modulators 879–880*t*
Serous otitis 822
Serum ascites albumin gradient 605
        CA 19-9, 631, 637
        ferritin 286
        haptoglobin 295
Sexually transmitted disease (STD) 101,
        573–574
Sézary syndrome 866
Shigella 570
Shingles, vaccination for 118–119
Short QT syndrome 240
Shoulder impingement syndrome 699
Shoulder pain 699–703. *See also*
        Musculoskeletal complaints
    clinical presentation 700–702
    diagnostic testing 702
    general principles 699–700
    treatment of 702–703
Shunts, systemic-to-pulmonary 385
Shwachman syndrome 362
Sialolithiasis 838–839
    diagnosis 838–839
    general principles 838
    treatment of 839

Sickle cell diseases 297–300
  clinical presentation of 297
  complications 300
  diagnostic testing 299
  sickle cell diseases 297
  treatment of 299
Sickle cell trait 297
Sigmoidoscopy 597, 600
Sildenafil 80
Silodosin 75
Simvastatin 256t
Sinus node dysfunction 237
Sinus tachycardia 220, 224
Sirolimus (SRL) 635
Sjögren's syndrome 679–680
Skin and soft tissue infections 535–543
  abscesses 538
  animal and human bite wounds
      540–541
  carbuncles 538
  cellulitis 535–537
  erysipelas 535–537
  fungal skin infections 860–862
    candidiasis 860
    onychomycosis 861
    tinea capitis 860
    tinea corporis 861
    tinea cruris 861
    tinea pedis 861
    tinea versicolor 860
  furuncles 538
  herpes zoster 543
  impetigo 539
  necrotizing fasciitis 539–540
  spider bites 541–542
Skin cancer prevention 845–846
Skin infestations 863
Skin neoplasms 845–846. *See also* Cancer
  acrochordon 846
  actinic keratosis 847
  basal cell carcinoma 848
  cherry angioma 847
  keratinous cyst 847
  lipoma 847
  melanocytic nevus 847
  melanoma 848–849
  seborrheic keratosis 846
  skin cancer prevention 845–846
  skin tag 846
  solar lentigo 847
  squamous cell carcinoma 848
Skin sweat testing 362
Skin tag 846
Sleep disorders 389–397
  insomnia 393–396
  obstructive sleep apnea 389–392
  restless legs syndrome 396–397
Small-cell lung cancer (SCLC) 733, 742
Smoking cessation 956–967

benefits of 349
  in chronic heart failure patients 196
  counseling 957–958
  in diabetic patients 424
  general principles 956
  guidelines 956
  medications 959–967
    bupropion 965–966
    clonidine 966
    nicotine replacement therapy 965–966
    nortriptyline 966
    varenicline 966
  Prochaska model of stages of change 958
  recommendations 956–957
  weight gain 958
Sodium-glucose cotransporter 2 (SGLT2)
      inhibitor 418
Solar lentigo 847
Solifenacin 782
Sotalol 223t
Southern tick-associated rash 557
Spasmodic dysphonia 838
Specific gravity 481
Spermatocele 82
Spherocytes 296
Spider bites 541–542
Spinal cord compression 740
Spinal manipulation 697
Spinal stenosis 691, 693
Spirometry 343, 344t
Spironolactone 141, 453
Splenectomy
  of IgM-mediated disease 297
  thalassemia 290
Splenic vein thrombosis 637
Splenomegaly 602
Spondyloarthropathies, seronegative
      676–678
  clinical presentation 677
  diagnostic testing 678
  general principles 676–677
  treatment of 678
Spondylolisthesis 691
Spondylosis 687, 691
Spontaneous bacterial peritonitis (SBP)
      632–633
Sporothrix schenckii 553
Sporotrichosis 553
Sputum 333
Sputum cultures 363, 364
Squamous cell carcinoma 848
Squamous epithelial cells 483
St. John's wort 34
Staphylococcus aureus 704
Stasis dermatitis 850
Statin therapy 175
Statins 20, 256t, 258–259
Steatorrhea 637
Stem cell donor, counseling 306

Stenosing tenosynovitis 706
Stereotactic body radiation therapy (SBRT) 409
Steroids 745t, 769
  adjunctive use of 572
  epidural injections 698
  of IgM-mediated disease 297
  intra-articular 665
  long-term use of 795
  nonresponders 269
  oral 672, 945
  systemic 856, 857
  topical 609, 844–845
Stevens-Johnson syndrome 856
Stimulant laxatives 599
Stomatitis 744–745
Stress echocardiography 211
Stress incontinence 781
Stress testing 146, 166–167
Stroke 298
  clinical presentation 930
  definition of 929
  diagnostic testing 930
  differential diagnosis 930
  general principles 929–930
  hypertension and 139
  treatment of 930–932
Struvite stones 513, 516
Stucco keratoses 846
Student's elbow 704
Subacute cutaneous lupus erythematosus 863
Subendocardial ischemia 165
Subungual hematoma 707
Sucralose 460t
Sudden cardiac death (SCD) 235–236
Sudden sensorineural hearing loss 831
Sugar substitutes 459
Suicidal behavior 882–884
Sulfadiazine 573
Sulfamethoxazole 521
Sulfasalazine 668, 678
Sulfonylureas 417
Superficial fungal infections 553–554
Superficial thrombophlebitis 311, 318
Superficial vein thrombosis (SVT) 318
Superior vena cava obstruction 740
Surgical patients 11–38
  elective vs. emergent surgery 11
  general vs. regional anesthesia 13
  medication adjustments in perioperative
    period 33–34
    anticonvulsants 33
    herbal medications 34
    psychiatric medications 33–34
  overview 11
  perioperative antiplatelet/anticoagulation
    management 30–31
  perioperative considerations in
    diabetes mellitus 28–30

    kidney disease 28
    liver disease 27–28
  perioperative corticosteroid management
    31–33
  preoperative cardiovascular risk assessment
    13–21
  preoperative laboratory testing 11–13
    coagulation studies 12
    complete blood count 12
    renal function tests 12
    serum electrolytes 12
    urinalysis 12–13
  preoperative pulmonary evaluation 23–27
Sweet syndrome 866
Sympathomimetic agents 802
Syncope 241–242
Syndrome of inappropriate antidiuretic
    hormone (SIADH) 741
Synovial fluid 663
Syphilis 570, 575–577
  latent syphilis 576
  primary syphilis 575
  secondary syphilis 575
Systemic lupus erythematosus 496, 674–676
  criteria for 675t
  diagnosis of 674–675
  general principles 674
  treatment of 676

T

Tachyarrhythmias 219
Tachycardia, narrow-complex 219–230
  atrial fibrillation 224–227
  atrial flutter 227
  atrial tachycardia 229
  multifocal atrial tachycardia 230, 230f
  reentrant supraventricular tachycardia
    227–229, 228f
  sinus tachycardia 220, 224
Tadalafil 80
Takayasu arteritis 681
Tamoxifen 732
Tamponade, cardiac 203
Tamsulosin 75
Tdap vaccine 108–109
Tegaserod 654
Telangiectasia 333
Telogen effluvium 858
Temporal arteritis 945
Tendinosis 704
Tendon xanthomas 867
Tendonitis
  Achilles 716
  bicipital 699
  calcific 699
  rotator cuff 699
Tennis elbow 703

Tension-type headache 906, 908*t*
Terazosin 74
Terbinafine 860, 861
Teriparatide 52
Terson syndrome 946
Testicular cancer 82, 735
Testicular disorders 450
Testicular masses 82–84
  clinical presentation 83
  diagnostic testing 83–84
  hydrocele 82–84
  malignant masses 84
  spermatocele 82
  treatment 84
  varicocele 82–84
Testosterone 79, 452
Tetanus vaccines 108–110, 109*f*
Tetrahydrocannabinol/dronabinol 788
Thalassemia 288–290
  classification of 288–289
  clinical presentation of 289
  diagnostic testing 289
  general principles 288
  history 289
  intermedia 288
  major 288
  minor (trait) 288
  physical examination 289
  surgical management 290
  treatment of 289
Thalidomide 739
Therapeutic lifestyle change (TLC) 144,
    254, 255*t*
Thiamine 461*t*
Thiazide 138, 140–141
Thiazide diuretics 188*t*
Thiazolidinediones 418
Thienopyridines 276
Thionamides 436–437
Thoracentesis 401–404
  indications for 401*t*
  therapeutic 405
Thoracoscopy 404
Thrombin inhibitor, direct 316–317
Thrombin time 267
Thrombocytopenia
  chemotherapy-induced 275
  classification of 268*t*
  drug-induced 270–271
  familial 275
  gestational 275
  heparin-induced 273–274
  to liver disease 275
Thrombocytosis 742
  secondary 302
Thrombophlebitis 309, 311, 318
Thromboprophylaxis 36*t*
Thrombotic microangiopathies (TMA) 498

Thrombotic thrombocytopenic purpura (TTP)
    271–272
Thyroid disease 136*t*
  screening for 100
  skin signs of 866
Thyroid nodules 440
Thyroidectomy, subtotal 438
Thyroid-stimulating hormone (TSH) 47, 431
Thyroxine 431, 434
Thyroxine-binding globulin (TBG) 431
Tibial tubercle apophysitis 712
Tick paralysis 557
Tick-borne disease 557–561
  anaplasmosis 560
  babesiosis 560–561
  ehrlichiosis 560
  Lyme disease 558–559
  Rocky Mountain spotted fever 559
Tick-borne relapsing fever 557
Tinea capitis 860
Tinea corporis 861
Tinea cruris 861
Tinea pedis 861
Tinea unguium 861
Tinea versicolor 553–554, 860
  candidal infections 553–554
  candidal vaginitis 554
  candiduria 554
  infections by dermatophytes 553
  oral candidiasis 554
  sporotrichosis 553
Tinnitus 824–826
  causes of 825*t*
  diagnosis 824
  general principles 824
  objective 824
  subjective 824
  treatment of 824–826
Tiotropium 346*t*
Tirofiban 276
Tobacco use and cessation 146. *See also* Smoking
    and cessation
Tofacitinib 669
Tolterodine 782
Topical estrogen 783
Topiramate 476, 910, 916*t*
Torsade de pointes 233–234
Toxic epidermolysis necrosis (TEN) 856
Toxic megacolon 642
Toxic multinodal goiter (MNG) 435
Toxoplasma gondii 572
Toxoplasmas 572–573
Tracheal stenosis 328
Tracheotomy 392
Tramadol 696, 764
Transarterial chemoembolization (TACE) 630
Transarterial radioembolization (TARE) 630
Transbronchial biopsies 375

Transcutaneous electrical nerve stimulation (TENS) 698
Transfats 458
Transferrin 286
Transjugular intrahepatic portosystemic shunt (TIPS) 632
Transsphenoidal surgery 449
Transudative pleural effusion 400, 404
Transurethral resection of prostate (TURP) 76
Trastuzumab 732
Traumatic brain injury (TBI) 932–933
Traumatic iris 951
Travel medicine 544–547
  malaria 547
  pretravel consultation 544
  returning traveler 544–546
  traveler's diarrhea 546–547
Traveler's diarrhea 546–547
Trendelenburg gait 710
Trichloroacetic acid 580
Trichomonas vaginalis 60–61
Trichomoniasis 575
Trichophyton spp., 553
Trichotillomania 858
Tricyclic antidepressants (TCAs) 33, 655–656, 768, 807, 880–881*t*
Trigeminal neuralgia 921
Trigger finger 707
Trigger point injection 697
Triglycerides 404
Trimethoprim 521
Trimethoprim-sulfamethoxazole (TMP-SMX) 568
Triptans 909
Tropical pancreatitis 636
Trospium 782
Tryptase 793
Tuberculosis (TB) 526–528
  clinical presentation 526
  diagnostic testing 526
  general principles 526
  HIV infection and 571
  latent 528–529
  monitoring 528
  treatment 526–528
Tularemia 557
Tumor lysis syndrome 743
Tumor necrosis factor (TNF) 562
Tylectomy 732
Tympanocentesis 823
Type 1 diabetes mellitus 29, 412
  diagnostic criteria for 414
  insulin for 420
Type 2 diabetes mellitus 29–30, 412–413
  diet-controlled diabetes 29
  insulin for 30, 420
  oral therapy for 29–30

U

Ulcerative colitis 642, 643*t*, 677
Ulcers 854
  aphthous 644
  genital 575–579
  Marjolin 848
  pressure
    classification of 784
    complications 786
    definition 784
    diagnosis 785
    prevention 784–785
    risk factors 784
    treatment 785–786
  venous 854
Ulnar nerve entrapment 704, 706, 921
Ultrasound 636
Undernutrition 477–478
  clinical presentation 477
  diagnostic testing 478
  general principles 477
Unfractionated heparins (UFHs) 315
Upper airway cough syndrome 332
Upper gastrointestinal bleeding 632
Urethritis 574–575
Urge incontinence 781
Uric acid stones 512, 515
Urinalysis 72, 480–483
  macroscopic examination 480
  microscopic examination 480, 482–483
  specimen collection 480
  testing procedure 480
Urinary incontinence 781–783
  causes of 781
  clinical presentation 781–782
  diagnostic testing 782
  general principles 781
  treatment of 782–783
  types of 781
Urinary tract infections
  complicated 533–534
  uncomplicated
    in men 532–533
    in women 530–532
Urine 480–483
  casts 483
  clarity 481
  color 480
  crystals in 483
  epithelial cells in 483
  glucose in 481
  hemoglobin in 482
  leukocyte esterase in 482
  nitrites 482
  odor 481
  organisms in 483
  pH 481
  protein in 481–482

red blood cells in 482
specific gravity 481
white blood cells in 482
Urine albumin-creatinine 487
Urine protein-creatinine ratio 487
Ursodeoxycholic acid 636
Urticaria 805–807
  acute 805
  chronic 805
  clinical presentation 806
  diagnostic testing 806–807
  etiology 805–806
  idiopathic 805
  immunologic 806
  nonimmunologic 806
  pathophysiology 806
  treatment 807
Uveitis 645
Uvulopalatopharyngoplasty 392
Uvulopalatoplasty, laser-assisted 392

V

Vaccinations 365. *See also* Immunizations, adult
Vaccine Adverse Events Reporting System
    (VAERS) 103
Vaginitis 59, 575
Valganciclovir 569
Valproic acid 910, 915*t*
Valvular heart disease
  anticoagulation 216–217
  aortic regurgitation 209–210
  aortic stenosis 206–209
  endocarditis prophylaxis 215–216
  mitral regurgitation
    degenerative 212–214
    functional 214–215
  mitral stenosis 210–212
  perioperative considerations for 22
Vancomycin 552
Vardenafil 80
Varenicline 966
Varicella-Zoster virus (VZV) 117–118,
    543, 569
Varicocele 82–84
Vascular dementia 928
Vascular exam 134
Vasculitic neuropathy 921, 923
Vasculitis 666, 680–682, 864–865
  cutaneous 681
  secondary 681
Vasodilators 144
Vasomodulators 383–385, 384*t*
Vasoocclusive complications 298
Venlafaxine 923
Venography 312
Venom hypersensitivity. *See also* Allergy
  diagnosis 804

general principles 803–804
  treatment 804–805
Venous thromboembolism (VTE) 309–323
  anatomy of 309
  clinical presentation 311
  definition of 309
  diagnostic testing 311–314
    D-dimer 311
    hypercoagulability testing 312
  differential diagnosis of 311
  etiology/pathophysiology of 309
  general principles 309
  prevention of 310
  prophylaxis 34
  risk factors 310
Venous ulcers 854
Ventricular arrhythmias
  acute myocardial infarction 233
  general principles 232
  idiopathic 233
  nonsustained 232
  polymorphic 233
  premature ventricular contractions 232
  sudden cardiac death in 235–236
  sustained 232–233
  torsade de pointes 233–234
  treatment of 233
  Wolff-Parkinson-White syndrome 234–235
Ventricular fibrillation 234
Ventricular tachycardia 230–231, 231*f*
  idiopathic 233
Verapamil 223*t*
Verruca plana 862
Verruca vulgaris 862
Vertebrobasilar ischemia 934
Vertiginous migraine 934
Vertigo 826–831, 933–934
  benign paroxysmal positional 827
  causes of 827*t*
  central *vs.* peripheral 830*t*
  clinical features of 828–830*t*
  clinical presentation 826
  diagnostic testing 827
  general principles 826
  treatment 827
Vestibular neuritis 826, 827
Vestibular schwannoma 834
Vibrio sp. 550*t*
Video-assisted thorascopic surgery (VATS)
    375, 409
Vinblastine 737
Viral hepatitis
  hepatitis A 617
  hepatitis B 618, 619*t*, 620
  hepatitis C 620–621
Viral infection, chronic 631
Viral orchitis 450
Viral skin infections 862

Vision loss, acute 946–947
Vision loss, chronic 947–948
  age-related muscular degeneration 947
  cataracts 947
  glaucoma 947–948
Vision loss, transient 944
Visual acuity 940
Visual field defects 945–946
Visual fields 942
Vitamin(s) 459, 461–463t
Vitamin A 461t
Vitamin B$_1$ 461t
Vitamin B$_2$ 462t
Vitamin B$_3$ 462t
Vitamin B$_6$ 462t
Vitamin B$_{12}$ 290–291, 462t
Vitamin C 461t
Vitamin D 53, 461t, 504–505
Vitamin E 461t
Vitamin K 461t
Vitamin K deficiency 280
Vitiligo 859
Vitreous hemorrhage 946
Vomiting 586–589
  in cancer patients 745
  causes of 588t
  clinical presentation 586–587
  diagnostic testing 587
  treatment of 587, 589
von Willebrand disease 278–280.
    See also Hemostasis
  clinical presentation 279
  diagnostic testing 279
  general principles 278
  hemostasis test patterns in 279t
  treatment of 280
von Willebrand factor (vWF) 278
V/Q scanning 313
Vulvovaginal candidiasis 61, 575

W

Waldenström macroglobulinemia 296
Warfarin 317–318, 320, 322, 383, 931
Warm-antibody AIHA (WAIHA) 296–297
Warts 862
Water-soluble vitamins 462–463t
Waxy casts 483
WBC casts 483
Weber test, for hearing loss 832
Wegener's granulomatosis 497, 681

Weight gain 958
Weight reduction 145, 145t
Wheezing 328, 608
Whiff test 60
Whiplash (neck injury) 687, 690
Whipple procedure 637
White blood cells 482
  disorders 303–305
WHO pain ladder 760
Wide-complex tachycardias 230–232
Wilson disease 625–626
Wolff-Parkinson-White syndrome 226, 234–235
Women's health 46–61
  bacterial vaginosis 59–60
  breast masses 58–59
  cervical cancer screening 56–57
  menopause 54–56
  nipple discharge 57–58
  osteoporosis 46–54
  trichomonas vaginitis 60–61
  vaginitis 59
  vulvovaginal candidiasis 61
Wrist and hand pain 706–708
  clinical presentation 707–708
  diagnostic testing 708
  general principles 706–707
  treatment of 605, 708

X

Xa inhibitors, direct 316
Xanthelasma 867

Y

Yellow fever 545t
Yergason sign 702
Yersinia enterocolitica 877
Yocoum test 701
Young's modulus 362

Z

Zanamivir 522
Zinc 466t
Zoledronic acid 51, 446
Zolmitriptan 910
Zonisamide 916t
Zostavax 119
Zoster ophthalmicus 543